This book provides a comprehensive and critical overview of the immunological aspects of autoimmune neurological disease, with particular emphasis on recent research findings. Following introductory chapters on antigen recognition and self–non-self discrimination and on neuroimmunology, the chapters dealing with specific autoimmune neurological diseases are presented in a standardized format with sections on clinical features, genetics, neuropathology, pathophysiology, immunology (including immunopathology, pathogenesis and immunoregulation) and therapy. Each chapter has a concluding section, which summarizes the key points and suggests directions for future research. The diseases range from relatively common conditions such as multiple sclerosis, the Guillain–Barré syndrome and myasthenia gravis to rarer conditions such as the stiff-man syndrome. Animal models of autoimmmune neurological disease are covered in detail, because of their importance in understanding the human diseases. The widely studied experimental autoimmune encephalomyelitis is dealt with first, not only because it serves as a model for T-cell-mediated disease of the nervous system, especially multiple sclerosis, but also because it is the prototype of T-cell-mediated autoimmunity in general. This book is suitable for clinicians and neurologists managing patients with autoimmune neurological disease, and for immunologists, neuroscientists and neurologists investigating the pathogenesis and pathophysiology of these disorders.

Autoimmune neurological disease

CAMBRIDGE REVIEWS IN CLINICAL IMMUNOLOGY

Series editors:

D. B. G. OLIVIERA

Lister Institute Research Fellow, University of Cambridge, Addenbrooke's Hospital, Cambridge.

D. K. PETERS

Regius Professor of Physic, University of Cambridge, Addenbrooke's Hospital, Cambridge.

A. P. WEETMAN

Professor of Medicine, University of Sheffield Clinical Sciences Centre.

Recent advances in immunology, particularly at the molecular level, have led to a much clearer understanding of the causes and consequences of autoimmunity. The aim of this series is to make these developments accessible to clinicians who feel daunted by such advances and require a clear exposition of the scientific and clinical issues. The various clinical specialities will be covered in separate volumes, which will follow a fixed format: a brief introduction to basic immunology followed by a comprehensive review of recent findings in the autoimmune conditions which, in particular, will compare animal models with their human counterparts. Sufficient clinical detail, especially regarding treatment, will also be included to provide basic scientists with a better understanding of these aspects of autoimmunity. Thus each volume will be self-contained and comprehensible to a wide audience. Taken as a whole the series will provide an overview of all the important autoimmune disorders.

Autoimmune Endocrine Disease A. P. Weetman

Immunological Aspects of Renal Disease D. B. G. Oliveira

Immunological Aspects of the Vascular Endothelium Edited by C. O. S. Savage & J. D. Pearson

Gastrointestinal and Hepatic Immunology Edited by R. V. Heatley

Autoimmune neurological disease

MICHAEL P. PENDER
Reader in Medicine, The University of Queensland
Director of Neurology, Royal Brisbane Hospital

AND

PAMELA A. McCOMBE
Honorary Senior Lecturer in Medicine
Department of Medicine, The University of Queensland

CAMBRIDGE
UNIVERSITY PRESS

Published by the Press Syndicate of the University of Cambridge
The Pitt Building, Trumpington Street, Cambridge CB2 1RP
40 West 20th Street, New York, NY 10011-4211, USA
10 Stamford Road, Oakleigh, Melbourne 3166, Australia

First published 1995

A catalogue record for this book is available from the British Library

Library of Congress cataloguing in publication data

Autoimmune neurological disease/edited by Michael P. Pender and Pamela A. McCombe.
p. cm. – (Cambridge reviews in clinical immunology)
Includes index. 0-521-46113-8hc
1. Nervous system–Diseases–Immunological aspects. 2. Autoimmune diseases. 3. Neuroimmunology. I. Pender, Michael P. II. McCombe, Pamela A. III. Series.
[DNLM: 1. Nervous System Diseases. 2. Autoimmune Diseases. 3. Nervous System–immunology. WL 140 A939 1996]
RC346.5.A98 1996
616.8′0479–dc20
DNLM/DLC
for Library of Congress 95-8040 CIP

ISBN 0 521 46113 8 hardback

Transferred to digital printing 2003

PN

Contents

Preface

This book aims to provide a comprehensive overview of the immunological aspects of autoimmune neurological disease, with particular emphasis on recent research findings. Following introductory chapters on antigen recognition and self–non-self discrimination and on neuroimmunology, the chapters dealing with specific autoimmune neurological diseases are presented in a standardized format with sections on clinical features, genetics, neuropathology, pathophysiology, immunology (including immunopathology, pathogenesis and immunoregulation) and therapy. Each chapter has a concluding section which summarizes the key points and suggests directions for future research. Animal models of autoimmune neurological disease are covered in detail because of their importance in understanding the human diseases. The widely studied experimental autoimmune encephalomyelitis is dealt with first, not only because it serves as a model for T-cell-mediated disease of the nervous system, especially multiple sclerosis, but also because it is the prototype of T-cell-mediated autoimmunity in general. The chapters dealing with disorders of the central nervous system (Chapters 3–6), as well as Chapters 2 and 12, have been written by myself, whereas the chapters dealing with disorders of the peripheral nervous system and muscle (Chapters 7–11) and Chapter 13 have been written by Pamela McCombe. Chapter 1 has been written by Ian Frazer, Professor of Medicine, The University of Queensland, Princess Alexandra Hospital, Woolloongabba, Queensland.

The intended readership of this book includes neurologists involved in managing patients with autoimmune neurological disease, as well as basic and clinical researchers investigating the pathogenesis of these disorders. The references range from important early papers to work published in mid-1994.

Brisbane

Michael P. Pender

–1–
Antigen recognition and self–non-self discrimination

IAN H. FRAZER

In organ-specific autoimmune disease, immune destruction is focused on a limited range of tissues or cells, and the autoimmune response must persist to produce disease. These observations imply that continued specific recognition of some antigen or antigens is central to the process of organ-specific autoimmunity. This introductory chapter will examine current understanding of how a controlled antigen-specific immune response arises, with a particular focus on how the regulatory mechanisms could go wrong to allow persisting self-destructive immune responses or organ-specific autoimmunity to develop.

The mammalian immune system has evolved to maximize the survival potential of a long-lived, complex multicellular host in an environment which includes a multiplicity of rapidly evolving and potentially harmful micro-organisms. Since some micro-organisms may be beneficial to their host, the immune system appears first to have developed the ability to recognize, and contain or eliminate, the tissue damage caused by infection rather than the organisms themselves: indeed, it has been argued that this remains its primary task (Matzinger, 1994). The most primitive recognition systems are for bacterial cell wall components in the intracellular fluid or blood, and for products of necrotic host cells. Ability of cells to distinguish self from non-self is demonstrated in the most primitive multicellular organisms, namely corals and sponges, and is a basic requirement of a multicellular organism pursuing a sexual reproduction strategy. However, immune effector mechanisms need to recognize specific antigen, as opposed to generic 'non-self', as a target only if the immune system has memory. Immunological memory can be defined for a whole animal as the ability of an immune effector mechanism to respond more effectively to a repeat encounter with a specific antigen. Memory is the defining characteristic of the mammalian immune system, allowing focus of the immune effector response on an antigen even in the absence of tissue destruction. With memory, therefore, comes the potential for immune destruction of viable tissue, which may be harmful rather than beneficial.

Components of the immune system

The mammalian immune system appears to be a hybrid of many types of defence system. These include:

phagocytic cells, natural killer cells and the alternative complement pathway which have evolved to neutralize bacterial and viral infectious agents causing tissue damage, and dispose of damaged cells. These effector mechanisms do not display memory, and distinguish damaged from healthy tissue rather than self from non-self.

polymorphic cell membrane glycoproteins and corresponding glycoprotein ligands which prevent multicellular animals merging imperceptibly with their neighbours. Contact of a cell with a non-self cell can result in alteration of cell motility to allow withdrawal, in failure of cell–cell adhesion, or possibly in programmed cell death for an isolated non-self cell.

antigen-specific systems which have adapted components of the more primitive systems to increase the efficiency of eradication of infections by providing immunological memory.

With the development of mechanisms for specific recognition of antigen there comes a teleological 'requirement' for the immune system not to respond to self. To achieve this, there is a bias of the effector cells of the antigen-specific immune system towards non-response on recognition of cognate antigen. Thus, effector cells require multiple activation signals in addition to antigen recognition before a potentially destructive immune response is initiated (Smith, Farrah & Goodwin, 1994). Further, antigen-specific cytotoxic immune responses appear to be self limited, even in the presence of continued antigenic stimulus (Moskophidis *et al.*, 1993), presumably lest the immune response be worse for the host than the provoking agent.

Specific recognition of antigen

The immune system has few *antigen-specific* recognition mechanisms at its disposal. The major effectors of antigen-specific recognition and memory are two lineages of bone-marrow-derived recirculating long-lived cells, the $\alpha\beta$ T lymphocytes and the B lymphocytes. Each uses a membrane receptor of randomly generated specificity to survey the environment. The $\alpha\beta$ T cells survey the surface of other cells for peptides complexed with one of a series

Table 1.1. *Response to an immunocyte to cognate antigen*

Reset cell cycle programme	Replicate, or die
Reset receptor programme	Alter (positively or negatively) the cell's co-stimulatory requirements for further signalling by the same antigen
Alter adhesiveness/motility	Alter cell adhesion molecules so that the cell traffics to different tissues
Invoke effector functions	Signal cells in contact by expression of new surface molecule Secrete cytokines that affect adjacent cells, including immunocytes Secrete antibody[a] Kill cells in contact[b]

[a] B-cell-specific effector mechanism
[b] T-cell-specific effector mechanism

of polymorphic molecules, the major histocompatibility complex molecules (MHC), which have evolved for the specific function of antigen presentation. B cells survey the extracellular fluid for molecules displaying particular patterns of charge density termed epitopes. B and T cells respond to recognition of their cognate antigen with a similar range of possible outcomes (Table 1.1). It is worth noting that the majority of potentially antigen-specific cells in an inflammatory response, including an autoimmune inflammatory response, appear to be directed to the site of inflammation, not by recognition of their own specific antigen, but as effector cells non-specifically attracted to the site of an immune response.

The T cell antigen receptor

The molecular and cellular basis of the antigen recognition mechanisms of both B and T lymphocytes are now defined. Considering first the T cell repertoire, $\alpha\beta$ T lymphocytes express on their cell membranes a clonotypic heterodimeric protein termed the T cell receptor (TCR). Each receptor is able to interact with a specific peptide, or more commonly a small range of peptides, presented in the context of MHC on a cell membrane, and to signal the T cell through a linked membrane protein complex termed CD3 (Weiss & Littman, 1994). The TCR comprises clonotypic α and β chains, each of which has structural homology with other members of a family of cell surface signalling and adhesion molecules termed the immunoglobulin (Ig) superfamily, and at least four invariant chains which are involved in signal transduction. The genes encoding the α and β polypeptides of the TCR of each of the estimated 10^8 T cell lines that constitute the T cell repertoire are generated from the random joining of a constant region of the α and β chain genes to one from each of a family of minigenes termed V, D and J (Leiden, 1993), which encode much of the complementarity-determining protein sequence of the TCR. This somatic gene rearrangement occurs only in the T cell, as part of a co-ordinated programme of T cell maturation within the thymus. T cells, having rearranged their receptor genes to express a single receptor specificity, or on occasions two receptors with a common β chain and two discrete α chains (Padovan *et al.*, 1993), undergo a selection process in the thymus. Most TCRs generated at random cannot recognize the particular MHC molecules carried by host cells, or recognize them too well, and these cells are positively or negatively selected to die by apoptosis (programmed cell death) within the thymus. An immature T cell that engages 'self peptide + MHC' presented by thymic stromal cells is delivered a *lck*-dependent growth signal, without which the cell dies (von Boehmer, 1994); too efficient an engagement, on the other hand, delivers another signal allowing activation of suicide genes (Russell & Wang, 1993; Nossal, 1994). The T cell repertoire thus consists of clones of cells with receptors that are able to interact with intermediate affinity with the MHC/self-peptide complexes on thymic stromal cells (Ashton-Rickardt & Tonegawa, 1994).

T cell repertoire selection

The immune repertoire of an animal is shaped to some extent by the alleles of each MHC molecule expressed by that particular animal, and to some extent by the available Vβ chain repertoire. Most animals have multiple Vβ chains in their germline DNA for use in TCR gene assembly. However, some viral and bacterial antigens, termed 'superantigens', are able to bind to MHC and also to specific Vβ chains. A subset of these antigens, transmissible through the germline, can through expression in the thymus delete the entire subset of T cells that use their cognate Vβ gene (Held *et al.*, 1994). A remarkable diversity of repertoire can be maintained in animal species monomorphic for MHC, and even by animals transgenic for a TCR β chain gene which can therefore by a process of allelic exclusion express TCRs with only one Vβ chain. This diversity is supplemented by an apparent ability of one TCR to recognize multiple MHC/peptide complexes, an observation that may be the basis of allorecognition and of the activation of potentially self-reactive clones of T cells by environmental antigens. Early contact with environmental antigen also shapes the immune repertoire of an animal. This is exemplified by the NOD (non-obese diabetic) mouse, which is more diabetes prone if it is reared under germ-free conditions, and by some mice prone to experimental autoimmune encephalomyelitis (EAE), which are in contrast relatively more resistant to the induction of EAE if reared in a germ-free environment. The consequence for an individual T lymphocyte of TCR–ligand interaction depends in some way on the affinity of the sum of the approximately 5000 receptors on the T cell for the sum of the peptide/MHC complexes on the target cell, and the number of receptors engaged (Corr *et al.*, 1994). It also depends on the co-stimulatory signals delivered by the antigen-presenting cell or by local immunocytes, a topic that will be reviewed later in this chapter.

CD8$^+$ T cell function

The $\alpha\beta$ T cell population can be divided into two major groups, characterized by the expression on their membrane of one of a pair of cell surface glycoproteins of the Ig superfamily, termed CD4 and CD8. Immature T cells express both molecules, while mature T cells express one or other. A CD8 molecule on the cell membrane directs the receptor specificity of that T cell to peptide carried by a subset of the MHC molecules termed class I molecules, which are found on the membranes of nearly all cell types. Each MHC class I molecule transports an 8–9-mer peptide derived from within the cell to the cell membrane (Monaco, 1992). The peptide is located in a groove on the surface of the folded MHC polypeptide, which is complexed to β_2-microglobulin. The peptide is derived from an intracellular protein by proteasome-mediated proteolysis, and loaded onto the peptide-binding groove of the MHC molecule by peptide-transporter molecules (TAP 1 and TAP 2). The MHC molecule is only stable with a peptide in the groove; once in place the peptide is difficult to displace, and generally remains in the peptide-binding groove for the life of the MHC molecule. Thus, CD8$^+$ T cells survey peptides synthesized intracellularly. The vast majority of the peptides presented by MHC class I molecules have been demonstrated to be self peptides derived from a restricted range of self proteins. Virally encoded peptides are also presented by virus-infected cells. The TAP proteins, polymorphic in some species, convey some selectivity on the peptides presented. The MHC class I proteins are polymorphic in most species, and each allele of each of the polymorphic MHC class I loci is expressed, giving most mammals and humans a choice of up to six MHC class I molecules with which to present peptide. Each MHC class I molecule has a set of peptide sequences that it is best able to bind: generally the second and the last residue of the 8–9-mer peptide are critical and can tolerate few substitutions from the 'ideal' peptide ligand for that MHC molecule (Rammensee, Falk & Rötzschke, 1994). The molecular basis of this specificity has been clarified by the solution of the crystal structure of the MHC/peptide complex. A given protein antigen will thus be presented by different peptide/MHC complexes to the immune system in different people. However, there is little evidence that the response to any protein is limited by the availability of epitopes for a particular MHC background. Most proteins, in addition to an immunodominant epitope, generally have several sub-dominant epitopes (Sercarz *et al.*, 1993), which can be recognized by a different T cell clone if the dominant epitope is destroyed by mutation. The majority of $CD8^+$ cells appear to be effector cells for T-cell-mediated cytolysis (cytotoxic T cells). Cytotoxic T cells kill their cognate targets by a mechanism dependent on the secretion of perforin or the activation of *fas* (Kägi *et al.*, 1994).

$CD4^+$ T cell function

The receptor on $CD4^+$ T cells is directed by the CD4 molecule to interact with peptides presented by MHC class II molecules. MHC class II molecules are structurally similar to, but functionally quite different from, MHC class I molecules. They are present constitutively on a limited subset of bone-marrow-derived cells including dendritic cells, Langerhans cells and B cells, and can be induced by activation on T cells and monocytic cells, and by cytokines on some epithelial cells. They bind 10–20-mer peptides (Engelhard, 1994), which are generally derived by proteolysis of extracellular proteins, including phagocytosed micro-organisms and necrotic cells, within phagolysosomes (Cresswell, 1994). MHC class II molecules present whichever available peptide is of highest affinity for their antigen-binding groove. Like MHC class I molecules, MHC class II molecules have preferred binding sequences, but the peptide contact requirements are more relaxed than for class I, probably because as shown by the crystal structure the peptide-binding groove is open ended and the opportunities for peptide–MHC contact are greater (Brown *et al.*, 1993). The majority of $CD4^+$ T cells respond to signalling by release of pro-inflammatory and immunostimulatory cytokines and are termed T helper (T_H) cells, although $CD4^+$ T cells with direct cytotoxic function are also described.

Co-stimulation as a requirement for activation of T cells

$CD8^+$ T cells are generally unresponsive when first presented with their cognate ‘peptide + MHC’ specificity, and do not differentiate into mature effector cells unless they receive a series of co-stimulatory signals. These include growth-promoting cytokines (interleukin-2 [IL-2]) and activation of membrane receptors by molecules, such as B7.1 and B7.2 which are present on professional antigen-presenting cells including B cells and dendritic cells.

B7.1 is clearly a crucial co-stimulatory molecule, as its expression alone on an otherwise non-stimulatory target cell is sufficient to allow induction of a cytotoxic T cell response to a non-self peptide (Allison, 1994). A certain density of MHC/peptide complexes on the target cell is assumed to be necessary, and affinity of the effector cell for its target is clearly important. Further requirements for activation of naive $CD8^+$ cytotoxic T cells probably exist, including help from T_H cells. A crucial issue is whether, and by what mechanism, such help might be cognate, by analogy with the cognate help given by T_H cells to B cells. Help, if cognate, would require covalent linkage of the T_H epitope to the cytotoxic T cell epitope, and a requirement for cognate help for activation of cytotoxic T cell precursors would make autoimmunity stimulated through cross-reactivity between an autoantigen carrying a T_H and a cytotoxic T cell epitope and another protein expressing the same T_H and cytotoxic T cell epitope most unlikely. Unstimulated $CD8^+$ T cells traffic from blood to lymph node through the high-endothelial venules. The lymph node is probably the major site of priming of cytotoxic T cell precursors to responsiveness. In contrast, $CD8^+$ T cells which have been recently primed by exposure to antigen and cytokine in the lymph node can traffic into the tissues to carry out their effector functions without further priming.

$CD4^+$ T cells, like $CD8^+$ T cells, need co-stimulation before a cellular response follows TCR stimulation: such co-stimulation is constitutively provided by B7 and cytokines, including IL-1, secreted by professional antigen-presenting cells (APCs), but may not be available from non-professional APCs. Non-professional APCs are those cells on which expression of MHC class II molecules can be induced, and include keratinocytes and endothelial cells. Presentation of cognate peptide + MHC by these cells may lead to tolerogenic signalling of the T cell (Bal *et al.*, 1990). Co-stimulatory signalling requirements are tightly temporally linked to receptor activation by peptide/MHC complexes, which alter the expression and affinity of cytokine receptors on the cells. They are also altered by previous exposure of the T cell to antigen. T cells which have recently responded to their cognate antigen and which can be recognized as expressing the activation-associated isoforms (CD45RO) of the CD45 antigen (Lightstone & Marvel, 1993), together with the CD44 molecule, require less co-stimulation to respond positively to antigen. T_H cells start life as long-lived effector precursors (T_H0) which express adhesion molecules that allow them to circulate in the blood and through the lymphoid organs, awaiting stimulation by a professional APC. Upon such stimulation, and depending on the cytokine environment of the T cell at the time, these precursor cells differentiate to secrete different cytokines and become activated T_H effector cells. There appears to be a continuous spectrum of cytokine secretion patterns from activated T_H cells (Paul & Seder, 1994), the polar extremes of which have been termed T_H1 or T_H2 type responses. T_H1 cells produce pro-inflammatory and cytostatic cytokines, including tumour necrosis factor-β (TNF-β), interferon-γ (IFN-γ) and macrophage inflammatory protein-1α (MIP-1α), whereas T_H2 cells produce cytokines more geared to activate B cell proliferation and differentiation (IL-4, IL-5, IL-6 and IL-10). The major determinants of the cytokine profile produced in response to antigen is unknown; different mouse strains respond differently to the same antigen, suggesting that the explanation may rest with the APC rather than the T cell. Once an immune response is produced, the cytokines from one T_H polarity tend to inhibit production of those of the opposite polarity. Chronic antigen stimulation tends nevertheless to lead to a T_H2 bias to the immune response, regardless of organism, and the nature of the dominant cytokine secretion pattern may reflect some ability of the APC to process and dispose of the antigens of a particular pathogen. Activated T_H cells revert with time to express adhesion molecules more typical of T_H0 cells, but retain a memory function that is manifest as persistence of antigen-specific T cells, with a reduced or different requirement for co-stimulatory signals for activation, in the spleen and lymph nodes of the primed animal.

Peripheral T cell tolerance

While events in the thymus during T cell maturation are the primary determinant of the T cell repertoire, further mechanisms shape the responsiveness of effector T cells to antigen presented peripherally. T cells, unlike B cells, have no mechanism for somatic mutation to generate further antigen-driven receptor affinity. Therefore, T_H cells are in a unique position to control whether an effective immune response is generated against antigen, including self-antigen. This is best demonstrated in mice transgenic for proteins derived from micro-organisms, including hepatitis B virus and lymphocytic choriomeningitis virus (LCMV). Mice transgenic for LCMV gp120 in the pancreatic islet cells, and also transgenic for a TCR specific for a peptide from LCMV gp120 in the context of the appropriate MHC molecule, such that 'all' T cells in the mouse are specific for LCMV gp120, have healthy pancreatic islet cells unless challenged with live LCMV. On such challenge, LCMV-directed destruction of the pancreatic islet cells rapidly follows (Ohashi *et al.*, 1991). Therefore, autoreactive T cells can ignore peripherally expressed self antigen unless they are primed by a more immunogenic method of antigen presentation. There are more active means of tolerance than the 'ignorance' demonstrated by the LCMV transgenic mice. Presentation of antigen by fixed APCs, or by keratinocytes, to naive cytotoxic T cell precursors can lead to induction of tolerance to the antigen, an active state of non-responsiveness that can be permanent in face of immunogenic antigen challenge. The non-responsiveness to antigen of tolerized cells can sometimes be overcome by exogenous cytokine (Heath *et al.*, 1992). Peripheral tolerance can be a yet more active process, conveyed as antigen-specific tolerance to naive effector T cells, even in the absence of antigen, by specifically tolerized $CD4^+$ T cells, described in a model of induced 'infectious' tolerance to MLS antigen (Qin *et al.*, 1993). Tolerance through 'exhaustion' of clones of antigen-responsive cytotoxic T cells after antigen recognition is also recognized. Thus, there are many mechanisms for the maintenance of tolerance to self antigens even in the presence of potentially autoreactive T cell clones.

The B cell story

B cells 'see' antigen as a map of charge density on the surface of a molecule, utilizing a polymorphic membrane-bound receptor, immunoglobulin, which like the TCR is a member of the Ig supergene family. The genes coding for Ig have evolved the ability to encode proteins with similar antigen specificity but different properties, through selection of one of a choice of constant regions of the protein. While the prototypic antigen receptor, IgD, is membrane bound, individual B cells can differentiate into plasma cells, which produce Ig molecules destined for cross-linking of soluble antigen (IgM), complement activation (IgG1 and IgG3), secretion on mucosal surfaces (IgA), or mast cell activation (IgE). Receptor diversity is generated during B cell maturation by a process of somatic cell gene rearrangements resembling that found in T cells: the site and nature of the process of repertoire selection are less clear, but deletion or functional silencing of immature B cells by soluble or membrane-bound self antigen is well described. B cells, like T cells, generally require co-stimulation to become mature effector cells, though some B cells can respond to polyvalent polysaccharide antigens without such help. Co-stimulation is generally cognate, requiring interaction between the B cell and a T_H cell specific for a peptide from the antigen to which the B cell is responsive. The mechanism of this cognate help involves the B cell in its role as a professional APC – protein is ingested after binding to the Ig receptor on the B cell, and presented in the context of MHC class II molecules to a cognate T cell. This T_H cell, in addition to secreting appropriate cytokines (IL-2, IL-4), displays increased levels of CD40 antigen, which stimulates the B cell directly through a membrane receptor termed p39 (Laman, Claasen & Noelle, 1994). Stimulated B cells divide in the germinal centre of the lymph node in response to antigen, and during division undergo somatic mutation of the complementarity-determining regions of the Ig receptor. Thus, during an immune response B cells are selected with increasing affinity for the stimulating antigen, a process not observed in T cells undergoing similar antigen-driven proliferation. Analysis of autoreactive clones of B cells in patients with autoimmune disease demonstrates that the B cell IgG genes have mutated from the germline configuration, suggesting strongly that autoantibody secretion is antigen driven. A more primitive variety of B cells, termed B1 cells, are $CD5^+$ cells, which are derived from mesenchymal rather than bone marrow tissues and which secrete polyvalent low-affinity IgM antibody that often has autoreactive capacity (Kantor, 1991). The ability of these cells to undergo affinity maturation and class switching, and to secrete antibodies able to cause tissue damage, is currently under investigation.

The molecular and genetic basis of autoimmunity

Potentially autoreactive B and T cells exist in healthy individuals, but do not normally respond to self antigen. They can be deleted from the repertoire through artificially induced thymic expression of the appropriate antigens, which prevents expression of disease in animals otherwise prone to organ-specific autoimmune disease (Posselt *et al.*, 1993). T-cell-dependent autoimmunity is a puzzle: not only must an immune response be induced involving autoreactive T cell precursors, but several mechanisms of peripheral tolerance must be overcome, and finally the induced immune response must fail to switch off, or at least fail to switch to a predominantly T_H2 type response, as would generally occur in the course of a normal immune response. Autoimmunity must therefore be multifactorial, and may, like oncogenesis, involve different genetic events in different patients with the same disease. This is demonstrated by the impaired penetrance of most autoimmune diseases in identical twins (Shoenfeld & Isenberg, 1989), by the onset of these disorders in adult life, and by complex heritability patterns: an organ-specific autoimmune diathesis is inherited with the A1,B8,DR3 MHC haplotype, but in different individuals different target organs will be damaged, and kindred sharing the haplotype may have autoantibodies but no autoimmune disease.

Induction of the autoreactive immune response

Induction of the autoreactive immune response can be achieved if the cognate antigen or a cross-reacting antigen is presented correctly. The antigenic peptide may be presented in the context of inflammation, as a result of tissue destruction mediated by an infective process. Particular MHC types may convey the risk of autoimmune disease through their ability to present self peptides, or may allow common pathogens to present peptides cross-reactive with self antigens. With regard to induction of the immune response, it is worth noting that several T-cell-mediated autoimmune diseases have been transferred by bone marrow to patients without previous autoimmune disease (Marmont, 1994). Similarly, autoimmune disease has been cured by bone marrow transplantation, suggesting that at least one abnormality is in the marrow-derived APCs and that this lesion is dominant over the presence or absence of T cells able to respond to self antigen.

Failure of peripheral tolerance

A fundamental problem with antigen presentation may be suggested by the ability of TNF to induce autoimmunity in mice transgenic for expression of B7.1 on their islet cells, or by the induction of autoimmunity by the induced expression of B7 on islet cells transgenic for a viral glycoprotein in mice also transgenic for T cells specific for the viral protein (Harlan *et al.*, 1994).

Failure to switch off an induced immune response

Failure to switch off an induced immune response can have a single-gene heritable basis, as in autoimmunity-prone inbred mice. IL-10 can prevent autoimmune disease in otherwise prone animals (Rott, Fleischer & Cash, 1994), and failure to control cytokine expression correctly during an immune response may also be a mechanism for development of autoimmunity. Recurrence of disease may be a reflection of renewed antigen presentation, or conversely a new generation of immunocompetent T_H0 cells with relevant specificity may be recruited through the thymus to produce disease recurrence when antigen persists.

In conclusion, initiation and persistence of the autoimmune response remain enigmatic, but, given the presence of potentially autoreactive T cell clones in all animals, the challenge is probably to establish why every episode of tissue damage is not followed by the induction of a sustained tissue-destructive autoimmune response, rather than to explain why potentially autoreactive T cells are on occasion primed to produce disease (Peakman & Vergani, 1994).

References

Allison, J.P. (1994). CD28-B7 interactions in T-cell activation. *Current Opinion in Immunology*, **6**, 414–19.

Ashton-Rickardt, P.G. & Tonegawa, S. (1994). A differential avidity model for T-cell selection. *Immunology Today*, **15**, 362–6.

Bal, V., McIndoe, A., Denton, G., Hudson, D., Lombardi, G., Lamb, J. & Lechler, R. (1990). Antigen presentation by keratinocytes induces tolerance in human T cells. *European Journal of Immunology*, **20**, 1893–7.

Brown, J.H., Jardetzky, T.S., Gorga, J.C., Stern, L.J., Urban, R.G., Strominger, J.L. & Wiley, D.C. (1993). Three-dimensional structure of the human class II histocompatibility antigen HLA-DR1. *Nature*, **364**, 33–9.

Corr, M., Slanetz, A.E., Boyd, L.F., Jelonek, M.T., Khilko, S., Al-Ramadi, B.K., Kim, Y.S., Maher, S.E., Bothwell, A.L.M. & Margulies, D.H. (1994). T cell receptor-MHC class I peptide interactions: affinity, kinetics, and specificity. *Science*, **265**, 946–9.

Cresswell, P. (1994). Assembly, transport and function of MHC class II molecules. *Annual Review of Immunology*, **12**, 259–94.

Engelhard, V.H. (1994). Structure of peptides associated with class I and class II MHC molecules. *Annual Review of Immunology*, **12**, 181–208.

Harlan, D.M., Hengartner, H., Huang, M.L., Kang, Y.-H., Abe, R., Moreadith, R.W., Pircher, H., Gray, G.S., Ohashi, P.S., Freeman, G.J., Nadler, L.M., June, C.H. & Aichele, P. (1994). Mice expressing both B7–1 and viral glycoprotein on pancreatic beta cells along with glycoprotein-specific transgenic T cells develop diabetes due to a breakdown of T-lymphocyte unresponsiveness. *Proceedings of the National Academy of Sciences USA*, **91**, 3137–41.

Heath, W.R., Allison, J., Hoffmann, M.W., Schönrich, G., Hämmerling, G., Arnold, B. & Miller J.F.A.P. (1992). Autoimmune diabetes as a consequence of locally produced interleukin-2. *Nature*, **359**, 547–9.

Held, W., Acha-Orbea, H., MacDonald, H.R. & Waanders, G.A. (1994). Superantigens and retroviral infection: insights from mouse mammary tumor virus. *Immunology Today*, **15**, 184–90.

Kantor, A.B. (1991). The development and repertoire of B-1 cells (CD5 B cells). *Immunology Today*, **12**, 389–91.

Kägi, D., Vignaux, F., Ledermann, B., Bürki, K., Depraetere, V., Nagata, S., Hengartner, H. & Golstein, P. (1994). Fas and perforin pathways as major mechanisms of T cell-mediated cytotoxicity. *Science*, **265**, 528–30.

Laman, J.D., Claasen, E. & Noelle, R.J. (1994). Immunodeficiency due to a faulty interaction between T cells and B cells. *Current Opinion in Immunology*, **6**, 636–41.

Leiden, J.M. (1993). Transcriptional regulation of T cell receptor genes. *Annual Review of Immunology*, **11**, 539–70.

Lightstone, L. & Marvel, J. (1993). $CD45RA^+$ T cells: not simple virgins. *Clinical Science*, **85**, 515–19.

Marmont, A.M. (1994). Defining criteria for autoimmune diseases. *Immunology Today*, **15**, 388.

Matzinger, P. (1994). Tolerance, danger and the extended family. *Annual Review of Immunology*, **12**, 991–1045.

Monaco, J.J. (1992). A molecular model of MHC class-I-restricted antigen processing. *Immunology Today*, **13**, 173–9.

Moskophidis, D., Lechner, F., Pircher, H. & Zinkernagel, R.M. (1993). Virus persistence in acutely infected immunocompetent mice by exhaustion of antiviral cytotoxic effector T cells. *Nature*, **362**, 758–61.

Nossal, G.J.V. (1994). Negative selection of lymphocytes. *Cell*, **76**, 229–39.

Ohashi, P.S., Oehen, S., Buerki, K., Pircher, H., Ohashi, C.T., Odermatt, B., Malissen, B., Zinkernagel, R.M. & Hengartner, H. (1991). Ablation of 'tolerance' and induction of diabetes by virus infection in viral antigen transgenic mice. *Cell*, **65**, 305–17.

Padovan, E., Casorati, G., Dellabona, P., Meyer, S., Brockhaus, M. & Lanzavecchia, A. (1993). Expression of two T cell receptor alpha chains: dual receptor T cells. *Science*, **262**, 422–4.

Paul, W.E. & Seder, R.A. (1994). Lymphocyte responses and cytokines. *Cell*, **76**, 241–51.

Peakman, M. & Vergani, D. (1994). Autoimmune disease: etiology, therapy and regeneration. *Immunology Today*, **15**, 345–7.

Posselt, A.M., Barker, C.F., Friedman, A.L., Koeberlein, B., Tomaszewski, J.E., & Naji, A. (1993). Intrathymic inoculation of islets at birth prevents autoimmune diabetes and pancreatic insulitis in the BB rat. *Transplantation Proceedings*, **25**, 301–2.

Qin, S., Cobbold, S.P., Pope, H., Elliott, J., Kioussis, D., Davies, J. & Waldmann, H. (1993). 'Infectious' transplantation tolerance. *Science*, **259**, 974–7.

Rammensee, H., Falk, K. & Rötzschke, O. (1994). Peptides naturally presented by MHC class 1 molecules. *Annual Review of Immunology*, **11**, 213–44.

Rott, O., Fleischer, B. & Cash, E. (1994). Interleukin-10 prevents experimental allergic encephalomyelitis in rats. *European Journal of Immunology*, **24**, 1434–40.

Russell, J.H. & Wang, R. (1993). Autoimmune *gld* mutation uncouples suicide and cytokine/proliferation pathways in activated, mature T cells. *European Journal of Immunology*, **23**, 2379–82.

Sercarz, E.E., Lehmann, P.V., Ametani, A., Benichou, G., Miller, A. & Moudgil, K. (1993). Dominance and crypticity of T cell antigenic determinants. *Annual Review of Immunology*, **11**, 729–66.

Shoenfeld, Y. & Isenberg, D. (1989). The genetic components of autoimmunity. In *The Mosaic of Autoimmunity*, ed. Y. Shoenfeld & D. Isenberg, pp. 169–228. Amsterdam: Elsevier.

Smith, C.A., Farrah, T. & Goodwin, R.G. (1994). The TNF receptor superfamily of cellular and viral proteins: activation, costimulation and death. *Cell*, **76**, 959–62.

von Boehmer, H. (1994). Positive selection of lymphocytes. *Cell*, **76**, 219–28.

Weiss, A. & Littman, D.R. (1994). Signal transduction by lymphocyte antigen receptors. *Cell*, **76**, 263–74.

–2–

An introduction to neuroimmunology

MICHAEL P. PENDER

Classically the brain has been regarded as an 'immunologically privileged' site, because alien tissue grafts transplanted there survive longer than similar grafts in other sites (Barker & Billingham, 1977). The relative hospitality of the brain to foreign tissue has been attributed to a lack of lymphatic drainage, the presence of the blood–brain barrier, the lack of constitutive expression of major histocompatibility complex (MHC) molecules, and the possible presence of chemical substances that might inhibit lymphocyte traffic. However, recent studies indicate that, in general, immune responses proceed in the nervous system in a similar manner to that in other organs. Yet the nervous system still has a number of attributes that influence local immune responses and that may be relevant to the pathogenesis of autoimmune neurological disease.

Specialization of structure and function in the nervous system

Central and peripheral nervous system

The nervous system is subdivided into the central nervous system (CNS) and the peripheral nervous system (PNS). The CNS comprises the cerebral hemispheres, the cerebellum, the brainstem, the spinal cord, and the olfactory and optic nerves. The PNS comprises the cranial nerve roots and cranial nerves, the spinal nerve roots (dorsal and ventral), the dorsal root ganglia, the spinal nerves and the peripheral nerves. The junctions of the CNS and PNS are defined by transitional zones where the dorsal roots enter the spinal cord (dorsal root entry zones) and where the ventral roots exit from the spinal cord (ventral root exit zones) and where the third to twelfth cranial nerves enter or leave the brainstem. The autonomic nervous system is a functional subdivision of the nervous system which has components in both the CNS and the PNS.

Cellular components and subcellular specialization

The CNS is composed of neurones, glia, blood vessels and meninges. The neuronal population consists of subsets of highly specialized cells which express different cytoplasmic and cell surface proteins and which have different functions. Furthermore, the individual neurones exhibit subcellular specialization with dendritic, somatic, axonal and synaptic regions. The glial population consists of cells with a neuroectodermal origin (astrocytes, oligodendrocytes and ependymal cells) and cells that are derived from bone marrow (microglia). Oligodendrocytes form myelin sheaths around axons by the spiral compaction of their plasma membranes. The PNS is mainly composed of axons, Schwann cells (which form the myelin sheaths) and connective tissue elements. In the dorsal root ganglion region, neuronal cell bodies are also present.

Diversity of potential target antigens and clinical syndromes in autoimmune neurological disease

As a consequence of the diversity of specialized cells and subcellular components in the nervous system, there is a wide range of potential target antigens and clinical syndromes in autoimmune neurological disease. Even in the case of autoimmunity directed at a single specialized structure, such as the myelin sheath, there may be a wide range of clinical presentations, because of the segmental and topographical organization of the nervous system.

The blood–brain barrier and blood–nerve barrier

The blood–brain barrier is a barrier inhibiting the entry of intravenously administered dyes into the CNS parenchyma. Using horseradish peroxidase as a tracer, Reese & Karnovsky (1967) demonstrated that the barrier is located at the level of the CNS vascular endothelium. They concluded that the impermeability of the endothelium resulted from the presence of tight interendothelial junctions and a lack of micropinocytosis in the endothelial cells. Other elements, including the endothelial basement membrane and the perivascular glia limitans, contribute to the layered structure at the blood–brain interface, but do not appear to contribute significantly to the functional blood–brain barrier. In the PNS an analogous blood–nerve barrier is present in the peripheral nerve, but not in the spinal roots or dorsal root ganglia (Waksman, 1961; Olsson, 1968; Jacobs, MacFarlane & Cavanagh, 1976). These barriers limit the access of circulating antibodies to the nervous system, but do not appear to limit T cell access, as activated T cells of any specificity can enter the normal CNS parenchyma (see below).

Immunological surveillance of the nervous system by T cells

Studies on the migration of labelled T cells following intravenous injection have shown that activated T cells of any specificity enter the normal CNS parenchyma as early as 3 h after injection (Wekerle *et al.*, 1986; Hickey, Hsu & Kimura, 1991; Ludowyk, Willenborg & Parish, 1992). Thus, T cell traffic in the CNS appears to be governed by the same principle as applies to other organs, namely that activated T cells preferentially migrate from the blood into tissues, whereas resting cells exit in lymph node high-endothelial venules (Mackay, Marston & Dudler, 1990). Low numbers of T cells are consistently demonstrable in normal human and rat brains (Booss *et al.*, 1983; Lassmann *et al.*, 1986), indicating that the CNS is continuously patrolled by activated T cells (Wekerle *et al.*, 1986). This conclusion is also supported by studies in radiation bone marrow chimeras (Lassmann *et al.*, 1993).

MHC expression and antigen presentation in the nervous system

Having entered the nervous system, T cells will cause disease only if they recognize their specific antigens in the context of MHC molecules. $CD8^+$ T cells recognize antigen in the context of class I MHC molecules, and $CD4^+$ T cells recognize antigen in the context of class II MHC (Ia) molecules. Compared to other organs, the CNS exhibits a low level of MHC antigen expression (Pizarro *et al.*, 1961; Wong *et al.*, 1984).

Neurones

Neurones do not express MHC class I or class II antigens either *in situ* or after exposure to interferon-γ (IFN-γ) *in vitro* (Wong *et al.*, 1984; Bartlett, Kerr & Bailey, 1989). The absence of such MHC antigen expression indicates that neurones cannot be targets of a conventional MHC-restricted specific T cell attack. However, neurones can be destroyed by natural killer cells through an unknown targeting mechanism (Hickey *et al.*, 1992*a*).

Astrocytes

Astrocytes do not normally express MHC antigens *in situ* but can be induced to express both class I and class II antigens after exposure to IFN-γ *in vitro* (Wong *et al.*, 1984). After being induced to express class II antigen, rat astrocytes are capable of presenting myelin basic protein (MBP) to MBP-specific $CD4^+$ T cells and inducing the proliferation of these T cells *in vitro* (Fontana, Fierz & Wekerle, 1984; Fierz *et al.*, 1985). However, Sedgwick *et al.* (1991*a*) have shown that the *in vitro* antigen-presenting capacity of rat astrocytes does not apply for naive $CD4^+$ T cells. Although human astrocytes expressing class II antigen can present MBP to MBP-specific T cells, they do not induce T cell proliferation but inhibit it (Weber *et al.*, 1994). Despite these *in vitro* findings, it is doubtful whether astrocytes have an antigen-presenting role *in vivo*, because they do not express detectable MHC class II antigen in inflammatory lesions (Matsumoto, Ohmori & Fujiwara, 1992).

Oligodendrocytes

Oligodendrocytes do not express MHC antigens *in situ* (Wong *et al.*, 1984). Under standard *in vitro* conditions, oligodendrocytes can be induced by IFN-γ to express class I but not class II antigen (Wong *et al.*, 1984; Turnley, Miller & Bartlett, 1991); however, in the presence of glucocorticoid, IFN-γ induces the expression of class II MHC molecules (Bergsteinsdottir *et al.*, 1992).

Schwann cells

Exposure of Schwann cells to IFN-γ *in vitro* increases the expression of class I MHC antigen and induces the expression of class II antigen (Armati, Pollard & Gatenby, 1990). Furthermore, Schwann cells expressing class II antigen can present the P_2 myelin protein to P_2-specific $CD4^+$ T cell lines (Argall *et al.*, 1992).

Endothelial cells

In the normal CNS, vascular endothelial cells express MHC class I antigen but not class II antigen (Lassmann *et al.*, 1991; Graeber *et al.*, 1992), except in the guinea pig, where occasional endothelial cells express class II antigen (Sobel *et al.*, 1984). After being induced to express Ia antigen by IFN-γ, murine cerebral vascular endothelial cells can present MBP to MBP-sensitized T cells *in vitro* (McCarron *et al.*, 1985, 1986).

Microglia

Microglia are bone-marrow-derived cells that are resident in the CNS parenchyma and that phenotypically resemble monocytes and tissue macrophages (Perry, Hume & Gordon, 1985). However, in the mature animal there is no major turnover or replacement of resident microglia by bone-marrow-derived cells, even after severe CNS inflammation (Matsumoto & Fujiwara, 1987; Lassmann *et al.*, 1993). Microglia have a dendritic or ramified morphology and are present throughout the grey and white matter. Microglial cell processes are also a minor component of the perivascular glia limitans, which mainly consists of astrocytic foot processes (Lassmann *et al.*, 1991).

In general, class II MHC antigen expression is undetectable on microglia in the normal rat CNS, whereas it is readily detectable on morphologically similar dendritic cells in the interstitial connective tissues of a wide range of other organs (Hart & Fabre, 1981; Lassmann *et al.*, 1986). However, some degree of class II antigen expression can be detected on microglia in the normal Brown Norway rat (Sedgwick *et al.*, 1993) and in the normal human CNS (Hayes, Woodroofe & Cuzner, 1987; Graeber *et al.*, 1992). There is also some expression of MHC class I antigen on microglia in the normal human CNS (Graeber *et al.*, 1992). In experimental animals, an upregulation of microglial class I and class II antigen expression occurs following various insults to the nervous system, including experimental autoimmune encephalomyelitis (EAE) (Matsumoto *et al.*, 1986; Vass *et al.*, 1986; McCombe *et al.*, 1992; Gehrmann *et al.*, 1993), peripheral nerve transection (Streit, Graeber & Kreutzberg, 1989*a*,*b*), ischaemia (Gehrmann *et al.*, 1992) and experimental autoimmune neuritis (Gehrmann *et al.*, 1993). After such insults microglia also become activated to proliferate (Graeber *et al.*, 1988*b*; Sedgwick *et al.*, 1991*b*; McCombe, de Jersey & Pender, 1994), upregulate the expression of complement receptor type 3 (CR3) (Graeber, Streit & Kreutzberg, 1988*a*) and express other macrophage markers, such as ED1 (Graeber *et al.*, 1990; Lassmann *et al.*, 1993). Upregulated microglial class II MHC antigen expression has also been found in a wide range of human disorders, including multiple sclerosis, Alzheimer's disease and Parkinson's disease (Hayes *et al.*, 1987; McGeer, Itagaki & McGeer, 1988). Reid *et al.* (1993) have shown that microglia can be activated and induced to proliferate and/or undergo apoptosis (programmed cell death) by stimulation of CR3.

The similarities between microglia and macrophages have raised the possibility that microglia may act as antigen-presenting cells. After being induced to express class II MHC antigen by IFN-γ, microglia have been reported to be capable of presenting antigen to T cells *in vitro* (Frei *et al.*,

1987; Matsumoto *et al.*, 1992), although in the experiments of Matsumoto *et al.* (1992) T cell proliferation was inhibited when higher numbers of microglial cells were used. The presence of class II antigen expression does not necessarily indicate an ability to upregulate the immune response, as there is evidence that such expression on non-specialized antigen-presenting cells may serve as an extrathymic mechanism for maintaining self tolerance (Markmann *et al.*, 1988). Whether parenchymal microglia have an upregulatory or downregulatory effect on the immune response *in vivo* is unknown at present.

Perivascular and meningeal macrophages

Recent studies have indicated that perivascular macrophages and meningeal macrophages are the major antigen-presenting cells in the CNS. The term 'perivascular macrophages' refers to cells that constitutively express class I and class II MHC antigens and standard macrophage markers and that are located in the Virchow–Robin perivascular space between the vascular basement membrane and the parenchymal basement membrane of the glia limitans (Graeber, Streit & Kreutzberg, 1989; Graeber *et al.*, 1992; Hickey, Vass & Lassmann, 1992*b*). These are the same cells that Hickey & Kimura (1988) called 'perivascular microglia'. They are distinguishable from parenchymal microglia by their location, morphology and constitutive expression of standard macrophage markers. Similar macrophages are also present in the leptomeninges (Hickey & Kimura, 1988; Graeber *et al.*, 1989).

Studies on F_1-to-parent bone marrow chimeras as recipients of MBP-specific T cells have shown that histocompatibility between the recipient's bone-marrow-derived cells and the donor T cells is sufficient for the induction of EAE (Hinrichs, Wegmann & Dietsch, 1987; Hickey & Kimura, 1988; Myers, Dougherty & Ron, 1993). In these chimeras the histocompatible bone-marrow-derived cells in the CNS are virtually confined to the perivascular and meningeal macrophage populations, as there is minimal settlement of these cells into the parenchymal microglial population (Hickey & Kimura, 1988). Therefore, these studies indicate that the perivascular macrophages and meningeal macrophages are major antigen-presenting cells in the CNS. Studies using parent-to-F_1 bone marrow chimeras as recipients of MBP-specific T cells have indicated that EAE can also be induced, albeit less efficiently, when there is histocompatibility only between the recipient's resident parenchymal cells and the donor T cells (Myers *et al.*, 1993). These studies were interpreted as indicating that endothelial cells or astrocytes can act as antigen-presenting cells *in vivo*; however, it remains possible that radiation-resistant parenchymal microglia may be the antigen-presenting cells in this model.

Adhesion molecule expression and cytokine production in the nervous system

Adhesion molecule expression and cytokine production are important in the evolution of an immune response; however, the nervous system does not appear to differ from other organs in these respects (Fabry, Raine & Hart, 1994).

Access of circulating antibody to the intact nervous system

It is widely believed that the blood–brain barrier and blood–nerve barrier limit the access of circulating antibody to the normal nervous system. However, Reid *et al.* (1993) have recently reported that an anti-CR3 antibody readily gains access to the normal CNS through an unknown mechanism. Levine *et al.* (1991) found that circulating anti-viral antibody can enter the CNS and mediate the clearance of alphavirus infection from neurones in the absence of specific cell-mediated immunity but it was unknown whether the blood–brain barrier was intact.

Lymphatic drainage of the nervous system

Classically, the nervous system has been considered to lack lymphatic drainage; however, recent studies indicate that the magnitude of outflow of labelled protein from the CNS to the deep cervical lymph is much greater than was previously appreciated (Cserr & Knopf, 1992). Gordon, Knopf & Cserr (1992) have shown that, under conditions of normal blood–brain barrier permeability, ovalbumin evokes a greater serum antibody response when introduced into the brain or cerebrospinal fluid than when introduced into extracerebral sites. Prineas (1979) observed that thin-walled channels resembling lymphatic capillaries and containing lymphocytes and macrophages were present within the perivascular spaces of the CNS of patients with various neurological disorders. He suggested that the perivascular spaces may serve the same function in the CNS as lymphatic vessels serve in other tissues and that lymphocytes may normally circulate through these channels. However, it is unknown whether the channels ultimately drain into the cervical lymph nodes.

Downregulation of the immune attack within the nervous system

Downregulation within the nervous system itself may play an important role in limiting the immune attack (Wekerle, 1988). Apoptosis of T cells occurs in the CNS in acute EAE and may contribute to the subsidence of inflammation during spontaneous recovery (Pender *et al.*, 1991, 1992; Schmied *et al.*, 1993). Furthermore, there is evidence that the apoptotic process selectively eliminates autoreactive T cells from the CNS during clinical recovery (Tabi, McCombe & Pender, 1994). The mechanism for this selective elimination is unknown, but one possibility is activation-induced T cell death resulting from interaction with non-specialized antigen-presenting cells that fail to deliver the co-stimulatory signal (Pender, 1993; Tabi *et al.*, 1994). Ohmori *et al.* (1992) found that there is little T cell proliferation within the CNS in acute EAE. As cells expressing the interleukin-2 receptor outnumbered proliferating T cells, they concluded that a state of T cell anergy is induced by interaction with glial cells expressing class II MHC antigen. However, as T cells undergoing apoptosis can still express cell surface molecules (Pender *et al.*, 1992), their results could also be explained by activation-induced T cell apoptosis. It has been hypothesized that T cell apoptosis in the target organ may also occur in other self-limited, T-cell-mediated autoimmune diseases and that it may be a general mechanism for maintaining extrathymic tolerance (Pender *et al.*, 1992; Pender, 1993). Macrophage apoptosis also occurs in the CNS in EAE and may contribute to the downregulation of this autoimmune disease (Nguyen, McCombe & Pender, 1994).

Conclusions

Although the brain is classically regarded as an immunologically privileged site that is exempt from immune surveillance, recent studies indicate that immune responses in the nervous system proceed in a similar manner to those in other organs. As a consequence of the diversity of specialized cells and subcellular components in the nervous system, there is a wide range of potential target antigens and clinical syndromes in autoimmune neurological disease. Despite the blood–brain barrier, the CNS is continuously patrolled by activated T cells and may be accessed by certain circulating antibodies. Perivascular macrophages and meningeal macrophages appear to be the main antigen-presenting cells. Although parenchymal microglia can be readily induced to express class II MHC antigen *in vivo* after a variety of insults, it is unknown whether they upregulate or indeed downregulate the immune response in the CNS. Finally, autoreactive T cells may be selectively eliminated from the CNS by apoptosis during spontaneous recovery from EAE. It has been hypothesized that T cell apoptosis in the target organ may be a general protective mechanism that also operates in other self-limited T-cell-mediated autoimmune diseases.

References

Argall, K.G., Armati, P.J., Pollard, J.D., Watson, E. & Bonner, J. (1992). Interactions between CD4+ T-cells and rat Schwann cells *in vitro*. 1. Antigen presentation by Lewis rat Schwann cells to P2-specific CD4+ T-cell lines. *Journal of Neuroimmunology*, **40**, 1–18.

Armati, P.J., Pollard, J.D. & Gatenby, P. (1990). Rat and human Schwann cells *in vitro* can synthesize and express MHC molecules. *Muscle and Nerve*, **13**, 106–16.

Barker, C.F. & Billingham, R.E. (1977). Immunologically privileged sites. *Advances in Immunology*, **25**, 1–54.

Bartlett, P.F., Kerr, R.S.C. & Bailey, K.A. (1989). Expression of MHC antigens in the central nervous system. *Transplantation Proceedings*, **21**, 3163–5.

Bergsteinsdottir, K., Brennan, A., Jessen, K.R. & Mirsky, R. (1992). In the presence of dexamethasone, gamma interferon induces rat oligodendrocytes to express major histocompatibility complex class II molecules. *Proceedings of the National Academy of Sciences USA*, **89**, 9054–8.

Booss, J., Esiri, M.M., Tourtellotte, W.W. & Mason, D.Y. (1983). Immunohistological analysis of T lymphocyte subsets in the central nervous system in chronic progressive multiple sclerosis. *Journal of the Neurological Sciences*, **62**, 219–32.

Cserr, H.F. & Knopf, P.M. (1992). Cervical lymphatics, the blood–brain barrier and the immunoreactivity of the brain: a new view. *Immunology Today*, **13**, 507–12.

Fabry, Z., Raine, C.S. & Hart, M.N. (1994). Nervous tissue as an immune compartment: the dialect of the immune response in the CNS. *Immunology Today*, **15**, 218–24.

Fierz, W., Endler, B., Reske, K., Wekerle, H. & Fontana, A. (1985). Astrocytes as antigen-presenting cells. I. Induction of Ia antigen expression on astrocytes by T cells via immune interferon and its effect on antigen presentation. *Journal of Immunology*, **134**, 3785–93.

Fontana, A., Fierz, W. & Wekerle, H. (1984). Astrocytes present myelin basic protein to encephalitogenic T-cell lines. *Nature*, **307**, 273–6.

Frei, K., Siepl, C., Groscurth, P., Bodmer, S., Schwerdel, C. & Fontana, A. (1987). Antigen presentation and tumor cytotoxicity by interferon-gamma-treated microglial cells. *European Journal of Immunology*, **17**, 1271–8.

Gehrmann, J., Bonnekoh, P., Miyazawa, T., Hossmann, K.A. & Kreutzberg, G.W. (1992). Immunocytochemical study of an early microglial activation in ischemia. *Journal of Cerebral Blood Flow and Metabolism*, **12**, 257–69.

Gehrmann, J., Gold, R., Linington, C., Lannes Vieira, J., Wekerle, H. & Kreutzberg, G.W. (1993). Microglial involvement in experimental autoimmune inflammation of the central and peripheral nervous system. *Glia*, **7**, 50–9.

Gordon, L.B., Knopf, P.M. & Cserr, H.F. (1992). Ovalbumin is more immunogenic when introduced into brain or cerebrospinal fluid than into extracerebral sites. *Journal of Neuroimmunology*, **40**, 81–7.

Graeber, M.B., Streit, W.J., Buringer, D., Sparks, D.L. & Kreutzberg, G.W. (1992). Ultrastructural location of major histocompatibility complex (MHC) class II positive perivascular cells in histologically normal human brain. *Journal of Neuropathology and Experimental Neurology*, **51**, 303–11.

Graeber, M.B., Streit, W.J., Kiefer, R., Schoen, S.W. & Kreutzberg, G.W. (1990). New expression of myelomonocytic antigens by microglia and perivascular cells following lethal motor neuron injury. *Journal of Neuroimmunology*, **27**, 121–32.

Graeber, M.B., Streit, W.J. & Kreutzberg, G.W. (1988*a*). Axotomy of the rat facial nerve leads to increased CR3 complement receptor expression by activated microglial cells. *Journal of Neuroscience Research*, **21**, 18–24.

Graeber, M.B., Streit, W.J. & Kreutzberg, G.W. (1989). Identity of ED2-positive perivascular cells in rat brain. *Journal of Neuroscience Research*, **22**, 103–6.

Graeber, M.B., Tetzlaff, W., Streit, W.J. & Kreutzberg, G.W. (1988*b*). Microglial cells but not astrocytes undergo mitosis following rat facial nerve axotomy. *Neuroscience Letters*, **85**, 317–21.

Hart, D.N.J. & Fabre, J.W. (1981). Demonstration and characterization of Ia-positive dendritic cells in the interstitial connective tissues of rat heart and other tissues, but not brain. *Journal of Experimental Medicine*, **154**, 347–61.

Hayes, G.M., Woodroofe, M.N. & Cuzner, M.L. (1987). Microglia are the major cell type expressing MHC class II in human white matter. *Journal of the Neurological Sciences*, **80**, 25–37.

Hickey, W.F., Hsu, B.L. & Kimura, H. (1991). T-lymphocyte entry into the central nervous system. *Journal of Neuroscience Research*, **28**, 254–60.

Hickey, W.F. & Kimura, H. (1988). Perivascular microglial cells of the CNS are bone marrow-derived and present antigen *in vivo*. *Science*, **239**, 290–2.

Hickey, W.F., Ueno, K., Hiserodt, J.C. & Schmidt, R.E. (1992*a*). Exogenously-induced, natural killer cell-mediated neuronal killing: a novel pathogenetic mechanism. *Journal of Experimental Medicine*, **176**, 811–17.

Hickey, W.F., Vass, K. & Lassmann, H. (1992*b*). Bone marrow-derived elements in the central nervous system: an immunohistochemical and ultrastructural survey of rat chimeras. *Journal of Neuropathology and Experimental Neurology*, **51**, 246–56.

Hinrichs, D.J., Wegmann, K.W. & Dietsch, G.N. (1987). Transfer of experimental allergic encephalomyelitis to bone marrow chimeras. Endothelial cells are not a restricting element. *Journal of Experimental Medicine*, **166**, 1906–11.

Jacobs, J.M., MacFarlane, R.M. & Cavanagh, J.B. (1976). Vascular leakage in the dorsal root ganglia of the rat, studied with horseradish peroxidase. *Journal of the Neurological Sciences*, **29**, 95–107.

Lassmann, H., Schmied, M., Vass, K. & Hickey, W.F. (1993). Bone marrow derived elements and resident microglia in brain inflammation. *Glia*, **7**, 19–24.

Lassmann, H., Vass, K., Brunner, C. & Seitelberger, F. (1986). Characterization of inflammatory infiltrates in experimental allergic encephalomyelitis. *Progress in Neuropathology*, **6**, 33–62.

Lassmann, H., Zimprich, F., Vass, K. & Hickey, W.F. (1991). Microglial cells are a component of the perivascular glia limitans. *Journal of Neuroscience Research*, **28**, 236–43.

Levine, B., Hardwick, J.M., Trapp, B.D., Crawford, T.O., Bollinger, R.C. & Griffin, D.E. (1991). Antibody-mediated clearance of alphavirus infection from neurons. *Science*, **254**, 856–60.

Ludowyk, P.A., Willenborg, D.O. & Parish, C.R. (1992). Selective localisation of neuro-specific T lymphocytes in the central nervous system. *Journal of Neuroimmunology*, **37**, 237–50.

Mackay, C.R., Marston, W.L. & Dudler, L. (1990). Naive and memory T cells show distinct pathways of lymphocyte recirculation. *Journal of Experimental Medicine*, **171**, 801–17.

Markmann, J., Lo, D., Naji, A., Palmiter, R.D., Brinster, R.L. & Heber Katz, E. (1988). Antigen presenting function of class II MHC expressing pancreatic beta cells *Nature*, **336**, 476–9.

Matsumoto, Y. & Fujiwara, M. (1987). Absence of donor-type major histocompatibility complex class I antigen-bearing microglia in the rat central nervous system of radiation bone marrow chimeras. *Journal of Neuroimmunology*, **17**, 71–82.

Matsumoto, Y., Hara, N., Tanaka, R. & Fujiwara, M. (1986). Immunohistochemical analysis of the rat central nervous system during experimental allergic encephalomyelitis, with special reference to Ia-positive cells with dendritic morphology. *Journal of Immunology*, **136**, 3668–76.

Matsumoto, Y., Ohmori, K. & Fujiwara, M. (1992). Immune regulation by brain cells in the central nervous system: microglia but not astrocytes present myelin basic protein to encephalitogenic T cells under *in vivo*-mimicking conditions. *Immunology*, **76**, 209–16.

McCarron, R.M., Kempski, O., Spatz, M. & McFarlin, D.E. (1985). Presentation of myelin basic protein by murine cerebral vascular endothelial cells. *Journal of Immunology*, **134**, 3100–3.

McCarron, R.M., Spatz, M., Kempski, O., Hogan, R.N., Muehl, L. & McFarlin, D.E. (1986). Interaction between myelin basic protein-sensitized T lymphocytes and murine cerebral vascular endothelial cells. *Journal of Immunology*, **137**, 3428–35.

McCombe, P.A., de Jersey, J. & Pender, M.P. (1994). Inflammatory cells, microglia and MHC class II antigen positive cells in the spinal cord of Lewis rats with acute and chronic relapsing experimental autoimmune encephalomyelitis. *Journal of Neuroimmunology*, **51**, 153–67.

McCombe, P.A., Fordyce, B.W., de Jersey, J., Yoong, G. & Pender, M.P. (1992). Expression of CD45RC and Ia antigen in the spinal cord in acute experimental allergic encephalomyelitis: an immunocytochemical and flow cytometric study. *Journal of the Neurological Sciences*, **113**, 177–86.

McGeer, P.L., Itagaki, S. & McGeer, E.G. (1988). Expression of the histocompatibility glycoprotein HLA-DR in neurological disease. *Acta Neuropathologica (Berlin)*, **76**, 550–7.

Myers, K.J., Dougherty, J.P. & Ron, Y. (1993). *In vivo* antigen presentation by both brain parenchymal cells and hematopoietically derived cells during the induction of experimental autoimmune encephalomyelitis. *Journal of Immunology*, **151**, 2252–60.

Nguyen, K.B., McCombe, P.A. & Pender, M.P. (1994). Macrophage apoptosis in the central nervous system in experimental autoimmune encephalomyelitis. *Journal of Autoimmunity*, **7**, 145–52.

Ohmori, K., Hong, Y., Fujiwara, M. & Matsumoto, Y. (1992). *In situ* demonstration of proliferating cells in the rat central nervous system during experimental autoimmune encephalomyelitis. Evidence suggesting that most infiltrating T cells do not proliferate in the target organ. *Laboratory Investigation*, **66**, 54–62.

Olsson, Y. (1968). Topographical differences in the vascular permeability of the peripheral nervous system. *Acta Neuropathologica*, **10**, 26–33.

Pender, M.P. (1993). Apoptosis in the target organ of an autoimmune disease. In *Programmed Cell Death: The Cellular and Molecular Biology of Apoptosis*, ed. M. Lavin & D. Watters, pp. 235–44. Chur, Switzerland: Harwood Academic Publishers.

Pender, M.P., McCombe, P.A., Yoong, G. & Nguyen, K.B. (1992). Apoptosis of $\alpha\beta$ T lymphocytes in the nervous system in experimental autoimmune encephalomyelitis: its possible implications for recovery and acquired tolerance. *Journal of Autoimmunity*, **5**, 401–10.

Pender, M.P., Nguyen, K.B., McCombe, P.A. & Kerr, J.F.R. (1991). Apoptosis in the nervous system in experimental allergic encephalomyelitis. *Journal of the Neurological Sciences*, **104**, 81–7.

Perry, V.H., Hume, D.A. & Gordon, S. (1985). Immunohistochemical localization of macrophages and microglia in the adult and developing mouse brain. *Neuroscience*, **15**, 313–26.

Pizarro, O., Hoecker, G., Rubinstein, P. & Ramos, A. (1961). The distribution in the tissues and the development of H-2 antigens of the mouse. *Proceedings of the National Academy of Sciences USA*, **47**, 1900–7.

Prineas, J.W. (1979). Multiple sclerosis: presence of lymphatic capillaries and lymphoid tissue in the brain and spinal cord. *Science*, **203**, 1123–5.

Reese, T.S. & Karnovsky, M.J. (1967). Fine structural localization of a blood–brain barrier to exogenous peroxidase. *Journal of Cell Biology*, **34**, 207–17.

Reid, D.M., Perry, V.H., Andersson, P.B. & Gordon, S. (1993). Mitosis and apoptosis of microglia *in vivo* induced by an anti-CR3 antibody which crosses the blood–brain barrier. *Neuroscience*, **56**, 529–33.

Schmied, M., Breitschopf, H., Gold, R., Zischler, H., Rothe, G., Wekerle, H. & Lassmann, H. (1993). Apoptosis of T lymphocytes in experimental autoimmune encephalomyelitis. Evidence for programmed cell death as a mechanism to control inflammation in the brain. *American Journal of Pathology*, **143**, 446–52.

Sedgwick, J.D., Mossner, R., Schwender, S. & ter Meulen, V. (1991*a*). Major histocompatibility complex-expressing nonhematopoietic astroglial cells prime only CD8+ T lymphocytes: astroglial cells as perpetuators but not initiators of CD4+ T cell responses in the central nervous system. *Journal of Experimental Medicine*, **173**, 1235–46.

Sedgwick, J.D., Schwender, S., Gregersen, R., Dorries, R. & ter Meulen, V. (1993). Resident macrophages (ramified microglia) of the adult Brown Norway rat central nervous system are constitutively major histocompatibility complex class II positive. *Journal of Experimental Medicine*, **177**, 1145–52.

Sedgwick, J.D., Schwender, S., Imrich, H., Dorries, R., Butcher, G.W. & ter Meulen, V. (1991*b*). Isolation and direct characterization of resident microglial cells from the normal and inflamed central nervous system. *Proceedings of the National Academy of Sciences USA*, **88**, 7438–42.

Sobel, R.A., Blanchette, B.W., Bhan, A.K. & Colvin, R.B. (1984) The immunopathology of experimental allergic encephalomyelitis. II. Endothelial cell Ia increases prior to inflammatory cell infiltration. *Journal of Immunology*, **132**, 2402–7.

Streit, W.J., Graeber, M.B. & Kreutzberg, G.W. (1989*a*). Peripheral nerve lesion produces increased levels of major histocompatibility complex antigens in the central nervous system. *Journal of Neuroimmunology*, **21**, 117–23.

Streit, W.J., Graeber, M.B. & Kreutzberg, G.W. (1989*b*). Expression of Ia antigen on perivascular and microglial cells after sublethal and lethal motor neuron injury. *Experimental Neurology*, **105**, 115–26.

Tabi, Z., McCombe, P.A. & Pender, M.P. (1994). Apoptotic elimination of $V\beta 8.2^+$ cells from the central nervous system during recovery from experimental autoimmune encephalomyelitis induced by the passive transfer of $V\beta 8.2^+$ encephalitogenic T cells. *European Journal of Immunology*, **24**, 2609–17.

Turnley, A.M., Miller, J.F.A.P. & Bartlett, P.F. (1991). Regulation of MHC molecules on MBP positive oligodendrocytes in mice by IFN-γ and TNF-α. *Neuroscience Letters*, **123**, 45–8.

Vass, K., Lassmann, H., Wekerle, H. & Wisniewski, H.M. (1986). The distribution of Ia antigen in the lesions of rat acute experimental allergic encephalomyelitis. *Acta Neuropathologica (Berlin)*, **70**, 149–60.

Waksman, B.H. (1961). Experimental study of diphtheritic polyneuritis in the rabbit and guinea pig. III. The blood–nerve barrier in the rabbit. *Journal of Neuropathology and Experimental Neurology*, **20**, 35–77.

Weber, F., Meinl, E., Aloisi, F., Nevinny Stickel, C., Albert, E., Wekerle, H. & Hohlfeld, R. (1994). Human astrocytes are only partially competent antigen presenting cells. Possible implications for lesion development in multiple sclerosis. *Brain*, **117**, 59–69.

Wekerle, H. (1988). Intercellular interactions in myelin-specific autoimmunity. *Journal of Neuroimmunology*, **20**, 211–16.

Wekerle, H., Linington, C., Lassmann, H. & Meyermann, R. (1986). Cellular immune reactivity within the CNS. *Trends in Neurosciences*, **9**, 271–7.

Wong, G.H.W., Bartlett, P.F., Clark-Lewis, I., Battye, F. & Schrader, J.W. (1984). Inducible expression of H-2 and Ia antigens on brain cells. *Nature*, **310**, 688–91.

–3–
Experimental autoimmune encephalomyelitis

MICHAEL P. PENDER

Introduction

Shortly after the introduction of the anti-rabies vaccine by Pasteur in 1885, there appeared reports of neurological complications in some of the patients vaccinated. The complications developed after a latent period and consisted of weakness and sensory disturbance in the limbs, sphincter dysfunction and cranial nerve involvement. The clinical picture differed from the typical one of rabies. The pathological findings also were different from those of rabies and consisted of perivascular inflammation and demyelination in the central nervous system (CNS) (Bassoe & Grinker, 1930).

Considerable controversy arose as to the cause of these 'neuroparalytic accidents', as they were called. Pasteur's vaccination involved a series of subcutaneous injections of suspensions of desiccated spinal cords of rabbits that had been infected with rabies virus. Theories put forward to explain the neuroparalytic accidents included vaccine transmission of attenuated rabies virus (cited by Bassoe & Grinker, 1930) and a toxic effect of a foreign nerve substance (Müller, 1908).

To elucidate the problem, the effect of injections of nervous tissue in experimental animals was studied. In 1898 Centanni reported that rabbits tolerated injections of brain substance poorly; the resulting weakness, emaciation and abscess formation were not due to infection at inoculation but were attributed to toxins produced by the decomposition of the injected material. Similar observations were made by other investigators in rabbits as well as in other animals. Koritschoner & Schweinburg (1925) inoculated rabbits subcutaneously for 14 days with normal human spinal cord tissue. The rabbits lost weight and some developed a flaccid paralysis of the hindlimbs or of all four limbs, which usually proved fatal. Histological examination revealed hyperaemia and oedema of the spinal cord, degenerative changes in the nerve cells with neuronophagia, small haemorrhages predominantly in the grey matter, and sometimes perivascular infiltration with small round mononuclear cells. They concluded that the nervous tissue administered was responsible for the post-rabies vaccination paralysis in humans.

Rivers, Sprunt & Berry (1933) gave repeated intramuscular injections of brain extracts and brain emulsions into eight monkeys, two of which developed ataxia and weakness and were found to have perivascular inflammatory and demyelinated lesions in the CNS. Rivers & Schwentker (1935) and Ferraro & Jervis (1940) confirmed and extended these studies. Ferraro & Jervis noted the close pathological similarities of the experimental disease and post-rabies vaccination encephalomyelitis, the various encephalitides which occasionally followed vaccinia or exanthematic disease of childhood, and also certain cases of acute multiple sclerosis. They suggested that an investigation of the mechanism operating in the experimental disease might give a clue to the cause of 'exanthematic encephalitis'.

The introduction of adjuvants into the inoculum greatly facilitated the induction and thus the study of the experimental disease. By the addition of complete Freund's adjuvant (CFA) (mycobacteria in mineral oil) to the emulsions of nervous tissue, acute disseminated encephalomyelitis was produced in monkeys (Morgan, 1947; Kabat, Wolf & Bezer, 1947), rabbits (Morrison, 1947) and guinea pigs (Freund, Stern & Pisani, 1947) with a much reduced latent period after a single injection or only a few injections of homologous CNS tissue. Since then the disease has been induced in rats, mice, cats, dogs, sheep, goats, pigs, pigeons and chickens (reviewed by Waksman [1959]). It is now well established that the experimental disease is mediated by T cells directed at myelin antigens, and it has become known as experimental autoimmune (allergic) encephalomyelitis (EAE). EAE is the prototype for cell-mediated autoimmune disease in general, and is the best available animal model of human CNS inflammatory demyelinating disease. It has three forms, which vary in clinical course and neuropathology: acute EAE, hyperacute EAE and chronic relapsing EAE. Acute EAE and hyperacute EAE are monophasic diseases which resemble the human diseases, acute disseminated encephalomyelitis and acute haemorrhagic leukoencephalitis, respectively. Chronic relapsing EAE has a chronic relapsing course and resembles the human disease, multiple sclerosis.

Induction and the role of genetic factors

EAE can be induced by inoculation with homogenized CNS tissue, purified CNS myelin or specific CNS myelin antigens together with CFA. Two myelin proteins have been shown to be encephalitogenic: myelin basic protein (MBP) (Laatsch *et al.*, 1962) and myelin proteolipid protein (PLP) (Williams *et al.*, 1982). The region of the protein responsible for inducing

EAE varies with the species and the major histocompatibility complex (MHC) class II haplotype. The 113–121 sequence of bovine MBP is encephalitogenic in the guinea pig (Eylar *et al.*, 1970) while the 153–166 sequence is encephalitogenic in the rhesus monkey (Karkhanis *et al.*, 1975). In the SJL/J (H-2^s) mouse, the 89–101 sequence of rat MBP is encephalitogenic and is restricted by I-A (Sakai *et al.*, 1988); in the PL/J (H-2^u) mouse, the acetyl(Ac)1–11 (Zamvil *et al.*, 1987) and 35–47 sequences (Zamvil *et al.*, 1988*b*) are encephalitogenic and are restricted by I-A and I-E, respectively; and in the A.CA (H-2^f) mouse the 1–11, 9–20 and 87–99 are encephalitogenic (Rajan *et al.*, 1993). The importance of the I-A haplotype of the antigen-presenting cell in determining the encephalitogenic epitope of MBP has been clearly shown in (SJL × PL)F_1 mice (McCarron & McFarlin, 1988). Furthermore, in these mice the minimum structural requirements for an inoculated *N*-terminal peptide to be capable of inducing EAE have been defined as a sequence of six amino acids containing five of the native residues (1,3,4,5,6) (Gautam *et al.*, 1994). In the Lewis rat (RT1^l) the sequences 72–89 and 87–99 of rat MBP are encephalitogenic and are restricted by I-A and I-E, respectively (Offner *et al.*, 1989); in the Buffalo rat (RT1^b) the sequence 87–99 is encephalitogenic (Jones *et al.*, 1992). With regard to PLP the encephalitogenic sequences are 103–116 in SWR (H-2^q) mice (Tuohy *et al.*, 1988), 139–151 (Tuohy *et al.*, 1989) and 178–191 (Greer *et al.*, 1992) in SJL/J mice, 215–232 in C3H/He (H-2^k) mice (Endoh *et al.*, 1990), 43–64 in PL/J mice (Whitham *et al.*, 1991), and 56–70 in Biozzi AB/H (H-2^{dq1}) and the MHC-similar non-obese diabetic (H-2^{Anod}) mice (Amor *et al.*, 1993). The 91–110 sequence of PLP is encephalitogenic in the New Zealand White rabbit (Linington, Gunn & Lassmann, 1990) while the 217–240 sequence is encephalitogenic in the Lewis rat (Zhao *et al.*, 1994).

The genetic susceptibility to EAE is also determined by non-MHC genes. Studies in the EAE-susceptible SJL/J mouse and the EAE-resistant B10.S mouse, which share the H-2^s haplotype, have indicated that disease susceptibility is determined by the intrinsic ability of prethymic cells in the bone marrow to develop into encephalitogenic T cells (Binder *et al.*, 1993). Goverman *et al.* (1993) have shown that transgenic mice expressing genes encoding a rearranged T cell receptor (TCR) specific for MBP spontaneously develop EAE when housed in a non-sterile facility but not when housed in a sterile, specific-pathogen-free facility. This transgenic model demonstrates the role of TCR genes and environmental factors in the development of EAE. The gene encoding *Bordetella-pertussis*-induced histamine sensitization, which maps distal to the TCR β-chain gene on mouse chromosome 6 (Sudweeks *et al.*, 1993), also appears to contribute to susceptibility to EAE, as the administration of pertussis toxin, which increases vascular permeability, is required to induce acute EAE in the mouse and hyperacute EAE in the rat. Genetically determined target organ factors may also play a role in the susceptibility to EAE (Mostarica Stojkovic *et al.*, 1992).

EAE can also be induced by the passive transfer of T cells specific for MBP, PLP or the appropriate encephalitogenic peptides. Passive EAE was first induced by the direct intravenous transfer of lymph node cells from animals sensitized to whole CNS tissue (Paterson, 1960). Techniques were later developed for the *in vitro* augmentation of donor lymphocyte activity by incubation with concanavalin A (Panitch & McFarlin, 1977) or specific antigen (Richert *et al.*, 1979), and these have ultimately led to the development of MBP-specific and PLP-specific T cell lines and clones that are capable of transferring disease in low doses (Ben Nun, Wekerle & Cohen, 1981*a*; Zamvil *et al.*, 1985; Satoh *et al.*, 1987; van der Veen *et al.*, 1990). Linington *et al.* (1993) have shown that EAE can also be induced in the Lewis rat by transferring both T cells and antibody specific for myelin/oligodendrocyte glycoprotein (MOG).

Acute EAE

In general, induction of EAE by active or passive immunization results in acute EAE, a monophasic illness that is usually followed by spontaneous recovery. Hyperacute EAE or chronic relapsing EAE can be induced by altering the adjuvant, the animal strain or the age of the animal at the time of sensitization, or by treatment with immunosuppressants.

Hyperacute EAE

Hyperacute EAE has a shorter latent period, a more rapidly progressive clinical course and a higher mortality than acute EAE. It can be induced in Lewis rats by inoculation with a mixture of aqueous spinal cord homogenate and aqueous pertussis vaccine (Levine & Wenk, 1965). In contrast, when Lewis rats are inoculated with spinal cord homogenate and CFA, acute EAE develops. Hyperacute EAE can also be induced in the rhesus monkey by inoculation with whole spinal cord tissue and CFA (Ravkina *et al.*, 1979).

Chronic relapsing EAE

Chronic relapsing EAE is characterized by recurrent clinical attacks (relapses) followed by periods of partial or complete clinical recovery (remissions). It can be induced in immature strain 13 and Hartley guinea pigs by a single inoculation with homogenized spinal cord tissue and complete Freund's adjuvant (Wisniewski & Keith, 1977); inoculation of older animals in the same manner results in acute EAE in most animals (Lassmann & Wisniewski, 1979*a*). In the SJL/J mouse, chronic relapsing EAE can be induced by two injections of spinal cord homogenate in CFA, one week apart (Brown & McFarlin, 1981; Brown, McFarlin & Raine, 1982), or by the passive transfer of MBP-sensitized lymph node cells (Raine, Mokhtarian & McFarlin, 1984; Mokhtarian, McFarlin & Raine, 1984) or PLP-sensitized lymph node cells (van der Veen *et al.*, 1989) in the absence of a peripheral antigen depot. In the Lewis rat, acute EAE can be converted into chronic relapsing EAE by treatment with low-dose cyclosporin A after inoculation with spinal cord tissue and CFA (Polman *et al.*, 1988; Pender *et al.*, 1990).

Clinical features

After a latent period following active or passive immunization, the animals lose weight and develop neurological signs. In acute EAE the animals either die, or recover and have no further attacks. In chronic relapsing EAE typically the animals recover from the first attack and have subsequent relapses, which are separated by periods of partial or complete clinical recovery; however, within a group of animals developing chronic relapsing EAE, some of the inoculated animals may exhibit a chronic persistent or chronic progressive neurological deficit continuing from the first attack or from subsequent attacks (Pender *et al.*, 1990). Hyperacute EAE differs clinically from acute EAE in having a shorter latent period, a more rapidly progressive course and a higher mortality (Levine & Wenk, 1965; Hansen & Pender, 1989).

The latent period after immunization varies according to species and method of immunization. For example, in Lewis rats with acute EAE induced by inoculation with spinal cord tissue or MBP in CFA the latent period is 8–14 days (Pender, 1988*a*,*b*) whereas the latent period is reduced to four days when EAE is induced by the passive transfer of MBP-sensitized lymphocytes (Pender, Nguyen & Willenborg, 1989). The latent period for hyperacute EAE in the Lewis rat is 6–7 days (Hansen & Pender, 1989). For each species the neurological signs are usually the same, whether the animal has acute EAE, hyperacute EAE or chronic relapsing EAE. In the monkey the neurological signs consist of visual loss, optic disc oedema, optic atrophy, ptosis, facial weakness, nystagmus, tremor, limb weakness (including hemiplegia), spasticity and ataxia (Rivers *et al.*, 1933; Rivers & Schwentker, 1935; Ferraro & Jervis, 1940; Morgan, 1947; Kabat *et al.*, 1947; Hayreh *et al.*, 1981). Rabbits exhibit lateral splaying and ataxia of the hindlimbs followed by similar involvement of the forelimbs, areflexia, impaired limb nociception, limb weakness, paradoxical breathing, slowing of respiration and hypothermia (Pender & Sears, 1984). In the guinea pig, mouse and rat the main neurological signs are tail (in the mouse and rat) and limb weakness. Lewis rats display a striking ascending paralysis, commencing in the distal tail and extending to the whole tail, hindlimbs and sometimes the forelimbs (Simmons *et al.*, 1982; Pender, 1986*a*); the tail weakness is accompanied by an ascending impairment of tail nociception (Pender, 1986*a*). Another characteristic feature in the Lewis rat is rapid clinical recovery, especially from EAE induced by active or passive sensitization to MBP (Simmons *et al.*, 1981; Pender, 1988*a*; Pender *et al.*, 1989); in such cases hindlimb weakness may last for three days or less.

Neuropathology

The characteristic histological features of EAE are meningeal infiltration with mononuclear cells, perivascular cuffing with mononuclear cells, parenchymal infiltration with mononuclear cells and a variable degree of primary demyelination in the CNS. Primary demyelination refers to a loss of myelin from intact axons (nerve fibres), as opposed to secondary demyelination where the loss of myelin results from axonal degeneration. In this chapter the term 'demyelination' will always indicate primary demyelination. The distribution of lesions within the CNS varies according to the animal species and the stage of the disease: in monkeys with acute EAE, the cerebrum, brainstem, cerebellum and optic nerve are principally involved (Morgan, 1947; Hayreh *et al.*, 1981); in rabbits and rats with acute EAE the spinal cord and brainstem are the main sites of involvement (Pender & Sears, 1984, 1986) while in rats with chronic relapsing EAE there is also prominent involvement of the cerebellum (Pender *et al.*, 1990); in guinea pigs and SJL/J mice with chronic relapsing EAE there is prominent involvement of the cerebrum, brainstem, cerebellum, optic nerves and spinal cord (Lassmann & Wisniewski, 1979*b*; Raine *et al.*, 1984). In guinea pigs with chronic relapsing EAE it has been noted that higher regions of the neuraxis are affected with increasing duration of disease (Lassmann & Wisniewski, 1978).

The peripheral nervous system (PNS) is also involved when EAE is induced by sensitization to whole CNS tissue or MBP. This PNS involvement is explained by the fact that the P_1 protein from the PNS is identical to CNS MBP (Brostoff & Eylar, 1972; Greenfield *et al.*, 1973). PNS involvement occurs in acute EAE in the monkey (Ferraro & Roizin, 1954), rabbit (Waksman & Adams, 1955; Wisniewski, Prineas & Raine, 1969; Pender & Sears, 1984), guinea pig (Freund *et al.*, 1947; Waksman & Adams, 1956), mouse (Waksman & Adams, 1956) and rat (Pender & Sears, 1986; Pender, 1988*a*; Pender *et al.*, 1989). It also occurs in chronic relapsing EAE in guinea pigs (Madrid & Wisniewski, 1978), mice (Brown *et al.*, 1982) and rats (Lassmann, Kitz & Wisniewski, 1980; Pender *et al.*, 1990). In Lewis rats there is active PNS involvement in the early stages of chronic relapsing EAE but not in the later stages, when there is still active CNS involvement (Pender *et al.*, 1990). In general, the PNS disease occurs mainly in the spinal roots and ganglia and there is little involvement of the peripheral nerves (Pender & Sears, 1984, 1986; Pender, 1988*a*); however, in the guinea pig the peripheral nerves are particularly affected (Waksman & Adams, 1956). In contrast to when EAE is induced by immunization with whole CNS tissue or MBP, the PNS is not involved when EAE is induced by sensitization to PLP (Chalk *et al.*, 1994*b*). Sparing of the PNS in PLP-induced EAE is expected, because of the absence of PLP in the PNS (Finean, Hawthorne & Patterson, 1957; Folch, Lees & Carr, 1958).

The type of lesion also varies with the animal species, the sensitizing neuroantigen(s) and the adjuvant used. Typically the inflammatory infiltrate consists predominantly of mononuclear cells (lymphocytes and macrophages) although some polymorphonuclear cells may be present. Generally the white matter is more severely involved than the grey matter, but severe grey matter inflammation is not unusual in acute EAE. Some oedema and erythrocyte extravasation may also occur in acute EAE. In hyperacute EAE in the Lewis rat and monkey, the lesions are characterized by a major neutrophilic infiltrate, prominent oedema, fibrin deposition, haemorrhage, vascular and parenchymal necrosis and vascular thrombosis (Levine & Wenk, 1965; Ravkina *et al.*, 1979). In chronic relapsing EAE the inflammatory infiltrate is maximal during clinical attacks and minimal during clinical remission (Pender *et al.*, 1990).

The degree of primary demyelination varies according to the animal species, sensitizing neuroantigen(s) and stage of disease. In acute MBP-induced EAE (MBP-EAE) in the Lewis rat the CNS demyelination is mainly limited to the dorsal root entry and ventral root exit zones of the spinal cord while there is prominent demyelination in the PNS, namely the spinal roots (Pender, 1988*a,c*; Pender *et al.*, 1989). Extensive CNS demyelination can be induced by the intravenous or intraperitoneal administration of a monoclonal antibody against MOG in rats that have been inoculated with MBP and CFA or that have received transferred MBP-specific T cells (Schluesener *et al.*, 1987; Linington *et al.*, 1988; Lassmann *et al.*, 1988). On the other hand prominent CNS demyelination can be induced in the Buffalo rat by the passive transfer of MBP-specific T cells without the administration of demyelinating antibody (Jones *et al.*, 1990). Inoculation of Lewis rats with whole CNS tissue or PLP and CFA also results in more extensive CNS demyelination than occurs in MBP-EAE (Pender & Sears, 1986; Chalk *et al.*, 1994*b*). Extensive CNS demyelination can also be induced in Lewis rats by the combined transfer of MOG-specific T cells and anti-MOG antibody, whereas transfer of MOG-specific T cells alone results in severe CNS inflammation without demyelination (Linington *et al.*, 1993). In Lewis rats with chronic relapsing EAE induced by inoculation with whole CNS tissue, there is prominent spinal cord demyelination in the first attack and extensive spinal cord demyelination at later stages (Pender *et al.*, 1990). In guinea pigs with acute EAE induced by inoculation with MBP and CFA, there is limited CNS demyelination but large demyelinated lesions occur in the spinal cord when the animals are pretreated by immunization with ovalbumin and muramyl dipeptide and a second injection of ovalbumin (Colover, 1980). Confluent demyelinated plaques in the optic nerve, cerebrum, cerebellum and spinal cord are a characteristic feature of chronic relapsing EAE in guinea pigs (Lassmann & Wisniewski, 1979*b*). After clinical recovery from acute EAE and the attacks of chronic relapsing EAE, there is CNS remyelination by oligodendrocytes and PNS remyelination by Schwann cells (Pender, 1989; Pender *et al.*, 1989, 1990). In chronic relapsing EAE, shadow plaques representing extensive areas of CNS remyelination can be found (Lassmann & Wisniewski, 1979*b*; Pender *et al.*, 1990).

Other typical features of EAE are the presence of macrophages laden with myelin debris in regions of active demyelination, and, in chronic relapsing EAE, the occurrence of astrocytic gliosis (Lassmann & Wisniewski, 1979*b*; Raine *et al.*, 1984; Pender *et al.*, 1990). Although primary demyelination is the predominant type of parenchymal damage in EAE, axonal degeneration and loss are also important components of the pathology in the later stages of chronic relapsing EAE (Lassmann & Wisniewski, 1979*b*; Raine *et al.*, 1984; Pender *et al.*, 1990). Axonal damage and degeneration are well recognized features of hyperacute EAE (Lampert, 1967; Hansen & Pender, 1989) and may also occur to a limited extent in acute EAE (Lampert & Kies, 1967; Pender, 1989).

Of all the forms of EAE that have been described, chronic relapsing EAE in the guinea pig most closely resembles multiple sclerosis in neuropathology (Lassmann & Wisniewski, 1979*b*).

Pathophysiology

What causes the neurological signs in EAE and what is the mechanism for the clinical recovery? Conduction block due to primary demyelination is likely to be the main cause of neurological signs (Pender, 1987). The role of demyelination in the production of neurological signs has been clearly demonstrated by the fact that MOG-specific T cells induce severe CNS inflammation and disruption of the blood–brain barrier but no demyelination or neurological signs, while the additional intravenous administration of anti-MOG antibody induces extensive CNS demyelination and severe neurological signs (Linington *et al.*, 1993). When considering the relationship between the clinical and neuropathological features of EAE, it is important to know the extent of neuropathology in the PNS as well as in the

CNS. For example, in rabbits with EAE induced by inoculation with whole spinal cord and CFA, demyelination-induced conduction block in the PNS, specifically the dorsal root ganglia, accounts for the ataxia and areflexia (Pender & Sears, 1982, 1984, 1985). In Lewis rats with MBP-EAE, conduction block due to demyelination in the spinal roots is a major cause of the neurological signs, although significant conduction block also occurs in the dorsal columns of the spinal cord (Pender, 1986*a*, 1988*a*,*c*; Chalk, McCombe & Pender, 1994*a*). Conduction abnormalities attributed to demyelination have also been demonstrated in the spinal roots and spinal cord in rats with EAE induced by the passive transfer of MBP-specific T line cells (Heininger *et al.*, 1989). In contrast to the findings in MBP-EAE, demyelination and nerve conduction abnormalities are restricted to the CNS in PLP-EAE (Chalk *et al.*, 1994*a*). In acute or chronic relapsing EAE induced in the rat by inoculation with whole CNS tissue, conduction block due to CNS demyelination is an important cause of the neurological deficit, although demyelination-induced nerve conduction abnormalities also occur in the proximal PNS (Pender, 1986*b*, 1988*b*; Stanley & Pender, 1991).

The rapid clinical recovery from acute EAE in the Lewis rat is explained by restoration of conduction due to CNS remyelination by oligodendrocytes and PNS remyelination by Schwann cells (Pender, 1989; Pender *et al.*, 1989). Restoration of conduction by CNS and PNS remyelination also accounts for clinical recovery after attacks of chronic relapsing EAE (Stanley & Pender, 1991). Axonal damage is also likely to be an important factor contributing to the neurological signs in some forms of EAE. It is probable that axonal degeneration is a major cause of the persistent conduction failure occurring in chronic relapsing EAE (Stanley & Pender, 1991). Selective bulbospinal monoamine axon damage may also contribute to the neurological signs of EAE (White & Bowker, 1988; Bieger & White, 1981). Oedema is unlikely to cause neurological signs, except when it occurs in a confined space and leads to vascular compression and secondary ischaemia, for example in the optic canal.

Immunopathology of the CNS and PNS lesions

Characteristics of the inflammatory infiltrate

Immunocytochemical studies have shown that the inflammatory infiltrate in both acute EAE and chronic relapsing EAE is composed predominantly of $CD4^+$ T lymphocytes and macrophages with a smaller proportion of $CD8^+$ T lymphocytes and B lymphocytes (Traugott *et al.*, 1981; Sriram *et al.*, 1982; Hickey *et al.*, 1983; Sobel *et al.*, 1984*b*; Traugott, Raine & McFarlin, 1985; Traugott, McFarlin & Raine, 1986; Matsumoto & Fujiwara, 1987;

McCombe *et al.*, 1992; McCombe, de Jersey & Pender, 1994). Similar results have been obtained using flow cytometry to assess cells extracted from the spinal cord (Lyman, Abrams & Raine, 1989*a*; Jensen *et al.*, 1992; McCombe *et al.*, 1992, 1994). The number of infiltrating T cells declines substantially during clinical remission (McCombe *et al.*, 1994). The majority of T cells use the $\alpha\beta$ TCR and a minority use the $\gamma\delta$ TCR (Sobel & Kuchroo, 1992). An important finding not evident in conventional histological sections is that T cells infiltrate diffusely into the CNS parenchyma and are not restricted to perivascular infiltrates (Sobel *et al.*, 1984*b*; Matsumoto & Fujiwara, 1987). PNS inflammatory infiltrates also are mainly composed of T cells and monocytes/macrophages (Lassmann *et al.*, 1986). Within the CNS in EAE, there is an enrichment of activated $CD4^+$ T cells expressing the interleukin-2 receptor (IL-2R) and of memory ($CD45RC^-$) $CD4^+$ T cells, suggesting that such T cells selectively enter the CNS (Jensen *et al.*, 1992; McCombe *et al.*, 1992, 1994). In chronic relapsing EAE, plasma cells are prominent in tissue sections (Bernheimer, Lassmann & Suchanek, 1988) and the relative proportion of B cells/plasma cells increases in cells extracted from the spinal cord (McCombe *et al.*, 1994).

MHC class II (Ia) antigen expression in the nervous system

In the normal CNS, Ia antigen expression is limited to stellate cells in the meninges and to some perivascular mononuclear cells (Matsumoto & Fujiwara, 1986; Vass *et al.*, 1986). In the guinea pig, there is also occasional Ia expression on CNS endothelial cells (Sobel *et al.*, 1984*a*). In guinea pigs with EAE there is enhancement of Ia expression on CNS endothelial cells prior to detectable inflammatory cell infiltration (Sobel *et al.*, 1984*a*; Sobel, Natale & Schneeberger, 1987). However, in the rat, endothelial Ia expression does not occur in EAE (Matsumoto *et al.*, 1986; Vass *et al.*, 1986). In all species, Ia expression is observed on infiltrating leukocytes (activated T cells, B cells and macrophages) (Hickey *et al.*, 1983; Sobel *et al.*, 1984*b*; Traugott *et al.*, 1985; Vass *et al.*, 1986; Sobel *et al.*, 1987; McCombe *et al.*, 1992, 1994). A striking feature is the prominent expression of Ia antigen on microglia diffusely throughout the CNS parenchyma; such microglial Ia expression commences prior to the onset of neurological signs, spreads during the clinical attack and persists after recovery (Matsumoto *et al.*, 1986; Vass *et al.*, 1986; Konno *et al.*, 1989; McCombe *et al.*, 1992, 1994; Uitdehaag *et al.*, 1993). In contrast to the Ia expression on microglia, there is no detectable expression of Ia by astrocytes or oligodendrocytes (Matsumoto *et al.*, 1986; Vass *et al.*, 1986). The PNS lesions of EAE are characterized by Ia expression on infiltrating mononuclear cells but not on endothelial cells (at least in the rat), Schwann cells or axons (Lassmann *et al.*, 1986).

Pathogenesis

T cell entry into the CNS, and adhesion molecule expression

How do T cells enter the CNS in EAE? Activated T cells of any specificity can cross the intact blood–brain barrier, but only those cells with specificity for CNS antigens accumulate in the CNS (Wekerle *et al.*, 1986; Hickey, Hsu & Kimura, 1991; Ludowyk, Willenborg & Parish, 1992). Immunocytochemical studies have demonstrated the upregulated co-expression of intercellular adhesion molecule-1 (ICAM-1; CD54) and the addressin MECA-325 (a marker of lymph node high-endothelial venules) on CNS endothelial cells during clinical attacks of EAE with downregulation in remission (Cannella, Cross & Raine, 1990; Raine *et al.*, 1990; Wilcox *et al.*, 1990; O'Neill *et al.*, 1991). Baron *et al.* (1993) found that anti-ICAM-1 antibody effectively inhibits passively transferred EAE; however, others have found that it has little or no effect on passively transferred EAE, but can inhibit actively induced EAE, possibly by interfering with sensitization (Archelos *et al.*, 1993; Cannella, Cross & Raine, 1993; Willenborg *et al.*, 1993). An interaction between the $\alpha4$ integrin, very late antigen-4 (VLA-4), on encephalitogenic T cells and its ligand, vascular cell adhesion molecule-1 (VCAM-1), is necessary for T cell entry into the CNS in EAE (Yednock *et al.*, 1992; Baron *et al.*, 1993). Anti-VLA-4 inhibits the binding of lymphocytes and monocytes to inflamed EAE brain vessels *in vitro* and effectively prevents the accumulation of leukocytes in the CNS *in vivo* and the development of EAE (Yednock *et al.*, 1992). Furthermore, a high level of expression of VLA-4 is essential for the encephalitogenicity of MBP-specific T cell clones, anti-VCAM-1 delays the onset of passively transferred EAE, and VCAM-1 is expressed on CNS endothelium where perivascular cuffs are present (Baron *et al.*, 1993). VLA-4 expression is also required for PLP-specific T cells to be encephalitogenic, although this requirement can be bypassed by pretreating the recipient with pertussis vaccine and irradiation, which probably act by increasing vascular permeability and facilitating entry into the CNS (Kuchroo *et al.*, 1993). One proposed scenario for T cell entry into the CNS in EAE is as follows. Once the activated CNS-antigen-specific T cell binds to the endothelium, whether it be by a lymphocyte function associated molecule-1 (LFA-1)/ICAM-1 interaction or by selectin binding, the T cell induces upregulation of VCAM-1 on the endothelium by producing interferon-γ (IFN-γ) and tumour necrosis factor (TNF), and then the VLA-4-expressing T cell binds to the newly induced VCAM-1 and enters the CNS (Baron *et al.*, 1993).

Antigen-presenting cells in the CNS

An important question is what cells present CNS antigens to the encephalitogenic T cells so that the latter can accumulate in the CNS and exert their effector function. After being induced to express Ia antigen by IFN-γ, astrocytes (Fontana, Fierz & Wekerle, 1984; Fierz *et al.*, 1985) and cerebral vascular endothelial cells (McCarron *et al.*, 1985, 1986) are capable of presenting MBP to MBP-specific T cells *in vitro*; however, it is doubtful whether these cells have an antigen-presenting role *in vivo* in EAE. MHC class II (Ia) antigen expression is required for a cell to present antigen to the $CD4^+$ T cells that mediate EAE. As discussed above, astrocytes do not express detectable levels of Ia antigen in EAE, and endothelial cells express Ia antigen in guinea pigs but not in rats. On the other hand, microglia exhibit prominent expression of Ia antigen in EAE. Some authors have interpreted the microglial Ia expression as a mechanism upregulating the immune response by antigen presentation (Matsumoto *et al.*, 1986); others have interpreted it as indicating a reparative role for microglia (Konno *et al.*, 1989) or as a mechanism downregulating the immune response (McCombe *et al.*, 1992; Uitdehaag *et al.*, 1993). After being induced to express Ia antigen by IFN-γ, microglia have been reported to be capable of presenting antigen to T cells *in vitro* (Frei *et al.*, 1987; Matsumoto, Ohmori & Fujiwara, 1992), although in the experiments of Matsumoto *et al.*, T cell proliferation was inhibited when higher numbers of microglial cells were used. Further studies are needed to determine whether microglia upregulate or downregulate the inflammatory response in EAE. One study reported that the inducibility of Ia antigen expression on astrocytes correlates positively with susceptibility to EAE (Massa, ter Meulen & Fontana, 1987) but this was not confirmed by subsequent studies (Matsumoto, Kawai & Fujiwara, 1989; Barish & Raissdana, 1990).

Studies using F_1-to-parent bone marrow chimeras as recipients of MBP-specific T cells have demonstrated that bone-marrow-derived cells can serve as the only antigen-presenting cells within the CNS in EAE (Hinrichs, Wegmann & Dietsch, 1987; Hickey & Kimura, 1988; Myers, Dougherty & Ron, 1993). In these chimeras the bone-marrow-derived cells in the CNS are essentially restricted to the perivascular and meningeal macrophage populations, as there is minimal settlement of these cells into the parenchymal microglial population (Hickey & Kimura, 1988). Therefore, these studies indicate that the perivascular and meningeal macrophages are major antigen-presenting cells in the CNS in EAE. Further evidence that bone-marrow-derived cells can serve as the sole antigen-presenting cells within the CNS comes from passive transfer studies in severe combined immunodeficient (SCID) mice. EAE can be transferred by encephalitogenic T cells to SCID mice reconstituted with allogeneic or xenogeneic haematopoietic stem cells from the same source as the donor T cells (Jones *et al.*, 1993). Studies using parent-to-F_1 bone marrow chimeras as recipients of MBP-specific T cells have indicated that EAE can also be induced, albeit less efficiently, when there is histocompatibility between only the recipient's resident parenchymal cells and the donor T cells (Myers *et al.*, 1993). These studies were interpreted as indicating that endothelial cells or astrocytes can act as antigen-presenting cells *in vivo*; however, it remains possible that radiation-resistant parenchymal microglia may be the antigen-presenting cells in this model.

Roles of $CD4^+$ T cells and $CD8^+$ T cells in EAE

The passive transfer of EAE by MBP-specific lymph node cells requires the presence of $CD4^+$ T cells in the transferred population (Pettinelli & McFarlin, 1981). EAE can be passively transferred by MBP-specific or PLP-specific $CD4^+$ T cell clones (Zamvil *et al.*, 1985; van der Veen *et al.*, 1990) but to date has not been transferrable by $CD8^+$ T cells. Such passive transfer studies do not rule out a role for $CD8^+$ T cells as effectors or regulators in EAE, as the recipients' $CD8^+$ T cells may have been involved. Experiments employing antibody-mediated *in vivo* depletion of $CD8^+$ T cells have yielded conflicting results, possibly due to interspecies differences or differences in the degree of depletion achieved. In the Lewis rat, long-term depletion of $CD8^+$ T cells was found not to influence the course of actively or passively induced EAE (Sedgwick, 1988). In the mouse, depletion of $CD8^+$ T cells had no effect on acute or chronic relapsing EAE in one study (Sriram & Carroll, 1988), and in another study $CD8^+$ T cell depletion had no effect on the severity of acute EAE induced by inoculation with *N*-terminal MBP nonapeptide but eliminated the normal resistance to reinduction of EAE (Jiang, Zhang & Pernis, 1992). Mutant mice completely lacking in CD8 ($CD8^{-/-}$) have less severe acute EAE and a higher incidence of relapses when inoculated with MBP than do control mice, indicating that $CD8^+$ T cells may participate as both effectors and regulators in EAE (Koh *et al.*, 1992). Jiang *et al.* (1992) suggested that the lack of effect of $CD8^+$ T cell depletion on the severity of EAE in their study was probably due to an inability of the *N*-terminal MBP nonapeptide to bind to class I MHC molecules and provide a target for pathogenic $CD8^+$ T cells. The immunoregulation of EAE will be discussed in detail later in this chapter.

TCR Vβ gene usage of T cells in EAE

MBP-specific encephalitogenic $CD4^+$ T cell clones derived from B10.PL (H-2^u) and PL/J (H-2^u) mice have a markedly restricted usage of TCR Vβ

genes and, to a lesser extent, of Vα genes: approximately 80% of T cell clones reactive to the immunodominant *N*-terminal MBP nonapeptide use Vβ8.2 (Urban *et al.*, 1988; Acha Orbea *et al.*, 1988; Zamvil *et al.*, 1988*a*). In the Lewis rat it was initially found that 100% of T cell clones reactive to the immunodominant 72–89 MBP peptide use Vβ8.2 (Burns *et al.*, 1989; Chluba *et al.*, 1989); however, more recently it has been shown that these T cells also use other Vβ genes and that their TCR usage is influenced by the type of antigen-presenting cell (Sun, Le & Coleclough, 1993). Lewis rat T cells reactive to the encephalitogenic 87–99 MBP peptide demonstrate heterogeneous usage of TCR Vβ genes (Sun *et al.*, 1992*b*). In the SJL/J mouse (H-2^s), T cell clones specific for the encephalitogenic 91–103 MBP peptide or the encephalitogenic 139–151 PLP peptide exhibit a diverse usage of TCR Vβ genes (Su & Sriram, 1992; Kuchroo *et al.*, 1992).

The expression of Vβ genes has also been studied in the CNS during the course of EAE. In the Lewis rat there is a selective accumulation of Vβ8.2$^+$ T cells in the CNS during the early clinical phase of EAE induced by inoculation with MBP (Offner *et al.*, 1993; Tsuchida *et al.*, 1993) or by the passive transfer of a Vβ8.2$^+$ T cell clone specific for the 72–89 MBP peptide (Tabi, McCombe & Pender, 1994). At the peak of clinical disease the majority of the infiltrating Vβ8.2$^+$ cells are found in the parenchyma as opposed to the perivascular space (Tsuchida *et al.*, 1993). During clinical recovery the proportion of Vβ8.2$^+$ cells in the CNS declines as a result of selective apoptotic elimination (Tabi *et al.*, 1994). In (PL/J × SJL/J)F_1 mice with EAE induced by a transferred Vβ8.2$^+$ T cell clone specific for the Ac1–16 peptide of MBP, the great majority of lymphocytes in the CNS were reported to be Vβ8.2$^+$ (Baron *et al.*, 1993). In contrast, Bell *et al.* (1993) did not detect preferential utilization of a single TCR Vβ gene in the CNS at any time during the course of EAE induced in the same mice by inoculation with the Ac1–11 MBP peptide, despite the fact that this epitope is recognized mainly by Vβ8$^+$ T cells. One possible explanation for this discrepancy is that Vβ8 may not be dominant for recognition of Ac1–11 *in vivo*. Sobell & Kuchroo (1992) found a diverse TCR Vβ gene usage in the CNS of SJL/J mice with EAE induced by immunization with the 139–151 PLP peptide, but this is not surprising, as T cells specific for this peptide use diverse Vβ genes (Kuchroo *et al.*, 1992). Although they did not find preferential utilization of a single TCR Vβ gene in the CNS when EAE was induced by the passive transfer of T cell clones using a single TCR Vβ gene, the CNS was not examined early in the course of clinical disease and a selective accumulation of cells using the appropriate gene may have been missed (Sobel & Kuchroo, 1992).

In conclusion, it appears that in the early stages of EAE induced by the transfer of T cell clones there is a selective accumulation in the CNS of T cells using the Vβ gene transcribed by the clone. A similar selective accumulation occurs in actively induced EAE when the immunogen is recognized *in vivo* mainly by T cells using a single Vβ gene, but not when the immunogen is recognized by T cells using a variety of Vβ genes.

Specificity of T cells within the CNS in EAE

Studies on the proportion of myelin antigen-specific T cells in the CNS in EAE have yielded conflicting results. Sedgwick, Brostoff & Mason (1987) concluded that MBP-specific T cells constitute only a small minority of the infiltrating cells in the CNS of Lewis rats with passively transferred MBP-EAE. Their conclusion depended on the assumption that all MBP-specific T cells in the CNS are IL-2R$^+$; however, this may underestimate the proportion of MBP-specific T cells, as the expression of this receptor is transient. A similar conclusion was reached in a study that employed [^{14}C]thymidine-labelled MBP-sensitized lymphocytes in the SJL/J mouse: labelled cells constituted a minority (1–4%) of the inflammatory cells in the CNS in the acute and early chronic phases of the disease and could not be found in the CNS in relapses (Cross *et al.*, 1990). In contrast, another laboratory studying the same model, but using a different label, found that labelled cells constituted about 45% of infiltrating CD4$^+$ T cells at the time of onset of neurological signs (Zeine & Owens, 1992). One variable that could account for the difference in these results is the extent to which the label is lost after the donor T cell proliferation that occurs in the lymphoid organs of the recipients prior to the development of EAE (Matsumoto, Kawai & Fujiwara, 1988; Ohmori *et al.*, 1992).

This problem can be avoided by employing methods that do not require the use of an exogenous label. In one study, MBP-activated spleen cells were injected into bone marrow chimeras, and a monoclonal antibody directed against chimera-specific MHC antigens was used to determine the origin of the infiltrating T cells: donor T cells accounted for 46% of the total inflammatory cells at the preclinical stage, 23% at the clinical stage and 37% after recovery (Matsumoto & Fujiwara, 1988). At all stages of disease, donor T cells constituted the majority of the T cells infiltrating the CNS parenchyma. Using Thy-1 congenic SJL/J mice as recipients of MBP-activated lymph node cells, Skundric *et al.* (1993) found that donor cells constituted 7–10% of the CNS-infiltrating cells during the early attacks of chronic relapsing EAE and 2–5% of the infiltrate at later stages (up to ten relapses). However, in this study and the previous ones, it is likely that only a small proportion of the donor T cells were MBP-specific, as bulk cultures rather than lines or clones were used. The selective accumulation of Vβ8.2$^+$ T cells in the CNS in the early clinical phase of EAE induced by the transfer of MBP-specific Vβ8.2$^+$ T cells (Tabi *et al.*, 1994) (see above) strongly suggests that these infiltrating cells are MBP-specific, but does not prove it, as recipient-derived cells of other specificities may also use Vβ8.2. In conclusion, although all the above studies have limitations, it would appear that a significant proportion of the T cells infiltrating the CNS in the early clinical phase of EAE are specific for myelin antigens.

The functional state of the T cells in the CNS also needs to be considered. Cells recovered from the spinal cord of Lewis rats with EAE can transfer EAE after *in vitro* activation with MBP (Hayosh & Swanborg, 1986). Limiting dilution analysis indicates a marked enrichment of MBP-reactive T cells in the spinal cord compared to the lymph nodes and spleen of Lewis rats in the early clinical phase of actively or passively induced MBP-EAE (Mor & Cohen, 1992; Tabi *et al.*, 1994). The frequency of MBP-reactive T cells in the CNS declines markedly during clinical recovery. This loss of function can be explained by selective apoptosis (programmed cell death) of these cells in the CNS (Tabi *et al.*, 1994). Mor & Cohen (1992) also found that T cells reactive to the 65-kDa heat shock protein (hsp65) were enriched in the spinal cord and they suggested that these cells may recognize hsp65 in the CNS.

Spreading of T-cell autoimmunity to additional antigenic determinants

By measuring T cell proliferative responses in the spleen, Lehmann *et al.* (1992) have shown that in (SJL × B10.PL)F_1 mice inoculated with MBP there is immune dominance of a single determinant of MBP, Ac1–11, in the inductive phase of EAE, but that in later stages of chronic EAE there is spreading of the T cell response to cryptic MBP determinants, namely MBP peptides 35–47, 81–100 and 121–140. Furthermore, similar determinant spreading occurred in mice with EAE induced by immunization with the Ac1–11 MBP peptide, and there was an apparent hierarchy of responsiveness to the cryptic determinants. Lehmann *et al.* concluded that priming to these additional determinants had occurred in the inflamed CNS during the course of EAE. Spreading of the autoimmune T cell response to PLP has been observed in (SJL/J × PL/J)F_1 mice with chronic relapsing EAE induced by immunization with MBP (Perry, Barzaga Gilbert & Trotter, 1991). Further studies are required to determine whether intramolecular and extramolecular determinant spreading contributes to the progression of disease in the CNS.

The role of cytokines in EAE

$CD4^+$ T cells can be divided into two subsets, based on the pattern of lymphokine secretion – T helper 1 (T_H1) and T helper 2 (T_H2) cells. T_H1 cells produce IL-2 and IFN-γ and have a role in cell-mediated immunity;

T_H2 cells produce IL-4, IL-5 and IL-10 and help in antibody production. Encephalitogenic MBP-specific T cells are of the T_H1 subset, as they secrete IL-2, IFN-γ and TNF-α and/or -β, but not IL-4, and they do not help antibody production by MBP-primed B cells *in vitro* (Ando *et al.*, 1989; Baron *et al.*, 1993). Encephalitogenic T cells specific for the 139–151 PLP peptide are also of the T_H1 subset (Kuchroo *et al.*, 1993; van der Veen, Kapp & Trotter, 1993), while non-encephalitogenic T_H2 cells recognizing the same peptide inhibit the *in vitro* proliferation of the encephalitogenic cells by secreting IL-10, which interferes with the function of antigen-presenting cells (van der Veen & Stohlman, 1993).

A role for IL-2 in the pathogenesis of EAE is indicated by the inhibitory effects of anti-IL-2 antibody and anti-IL-2R antibody on passively transferred EAE, although these antibodies have little effect on actively induced EAE (Engelhardt, Diamantstein & Wekerle, 1989; Duong *et al.*, 1992). The *in vivo* administration of IL-2 enhances passively transferred EAE (Schluesener & Lassmann, 1986). IL-1 has a pathogenic role as indicated by the aggravation of EAE by IL-1α and the inhibition by soluble IL-1 receptor, an IL-1 antagonist (Jacobs *et al.*, 1991). It has been reported that the encephalitogenicity of MBP-specific T cell clones is strongly correlated with the production of TNF-α/β but not with that of IL-2 or IFN-γ (Powell *et al.*, 1990). Anti-TNF antibody inhibits passively transferred EAE (Ruddle *et al.*, 1990; Selmaj, Raine & Cross, 1991), and, when given just before the time of clinical onset, also inhibits actively induced EAE (Santambrogio *et al.*, 1993). It may act by antagonizing TNF-induced endothelial adhesion molecule expression or parenchymal damage. *In vitro*, TNF induces myelin sheath dilatation and oligodendrocyte death in myelinated mouse spinal cord tissue (Selmaj & Raine, 1988). With regard to IFN-γ, anti-IFN-γ antibody therapy aggravates EAE, and IFN-γ therapy inhibits EAE (Billiau *et al.*, 1988; Voorthuis *et al.*, 1990; Duong *et al.*, 1992). These findings indicate that IFN-γ has a disease-limiting role, which might be explained by the induction of T cell apoptosis (Liu & Janeway, 1990; Groux *et al.*, 1993). Transforming growth factor-β (TGF-β) also has an inhibitory role in EAE. EAE is inhibited by TGF-β1 and TGF-β2 (Kuruvilla *et al.*, 1991; Johns *et al.*, 1991; Racke *et al.*, 1991, 1993; Santambrogio *et al.*, 1993) and aggravated by anti-TGF-β antibody (Racke *et al.*, 1992; Johns & Sriram, 1993; Santambrogio *et al.*, 1993). TGF-β1 and TGF-β2 inhibit the activation of encephalitogenic T cells *in vitro* (Schluesener & Lider, 1989); however, the inhibitory effect of TGF-β *in vivo* in EAE has been attributed to antagonism of TNF production and antagonism of the actions of TNF on the CNS vascular endothelium and parenchyma, rather than to inhibition of T cell activation (Santambrogio *et al.*, 1993). IL-10 also inhibits the development of EAE (Rott, Fleischer & Cash, 1994).

The expression of cytokines in the CNS in EAE has been studied with the reverse transcriptase/polymerase chain reaction technique to detect cytokine mRNA or with immunocytochemistry to detect the actual cytokines. During clinical attacks of EAE there is increased expression of IL-1, IL-2, IFN-γ, TNF-α, perforin (pore-forming protein) and IL-6 in the CNS, while during clinical remission there is a decline in the expression of these cytokines (Kennedy *et al.*, 1992; Khoury, Hancock & Weiner, 1992; Merrill *et al.*, 1992; Bauer *et al.*, 1993; Held *et al.*, 1993; Stoll *et al.*, 1993; Renno *et al.*, 1994) and increased expression of IL-10 (Kennedy *et al.*, 1992) and TGF-β (Khoury *et al.*, 1992). Increased IL-4 expression has also been detected in the CNS in EAE but there is conflicting evidence on whether it is maximal during the clinical attack or during clinical remission (Kennedy *et al.*, 1992; Khoury *et al.*, 1992; Merrill *et al.*, 1992). During clinical attacks of EAE there is also increased expression in the CNS of factors associated with the growth, differentiation and chemotaxis of cells of the monocyte/macrophage series, namely colony stimulating factor-1, its receptor c-fms, and macrophage chemotactic factor-1 (Hulkower *et al.*, 1993).

In conclusion, it would appear that IL-1, IL-2 and TNF have important roles in promoting the development of EAE, whereas IFN-γ, TGF-β and IL-10 have disease-limiting roles. The roles of IL-4, IL-5 and IL-6 have yet to be clarified.

The role of B cells and antibody in EAE

Intact B cell function is required for the induction of EAE by active immunization (Gausas *et al.*, 1982; Willenborg & Prowse, 1983; Myers *et al.*, 1992) but is not necessary for the development of EAE after passive transfer (Willenborg, Sjollema & Danta, 1986). These findings indicate a role for B cells as antigen-presenting cells in the activation of encephalitogenic T cells in peripheral lymphoid organs. However, the antigen-presenting role of the B cell is a complex one, as the simultaneous intravenous injection of encephalitogenic MBP peptide covalently coupled to anti-IgD monoclonal antibody (a strategy aimed at targeting the autoantigen to B cells) prevents EAE in rats immunized with MBP in CFA (Day *et al.*, 1992). The B cell depletion studies of Willenborg *et al.* (1986) suggest that antibody is not essential in the effector phase of EAE, a conclusion supported by the observation that EAE can be passively transferred by MBP-specific T_H1 cells that do not provide helper function for anti-MBP antibody production (Ando *et al.*, 1989). However, Myers *et al.* (1992) have shown that anti-MBP antibodies enhance the induction of EAE by passively transferred MBP-specific T cells and have proposed that the antibodies increase the presentation of myelin antigens in the CNS to the encephalitogenic T cells. Other studies also indicate that antibody has an important role in amplifying both the clinical disability and the neuropathological lesions of EAE. The administration of a monoclonal antibody against MOG increases the severity of neurological signs and greatly augments CNS demyelination in rats with actively or passively induced MBP-EAE (Schluesener *et al.*, 1987; Lassmann *et al.*, 1988; Linington *et al.*, 1988). The intravenous injection of anti-MOG antibody also induces severe neurological signs and extensive CNS demyelination in rats with CNS inflammation produced by the transfer of MOG-specific T cells (Linington *et al.*, 1993). Injection of anti-MOG into SJL/J mice recovering from an attack of chronic relapsing EAE induces fatal relapses (Schluesener *et al.*, 1987).

The sera of guinea pigs with acute or chronic relapsing EAE induced by inoculation with whole CNS tissue can induce CNS demyelination *in vitro* or *in vivo* when injected into the subarachnoid space; this demyelinating activity is complement-dependent and antibody-mediated and correlates well with the antibody titre to MOG (also known as M2), a surface glycoprotein restricted to CNS myelin and oligodendrocytes (Lebar *et al.*, 1976, 1986; Lassmann, Kitz & Wisniewski, 1981; Lassmann *et al.*, 1983; Linington & Lassmann, 1987). Anti-M2 antibodies are present in the CNS tissue of guinea pigs with chronic EAE, the amount of these antibodies being related to the severity of disease (Lebar, Baudrimont & Vincent, 1989). These findings indicate an important role for these antibodies in the development of demyelinating lesions in this form of EAE. Saida *et al.* (1979) found that the sera of rabbits with acute EAE induced by inoculation with whole CNS tissue and CFA induce PNS demyelination *in vivo* following intraneural injection and suggested that anti-galactocerebroside antibodies may contribute to the PNS and CNS demyelination in this form of EAE. The sera of guinea pigs and rats with chronic EAE also induce PNS demyelination *in vivo* (Lassmann *et al.*, 1983). Although circulating demyelinating antibodies can enter the CNS or PNS through damaged blood–brain or blood–nerve barriers, antibody produced locally by plasma cells within the CNS may also contribute to the development of demyelination (Bernheimer *et al.*, 1988). B cells within the CNS may also act as antigen-presenting cells and thus help to diversify the T cell immune response against CNS antigens (McCombe *et al.*, 1994).

Anti-myelin antibodies could exert their demyelinating effect in EAE by complement-dependent antibody-mediated demyelination or antibody-dependent cell-mediated demyelination. The ability of anti-MOG antibodies to induce demyelination in EAE is related to their ability to fix complement (Piddlesden *et al.*, 1993). However, in rats with MBP-EAE receiving anti-MOG antibody, decomplementation with cobra venom factor abolishes C9 deposition within the CNS but has no effect on the augmentative action of the antibody on the neurological signs or CNS demyelination (Piddlesden *et al.*, 1991). This indicates that the antibody-mediated demyelination is independent of the formation of complement membrane attack complex and results from an antibody-dependent cell-mediated immune attack, which might be enhanced by the action of complement. One mechanism for antibody-dependent cell-mediated demyelination is the opsonization of myelin for phagocytosis by macrophages. When preincubated with CNS myelin, sera or cerebrospinal fluid (CSF) derived from animals with EAE and containing anti-myelin antibodies can induce phagocytosis of the myelin by cultured macrophages or microglia (Sadler *et al.*, 1991; Sommer, Forno & Smith, 1992; Smith, 1993). In an immunocytochemical study of the CNS in acute EAE, IgG was occasionally demonstrated in macrophage clathrin-coated pits containing myelin droplets, suggesting that IgG may act as a ligand for receptor-mediated phagocytosis of myelin (Moore & Raine, 1988). Another possible mechanism for antibody-dependent cell-mediated demyelination involves natural killer cells. As natural killer cells have Fc receptors, anti-myelin antibody may target natural killer cells to oligodendrocytes or Schwann cells, which might then be induced to die by apoptosis.

In conclusion, B cells have a role in EAE as antigen-presenting cells in the peripheral lymphoid organs and possibly also in the CNS. They also produce myelin-specific antibodies, which augment demyelination by enhancing phagocytosis of myelin.

Mechanism of demyelination in EAE

It is generally held that myelin, not the oligodendrocyte, is the primary target in EAE (Itoyama & Webster, 1982; Moore, Traugott & Raine, 1984; Sternberger *et al.*, 1984; Webster, Shii & Lassmann, 1985). The initial myelin damage is usually attributed to delayed-type hypersensitivity with activated macrophages releasing such toxic products as proteolytic enzymes (Banik, 1992), TNF-α (see above) and oxygen- and nitrogen-derived free radicals. The altered myelin is then phagocytosed by macrophages and possibly microglia. Mononuclear and polymorphonuclear leukocytes isolated from the CNS of rats with hyperacute EAE secrete increased amounts of oxygen- and nitrogen-derived free radicals (MacMicking *et al.*, 1992), and nitric oxide has been demonstrated in the spinal cords of mice with EAE by electron paramagnetic resonance spectroscopy (Lin *et al.*, 1993). When present, anti-myelin antibodies may opsonize myelin for phagocytosis by macrophages, as discussed above. An essential role for macrophages in the CNS in EAE has been demonstrated by the observation that EAE can be inhibited by the depletion of CNS-infiltrating macrophages by the intravenous injection of mannosylated liposomes containing dichloromethylene diphosphonate (Huitinga *et al.*, 1990). Furthermore, treatment with antibodies to the type 3 complement receptor, which is expressed by macrophages and involved in their recruitment to inflammatory sites, inhibits

EAE (Huitinga *et al.*, 1993). However, these findings do not indicate whether the role of CNS macrophages depends on their function as antigen-presenting cells or as primary effector cells.

The possibility that the oligodendrocyte is the primary target in EAE has not been excluded. It has been suggested that some of the apoptotic cells present in the CNS in EAE may be oligodendrocytes (Pender *et al.*, 1991) but this has not been established by immunocytochemistry, which is needed for definitive identification. Oligodendrocyte apoptosis would be expected to lead to phagocytosis of the apoptotic oligodendrocyte and of the myelin it supports (Pender *et al.*, 1991). Hence, invasion of the myelin sheath by macrophages does not necessarily indicate that myelin is the primary target. One study using a silver impregnation technique reported depletion of oligodendrocytes in otherwise normal-appearing white matter as well as in demyelinated regions, and concluded that the oligodendrocyte is the primary target (Ohkawa, 1989).

T cell cytotoxicity is one mechanism that could result in primary oligodendrocyte destruction in EAE. Encephalitogenic MBP-specific $CD4^+$ T cells have a cytotoxic capacity *in vitro* against MBP-pulsed astrocytes (Sun & Wekerle, 1986), macrophages (Fallis & McFarlin, 1989) and cerebral vascular endothelial cells (Sedgwick *et al.*, 1990; McCarron *et al.*, 1991). As this cytotoxicity is restricted by class II MHC antigens, it would be anticipated that class II MHC expression by oligodendrocytes would be a prerequisite for oligodendrocyte-directed cytotoxicity. Under standard *in vitro* conditions, oligodendrocytes can be induced by IFN-γ to express class I MHC antigen but are refractory to class II induction (Turnley, Miller & Bartlett, 1991); however, in the presence of glucocorticoid, IFN-γ induces the expression of MHC class II molecules (Bergsteinsdottir *et al.*, 1992). Encephalitogenic MBP-specific $CD4^+$ T cell lines have been reported to be cytotoxic to oligodendrocytes *in vitro*, but only with the addition of antigen-presenting cells and MBP (Kawai & Zweiman, 1988, 1990); it was unclear whether the cytotoxicity was MHC-restricted. When MBP-specific T cell hybridoma cells were used instead of lines, oligodendrocytes were killed in the absence of other cell populations and added MBP (Kawai, Heber Katz & Zweiman, 1991). Although the hybridoma cells were MHC class II-restricted in their response to MBP, the oligodendrocytes did not express detectable class II MHC molecules and the cytotoxicity was not inhibited by antibodies against MHC class II or I antigens (Kawai *et al.*, 1991). Oligodendrocyte killing without conventional MHC restriction has also been observed with an oligodendrocyte-specific $CD8^+$ $CD4^-$ $TCR\alpha\beta^+$ T cell clone probably recognizing a MOG (M2) epitope (Jewtoukoff, Lebar & Bach, 1989). Non-MHC-restricted oligodendrocyte killing might also be effected by natural killer cells targeted through their Fc receptors to antibody-coated oligodendrocytes, but this possibility has not yet been examined. Studies in bone marrow chimeras and SCID mice indicate that EAE can be transferred by encephalitogenic T cells without the need for syngeneic MHC expression by oligodendrocytes (Hinrichs *et al.*, 1987; Hickey & Kimura, 1988; Myers *et al.*, 1993; Jones *et al.*, 1993). Further studies are needed to determine whether primary oligodendrocyte destruction is a significant mechanism of demyelination *in vivo* in EAE.

The blood–brain barrier in EAE

The blood–brain barrier is a layered structure consisting of the following components: cerebral vascular endothelial cells, which have tight intercellular junctions; the endothelial basement membrane; and the perivascular glia limitans, composed predominantly of astrocytic foot processes but also incorporating parenchymal microglia. As discussed above, activated T cells of any specificity can cross the intact blood–brain barrier, but only those that recognize their specific antigen accumulate in the CNS. In EAE, there is a breakdown of the blood–brain barrier (increased vascular permeability) manifested by exudation of plasma components and leakage of circulating exogenous tracers into the CNS parenchyma. The breakdown occurs concomitantly with, not prior to, the infiltration of mononuclear phagocytes (Ackermann, Ulrich & Heitz, 1981; Simmons *et al.*, 1987). The increased vascular permeability is attributed to the action of cytokines released by the activated T cells. Complement activation may also contribute. In chronic relapsing EAE, the damage to the blood–brain barrier is localized to demyelinating plaques and the vicinity of inflamed blood vessels; actively demyelinating lesions show a massive increase in blood–brain barrier permeability, whereas in inactive or remyelinated lesions the damage is minimal or absent (Kitz *et al.*, 1984). Elevated CSF albumin is a reliable indicator of blood–brain barrier breakdown in lesions located near the inner or outer surface of the brain and spinal cord; however, single lesions with barrier damage located in the depth of the CNS parenchyma may not be accompanied by an increase in the level of CSF albumin (Kitz *et al.*, 1984). The increase in the blood–brain barrier permeability in EAE is due to an increase in transendothelial active vesicular transport in the capillary bed (Lossinsky *et al.*, 1989; Claudio *et al.*, 1989) and also an increase in passive transfer across inflamed venules through the interendothelial cellular junctions and alongside migrating inflammatory cells (Claudio *et al.*, 1990).

Magnetic resonance imaging

Magnetic resonance imaging of the accumulation of intravenously administered gadolinium in the CNS (gadolinium enhancement) is a non-invasive method for serially recording changes in the blood–brain barrier. In chronic relapsing EAE, regions of gadolinium enhancement correspond to sites of blood–brain barrier breakdown, as detected by traditional tracer methods (Hawkins *et al.*, 1990). Furthermore, in regions of spinal cord showing gadolinium enhancement, there is evidence of active vesicular transendothelial transport as a mechanism for the blood–brain barrier breakdown (Hawkins *et al.*, 1992). In the guinea pig, the extent and time course of gadolinium enhancement were found to correlate well with the clinical course of chronic relapsing EAE (Hawkins *et al.*, 1991). Moreover, it was found that the pattern of blood–brain barrier breakdown evolves from a diffuse shortlived disturbance in acute EAE to a more focal and prolonged breakdown in animals with chronic relapsing and progressive disease. Seeldrayers *et al.* (1993) found evidence of a breakdown in the blood–CSF barrier as early as 4–8 h after the passive transfer of an MBP-specific T cell line and suggested that this might represent the early and privileged passage of the activated T cells through the more permeable meningeal vessels. They observed a similar but less severe change after the passive transfer of an ovalbumin-specific T cell line, indicating that this early phenomenon is not entirely antigen-specific.

Immunological findings in the peripheral blood and CSF

Peripheral blood

While T cell responses to myelin antigens have been studied extensively in the lymph nodes and spleen in EAE, little attention has been given to peripheral blood T cell responses to these antigens. Massacesi *et al.* (1992) found increased peripheral blood T cell proliferative responses to brain homogenate, MBP and occasionally to PLP in cynomolgus monkeys with acute fatal EAE or chronic relapsing EAE induced by inoculation with human brain white matter homogenate and CFA.

Cerebrospinal fluid

In acute EAE there is a CSF mononuclear pleocytosis that commences one day before the onset of neurological signs and decreases during clinical recovery. On the day of clinical onset the cells consist predominantly of $CD45RC^{-}CD4^{+}$ and $CD45RC^{-}CD8^{+}$ T cells, which are enriched for $IL\text{-}2R^{+}$ cells compared to the peripheral blood and lymph nodes (Offner *et al.*, 1993). In Lewis rats with acute EAE induced by active immunization with MBP there is an over-representation of $V\beta8.2^{+}$ T cells in the CSF at and just prior to clinical onset, but the proportion of $V\beta8.2^{+}$ cells declines as the disease progresses (Offner *et al.*, 1993). These findings parallel the changes in the Vβ8.2$^+$ population in the spinal cord. IL-2 and IFN-γ mRNA levels are also increased in CSF cells during EAE and correlate with those in whole CNS tissue (Renno *et al.*, 1994).

By electrophoresis with isoelectric focusing, oligoclonal IgG bands are detected in brain extracts and CSF of guinea pigs with chronic relapsing EAE (Mehta, Lassmann & Wisniewski, 1981). However, unlike in multiple sclerosis, identical oligoclonal IgG band patterns are found in the serum and CSF, and hence these findings do not indicate intrathecal synthesis of IgG (Suckling *et al.*, 1983; Mehta *et al.*, 1985*a*). This may be due to a more severe breakdown of the blood–brain barrier in EAE. The CSF IgG index (also an indicator of intrathecal IgG synthesis) is normal in animals with actively demyelinating lesions and a high CSF albumin quotient (Q-albumin – an indicator of breakdown in the blood–brain barrier), and elevated in animals with inactive lesions and a normal Q-albumin (Kitz *et al.*, 1984). Another study also found that intrathecal IgG synthesis was greatest in guinea pigs with little blood–brain barrier damage (Walls, Suckling & Rumsby, 1989).

With regard to the specificity of the oligoclonal IgG bands in the guinea pig, there is equal reactivity to spinal cord tissue and *Mycobacterium tuberculosis* in the first remission of chronic relapsing EAE and after recovery from acute EAE, and predominant reactivity against spinal cord during and after the first relapse of chronic relapsing EAE (Mehta, Patrick & Wisniewski, 1985*b*). The reactivity against spinal cord tissue is directed predominantly against MBP and weakly against PLP, with some reactivity to lipid or non-myelin protein (Mehta *et al.*, 1987). However, there is no evidence of intrathecal synthesis of antibody specific for neuroantigens or adjuvant, as the relative antibody levels to whole spinal cord homogenate, MBP and *Mycobacterium tuberculosis* were found to be lower in the CSF than in the serum (Walls *et al.*, 1989). Indeed, the CSF/serum ratios for each specific antibody were inversely correlated with total intrathecal IgG synthesis, indicating that much of the antibody production within the CNS is the result of polyclonal B cell activation.

Immunoregulation

Spontaneous clinical recovery and resistance to reinduction of EAE

Lewis rats demonstrate rapid spontaneous clinical recovery from actively and passively induced acute EAE. This recovery is dependent on the endogenous release of corticosterone, which causes antigen-nonspecific immunosuppression (Levine, Sowinski & Steinetz, 1980; MacPhee, Antoni

& Mason, 1989). Rats that have recovered from acute EAE induced by active immunization with MBP also acquire tolerance to MBP, as evidenced by resistance to active reinduction of EAE (Willenborg, 1979; Hinrichs, Roberts & Waxman, 1981). Unlike the recovery phase of acute EAE, this refractory phase is not associated with elevated corticosterone levels in the blood (MacPhee *et al.*, 1989). As spleen cells from convalescent rats can be used to reconstitute the lymphomyeloid apparatus of lethally irradiated recipients which then develop EAE normally after active immunization, it has been concluded that an active suppressive mechanism and not clonal deletion is responsible for the resistance to active reinduction (Willenborg, 1979). This conclusion has been supported by the finding that spleen cells from tolerant convalescent rats can transfer EAE after *in vitro* stimulation with MBP (Holda & Swanborg, 1981). However, these studies have not excluded the possibility that there is a significant depletion of MBP-specific T cells in the lymphoid organs of convalescent rats and that this contributes to the tolerant state. Although convalescent rats do not develop clinical signs after reimmunization, they have a higher incidence of cerebellar lesions than naive controls, suggesting that the tolerance is incomplete and that local CNS factors may contribute to the resistance to active reinduction (Levine & Sowinski, 1980). Furthermore, convalescent rats are fully susceptible to the induction of EAE by the passive transfer of MBP-specific lymphocytes (Willenborg, 1979; Hinrichs *et al.*, 1981), although the convalescent rats develop more cerebellar lesions (Willenborg, 1979). The resistance to active reinduction of EAE appears to be antigen-specific as the convalescent rats develop experimental autoimmune neuritis after immunization with the neuritogenic peptide of PNS P_2 protein (Day, Tse & Mason, 1991). The results of experiments involving preimmunization with MBP or P_2 peptide followed by challenge with a mixture of both suggest that the refractoriness to reinduction, although specific in its induction, is nonspecific in its effect (Day *et al.*, 1991). Rats that have recovered from passively transferred MBP-EAE have been reported to be partially (Welch, Holda & Swanborg, 1980; Ben Nun & Cohen, 1981) or fully susceptible (Hinrichs *et al.*, 1981) to the reinduction of MBP-EAE by active means, and fully susceptible to the reinduction of MBP-EAE by passive means (Hinrichs *et al.*, 1981; Ben Nun & Cohen, 1981).

Effects of immunosuppressant drugs on susceptibility to induction, reinduction and relapse

Low-dose cyclophosphamide treatment prior to inoculation potentiates the development of EAE in resistant rat strains (Mostarica Stojkovic, Petrovic & Lukic, 1982; Kallen, Dohlsten & Klementsson, 1986) and abrogates induced resistance to EAE in mice (Lando, Teitelbaum & Arnon, 1979).

These effects have been attributed to the selective elimination of suppressor cells by cyclophosphamide. A single injection of cyclophosphamide precipitates a relapse in rats that have recovered from actively induced EAE (Minagawa *et al.*, 1987). Whereas high-dose cyclosporin A suppresses the development of EAE (Bolton *et al.*, 1982), low-dose cyclosporin A therapy converts acute EAE into chronic relapsing EAE (Polman *et al.*, 1988; Pender *et al.*, 1990). As cyclosporin A inhibits activation-induced T cell apoptosis (Shi, Sahai & Green, 1989), it may lead to relapses by preventing the apoptotic elimination of encephalitogenic T cells in the CNS or in peripheral lymphoid organs or possibly of their precursors in the thymus (Pender, 1993). Alternatively, low-dose cyclosporin A may selectively inhibit suppressor T cells. Further studies are required to determine how low-dose cyclosporin A causes relapses.

Suppressor or regulatory cells

Lymph node or spleen cells of rats and spleen cells of mice rendered resistant to EAE by injections of MBP in incomplete Freund's adjuvant can passively transfer the state of unresponsiveness to normal recipients (Swierkosz & Swanborg, 1975, 1977; Bernard, 1977). The cells responsible for the transfer of unresponsiveness have been shown to be T cells and have been termed 'suppressor T cells' (Welch & Swanborg, 1976). However, there has been considerable controversy concerning the use of the term 'suppressor T cell', and some authors use the term 'regulatory T cell' to refer to cells with similar functions. Suppressor T cells have also been isolated from rats during and after recovery from actively induced EAE (Adda, Beraud & Depieds, 1977; Welch *et al.*, 1980).

$CD4^+$ suppressor or regulatory T cells

Nylon-adherent $CD4^+$ suppressor T cells isolated from the spleens of post-recovery rats inhibit, in an antigen-specific manner, the *in vitro* production of IFN-γ, but not IL-2, by EAE effector cells (McDonald & Swanborg, 1988; Karpus & Swanborg, 1989). This inhibitory effect is mediated through the secretion of TGF-β by the suppressor cells (Karpus & Swanborg, 1991*a*). It has also been shown that $CD4^+$ suppressor T cells recognize a determinant associated with the TCR on the surface of EAE effector cells and respond by secreting IL-4 (Karpus, Gould & Swanborg, 1992). However, both $CD4^+$ suppressor T cells and MBP-primed B cells are required to transfer protection against actively induced EAE (Karpus & Swanborg, 1991*b*). Ellerman, Powers & Brostoff (1988) have isolated $CD4^+$ suppressor T cell lines from rats that have recovered from EAE. When admixed with MBP-specific T helper cells, these lines prevent the passive transfer of EAE;

however, they do not transfer protection against actively induced EAE. Interestingly, Kumar & Sercarz (1993) have isolated $CD4^+$ regulatory T cells from the spleens of B10.PL mice recovering from actively induced MBP-EAE; these cells proliferate in response to a single immunodominant TCR peptide from the $V\beta8.2$ chain used by most of the encephalitogenic T cells, indicating natural priming during the course of the disease. Furthermore, when cloned and passively transferred, these regulatory T cells specifically downregulate the proliferative response to the encephalitogenic Ac1–9 MBP peptide in MBP-immunized mice and protect against the active induction of MBP-EAE. Kumar & Sercarz (1993) have suggested that this downregulation offers a mechanism for antigen-specific, network-induced recovery from autoimmune disease. As mentioned earlier, Van der Veen & Stohlman (1993) have isolated a T_H2 clone which is specific for the 139–151 PLP peptide and which inhibits the proliferation of a T_H1 encephalitogenic clone specific for the same peptide by secreting IL-10.

$CD8^+$ suppressor or regulatory T cells

Sun *et al.* (1988*b*) have isolated $CD8^+$ suppressor T cell lines from the spleens of Lewis rats that have recovered from EAE induced by the passive transfer of an MBP-specific $CD4^+$ T cell line. These suppressor cells specifically respond to determinants on the encephalitogenic line but not to MBP, selectively lyse the encephalitogenic line *in vitro* and efficiently neutralize its encephalitogenic capacity *in vivo*. Similar $CD8^+$ suppressor T cells can be isolated from rats rendered resistant to the passive transfer of EAE by pretreatment with injections of attenuated encephalitogenic line cells (Sun, Ben Nun & Wekerle, 1988*a*). *In vivo* elimination of the $CD8^+$ T cell subset, by thymectomy and OX-8 antibody injection before the initial cell transfer, totally blocked the induction of resistance, indicating that $CD8^+$ suppressor T cells are responsible for the induced resistance to passively transferred EAE (Sun *et al.*, 1988*a*). $CD4^-CD8^-$ splenic T cells also proliferate in response to the respective encephalitogenic line cells; after stimulation with these, a significant proportion of the double negative T cells become $CD8^+$ and have strong cytolytic activity towards the encephalitogenic line cells (Sun *et al.*, 1991). Lider *et al.* (1988) have also isolated $CD8^+$ suppressor T cells from the draining lymph nodes of rats vaccinated against EAE by a subencephalitogenic dose of an MBP-specific T cell clone. Such T cell vaccination induces resistance to EAE passively transferred by an encephalitogenic dose of the same clone. The suppressor cells are specifically responsive to the MBP-specific T cell clone and suppress the response of the clone to MBP. Hence, it has been concluded that T cell vaccination induces resistance to passively transferred EAE by activating an anti-idiotypic network (Lider *et al.*, 1988).

$CD8^+$ suppressor T cells have been isolated from the spleens and mesenteric lymph nodes of rats protected against actively induced EAE by the oral administration of MBP (oral tolerance) (Lider *et al.*, 1989). These suppressor cells passively transfer protection against actively induced EAE and inhibit *in vitro* proliferative responses of MBP-specific T cells to MBP. Their suppressive effects both *in vitro* and *in vivo* appear to be mediated by the release of TGF-β after specific triggering by non-encephalitogenic MBP epitopes (Miller, Lider & Weiner, 1991; Miller *et al.*, 1992, 1993). In contrast, Whitacre *et al.* (1991), using a higher dose of oral MBP, found no compelling evidence for a role of suppressor T cells in the induction of oral tolerance to MBP in the Lewis rat.

In conclusion, $CD4^+$ and $CD8^+$ suppressor or regulatory T cells have been described which are reactive to encephalitogenic T cells or to myelin proteins, and which can act on the induction or effector phase of EAE. However, further studies are required to determine the role of suppressor or regulatory T cells in the development of antigen-specific tolerance after recovery from actively induced EAE and in the prevention of relapses.

Clonal deletion in the thymus

Except in transgenic mice expressing genes encoding a rearranged TCR specific for MBP (Goverman *et al.*, 1993), EAE does not develop spontaneously but requires induction by active or passive immunization, despite the fact that autoaggressive encephalitogenic T cell lines can be established from unprimed normal Lewis rat lymph node populations (Schluesener & Wekerle, 1985). Clearly, such autoaggressive T cells have avoided clonal deletion by activation-induced apoptosis in the thymus, a process that is important in the normal neonatal development of tolerance (Smith *et al.*, 1989; Murphy, Heimberger & Loh, 1990). Encephalitogenic T cells may escape this tolerance mechanism because of the relatively late formation of CNS myelin during ontogeny and because of sequestration of myelin antigens within the CNS. Longlasting MBP-specific tolerance can be induced in Lewis rats by injecting them with high doses of MBP in the early neonatal period (Qin *et al.*, 1989). Neonatally tolerized rats are completely resistant to the induction of EAE by immunization with MBP and CFA in adult life. This tolerance appears to be due to the deletion of MBP-specific T cells, and there is no evidence for the involvement of suppressor cells (Qin *et al.*, 1989). Neonatal tolerance can also be induced to the dominant T cell determinant of MBP in B10.PL mice (Clayton *et al.*, 1989). The thymus may also play a role in acquired tolerance in the adult. The intrathymic injection of MBP 48 h prior to immunization with MBP and adjuvants protects Lewis rats from the development of EAE and reduces the lymphocyte proliferative response to MBP (Khoury *et al.*, 1993). Furthermore, the intrathymic injection of the major encephalitogenic 71–90 MBP peptide but not the non-encephalitogenic 21–40 peptide also protects against the development of EAE (Khoury *et al.*, 1993). This effect may be due to the deletion of encephalitogenic T cells circulating through the thymus.

Downregulation within the CNS

The spontaneous clinical recovery that occurs after attacks of EAE is associated with a major reduction in the T cell infiltrate in the CNS (McCombe *et al.*, 1992, 1994; Zeine & Owens, 1993). Such a reduction in the number of infiltrating T cells could be due either to the emigration of T cells from the CNS or to death of T cells within the CNS. Apoptosis (programmed cell death) of T cells occurs in the CNS in Lewis rats with acute EAE and may contribute to the resolution of inflammation in the CNS and the spontaneous clinical recovery (Pender *et al.*, 1992). Schmied *et al.* (1993) have shown that T cell apoptosis in the CNS in EAE reaches a peak during clinical recovery. Recent evidence indicates that the apoptotic process in the CNS may selectively involve the encephalitogenic T cells. Tabi *et al.* (1994) have shown that $V\beta8.2^+$ T cells selectively undergo apoptosis in the CNS in Lewis rats with EAE induced by the passive transfer of cloned $V\beta8.2^+$ T cells specific for the 72–89 MBP peptide. The selective apoptotic elimination of these cells explains the selective decrease in the number and proportion of $V\beta8.2^+$ T cells in the CNS during the clinical course of EAE and the decline in the frequency of CNS-infiltrating cells that proliferate in response to the 72–89 MBP peptide. Furthermore, when a T cell clone specific for a non-CNS antigen (ovalbumin) is co-transferred with the MBP-specific T cell clone, the proliferative response of the CNS-infiltrating cells to ovalbumin is very high at a time when there is no detectable response to the 72–89 MBP peptide (at the peak of clinical disease), indicating that the apoptotic process is antigen-specific (Tabi *et al.*, 1994).

The mechanism responsible for T cell apoptosis in the CNS is unclear, but one possibility is activation-induced cell death occurring as a result of reactivation of the encephalitogenic cells in the CNS by non-specialized antigen-presenting cells that fail to provide the co-stimulatory signal (Pender *et al.*, 1992; Tabi *et al.*, 1994). The astrocyte is a possible candidate for such a downregulatory antigen-presenting cell, although the Ia expression required for antigen presentation to $CD4^+$ T cells has not been detected on astrocytes in EAE (see above). On the other hand, microglia exhibit prominent expression of Ia antigen persisting after clinical recovery (see above) and might serve as downregulatory antigen-presenting cells. Interestingly, rat strains resistant to the induction of EAE have a greater degree of constitutive Ia expression on microglia than do rats susceptible to EAE (Sedgwick *et al.*, 1993). As glucocorticoids can induce apoptosis in mature T cells (Zubiaga, Munoz & Huber, 1992), the endogenous corticosterone release that occurs during the course of EAE in the Lewis rat (MacPhee *et al.*, 1989) may also contribute to the T cell apoptosis in the CNS (Pender *et al.*, 1992).

Ohmori *et al.* (1992) have shown that there is little T cell proliferation within the CNS in EAE. As IL-2R$^+$ cells outnumbered proliferating T cells, it was concluded that a state of T cell anergy had been induced by interaction with glial cells expressing Ia antigen. However, as T cells undergoing apoptosis can still express cell surface molecules (Pender *et al.*, 1992), these results could also be explained by activation-induced T cell apoptosis. It has also been suggested that downregulation of the immune response in the CNS in EAE could result from the release of immunosuppressive factors by activated astrocytes (Matsumoto *et al.*, 1993). Apoptosis of macrophages occurs in the CNS in EAE and may contribute to the resolution of inflammation (Nguyen, McCombe & Pender, 1994).

In conclusion, T cell apoptosis in the CNS is likely to play an important role in the downregulation of the immune response during spontaneous recovery from EAE. Interestingly, a local CNS mechanism(s) may also contribute to the resistance to induction (Mostarica Stojkovic *et al.*, 1992) and reinduction of EAE (Levine & Sowinski, 1980). Further studies are needed to determine whether T cell apoptosis, for example triggered by antigen presentation by Ia$^+$ microglia, is such a mechanism.

Therapy

Therapy with myelin antigens

EAE can be inhibited by the injection of myelin antigens without mycobacteria, by the injection of spleen cells coupled to myelin antigens, and by the oral or intranasal administration of myelin antigens.

Injection of myelin antigens without mycobacteria

Chronic relapsing EAE can be permanently suppressed in guinea pigs by a single series of injections of MBP in incomplete Freund's adjuvant (Raine, Traugott & Stone, 1978). In the rhesus monkey, chronic progressive EAE is suppressed by the injection of an emulsion of spinal cord tissue with incomplete Freund's adjuvant (Ravkina, Rogova & Lazarenko, 1978). Injections of MBP or MBP peptide without mycobacteria also suppress MBP-EAE in the rhesus monkey (Eylar, Jackson & Kniskern, 1979). In the

Lewis rat, intraperitoneal injections of the encephalitogenic 68–88 peptide of MBP confer protection against the induction of EAE by immunization with the peptide and CFA (Chou *et al.*, 1980). Furthermore, repeated intravenous injections of large doses of MBP or encephalitogenic MBP peptide can inhibit the development of passively transferred MBP-EAE in mice (Critchfield *et al.*, 1994). However, in Biozzi AB/H mice with chronic relapsing EAE, treatment with CNS antigens in incomplete Freund's adjuvant after recovery from the first attack precipitates relapses (O'Neill, Baker & Turk, 1992). The protective effect of the injection of myelin antigens without mycobacteria has been attributed to the involvement of suppressor T cells (Bernard, 1977; O'Neill *et al.*, 1992) or to the induction of anergy (Gaur *et al.*, 1992) or apoptosis in the encephalitogenic T cells (Critchfield *et al.*, 1994).

Injection of spleen cells coupled to myelin antigens

Sriram, Schwartz & Steinman (1983) found that the intravenous administration of syngeneic spleen cells coupled to MBP prevents acute EAE induced in SJL/J mice by immunization with spinal cord homogenate and adjuvants. A similar pretreatment suppresses the active induction of acute MBP-EAE in Lewis rats (McKenna *et al.*, 1983). Kennedy *et al.* (1988; 1990) found that chronic relapsing EAE induced in SJL/J mice by immunization with spinal cord homogenate could be inhibited by the intravenous administration of syngeneic spleen cells coupled to spinal cord homogenate, PLP or PLP encephalitogenic peptide, but not MBP. This method of treatment was also effective when commenced after the onset of EAE. When splenocytes coupled to spinal cord homogenate were injected after the first episode but before the first relapse of chronic relapsing EAE transferred by MBP-specific T cells, all subsequent relapses were inhibited, whereas treatment with splenocytes coupled to MBP inhibited the first relapse but not subsequent ones (Tan *et al.*, 1991). These results suggest that in the later relapses there is involvement of T cells with specificities different from that of the T cells inducing the first episode (Tan *et al.*, 1991). Passively transferred MBP-EAE in the Lewis rat can be prevented by the intravenous injection of syngeneic splenocytes coupled to MBP or to the encephalitogenic 68–86 MBP peptide two days after the transfer of the MBP-specific T cells (Pope, Paterson & Miller, 1992). The effect is dose-dependent, dependent on the intravenous route of administration of the antigen-coupled splenocytes, antigen-specific and dependent on the use of the carbodiimide coupling reagent (Pope *et al.*, 1992). This form of tolerance may be due to activation-induced apoptosis of the encephalitogenic T cells following interaction with antigen-presenting cells that, because of chemical fixation, do not produce the co-stimulatory signal.

Oral or intranasal administration of myelin antigens

The oral administration of MBP protects Lewis rats from actively induced acute EAE (Bitar & Whitacre, 1988; Higgins & Weiner, 1988). The relapses of chronic relapsing EAE in the Lewis rat and the guinea pig can also be suppressed by the oral administration of myelin after recovery from the first attack (Brod *et al.*, 1991). As discussed above, oral tolerance has been attributed by some workers to the action of $CD8^+$ suppressor T cells (Lider *et al.*, 1989; Miller *et al.*, 1991, 1992). However, using a higher dose of oral MBP, Whitacre *et al.* (1991) found a profound decrease in MBP-reactive IL-2-secreting T cells in the lymph nodes of orally tolerant rats challenged by immunization with MBP and CFA, compared to control animals similarly challenged. They concluded that the tolerant state was due to clonal anergy or clonal deletion and found no evidence for a role of suppressor cells. A likely explanation for this discrepancy has been provided by studies on oral tolerance to S-antigen in experimental autoimmune uveoretinitis: low-dose therapy was found to be mediated by suppressor T cells and high-dose therapy to be mediated by clonal anergy (or deletion) (Gregerson, Obritsch & Donoso, 1993). It has also been reported that the intranasal administration of encephalitogenic MBP peptide prior to disease induction inhibits the development of EAE in mice (Metzler & Wraith, 1993).

Vaccination with T cells, and anti-TCR therapy

Vaccination with T cells

The intravenous injection of MBP-specific T cell lines attenuated by treatment with mitomycin C or irradiation protects Lewis rats from actively induced MBP-EAE (Ben Nun, Wekerle & Cohen, 1981*b*). Furthermore, vaccination with a subencephalitogenic dose of an MBP-specific T cell clone induces resistance to EAE passively transferred by an encephalitogenic dose of the same clone (Lider *et al.*, 1988). Studies using different MBP-specific T cell lines have shown that the protection is specific for the particular MBP determinant, suggesting the involvement of a regulatory mechanism directed against the TCR (Holoshitz *et al.*, 1983). As discussed above, further studies have led to the conclusion that anti-idiotypic $CD8^+$ suppressor T cells specifically reactive to the vaccinating clone are responsible for the protective effect of T cell vaccination (Lider *et al.*, 1988). Anti-ergotypic T cells (T cells that recognize and respond to the state of activation of other T cells) may also contribute (Lohse *et al.*, 1989).

Anti-TCR therapy

The observation of restricted TCR $V\beta$ gene usage by MBP-specific T cells led to the finding that anti-$V\beta8$ monoclonal antibodies prevent and reverse

EAE in mice (Acha Orbea *et al.*, 1988; Urban *et al.*, 1988). In the Lewis rat, a monoclonal antibody specific for MBP-specific T cells was found to abrogate actively induced MBP-EAE (Owhashi & Heber Katz, 1988). Furthermore, an anti-idiotypic antibody directed against an antibody to the Ac1–9 MBP peptide inhibits the development of passively transferred EAE in mice by cross-reacting with an idiotype on the TCR of encephalitogenic T cells specific for this peptide (Zhou & Whitaker, 1993). Vaccination with TCR peptides from the regions used by encephalitogenic T cells has also been found to inhibit the induction of EAE (Howell *et al.*, 1989; Vandenbark, Hashim & Offner, 1989), although some authors have found that it enhances EAE (Desquenne Clark *et al.*, 1991; Sun, 1992). Vandenbark *et al.* (1989) found that immunization of Lewis rats with a synthetic peptide (39–59) representing the hypervariable region of the TCR Vβ8 molecule prevents the active induction of MBP-EAE. They reported that T cells specific for the TCR Vβ8 peptide could be isolated from the lymph nodes of the protected rats and could passively transfer protection against actively induced MBP-EAE (Vandenbark *et al.*, 1989). Immunization with this peptide also generated peptide-specific antibodies that suppressed EAE induced by active immunization with encephalitogenic MBP peptide and CFA (Hashim *et al.*, 1990). Moreover, the intradermal injection of the TCR Vβ8 peptide in saline commencing on the day of onset of clinical signs was found to reduce the severity of EAE induced by immunization with MBP and CFA; this effect was attributed to the boosting of anti-Vβ8 T cells and antibodies raised naturally in response to encephalitogenic V$\beta 8^+$ T cells (Offner, Hashim & Vandenbark, 1991). In contrast, Sun (1992) found that immunization of Lewis rats with the same TCR Vβ8(39–59) peptide did not induce the production of regulatory T cells reactive to the intact TCR Vβ8 region on encephalitogenic T cells. Furthermore, he found that rats that had recovered from actively induced or passively transferred EAE did not generate regulatory T cells recognizing this peptide, and that the transfer of large doses of peptide-specific T cells did not protect the animals from EAE. Sun concluded that the Vβ8(39–59) peptide may comprise cryptic epitopes that function as immunogens only when dissociated from large protein complexes (Sun, 1992). Jung *et al.* (1993) found similar results to those of Sun. In the mouse the inhibitory effect of TCR peptide vaccination on the T cell response to a non-CNS-immunogen (sperm whale myoglobin) has been attributed to the induction of T cell clonal anergy and is dependent on the presence of CD8$^+$ T cells (Gaur *et al.*, 1993).

In conclusion, antibodies specific for the TCR used by encephalitogenic T cells can inhibit disease mediated by these cells. TCR peptide vaccination can also inhibit the development of EAE; however, as it may also enhance EAE, it is of doubtful therapeutic value. The mechanism responsible for any inhibitory effect of TCR peptide therapy remains unclear.

Therapy with peptides binding to MHC

It has been proposed that peptides that bind with high affinity to disease-associated MHC restriction elements but that do not activate encephalitogenic T cells may block the interaction of MHC with the encephalitogenic TCR and be useful in the therapy of EAE (Wraith *et al.*, 1989). In mice, synthetic peptides that bind with high affinity to the appropriate MHC and that are structurally related to an autoantigenic sequence of MBP inhibit EAE when co-immunized with the encephalitogenic MBP peptide (Wraith *et al.*, 1989; Sakai *et al.*, 1989; Smilek *et al.*, 1991). However, in at least one case, inhibition appeared not to be entirely due to binding to the restricting MHC molecules (Wraith *et al.*, 1989; Smilek *et al.*, 1991). Thus, disease inhibition by structurally related peptides may have been achieved through antigen-specific or other regulatory mechanisms. Involvement of antigen-specific regulatory mechanisms as well as competitive MHC blockade has been demonstrated in another study using peptide analogues of disease-associated epitopes (Wauben *et al.*, 1992). Inhibition of EAE in mice has been observed when a structurally unrelated peptide with high-affinity MHC binding is co-immunized with an encephalitogenic PLP peptide; however, as the inhibitory peptide was immunogenic, the possibility that clonal immunodominance contributed to the inhibition of EAE could not be excluded (Lamont *et al.*, 1990). Further studies have shown that EAE can be inhibited by co-immunization with a non-immunogenic structurally unrelated peptide that binds to the relevant MHC molecule, indicating that peptide binding to MHC can itself inhibit EAE (Gautam *et al.*, 1992). EAE can also be suppressed in mice by the intravenous administration of soluble complexes of MHC class II molecules and encephalitogenic MBP or PLP peptide, but the mechanism of this inhibition remains to be elucidated (Sharma *et al.*, 1991).

Anti-CD4 antibody, anti-CD5 antibody and anti-TCR$\alpha\beta$ antibody

Anti-CD4 antibody given by intraperitoneal injection commencing on the day of onset of clinical signs inhibits the progression of disease and accelerates clinical recovery from actively induced acute EAE in the rat and mouse (Brostoff & Mason, 1984; Waldor *et al.*, 1985). Anti-CD4 therapy also reduces the incidence of relapses when commenced after the onset of chronic relapsing EAE in mice (Sriram & Roberts, 1986). The suppressive effect of anti-CD4 therapy in chronic relapsing EAE correlates with the inhibition of MBP-specific and PLP-specific T cell proliferative and delayed-type hypersensitivity responses (Kennedy *et al.*, 1987). Studies in the Lewis rat have shown that the immunoglobulin isotype of the anti-CD4 antibody influences the effectiveness of the therapy (Waldor *et al.*, 1987), and that a major depletion of $CD4^+$ cells is not necessary for the therapy to be effective (Brostoff & Mason, 1984; Brostoff & White, 1986; Waldor *et al.*, 1987). However, as CD4 is also expressed by macrophages in the rat, these findings are difficult to interpret. Studies in the mouse have confirmed that immunoglobulin isotype is important, but have shown that therapeutic efficacy correlates with the depletion of $CD4^+$ T cells (Alters *et al.*, 1990). The depletion of $CD4^+$ T cells *in vivo* does not correlate with the ability of the antibody to mediate complement-dependent cytotoxicity or antibody-dependent cell-mediated cytotoxicity *in vitro*, indicating that additional antibody-dependent cytotoxicity mechanisms are operative *in vivo* (Alters *et al.*, 1990). One possible mechanism is activation-induced T cell apoptosis, which can result from ligation of CD4 prior to T cell activation (Newell *et al.*, 1990). Mannie, Morrison Plummer & McConnell (1993) have provided evidence that anti-CD4 antibody may inhibit the transduction of co-stimulatory signals that are required for the initiation of IL-2 production. EAE can also be inhibited by the administration of a synthetic CD4 analogue (Jameson *et al.*, 1994), anti-CD5 antibody (Sun, Branum & Sun, 1992*a*) or antibody against the $\alpha\beta$ TCR (Matsumoto *et al.*, 1994).

Antibody to class II MHC (Ia) antigen or to antigen–Ia complex

The administration of antibody against the appropriate MHC class II restriction element accelerates recovery from actively induced acute EAE and suppresses chronic relapsing EAE in the mouse (Sriram & Steinman, 1983). In contrast, anti-Ia antibody treatment has no effect on actively induced acute EAE in the Lewis rat (Brostoff & White, 1986). Monoclonal antibodies directed specifically against the MBP–Ia complex inhibit EAE in the mouse and offer a more selective form of immunotherapy than anti-Ia antibodies (Aharoni *et al.*, 1991).

Modulation of cytokine and integrin/adhesion molecule function

The inhibitory effects of soluble IL-1 receptor, TGF-β1, TGF-β2, anti-IL-2, anti-IL-2R and anti-TNF on EAE have already been discussed above (page 42), while the inhibitory effects of antibodies to VLA-4, VCAM-1 and ICAM-1 have been dealt with on page 36.

Chimeric cytotoxin IL-2–PE40

By constructing a chimeric protein by fusing IL-2 and *Pseudomonas* exotoxin (PE) with its cell-binding domain deleted (PE40), a cytotoxin can be selectively targeted to T cells expressing IL-2R (Beraud *et al.*, 1991). In the Lewis rat, treatment with IL-2R–PE40 dramatically prevents EAE passively transferred by an MBP-specific T cell line and also inhibits actively induced MBP-EAE (Beraud *et al.*, 1991).

Cop 1

Cop 1 is a synthetic basic random copolymer of L-alanine, L-glutamic acid, L-lysine and L-tyrosine with a molecular weight of 21 000 and with immunological cross-reactivity with MBP (Teitelbaum *et al.*, 1991). It prevents acute EAE in the guinea pig when injected intradermally with incomplete Freund's adjuvant prior to inoculation with MBP and CFA (Teitelbaum *et al.*, 1971). It is also effective in preventing EAE when commenced after inoculation but before the onset of neurological signs, whether given intradermally with incomplete Freund's adjuvant or intravenously in isotonic saline (Teitelbaum *et al.*, 1971). Cop 1 also prevents chronic relapsing EAE in the guinea pig when given prior to induction, and suppresses this disease when commenced at the time of clinical onset (Keith *et al.*, 1979). The inhibitory effect of Cop 1 on EAE has been attributed to the selective stimulation of suppressor T cells (Lando *et al.*, 1979; Aharoni, Teitelbaum & Arnon, 1993) and to the specific inhibition of MBP-specific effector T cells (Teitelbaum *et al.*, 1988).

Bacterial superantigens

Some bacterial and viral proteins (superantigens) are potent activators of T cells with certain $V\beta$ TCR, and, when applied *in vivo*, can induce anergy or apoptosis in those T cells responding to them. As encephalitogenic MBP-specific T cells in the Lewis rat are $V\beta8.2^+$, bacterial superantigens have been tested for their effect on EAE (Rott, Wekerle & Fleischer, 1992). Staphylococcal enterotoxin E, which selectively interacts with $V\beta8.2$, completely abrogates susceptibility to actively induced MBP-EAE in the Lewis rat (Rott *et al.*, 1992). T cells from the protected animals do not respond to MBP in proliferation studies. However, when given after the induction of MBP-EAE, staphylococcal enterotoxins precipitate relapses in mice that are in clinical remission after an initial attack, and induce attacks in those with subclinical disease (Brocke *et al.*, 1993; Schiffenbauer *et al.*, 1993). Matsumoto & Fujiwara (1993) found that staphylococcal enterotoxin D inhibits actively induced MBP-EAE in rats when given prior to immunization and enhances disease when given after immunization. The ability of superantigens to enhance EAE by activating encephalitogenic T cells using certain $V\beta$ TCR provides a mechanism by which bacterial or viral infections may trigger attacks of multiple sclerosis.

Sulphated polysaccharides

Heparin and fucoidan, which are sulphated polysaccharides, completely inhibit passively transferred EAE in rats, even when treatment is commenced three days after cell transfer (Willenborg & Parish, 1988). A heparin preparation devoid of anticoagulant activity also partially inhibits EAE, indicating that the inhibitory effect is not solely dependent on such activity. Heparin treatment also delays the onset of actively induced EAE. These therapeutic effects of sulphated polysaccharides have been attributed to the inhibition of the enzyme-dependent movement of lymphocytes across the CNS vascular endothelium (Willenborg & Parish, 1988).

ACTH and corticosteroids

Adrenocorticotrophic hormone (ACTH) prevents acute EAE in guinea pigs when administered after inoculation and before the time of onset of neurological signs (Moyer *et al.*, 1950). When given after the onset of neurological signs, it reverses paralysis, although relapse may occur following cessation of therapy (Gammon & Dilworth, 1953). The corticosteroid, methylprednisolone, suppresses acute EAE in the rabbit when given prior to the onset of neurological signs; however, when the dose is reduced, the clinical signs of EAE emerge (Kibler, 1965). When administered after the onset of neurological signs, methylprednisolone reverses neurological signs, but most animals relapse when treatment is withdrawn (Vogel, Paty & Kibler, 1972).

Immunosuppressants

Cyclophosphamide

Cyclophosphamide (5 mg/kg per day by intraperitoneal injection) commencing after the onset of neurological signs is effective in promoting recovery from EAE in the Lewis rat (Paterson & Drobish, 1969). In the rabbit, the same dose of cyclophosphamide has little clinical effect when commenced on the day of onset of neurological signs; however, a dose of 20 mg/kg per day is effective (Vogel *et al.*, 1972). It is important to note that cyclophosphamide can also aggravate EAE. A single injection of cyclophosphamide (20–40 mg/kg) two days prior to inoculation potentiates the development of EAE in resistant rat strains (Mostarica Stojkovic *et al.*, 1982; Kallen *et al.*, 1986) and abrogates induced resistance to EAE in mice (Lando *et al.*, 1979). These effects have been attributed to the selective elimination of suppressor cells by cyclophosphamide. A single injection of cyclophosphamide (100 mg/kg) precipitates a relapse in rats that have recovered from actively induced EAE (Minagawa *et al.*, 1987).

Cyclosporin A

Cyclosporin A prevents actively induced EAE in the rat, guinea pig and monkey (Bolton *et al.*, 1982). It is also effective in suppressing EAE when commenced after the onset of clinical signs, although the signs may recur when treatment is stopped. Interestingly, low-dose cyclosporin A converts acute EAE into chronic relapsing EAE with prominent CNS demyelination, as discussed above (Polman *et al.*, 1988; Pender *et al.*, 1990).

FK506 and rapamycin

FK506, when given intramuscularly for 5–12 days from the time of immunization, prevents the development of actively induced EAE in the rat (Inamura *et al.*, 1988). In contrast, the oral administration of FK506 for 12 days after immunization delays the onset of EAE and converts it from an acute to a chronic relapsing form (Deguchi *et al.*, 1991). Rapamycin, a potent immunosuppressive agent with a mechanism of action different from that of cyclosporin A or FK506, also inhibits EAE (Carlson *et al.*, 1993).

Immunosuppression followed by syngeneic bone marrow transplantation

Acute immunosuppression by total body irradiation or a single high dose of cyclophosphamide, followed by syngeneic bone marrow transplantation, six days after immunization with spinal cord homogenate and adjuvants, prevents the development of EAE in mice (Karussis *et al.*, 1992). Furthermore, mice treated with cyclophosphamide and syngeneic bone marrow transplantation become resistant to rechallenge with the same encephalitogenic inoculum, apparently as a result of the specific tolerization of newly developing lymphocytes to the immunizing antigens (Karussis *et al.*, 1992). When applied after the onset of clinical disease, the same therapeutic regimen facilitated recovery from the first attack and prevented spontaneous relapses in mice with chronic relapsing EAE induced by the passive transfer of MBP-sensitized lymph node cells (Karussis *et al.*, 1993*c*). It also reduced the incidence and delayed the onset of relapses provoked by immunization with MBP and CFA 78 days after the passive induction of chronic relapsing EAE.

Other agents

ET-18-OCH3 is an alkyllysophospholipid that is a synthetic analogue of the naturally occurring 2-lysophosphatidylcholine and that possesses a high immunomodulatory and antineoplastic capacity. It suppresses actively induced acute MBP-EAE in the rat (Klein Franke & Munder, 1992). SRI 62–834, a cyclic ether analogue of ET-18-OCH3, suppresses chronic relapsing EAE in the Lewis rat when administered from the time of the first remission on day 15 until day 31 (Chabannes, Ryffel & Borel, 1992). Withdrawal of SRI 62–834 on day 31 did not lead to a relapse in contrast to withdrawal of cyclosporin A. The oral administration of linomide, an immunomodulating agent that stimulates natural killer cell activity, inhibits acute and chronic relapsing EAE (Karussis *et al.*, 1993*a*,*b*). EAE can also be inhibited by Δ^9-tetrahydrocannabinol, an active component of marijuana (Lyman *et al.*, 1989*b*), and by pentoxifylline, a phosphodiesterase inhibitor that inhibits TNF and to a lesser extent IL-2 production in activated T cells (Nataf *et al.*, 1993; Rott, Cash & Fleischer, 1993).

Conclusions

EAE is an autoimmune demyelinating disease that can be induced by active immunization with myelin antigens and adjuvants. It can also be induced by the passive transfer of T cells specific for MBP, T cells specific for PLP, or a combination of T cells and antibodies specific for MOG. Despite the fact that autoaggressive encephalitogenic T cell lines can be established from unprimed normal rat lymph node populations, EAE does not develop spontaneously, except in transgenic mice expressing genes encoding a rearranged TCR specific for MBP. In MBP-EAE, inflammation and demyelination occur in the CNS and the proximal PNS, whereas in PLP-EAE and MOG-EAE, the inflammation and demyelination are restricted to the CNS. EAE generally has an acute monophasic clinical course followed by spontaneous recovery; however, in some animal strains a chronic relapsing form develops. The acute form of EAE resembles the human disease, acute disseminated encephalomyelitis, while the chronic relapsing form resembles multiple sclerosis. Studies on EAE have yielded valuable information about possible disease mechanisms and therapy for multiple sclerosis and also information about the pathogenesis and immunoregulation of T-cell-mediated autoimmune disease in general. Major unanswered questions are what regulatory mechanisms control the potentially encephalitogenic T cells that are present in normal animals and what mechanisms prevent the development of relapses in most animals with EAE? Possible mechanisms include the action of suppressor or regulatory T cells and the occurrence of apoptosis of autoreactive T cells in the CNS and possibly in the thymus. Further studies are also required to determine whether intramolecular and extramolecular antigenic determinant spreading contributes to the progression of disease in the CNS in EAE.

References

Acha Orbea, H., Mitchell, D.J., Timmermann, L., Wraith, D.C., Tausch, G.S., Waldor, M.K., Zamvil, S.S., McDevitt, H.O. & Steinman, L. (1988). Limited heterogeneity of T cell receptors from lymphocytes mediating autoimmune encephalomyelitis allows specific immune intervention. *Cell*, **54**, 263–73.

Ackermann, H.P., Ulrich, J. & Heitz, P.U. (1981). Experimental allergic encephalomyelitis. Exudate and cellular infiltrates in the spinal cord of Lewis rats. *Acta Neuropathologica*, **54**, 149–52.

Adda, D.H., Beraud, E. & Depieds, R. (1977). Evidence for suppressor cells in Lewis rats' experimental allergic encephalomyelitis. *European Journal of Immunology*, **7**, 620–3.

Aharoni, R., Teitelbaum, D. & Arnon, R. (1993). T suppressor hybridomas and interleukin-2-dependent lines induced by copolymer 1 or by spinal cord homogenate down-regulate experimental allergic encephalomyelitis. *European Journal of Immunology*, **23**, 17–25.

Aharoni, R., Teitelbaum, D., Arnon, R. & Puri, J. (1991). Immunomodulation of experimental allergic encephalomyelitis by antibodies to the antigen-Ia complex. *Nature*, **351**, 147–50.

Alters, S.E., Sakai, K., Steinman, L. & Oi, V.T. (1990). Mechanisms of anti-CD4-mediated depletion and immunotherapy. A study using a set of chimeric anti-CD4 antibodies. *Journal of Immunology*, **144**, 4587–92.

Amor, S., Baker, D., Groome, N. & Turk, J.L. (1993). Identification of a major encephalitogenic epitope of proteolipid protein (residues 56–70) for the induction of experimental allergic encephalomyelitis in Biozzi AB/H and nonobese diabetic mice. *Journal of Immunology*, **150**, 5666–72.

Ando, D.G., Clayton, J., Kono, D., Urban, J.L. & Sercarz, E.E. (1989). Encephalitogenic T cells in the B10.PL model of experimental allergic encephalomyelitis (EAE) are of the Th-1 lymphokine subtype. *Cellular Immunology*, **124**, 132–43.

Archelos, J.J., Jung, S., Maurer, M., Schmied, M., Lassmann, H., Tamatani, T., Miyasaka, M., Toyka, K.V. & Hartung, H.P. (1993). Inhibition of experimental autoimmune encephalomyelitis by an antibody to the intercellular adhesion molecule ICAM-1. *Annals of Neurology*, **34**, 145–54.

Banik, N.L. (1992). Pathogenesis of myelin breakdown in demyelinating diseases: role of proteolytic enzymes. *Critical Reviews in Neurobiology*, **6**, 257–71.

Barish, M.E. & Raissdana, S.S. (1990). Induction of class II major histocompatibility complex antigens on a population of astrocytes from a mouse strain (BALB/c) resistant to experimental allergic encephalomyelitis. *Brain Research*, **510**, 329–34.

Baron, J.L., Madri, J.A., Ruddle, N.H., Hashim, G. & Janeway, C.A.J. (1993). Surface expression of alpha 4 integrin by CD4 T cells is required for their entry into brain parenchyma. *Journal of Experimental Medicine*, **177**, 57–68.

Bassoe, P. & Grinker, R.R. (1930). Human rabies and rabies vaccine encephalomyelitis. A clinicopathologic study. *Archives of Neurology and Psychiatry*, **23**, 1138–60.

Bauer, J., Berkenbosch, F., Van Dam, A.M. & Dijkstra, C.D. (1993). Demonstration of interleukin-1 beta in Lewis rat brain during experimental allergic encephalomyelitis by immunocytochemistry at the light and ultrastructural level. *Journal of Neuroimmunology*, **48**, 13–21.

Bell, R.B., Lindsey, J.W., Sobel, R.A., Hodgkinson, S. & Steinman, L. (1993). Diverse T cell receptor V beta gene usage in the central nervous system in experimental allergic encephalomyelitis. *Journal of Immunology*, **150**, 4085–92.

Ben Nun, A. & Cohen, I.R. (1981). Vaccination against autoimmune encephalomyelitis (EAE): attenuated autoimmune T lymphocytes confer resistance to induction of active EAE but not to EAE mediated by the intact T lymphocyte line. *European Journal of Immunology*, **11**, 949–52.

Ben Nun, A., Wekerle, H. & Cohen, I.R. (1981*a*). The rapid isolation of clonable antigen-specific T lymphocyte lines capable of mediating autoimmune encephalomyelitis. *European Journal of Immunology*, **11**, 195–9.

Ben Nun, A., Wekerle, H. & Cohen, I.R. (1981*b*). Vaccination against autoimmune encephalomyelitis with T-lymphocyte line cells reactive against myelin basic protein. *Nature*, **292**, 60–1.

Beraud, E., Lorberboum Galski, H., Chan, C.C., FitzGerald, D., Pastan, I. & Nussenblatt, R.B. (1991). Immunospecific suppression of encephalitogenic-activated T lymphocytes by chimeric cytotoxin IL-2-PE40. *Cellular Immunology*, **133**, 379–89.

Bergsteinsdottir, K., Brennan, A., Jessen, K.R. & Mirsky, R. (1992). In the presence of dexamethasone, gamma interferon induces rat oligodendrocytes to express major histocompatibility complex class II molecules. *Proceedings of the National Academy of Sciences USA*, **89**, 9054–8.

Bernard, C.C. (1977). Suppressor T cells prevent experimental autoimmune encephalomyelitis in mice. *Clinical and Experimental Immunology*, **29**, 100–9.

Bernheimer, H., Lassmann, H. & Suchanek, G. (1988). Dynamics of IgG+, IgA+, and IgM+ plasma cells in the central nervous system of guinea pigs with chronic relapsing experimental allergic encephalomyelitis. *Neuropathology and Applied Neurobiology*, **14**, 157–67.

Bieger, D. & White, S.R. (1981). Anatomical evidence for bulbospinal monoamine axon damage in rats with experimental allergic encephalomyelitis. *Neuroscience*, **6**, 1745–52.

Billiau, A., Heremans, H., Vandekerckhove, F., Dijkmans, R., Sobis, H., Meulepas, E. & Carton, H. (1988). Enhancement of experimental allergic encephalomyelitis in mice by antibodies against IFN-gamma. *Journal of Immunology*, **140**, 1506–10.

Binder, T.A., Greiner, D.L., Grunnet, M. & Goldschneider, I. (1993). Relative susceptibility of SJL/J and B10.S mice to experimental allergic encephalomyelitis (EAE) is determined by the ability of prethymic cells in bone marrow to develop into EAE effector T cells. *Journal of Neuroimmunology*, **42**, 23–32.

Bitar, D.M. & Whitacre, C.C. (1988). Suppression of experimental autoimmune encephalomyelitis by the oral administration of myelin basic protein. *Cellular Immunology*, **112**, 364–70.

Bolton, C., Borel, J.F., Cuzner, M.L., Davison, A.N. & Turner, A.M. (1982). Immunosuppression by cyclosporin A of experimental allergic encephalomyelitis. *Journal of the Neurological Sciences*, **56**, 147–53.

Brocke, S., Gaur, A., Piercy, C., Gautam, A., Gijbels, K., Fathman, C.G. & Steinman, L. (1993). Induction of relapsing paralysis in experimental autoimmune encephalomyelitis by bacterial superantigen. *Nature*, **365**, 642–4.

Brod, S.A., al Sabbagh, A., Sobel, R.A., Hafler, D.A. & Weiner, H.L. (1991). Suppression of experimental autoimmune encephalomyelitis by oral administration of myelin antigens: IV. Suppression of chronic relapsing disease in the Lewis rat and strain 13 guinea pig. *Annals of Neurology*, **29**, 615–22.

Brostoff, S.W. & Eylar, E.H. (1972). The proposed amino acid sequence of the P1 protein of rabbit sciatic nerve myelin. *Archives of Biochemistry and Biophysics*, **153**, 590–8.

Brostoff, S.W. & Mason, D.W. (1984). Experimental allergic encephalomyelitis: successful treatment *in vivo* with a monoclonal antibody that recognizes T helper cells. *Journal of Immunology*, **133**, 1938–42.

Brostoff, S.W. & White, T.M. (1986). Treatment of clinical experimental allergic encephalomyelitis in the rat with monoclonal antibodies. *Journal of Neuroimmunology*, **13**, 233–40.

Brown, A., McFarlin, D.E. & Raine, C.S. (1982). Chronologic neuropathology of relapsing experimental allergic encephalomyelitis in the mouse. *Laboratory Investigation*, **46**, 171–85.

Brown, A.M. & McFarlin, D.E. (1981). Relapsing experimental allergic encephalomyelitis in the SJL/J mouse. *Laboratory Investigation*, **45**, 278–84.

Burns, F.R., Li, X.B., Shen, N., Offner, H., Chou, Y.K., Vandenbark, A.A. & Heber Katz, E. (1989). Both rat and mouse T cell receptors specific for the encephalitogenic determinant of myelin basic protein use similar V alpha and V beta chain genes even though the major histocompatibility complex and encephalitogenic determinants being recognized are different. *Journal of Experimental Medicine*, **169**, 27–39.

Cannella, B., Cross, A.H. & Raine, C.S. (1990). Upregulation and coexpression of adhesion molecules correlate with relapsing autoimmune demyelination in the central nervous system. *Journal of Experimental Medicine*, **172**, 1521–4.

Cannella, B., Cross, A.H. & Raine, C.S. (1993). Anti-adhesion molecule therapy in experimental autoimmune encephalomyelitis. *Journal of Neuroimmunology*, **46**, 43–55.

Carlson, R.P., Hartman, D.A., Tomchek, L.A., Walter, T.L., Lugay, J.R., Calhoun, W., Sehgal, S.N. & Chang, J.Y. (1993). Rapamycin, a potential disease-modifying antiarthritic drug. *Journal of Pharmacology and Experimental Therapeutics*, **266**, 1125–38.

Centanni, E. (1898). Sui prodotti tossici secondarii nelle infezioni. *Riforma Medica*, **3**, 637–44.

Chabannes, D., Ryffel, B. & Borel, J.F. (1992). SRI 62–834, a cyclic ether analogue of the phospholipid ET-18-OCH3, displays long-lasting beneficial effect in chronic relapsing experimental allergic encephalomyelitis in the Lewis rat. Comparison with cyclosporin and (Val2)-dihydrocyclosporin effects in clinical, functional and histological studies. *Journal of Autoimmunity*, **5**, 199–211.

Chalk, J.B., McCombe, P.A. & Pender, M.P. (1994*a*). Conduction abnormalities are restricted to the central nervous system in experimental autoimmune encephalomyelitis induced by inoculation with proteolipid protein but not with myelin basic protein. *Brain*, **117**, 975–86.

Chalk, J.B., McCombe, P.A., Smith, R. & Pender, M.P. (1994*b*). Clinical and histological findings in proteolipid protein-induced experimental autoimmune encephalomyelitis (EAE) in the Lewis rat. Distribution of demyelination differs from that in EAE induced by other antigens. *Journal of the Neurological Sciences*, **123**, 154–61.

Chluba, J., Steeg, C., Becker, A., Wekerle, H. & Epplen, J.T. (1989). T cell receptor beta chain usage in myelin basic protein-specific rat T lymphocytes. *European Journal of Immunology*, **19**, 279–84.

Chou, F.C., Chou, C.H., Fritz, R.B. & Kibler, R.F. (1980). Prevention of experimental allergic encephalomyelitis in Lewis rats with peptide 68–88 of guinea pig myelin basic protein. *Annals of Neurology*, **7**, 336–9.

Claudio, L., Kress, Y., Factor, J. & Brosnan, C.F. (1990). Mechanisms of edema formation in experimental autoimmune encephalomyelitis. The contribution of inflammatory cells. *American Journal of Pathology*, **137**, 1033–45.

Claudio, L., Kress, Y., Norton, W.T. & Brosnan, C.F. (1989). Increased vesicular transport and decreased mitochondrial content in blood–brain barrier endothelial cells during experimental autoimmune encephalomyelitis. *American Journal of Pathology*, **135**, 1157–68.

Clayton, J.P., Gammon, G.M., Ando, D.G., Kono, D.H., Hood, L. & Sercarz, E.E. (1989). Peptide-specific prevention of experimental allergic encephalomyelitis. Neonatal tolerance induced to the dominant T cell determinant of myelin basic protein. *Journal of Experimental Medicine*, **169**, 1681–91.

Colover, J. (1980). A new pattern of spinal-cord demyelination in guinea pigs with acute experimental allergic encephalomyelitis mimicking multiple sclerosis. *British Journal of Experimental Pathology*, **61**, 390–400.

Critchfield, J.M., Racke, M.K., Zuniga Pflucker, J.C., Cannella, B., Raine, C.S., Goverman, J. & Lenardo, M.J. (1994). T cell deletion in high antigen dose therapy of autoimmune encephalomyelitis. *Science*, **263**, 1139–43.

Cross, A.H., Cannella, B., Brosnan, C.F. & Raine, C.S. (1990). Homing to central nervous system vasculature by antigen-specific lymphocytes. I. Localization of 14C-labeled cells during acute, chronic, and relapsing experimental allergic encephalomyelitis. *Laboratory Investigation*, **63**, 162–70.

Day, M.J., Tse, A. & Mason, D.W. (1991). The refractory phase of experimental allergic encephalomyelitis in the Lewis rat is antigen specific in its induction but not in its effect. *Journal of Neuroimmunology*, **34**, 197–203.

Day, M.J., Tse, A.G., Puklavec, M., Simmonds, S.J. & Mason, D.W. (1992). Targeting autoantigen to B cells prevents the induction of a cell-mediated autoimmune disease in rats. *Journal of Experimental Medicine*, **175**, 655–9.

Deguchi, K., Takeuchi, H., Miki, H., Yamada, A., Touge, T., Terada, S. & Nishioka, M. (1991). Effects of FK 506 on acute experimental allergic encephalomyelitis. *Transplantation Proceedings*, **23**, 3360–2.

Desquenne Clark, L., Esch, T.R., Otvos, L.J. & Heber Katz, E. (1991). T-cell receptor peptide immunization leads to enhanced and chronic experimental allergic encephalomyelitis. *Proceedings of the National Academy of Sciences USA*, **88**, 7219–23.

Duong, T.T., St. Louis, J., Gilbert, J.J., Finkelman, F.D. & Strejan, G.H. (1992). Effect of anti-interferon-gamma and anti-interleukin-2 monoclonal antibody treatment on the development of actively and passively induced experimental allergic encephalomyelitis in the SJL/J mouse. *Journal of Neuroimmunology*, **36**, 105–15.

Ellerman, K.E., Powers, J.M. & Brostoff, S.W. (1988). A suppressor T-lymphocyte cell line for autoimmune encephalomyelitis. *Nature*, **331**, 265–7.

Endoh, M., Kunishita, T., Nihei, J., Nishizawa, M. & Tabira, T. (1990). Susceptibility to proteolipid apoprotein and its encephalitogenic determinants in mice. *International Archives of Allergy and Applied Immunology*, **92**, 433–8.

Engelhardt, B., Diamantstein, T. & Wekerle, H. (1989). Immunotherapy of experimental autoimmune encephalomyelitis (EAE): differential effect of anti-IL-2 receptor antibody therapy on actively induced and T-line mediated EAE of the Lewis rat. *Journal of Autoimmunity*, **2**, 61–73.

Eylar, E.H., Caccam, J., Jackson, J.J., Westall, F.C. & Robinson, A.B. (1970). Experimental allergic encephalomyelitis: synthesis of disease-inducing site of the basic protein. *Science*, **168**, 1220–3.

Eylar, E.H., Jackson, J.J. & Kniskern, P.J. (1979). Suppression and reversal of allergic encephalomyelitis in rhesus monkeys with basic protein and peptides. *Neurochemical Research*, **4**, 249–58.

Fallis, R.J. & McFarlin, D.E. (1989). Chronic relapsing experimental allergic encephalomyelitis. Cytotoxicity effected by a class II restricted T cell line specific for an encephalitogenic epitope. *Journal of Immunology*, **143**, 2160–5.

Ferraro, A. & Jervis, G.A. (1940). Experimental disseminated encephalopathy in the monkey. *Archives of Neurology and Psychiatry*, **43**, 195–209.

Ferraro, A. & Roizin, L. (1954). Neuropathologic variations in experimental allergic encephalomyelitis. Hemorrhagic encephalomyelitis, perivenous encephalomyelitis, diffuse encephalomyelitis, patchy gliosis. *Journal of Neuropathology and Experimental Neurology*, **13**, 60–89.

Fierz, W., Endler, B., Reske, K., Wekerle, H. & Fontana, A. (1985). Astrocytes as antigen-presenting cells. I. Induction of Ia antigen expression on astrocytes by T cells via immune interferon and its effect on antigen presentation. *Journal of Immunology*, **134**, 3785–93.

Finean, J.B., Hawthorne, J.N. & Patterson, J.D.E. (1957). Structural and chemical differences between optic and sciatic nerve myelins. *Journal of Neurochemistry*, **1**, 256–9.

Folch, J., Lees, M. & Carr, S. (1958). Studies of the chemical composition of the nervous system. *Experimental Cell Research (Supplement)*, **5**, 58–71.

Fontana, A., Fierz, W. & Wekerle, H. (1984). Astrocytes present myelin basic protein to encephalitogenic T-cell lines. *Nature*, **307**, 273–6.

Frei, K., Siepl, C., Groscurth, P., Bodmer, S., Schwerdel, C. & Fontana, A (1987). Antigen presentation and tumor cytotoxicity by interferon-gamma-treated microglial cells. *European Journal of Immunology*, **17**, 1271–8.

Freund, J., Stern, E.R. & Pisani, T.M. (1947). Isoallergic encephalomyelitis and radiculitis in guinea pigs after one injection of brain and mycobacteria in water-in-oil emulsion. *Journal of Immunology*, **57**, 179–94.

Gammon, G.A. & Dilworth, M.J. (1953). Effect of corticotropin on paralysis of experimental allergic encephalomyelitis. *Archives of Neurology and Psychiatry* **69**, 649.

Gaur, A., Ruberti, G., Haspel, R., Mayer, J.P. & Fathman, C.G. (1993). Requirement for CD8+ cells in T cell receptor peptide-induced clonal unresponsiveness [published erratum appears in *Science* 1993 Apr 16;**260**(5106):preceding 281]. *Science*, **259**, 91–4.

Gaur, A., Wiers, B., Liu, A., Rothbard, J. & Fathman, C.G. (1992). Amelioration of autoimmune encephalomyelitis by myelin basic protein synthetic peptide-induced anergy. *Science*, **258**, 1491–4.

Gausas, J., Paterson, P.Y., Day, E.D. & Dal Canto, M.C. (1982). Intact B-cell activity is essential for complete expression of experimental allergic encephalomyelitis in Lewis rats. *Cellular Immunology*, **72**, 360–6.

Gautam, A.M., Lock, C.B., Smilek, D.E., Pearson, C.I., Steinman, L. & McDevitt, H.O. (1994). Minimum structural requirements for peptide presentation by major histocompatibility complex class II molecules: implications in induction of autoimmunity. *Proceedings of the National Academy of Sciences USA*, **91**, 767–71.

Gautam, A.M., Pearson, C.I., Sinha, A.A., Smilek, D.E., Steinman, L. & McDevitt, H.O. (1992). Inhibition of experimental autoimmune encephalomyelitis by a nonimmunogenic non-self peptide that binds to I-A^u. *Journal of Immunology*, **148**, 3049–54.

Goverman, J., Woods, A., Larson, L., Weiner, L.P., Hood, L. & Zaller, D.M. (1993). Transgenic mice that express a myelin basic protein-specific T cell receptor develop spontaneous autoimmunity. *Cell*, **72**, 551–60.

Greenfield, S., Brostoff, S., Eylar, E.H. & Morell, P. (1973). Protein composition of myelin of the peripheral nervous system. *Journal of Neurochemistry*, **20**, 1207–16.

Greer, J.M., Kuchroo, V.K., Sobel, R.A. & Lees, M.B. (1992). Identification and characterization of a second encephalitogenic determinant of myelin proteolipid protein (residues 178–191) for SJL mice. *Journal of Immunology*, **149**, 783–8.

Gregerson, D.S., Obritsch, W.F. & Donoso, L.A. (1993). Oral tolerance in experimental autoimmune uveoretinitis. Distinct mechanisms of resistance are induced by low dose vs high dose feeding protocols. *Journal of Immunology*, **151**, 5751–61.

Groux, H., Monte, D., Plouvier, B., Capron, A. & Ameisen, J.C. (1993). CD3-mediated apoptosis of human medullary thymocytes and activated peripheral T cells: respective roles of interleukin-1, interleukin-2, interferon-gamma and accessory cells. *European Journal of Immunology*, **23**, 1623–9.

Hansen, L.A. & Pender, M.P. (1989). Hypothermia due to an ascending impairment of shivering in hyperacute experimental allergic encephalomyelitis in the Lewis rat. *Journal of the Neurological Sciences*, **94**, 231–40.

Hashim, G.A., Vandenbark, A.A., Galang, A.B., Diamanduros, T., Carvalho, E., Srinivasan, J., Jones, R., Vainiene, M., Morrison, W.J. & Offner, H. (1990). Antibodies specific for VB8 receptor peptide suppress experimental autoimmune encephalomyelitis. *Journal of Immunology*, **144**, 4621–7.

Hawkins, C.P., Mackenzie, F., Tofts, P., du Boulay, E.P. & McDonald, W.I. (1991). Patterns of blood–brain barrier breakdown in inflammatory demyelination. *Brain*, **114**, 801–10.

Hawkins, C.P., Munro, P.M., Landon, D.N. & McDonald, W.I. (1992). Metabolically dependent blood–brain barrier breakdown in chronic relapsing experimental allergic encephalomyelitis. *Acta Neuropathologica (Berlin)*, **83**, 630–5.

Hawkins, C.P., Munro, P.M., Mackenzie, F., Kesselring, J., Tofts, P.S., du Boulay, E.P., Landon, D.N. & McDonald, W.I. (1990). Duration and selectivity of blood–brain barrier breakdown in chronic relapsing experimental allergic encephalomyelitis studied by gadolinium-DTPA and protein markers. *Brain*, **113**, 365–78.

Hayosh, N.S. & Swanborg, R.H. (1986). Autoimmune effector cells. VII. Cells isolated from thymus and spinal cord of rats with experimental allergic encephalomyelitis transfer disease. *American Journal of Pathology*, **122**, 218–22.

Hayreh, S.S., Massanari, R.M., Yamada, T. & Hayreh, S.M. (1981). Experimental allergic encephalomyelitis. I. Optic nerve and central nervous system manifestations. *Investigative Ophthalmology and Visual Science*, **21**, 256–69.

Heininger, K., Fierz, W., Schafer, B., Hartung, H.P., Wehling, P. & Toyka, K.V. (1989). Electrophysiological investigations in adoptively transferred experimental autoimmune encephalomyelitis in the Lewis rat. *Brain*, **112**, 537–52.

Held, W., Meyermann, R., Qin, Y. & Mueller, C. (1993). Perforin and tumor necrosis factor alpha in the pathogenesis of experimental allergic encephalomyelitis: comparison of auto-antigen induced and transferred disease in Lewis rats. *Journal of Autoimmunity*, **6**, 311–22.

Hickey, W.F., Gonatas, N.K., Kimura, H. & Wilson, D.B. (1983). Identification and quantitation of T lymphocyte subsets found in the spinal cord of the Lewis rat during acute experimental allergic encephalomyelitis. *Journal of Immunology*, **131**, 2805–9.

Hickey, W.F., Hsu, B.L. & Kimura, H. (1991). T-lymphocyte entry into the central nervous system. *Journal of Neuroscience Research*, **28**, 254–60.

Hickey, W.F. & Kimura, H. (1988). Perivascular microglial cells of the CNS are bone marrow-derived and present antigen *in vivo*. *Science*, **239**, 290–2.

Higgins, P.J. & Weiner, H.L. (1988). Suppression of experimental autoimmune encephalomyelitis by oral administration of myelin basic protein and its fragments. *Journal of Immunology*, **140**, 440–5.

Hinrichs, D.J., Roberts, C.M. & Waxman, F.J. (1981). Regulation of paralytic experimental allergic encephalomyelitis in rats: susceptibility to active and passive disease reinduction. *Journal of Immunology*, **126**, 1857–62.

Hinrichs, D.J., Wegmann, K.W. & Dietsch, G.N. (1987). Transfer of experimental allergic encephalomyelitis to bone marrow chimeras. Endothelial cells are not a restricting element. *Journal of Experimental Medicine*, **166**, 1906–11.

Holda, J.H. & Swanborg, R.H. (1981). Regulation of experimental allergic encephalomyelitis. III. Demonstration of effector cells in tolerant rats. *European Journal of Immunology*, **11**, 338–40.

Holoshitz, J., Frenkel, A., Ben Nun, A. & Cohen, I.R. (1983). Autoimmune encephalomyelitis (EAE) mediated or prevented by T lymphocyte lines directed against diverse antigenic determinants of myelin basic protein. Vaccination is determinant specific. *Journal of Immunology*, **131**, 2810–13.

Howell, M.D., Winters, S.T., Olee, T., Powell, H.C., Carlo, D.J. & Brostoff, S.W. (1989). Vaccination against experimental allergic encephalomyelitis with T cell receptor peptides [published erratum appears in *Science* 1990 Mar 9;**247**(4947):1167]. *Science*, **246**, 668–70.

Huitinga, I., Damoiseaux, J.G., Dopp, E.A. & Dijkstra, C.D. (1993). Treatment with anti-CR3 antibodies ED7 and ED8 suppresses experimental allergic encephalomyelitis in Lewis rats. *European Journal of Immunology*, **23**, 709–15.

Huitinga, I., van Rooijen, N., De Groot, C.J., Uitdehaag, B.M. & Dijkstra, C.D. (1990). Suppression of experimental allergic encephalomyelitis in Lewis rats after elimination of macrophages. *Journal of Experimental Medicine*, **172**, 1025–33.

Hulkower, K., Brosnan, C.F., Aquino, D.A., Cammer, W., Kukshrestha, S., Guida, M.P., Rapoport, D.A. & Berman, J.W. (1993). Expression of CSF-1, c-fms, and MCP-1 in the central nervous system of rats with experimental allergic encephalomyelitis. *Journal of Immunology*, **150**, 2525–33.

Inamura, N., Hashimoto, M., Nakahara, K., Nakajima, Y., Nishio, M., Aoki, H., Yamaguchi, I. & Kohsaka, M. (1988). Immunosuppressive effect of FK506 on experimental allergic encephalomyelitis in rats. *International Journal of Immunopharmacology*, **10**, 991–5.

Itoyama, Y. & Webster, H.D. (1982). Immunocytochemical study of myelin-associated glycoprotein (MAG) and basic protein (BP) in acute experimental allergic encephalomyelitis (EAE). *Journal of Neuroimmunology*, **3**, 351–64.

Jacobs, C.A., Baker, P.E., Roux, E.R., Picha, K.S., Toivola, B., Waugh, S. & Kennedy, M.K. (1991). Experimental autoimmune encephalomyelitis is exacerbated by IL-1 alpha and suppressed by soluble IL-1 receptor. *Journal of Immunology*, **146**, 2983–9.

Jameson, B.A., McDonnell, J.M., Marini, J.C. & Korngold, R. (1994). A rationally designed CD4 analogue inhibits experimental allergic encephalomyelitis. *Nature*, **368**, 744–6.

Jensen, M.A., Arnason, B.G., Toscas, A. & Noronha, A. (1992). Preferential increase of IL-2R$^+$ CD4$^+$ T cells and CD45RB$^-$ CD4$^+$ T cells in the central nervous system in experimental allergic encephalomyelitis. *Journal of Neuroimmunology*, **38**, 255–61.

Jewtoukoff, V., Lebar, R. & Bach, M.A. (1989). Oligodendrocyte-specific autoreactive T cells using an alpha/beta T-cell receptor kill their target without self restriction. *Proceedings of the National Academy of Sciences USA*, **86**, 2824–8.

Jiang, H., Zhang, S.I. & Pernis, B. (1992). Role of CD8+ T cells in murine experimental allergic encephalomyelitis. *Science*, **256**, 1213–15.

Johns, L.D., Flanders, K.C., Ranges, G.E. & Sriram, S. (1991). Successful treatment of experimental allergic encephalomyelitis with transforming growth factor-beta 1. *Journal of Immunology*, **147**, 1792–6.

Johns, L.D. & Sriram, S. (1993). Experimental allergic encephalomyelitis neutralizing antibody to TGF beta 1 enhances the clinical severity of the disease. *Journal of Neuroimmunology*, **47**, 1–7.

Jones, R.E., Bourdette, D.N., Offner, H. & Vandenbark, A.A. (1990). Myelin basic protein-specific T cells induce demyelinating experimental autoimmune encephalomyelitis in Buffalo rats. *Journal of Neuroimmunology*, **30**, 61–9.

Jones, R.E., Bourdette, D., Offner, H. & Vandenbark, A.A. (1992). The synthetic 87–99 peptide of myelin basic protein is encephalitogenic in Buffalo rats. *Journal of Neuroimmunology*, **37**, 203–12.

Jones, R.E., Bourdette, D.N., Whitham, R.H., Offner, H. & Vandenbark, A.A. (1993). Induction of experimental autoimmune encephalomyelitis in severe combined immunodeficient mice reconstituted with allogeneic or xenogeneic hematopoietic cells. *Journal of Immunology*, **150**, 4620–9.

Jung, S., Schluesener, H.J., Toyka, K.V. & Hartung, H.P. (1993). Modulation of EAE by vaccination with T cell receptor peptides: V beta 8 T cell receptor peptide-specific CD4$^+$ lymphocytes lack direct immunoregulatory activity. *Journal of Neuroimmunology*, **45**, 15–22.

Kabat, E.A., Wolf, A. & Bezer, A.E. (1947). The rapid production of acute disseminated encephalomyelitis in rhesus monkeys by injection of heterologous and homologous brain tissue with adjuvants. *Journal of Experimental Medicine*, **85**, 117–30.

Kallen, B., Dohlsten, M. & Klementsson, H. (1986). Effect of cyclophosphamide pretreatment on autoimmune encephalomyelitis in rats. *Acta Neurologica Scandinavica*, **73**, 338–44.

Karkhanis, Y.D., Carlo, D.J., Brostoff, S.W. & Eylar, E.H. (1975). Allergic encephalomyelitis. Isolation of an encephalitogenic peptide active in the monkey. *Journal of Biological Chemistry*, **250**, 1718–22.

Karpus, W.J., Gould, K.E. & Swanborg, R.H. (1992). CD4$^+$ suppressor cells of autoimmune encephalomyelitis respond to T cell receptor-associated determinants on effector cells by interleukin-4 secretion. *European Journal of Immunology*, **22**, 1757–63.

Karpus, W.J. & Swanborg, R.H. (1989). CD4$^+$ suppressor cells differentially affect the production of IFN-gamma by effector cells of experimental autoimmune encephalomyelitis. *Journal of Immunology*, **143**, 3492–7.

Karpus, W.J. & Swanborg, R.H. (1991*a*). CD4$^+$ suppressor cells inhibit the function of effector cells of experimental autoimmune encephalomyelitis through a mechanism involving transforming growth factor-beta. *Journal of Immunology*, **146**, 1163–8.

Karpus, W.J. & Swanborg, R.H. (1991*b*). Protection against experimental autoimmune encephalomyelitis requires both CD4$^+$ T suppressor cells and myelin basic protein-primed B cells. *Journal of Neuroimmunology*, **33**, 173–7.

Karussis, D.M., Lehmann, D., Slavin, S., Vourka Karussis, U., Mizrachi Koll, R., Ovadia, H., Ben Nun, A., Kalland, T. & Abramsky, O. (1993*a*). Inhibition of acute, experimental autoimmune encephalomyelitis by the synthetic immunomodulator linomide. *Annals of Neurology*, **34**, 654–60.

Karussis, D.M., Lehmann, D., Slavin, S., Vourka Karussis, U., Mizrachi Koll, R., Ovadia, H., Kalland, T. & Abramsky, O. (1993*b*). Treatment of chronic-relapsing experimental autoimmune encephalomyelitis with the synthetic immunomodulator linomide (quinoline-3-carboxamide). *Proceedings of the National Academy of Sciences USA*, **90**, 6400–4.

Karussis, D.M., Slavin, S., Lehmann, D., Mizrachi Koll, R., Abramsky, O. & Ben Nun, A. (1992). Prevention of experimental autoimmune encephalomyelitis and induction of tolerance with acute immunosuppression followed by syngeneic bone marrow transplantation. *Journal of Immunology*, **148**, 1693–8.

Karussis, D.M., Vourka Karussis, U., Lehmann, D., Ovadia, H., Mizrachi Koll, R., Ben Nun, A., Abramsky, O. & Slavin, S. (1993*c*). Prevention and reversal of adoptively transferred, chronic relapsing experimental autoimmune encephalomyelitis with a single high dose cytoreductive treatment followed by syngeneic bone marrow transplantation. *Journal of Clinical Investigation*, **92**, 765–72.

Kawai, K., Heber Katz, E. & Zweiman, B. (1991). Cytotoxic effects of myelin basic protein-reactive T cell hybridoma cells on oligodendrocytes. *Journal of Neuroimmunology*, **32**, 75–81.

Kawai, K. & Zweiman, B. (1988). Cytotoxic effect of myelin basic protein-reactive T cells on cultured oligodendrocytes. *Journal of Neuroimmunology*, **19**, 159–65.

Kawai, K. & Zweiman, B. (1990). Characteristics of *in vitro* cytotoxic effects of myelin basic protein-reactive T cell lines on syngeneic oligodendrocytes. *Journal of Neuroimmunology*, **26**, 57–67.

Keith, A.B., Arnon, R., Teitelbaum, D., Caspary, E.A. & Wisniewski, H.M. (1979). The effect of Cop 1, a synthetic polypeptide, on chronic relapsing experimental allergic encephalomyelitis in guinea pigs. *Journal of the Neurological Sciences*, **42**, 267–74.

Kennedy, M.K., Clatch, R.J., Dal Canto, M.C., Trotter, J.L. & Miller, S.D. (1987). Monoclonal antibody-induced inhibition of relapsing EAE in SJL/J mice correlates with inhibition of neuroantigen-specific cell-mediated immune responses. *Journal of Neuroimmunology*, **16**, 345–64.

Kennedy, M.K., Dal Canto, M.C., Trotter, J.L. & Miller, S.D. (1988). Specific immune regulation of chronic-relapsing experimental allergic encephalomyelitis in mice. *Journal of Immunology*, **141**, 2986–93.

Kennedy, M.K., Tan, L.J., Dal Canto, M.C., Tuohy, V.K., Lu, Z.J., Trotter, J.L. & Miller, S.D. (1990). Inhibition of murine relapsing experimental autoimmune encephalomyelitis by immune tolerance to proteolipid protein and its encephalitogenic peptides. *Journal of Immunology*, **144**, 909–15.

Kennedy, M.K., Torrance, D.S., Picha, K.S. & Mohler, K.M. (1992). Analysis of cytokine mRNA expression in the central nervous system of mice with experimental autoimmune encephalomyelitis reveals that IL-10 mRNA expression correlates with recovery. *Journal of Immunology*, **149**, 2496–505.

Khoury, S.J., Hancock, W.W. & Weiner, H.L. (1992). Oral tolerance to myelin basic protein and natural recovery from experimental autoimmune encephalomyelitis are associated with downregulation of inflammatory cytokines and differential upregulation of transforming growth factor beta, interleukin 4, and prostaglandin E expression in the brain. *Journal of Experimental Medicine*, **176**, 1355–64.

Khoury, S.J., Sayegh, M.H., Hancock, W.W., Gallon, L., Carpenter, C.B. & Weiner, H.L. (1993). Acquired tolerance to experimental autoimmune encephalomyelitis by intrathymic injection of myelin basic protein or its major encephalitogenic peptide. *Journal of Experimental Medicine*, **178**, 559–66.

Kibler, R.F. (1965). Large dose corticosteroid therapy of experimental and human demyelinating diseases. *Annals of the New York Academy of Sciences*, **122**, 469–79.

Kitz, K., Lassmann, H., Karcher, D. & Lowenthal, A. (1984). Blood–brain barrier in chronic relapsing experimental allergic encephalomyelitis: a correlative study between cerebrospinal fluid protein concentrations and tracer leakage in the central nervous system. *Acta Neuropathologica*, **63**, 41–50.

Klein Franke, A. & Munder, P.G. (1992). Alkyllysophospholipid prevents induction of experimental allergic encephalomyelitis. *Journal of Autoimmunity*, **5**, 83–91.

Koh, D.R., Fung Leung, W.P., Ho, A., Gray, D., Acha Orbea, H. & Mak, T.W. (1992). Less mortality but more relapses in experimental allergic encephalomyelitis in $CD8^{-/-}$ mice. *Science*, **256**, 1210–13.

Konno, H., Yamamoto, T., Iwasaki, Y., Saitoh, T., Suzuki, H. & Terunuma, H. (1989). Ia-expressing microglial cells in experimental allergic encephalomyelitis in rats. *Acta Neuropathologica (Berlin)*, **77**, 472–9.

Koritschoner, R. & Schweinburg, F. (1925). Klinische und experimentelle Beobachtungen über Lähmungen nach Wutschutzimpfung. *Zeitschrift für Immunitätsforschung und experimentelle Therapie*, **42**, 217–83.

Kuchroo, V.K., Martin, C.A., Greer, J.M., Ju, S.T., Sobel, R.A. & Dorf, M.E. (1993). Cytokines and adhesion molecules contribute to the ability of myelin proteolipid protein-specific T cell clones to mediate experimental allergic encephalomyelitis. *Journal of Immunology*, **151**, 4371–82.

Kuchroo, V.K., Sobel, R.A., Laning, J.C., Martin, C.A., Greenfield, E., Dorf, M.E. & Lees, M.B. (1992). Experimental allergic encephalomyelitis mediated by cloned T cells specific for a synthetic peptide of myelin proteolipid protein. Fine specificity and T cell receptor V beta usage. *Journal of Immunology*, **148**, 3776–82.

Kumar, V. & Sercarz, E.E. (1993). The involvement of T cell receptor peptide-specific regulatory CD4+ T cells in recovery from antigen-induced autoimmune disease. *Journal of Experimental Medicine*, **178**, 909–16.

Kuruvilla, A.P., Shah, R., Hochwald, G.M., Liggitt, H.D., Palladino, M.A. & Thorbecke, G.J. (1991). Protective effect of transforming growth factor β_1 on experimental autoimmune diseases in mice. *Proceedings of the National Academy of Sciences USA*, **88**, 2918–21.

Laatsch, R.H., Kies, M.W., Gordon, S. & Alvord, E.C. (1962). The encephalomyelitic activity of myelin isolated by ultracentrifugation. *Journal of Experimental Medicine*, **115**, 777–88.

Lamont, A.G., Sette, A., Fujinami, R., Colon, S.M., Miles, C. & Grey, H.M. (1990). Inhibition of experimental autoimmune encephalomyelitis induction in SJL/J mice by using a peptide with high affinity for IA^s molecules. *Journal of Immunology*, **145**, 1687–93.

Lampert, P. (1967). Electron microscopic studies on ordinary and hyperacute experimental allergic encephalomyelitis. *Acta Neuropathologica*, **9**, 99–126.

Lampert, P.W. & Kies, M.W. (1967). Mechanism of demyelination in allergic encephalomyelitis of guinea pigs: an electron microscopic study. *Experimental Neurology*, **18**, 210–23.

Lando, Z., Teitelbaum, D. & Arnon, R. (1979). Effect of cyclophosphamide on suppressor cell activity in mice unresponsive to EAE. *Journal of Immunology*, **123**, 2156–60.

Lassmann, H., Brunner, C., Bradl, M. & Linington, C. (1988). Experimental allergic encephalomyelitis: the balance between encephalitogenic T lymphocytes and demyelinating antibodies determines size and structure of demyelinated lesions. *Acta Neuropathologica (Berlin)*, **75**, 566–76.

Lassmann, H., Kitz, K. & Wisniewski, H.M. (1980). Chronic relapsing experimental allergic encephalomyelitis in rats and guinea pigs – a comparison. In *Search for the Cause of Multiple Sclerosis and other Chronic Diseases of the Central Nervous System*, ed. A. Boese, pp. 96–104. Weinheim: Verlag Chemie.

Lassmann, H., Kitz, K. & Wisniewski, H.M. (1981). *In vivo* effect of sera from animals with chronic relapsing experimental allergic encephalomyelitis on central and peripheral myelin. *Acta Neuropathologica*, **55**, 297–306.

Lassmann, H., Stemberger, H., Kitz, K. & Wisniewski, H.M. (1983). *In vivo* demyelinating activity of sera from animals with chronic experimental allergic encephalomyelitis. Antibody nature of the demyelinating factor and the role of complement. *Journal of the Neurological Sciences*, **59**, 123–37.

Lassmann, H., Vass, K., Brunner, C. & Wisniewski, H.M. (1986). Peripheral nervous system lesions in experimental allergic encephalomyelitis. Ultrastructural distribution of T cells and Ia-antigen. *Acta Neuropathologica (Berlin)*, **69**, 193–204.

Lassmann, H. & Wisniewski, H.M. (1978). Chronic relapsing EAE. Time course of neurological symptoms and pathology. *Acta Neuropathologica*, **43**, 35–42.

Lassmann, H. & Wisniewski, H.M. (1979*a*). Chronic relapsing experimental allergic encephalomyelitis: effect of age at the time of sensitization on clinical course and pathology. *Acta Neuropathologica*, **47**, 111–16.

Lassmann, H. & Wisniewski, H.M. (1979*b*). Chronic relapsing experimental allergic encephalomyelitis: clinicopathological comparison with multiple sclerosis. *Archives of Neurology*, **36**, 490–7.

Lebar, R., Baudrimont, M. & Vincent, C. (1989). Chronic experimental autoimmune encephalomyelitis in the guinea pig. Presence of anti-M2 antibodies in central nervous system tissue and the possible role of M2 autoantigen in the induction of the disease. *Journal of Autoimmunity*, **2**, 115–32.

Lebar, R., Boutry, J.M., Vincent, C., Robineaux, R. & Voisin, G.A. (1976). Studies on autoimmune encephalomyelitis in the guinea pig. II. An *in vitro* investigation on the nature, properties, and specificity of the serum-demyelinating factor. *Journal of Immunology*, **116**, 1439–46.

Lebar, R., Lubetzki, C., Vincent, C., Lombrail, P. & Boutry, J.M. (1986). The M2 autoantigen of central nervous system myelin, a glycoprotein present in oligodendrocyte membrane. *Clinical and Experimental Immunology*, **66**, 423–34.

Lehmann, P.V., Forsthuber, T., Miller, A. & Sercarz, E.E. (1992). Spreading of T-cell autoimmunity to cryptic determinants of an autoantigen. *Nature*, **358**, 155–7.

Levine, S. & Sowinski, R. (1980). Experimental allergic encephalomyelitis. Inhibition of clinical signs and paradoxical enhancement of lesions in second attacks. *American Journal of Pathology*, **101**, 375–85.

Levine, S., Sowinski, R. & Steinetz, B. (1980). Effects of experimental allergic encephalomyelitis on thymus and adrenal: relation to remission and relapse. *Proceedings of the Society for Experimental Biology and Medicine*, **165**, 218–24.

Levine, S. & Wenk, E.J. (1965). A hyperacute form of allergic encephalomyelitis. *American Journal of Pathology*, **47**, 61–88.

Lider, O., Reshef, T., Beraud, E., Ben Nun, A. & Cohen, I.R. (1988). Anti-idiotypic network induced by T cell vaccination against experimental autoimmune encephalomyelitis. *Science*, **239**, 181–3.

Lider, O., Santos, L.M., Lee, C.S., Higgins, P.J. & Weiner, H.L. (1989). Suppression of experimental autoimmune encephalomyelitis by oral administration of myelin basic protein. II. Suppression of disease and *in vitro* immune responses is mediated by antigen-specific CD8$^+$ T lymphocytes. *Journal of Immunology*, **142**, 748–52.

Lin, R.F., Lin, T.S., Tilton, R.G. & Cross, A.H. (1993). Nitric oxide localized to spinal cords of mice with experimental allergic encephalomyelitis: an electron paramagnetic resonance study. *Journal of Experimental Medicine*, **178**, 643–8.

Linington, C., Berger, T., Perry, L., Weerth, S., Hinze Selch, D., Zhang, Y., Lu, H.C., Lassmann, H. & Wekerle, H. (1993). T cells specific for the myelin oligodendrocyte glycoprotein mediate an unusual autoimmune inflammatory response in the central nervous system. *European Journal of Immunology*, **23**, 1364–72.

Linington, C., Bradl, M., Lassmann, H., Brunner, C. & Vass, K. (1988). Augmentation of demyelination in rat acute allergic encephalomyelitis by circulating mouse monoclonal antibodies directed against a myelin/oligodendrocyte glycoprotein. *American Journal of Pathology*, **130**, 443–54.

Linington, C., Gunn, C.A. & Lassmann, H. (1990). Identification of an encephalitogenic determinant of myelin proteolipid protein for the rabbit. *Journal of Neuroimmunology*, **30**, 135–44.

Linington, C. & Lassmann, H. (1987). Antibody responses in chronic relapsing experimental allergic encephalomyelitis: correlation of serum demyelinating activity with antibody titre to the myelin/oligodendrocyte glycoprotein (MOG). *Journal of Neuroimmunology*, **17**, 61–9.

Liu, Y. & Janeway, C.A. (1990). Interferon γ plays a critical role in induced cell death of effector T cell: a possible third mechanism of self-tolerance. *Journal of Experimental Medicine*, **172**, 1735–9.

Lohse, A.W., Mor, F., Karin, N. & Cohen, I.R. (1989). Control of experimental autoimmune encephalomyelitis by T cells responding to activated T cells. *Science*, **244**, 820–2.

Lossinsky, A.S., Badmajew, V., Robson, J.A., Moretz, R.C. & Wisniewski, H.M. (1989). Sites of egress of inflammatory cells and horseradish peroxidase transport across the blood–brain barrier in a murine model of chronic relapsing experimental allergic encephalomyelitis. *Acta Neuropathologica (Berlin)*, **78**, 359–71.

Ludowyk, P.A., Willenborg, D.O. & Parish, C.R. (1992). Selective localisation of neuro-specific T lymphocytes in the central nervous system. *Journal of Neuroimmunology*, **37**, 237–50.

Lyman, W.D., Abrams, G.A. & Raine, C.S. (1989*a*). Experimental autoimmune encephalomyelitis: isolation and characterization of inflammatory cells from the central nervous system. *Journal of Neuroimmunology*, **25**, 195–201.

Lyman, W.D., Sonett, J.R., Brosnan, C.F., Elkin, R. & Bornstein, M.B. (1989*b*). Δ^9-Tetrahydrocannabinol: a novel treatment for experimental autoimmune encephalomyelitis. *Journal of Neuroimmunology*, **23**, 73–81.

MacMicking, J.D., Willenborg, D.O., Weidemann, M.J., Rockett, K.A. & Cowden, W.B. (1992). Elevated secretion of reactive nitrogen and oxygen intermediates by inflammatory leukocytes in hyperacute experimental autoimmune encephalomyelitis: enhancement by the soluble products of encephalitogenic T cells. *Journal of Experimental Medicine*, **176**, 303–7.

MacPhee, I.A., Antoni, F.A. & Mason, D.W. (1989). Spontaneous recovery of rats from experimental allergic encephalomyelitis is dependent on regulation of the immune system by endogenous adrenal corticosteroids. *Journal of Experimental Medicine*, **169**, 431–45.

Madrid, R.E. & Wisniewski, H.M. (1978). Peripheral nervous system pathology in relapsing experimental allergic encephalomyelitis. *Journal of Neurocytology*, **7**, 265–81.

Mannie, M.D., Morrison Plummer, J. & McConnell, T.J. (1993). Differentiation of encephalitogenic T cells confers resistance to an inhibitory anti-CD4 monoclonal antibody. *Journal of Immunology*, **151**, 7293–306.

Massa, P.T., ter Meulen, V. & Fontana, A. (1987). Hyperinducibility of Ia antigen on astrocytes correlates with strain-specific susceptibility to experimental autoimmune encephalomyelitis. *Proceedings of the National Academy of Sciences USA*, **84**, 4219–23.

Massacesi, L., Joshi, N., Lee Parritz, D., Rombos, A., Letvin, N.L. & Hauser, S.L. (1992). Experimental allergic encephalomyelitis in cynomolgus monkeys. Quantitation of T cell responses in peripheral blood. *Journal of Clinical Investigation*, **90**, 399–404.

Matsumoto, Y. & Fujiwara, M. (1986). *In situ* detection of class I and II major histocompatibility complex antigens in the rat central nervous system during experimental allergic encephalomyelitis. An immunohistochemical study. *Journal of Neuroimmunology*, **12**, 265–77.

Matsumoto, Y. & Fujiwara, M. (1987). The immunopathology of adoptively transferred experimental allergic encephalomyelitis (EAE) in Lewis rats. Part 1. Immunohistochemical examination of developing lesions of EAE. *Journal of the Neurological Sciences*, **77**, 35–47.

Matsumoto, Y. & Fujiwara, M. (1988). Adoptively transferred experimental allergic encephalomyelitis in chimeric rats: identification of transferred cells in the lesions of the central nervous system. *Immunology*, **65**, 23–9.

Matsumoto, Y. & Fujiwara, M. (1993). Immunomodulation of experimental autoimmune encephalomyelitis by staphylococcal enterotoxin D. *Cellular Immunology*, **149**, 268–78.

Matsumoto, Y., Hanawa, H., Tsuchida, M. & Abo, T. (1993). *In situ* inactivation of infiltrating T cells in the central nervous system with autoimmune encephalomyelitis. The role of astrocytes. *Immunology*, **79**, 381–90.

Matsumoto, Y., Hara, N., Tanaka, R. & Fujiwara, M. (1986). Immunohistochemical analysis of the rat central nervous system during experimental allergic encephalomyelitis, with special reference to Ia-positive cells with dendritic morphology. *Journal of Immunology*, **136**, 3668–76.

Matsumoto, Y., Kawai, K. & Fujiwara, M. (1988). Hemorrhagic autoimmune encephalomyelitis induced by adoptive transfer of activated semiallogeneic spleen cells into irradiated rats. *American Journal of Pathology*, **133**, 306–15.

Matsumoto, Y., Kawai, K. & Fujiwara, M. (1989). *In situ* Ia expression on brain cells in the rat: autoimmune encephalomyelitis-resistant strain (BN) and susceptible strain (Lewis) compared. *Immunology*, **66**, 621–7.

Matsumoto, Y., Ohmori, K. & Fujiwara, M. (1992). Immune regulation by brain cells in the central nervous system: microglia but not astrocytes present myelin basic protein to encephalitogenic T cells under *in vivo*-mimicking conditions. *Immunology*, **76**, 209–16.

Matsumoto, Y., Tsuchida, M., Hanawa, H. & Abo, T. (1994). Successful prevention and treatment of autoimmune encephalomyelitis by short-term administration of anti-T-cell receptor $\alpha\beta$ antibody. *Immunology*, **81**, 1–7.

McCarron, R. & McFarlin, D.E. (1988). Adoptively transferred experimental autoimmune encephalomyelitis in SJL/J, PL/J, and (SJL/J × PL/J)F_1 mice. Influence of I-A haplotype on encephalitogenic epitope of myelin basic protein. *Journal of Immunology*, **141**, 1143–9.

McCarron, R.M., Kempski, O., Spatz, M. & McFarlin, D.E. (1985). Presentation of myelin basic protein by murine cerebral vascular endothelial cells. *Journal of Immunology*, **134**, 3100–3.

McCarron, R.M., Racke, M., Spatz, M. & McFarlin, D.E. (1991). Cerebral vascular endothelial cells are effective targets for *in vitro* lysis by encephalitogenic T lymphocytes. *Journal of Immunology*, **147**, 503–8.

McCarron, R.M., Spatz, M., Kempski, O., Hogan, R.N., Muehl, L. & McFarlin, D.E. (1986). Interaction between myelin basic protein-sensitized T lymphocytes and murine cerebral vascular endothelial cells. *Journal of Immunology*, **137**, 3428–35.

McCombe, P.A., de Jersey, J. & Pender, M.P. (1994). Inflammatory cells, microglia and MHC class II antigen positive cells in the spinal cord of Lewis rats with acute and chronic relapsing experimental autoimmune encephalomyelitis. *Journal of Neuroimmunology*, **51**, 153–67.

McCombe, P.A., Fordyce, B.W., de Jersey, J., Yoong, G. & Pender, M.P. (1992). Expression of CD45RC and Ia antigen in the spinal cord in acute experimental allergic encephalomyelitis: an immunocytochemical and flow cytometric study. *Journal of the Neurological Sciences*, **113**, 177–86.

McDonald, A.H. & Swanborg, R.H. (1988). Antigen-specific inhibition of immune interferon production by suppressor cells of autoimmune encephalomyelitis. *Journal of Immunology*, **140**, 1132–8.

McKenna, R.M., Carter, B.G., Paterson, J.A. & Sehon, A.H. (1983). The suppression of experimental allergic encephalomyelitis in Lewis rats by treatment with myelin basic protein-cell conjugates. *Cellular Immunology*, **81**, 391–402.

Mehta, P.D., Lassmann, H. & Wisniewski, H.M. (1981). Immunologic studies of chronic relapsing EAE in guinea pigs: similarities to multiple sclerosis. *Journal of Immunology*, **127**, 334–8.

Mehta, P.D., Patrick, B.A., Mehta, S.P. & Wisniewski, H.M. (1985*a*). Chronic relapsing EAE in guinea pigs: IgG index and oligoclonal bands in cerebrospinal fluid and sera. *Immunological Investigations*, **14**, 347–54.

Mehta, P.D., Patrick, B.A., Mehta, S.P. & Wisniewski, H.M. (1987). Specificity of oligoclonal IgG bands against myelin proteins in chronic relapsing EAE in guinea pigs. *Journal of Immunology*, **138**, 746–51.

Mehta, P.D., Patrick, B.A. & Wisniewski, H.M. (1985*b*). Specificity of oligoclonal IgG bands in sera from chronic relapsing experimental allergic encephalomyelitis guinea pigs. *Journal of Immunology*, **134**, 2338–42.

Merrill, J.E., Kono, D.H., Clayton, J., Ando, D.G., Hinton, D.R. & Hofman, F.M. (1992). Inflammatory leukocytes and cytokines in the peptide-induced disease of experimental allergic encephalomyelitis in SJL and B10.PL mice. *Proceedings of the National Academy of Sciences USA*, **89**, 574–8.

Metzler, B. & Wraith, D.C. (1993). Inhibition of experimental autoimmune encephalomyelitis by inhalation but not oral administration of the encephalitogenic peptide: influence of MHC binding affinity. *International Immunology*, **5**, 1159–65.

Miller, A., al Sabbagh, A., Santos, L.M., Das, M.P. & Weiner, H.L. (1993). Epitopes of myelin basic protein that trigger TGF-β release after oral tolerization are distinct from encephalitogenic epitopes and mediate epitope-driven bystander suppression. *Journal of Immunology*, **151**, 7307–15.

Miller, A., Lider, O., Roberts, A.B., Sporn, M.B. & Weiner, H.L. (1992). Suppressor T cells generated by oral tolerization to myelin basic protein suppress both *in vitro* and *in vivo* immune responses by the release of transforming growth factor β after antigen-specific triggering. *Proceedings of the National Academy of Sciences USA*, **89**, 421–5.

Miller, A., Lider, O. & Weiner, H.L. (1991). Antigen-driven bystander suppression after oral administration of antigens. *Journal of Experimental Medicine*, **174**, 791–8.

Minagawa, H., Takenaka, A., Itoyama, Y. & Mori, R. (1987). Experimental allergic encephalomyelitis in the Lewis rat. A model of predictable relapse by cyclophosphamide. *Journal of the Neurological Sciences*, **78**, 225–35.

Mokhtarian, F., McFarlin, D.E. & Raine, C.S. (1984). Adoptive transfer of myelin basic protein-sensitized T cells produces chronic relapsing demyelinating disease in mice. *Nature*, **309**, 356–8.

Moore, G.R. & Raine, C.S. (1988). Immunogold localization and analysis of IgG during immune-mediated demyelination. *Laboratory Investigation*, **59**, 641–8.

Moore, G.R., Traugott, U. & Raine, C.S. (1984). Survival of oligodendrocytes in chronic relapsing experimental autoimmune encephalomyelitis. *Journal of the Neurological Sciences*, **65**, 137–45.

Mor, F. & Cohen, I.R. (1992). T cells in the lesion of experimental autoimmune encephalomyelitis. Enrichment for reactivities to myelin basic protein and to heat shock proteins. *Journal of Clinical Investigation*, **90**, 2447–55.

Morgan, I.M. (1947). Allergic encephalomyelitis in monkeys in response to injection of normal monkey nervous tissue. *Journal of Experimental Medicine*, **85**, 131–40.

Morrison, L.R. (1947). Disseminated encephalomyelitis experimentally produced by the use of homologous antigen. *Archives of Neurology and Psychiatry*, **58**, 391–416.

Mostarica Stojkovic, M., Petrovic, M. & Lukic, M.L. (1982). Resistance to the induction of EAE in AO rats: its prevention by the pre-treatment with cyclophosphamide or low dose of irradiation. *Clinical and Experimental Immunology*, **50**, 311–17.

Mostarica Stojkovic, M., Vukmanovic, S., Ramic, Z. & Lukic, M.L. (1992). Evidence for target tissue regulation of resistance to the induction of experimental allergic encephalomyelitis in AO rats. *Journal of Neuroimmunology*, **41**, 97–104.

Moyer, A.W., Jervis, G.A., Black, J., Koprowski, H. & Cox, H.R. (1950). Action of adrenocorticotropic hormone (ACTH) in experimental allergic encephalomyelitis of the guinea pig. *Proceedings of the Society for Experimental Biology and Medicine*, **75**, 387–90.

Murphy, K.M., Heimberger, A.B. & Loh, D.Y. (1990). Induction by antigen of intrathymic apoptosis of $CD4^+CD8^+$ TCR^{lo} thymocytes *in vivo*. *Science*, **250**, 1720–3.

Müller, E. (1908). Über akute Paraplegien nach Wutschutzimpfungen. *Deutsche Zeitschrift für Nervenheilkunde*, **34**, 252–78.

Myers, K.J., Dougherty, J.P. & Ron, Y. (1993). *In vivo* antigen presentation by both brain parenchymal cells and hematopoietically derived cells during the induction of experimental autoimmune encephalomyelitis. *Journal of Immunology*, **151**, 2252–60.

Myers, K.J., Sprent, J., Dougherty, J.P. & Ron, Y. (1992). Synergy between encephalitogenic T cells and myelin basic protein-specific antibodies in the induction of experimental autoimmune encephalomyelitis. *Journal of Neuroimmunology*, **41**, 1–8.

Nataf, S., Louboutin, J.P., Chabannes, D., Feve, J.R. & Muller, J.Y. (1993). Pentoxifylline inhibits experimental allergic encephalomyelitis. *Acta Neurologica Scandinavica*, **88**, 97–9.

Newell, M.K., Haughn, L.J., Maroun, C.R. & Julius, M.H. (1990). Death of mature T cells by separate ligation of CD4 and the T-cell receptor for antigen. *Nature*, **347**, 286–9.

Nguyen, K.B., McCombe, P.A. & Pender, M.P. (1994). Macrophage apoptosis in the central nervous system in experimental autoimmune encephalomyelitis. *Journal of Autoimmunity*, **7**, 145–52.

O'Neill, J.K., Baker, D. & Turk, J.L. (1992). Inhibition of chronic relapsing experimental allergic encephalomyelitis in the Biozzi AB/H mouse. *Journal of Neuroimmunology*, **41**, 177–87.

O'Neill, J.K., Butter, C., Baker, D., Gschmeissner, S.E., Kraal, G., Butcher, E.C. & Turk, J.L. (1991). Expression of vascular addressins and ICAM-1 by endothelial cells in the spinal cord during chronic relapsing experimental allergic encephalomyelitis in the Biozzi AB/H mouse. *Immunology*, **72**, 520–5.

Offner, H., Buenafe, A.C., Vainiene, M., Celnik, B., Weinberg, A.D., Gold, D.P., Hashim, G. & Vandenbark, A.A. (1993). Where, when, and how to detect biased expression of disease-relevant $V\beta$ genes in rats with experimental autoimmune encephalomyelitis. *Journal of Immunology*, **151**, 506–17.

Offner, H., Hashim, G.A., Celnik, B., Galang, A., Li, X.B., Burns, F.R., Shen, N., Heber Katz, E. & Vandenbark, A.A. (1989). T cell determinants of myelin basic protein include a unique encephalitogenic I-E-restricted epitope for Lewis rats. *Journal of Experimental Medicine*, **170**, 355–67.

Offner, H., Hashim, G.A. & Vandenbark, A.A. (1991). T cell receptor peptide therapy triggers autoregulation of experimental encephalomyelitis. *Science*, **251**, 430–2.

Ohkawa, T. (1989). Experimental allergic encephalomyelitis. I. Oligodendroglial cell population in monkey brain at the acute stage. *Acta Pathologica Japonica*, **39**, 224–8.

Ohmori, K., Hong, Y., Fujiwara, M. & Matsumoto, Y. (1992). *In situ* demonstration of proliferating cells in the rat central nervous system during experimental autoimmune encephalomyelitis. Evidence suggesting that most infiltrating T cells do not proliferate in the target organ. *Laboratory Investigation*, **66**, 54–62.

Owhashi, M. & Heber Katz, E. (1988). Protection from experimental allergic encephalomyelitis conferred by a monoclonal antibody directed against a shared idiotype on rat T cell receptors specific for myelin basic protein. *Journal of Experimental Medicine*, **168**, 2153–64.

Panitch, H.S. & McFarlin, D.E. (1977). Experimental allergic encephalomyelitis: enhancement of cell-mediated transfer by concanavalin A. *Journal of Immunology*, **119**, 1134–7.

Paterson, P.Y. (1960). Transfer of allergic encephalomyelitis in rats by means of lymph node cells. *Journal of Experimental Medicine*, **111**, 119–36.

Paterson, P.Y. & Drobish, D.G. (1969). Cyclophosphamide: effect on experimental allergic encephalomyelitis in Lewis rats. *Science*, **165**, 191–2.

Pender, M.P. (1986*a*). Ascending impairment of nociception in rats with experimental allergic encephalomyelitis. *Journal of the Neurological Sciences*, **75**, 317–28.

Pender, M.P. (1986*b*). Conduction block due to demyelination at the ventral root exit zone in experimental allergic encephalomyelitis. *Brain Research*, **367**, 398–401.

Pender, M.P. (1987). Demyelination and neurological signs in experimental allergic encephalomyelitis. *Journal of Neuroimmunology*, **15**, 11–24.

Pender, M.P. (1988*a*). The pathophysiology of myelin basic protein-induced acute experimental allergic encephalomyelitis in the Lewis rat. *Journal of the Neurological Sciences*, **86**, 277–89.

Pender, M.P. (1988*b*). The pathophysiology of acute experimental allergic encephalomyelitis induced by whole spinal cord in the Lewis rat. *Journal of the Neurological Sciences*, **84**, 209–22.

Pender, M.P. (1988*c*). Demyelination of the peripheral nervous system causes neurologic signs in myelin basic protein-induced experimental allergic encephalomyelitis: implications for the etiology of multiple sclerosis. *Annals of the New York Academy of Sciences*, **540**, 732–4.

Pender, M.P. (1989). Recovery from acute experimental allergic encephalomyelitis in the Lewis rat: early restoration of nerve conduction and repair by Schwann cells and oligodendrocytes. *Brain*, **112**, 393–416.

Pender, M.P. (1993). Apoptosis in the target organ of an autoimmune disease. In *Programmed Cell Death: The Cellular and Molecular Biology of Apoptosis*, ed. M. Lavin & D. Watters, pp. 235–44. Chur, Switzerland: Harwood Academic Publishers.

Pender, M.P., McCombe, P.A., Yoong, G. & Nguyen, K.B. (1992). Apoptosis of $\alpha\beta$ T lymphocytes in the nervous system in experimental autoimmune encephalomyelitis: its possible implications for recovery and acquired tolerance. *Journal of Autoimmunity*, **5**, 401–10.

Pender, M.P., Nguyen, K.B., McCombe, P.A. & Kerr, J.F.R. (1991). Apoptosis in the nervous system in experimental allergic encephalomyelitis. *Journal of the Neurological Sciences*, **104**, 81–7.

Pender, M.P., Nguyen, K.B. & Willenborg, D.O. (1989). Demyelination and early remyelination in experimental allergic encephalomyelitis passively transferred with myelin basic protein-sensitized lymphocytes in the Lewis rat. *Journal of Neuroimmunology*, **25**, 125–42.

Pender, M.P. & Sears, T.A. (1982). Conduction block in the peripheral nervous system in experimental allergic encephalomyelitis. *Nature*, **296**, 860–2.

Pender, M.P. & Sears, T.A. (1984). The pathophysiology of acute experimental allergic encephalomyelitis in the rabbit. *Brain*, **107**, 699–726.

Pender, M.P. & Sears, T.A. (1985). Vulnerability of the dorsal root ganglion in experimental allergic encephalomyelitis. *Clinical and Experimental Neurology*, **21**, 211–23.

Pender, M.P. & Sears, T.A. (1986). Involvement of the dorsal root ganglion in acute experimental allergic encephalomyelitis in the Lewis rat – a histological and electrophysiological study. *Journal of the Neurological Sciences*, **72**, 231–42.

Pender, M.P., Stanley, G.P., Yoong, G. & Nguyen, K.B. (1990). The neuropathology of chronic relapsing experimental allergic encephalomyelitis induced in the Lewis rat by inoculation with whole spinal cord and treatment with cyclosporin A. *Acta Neuropathologica (Berlin)*, **80**, 172–83.

Perry, L.L., Barzaga Gilbert, E. & Trotter, J.L. (1991). T cell sensitization to proteolipid protein in myelin basic protein-induced relapsing experimental allergic encephalomyelitis. *Journal of Neuroimmunology*, **33**, 7–15.

Pettinelli, C.B. & McFarlin, D.E. (1981). Adoptive transfer of experimental allergic encephalomyelitis in SJL/J mice after *in vitro* activation of lymph node cells by myelin basic protein: requirement for Lyt $1^+ 2^-$ T lymphocytes. *Journal of Immunology*, **127**, 1420–3.

Piddlesden, S., Lassmann, H., Laffafian, I., Morgan, B.P. & Linington, C. (1991). Antibody-mediated demyelination in experimental allergic encephalomyelitis is independent of complement membrane attack complex formation. *Clinical and Experimental Immunology*, **83**, 245–50.

Piddlesden, S.J., Lassmann, H., Zimprich, F., Morgan, B.P. & Linington, C. (1993). The demyelinating potential of antibodies to myelin oligodendrocyte glycoprotein is related to their ability to fix complement. *American Journal of Pathology*, **143**, 555–64.

Polman, C.H., Matthaei, I., De Groot, C.J., Koetsier, J.C., Sminia, T. & Dijkstra, C.D. (1988). Low-dose cyclosporin A induces relapsing remitting experimental allergic encephalomyelitis in the Lewis rat. *Journal of Neuroimmunology*, **17**, 209–16.

Pope, L., Paterson, P.Y. & Miller, S.D. (1992). Antigen-specific inhibition of the adoptive transfer of experimental autoimmune encephalomyelitis in Lewis rats. *Journal of Neuroimmunology*, **37**, 177–89.

Powell, M.B., Mitchell, D., Lederman, J., Buckmeier, J., Zamvil, S.S., Graham, M., Ruddle, N.H. & Steinman, L. (1990). Lymphotoxin and tumor necrosis factor-alpha production by myelin basic protein-specific T cell clones correlates with encephalitogenicity. *International Immunology*, **2**, 539–44.

Qin, Y.F., Sun, D.M., Goto, M., Meyermann, R. & Wekerle, H. (1989). Resistance to experimental autoimmune encephalomyelitis induced by neonatal tolerization to myelin basic protein: clonal elimination vs. regulation of autoaggressive lymphocytes. *European Journal of Immunology*, **19**, 373–80.

Racke, M.K., Cannella, B., Albert, P., Sporn, M., Raine, C.S. & McFarlin, D.E. (1992). Evidence of endogenous regulatory function of transforming growth factor-$\beta 1$ in experimental allergic encephalomyelitis. *International Immunology*, **4**, 615–20.

Racke, M.K., Dhib Jalbut, S., Cannella, B., Albert, P.S., Raine, C.S. & McFarlin, D.E. (1991). Prevention and treatment of chronic relapsing experimental allergic encephalomyelitis by transforming growth factor-β_1. *Journal of Immunology*, **146**, 3012–17.

Racke, M.K., Sriram, S., Carlino, J., Cannella, B., Raine, C.S. & McFarlin, D.E. (1993). Long-term treatment of chronic relapsing experimental allergic encephalomyelitis by transforming growth factor-$\beta 2$. *Journal of Neuroimmunology*, **46**, 175–83.

Raine, C.S., Cannella, B., Duijvestijn, A.M. & Cross, A.H. (1990). Homing to central nervous system vasculature by antigen-specific lymphocytes. II. Lymphocyte/endothelial cell adhesion during the initial stages of autoimmune demyelination. *Laboratory Investigation*, **63**, 476–89.

Raine, C.S., Mokhtarian, F. & McFarlin, D.E. (1984). Adoptively transferred chronic relapsing experimental autoimmune encephalomyelitis in the mouse. Neuropathologic analysis. *Laboratory Investigation*, **51**, 534–46.

Raine, C.S., Traugott, U. & Stone, S.H. (1978). Suppression of chronic allergic encephalomyelitis: relevance to multiple sclerosis. *Science*, **201**, 445–8.

Rajan, A.J., Cross, A.H., Raine, C.S. & Diamond, B. (1993). Multiple encephalitogenic peptides of myelin basic protein in A.CA mice. *Cellular Immunology*, **147**, 378–87.

Ravkina, L., Harib, I., Manovitch, Z., Deconenko, E., Letchinskaja, E. & Papilova, E. (1979). Hyperacute experimental allergic encephalomyelitis in rhesus monkeys as a model of acute necrotizing hemorrhagic encephalomyelitis. *Journal of Neurology*, **221**, 113–25.

Ravkina, L., Rogova, V. & Lazarenko, L. (1978). Chronic experimental allergic encephalomyelitis in rhesus monkeys and its modification by treatment. *Journal of the Neurological Sciences*, **38**, 281–93.

Renno, T., Lin, J.Y., Piccirillo, C., Antel, J. & Owens, T. (1994). Cytokine production by cells in cerebrospinal fluid during experimental allergic encephalomyelitis in SJL/J mice. *Journal of Neuroimmunology*, **49**, 1–7.

Richert, J.R., Driscoll, B.F., Kies, M.W. & Alvord, E.C. Jr (1979). Adoptive transfer of experimental allergic encephalomyelitis: incubation of rat spleen cells with specific antigen. *Journal of Immunology*, **122**, 494–6.

Rivers, T.M. & Schwentker, F.F. (1935). Encephalomyelitis accompanied by myelin destruction experimentally produced in monkeys. *Journal of Experimental Medicine*, **61**, 689–702.

Rivers, T.M., Sprunt, D.M. & Berry, G.P. (1933). Observations on attempts to produce acute disseminated encephalomyelitis in monkeys. *Journal of Experimental Medicine*, **58**, 39–53.

Rott, O., Cash, E. & Fleischer, B. (1993). Phosphodiesterase inhibitor pentoxifylline, a selective suppressor of T helper type 1- but not type 2-associated lymphokine production, prevents induction of experimental autoimmune encephalomyelitis in Lewis rats. *European Journal of Immunology*, **23**, 1745–51.

Rott, O., Fleischer, B. & Cash, E. (1994). Interleukin-10 prevents experimental allergic encephalomyelitis in rats. *European Journal of Immunology*, **24**, 1434–40.

Rott, O., Wekerle, H. & Fleischer, B. (1992). Protection from experimental allergic encephalomyelitis by application of a bacterial superantigen. *International Immunology*, **4**, 347–53.

Ruddle, N.H., Bergman, C.M., McGrath, K.M., Lingenheld, E.G., Grunnet, M.L., Padula, S.J. & Clark, R.B. (1990). An antibody to lymphotoxin and tumor necrosis factor prevents transfer of experimental allergic encephalomyelitis. *Journal of Experimental Medicine*, **172**, 1193–200.

Sadler, R.H., Sommer, M.A., Forno, L.S. & Smith, M.E. (1991). Induction of anti-myelin antibodies in EAE and their possible role in demyelination. *Journal of Neuroscience Research*, **30**, 616–24.

Saida, T., Saida, K., Brown, M.J. & Silberberg, D.H. (1979). Peripheral nerve demyelination induced by intraneural injection of experimental allergic encephalomyelitis serum. *Journal of Neuropathology and Experimental Neurology*, **38**, 498–518.

Sakai, K., Zamvil, S.S., Mitchell, D.J., Hodgkinson, S., Rothbard, J.B. & Steinman, L. (1989). Prevention of experimental encephalomyelitis with peptides that block interaction of T cells with major histocompatibility complex proteins. *Proceedings of the National Academy of Sciences USA*, **86**, 9470–4.

Sakai, K., Zamvil, S.S., Mitchell, D.J., Lim, M., Rothbard, J.B. & Steinman, L. (1988). Characterization of a major encephalitogenic T cell epitope in SJL/J mice with synthetic oligopeptides of myelin basic protein. *Journal of Neuroimmunology*, **19**, 21–32.

Santambrogio, L., Hochwald, G.M., Saxena, B., Leu, C.H., Martz, J.E., Carlino, J.A., Ruddle, N.H., Palladino, M.A., Gold, L.I. & Thorbecke, G.J. (1993). Studies on the mechanisms by which transforming growth factor-beta (TGF-beta) protects against allergic encephalomyelitis. Antagonism between TGF-beta and tumor necrosis factor. *Journal of Immunology*, **151**, 1116–27.

Satoh, J., Sakai, K., Endoh, M., Koike, F., Kunishita, T., Namikawa, T., Yamamura, T. & Tabira, T. (1987). Experimental allergic encephalomyelitis mediated by murine encephalitogenic T cell lines specific for myelin proteolipid apoprotein. *Journal of Immunology*, **138**, 179–84.

Schiffenbauer, J., Johnson, H.M., Butfiloski, E.J., Wegrzyn, L. & Soos, J.M. (1993). Staphylococcal enterotoxins can reactivate experimental allergic encephalomyelitis. *Proceedings of the National Academy of Sciences USA*, **90**, 8543–6.

Schluesener, H.J. & Lassmann, H. (1986). Recombinant interleukin 2 (IL-2) promotes T cell line-mediated neuroautoimmune disease. *Journal of Neuroimmunology*, **11**, 87–91.

Schluesener, H.J. & Lider, O. (1989). Transforming growth factors beta 1 and beta 2: cytokines with identical immunosuppressive effects and a potential role in the regulation of autoimmune T cell function. *Journal of Neuroimmunology*, **24**, 249–58.

Schluesener, H.J., Sobel, R.A., Linington, C. & Weiner, H.L. (1987). A monoclonal antibody against a myelin oligodendrocyte glycoprotein induces relapses and demyelination in central nervous system autoimmune disease. *Journal of Immunology*, **139**, 4016–21.

Schluesener, H.J. & Wekerle, H. (1985). Autoaggressive T lymphocyte lines recognizing the encephalitogenic region of myelin basic protein: *in vitro* selection from unprimed rat T lymphocyte populations. *Journal of Immunology*, **135**, 3128–33.

Schmied, M., Breitschopf, H., Gold, R., Zischler, H., Rothe, G., Wekerle, H. & Lassmann, H. (1993). Apoptosis of T lymphocytes in experimental autoimmune encephalomyelitis. Evidence for programmed cell death as a mechanism to control inflammation in the brain. *American Journal of Pathology*, **143**, 446–52.

Sedgwick, J., Brostoff, S. & Mason, D. (1987). Experimental allergic encephalomyelitis in the absence of a classical delayed-type hypersensitivity reaction. Severe paralytic disease correlates with the presence of interleukin 2 receptor-positive cells infiltrating the central nervous system. *Journal of Experimental Medicine*, **165**, 1058–75.

Sedgwick, J.D. (1988). Long-term depletion of CD8+ T cells *in vivo* in the rat: no observed role for CD8+ (cytotoxic/suppressor) cells in the immunoregulation of experimental allergic encephalomyelitis. *European Journal of Immunology*, **18**, 495–502.

Sedgwick, J.D., Hughes, C.C., Male, D.K., MacPhee, I.A. & ter Meulen, V. (1990). Antigen-specific damage to brain vascular endothelial cells mediated by encephalitogenic and nonencephalitogenic CD4+ T cell lines *in vitro*. *Journal of Immunology*, **145**, 2474–81.

Sedgwick, J.D., Schwender, S., Gregersen, R., Dorries, R. & ter Meulen, V. (1993). Resident macrophages (ramified microglia) of the adult Brown Norway rat central nervous system are constitutively major histocompatibility complex class II positive. *Journal of Experimental Medicine*, **177**, 1145–52.

Seeldrayers, P.A., Syha, J., Morrissey, S.P., Stodal, H., Vass, K., Jung, S., Gneiting, T., Lassmann, H., Haase, A., Hartung, H.P. *et al.* (1993). Magnetic resonance imaging investigation of blood–brain barrier damage in adoptive transfer experimental autoimmune encephalomyelitis. *Journal of Neuroimmunology*, **46**, 199–206.

Selmaj, K., Raine, C.S. & Cross, A.H. (1991). Anti-tumor necrosis factor therapy abrogates autoimmune demyelination. *Annals of Neurology*, **30**, 694–700.

Selmaj, K.W. & Raine, C.S. (1988). Tumor necrosis factor mediates myelin and oligodendrocyte damage *in vitro*. *Annals of Neurology*, **23**, 339–46.

Sharma, S.D., Nag, B., Su, X.M., Green, D., Spack, E., Clark, B.R. & Sriram, S. (1991). Antigen-specific therapy of experimental allergic encephalomyelitis by soluble class II major histocompatibility complex–peptide complexes. *Proceedings of the National Academy of Sciences USA*, **88**, 11465–9.

Shi, Y., Sahai, B.M. & Green, D.R. (1989). Cyclosporin A inhibits activation-induced cell death in T-cell hybridomas and thymocytes. *Nature*, **339**, 625–6.

Simmons, R.D., Bernard, C.C., Ng, K.T. & Carnegie, P.R. (1981). Hind-limb motor ability in Lewis rats during the onset and recovery phases of experimental autoimmune encephalomyelitis. *Brain Research*, **215**, 103–14.

Simmons, R.D., Bernard, C.C., Singer, G. & Carnegie, P.R. (1982). Experimental autoimmune encephalomyelitis. An anatomically-based explanation of clinical progression in rodents. *Journal of Neuroimmunology*, **3**, 307–18.

Simmons, R.D., Buzbee, T.M., Linthicum, D.S., Mandy, W.J., Chen, G. & Wang, C. (1987). Simultaneous visualization of vascular permeability change and leukocyte egress in the central nervous system during autoimmune encephalomyelitis. *Acta Neuropathologica (Berlin)*, **74**, 191–3.

Skundric, D.S., Kim, C., Tse, H.Y. & Raine, C.S. (1993). Homing of T cells to the central nervous system throughout the course of relapsing experimental autoimmune encephalomyelitis in Thy-1 congenic mice. *Journal of Neuroimmunology*, **46**, 113–21.

Smilek, D.E., Wraith, D.C., Hodgkinson, S., Dwivedy, S., Steinman, L. & McDevitt, H.O. (1991). A single amino acid change in a myelin basic protein peptide confers the capacity to prevent rather than induce experimental autoimmune encephalomyelitis. *Proceedings of the National Academy of Sciences USA*, **88**, 9633–7.

Smith, C.A., Williams, G.T., Kingston, R., Jenkinson, E.J. & Owen, J.J.T. (1989). Antibodies to CD3/T-cell receptor complex induce death by apoptosis in immature T cells in thymic cultures. *Nature*, **337**, 181–4.

Smith, M.E. (1993). Phagocytosis of myelin by microglia *in vitro*. *Journal of Neuroscience Research*, **35**, 480–7.

Sobel, R.A., Blanchette, B.W., Bhan, A.K. & Colvin, R.B. (1984*a*). The immunopathology of experimental allergic encephalomyelitis. II. Endothelial cell Ia increases prior to inflammatory cell infiltration. *Journal of Immunology*, **132**, 2402–7.

Sobel, R.A., Blanchette, B.W., Bhan, A.K. & Colvin, R.B. (1984*b*). The immunopathology of experimental allergic encephalomyelitis. I. Quantitative analysis of inflammatory cells *in situ*. *Journal of Immunology*, **132**, 2393–401.

Sobel, R.A. & Kuchroo, V.K. (1992). The immunopathology of acute experimental allergic encephalomyelitis induced with myelin proteolipid protein. T cell receptors in inflammatory lesions. *Journal of Immunology*, **149**, 1444–51.

Sobel, R.A., Natale, J.M. & Schneeberger, E.E. (1987). The immunopathology of acute experimental allergic encephalomyelitis. IV. An ultrastructural immunocytochemical study of class II major histocompatibility complex molecule (Ia) expression. *Journal of Neuropathology and Experimental Neurology*, **46**, 239–49.

Sommer, M.A., Forno, L.S. & Smith, M.E. (1992). EAE cerebrospinal fluid augments *in vitro* phagocytosis and metabolism of CNS myelin by macrophages. *Journal of Neuroscience Research*, **32**, 384–94.

Sriram, S. & Carroll, L. (1988). *In vivo* depletion of Lyt-2 cells fails to alter acute and relapsing EAE. *Journal of Neuroimmunology*, **17**, 147–57.

Sriram, S. & Roberts, C.A. (1986). Treatment of established chronic relapsing experimental allergic encephalomyelitis with anti-L3T4 antibodies. *Journal of Immunology*, **136**, 4464–9.

Sriram, S., Schwartz, G. & Steinman, L. (1983). Administration of myelin basic protein-coupled spleen cells prevents experimental allergic encephalitis. *Cellular Immunology*, **75**, 378–82.

Sriram, S., Solomon, D., Rouse, R.V. & Steinman, L. (1982). Identification of T cell subsets and B lymphocytes in mouse brain experimental allergic encephalitis lesions. *Journal of Immunology*, **129**, 1649–51.

Sriram, S. & Steinman, L. (1983). Anti I-A antibody suppresses active encephalomyelitis: treatment model for diseases linked to IR genes. *Journal of Experimental Medicine*, **158**, 1362–7.

Stanley, G.P. & Pender, M.P. (1991). The pathophysiology of chronic relapsing experimental allergic encephalomyelitis in the Lewis rat. *Brain*, **114**, 1827–53.

Sternberger, N.H., McFarlin, D.E., Traugott, U. & Raine, C.S. (1984). Myelin basic protein and myelin-associated glycoprotein in chronic, relapsing experimental allergic encephalomyelitis. *Journal of Neuroimmunology*, **6**, 217–29.

Stoll, G., Muller, S., Schmidt, B., van der Meide, P., Jung, S., Toyka, K.V. & Hartung, H.P. (1993). Localization of interferon-gamma and Ia-antigen in T cell line-mediated experimental autoimmune encephalomyelitis. *American Journal of Pathology*, **142**, 1866–75.

Su, X.M. & Sriram, S. (1992). Analysis of TCR V beta gene usage and encephalitogenicity of myelin basic protein peptide p91–103 reactive T cell clones in SJL mice: lack of evidence for V gene hypothesis. *Cellular Immunology*, **141**, 485–95.

Suckling, A.J., Reiber, H., Kirby, J.A. & Rumsby, M.G. (1983). Chronic relapsing experimental allergic encephalomyelitis. Immunological and blood–cerebrospinal fluid barrier-dependent changes in the cerebrospinal fluid. *Journal of Neuroimmunology*, **4**, 35–45.

Sudweeks, J.D., Todd, J.A., Blankenhorn, E.P., Wardell, B.B., Woodward, S.R., Meeker, N.D., Estes, S.S. & Teuscher, C. (1993). Locus controlling *Bordetella pertussis*-induced histamine sensitization (*Bphs*), an autoimmune disease-susceptibility gene, maps distal to T-cell receptor beta-chain gene on mouse chromosome 6. *Proceedings of the National Academy of Sciences USA*, **90**, 3700–4.

Sun, D. (1992). Synthetic peptides representing sequence 39 to 59 of rat V beta 8 TCR fail to elicit regulatory T cells reactive with V beta 8 TCR on rat encephalitogenic T cells. *Cellular Immunology*, **141**, 200–10.

Sun, D., Ben Nun, A. & Wekerle, H. (1988*a*). Regulatory circuits in autoimmunity: recruitment of counter-regulatory CD8+ T cells by encephalitogenic CD4+ T line cells. *European Journal of Immunology*, **18**, 1993–9.

Sun, D., Branum, K. & Sun, Q. (1992*a*). Prevention of experimental autoimmune encephalomyelitis in Lewis rats by treatment with an anti-rat CD5 antibody (OX19). *Cellular Immunology*, **145**, 263–71.

Sun, D., Gold, D.P., Smith, L., Brostoff, S. & Coleclough, C. (1992*b*). Characterization of rat encephalitogenic T cells bearing non-V beta 8 T cell receptors. *European Journal of Immunology*, **22**, 591–4.

Sun, D., Le, J. & Coleclough, C. (1993). Diverse T cell receptor beta chain usage by rat encephalitogenic T cells reactive to residues 68–88 of myelin basic protein. *European Journal of Immunology*, **23**, 494–8.

Sun, D., Qin, Y., Chluba, J., Epplen, J.T. & Wekerle, H. (1988*b*). Suppression of experimentally induced autoimmune encephalomyelitis by cytolytic T–T cell interactions. *Nature*, **332**, 843–5.

Sun, D. & Wekerle, H. (1986). Ia-restricted encephalitogenic T lymphocytes mediating EAE lyse autoantigen-presenting astrocytes. *Nature*, **320**, 70–2.

Sun, D., Wekerle, H., Raper, K. & Gold, D.P. (1991). $CD4^-CD8^-$ splenic T cells from Lewis rats recovered from experimental autoimmune encephalomyelitis respond to encephalitogenic T cells that mediate this disorder. *Cellular Immunology*, **137**, 292–302.

Swierkosz, J.E. & Swanborg, R.H. (1975). Suppressor cell control of unresponsiveness to experimental allergic encephalomyelitis. *Journal of Immunology*, **115**, 631–3.

Swierkosz, J.E. & Swanborg, R.H. (1977). Immunoregulation of experimental allergic encephalomyelitis: conditions for induction of suppressor cells and analysis of mechanism. *Journal of Immunology*, **119**, 1501–6.

Tabi, Z., McCombe, P.A. & Pender, M.P. (1994). Apoptotic elimination of Vβ8.2$^+$ cells from the central nervous system during recovery from experimental autoimmune encephalomyelitis induced by the passive transfer of Vβ8.2$^+$ encephalitogenic T cells. *European Journal of Immunology*, **24**, 2609–17.

Tan, L.J., Kennedy, M.K., Dal Canto, M.C. & Miller, S.D. (1991). Successful treatment of paralytic relapses in adoptive experimental autoimmune encephalomyelitis via neuroantigen-specific tolerance. *Journal of Immunology*, **147**, 1797–802.

Teitelbaum, D., Aharoni, R., Arnon, R. & Sela, M. (1988). Specific inhibition of the T-cell response to myelin basic protein by the synthetic copolymer Cop 1. *Proceedings of the National Academy of Sciences USA*, **85**, 9724–8.

Teitelbaum, D., Aharoni, R., Sela, M. & Arnon, R. (1991). Cross-reactions and specificities of monoclonal antibodies against myelin basic protein and against the synthetic copolymer 1. *Proceedings of the National Academy of Sciences USA*, **88**, 9528–32.

Teitelbaum, D., Meshorer, A., Hirshfeld, T., Arnon, R. & Sela, M. (1971). Suppression of experimental allergic encephalomyelitis by a synthetic polypeptide. *European Journal of Immunology*, **1**, 242–8.

Traugott, U., McFarlin, D.E. & Raine, C.S. (1986). Immunopathology of the lesion in chronic relapsing experimental autoimmune encephalomyelitis in the mouse. *Cellular Immunology*, **99**, 395–410.

Traugott, U., Raine, C.S. & McFarlin, D.E. (1985). Acute experimental allergic encephalomyelitis in the mouse: immunopathology of the developing lesion. *Cellular Immunology*, **91**, 240–54.

Traugott, U., Shevach, E., Chiba, J., Stone, H.J. & Raine, C.S. (1981). Autoimmune encephalomyelitis: simultaneous identification of T and B cells in the target organ. *Science*, **214**, 1251–3.

Tsuchida, M., Matsumoto, Y., Hirahara, H., Hanawa, H., Tomiyama, K. & Abo, T. (1993). Preferential distribution of V beta 8.2-positive T cells in the central nervous system of rats with myelin basic protein-induced autoimmune encephalomyelitis. *European Journal of Immunology*, **23**, 2399–406.

Tuohy, V.K., Lu, Z.J., Sobel, R.A., Laursen, R.A. & Lees, M.B. (1988). A synthetic peptide from myelin proteolipid protein induces experimental allergic encephalomyelitis. *Journal of Immunology*, **141**, 1126–30.

Tuohy, V.K., Lu, Z., Sobel, R.A., Laursen, R.A. & Lees, M.B. (1989). Identification of an encephalitogenic determinant of myelin proteolipid protein for SJL mice. *Journal of Immunology*, **142**, 1523–7.

Turnley, A.M., Miller, J.F.A.P. & Bartlett, P.F. (1991). Regulation of MHC molecules on MBP positive oligodendrocytes in mice by IFN-γ and TNF-α. *Neuroscience Letters*, **123**, 45–8.

Uitdehaag, B.M., De Groot, C.J., Kreike, A., van der Meide, P.H., Polman, C.H. & Dijkstra, C.D. (1993). The significance of *in-situ* Ia antigen expression in the pathogenesis of autoimmune central nervous system disease. *Journal of Autoimmunity*, **6**, 323–35.

Urban, J.L., Kumar, V., Kono, D.H., Gomez, C., Horvath, S.J., Clayton, J., Ando, D.G., Sercarz, E.E. & Hood, L. (1988). Restricted use of T cell receptor V genes in murine autoimmune encephalomyelitis raises possibilities for antibody therapy. *Cell*, **54**, 577–92.

van der Veen, R.C., Kapp, J.A. & Trotter, J.L. (1993). Fine-specificity differences in the recognition of an encephalitogenic peptide by T helper 1 and 2 cells. *Journal of Neuroimmunology*, **48**, 221–6.

van der Veen, R.C. & Stohlman, S.A. (1993). Encephalitogenic Th1 cells are inhibited by Th2 cells with related peptide specificity: relative roles of interleukin (IL)-4 and IL-10. *Journal of Neuroimmunology*, **48**, 213–20.

van der Veen, R.C., Trotter, J.L., Clark, H.B. & Kapp, J.A. (1989). The adoptive transfer of chronic relapsing experimental allergic encephalomyelitis with lymph node cells sensitized to myelin proteolipid protein. *Journal of Neuroimmunology*, **21**, 183–91.

van der Veen, R.C., Trotter, J.L., Hickey, W.F. & Kapp, J.A. (1990). The development and characterization of encephalitogenic cloned T cells specific for myelin proteolipid protein. *Journal of Neuroimmunology*, **26**, 139–45.

Vandenbark, A.A., Hashim, G. & Offner, H. (1989). Immunization with a synthetic T-cell receptor V-region peptide protects against experimental autoimmune encephalomyelitis. *Nature*, **341**, 541–4.

Vass, K., Lassmann, H., Wekerle, H. & Wisniewski, H.M. (1986). The distribution of Ia antigen in the lesions of rat acute experimental allergic encephalomyelitis. *Acta Neuropathologica (Berlin)*, **70**, 149–60.

Vogel, C., Paty, D.W. & Kibler, R.F. (1972). Treatment of experimental allergic encephalomyelitis in the rabbit. *Archives of Neurology*, **26**, 366–73.

Voorthuis, J.A., Uitdehaag, B.M., De Groot, C.J., Goede, P.H., van der Meide, P.H. & Dijkstra, C.D. (1990). Suppression of experimental allergic encephalomyelitis by intraventricular administration of interferon-gamma in Lewis rats. *Clinical and Experimental Immunology*, **81**, 183–8.

Waksman, B.H. (1959). Experimental allergic encephalomyelitis and the 'auto-allergic' diseases. *International Archives of Allergy and Applied Immunology*, **14** (Suppl.), 1–87.

Waksman, B.H. & Adams, R.D. (1955). Allergic neuritis: an experimental disease of rabbits induced by the injection of peripheral nervous tissue and adjuvants. *Journal of Experimental Medicine*, **102**, 213–36.

Waksman, B.H. & Adams, R.D. (1956). A comparative study of experimental allergic neuritis in the rabbit, guinea pig and mouse. *Journal of Neuropathology and Experimental Neurology*, **15**, 293–333.

Waldor, M.K., Mitchell, D., Kipps, T.J., Herzenberg, L.A. & Steinman, L. (1987). Importance of immunoglobulin isotype in therapy of experimental autoimmune encephalomyelitis with monoclonal anti-CD4 antibody. *Journal of Immunology*, **139**, 3660–4.

Waldor, M.K., Sriram, S., Hardy, R., Herzenberg, L.A., Lanier, L., Lim, M. & Steinman, L. (1985). Reversal of experimental allergic encephalomyelitis with monoclonal antibody to a T-cell subset marker. *Science*, **227**, 415–17.

Walls, A.F., Suckling, A.J. & Rumsby, M.G. (1989). The origin and specificity of intrathecal IgG in chronic relapsing experimental allergic encephalomyelitis. *Autoimmunity*, **2**, 123–32.

Wauben, M.H., Boog, C.J., van der Zee, R., Joosten, I., Schlief, A. & van Eden, W. (1992). Disease inhibition by major histocompatibility complex binding peptide analogues of disease-associated epitopes: more than blocking alone. *Journal of Experimental Medicine*, **176**, 667–77.

Webster, H.D., Shii, H. & Lassmann, H. (1985). Immunocytochemical study of myelin-associated glycoprotein (MAG), basic protein (BP), and glial fibrillary acidic protein (GFAP) in chronic relapsing experimental allergic encephalomyelitis (EAE). *Acta Neuropathologica*, **65**, 177–89.

Wekerle, H., Linington, C., Lassmann, H. & Meyermann, R. (1986). Cellular immune reactivity within the CNS. *Trends in Neurosciences*, **9**, 271–7.

Welch, A.M., Holda, J.H. & Swanborg, R.H. (1980). Regulation of experimental allergic encephalomyelitis. II. Appearance of suppressor cells during the remission phase of the disease. *Journal of Immunology*, **125**, 186–9.

Welch, A.M. & Swanborg, R.H. (1976). Characterization of suppressor cells involved in regulation of experimental allergic encephalomyelitis. *European Journal of Immunology*, **6**, 910–12.

Whitacre, C.C., Gienapp, I.E., Orosz, C.G. & Bitar, D.M. (1991). Oral tolerance in experimental autoimmune encephalomyelitis. III. Evidence for clonal anergy. *Journal of Immunology*, **147**, 2155–63.

White, S.R. & Bowker, R.M. (1988). Retrograde transport of horseradish peroxidase is specifically impaired in bulbospinal serotonin axons during experimental allergic encephalomyelitis. *Journal of Neuroimmunology*, **18**, 75–86.

Whitham, R.H., Jones, R.E., Hashim, G.A., Hoy, C.M., Wang, R.Y., Vandenbark, A.A. & Offner, H. (1991). Location of a new encephalitogenic epitope (residues 43 to 64) in proteolipid protein that induces relapsing experimental autoimmune encephalomyelitis in PL/J and (SJL × PL)F1 mice. *Journal of Immunology*, **147**, 3803–8.

Wilcox, C.E., Ward, A.M., Evans, A., Baker, D., Rothlein, R. & Turk, J.L. (1990). Endothelial cell expression of the intercellular adhesion molecule-1 (ICAM-1) in the central nervous system of guinea pigs during acute and chronic relapsing experimental allergic encephalomyelitis. *Journal of Neuroimmunology*, **30**, 43–51.

Willenborg, D.O. (1979). Experimental allergic encephalomyelitis in the Lewis rat: studies on the mechanism of recovery from disease and acquired resistance to reinduction. *Journal of Immunology*, **123**, 1145–50.

Willenborg, D.O. & Parish, C.R. (1988). Inhibition of allergic encephalomyelitis in rats by treatment with sulfated polysaccharides. *Journal of Immunology*, **140**, 3401–5.

Willenborg, D.O. & Prowse, S.J. (1983). Immunoglobulin-deficient rats fail to develop experimental allergic encephalomyelitis. *Journal of Neuroimmunology*, **5**, 99–109.

Willenborg, D.O., Simmons, R.D., Tamatani, T. & Miyasaka, M. (1993). ICAM-1-dependent pathway is not critically involved in the inflammatory process of autoimmune encephalomyelitis or in cytokine-induced inflammation of the central nervous system. *Journal of Neuroimmunology*, **45**, 147–54.

Willenborg, D.O., Sjollema, P. & Danta, G. (1986). Immunoglobulin deficient rats as donors and recipients of effector cells of allergic encephalomyelitis. *Journal of Neuroimmunology*, **11**, 93–103.

Williams, R.M., Lees, M.B., Cambi, F. & Macklin, W.B. (1982). Chronic experimental allergic encephalomyelitis induced in rabbits with bovine white matter proteolipid apoprotein. *Journal of Neuropathology and Experimental Neurology*, **41**, 508–21.

Wisniewski, H., Prineas, J. & Raine, C.S. (1969). An ultrastructural study of experimental demyelination and remyelination. I. Acute experimental allergic encephalomyelitis in the peripheral nervous system. *Laboratory Investigation*, **21**, 105–18.

Wisniewski, H.M. & Keith, A.B. (1977). Chronic relapsing experimental allergic encephalomyelitis: an experimental model of multiple sclerosis. *Annals of Neurology*, **1**, 144–8.

Wraith, D.C., Smilek, D.E., Mitchell, D.J., Steinman, L. & McDevitt, H.O. (1989). Antigen recognition in autoimmune encephalomyelitis and the potential for peptide-mediated immunotherapy. *Cell*, **59**, 247–55.

Yednock, T.A., Cannon, C., Fritz, L.C., Sanchez Madrid, F., Steinman, L & Karin, N. (1992). Prevention of experimental autoimmune encephalomyelitis by antibodies against alpha 4 beta 1 integrin. *Nature*, **356**, 63–6.

Zamvil, S., Nelson, P., Trotter, J., Mitchell, D., Knobler, R., Fritz, R. & Steinman, L. (1985). T-cell clones specific for myelin basic protein induce chronic relapsing paralysis and demyelination. *Nature*, **317**, 355–8.

Zamvil, S.S., Mitchell, D.J., Lee, N.E., Moore, A.C., Waldor, M.K., Sakai, K., Rothbard, J.B., McDevitt, H.O., Steinman, L. & Acha Orbea, H. (1988*a*). Predominant expression of a T cell receptor V beta gene subfamily in autoimmune encephalomyelitis [published erratum appears in *J Exp Med* 1988 Jul 1;**168**(1):455]. *Journal of Experimental Medicine*, **167**, 1586–96.

Zamvil, S.S., Mitchell, D.J., Moore, A.C., Schwarz, A.J., Stiefel, W., Nelson, P.A., Rothbard, J.B. & Steinman, L. (1987). T cell specificity for class II (I-A) and the encephalitogenic N-terminal epitope of the autoantigen myelin basic protein. *Journal of Immunology*, **139**, 1075–9.

Zamvil, S.S., Mitchell, D.J., Powell, M.B., Sakai, K., Rothbard, J.B. & Steinman, L. (1988*b*). Multiple discrete encephalitogenic epitopes of the autoantigen myelin basic protein include a determinant for I-E class II-restricted T cells. *Journal of Experimental Medicine*, **168**, 1181–6.

Zeine, R. & Owens, T. (1992). Direct demonstration of the infiltration of murine central nervous system by Pgp-1/CD44^{high} CD45RB^{low} CD4^{+} T cells that induce experimental allergic encephalomyelitis. *Journal of Neuroimmunology*, **40**, 57–69.

Zeine, R. & Owens, T. (1993). Loss rather than downregulation of CD4+ T cells as a mechanism for remission from experimental allergic encephalomyelitis. *Journal of Neuroimmunology*, **44**, 193–8.

Zhao, W., Wegmann, K.W., Trotter, J.L., Ueno, K. & Hickey, W.F. (1994). Identification of an *N*-terminally acetylated encephalitogenic epitope in myelin proteolipid apoprotein for the Lewis rat. *Journal of Immunology*, **153**, 901–9.

Zhou, S.R. & Whitaker, J.N. (1993). Specific modulation of T cells and murine experimental allergic encephalomyelitis by monoclonal anti-idiotypic antibodies. *Journal of Immunology*, **150**, 1629–42.

Zubiaga, A.M., Munoz, E. & Huber, B.T. (1992). IL-4 and IL-2 selectively rescue Th cell subsets from glucocorticoid-induced apoptosis. *Journal of Immunology*, **149**, 107–12.

–4–
Multiple sclerosis

MICHAEL P. PENDER

Introduction

Multiple sclerosis (MS) is a chronic inflammatory demyelinating disease of the central nervous system (CNS). The lesions of MS were first depicted in 1835 by the Scotsman, Robert Carswell (Compston, 1988). The cause of MS became a matter of great interest and speculation. In 1940, Ferraro & Jervis noted the close pathological similarities between experimental autoimmune encephalomyelitis (EAE) and certain cases of acute MS. These similarities gave rise to the theory that MS is an autoimmune disease, a theory further supported by the remarkable similarities between chronic relapsing EAE and MS (Lassmann & Wisniewski, 1979). Advances in the understanding of the immunology of EAE have been rapidly applied to research on MS. Indeed, our current knowledge of the immunology of MS is largely based on studies inspired by insights obtained from research on EAE.

Clinical features

General clinical features

MS generally first presents itself clinically between the ages of 15 and 50 years, but may commence as early as three years (Hanefeld *et al.*, 1991) or as late as the seventh decade. It is about twice as common in females as in males. MS typically results in neurological symptoms and signs indicative of involvement of the white matter of the CNS. The most common clinical features are: monocular visual loss, due to optic neuritis; weakness of the lower limbs, with or without upper limb weakness; sensory loss or paraesthesiae of the limbs or trunk; sensory or cerebellar ataxia; cranial nerve symptoms and signs, such as diplopia, facial sensory disturbance, oscillopsia and nystagmus, due to brainstem involvement; bladder and bowel disturbance; and memory and cognitive impairment. The typical course is one of relapses and remissions, with clinical evidence of involvement of the same or different regions of the CNS in different attacks. This relapsing–remitting pattern often later changes to a gradually progressive pattern of neurological deficit (secondary progression). About one-third of patients follow a progressive course from the onset without experiencing any obvious discrete attacks or remissions (primary progression). Rarely, MS takes an acute fulminant monophasic course, leading to death within three weeks to six months after the onset of the first clinical signs (Marburg's disease) (Lassmann, Budka & Schnaberth, 1981; Lassmann, 1983; Johnson, Lavin & Whetsell, 1990).

Diagnosis

The clinical diagnosis of MS requires the demonstration of involvement of different regions of the CNS at different times (dissemination in time and place) in the absence of any better explanation for the clinical findings (Poser *et al.*, 1983). The history of the illness and the clinical neurological examination have key roles in the diagnostic process, and laboratory investigations are often also necessary to establish a diagnosis. Examination of the cerebrospinal fluid (CSF) by isoelectric focusing typically shows oligoclonal immunoglobulin G (IgG) bands, which are not present in the serum, although such a pattern is not specific for MS and may be present in any inflammatory CNS disease (McLean, Luxton & Thompson, 1990). A mild mononuclear pleocytosis may also be present in the CSF. Electrophysiological studies of signal transmission through visual, somatosensory, auditory and motor pathways (evoked potential studies) are useful in demonstrating subclinical involvement, but do not show changes specific for MS. Magnetic resonance imaging (MRI) of the brain and spinal cord is highly sensitive for detecting MS lesions, although non-specific, and may also be valuable in excluding other pathology (Ormerod *et al.*, 1987). The CSF and MRI findings in MS and the information they provide about MS pathogenesis are discussed in detail later in this chapter.

Association with other autoimmune diseases

MS has been reported to occur concurrently with other autoimmune diseases, including ankylosing spondylitis (Khan & Kushner, 1979; Seyfert *et al.*, 1990), rheumatoid arthritis (Baker *et al.*, 1972; De Keyser, 1988; Seyfert *et al.*, 1990), scleroderma (Trostle, Helfrich & Medsger, 1986), inflammatory bowel disease (Rang, Brooke & Hermon-Taylor, 1982; Sadovnick, Paty & Yannakoulias, 1989; Seyfert *et al.*, 1990), autoimmune thyroid disease, especially Graves' disease (Baker *et al.*, 1972; De Keyser, 1988; Seyfert *et al.*, 1990; McCombe, Chalk & Pender, 1990), type I diabetes mellitus (Wertman, Zilber & Abramsky, 1992), Addison's disease (Baker *et al.*, 1972), autoimmune gastritis (Baker *et al.*, 1972), myasthenia gravis (Somer, Muller & Kinnunen, 1989), pemphigus vulgaris (Baker *et al.*, 1972), psoriasis (Cendrowski, 1989), alopecia areata (Seyfert *et al.*, 1990) and primary biliary cirrhosis (Pontecorvo, Levinson & Roth, 1992). To determine whether the association of MS with other autoimmune diseases is higher than that expected to occur by chance, Seyfert *et al.* (1990) conducted a prospective case–control study of MS patients and healthy volunteers and found 13 of 101 MS patients and two of 97 controls with such diseases ($P = 0.009$). They also found that MS patients have a significantly increased overall frequency of a variety of serum autoantibodies, particularly anti-thyroid-microsomal antibodies, anti-TSH-receptor antibodies, anti-pituitary antibodies, anti-parietal-cell antibodies, anti-smooth-muscle antibodies, anti-nuclear antibodies, anti-double-stranded-DNA antibodies and rheumatoid factor (Seyfert *et al.*, 1990). Other studies have also found a significantly higher frequency of serum organ-specific (especially anti-thyroid) antibodies (Kiessling & Pflughaupt, 1980; De Keyser, 1988; Ioppoli *et al.*, 1990; Tomasevic *et al.*, 1990) and non-organ-specific antibodies (De Keyser, 1988; Tomasevic *et al.*, 1990) in MS patients than in patients with other neurological disorders. Wertman *et al.* (1992) found that the prevalence of type I diabetes mellitus was significantly higher in MS patients under the age of 30 years than in the general population of the same age group. An anti-DNA antibody idiotype termed 16/6, which occurs with high frequency in the sera of patients with systemic lupus erythematosus, is also present at an increased frequency in the sera of patients with MS and of patients with other autoimmune diseases (Shoenfeld *et al.*, 1988). Collectively, the increased occurrence of other autoimmune disease and of serum autoantibodies in MS indicate that MS is also an autoimmune disease.

Uveitis

Anterior and posterior uveitis occur in patients with MS more frequently than would be expected by chance (Archambeau, Hollenhorst & Rucker, 1965; Breger & Leopold, 1966; Porter, 1972; Bamford *et al.*, 1978; Lightman *et al.*, 1987; Meisler *et al.*, 1989; Graham *et al.*, 1989). The concurrence of uveitis and MS may simply be another example of two autoimmune diseases occurring in patients with a susceptibility to autoimmunity, as discussed above. However, the frequency of this association is considerably higher than the association of MS with other individual autoimmune diseases, suggesting that the concurrence of uveitis and MS may also be due to cross-reactivity between uveal and CNS antigens. This hypothesis is supported by the finding that uveitis occurs in pigs and rabbits with EAE induced by inoculation with CNS tissue (Fog & Bardram, 1953; Bullington & Waksman, 1958). Recently, circulating antibodies to the uveitogenic retinal protein, arrestin (S-antigen), and to the homologous brain protein, β-

arrestin 1, have been found in eight out of 14 patients with MS but not in normal controls or patients with other neurological diseases (Ohguro *et al.*, 1993). Furthermore, in two patients with MS, serum antibody titres were higher during relapse than in remission. Cross-reactivity between uveal and CNS antigens may explain the close temporal relationship between the onset of uveitis and the onset or exacerbation of MS in some patients (Archambeau *et al.*, 1965).

Involvement of the peripheral nervous system

MS has classically been considered a disease restricted to the CNS; however, there have been several studies demonstrating subtle electrophysiological or neuropathological evidence of peripheral nervous system (PNS) involvement in patients with typical MS (Waxman, 1993), as well as reports of the concurrence of MS with clinically apparent chronic inflammatory demyelinating polyradiculoneuropathy (CIDP) (Thomas *et al.*, 1987; Rubin, Karpati & Carpenter, 1987; Mendell *et al.*, 1987). Furthermore, PNS involvement is frequent in acute MS (Marburg's disease) (Lassmann, 1983). As discussed in Chapter 3, involvement of the PNS, especially the proximal PNS, is usual in EAE induced by inoculation with whole CNS tissue or myelin basic protein (MBP), but not with proteolipid protein (PLP). Based on the findings in EAE, it can be hypothesized that the degree of PNS involvement in MS depends on whether the autoimmune attack is directed only against antigens confined to the CNS (for example PLP and myelin/oligodendrocyte glycoprotein [MOG]) or against antigens present in both the CNS and the PNS (for example MBP, galactocerebroside and myelin-associated glycoprotein [MAG]). As with the concurrence of MS and uveitis, some cases of concurrent MS and CIDP may simply be due to the tendency for different autoimmune diseases to occur in the same susceptible individual.

Genetics

A major genetic component in the susceptibility to MS has been clearly demonstrated by a population-based study of MS in twins. The concordance rate for MS in monozygotic twins (25.9%) was found to be much higher than that in dizygotic twins (2.3%) and non-twin siblings (1.9%) (Ebers *et al.*, 1986). Multiple genes appear to be involved in this genetic susceptibility, including class II HLA genes and possibly T cell receptor (TCR) genes.

Class II HLA genes

In 1973 Jersild *et al.* reported that MS is associated with the cellular specificity HLA-Dw2. However, the subsequent widespread use of serological typing techniques, which fail to distinguish Dw2 from the other DR2 haplotypes, resulted in the impression that this association was confined to Caucasian populations originating from Northern Europe (Hillert & Olerup, 1993). With the introduction of genomic typing techniques, it has now become clear that the DRw15,DQw6,Dw2 (DRB1*1501-DQA1*0102-DQB1*0602) haplotype is associated with MS, irrespective of ethnic origin (Olerup *et al.*, 1989; Hao *et al.*, 1992; Serjeantson *et al.*, 1992; Hillert & Olerup, 1993). The Dw2 haplotype segregates closely with MS in multiplex MS families, indicating that it plays an important role in determining susceptibility to MS (Hillert *et al.*, 1994). The relative contributions of the DR and DQ loci remain unclear; however, studies in Hong Kong Chinese (Serjeantson *et al.*, 1992) and French Canadians (Haegert & Francis, 1992) have implicated DQB1*0602 as a susceptibility allele. It has been suggested that DQ β chain polymorphisms at a single residue (26) contribute to the development of MS in the latter population (Haegert & Francis, 1992).

In Swedish and Norwegian patients there is evidence of immunogenetic heterogeneity between the relapsing–remitting and the primary progressive forms of MS. Whereas both clinical forms are associated with the DRw15,DQw6,Dw2 haplotype, the relapsing–remitting form is also associated with the DQB1 allelic pattern observed in the DRw17,DQw2 haplotype (Olerup *et al.*, 1989; Hillert *et al.*, 1992*a*).

TCR genes

A linkage between MS and the TCR β chain complex was found in one study of American MS multiplex families (Seboun *et al.*, 1989) but not in another family study (Lynch *et al.*, 1991). Population studies of North American Caucasian MS patients have indicated the existence of an MS susceptibility gene(s) within the region of the TCR β chain gene complex (Beall *et al.*, 1989) and more specifically within the TCR Vβ region (Beall *et al.*, 1993). In the latter study the TCR Vβ subhaplotype frequencies differed significantly from the control population only in the DR2$^+$ MS patients and not in the DR2$^-$ MS patients, providing the first evidence for gene complementation between an HLA class II gene and TCR Vβ gene(s) in conferring susceptibility to MS (Beall *et al.*, 1993). There is also evidence for an association with TCR Vβ and Cβ genes in French (Briant *et al.*, 1993) and Spanish (Martinez Naves *et al.*, 1993) MS patients. On the other hand, population studies of Scandinavian MS patients have not found an association between susceptibility to MS and TCR β chain haplotypes (Fugger *et al.*, 1990; Hillert, Leng & Olerup, 1991). An association between MS and a restriction fragment length polymorphism of the TCR Vα and Cα gene segments has also been reported (Oksenberg *et al.*, 1989; Sherritt *et al.*, 1992), but this was not confirmed by another study which found evidence that the seemingly polymorphic fragments may have resulted from incomplete cleavage of DNA by the restriction enzyme (Hillert, Leng & Olerup, 1992*b*).

Familial occurrence of MS with other autoimmune diseases: evidence for a primary autoimmune gene

In the families of patients with MS there appears to be an increased occurrence of other autoimmune diseases, including systemic lupus erythematosus, scleroderma, thyroid disease and inflammatory bowel disease (Trostle *et al.*, 1986; Minuk & Lewkonia, 1986; Bias *et al.*, 1986; Sloan *et al.*, 1987; Sadovnick *et al.*, 1989; McCombe *et al.*, 1990; Doolittle *et al.*, 1990). On the basis of a genetic analysis of 18 autoimmune kindreds (three containing a member with MS), Bias *et al.* (1986) have proposed that autoimmunity is inherited as an autosomal dominant trait with secondary genes, including HLA genes, determining the specific type of autoimmune disease.

Other genes

Evidence has been presented that an MBP gene or some other MBP-linked locus influences susceptibility to MS (Boylan *et al.*, 1990; Tienari *et al.*, 1992); however, another study did not demonstrate linkage between MS and the MBP gene (Rose *et al.*, 1993). In contrast to earlier studies, Walter *et al.* (1991) and Hillert (1993) found no evidence that Ig constant region genes confer susceptibility to MS. However, Walter *et al.* (1991) found an association between MS and an Ig heavy chain variable region gene segment. There is also a report of a significant association between MS and the M3 allele of α-1 antitrypsin, the major circulating protease inhibitor (McCombe *et al.*, 1985). Harding *et al.* (1992) have reported the occurrence of an MS-like illness in women with a mitochondrial DNA mutation found in Leber's hereditary optic neuropathy and have suggested that mitochondrial genes may contribute to susceptibility to MS.

In conclusion, the only confirmed genetic factor predisposing to MS is the HLA-DR-DQ haplotype DRw15,DQw6,Dw2. There is suggestive evidence of roles for the TCR β chain genes and a primary autoimmune gene in determining disease susceptibility, but further studies are needed to confirm their roles.

Neuropathology

Primary demyelination is the key morphological feature of the MS lesion (Périer & Grégoire, 1965; Prineas, 1985). Primary demyelination is a process resulting in loss of the myelin sheath with preservation of the underlying axon, in contrast to secondary demyelination, where myelin loss is a consequence of axonal loss. Other important characteristics of MS lesions are a mononuclear inflammatory infiltrate (see below), the presence of myelin breakdown products within macrophages, and astrocytic gliosis. The lesions of MS can occur virtually anywhere within the CNS, but the most common sites of involvement are the optic nerves, spinal cord and periventricular regions of the cerebral hemispheres. An essential feature is the occurrence of lesions of different ages, as indicated by varying degrees of inflammation, ongoing demyelination, remyelination and gliosis.

An important question concerning the pathogenesis of MS is whether the primary demyelination results from direct damage to the myelin sheath itself or whether it results from destruction of the oligodendrocyte, the cell that produces and maintains myelin. It is generally agreed that the oligodendrocyte is lost in the longstanding MS lesion, but there has been controversy concerning its fate in the early lesion. However, Prineas *et al.* have recently presented evidence that there is oligodendrocyte loss in the early lesion (Prineas *et al.*, 1989, 1993*a*).

Contrary to previous opinion, significant remyelination by oligodendrocytes does occur in MS (Lassmann, 1983; Prineas *et al.*, 1984, 1993*a*). Remyelination has been observed ten weeks after clinical onset (Prineas *et al.*, 1993*a*). It may well commence much earlier, as in rats with acute EAE it commences as early as six days after clinical onset (Pender, 1989; Pender, Nguyen & Willenborg, 1989). Remyelination of a demyelinating CNS lesion (possibly due to MS) has been observed in a brain biopsy from a 15-year-old boy about two weeks after the onset of neurological symptoms (Ghatak *et al.*, 1989). Prineas *et al.* (1993*a*) have suggested that new MS lesions normally remyelinate unless interrupted by recurrent disease activity. It is likely that shadow plaques (groups of thinly myelinated fibres) represent remyelination after a single previous episode of focal demyelination (Lassmann, 1983; Prineas *et al.*, 1993*a*). The finding that new demyelinating lesions may be superimposed on old shadow plaques supports the MRI evidence (see below) that local recurrence may be at least as important as progressive edge activity in determining plaque growth (Prineas *et al.*, 1993*b*). It also indicates that recurrent demyelination of the same area may be a factor underlying failed remyelination in MS.

Although primary demyelination is the hallmark of MS, axonal loss also occurs and may be severe in longstanding lesions (Barnes *et al.*, 1991). Occasionally, frank necrosis occurs. As mentioned earlier, PNS demyelination sometimes develops in patients with MS. All the above morphological features of MS are observed in chronic relapsing EAE (Lassmann & Wisniewski, 1979; Lassmann, 1983; see Chapter 3).

Pathophysiology

Evoked potential studies of signal transmission through visual, auditory, somatosensory and motor pathways reveal functional abnormalities in patients with MS. Although these studies are useful for clinical diagnosis, their contribution to understanding the pathophysiology of MS is limited by difficulties in interpretation. The typical evoked potential findings in MS are a prolongation of latency and a reduction in amplitude. In peripheral nerve conduction studies, a prolongation of latency indicates conduction slowing, whereas a reduction in amplitude (without temporal dispersion) indicates focal conduction block or complete conduction failure. However, evoked potential studies of CNS function are dependent on signal transmission through pathways containing one or more synapses where signals are normally delayed, integrated and amplified. Hence, prolongation of the latency of an evoked potential may be caused by increased synaptic delays due to presynaptic axonal conduction block as well as by conduction slowing. Furthermore, a reduction in the amplitude of the evoked postsynaptic field potential is an unreliable indicator of presynaptic axonal conduction block (Stanley, McCombe & Pender, 1992). Therefore, at present our understanding of the pathophysiology of MS has to rely mainly on experimental studies of demyelination in animals.

It is highly likely that the main mechanism producing neurological symptoms and signs in the early stages of MS is nerve conduction block due to primary demyelination. It is well established that primary demyelination *per se* in the CNS causes focal conduction block or conduction slowing at the site of demyelination (McDonald & Sears, 1970). Neurological symptoms and signs will result if conduction block occurs simultaneously in a significant proportion of fibres within a given pathway. In clinical attacks of EAE there is CNS conduction block due to demyelination (see Chapter 3).

Conduction slowing due to demyelination may have no significant clinical consequences, although it is possible that slowing of conduction in presynaptic axons may alter spatiotemporal integration in postsynaptic neurones and thus produce clinically apparent disturbances of function. However, because conduction is insecure in slowly conducting fibres, intermittent conduction block may occur and lead to neurological symptoms. For example, demyelinated fibres may be able to transmit signals at low frequencies but not at higher frequencies (McDonald & Sears, 1970), owing to an increase in threshold through the hyperpolarizing effect of the electrogenic Na^+/K^+ pump (Bostock & Grafe, 1985). An inability to sustain high-frequency transmission may contribute to the fading out of vision after looking at an object continuously for several seconds, and to the fatiguability of muscle strength experienced by some patients with MS. Conduction in demyelinated fibres is also susceptible to small changes in body temperature. A temperature increase of 0.5 °C can reversibly induce conduction block in demyelinated fibres by shortening the duration of the action potential and thus reducing the current available to excite the demyelinated region (Rasminsky, 1973). Cooling has the opposite effect. Reversible conduction block accounts for the temporary clinical deterioration that occurs in patients with MS with an increase in body temperature, for example due to fever. Demyelinated fibres may also generate ectopic impulses, either spontaneously or after mechanical stimulation (Smith & McDonald, 1982). Ephaptic transmission (lateral spread of excitation from one axon into an adjacent one) occurs in the congenitally dysmyelinated spinal root fibres of the dystrophic mouse (Rasminsky, 1980) and may possibly occur in demyelinated CNS fibres. Ectopic impulse generation and ephaptic transmission are likely to contribute to the paroxysmal phenomena that occur in MS, namely Lhermitte's sign, trigeminal neuralgia, painful tonic seizures and paroxysmal dysarthria.

Conduction can be restored in demyelinated CNS fibres by remyelination, although conduction is slow and insecure until the remyelination is well established (Smith, Blakemore & McDonald, 1981). However, remyelination is not essential to restore nerve conduction: nerve conduction can be restored in fibres that are still demyelinated, possibly by alterations in the distribution of Na^+ channels within the demyelinated axolemma, by reduction in the diameter of demyelinated axons or by glial ensheathment (Bostock & Sears, 1978; Smith, Bostock & Hall, 1982; Waxman *et al.*, 1989; Shrager & Rubinstein, 1990). During clinical recovery from EAE there is restoration of CNS conduction due to glial ensheathment and remyelination (see Chapter 3). The extent to which remyelination contributes to clinical recovery after attacks of MS remains to be determined.

It is possible that cytokines or other inflammatory mediators may also contribute to acute neural dysfunction in MS, but there is little evidence to support this suggestion. Oedema is unlikely to contribute to the neurological deficit, except when it occurs within a confined space, for example the optic canal, where it may result in secondary ischaemia. Axonal loss is likely to be an important cause of persistent neurological dysfunction in MS (Barnes *et al.*, 1991), as it is in chronic relapsing EAE (Stanley & Pender, 1991).

Magnetic resonance imaging and spectroscopy

Magnetic resonance imaging is a sensitive technique for the detection of CNS lesions in MS. The typical findings are regions of increased signal on T_2-weighted images, which correspond with histologically defined plaques (Ormerod *et al.*, 1987). It is likely that this increased signal is due to oedema in acute lesions and to gliosis in chronic lesions; demyelination per se is unlikely to make an important contribution (Ormerod *et al.*, 1987). Enhancement of T_1-weighted images after the intravenous administration of gadolinium diethylenetriaminepentaacetic acid (gadolinium) reflects breakdown of the blood–brain barrier and is a useful indicator of disease activity (Miller *et al.*, 1988). Serial studies have shown that gadolinium enhancement of T_1-weighted images precedes other MRI abnormalities in the evolving new lesion (Kermode *et al.*, 1990) and that enhancement can also occur in old lesions that have been non-enhancing on previous scans (Miller *et al.*, 1988). Although disease activity as indicated by gadolinium enhancement is usually asymptomatic, clinical deterioration in patients with relapsing–remitting MS is significantly associated with increased frequency and area of gadolinium-enhancing lesions (Smith *et al.*, 1993). Similar changes in gadolinium enhancement on MRI also occur in chronic relapsing EAE (see Chapter 3).

Serial MRI studies of MS have indicated a difference in the dynamics of disease activity between secondary progressive MS and primary progressive MS, particularly in relation to the inflammatory component of the lesions (Thompson *et al.*, 1991). Patients in the secondary progressive group had 18.2 new lesions per patient per year and 87% of these enhanced. Enhancement also occurred within and at the edge of pre-existing lesions. In contrast, patients in the primary progressive group had only 3.3 new lesions per patient per year and only 5% of these enhanced (Thompson *et al.*, 1991). MRI studies have demonstrated considerable expansion of the extracellular space in longstanding lesions, which probably reflects axonal loss (Barnes *et al.*, 1991).

Although MRI has provided important information about the temporal profile of inflammation in MS, it has not yielded information about the time course of demyelination, because it does not reveal normal myelin or myelin breakdown products. Proton magnetic resonance spectroscopy (MRS) can detect increased lipid resonances at 0.9 and 1.3 parts per million which probably indicates myelin breakdown products (Davie *et al.*, 1993, 1994; Koopmans *et al.*, 1993). Serial proton MRS of acute MS lesions has demonstrated such increased resonances in lesions which had been enhancing with gadolinium for less than one month, indicating that myelin breakdown occurs during the initial inflammatory stage of lesion development (Davie *et al.*, 1994). Increased choline signals also occur in MS lesions (Arnold *et al.*, 1992; Davie *et al.*, 1994) and were initially attributed to recent demyelination; however, a study on EAE has indicated that such an increase can be produced by the increased membrane turnover associated with inflammation in the absence of demyelination (Brenner *et al.*, 1993). Proton MRS of MS lesions has also demonstrated decreased *N*-acetylaspartate signals, which have been attributed to neuronal or axonal damage (Arnold *et al.*, 1992), although this change is partially reversible over 4–8 months and therefore cannot be explained solely by axonal loss (Davie *et al.*, 1994).

Immunopathology of the CNS lesions

Characteristics of the inflammatory infiltrate in the CNS

Immunocytochemical studies of CNS tissue sections from patients with MS have shown that the perivascular inflammatory cell cuffs and the parenchymal inflammatory cell infiltrate consist predominantly of T lymphocytes and macrophages (Traugott, Reinherz & Raine, 1983*a*,*b*; Booss *et al.*, 1983; Hauser *et al.*, 1986; Woodroofe *et al.*, 1986; Esiri & Reading, 1987; McCallum *et al.*, 1987; Sobel *et al.*, 1988; Boyle & McGeer, 1990). Generally $CD8^+$ T cells have been found to be more frequent than $CD4^+$ T cells (Booss *et al.*, 1983; Hauser *et al.*, 1986; Woodroofe *et al.*, 1986; McCallum *et al.*, 1987; Hayashi *et al.*, 1988), although one study found that $CD4^+$ T cells outnumbered $CD8^+$ T cells in the normal-appearing white matter adjacent to active chronic lesions (Traugott *et al.*, 1983*a*) and another found that there were slightly more $CD4^+$ T cells than $CD8^+$ T cells in plaques as well as in the adjacent white matter (Sobel *et al.*, 1988). The variations in cellular composition of MS lesions are likely to be due to variations in the pathological stage of the lesions studied (Sobel *et al.*, 1988). The preponderance of $CD8^+$ T cells over $CD4^+$ T cells in MS lesions is in contrast to the findings in EAE lesions, where $CD4^+$ T cells predominate (see Chapter 3). The numbers of both $CD4^+$ T cells and $CD8^+$ T cells are maximal at the borders of MS plaques, with the numbers falling off inside the plaque and in the adjacent normal-appearing white matter (McCallum *et al.*, 1987). Some of the infiltrating cells express the interleukin-2 receptor (IL-2R), indicating that they are activated T cells (Bellamy *et al.*, 1985; Hofman *et al.*, 1986; Sobel *et al.*, 1988). Compared with the lesions of viral encephalitis, the lesions of MS have a selective reduction in the number of cells expressing CD45RA, which is found on naive T cells (Sobel *et al.*, 1988).

$\gamma\delta$ T cells are also present in chronic MS lesions, where they co-localize with immature oligodendrocytes expressing the 65-kDa heat shock protein (hsp65) (Selmaj, Brosnan & Raine, 1991), and in acute lesions where hsp60 is present in foamy macrophages and hsp90 in reactive astrocytes (Wucherpfennig *et al.*, 1992*b*). Human $\gamma\delta$ T cells have been shown to lyse human oligodendrocytes *in vitro*, possibly by targeting hsp which are differentially expressed by oligodendrocytes compared to astrocytes and which can be recognized by $\gamma\delta$ T cells (Freedman *et al.*, 1991, 1992). It has been proposed that, after initiation of the inflammatory process in the CNS by $\alpha\beta$ T cells reactive with a myelin antigen(s), hsp may be overexpressed at the inflammatory site with resultant recruitment of $\gamma\delta$ T cells that induce demyelination (Wucherpfennig *et al.*, 1992*b*).

In some cases of MS there is a prominent accumulation of plasma cells in the perivascular spaces of the CNS, and plasma cells are also present in the parenchyma (Prineas & Wright, 1978). Esiri (1980) found that immunoglobulin-containing cells (the great majority of which were considered likely to be immunoglobulin-producing) are numerous in MS plaques. In recent plaques these cells were commonly found within the parenchyma as well as in perivascular cuffs, while in chronic plaques and normally myelinated tissue they were almost entirely confined to the perivascular spaces (Esiri, 1980). Using an MBP–enzyme conjugate technique, Gerritse *et al.* (1994) found B cells forming anti-MBP antibody in the brains of five out of 12 MS patients. Prineas & Graham (1981) found capping of surface IgG on macrophages contacting myelin sheaths and interpreted this as evidence that anti-myelin antibody opsonizes myelin for phagocytosis by macrophages. Granular deposits of the C9 component of complement and of the terminal complement complex have been demonstrated immunocytochemically in association with capillary endothelial cells, predominantly within plaques and adjacent white matter from MS patients but not from controls (Compston *et al.*, 1989). With the exception of the apparent predominance of $CD8^+$ T cells over $CD4^+$ T cells, the findings in MS are similar to those in EAE (see Chapter 3).

Major histocompatibility complex (MHC) class II antigen expression in the CNS

It is well established that MHC class II antigen is expressed on macrophages and microglia in MS lesions (Traugott & Raine, 1985; Woodroofe *et al.*, 1986; Hayes, Woodroofe & Cuzner, 1987; Cuzner *et al.*, 1988; McGeer, Itagaki & McGeer, 1988; Boyle & McGeer, 1990; Lee *et al.*, 1990; Bö *et al.*, 1994). Using double-labelling techniques and confocal microscopy, Bö *et al.* (1994) found that class II antigen is expressed not only by parenchymal macrophages within the CNS lesions but also by macrophages within the perivascular spaces (perivascular macrophages) of blood vessels both inside and outside the lesions. MHC class II antigen expression by microglia is found in many non-inflammatory neurological diseases (McGeer *et al.*, 1988), indicating that it represents a non-specific reactive phenomenon. Astrocytes in MS lesions have been reported to express MHC class II antigen (Traugott & Raine, 1985; Traugott, Scheinberg & Raine, 1985; Hofman *et al.*, 1986; Traugott & Lebon, 1988; Lee *et al.*, 1990); however, Boyle & McGeer (1990) and Bö *et al.* (1994) could not confirm this. Oligodendrocytes do not express MHC class II antigen in MS lesions (Lee & Raine, 1989; Lee *et al.*, 1990). Vascular endothelial cells have been reported to express MHC class II antigen (Traugott & Raine, 1985; Traugott *et al.*, 1985) but this was not confirmed by Bö *et al.* (1994).

In conclusion, it would appear that in MS lesions MHC class II antigen is expressed by microglia and macrophages but not by astrocytes, oligodendrocytes or endothelial cells. A similar cellular distribution of MHC class II antigen expression is found in EAE (see Chapter 3). As perivascular macrophages are the only MHC class II-positive cells in MS lesions that contain abundant cytoplasmic MHC class II immunoreactivity, it is likely that they act as antigen-presenting cells in MS (Bö *et al.*, 1994), as they do in EAE (see Chapter 3). At present it is unknown whether microglia upregulate or downregulate the immune response in MS.

Adhesion molecule and cytokine expression in the CNS

In MS lesions there is increased expression of intercellular adhesion molecule-1 (ICAM-1), vascular cell adhesion molecule-1 and E-selectin on CNS vascular endothelium (Sobel, Mitchell & Fondren, 1990; Washington *et al.*, 1994), indicating that adhesion molecules may play a role in T cell entry to the CNS, as in the case of EAE (see Chapter 3). ICAM-1 is also expressed on some glial cells, raising the possibility that inflammatory cells expressing the ICAM-1 ligand, lymphocyte function-associated molecule-1 (LFA-1), may also interact with glial cells through LFA-1/ICAM-1 binding (Sobel *et al.*, 1990).

Cells expressing tumour necrosis factor (TNF) are present in the brain lesions of MS but have not been detected in the normal brain (Hofman *et al.*, 1989). Studies using the polymerase chain reaction detected IL-1 mRNA in the majority of acute and subacute MS plaques, and IL-2 and IL-4 mRNA in some acute lesions (Wucherpfennig *et al.*, 1992*a*).

TCR gene usage in the CNS

Following the demonstration of restricted TCR Vβ gene usage by MBP-specific T cells in mice and rats (see Chapter 3) and in some patients with MS (see below), TCR gene usage by infiltrating T cells has been studied in MS brain tissue by the polymerase chain reaction to determine whether there is restricted usage, which might indicate a specific autoreactive response. Oksenberg *et al.* (1990) reported restricted TCR Vα gene usage in MS brain tissue, but a subsequent more detailed study demonstrated heterogeneous TCR Vα and Vβ gene usage in active MS lesions (Wucherpfennig *et al.*, 1992*a*). Some of the infiltrating T cells use Vβ5.2 (Oksenberg *et al.*, 1993), which has been reported by one group, but not others, to be selectively used by MBP-specific human T cells (see below). Interestingly, 40% of the TCR Vβ5.2 N(D)N rearrangements in the lesions of MS patients with the HLA-DRB1*1501-DQA1*0102-DQB1*0602-DPB1*0401 haplotype have been found to comprise VDJ sequences used by a cytotoxic T cell clone specific for MBP peptide 89–106 from an MS patient with this HLA haplotype or by encephalitogenic rat T cells specific for MBP peptide 87–99, suggesting that pathogenic MBP-specific T cells may be present in MS brain tissue (Oksenberg *et al.*, 1993). Further studies will be needed to determine whether this is a common and specific finding in MS lesions. It also remains possible that the infiltrating T cells using these Vβ-Dβ-Jβ sequences do not recognize MBP but other antigens.

Wucherpfennig *et al.* (1992*b*) found an accumulation of $\gamma\delta$ T cells that predominantly use the Vδ1 and Vδ2 gene segments in acute MS lesions. They concluded that $\gamma\delta$ T cells appeared to have undergone clonal expansion following recognition of a specific CNS ligand, possibly hsp. Hvas *et al.* (1993) found that the majority of $\gamma\delta$ T cells in chronic MS lesions express the Vγ2 and Vδ2 chains, but in a clonality assessment of brain samples from two patients did not find evidence of an MS-specific expansion of clones using particular types of $\gamma\delta$ TCR.

Immunological findings in the peripheral blood

Non-specific T cell findings

CD4 and CD8 expression

In the peripheral blood of MS patients, particularly those with chronic progressive MS, the $CD8^+$ T cell subset is decreased and the $CD4^+/CD8^+$ ratio is increased (Brinkman, Nillesen & Hommes, 1983; Hughes, Kirk & Compston, 1989; Trotter *et al.*, 1989; Ilonen *et al.*, 1990). In one study the $CD11b^+CD8^+$ subset (reportedly suppressor cells) (Hughes *et al.*, 1989) was found to be reduced but in another study the $CD11b^-CD8^+$ subset (reportedly cytotoxic) showed the more marked decrease (Ilonen *et al.*, 1990). CD8 and CD4 are released in soluble form upon T cell activation. In one study, soluble CD8 but not soluble CD4 was found to be significantly increased in the peripheral blood of MS patients, with the soluble CD8 level being higher in exacerbation than in remission (Tsukada *et al.*, 1991); however, in another study the soluble CD8 level was not elevated (Maimone & Reder, 1991). Munschauer *et al.* (1993) found that MS patients have a significantly greater population of circulating $CD3^+CD4^+CD8^+$ T cells than do healthy controls. The significance of these changes in CD4 and CD8 expression in the peripheral blood of MS patients is unknown.

Expression of T cell activation markers

CD45RA, the high molecular weight isoform of leukocyte common antigen, is expressed on naive T cells but not memory T cells. Patients with clinically active MS have generally been found to exhibit a selective decrease in the $CD4^+CD45RA^+$ subset in the peripheral blood compared with patients with clinically inactive MS and controls (Rose *et al.*, 1985, 1988; Morimoto *et al.*, 1987; Zaffaroni *et al.*, 1990; Porrini, Gambi & Malatesta, 1992; Eoli *et al.*, 1993). Serial studies on the same MS patients have shown that the peripheral blood $CD4^+CD45RA^-/CD4^+CD45RA^+$ ratio increases at the time of relapse (Rose *et al.*, 1988; Corrigan, Hutchinson & Feighery, 1990): in one study this increase usually resulted from a simultaneous decrease in $CD4^+CD45RA^+$ cells and increase in $CD4^+CD45RA^-$ cells (Rose *et al.*, 1988), whereas in another study there was no significant alteration in the $CD4^+CD45RA^+$ population but an increase in the $CD4^+CD45RA^-$ population (Corrigan *et al.*, 1990). These findings suggest that clinical disease activity is accompanied by a conversion of naive T cells to memory T cells (Corrigan *et al.*, 1990; Zaffaroni *et al.*, 1990).

$CD4^+CD29^+$ T cells (reportedly memory cells) have been found to be increased in the peripheral blood of MS patients (Gambi *et al.*, 1991). This was associated with an increase in circulating $CD4^+CD45RA^-$ cells and a decrease in $CD4^+CD29^-$ cells and hypothesized to be related to B cell activation (Gambi *et al.*, 1991). IL-2R (CD25) expression is a marker of T cell activation. Several studies have reported an increased proportion of $IL\text{-}2R^+$ cells in the peripheral blood of patients with MS (Bellamy *et al.*, 1985; Selmaj *et al.*, 1986; Konttinen *et al.*, 1987; Porrini *et al.*, 1992; Scolozzi *et al.*, 1992), but other studies have not found such an increase (Hafler *et al.*, 1985*b*; Crockard *et al.*, 1988). CD44 (Ta1) is also a marker of T cell activation. An increase in the proportion of $CD44^+$ cells in the peripheral blood of MS patients has been reported (Hafler *et al.*, 1985*b*) but this was not confirmed in another study (Crockard *et al.*, 1988).

Suppressor cell function

Non-specific suppressor cell function has been assessed in MS by determining the ability of peripheral blood mononuclear cells, after activation by concanavalin A and treatment with mitomycin C, to suppress the proliferative response of autologous cells to concanavalin A (Antel, Arnason & Medof, 1979). Antel *et al.* (1979) have shown that such activated suppressor cell function is reduced in patients with clinically active MS compared with patients with clinically stable MS, patients recovering from an exacerbation and normal controls. It is significantly higher in patients with progressive MS and severe disability than in those with progressive MS and moderate disability (Antel *et al.*, 1989). The functional suppressor deficit involves the $CD8^+$ T cell subset (J.P. Antel *et al.*, 1986*a*) and is also exhibited by $CD8^+$ T cell lines derived from the peripheral blood of patients with progressive MS and, to a lesser degree, stable MS (J. Antel *et al.*, 1986, 1988). *In vitro* pokeweed mitogen-induced IgG secretion by peripheral blood mononuclear cells (used as an indirect measure of $CD8^+$ T cell suppressor function) is increased in progressive MS, whereas alloantigen-directed cytotoxicity (a predominantly $CD8^+$ T cell function) is normal, suggesting a selective defect of suppressor cell function in MS rather than a generalized dysfunction of $CD8^+$ T cells (J.P. Antel *et al.*, 1986*b*). Other groups have confirmed the defect of peripheral blood suppressor cell function in active MS (Morimoto *et al.*, 1987; Chofflon *et al.*, 1988; O'Gorman, Aziz & Oger, 1989; Trotter *et al.*, 1989; Baxevanis, Reclos & Papamichail, 1990). Chofflon *et al.* (1988) found that the decrease in functional suppression in MS is linked to the decrease in circulating $CD4^+CD45RA^+$ T cells (previously called 'suppressor–inducer' cells); however, Baxevanis *et al.* (1990) concluded that it is due to the deficient expression of DR antigen on monocytes.

Autologous mixed lymphocyte reaction

The autologous mixed lymphocyte reaction (AMLR), which measures the T cell proliferative response to antigens on the surface of autologous non-T cells, is reduced in patients with MS compared to controls (Hafler, Buchsbaum & Weiner, 1985*a*; Hirsch, 1986). $CD4^+$ T cells from MS patients also exhibit a decreased AMLR (Baxevanis *et al.*, 1988; Hafler *et al.*, 1991). Hirsch (1986) attributed the decreased AMLR to a functional defect in a subpopulation of $CD4^+$ T cells, and Chofflon *et al.* (1988) concluded that both the decrease in the AMLR and the decrease in functional suppression are tightly linked to decreases in the $CD4^+CD45RA^+$ cells. However, Baxevanis *et al.* (1988) have provided evidence that the decreased AMLR is due to a monocyte functional (stimulatory) defect. Decreased secretion of IL-1, which is produced by monocytes as well as by other cells, has also been implicated in the decreased AMLR by the finding that IL-1 corrects the defective AMLR in MS patients but has no effect on the AMLR in controls (Hafler *et al.*, 1991). Moreover, the magnitude of the AMLR corresponded to the level of IL-1 secretion induced by lipopolysaccharide in the non-T-cell population (Hafler *et al.*, 1991).

β-adrenergic receptor expression

The density of high-affinity β-adrenergic receptors on $CD8^+CD28^-$ (reportedly suppressor cells) T cells is increased in progressive MS (Karaszewski *et al.*, 1990, 1991, 1993). Basal and isoproterenol-stimulated cyclic AMP levels in $CD8^+$ cells are also increased in patients with progressive MS (Karaszewski *et al.*, 1993). Karaszewski *et al.* (1990) have suggested that the increased β-adrenergic receptor density and the decreased suppressor cell function may be due to reduced sympathetic nervous system activity as a result of lesions in progressive MS. However, Zoukos *et al.* (1992) have found an increased density of β-adrenergic receptors on peripheral blood mononuclear cells from patients with chronic active rheumatoid arthritis as well as from patients with MS, indicating that the receptor upregulation can occur in the absence of nervous system disease. A possible role for cortisol and IL-1 was suggested by the finding that hydrocortisone or IL-1 upregulated β-adrenergic receptors on peripheral blood mononuclear cells from normal controls but not from patients with MS (Zoukos *et al.*, 1992).

Specific T cell findings

T cell reactivity to myelin basic protein

As MBP is encephalitogenic in laboratory animals (see Chapter 3), it has been proposed that it may be a target antigen in MS. Standard T cell proliferation assays have demonstrated MBP-reactive T cells in the peripheral blood of a minority of MS patients and also occasionally in healthy controls and patients with other neurological diseases (Lisak & Zweiman, 1977; Brinkman *et al.*, 1982; Johnson *et al.*, 1986; Vandenbark *et al.*, 1989; Trotter *et al.*, 1991; Kerlero de Rosbo *et al.*, 1993; Y. Zhang *et al.*, 1993). MBP reactivity appears to be more common in patients with clinically active MS than in those with clinically stable MS (Johnson *et al.*, 1986). In some studies but not others, group analysis has shown that the reactivity to MBP is significantly greater in MS patients than in normal controls or patients with other neurological diseases. Baxevanis *et al.* (1989*b*) found that all patients with severe progressive MS had significant proliferation of peripheral blood T cells in response to peptide fragment 45–89 of human MBP and also to synthetic peptides 15–31, 75–96 and 83–96 but not to 131–141. Normal controls and patients with other neurological diseases only occasionally showed significant proliferation in response to these peptides. The responding T cells from MS patients were $CD4^+$ and were dependent on monocytes and HLA-DR molecules for their activation (Baxevanis *et al.*, 1989*b*). Frick (1989) has reported increased $CD8^+$ T cell cytotoxicity towards cells coated with bovine MBP or human MBP peptide 114–122 in patients with MS. The results of Baxevanis *et al.* and of Frick require confirmation.

On the basis that mutant T cells represent a population enriched with dividing cells, Allegretta *et al.* (1990) isolated hypoxanthine guanine phosphoribosyltransferase-mutant T cell clones from the peripheral blood of patients with chronic progressive MS to determine their reactivity to MBP. Eleven of 258 mutant T cell clones from five of six MS patients proliferated in response to human MBP without prior *in vitro* exposure to this antigen, but no wild-type clones from these patients nor any mutant or wild-type clones from three normal controls responded to MBP. These results indicate that there are circulating activated MBP-specific T cells in patients with MS. A similar conclusion was reached by Ofosu Appiah *et al.* (1991) who used the limiting dilution technique to generate clones from *in vivo*-activated IL-2-responsive T cells in the peripheral blood of MS patients. Seven (three $CD4^+$ and four $CD8^+$) of 20 clones from ten MS patients but none of eight clones from five normal controls proliferated specifically in response to MBP. Using the limiting dilution assay, Chou *et al.* (1992) found an increased frequency of MBP-reactive T cells in the peripheral blood of MS patients compared with normal subjects and patients with other neurological diseases. In contrast, Zhang *et al.* (1992*a*) found no significant difference in the precursor frequency of MBP-reactive T cells in the peripheral blood of MS patients and normal controls; however, after primary culture with IL-2 the frequency of MBP-reactive T cells was significantly higher in MS patients than in normal individuals (Zhang *et al.*, 1994). Increased frequencies of T cells reactive to MBP and MBP peptides have been found in the peripheral blood of MS patients by counting the number of cells secreting interferon-γ (IFN-γ) in response to antigen in short-term cultures (Olsson *et al.*, 1990*b*, 1992); however, these results are difficult to interpret, because of the high background response. Using *in situ* hybridization with radiolabelled complementary DNA oligonucleotide probes, Link *et al.* (1994*a*,*b*) have demonstrated that, compared with patients with other neurological diseases, MS patients have increased numbers of peripheral blood mononuclear cells expressing IFN-γ, IL-4 and transforming growth factor-β mRNA after short-term culture in the presence of MBP.

A number of laboratories have isolated MBP-specific T cell lines or clones from the peripheral blood of MS patients and controls (Weber & Buurman, 1988; Vandenbark *et al.*, 1989; Martin *et al.*, 1990; Ota *et al.*, 1990; Pette *et al.*, 1990*a*; Liblau *et al.*, 1991; Burns *et al.*, 1991). Generally the MBP-specific T cell lines and clones are $CD4^+$ and restricted by HLA-DR molecules. The majority of the long-term lines and clones have been cytotoxic towards MBP-coated target cells (Weber & Buurman, 1988; Martin *et al.*, 1990; Zhang *et al.*, 1990) and have secreted substantial amounts of IFN-γ (Martin *et al.*, 1990). Multiple immunogenic regions of the MBP molecule have been identified by this approach but two regions are immunodominant, one in the middle of the molecule (87–106) (Martin *et al.*, 1990; Ota *et al.*, 1990; Zhang *et al.*, 1992*a*), and the other at the C-terminal region (154–172) (Martin *et al.*, 1990; Ota *et al.*, 1990; Zhang *et al.*, 1990, 1992*a*; Liblau *et al.*, 1991). Within the 87–106 region there are several nested immunogenic epitopes (Martin *et al.*, 1992). It is important to note that the 87–106 region includes peptides encephalitogenic in the SJL/J mouse (Sakai *et al.*, 1988) and in the Lewis and Buffalo rats (Offner *et al.*, 1989; Jones *et al.*, 1992), and that the 154–172 sequence includes the region that is encephalitogenic in monkeys (Karkhanis *et al.*, 1975). Ota *et al.* (1990) found that the proportion of MBP-specific T cell lines reacting with peptide 84–102 was higher in MS patients than in controls. Voskuhl *et al.* (1993*b*) reported that MS patients have a higher frequency of T cell lines specific for epitopes within isoforms of MBP expressed mainly during myelination, raising the possibility that the epitopes could be targeted during the remyelination that commonly occurs in MS.

Martin *et al.* (1990, 1991) found that the 87–106 peptide is recognized by cytotoxic T cells in the context of DR2, DR4 and DR6 and the 154–172 peptide is recognized in the context of DR1, DR4 and DR6. Furthermore, the DR2 molecule is capable of restricting T cell responses to multiple MBP epitopes (Chou *et al.*, 1989, 1991; Martin *et al.*, 1990; Jaraquemada *et al.*, 1990; Pette *et al.*, 1990*b*). In DR2$^+$ MS patients, both the DR2a and DR2b products function as restriction elements for MBP (Jaraquemada *et al.*, 1990; Pette *et al.*, 1990*b*). Valli *et al.* (1993) determined the binding of synthetic peptides spanning the entire human MBP sequence to ten purified HLA-DR molecules. All the peptides tested showed binding affinity for at least one of the DR molecules analysed, but three peptides (included in sequences 13–32, 84–103 and 144–163) were capable of binding to three or more DR molecules. Peptide 84–103 was the most degenerate in binding, in that it bound to eight out of the ten DR molecules tested. Notably it bound with highest affinity to DRB1*1501 and DRB1*0401 molecules. As DRB1*1501 is associated with an increased susceptibility to MS, Valli *et al.* concluded that their findings were consistent with a role for the 84–103 MBP peptide in the pathogenesis of MS. To correlate the binding pattern of MBP peptides to DR molecules with their recognition by T cells, they established MBP-specific T cell lines from the peripheral blood of MS patients, who were homozygous, heterozygous or negative for DRB1*1501. There was a good correlation between the binding data and T cell proliferation to MBP peptides. Although virtually all MBP peptides tested could be recognized by at least one T cell line from MS patients, there were three immunodominant epitopes, corresponding exactly to the peptides capable of binding to several DR molecules. These immunodominant epitopes correspond to the two demonstrated in earlier studies (see above) and a third previously suggested but undefined epitope in the N-terminal region (Martin *et al.*, 1990). No major difference was detected in the recognition of immunodominant MBP peptides by the lines from DRB1*1501 positive or negative MS patients (Valli *et al.*, 1993). Wucherpfennig *et al.* (1994) found that the 84–102 MBP peptide binds with high affinity to the DRB1*1501 and the DRB5*0101 molecules of the DRw15 haplotype, but that only DRB1 molecules served as restriction elements for a panel of T cell clones from two MS patients, suggesting that the complex of the 84–102 MBP peptide and DRB1 molecules is more immunogenic for MBP-reactive T cells. In a study on a multiplex family with MS, Voskuhl, Martin & McFarland (1993*a*) found no difference in the estimated precursor frequencies of MBP-specific T cell lines or peptide specificity of T cell lines when affected and unaffected siblings were compared. However, MBP-specific T cell lines from affected siblings were restricted to DRw15/DQw6 significantly more frequently than were those from unaffected siblings. A study of monozygotic twins discordant for MS revealed no significant differences in the frequency or HLA restriction patterns of MBP-specific T cells in affected and normal individuals but showed some differences in peptide specificity, indicating that, despite genetic identity, the MBP-specific T cell repertoire may be shaped differently (Martin *et al.*, 1993).

The finding of restricted TCR Vβ gene usage by encephalitogenic MBP-specific T cells in EAE (see Chapter 3) prompted studies to determine whether there was a similar restricted usage by MBP-specific T cells in MS, which could be exploited by selective anti-TCR therapy. Conflicting results have been obtained by different laboratories. Wucherpfennig *et al.* (1990) found that Vβ17 and to a lesser extent Vβ12 were frequently used by T cell lines reactive with the 84–102 peptide in different individuals, while Kotzin *et al.* (1991) reported a biased usage of Vβ5.2 and to a lesser extent Vβ6.1 by MBP-specific clones from MS patients but not controls. On the other hand, Ben Nun *et al.* (1991) demonstrated heterogeneous TCR Vβ gene usage among MBP-specific T cell clones from different individuals but a restricted usage among MBP-specific T cell clones of the same individual. Other studies have reported that the TCR Vα and Vβ gene usage by MBP-specific T cells in humans is highly heterogeneous, even among T cells that recognize the same region of MBP in association with the same DR molecule in the same individual (Richert *et al.*, 1991; Martin *et al.*, 1992; Giegerich *et al.*, 1992). An interesting recent finding is that identical twins discordant for MS use different Vα chains in the T cell recognition of MBP or tetanus toxoid, whereas twins concordant for MS and control twin sets use similar Vα chains (Utz *et al.*, 1993). The different Vα chain usage in twins discordant for MS was not due to a gap in the T cell repertoire, but could be due to skewing of the repertoire by either an environmental factor or the disease itself. As only two twin sets in each category were examined, further studies on other monozygotic twins will be needed to determine whether this is generally true.

In conclusion there is an increased frequency of activated MBP-specific T cells in the peripheral blood of MS patients. It is unknown whether these T cells are pathogenic, although the high-affinity binding of the immunodominant 84–102 MBP peptide to the MS-associated HLA-DRB1*1501 molecule supports a role for MBP-specific T cells in the pathogenesis of MS.

T cell reactivity to myelin proteolipid protein

As PLP is also encephalitogenic in laboratory animals (see Chapter 3), studies have been undertaken to determine whether autoreactivity to PLP contributes to the pathogenesis of MS. Trotter *et al.* (1991) have demonstrated significant T cell proliferative responses to PLP in the peripheral blood of six of 16 patients with rapid chronic progressive MS, three of 15 patients with clinically stable relapsing–remitting MS, none of 12 normal controls and one of ten patients with other neurological disease. T cells from the MS patients with positive responses to the whole protein also proliferated significantly in response to one or more of the PLP peptides 88–108, 103–116 and 139–154, which correspond to regions encephalitogenic in the rabbit (Linington, Gunn & Lassmann, 1990), SWR mouse (Tuohy *et al.*, 1988) and SJL/J mouse (Tuohy *et al.*, 1989). The findings of Trotter *et al.* (1991) are in contrast to those obtained in an earlier study, which demonstrated no significant T cell proliferative response to PLP in patients with active MS or normal controls, but significant responses in six of 16 patients with other neurological disease (Johnson *et al.*, 1986). Kerlero de Rosbo *et al.* (1993) did not find a significant increase in the T cell proliferative response to PLP in the peripheral blood of MS patients.

Using the limiting dilution assay, Chou *et al.* (1992) found no significant increase in the frequency of T cells reactive to PLP peptide 139–151 in the peripheral blood of MS patients. However, Zhang *et al.* (1994) demonstrated that after primary culture with IL-2 the frequency of PLP-reactive T cells was significantly higher in MS patients than in normal individuals, indicating that MS patients have an increased frequency of circulating *in vivo*-activated PLP-specific T cells. An increased frequency of T cells secreting IFN-γ in response to PLP has been found in the peripheral blood of MS patients compared to normal controls; however, these results are difficult to interpret, because of the relatively high background response and because no significant difference was found between MS patients and patients with other neurological diseases (J.B. Sun *et al.*, 1991). Using *in situ* hybridization with radiolabelled complementary DNA oligonucleotide probes, Link *et al.* (1994*a*,*b*) have demonstrated that, compared with patients with other neurological diseases, MS patients have increased numbers of peripheral blood mononuclear cells expressing IFN-γ, IL-4 and transforming growth factor-β mRNA after short-term culture in the presence of PLP. Pelfrey *et al.* (1993) used synthetic PLP peptides to generate T cell lines from the peripheral blood of MS patients. The lines were predominantly specific for the 40–60 PLP peptide and were CD4$^+$, cytotoxic and restricted by class II MHC molecules.

In conclusion, there is some evidence of increased T cell reactivity to PLP in the peripheral blood of MS patients, but further studies, particularly with synthetic peptides, are needed.

T cell reactivity to myelin/oligodendrocyte glycoprotein

The findings that antibodies against MOG augment demyelination in EAE, and that EAE can be transferred by a combination of MOG-specific T cells and MOG-specific antibodies (see Chapter 3) raise the possibility that MOG may be a target antigen in MS. J. Sun *et al.* (1991) found an increased frequency of T cells secreting IFN-γ in response to MOG in the peripheral blood of MS patients compared to controls. Kerlero de Rosbo *et al.* (1993) reported that the T cell proliferative response to MOG, but not to MBP, PLP or MAG, was significantly increased in the peripheral blood of MS patients compared to controls. Further studies are required to determine the role of MOG-specific T cells in the pathogenesis of MS.

T cell reactivity to myelin-associated glycoprotein

Johnson *et al.* (1986) demonstrated increased T cell proliferative responses to MAG in the peripheral blood of nine of 30 patients with active MS, two of ten patients with stable MS, one of seven patients with other neurological diseases and none of ten normal controls. Y. Zhang *et al.* (1993) found increased T cell proliferative responses to MAG in the peripheral blood of seven of 11 patients with MS and none of ten normal controls. In contrast, Kerlero de Rosbo *et al.* (1993) found no evidence of increased T cell proliferative responses to MAG in the peripheral blood of MS patients. Link *et al.* (1992) found a significantly increased frequency of peripheral blood T cells secreting IFN-γ in response to MAG in patients with MS compared to those with other neurological diseases but not compared to patients with tension headache. Further studies are needed to establish whether MAG-specific T cells have a role in the pathogenesis of MS.

T cell reactivity to other autoantigens

Cell-mediated immunity to human brain gangliosides as determined by the leukocyte migration inhibition test is significantly increased in the peripheral blood of patients with attacks of MS as compared to clinically stable MS patients, patients with other neurological diseases and normal controls (Beraud *et al.*, 1990). Increased $CD8^+$ T cell cytotoxicity towards cells coated with bovine brain gangliosides or cerebrosides has also been observed in patients with active MS compared to those with inactive MS (Frick, 1989).

Heat shock proteins are potential autoantigens because of their evolutionary conservation and immunogenicity. Peripheral blood T cell proliferative responses to mycobacterial hsp70, but not hsp65, are significantly more frequent in patients with MS than in patients with other neurological diseases or normal subjects (Salvetti *et al.*, 1992). Furthermore, the proportion of purified protein derivative-specific T cell lines that proliferate in response to hsp70 was found to be significantly higher in MS patients than in normal controls. $\gamma\delta$ T cells formed only a minority in nearly all the lines.

Specific suppressor or regulatory T cells

Zhang *et al.* (1992*b*) have generated, from MS patients, suppressor T cell lines specific for MBP-specific helper T cell clones. Most of the suppressor T cell lines were $CD4^+$ but one was $CD8^+$. The lines exhibited potent antigen-specific suppressor activity on the proliferation of MBP-specific T helper clones but not on T cell lines with other antigen specificity. The suppressor lines were weakly responsive to MBP and required the presence of autologous peripheral blood mononuclear cells for proliferation: the proliferation of $CD4^+$ suppressor lines was restricted by HLA-DR molecules, whereas that of the $CD8^+$ line was restricted by HLA class I molecules (Zhang *et al.*, 1992*b*). Further studies are required to determine whether such specific suppressor T cell activity differs in MS patients and controls. Anti-clonotypic cytotoxic $CD8^+$ T cells specific for MBP-reactive T cells have been isolated from the peripheral blood of MS patients vaccinated with irradiated autologous MBP-reactive T cells, but not from the blood of non-vaccinated MS patients (J. Zhang *et al.*, 1993). Furthermore, cytotoxic $CD4^+$ T cells specific for the TCR β chain of an autologous MBP-reactive T cell clone have been isolated from a normal subject (Saruhan Direskeneli *et al.*, 1993). Further studies are required to determine what function specific regulatory T cells have *in vivo*. Specific suppressor or regulatory T cells have also been isolated from rats recovering from EAE or protected against EAE by T cell vaccination or oral tolerance (see Chapter 3).

Antibody/B cell findings

Using a nitrocellulose immunospot assay, Olsson *et al.* (1990*a*) found no B cells producing antibodies against myelin or MBP in the peripheral blood of MS patients, although such cells were found in the CSF. With a different technique, Zhang *et al.* (1991) also found that the frequency of B cells producing anti-MBP antibodies was not increased in MS patients, although the frequency of B cells producing antibodies against measles virus was significantly increased. Patients with MS have a significantly higher frequency of peripheral blood cells producing anti-PLP IgG antibodies in the nitrocellulose immunospot assay compared to normal controls but not patients with other neurological diseases (J.B. Sun *et al.*, 1991). This assay has also shown an increased frequency of cells producing anti-MOG IgG antibodies in the peripheral blood of MS patients compared to controls (J. Sun *et al.*, 1991). Anti-MOG IgG antibodies have not been detected by enzyme-linked immunosorbent assay in the plasma of MS patients, although they are present in the CSF of some patients (Xiao, Linington & Link, 1991). Cells secreting IgG antibodies against MAG have been found in the peripheral blood of 20% of MS patients and only occasionally in controls (Baig *et al.*, 1991). With a sensitive solid-phase radioimmunoassay, Moller *et al.* (1989) could not detect an increase in anti-MAG antibodies in the sera of MS patients, although they found elevated levels in the CSF. Using an indirect immunofluorescence assay, Henneberg, Mayle & Kornhuber (1991) found antibodies to brain white matter in the sera of 33% of MS patients (73% of patients with active chronic progressive MS) and 3% of controls; however, the specific antigen(s) recognized by these antibodies was not determined. As mentioned earlier, circulating antibodies to the brain protein, β-arrestin 1, have been found in patients with MS, but not in controls (Ohguro *et al.*, 1993). Increased serum levels of IgG antibodies against endothelial cells have also been demonstrated in patients with MS, especially during an exacerbation (Tanaka *et al.*, 1987). Evidence for a more general systemic B cell activation in MS has been provided by the finding that patients without known intercurrent infection have higher numbers of antibody-secreting cells in both the bone marrow and the peripheral blood compared to normal controls (Fredrikson, Baig & Link, 1991).

Immune complexes

Serum immune complexes are increased in patient with MS, especially in those with active disease (Tanaka *et al.*, 1987; Procaccia *et al.*, 1988). The complexes have been found to contain IgG, IgM, IgA, complement components, β_2-microglobulin, anti-viral antibodies and sometimes viral antigens, and antibodies reactive to galactocerebroside and ganglioside (Coyle & Procyk Dougherty, 1984; Procaccia *et al.*, 1988). MBP or anti-MBP antibodies were found in the serum immune complexes of some MS patients in one study (Coyle & Procyk Dougherty, 1984), but MBP was not found in another study (Geffard, Boullerne & Brochet, 1993).

Monocytes

Baxevanis *et al.* (1989*a*) have found reduced HLA-DR antigen expression on peripheral blood monocytes from MS patients, especially those with active disease, and have concluded that this is responsible for the reduced AMLR (Baxevanis *et al.*, 1988) and reduced suppressor T cell activity

(Baxevanis *et al.*, 1990). In contrast, Armstrong *et al.* (1991) found normal HLA-DR antigen expression and increased HLA-DP and HLA-DQ antigen density on monocytes from patients with active MS. Increased HLA-DR expression has been demonstrated on blood monocytes from patients experiencing an increased frequency of exacerbations after intravenous administration of IFN-γ (Panitch *et al.*, 1987*b*). Other reported abnormalities of blood monocytes from patients with active MS include: an increased production of prostaglandin E in tissue culture (Dore Duffy *et al.*, 1986); increased levels of cellular cyclic AMP and reduced sensitivity to agents that stimulate prostaglandin E synthesis (Dore Duffy & Donovan, 1991); increased expression of the monocyte activation antigen Mo3 without increased HLA-DR expression (Dore Duffy, Donovan & Todd, 1992); increased spontaneous IL-6 secretion and intracellular IL-1β synthesis, and increased secretion of IL-1β after stimulation with T-cell-derived cytokines (Maimone, Reder & Gregory, 1993); and increased production of TNF-α, IL-1α, IL-1β and IL-6 after stimulation with lipopolysaccharide or phorbol ester (Imamura *et al.*, 1993). Reder *et al.* (1991) have suggested that prostaglandins secreted by monocytes may be responsible for the impairment of function of CD2 (the sheep red blood cell receptor) in peripheral blood T cells from MS patients. It is unclear whether the above changes in monocyte function are secondary to specific T cell activation or whether they are due to a primary abnormality of the monocyte.

Cytokines and adhesion molecules

Serum IL-2 levels are increased in patients with active MS, indicating systemic T cell activation (Gallo *et al.*, 1988, 1989*a*; Trotter *et al.*, 1988; Adachi, Kumamoto & Araki, 1989; Trotter, van der Veen & Clifford, 1990). However, serial studies on individual patients have shown no correlation between the level of serum IL-2 and clinical disease activity (Gallo *et al.*, 1991). Periodic bursts of increased serum IL-2 levels have been observed in patients with chronic progressive MS without associated sudden clinical worsening (Trotter *et al.*, 1990). Soluble IL-2R is released when T cells are activated and can be used as an index of T cell activation. Serum levels of soluble IL-2R are increased in patients with active MS (Adachi *et al.*, 1989; Gallo *et al.*, 1989*a*; Adachi, Kumamoto & Araki, 1990; Hartung *et al.*, 1990; Weller *et al.*, 1991; Chalon, Sindic & Laterre, 1993). However, serial studies on individual patients have shown no correlation between the serum level and clinical disease activity (Gallo *et al.*, 1991).

IL-6, a cytokine that promotes differentiation of B cells to antibody-secreting cells, is elevated in the sera of patients with MS, indicating systemic B cell activation (Frei *et al.*, 1991; Weller *et al.*, 1991; Shimada, Koh & Yanagisawa, 1993). Serum levels of soluble ICAM-1 are increased in

MS patients with clinically active disease or enhancing lesions on MRI, supporting a role for this adhesion molecule in the pathogenesis of MS (Hartung *et al.*, 1993; Tsukada *et al.*, 1993). Furthermore, in patients with an exacerbation of MS there is a positive correlation between serum soluble ICAM-1 and serum TNF-α levels (Tsukada *et al.*, 1993).

Immunological findings in the CSF

Non-specific T cell findings

A mild to moderate mononuclear pleocytosis is often present in the CSF in MS. The majority (80–90%) of cells are T lymphocytes (Brinkman *et al.*, 1983; Hauser *et al.*, 1983*b*). The proportion of T cells in the CSF is slightly increased compared to that in the peripheral blood, as it also is in normal controls (Hedlund, Sandberg Wollheim & Sjogren, 1989).

CD4 and CD8 expression

The $CD4^+$:$CD8^+$ ratio in the CSF in MS patients is about 2:1 (Brinkman *et al.*, 1983; Hauser *et al.*, 1983*b*). The proportion of $CD4^+$ T cells is increased and the proportion of $CD8^+$ T cells is decreased in the CSF compared to the peripheral blood (Antonen *et al.*, 1987; Matsui *et al.*, 1988; Hedlund *et al.*, 1989; Salmaggi *et al.*, 1989; Mix *et al.*, 1990; Scolozzi *et al.*, 1992). It appears that a similar difference in the proportions of $CD4^+$ T cells in the CSF and peripheral blood occurs in normal controls, but it is less clear whether this also applies to the difference in the proportions of $CD8^+$ T cells (Hedlund *et al.*, 1989). It is apparent that the decline in $CD8^+$ T cells in the peripheral blood (see above) is not accompanied by a sequestration of these cells in the CSF (Hauser *et al.*, 1983*b*). It has also been found that the proportion of $CD8^+$ T cells that are $CD11b^+$ (reportedly suppressor cells) is reduced in the CSF compared to the peripheral blood in active MS and non-inflammatory neurological diseases and compared to the CSF in other inflammatory neurological diseases (Salonen *et al.*, 1989; Matsui, Mori & Saida, 1990). Most of the $CD8^+$ T cells in the CSF in active MS are $CD11b^-$ (reportedly cytotoxic cells) (Salonen *et al.*, 1989). Soluble CD8 levels in the CSF are increased in MS compared to non-inflammatory neurological diseases, and the amount of soluble CD8 per CSF leukocyte is higher in MS than in other inflammatory neurological diseases (Maimone & Reder, 1991).

Expression of T cell activation markers

The proportion of $CD4^+$ cells that are $CD45RA^+$ (naive cells) is reduced in the CSF compared to the peripheral blood in patients with MS (Chofflon *et al.*, 1989; Hedlund *et al.*, 1989; Salonen *et al.*, 1989; Matsui *et al.*, 1990; Zaffaroni *et al.*, 1991); however, this CSF/peripheral blood differential is also found in patients with other neurological diseases and normal controls (Hedlund *et al.*, 1989; Salonen *et al.*, 1989; Matsui *et al.*, 1990). The fall in the proportion of $CD4^+CD45RA^+$ cells occurs in parallel with an increase in the proportion of $CD4^+CD45RO^+$ (memory) cells in the CSF compared with the peripheral blood (Hedlund *et al.*, 1989). Indeed, the majority of T cells in the CSF in MS patients, aseptic meningitis patients and healthy subjects are $CD45RO^+$ (Svenningsson *et al.*, 1993). An enrichment of memory cells has also been found in the CNS parenchyma in MS (Sobel *et al.*, 1988) and in EAE (see Chapter 3). T lymphocytes move rapidly from the peripheral blood into the CSF in progressive MS, as shown by the finding that 70% of T cells in the CSF are labelled by anti-CD2 monoclonal antibody 72–96 h after *in vivo* labelling of peripheral blood T cells with this antibody (Hafler & Weiner, 1987).

An increase in the proportion of $CD4^+CD29^+$ cells (reportedly memory cells) in the CSF compared to the peripheral blood has been found in parallel with the decrease in the proportion of $CD4^+CD45RA^+$ cells in the CSF compared to the peripheral blood in patients with MS and in normal controls (Chofflon *et al.*, 1989; Hedlund *et al.*, 1989). However, in one study it was found that there were decreases in the proportions of both $CD4^+CD29^+$ cells and $CD4^+CD45RA^+$ cells in the CSF in patients having exacerbations of MS compared to those with stable MS or non-inflammatory neurological disease (Marrosu, 1991).

Using flow cytometry to assess cell-cycle phase, Noronha *et al.* (1980, 1985) demonstrated activated cells and in particular activated $CD4^+$ T cells in the CSF in MS. Moreover, IL-$2R^+$ cells are enriched in the CSF compared to the peripheral blood (Bellamy *et al.*, 1985; Tournier Lasserve *et al.*, 1987; Scolozzi *et al.*, 1992). The proportion of T cells expressing HLA-DR molecules (a marker of T cell activation) is increased in the CSF compared to the peripheral blood in MS patients and normal controls (with tension headache) (Mix *et al.*, 1990). CSF T cells also express higher levels of very late activation antigens 3–6, LFA-1, LFA-3, CD2, CD26 and CD44 than do T cells in the peripheral blood in MS patients, aseptic meningitis patients and normal subjects, indicating that activated T cells selectively migrate to the CSF under both pathological and normal conditions (Svenningsson *et al.*, 1993).

Oligoclonal T cells (including $\gamma\delta$ cells)

Analysis of the rearranged TCR β chain and γ chain genes of T cells cloned from the CSF before *in vitro* expansion has shown oligoclonal T cells in some but not all patients with MS, but not in any patients with other neurological diseases (Hafler *et al.*, 1988*a*; Lee *et al.*, 1991). There was common usage of the TCR Vβ12 gene segment among four oligoclonal T cell populations derived from three patients with MS, suggesting that oligoclonal T cells might share similar specificities and that clonal expansion might have resulted from specific stimulation by an antigen. Furthermore, identical clones were found in the blood and CSF in three of nine patients (Lee *et al.*, 1991). Shimonkevitz *et al.* (1993) found clonal expansion of oligoclonal $\gamma\delta$ T cells in the CSF of patients with recent-onset MS, but not of patients with chronic MS or other neurological diseases.

Specific T cell findings

T cell reactivity to MBP

The proliferative response of CSF lymphocytes to MBP is increased in patients with clinically active MS compared to those with stable MS or patients with other neurological diseases (Lisak & Zweiman, 1977). Interestingly, the response of CSF lymphocytes to MBP is greater than that of peripheral blood lymphocytes in patients with clinically active MS, but not in patients with acute disseminated encephalomyelitis (Lisak & Zweiman, 1977). Chou *et al.* (1992) have found that 24% of IL-2/IL-4-reactive T cell isolates from the CSF of MS patients are MBP-specific compared to 3% of the corresponding isolates of patients with other neurological diseases. They also found that the frequency of MBP-reactive T cells in the CSF of MS patients is much higher than in the peripheral blood. Using limiting dilution analysis the same group found that, in contrast to the reactivity to intact MBP, the frequency in the CSF of T cells reactive to 'cryptic' epitopes of MBP is similar in MS and other neurological diseases (Satyanarayana *et al.*, 1993). Zhang *et al.* (1994) found that after culture with IL-2 the frequency of MBP-reactive T cells in the CSF of MS patients was more than tenfold higher than in the peripheral blood of the same patients. MBP-reactive T cells accounted for 7% of the IL-2-responsive cells in the CSF of MS patients but could not be detected among the IL-2-responsive cells in the CSF of patients with other neurological diseases (Zhang *et al.*, 1994). These T cells predominantly recognized MBP peptides 84–102 and 143–168. Increased frequencies of T cells secreting IFN-γ in response to MBP and MBP peptides have been found in the CSF of MS patients compared to the peripheral blood of MS patients and compared to the CSF of controls (Olsson *et al.*, 1990*b*; Soderstrom *et al.*, 1993); however, these results are confounded by the high background response. Cells expressing IFN-γ, IL-4 and transforming growth factor-β mRNA after short-term culture in the presence of MBP were found to be enriched in the CSF compared to the peripheral blood of MS patients; however, no comparison was made with CSF cells from controls (Link *et al.*, 1994*a*,*b*).

In conclusion, *in vivo*-activated MBP-specific T cells are enriched in the CSF of MS patients and occur at a substantially higher frequency than in patients with other neurological diseases. These findings are highly suggestive of a role for MBP-specific T cells in the pathogenesis of MS.

T cell reactivity to PLP

Chou *et al.* (1992) found that 13% of IL-2/IL-4-reactive T cell isolates from the CSF of MS patients recognized the PLP peptide 139–151 compared to 2% of the corresponding isolates of patients with other neurological diseases. They also found that the frequency of these T cells in the CSF of MS patients was much higher than in the peripheral blood. J.B. Sun *et al.* (1991) found an increased frequency of T cells secreting IFN-γ in response to PLP in the CSF of MS patients compared to the CSF of controls and compared to the peripheral blood of MS patients, but the high background response renders interpretation difficult. Cells expressing IFN-γ, IL-4 and transforming growth factor-β mRNA after short-term culture in the presence of PLP were found to be enriched in the CSF compared to the peripheral blood of MS patients; however, no comparison was made with CSF cells from controls (Link *et al.*, 1994*a*,*b*). These findings are suggestive of a role for PLP-reactive T cells in the pathogenesis of MS, but further studies are needed to establish this.

T cell reactivity to MOG, MAG and mycobacterial antigens

By counting cells secreting IFN-γ in response to antigen in short-term cultures, increased frequencies of MOG-reactive T cells and MAG-reactive T cells have been found in the CSF of MS patients compared to controls and compared to the peripheral blood of MS patients (J. Sun *et al.*, 1991; Link *et al.*, 1992). T cells proliferating in response to mycobacterial antigens are also enriched in the CSF of patients with MS, particularly those with disease of recent onset (Birnbaum, Kotilinek & Albrecht, 1993).

Non-specific antibody/B cell findings

A classical finding in the CSF in MS is the presence of oligoclonal IgG bands, which are not present in the serum (Link & Müller, 1971). This also occurs in other inflammatory diseases of the nervous system and indicates intrathecal synthesis of IgG. Intrathecal synthesis of IgG has also been demonstrated by calculating quantitative indices based on CSF and serum levels of albumin and IgG, but the most sensitive and specific method is isoelectric focusing, which detects oligoclonal IgG bands in 95% of cases of clinically definite MS (McLean *et al.*, 1990). Serial studies have indicated that the oligoclonal banding pattern in the CSF in MS remains stable over long periods (Walsh & Tourtellotte, 1986). The oligoclonal IgG is predominantly of the IgG1 subclass, but may also be of the IgG3, IgG2 and IgG4 subclasses in order of decreasing frequency (Losy, Mehta & Wisniewski, 1990). Intrathecal production of IgA and IgM also occurs in MS, as demonstrated by quantitative studies or by the detection of oligoclonal bands (Grimaldi *et al.*, 1985; Lolli, Halawa & Link, 1989; Sharief, Keir & Thompson, 1990; Sindic *et al.*, 1994). Oligoclonal IgM bands are more reliable than quantitative indices for detecting intrathecal production of IgM (Sharief *et al.*, 1990). Intrathecal synthesis of IgD has also been demonstrated in MS by calculation of index values (Lolli *et al.*, 1989; Sharief & Hentges, 1991*a*). The intrathecal synthesis of IgM and that of IgD have been found to correlate positively with MS relapse activity, CSF pleocytosis, and CSF/serum ratios of IL-2 and of soluble IL-2R (Sharief & Thompson, 1991; Sharief & Hentges, 1991*a*; Sharief, Hentges & Thompson, 1991). Furthermore, oligoclonal free kappa and free lambda light chains can be detected in the CSF by isoelectric focusing and immunoblotting in the majority of patients with MS and other inflammatory neurological disorders (Gallo *et al.*, 1989*b*; Sindic & Laterre, 1991).

The specificity of the major portion of the oligoclonal IgG in the CSF in MS has not been determined. In chronic relapsing EAE, oligoclonal IgG bands are present in the CSF; however, in contrast to the usual situation in MS, identical oligoclonal IgG band patterns are also found in the serum (see Chapter 3). This difference may be due to a more severe breakdown of the blood–brain barrier in EAE. In chronic relapsing EAE the predominant reactivity of the oligoclonal IgG is against CNS antigens, particularly MBP, whereas in MS there is little or no reactivity of oligoclonal IgG to CNS antigens (Mehta *et al.*, 1987; Cruz *et al.*, 1987).

The proportion of B cells that are $CD5^+$ (reportedly activated B cells) is significantly increased in the CSF of patients with relapsing–remitting MS compared to patients with chronic progressive MS and to patients with tension headache, but not compared to those with aseptic meningitis (Correale *et al.*, 1991). This proportion is higher in the CSF than in the peripheral blood of MS patients. It has been suggested that $CD5^+$ B cells in the CSF are responsible for the production of autoantibodies (Correale *et al.*, 1991).

Specific antibody/B cell findings

B cell reactivity to MBP

Cruz *et al.* (1987) found oligoclonal IgG antibody bands against MBP in the CSF of 32% of MS patients but not in the CSF of patients with other neurological diseases. Warren *et al.* (1994) detected elevated CSF anti-MBP antibodies in the vast majority of MS patients with clinically active disease and in a minority of MS patients in clinical remission. They also found anti-MBP antibodies in extracts from MS cerebral tissue and concluded that the most likely epitope of anti-MBP antibodies is located between residues 84 and 95 of human MBP (Warren & Catz, 1993).

However, studies of antibody levels in biological fluids, such as the CSF, may not accurately reflect a B cell response, as autoantibodies may bind to their target antigens, and catabolism *in vivo* may limit their detection. A new approach to studying the B cell response in MS has been provided by the use of the nitrocellulose immunospot assay. With this technique Olsson *et al.* (1990*a*) found that 79% of MS patients had CSF cells producing IgG antibodies against myelin, and 57% had CSF cells producing IgG antibodies against MBP. These cells comprised a large proportion of the total IgG-producing cells but were not detected in the peripheral blood. Cells producing IgG antibodies against myelin and MBP occurred at significantly lower frequencies in the CSF of patients with aseptic meningoencephalitis. The same group found a significantly higher frequency of cells secreting IgG antibodies against guinea pig MBP peptide 70–89, but not against three other MBP peptides or (in contrast to their earlier study) myelin, in the CSF of MS patients compared to patients with other neurological diseases, and concluded that the 70–89 peptide is an immunodominant B cell epitope in MS (Martino *et al.*, 1991). Cash *et al.* (1992) reported that CSF mononuclear cells from five of 11 patients with acute exacerbations of MS produced anti-MBP antibodies *in vitro* after stimulation with pokeweed mitogen, but did not find such reactivity in 20 patients with other neurological diseases.

Overall, these findings suggest that B cells producing anti-MBP antibodies in the CNS may play a role in the pathogenesis of MS.

B cell reactivity to PLP

Warren *et al.* (1994) found that a small percentage of patients with clinically active MS have an increase in anti-PLP antibodies, but not anti-MBP antibodies, in the CSF. J.B. Sun *et al.* (1991) found cells secreting IgG antibodies against PLP in the CSF of 82% of patients with MS. The frequency of these cells was significantly lower in patients with aseptic meningitis and other neurological diseases. In MS patients the cells were highly enriched in the CSF compared to the peripheral blood.

B cell reactivity to MOG

Anti-MOG IgG antibodies have been detected by enzyme-linked immunosorbent assay in the CSF (but not the plasma) of some patients with MS and less frequently in the CSF of patients with other neurological diseases (Xiao *et al.*, 1991). J. Sun *et al.* (1991) found cells secreting IgG antibodies against MOG in the CSF of eight of ten patients with MS. These cells occurred at a significantly higher frequency than in the CSF of controls. In MS patients they were highly enriched in the CSF compared to the peripheral blood.

B cell reactivity to MAG

Moller *et al.* (1989) observed a significant elevation of anti-MAG antibodies in the CSF, but not the serum, of patients with MS compared to patients with other neurological diseases and normal controls. Baig *et al.* (1991) found cells secreting IgG antibodies against MAG in the CSF of 48% of patients with MS. The frequency of these cells in the CSF in MS was higher than in other inflammatory and non-inflammatory neurological diseases and was higher than in the peripheral blood of MS patients. In the CSF from two of ten MS patients, anti-MAG and anti-MBP IgG-secreting cells were present concurrently (Baig *et al.*, 1991).

Antibodies to other autoantigens

Elevated levels of anti-galactocerebroside antibodies have been found in the CSF of 70% of MS patients and 50% of patients with other neurological diseases (Ichioka *et al.*, 1988). Zanetta *et al.* (1990) detected antibodies to the endogenous mannose-binding protein, cerebellar soluble lectin, in the CSF of 92% of MS patients and 16% of patients with other neurological diseases. Elevated levels of antibodies against many autoantigens expressed in non-neural tissues have also been found in the CSF of MS patients compared with normal controls and patients with other neurological diseases (Matsiota *et al.*, 1988).

Complement

Morgan, Campbell & Compston (1984) found a significant reduction in the level of C9 (terminal component of complement) in the CSF of patients with MS compared to controls with other neurological diseases, and concluded that this indicates intrathecal consumption of C9 due to formation of membrane attack complexes, which could contribute to CNS tissue damage in MS. In contrast, another study, which calculated the C9 index ([CSF C9/plasma C9] : [CSF albumin/plasma albumin]), concluded that there was intrathecal consumption of C9 in aseptic meningitis but not in MS (Halawa, Lolli & Link, 1989). Sanders *et al.* (1986) detected fluid-phase complement C5b–9 complexes in the CSF of 16 of 21 patients with MS and 13 of 14 patients with the Guillain–Barré syndrome and, at low concentrations, in the CSF of three of 11 patients with non-inflammatory CNS diseases. They suggested that terminal complement components may participate in nervous tissue damage in MS and the Guillain–Barré syndrome.

Cytokines

CSF levels of IL-2 are increased in patients with acute exacerbations of MS, compared to patients in remission, patients with chronic progressive MS and normal controls (Gallo *et al.*, 1988, 1989*a*; Sharief *et al.*, 1991; Sharief & Thompson, 1993). In patients with acute exacerbations of MS, the level of IL-2 is significantly higher in the CSF than in the serum, indicating intrathecal production (Sharief *et al.*, 1991). CSF/serum ratios of IL-2 correlate with intrathecal synthesis of IgM and that of IgD but not with that of IgG or IgA (Sharief *et al.*, 1991). There is conflicting evidence concerning the level of soluble IL-2R in the CSF in MS, with some groups reporting an increase, particularly in patients with acute exacerbations (Adachi *et al.*, 1990; Kittur *et al.*, 1990; Sharief *et al.*, 1991; Sharief & Thompson, 1993), and others finding it normal in all or nearly all patients (Gallo *et al.*, 1989*a*, 1991; Peter, Boctor & Tourtellotte, 1991; Fesenmeier *et al.*, 1991; Weller *et al.*, 1991; Chalon *et al.*, 1993). There are also conflicting reports regarding the level of IL-1β in the CSF, with one group detecting it in 53% of cases of active MS (Hauser *et al.*, 1990) and others finding it rarely or not at all (Maimone *et al.*, 1991; Peter *et al.*, 1991). CSF IL-6 levels are significantly higher in patients with MS than in normal controls and patients with non-inflammatory neurological diseases, but not than in patients with other inflammatory neurological diseases (Weller *et al.*, 1991; Maimone *et al.*, 1991; Frei *et al.*, 1991; Shimada *et al.*, 1993). Interestingly, Frei *et al.* (1991) found that MS patients had much higher levels of IL-6 in the plasma than in the CSF, but that patients with acute meningoencephalitis had much higher levels in the CSF than in the plasma.

TNF is increased in the CSF in MS compared to non-inflammatory neurological diseases (Hauser *et al.*, 1990; Maimone *et al.*, 1991; Sharief & Hentges, 1991*b*). The CSF level of TNF-α is significantly higher in chronic progressive MS than in stable MS (Sharief & Hentges, 1991*b*). In chronic progressive MS it is also significantly higher than the corresponding serum level, and correlates with the degree of disability and the rate of clinical progression (Sharief & Hentges, 1991*b*). These findings suggest that TNF-α is produced in the CNS in MS and that it may contribute to CNS tissue damage. TNF$^+$ cells have been detected in MS brain but not in normal brain (Hofman *et al.*, 1989).

In conclusion, IL-2 and TNF are likely to have important roles in promoting inflammation in MS, as is the case in EAE (see Chapter 3). The increased levels of IL-6 are consistent with the increased antibody production in MS.

Myelin basic protein

Antigenic material that is cross-reactive with MBP can be detected by radioimmunoassay in the CSF of patients with active myelin destruction caused by MS or other processes, such as CNS infarction (Cohen, Herndon & McKhann, 1976; Whitaker, 1977). MS patients with acute exacerbations have the highest levels, those with chronic progressive MS have slightly increased or normal levels, and clinically stable patients have normal levels (Cohen *et al.*, 1976; Whitaker, 1977; Whitaker & Herman, 1988). As the level of immunoreactive MBP in the CSF is a reliable indicator of active demyelination in MS, it may be used to monitor response to therapy. The sensitivity of the radioimmunoassay has been improved by using human MBP synthetic peptide 69–89 as a radioligand (Whitaker & Herman, 1988). An epitope in peptide 80–89 that shares a conformation with intact MBP appears to be a dominant epitope of MBP-like material in the CSF after CNS myelin injury (Whitaker & Herman, 1988). MBP-like material is also increased in the CSF during attacks of EAE (Rauch *et al.*, 1987). As MBP is also expressed in the PNS, the spinal root demyelination that commonly occurs in EAE (see Chapter 3) may contribute to this increase.

Transfer of neurological signs and CNS lesions to severe combined immunodeficiency mice

Saeki *et al.* (1992) transferred a disease characterized by paralysis, ataxia and inflammatory necrotic CNS lesions into severe combined immunodeficiency mice by the intracisternal injection of CSF cells from MS patients during exacerbation but not from MS patients during remission or from patients with cervical spondylosis. However, Hao *et al.* (1994) were unable to confirm this finding.

The role of viral and bacterial infection

For many years viruses have been incriminated in the pathogenesis of MS. No virus has been consistently isolated from the CNS of patients with MS and there is no convincing evidence that viral infection of the CNS itself plays a role in the development of MS. However, viral infection outside the nervous system might have a pathogenic role in MS by leading to the polyclonal activation of autoreactive T and/or B cells or, through molecular mimicry, to cross-reactivity against CNS autoantigens. Sibley, Bamford & Clark (1985) found that the exacerbation rate of MS was almost threefold higher at the time of common viral infections (two weeks before the onset of infection until five weeks afterwards) than at other times. This finding suggests that viral infections may trigger attacks of MS. Increased immune responses to a number of viruses have been reported in MS.

Measles virus

Anti-measles virus antibodies are produced intrathecally in MS (Norrby, 1978; Salmi *et al.*, 1983; Felgenhauer *et al.*, 1985; Dhib Jalbut *et al.*, 1990; Schadlich *et al.*, 1990). The intrathecal anti-viral response is not restricted to measles virus but is also directed against other viruses, including rubella, herpes zoster, parainfluenza, influenza, mumps and respiratory syncytial viruses (Norrby, 1978; Salmi *et al.*, 1983; Felgenhauer *et al.*, 1985; Schadlich *et al.*, 1990). Using the nitrocellulose immunospot assay, Baig *et al.* (1989) found cells secreting anti-measles virus IgG in the CSF of 88% of MS patients. They found a similar incidence and frequency of cells secreting IgG against herpes simplex virus in the CSF, but could not detect any cells secreting antibodies against these two viruses in the peripheral blood. However, using a different techique, another group found an increased frequency of peripheral blood B cells producing antibodies against measles virus in patients with MS (Zhang *et al.*, 1991). Dhib Jalbut *et al.* (1990) studied the antibody reactivity to purified measles virus polypeptides and concluded that the results were consistent with polyclonal B cell activation within the CNS, although a heightened response to the fusion polypeptide might also reflect cross-reactivity with a CNS autoantigen.

An unexplained finding in MS is the decreased generation, from the peripheral blood, of measles virus-specific and herpes simplex virus-specific cytotoxic T cells, which are predominantly restricted by HLA class II molecules (Jacobson, Flerlage & McFarland, 1985; de Silva & McFarland, 1991). In contrast, the generation of influenza virus-specific and mumps virus-specific cytotoxic T cell responses, which have large HLA class I-restricted components, is normal in MS (Jacobson *et al.*, 1985; Goodman, Jacobson & McFarland, 1989). Increased numbers of T cells secreting IFN-γ in response to measles virus and mumps virus have been found in the CSF, but not the blood, in MS compared to other neurological diseases (Link *et al.*, 1992); however, because of the high background response, these results are difficult to interpret.

Compston *et al.* (1986) reported that patients with inflammatory demyelinating diseases of the CNS had measles at a later age than HLA-DR matched normal controls, but the significance of this finding is unclear. Using the nested reverse transcription polymerase chain reaction, Godec *et al.* (1992) did not find measles virus genomic sequences in the brain of any of 19 MS patients. Another study using the polymerase chain reaction failed to detect measles virus genomic sequences in the peripheral blood lymphocytes of patients with MS (Bates *et al.*, 1993).

Epstein–Barr virus

The seropositivity rate and the titre of serum antibodies to Epstein–Barr virus (EBV) antigens is significantly higher in MS patients than in controls (Bray *et al.*, 1983; Larsen, Bloomer & Bray, 1985; Sumaya *et al.*, 1985). Larsen *et al.* (1985) found that the seropositivity rate was 100% in MS patients compared to 84% in controls. Furthermore, 85% of MS patients had CSF antibodies against EBV nuclear antigen-1 compared to 13% of EBV-seropositive controls (Bray *et al.*, 1992). A search of a protein sequence database revealed two pentapeptide identities between EBV nuclear antigen-1 and MBP; none of more than 32 000 other proteins in the database contained both pentapeptides (Bray *et al.*, 1992). This raises the possibility that EBV-specific T cells and antibodies might cross-react with MBP and contribute to the CNS tissue damage in MS. In a case–control study of 214 MS patients, recall of infectious mononucleosis in subjects seropositive for EBV capsid antigen was associated with a relative risk of 2.9 (Martyn, Cruddas & Compston, 1993). Those who reported having infectious mononucleosis before the age of 18 years had a relative risk of MS of 7.9. These epidemiological findings suggest that an age-dependent host response to EBV infection may have a role in the pathogenesis of MS.

Rubella virus

Anti-rubella virus antibodies are produced intrathecally in patients with MS (Norrby, 1978; Salmi *et al.*, 1983; Felgenhauer *et al.*, 1985; Schadlich *et al.*, 1990). As in the case of intrathecally produced anti-measles virus antibodies, this most probably represents polyclonal B cell activation within the CNS. However, Nath & Wolinsky (1990) found a relatively decreased IgG response to the rubella virus surface glycoprotein E1 and a relatively increased response to the surface glycoprotein E2 in the sera of MS patients compared to controls, and concluded that the response in MS is not simply due to polyclonal B cell activation. Patients with inflammatory CNS demyelinating disease were found to have had rubella at a later age than HLA-DR matched controls (Compston *et al.*, 1986), but the significance of this is unclear. Using the nested reverse transcription polymerase chain reaction, Godec *et al.* (1992) did not detect rubella viral genomic sequences in the brain of any of 19 MS patients.

Other viruses and bacteria

Koprowski *et al.* (1985) incriminated a retrovirus related to the human T cell lymphotropic viruses in the pathogenesis of MS. However, subsequent studies have found no evidence for a role of such a retrovirus in MS (Nishimura *et al.*, 1990; Ehrlich *et al.*, 1991). Although antibodies to human T cell lymphotropic virus-1 are slightly elevated in the sera of some patients with MS, this occurs in the absence of viral antigen and thus appears to be due to cross-reactivity (Shirazian *et al.*, 1993). A significant proportion of MS patients have CSF antibodies to the paramyxovirus, simian virus 5, but this is not specific for MS, as similar reactivity occurs in other neurological diseases where CSF oligoclonal banding is present (Goswami *et al.*, 1987; McLean & Thompson, 1989). Antibodies to human herpesvirus 6 are elevated in the sera of patients with MS, but viral DNA is rarely detected (Sola *et al.*, 1993; Wilborn *et al.*, 1994). Murray *et al.* (1992) detected coronavirus RNA by *in situ* hybridization in 12 of 22 MS brain samples and found coronavirus antigen by immunohistochemistry in two patients with rapidly progressive MS. However, the number of sections that were positive for coronavirus RNA was low (11%) and coronavirus RNA was also found in two of 21 controls. Further studies will be needed to confirm their findings and to determine how specific they are for MS.

Bacterial infections may also have a role in the pathogenesis of MS. Bacterial superantigens bind to certain TCR Vβ chains and MHC molecules and can thereby activate T cells using the fitting Vβ chains. Burns *et al.* (1992) showed that superantigenic staphylococcal toxins can activate human MBP-specific T cells and PLP-specific T cells, and suggested that toxins produced during bacterial infections may thereby contribute to the induction or exacerbation of MS. Staphylococcal superantigens can trigger relapses of EAE by activating MBP-specific T cells (see Chapter 3).

In conclusion, there is epidemiological evidence that viral infections may contribute to the pathogenesis of MS; however, there is no convincing evidence that viral infection of the CNS itself is involved. The elevation of anti-viral antibody levels in the sera or CSF appears to be mainly due to polyclonal activation resulting from the MS disease process or perhaps to an underlying disorder of immunoregulation. Viral infections may induce anti-viral immune responses that cross-react with myelin antigens, but the extent to which this contributes to the pathogenesis of MS is unclear. Conversely, some apparent anti-viral responses may actually represent cross-reactive responses driven by myelin antigens. Viral infections may trigger attacks of MS by non-specifically activating the immune system or by interfering with immunoregulation, but there is no direct evidence to support these hypotheses. An interesting possibility requiring further study is that bacterial infections may trigger attacks of MS through superantigenic activation of autoreactive T cells.

Therapy

Therapy in MS may be divided into (1) therapy of the disease process and (2) symptomatic therapy. Symptomatic therapy has an important role in the management of patients with MS and entails the use of drugs for the treatment of such problems as spasticity, pain, paroxysmal phenomena, tremor and urinary difficulties (Pender, 1992). It will not be discussed further here. Therapy of the disease process is directed at inhibiting the immune attack on the nervous system, and embraces a range of different approaches which generally have been inspired by research findings in EAE.

Oral administration of myelin

As the oral administration of MBP or myelin prevents EAE (oral tolerance) (see Chapter 3), Weiner *et al.* (1993) conducted a double-blind pilot study of oral myelin therapy in relapsing–remitting MS. The proportion of patients having exacerbations was lower in the myelin-treated group than in the placebo-treated group. However, in view of the small number of patients studied, conclusions about efficacy cannot be drawn from these data, and a more extensive clinical trial will be required to evaluate this treatment.

Vaccination with T cells, and anti-TCR therapy

As vaccination with attenuated MBP-specific T cells protects animals against EAE (see Chapter 3), preliminary studies of this therapy have been conducted in patients with MS. Subcutaneous inoculation of MS patients with irradiated autologous MBP-reactive T cells was found to induce a proliferative T cell response to the inoculates and a correlated decrease in the frequency of MBP-reactive T cells (J. Zhang *et al.*, 1993). T cells that specifically inhibited the proliferative response of the inoculates to MBP could be detected in the vaccinated MS patients but not in non-vaccinated ones. The majority of T cell lines responding to the inoculates were $CD8^+$, with a minority being $CD4^+$. The $CD8^+$ lines were specifically cytotoxic for the inoculates in an HLA class I-restricted manner. J. Zhang *et al.* (1993) concluded that clonotypic interactions regulating autoreactive T cells can be induced in humans by T cell vaccination. It will be important to determine whether this therapy can inhibit clinical disease activity in MS.

The observation of restricted TCR $V\beta$ gene usage by MBP-specific T cells in mice and rats led to the finding that anti-$V\beta8$ monoclonal antibodies or immunization with a synthetic TCR $V\beta8$ peptide can inhibit EAE (see Chapter 3). On the basis of the observation that there is a preferential usage of TCR $V\beta5.2$ and $V\beta6.1$ genes by MBP-reactive T cells in some patients with MS, MS patients have been immunized with synthetic peptides encompassing the second complementarity-determining regions of Vβ5.2 and Vβ6.1 (Bourdette *et al.*, 1994; Chou *et al.*, 1994). Some of the inoculated patients developed a T cell response to the TCR peptides. Further studies will be needed to determine whether this therapy has any effect on disease activity. Potential limitations of this approach are suggested by the generally heterogeneous TCR Vβ gene usage by human MBP-specific T cells (see above) and the finding that TCR peptide therapy can also aggravate EAE (Desquenne Clark *et al.*, 1991; Sun, 1992).

Anti-CD4 antibody

As anti-CD4 antibody therapy inhibits EAE (see Chapter 3), preliminary studies of this therapy have been conducted in MS (Hafler *et al.*, 1988*b*). Anti-CD4 or anti-CD2 murine monoclonal antibody infusions were found to inhibit *in vitro* immune responses; however, repeated infusions induced anti-mouse antibodies with anti-idiotypic-like activity that could block binding of the anti-T-cell monoclonal antibody to the T cell surface (Hafler *et al.*, 1988*b*).

Cop 1

Cop 1 is a synthetic basic random copolymer of L-alanine, L-glutamic acid, L-lysine and L-tyrosine with a molecular weight of 21 000 and with immunological cross-reactivity with MBP (Teitelbaum *et al.*, 1991). As it inhibits EAE (see Chapter 3), it has been suggested as a possible therapy for MS. In a double-blind, randomized, placebo-controlled pilot trial, Bornstein *et al.* (1987) observed that subcutaneous cop 1 reduced the number of exacerbations in relapsing–remitting MS. A more extensive clinical trial is in progress. Cop 1 has been observed to inhibit the responses of MBP-specific human T cell lines and clones to MBP, suggesting that it can compete with MBP for the binding to human HLA molecules (Teitelbaum *et al.*, 1992; Racke *et al.*, 1992); however, in another study it had no such effect (Burns & Littlefield, 1991).

ACTH and corticosteroids

In 1950 Moyer *et al.* found that adrenocorticotrophic hormone (ACTH) prevented acute EAE when administered after inoculation and before the onset of neurological signs. The corticosteroid, methylprednisolone has a similar effect (Kibler, 1965). Furthermore, ACTH and methylprednisolone each reverse the neurological signs of EAE when administered after the onset of signs (Gammon & Dilworth, 1953; Vogel, Paty & Kibler, 1972).

Moyer *et al.* (1950) suggested that ACTH or a corticosteroid might have a beneficial effect in the human diseases, post-vaccination encephalitis and acute MS. It was subsequently shown that, compared with placebo, intramuscular ACTH hastens neurological improvement after a relapse of MS (Rose *et al.*, 1970). High-dose intravenous methylprednisolone therapy accelerates recovery from relapses (Durelli *et al.*, 1986; Milligan, Newcombe & Compston, 1987) and is as effective as intramuscular ACTH (Thompson *et al.*, 1989). Although oral corticosteroids are often used in clinical practice to treat attacks of MS, they have not been demonstrated by placebo-controlled trials to be effective. Indeed, in acute optic neuritis, oral prednisone therapy was found to have no beneficial effect and appeared to increase the risk of new episodes of optic neuritis when compared to placebo, whereas high-dose intravenous methylprednisolone followed by a short course of oral prednisone accelerated recovery, resulted in slightly better vision six months later and had no effect on the recurrence of optic neuritis (Beck *et al.*, 1992). Interestingly, high-dose intravenous methylprednisolone therapy followed by a short course of oral prednisone for acute optic neuritis was also found to reduce the rate of development of MS over a two-year period (Beck *et al.*, 1993). Further studies are needed to determine whether this important observation can be confirmed. Long-term treatment with ACTH or corticosteroids has not been shown to have a beneficial effect on the course of MS.

High-dose intravenous methylprednisolone therapy reduces intrathecal IgG synthesis, the level of MBP in the CSF, and gadolinium enhancement of MRI brain lesions, but has no effect on the oligoclonal IgG pattern in the CSF (Durelli *et al.*, 1986; Warren *et al.*, 1986; Wajgt *et al.*, 1989; Burnham *et al.*, 1991; Barkhof *et al.*, 1992; Frequin *et al.*, 1992). As the MRI appearance of increased water content in normal-appearing white matter is also reduced by this therapy, it has been suggested that the clinical improvement is due to resolution of oedema (Kesselring *et al.*, 1989). However, an alternative explanation for the beneficial clinical effect is inhibition of immune-mediated demyelination (Pender, 1992), as indicated by the reduction in the level of MBP in the CSF.

Immunosuppressants

Cyclophosphamide

Treatment with high-dose intravenous cyclophosphamide plus ACTH has been reported to stabilize or improve progressive MS (Hauser *et al.*, 1983*a*), although a randomized, placebo-controlled, single-masked trial found that therapy with intravenous cyclophosphamide plus oral prednisone had no such effect (Canadian Cooperative Multiple Sclerosis Study Group, 1991).

Intensive immunosuppression with cyclophosphamide in combination with prednisone has been reported to decrease the level of MBP in the CSF in chronic progressive MS, indicating that it may inhibit demyelination (Lamers *et al.*, 1988). This therapy or high-dose cyclophosphamide alone was also found to decrease intrathecal IgG synthesis (Lamers *et al.*, 1988; Wajgt *et al.*, 1989). As cyclophosphamide can aggravate EAE as well as inhibit it (see Chapter 3), it is possible that cyclophosphamide may aggravate MS in some patients.

Cyclosporin A

Long-term cyclosporin A therapy has been found to have a modest effect in delaying disease progression in patients with moderately severe progressive MS (Multiple Sclerosis Study Group, 1990). However, this therapy has a high incidence of severe adverse effects, particularly renal impairment and hypertension, and its use requires close supervision. As low-dose cyclosporin A therapy converts acute EAE into chronic relapsing EAE (Polman *et al.*, 1988; Pender *et al.*, 1990), the possibility that cyclosporin A may aggravate MS in some patients needs to be considered (Pender, 1991).

Azathioprine

Long-term azathioprine therapy appears to have a small beneficial effect on MS, but the effect is so small that adverse effects preclude its routine use (British and Dutch Multiple Sclerosis Azathioprine Trial Group, 1988).

Total lymphoid irradiation

In a randomized double-blind study, patients with chronic progressive MS treated with total lymphoid irradiation (1980 cGy) had significantly less functional decline than those receiving sham-irradiation (Cook *et al.*, 1986). There was a significant relationship between the absolute blood lymphocyte count in the first year after total lymphoid irradiation and the subsequent course, patients with higher lymphocyte counts generally having a worse prognosis.

Interferon-γ

Intravenous IFN-γ therapy increases the exacerbation rate in MS and is therefore unsuitable for the treatment of this disease (Panitch *et al.*, 1987*a*). The number of circulating monocytes expressing HLA-DR molecules increased during therapy, particularly in those patients who had exacerbations. In contrast to MS, EAE is inhibited by IFN-γ and aggravated by anti-

IFN-γ therapy (see Chapter 3). Why IFN-γ has different effects on MS and EAE is unknown.

Interferon-β

In a randomized, double-blind, placebo-controlled trial, long-term subcutaneous IFN-β therapy significantly reduced the exacerbation rate in relapsing–remitting MS compared with placebo (IFNB Multiple Sclerosis Study Group, 1993). As there was little change in disability from baseline in both the placebo and treatment arms of the trial, it could not be determined whether IFN-β therapy had any effect on disability. A concomitant study found a significant reduction in disease activity as determined by MRI and a significant reduction in MRI-detected burden of disease in the patients receiving IFN-β compared to those receiving placebo (Paty *et al.*, 1993). Further studies are required to determine whether IFN-β therapy has any effect on clinical disability in relapsing–remitting MS and whether it has any beneficial effect on chronic progressive MS. IFN-β significantly augments *in vitro* non-specific suppressor cell function in progressive MS and in normal subjects (Noronha, Toscas & Jensen, 1990, 1992). IFN-α has a similar effect, whereas IFN-γ has no effect (Noronha *et al.*, 1992). IFN-β has also been reported to inhibit IFN-γ-induced HLA-DR gene transcription in a human astrocytoma cell line, but not to inhibit IFN-γ-induced HLA-DR expression in human monocytes (Ransohoff *et al.*, 1991). Furthermore, *in vitro* IFN-β inhibits mitogen-induced proliferation, IL-2R expression and IFN-γ production by peripheral blood mononuclear cells of MS patients and normal controls (Noronha, Toscas & Jensen, 1993; Rudick *et al.*, 1993). In a pilot study it was found that mitogen-driven IL-2R expression on peripheral blood T cells was reduced in patients with relapsing–remitting MS after IFN-β therapy but not after placebo (Rudick *et al.*, 1993). These actions of IFN-β may account for the beneficial clinical effect in relapsing–remitting MS. Alternatively, the anti-viral action of IFN-β may be responsible for the beneficial effect, as viral infections may trigger attacks of MS (Sibley *et al.*, 1985).

Conclusions

There is now convincing evidence that MS is an autoimmune disease. It has been clearly demonstrated by twin studies that there is a major genetic contribution to MS susceptibility, although at present the only confirmed genetic factor predisposing to MS is the HLA-DR-DQ haplotype DRw15,DQw6,Dw2 (DRB1*1501-DQA1*0102-DQB1*0602). The increased association of MS with other autoimmune diseases in the same individual and in family members suggests that a primary autoimmune gene(s) may also be involved, but further studies are needed to determine this. The CNS lesions of MS are characterized by primary demyelination and infiltration by T cells, macrophages and B cells, as is the case in EAE. As MBP, PLP and MOG are target antigens in EAE, immune responses to these antigens have been studied in patients with MS. There is good evidence that the frequency of *in vivo*-activated MBP-specific T cells is increased in both the peripheral blood and CSF and that MBP-specific B cell reactivity is increased in the CSF of MS patients. However, it is unknown whether these increased immune responses are pathogenic. There is also some evidence of increased T cell and B cell reactivity to PLP, MOG and MAG. A major question is whether the target antigen in MS is the same in all patients and at all stages of disease. It is possible that the initial target antigen may differ among patients and that additional antigens may be targeted in the same patient as the disease progresses. If the autoimmune process in MS is driven by a single antigen, it may be possible to treat the disease by tolerization with the appropriate antigen. However, at present there is no therapy that has been proven to prevent the progression of disability in MS. Further advances in the understanding of the pathogenesis of MS and autoimmunity in general may lead to the development of such a therapy.

References

Adachi, K., Kumamoto, T. & Araki, S. (1989). Interleukin-2 receptor levels indicating relapse in multiple sclerosis. *Lancet*, **1**, 559–60.

Adachi, K., Kumamoto, T. & Araki, S. (1990). Elevated soluble interleukin-2 receptor levels in patients with active multiple sclerosis. *Annals of Neurology*, **28**, 687–91.

Allegretta, M., Nicklas, J.A., Sriram, S. & Albertini, R.J. (1990). T cells responsive to myelin basic protein in patients with multiple sclerosis. *Science*, **247**, 718–21.

Antel, J., Bania, M., Noronha, A. & Neely, S. (1986). Defective suppressor cell function mediated by T8+ cell lines from patients with progressive multiple sclerosis. *Journal of Immunology*, **137**, 3436–9.

Antel, J., Brown, M., Nicholas, M.K., Blain, M., Noronha, A. & Reder, A. (1988). Activated suppressor cell function in multiple sclerosis – clinical correlations. *Journal of Neuroimmunology*, **17**, 323–30.

Antel, J.P., Arnason, B.G.W. & Medof, M.E. (1979). Suppressor cell function in multiple sclerosis: correlation with clinical disease activity. *Annals of Neurology*, **5**, 338–42.

Antel, J.P., Bania, M.B., Reder, A. & Cashman, N. (1986*a*). Activated suppressor cell dysfunction in progressive multiple sclerosis. *Journal of Immunology*, **137**, 137–41.

Antel, J.P., Freedman, M.S., Brodovsky, S., Francis, G.S. & Duquette, P. (1989). Activated suppressor cell function in severely disabled patients with multiple sclerosis. *Annals of Neurology*, **25**, 204–7.

Antel, J.P., Nicholas, M.K., Bania, M.B., Reder, A.T., Arnason, B.G. & Joseph, L. (1986*b*). Comparison of T8+ cell-mediated suppressor and cytotoxic functions in multiple sclerosis. *Journal of Neuroimmunology*, **12**, 215–24.

Antonen, J., Syrjala, P., Oikarinen, R., Frey, H. & Krohn, K. (1987). Acute multiple sclerosis exacerbations are characterized by low cerebrospinal fluid suppressor/cytotoxic T-cells. *Acta Neurologica Scandinavica*, **75**, 156–60.

Archambeau, P.L., Hollenhorst, R.W. & Rucker, C.W. (1965). Posterior uveitis as a manifestation of multiple sclerosis. *Mayo Clinic Proceedings*, **40**, 544–51.

Armstrong, M.A., Crockard, A.D., Hawkins, S.A., Gamble, L.A., Shah, S. & Bell, A.L. (1991). Class II major histocompatibility complex antigen expression on unstimulated and gamma-interferon stimulated monocytes from patients with multiple sclerosis, rheumatoid arthritis and normal controls. *Autoimmunity*, **9**, 261–8.

Arnold, D.L., Matthews, P.M., Francis, G.S., O'Connor, J. & Antel, J.P. (1992). Proton magnetic resonance spectroscopic imaging for metabolic characterization of demyelinating plaques. *Annals of Neurology*, **31**, 235–41.

Baig, S., Olsson, O., Olsson, T., Love, A., Jeansson, S. & Link, H. (1989). Cells producing antibody to measles and herpes simplex virus in cerebrospinal fluid and blood of patients with multiple sclerosis and controls. *Clinical and Experimental Immunology*, **78**, 390–5.

Baig, S., Olsson, T., Yu Ping, J., Hojeberg, B., Cruz, M. & Link, H. (1991). Multiple sclerosis: cells secreting antibodies against myelin-associated glycoprotein are present in cerebrospinal fluid. *Scandinavian Journal of Immunology*, **33**, 73–9.

Baker, H.W.G., Balla, J.I., Burger, H.G., Ebeling, P. & Mackay, I.R. (1972). Multiple sclerosis and autoimmune diseases. *Australian and New Zealand Journal of Medicine*, **2**, 256–60.

Bamford, C.R., Ganley, J.P., Sibley, W.A. & Laguna, J.F. (1978). Uveitis, perivenous sheathing and multiple sclerosis. *Neurology*, **28**, 119–24.

Barkhof, F., Frequin, S.T.F.M., Hommes, O.R., Lamers, K., Scheltens, P., van Geel, W.J.A. & Valk, J. (1992). A correlative triad of gadolinium-DTPA MRI, EDSS, and CSF-MBP in relapsing multiple sclerosis patients treated with high-dose intravenous methylprednisolone. *Neurology*, **42**, 63–7.

Barnes, D., Munro, P.M., Youl, B.D., Prineas, J.W. & McDonald, W.I. (1991). The longstanding MS lesion. A quantitative MRI and electron microscopic study. *Brain*, **114**, 1271–80.

Bates, P.R., McCombe, P.A., Sheean, G.L., Cooksley, W.G.E. & Pender, M.P. (1993). Failure to detect measles virus sequences in lymphocytes of patients with multiple sclerosis. *Australian and New Zealand Journal of Medicine*, **23**, 55.

Baxevanis, C.N., Reclos, G.J., Arsenis, P., Anastasopoulos, E., Katsiyiannis, A., Lymberi, P., Matikas, N. & Papamichail, M. (1989*a*). Decreased expression of HLA-DR antigens on monocytes in patients with multiple sclerosis. *Journal of Neuroimmunology*, **22**, 177–83.

Baxevanis, C.N., Reclos, G.J., Arsenis, P., Katsiyiannis, A., Matikas, N. & Papamichail, M. (1988). Monocyte defect causes decreased autoMLR in multiple sclerosis patients. *Advances in Experimental Medicine and Biology*, **237**, 839–42.

Baxevanis, C.N., Reclos, G.J. & Papamichail, M. (1990). Decreased HLA-DR antigen expression on monocytes causes impaired suppressor cell activity in multiple sclerosis. *Journal of Immunology*, **144**, 4166–71.

Baxevanis, C.N., Reclos, G.J., Servis, C., Anastasopoulos, E., Arsenis, P., Katsiyiannis, A., Matikas, N., Lambris, J.D. & Papamichail, M. (1989*b*). Peptides of myelin basic protein stimulate T lymphocytes from patients with multiple sclerosis. *Journal of Neuroimmunology*, **22**, 23–30.

Beall, S.S., Biddison, W.E., McFarlin, D.E., McFarland, H.F. & Hood, L.E. (1993). Susceptibility for multiple sclerosis is determined, in part, by inheritance of a 175-kb region of the TcR V beta chain locus and HLA class II genes. *Journal of Neuroimmunology*, **45**, 53–60.

Beall, S.S., Concannon, P., Charmley, P., McFarland, H.F., Gatti, R.A., Hood, L.E., McFarlin, D.E. & Biddison, W.E. (1989). The germline repertoire of T cell receptor beta-chain genes in patients with chronic progressive multiple sclerosis. *Journal of Neuroimmunology*, **21**, 59–66.

Beck, R.W., Cleary, P.A., Anderson, M.M.J., Keltner, J.L., Shults, W.T., Kaufman, D.I., Buckley, E.G., Corbett, J.J., Kupersmith, M.J., Miller, N.R. *et al.* (1992). A randomized, controlled trial of corticosteroids in the treatment of acute optic neuritis. *New England Journal of Medicine*, **326**, 581–8.

Beck, R.W., Cleary, P.A., Trobe, J.D., Kaufman, D.I., Kupersmith, M.J., Paty, D.W., Brown, C.H. & the Optic Neuritis Study Group (1993). The effect of corticosteroids for acute optic neuritis on the subsequent development of multiple sclerosis. *New England Journal of Medicine*, **329**, 1764–9.

Bellamy, A.S., Calder, V.L., Feldmann, M. & Davison, A.N. (1985). The distribution of interleukin-2 receptor bearing lymphocytes in multiple sclerosis: evidence for a key role of activated lymphocytes. *Clinical and Experimental Immunology*, **61**, 248–56.

Ben Nun, A., Liblau, R.S., Cohen, L., Lehmann, D., Tournier Lasserve, E., Rosenzweig, A., Zhang, J.W., Raus, J.C. & Bach, M.A. (1991). Restricted T-cell receptor V beta gene usage by myelin basic protein-specific T-cell clones in multiple sclerosis: predominant genes vary in individuals. *Proceedings of the National Academy of Sciences USA*, **88**, 2466–70.

Beraud, E., Golstein, M.M., Viallet, F., Sela, B.A., Galibert, R., Durbec, J.P., Khalil, R., Gastaut, J.L., Richard, P., Roux, H. *et al.* (1990). Multiple sclerosis: cell-mediated immunity to human brain gangliosides. *Autoimmunity*, **6**, 13–21.

Bias, W.B., Reveille, J.D., Beaty, T.H., Meyers, D.A. & Arnett, F.C. (1986). Evidence that autoimmunity in man is a mendelian dominant trait. *American Journal of Human Genetics*, **39**, 584–602.

Birnbaum, G., Kotilinek, L. & Albrecht, L. (1993). Spinal fluid lymphocytes from a subgroup of multiple sclerosis patients respond to mycobacterial antigens. *Annals of Neurology*, **34**, 18–24.

Booss, J., Esiri, M.M., Tourtellotte, W.W. & Mason, D.Y. (1983). Immunohistological analysis of T lymphocyte subsets in the central nervous system in chronic progressive multiple sclerosis. *Journal of the Neurological Sciences*, **62**, 219–32.

Bornstein, M.B., Miller, A., Slagle, S., Weitzman, M., Crystal, H., Drexler, E., Keilson, M., Merriam, A., Wassertheil Smoller, S., Spada, V. *et al.* (1987). A pilot trial of Cop 1 in exacerbating-remitting multiple sclerosis. *New England Journal of Medicine*, **317**, 408–14.

Bostock, H. & Grafe, P. (1985). Activity-dependent excitability changes in normal and demyelinated rat spinal root axons. *Journal of Physiology*, **365**, 239–57.

Bostock, H. & Sears, T.A. (1978). The internodal axon membrane: electrical excitability and continuous conduction in segmental demyelination. *Journal of Physiology*, **280**, 273–301.

Bourdette, D.N., Whitham, R.H., Chou, Y.K., Morrison, W.J., Atherton, J., Kenny, C., Liefeld, D., Hashim, G.A., Offner, H. & Vandenbark, A.A. (1994). Immunity to TCR peptides in multiple sclerosis. I. Successful immunization of patients with synthetic V beta 5.2 and V beta 6.1 CDR2 peptides. *Journal of Immunology*, **152**, 2510–19.

Boylan, K.B., Takahashi, N., Paty, D.W., Sadovnick, A.D., Diamond, M., Hood, L.E. & Prusiner, S.B. (1990). DNA length polymorphism 5′ to the myelin basic protein gene is associated with multiple sclerosis. *Annals of Neurology*, **27**, 291–7.

Boyle, E.A. & McGeer, P.L. (1990). Cellular immune response in multiple sclerosis plaques. *American Journal of Pathology*, **137**, 575–84.

Bö, L., Mörk, S., Kong, P.A., Nyland, H., Pardo, C.A. & Trapp, B.D. (1994). Detection of MHC class II-antigens on macrophages and microglia, but not on astrocytes and endothelia in active multiple sclerosis lesions. *Journal of Neuroimmunology*, **51**, 135–46.

Bray, P.F., Bloomer, L.C., Salmon, V.C., Bagley, M.H. & Larsen, P.D. (1983). Epstein–Barr virus infection and antibody synthesis in patients with multiple sclerosis. *Archives of Neurology*, **40**, 406–8.

Bray, P.F., Luka, J., Culp, K.W. & Schlight, J.P. (1992). Antibodies against Epstein–Barr nuclear antigen (EBNA) in multiple sclerosis CSF, and two pentapeptide sequence identities between EBNA and myelin basic protein. *Neurology*, **42**, 1798–804.

Breger, B.C. & Leopold, I.H. (1966). The incidence of uveitis in multiple sclerosis. *American Journal of Ophthalmology*, **62**, 540–5.

Brenner, R.E., Munro, P.M., Williams, S.C., Bell, J.D., Barker, G.J., Hawkins, C.P., Landon, D.N. & McDonald, W.I. (1993). The proton NMR spectrum in acute EAE: the significance of the change in the Cho:Cr ratio. *Magnetic Resonance in Medicine*, **29**, 737–45.

Briant, L., Avoustin, P., Clayton, J., McDermott, M., Clanet, M., Cambon Thomsen, A. & the French Group on Multiple Sclerosis (1993). Multiple sclerosis susceptibility: population and twin study of polymorphisms in the T-cell receptor β and γ genes region. *Autoimmunity*, **15**, 67–73.

Brinkman, C.J., Nillesen, W.M. & Hommes, O.R. (1983). T-cell subpopulations in blood and cerebrospinal fluid of multiple sclerosis patients: effect of cyclophosphamide. *Clinical Immunology and Immunopathology*, **29**, 341–8.

Brinkman, C.J., Nillesen, W.M., Hommes, O.R., Lamers, K.J., de Pauw, B.E. & Delmotte, P. (1982). Cell-mediated immunity in multiple sclerosis as determined by sensitivity of different lymphocyte populations to various brain tissue antigens. *Annals of Neurology*, **11**, 450–5.

British and Dutch Multiple Sclerosis Azathioprine Trial Group (1988). Double-masked trial of azathioprine in multiple sclerosis. *Lancet*, **2**, 179–83.

Bullington, S.J. & Waksman, B.H. (1958). Uveitis in rabbits with experimental allergic encephalomyelitis. Results produced by injection of nervous tissue and adjuvants. *Archives of Ophthalmology*, **59**, 435–45.

Burnham, J.A., Wright, R.R., Dreisbach, J. & Murray, R.S. (1991). The effect of high-dose steroids on MRI gadolinium enhancement in acute demyelinating lesions. *Neurology*, **41**, 1349–54.

Burns, J. & Littlefield, K. (1991). Failure of copolymer I to inhibit the human T-cell response to myelin basic protein. *Neurology*, **41**, 1317–19.

Burns, J., Littlefield, K., Gill, J. & Trotter, J.L. (1992). Bacterial toxin superantigens activate human T lymphocytes reactive with myelin autoantigens. *Annals of Neurology*, **32**, 352–7.

Burns, J., Littlefield, K., Gomez, C. & Kumar, V. (1991). Assessment of antigenic determinants for the human T cell response against myelin basic protein using overlapping synthetic peptides. *Journal of Neuroimmunology*, **31**, 105–13.

Canadian Cooperative Multiple Sclerosis Study Group (1991). The Canadian cooperative trial of cyclophosphamide and plasma exchange in progressive multiple sclerosis. *Lancet*, **337**, 441–6.

Cash, E., Weerth, S., Voltz, R. & Kornhuber, M. (1992). Cells of cerebrospinal fluid of multiple sclerosis patients secrete antibodies to myelin basic protein *in vitro*. *Scandinavian Journal of Immunology*, **35**, 695–701.

Cendrowski, W. (1989). [Multiple sclerosis and psoriasis]. *Wiadomosci Lekarskie*, **42**, 575–8.

Chalon, M.P., Sindic, C.J. & Laterre, E.C. (1993). Serum and CSF levels of soluble interleukin-2 receptors in MS and other neurological diseases: a reappraisal. *Acta Neurologica Scandinavica*, **87**, 77–82.

Chofflon, M., Weiner, H.L., Morimoto, C. & Hafler, D.A. (1988). Loss of functional suppression is linked to decreases in circulating suppressor inducer (CD4+ 2H4+) T cells in multiple sclerosis. *Annals of Neurology*, **24**, 185–91.

Chofflon, M., Weiner, H.L., Morimoto, C. & Hafler, D.A. (1989). Decrease of suppressor inducer (CD4+2H4+) T cells in multiple sclerosis cerebrospinal fluid. *Annals of Neurology*, **25**, 494–9.

Chou, Y.K., Bourdette, D.N., Offner, H., Whitham, R., Wang, R.Y., Hashim, G.A. & Vandenbark, A.A. (1992). Frequency of T cells specific for myelin basic protein and myelin proteolipid protein in blood and cerebrospinal fluid in multiple sclerosis. *Journal of Neuroimmunology*, **38**, 105–13.

Chou, Y.K., Henderikx, P., Vainiene, M., Whitham, R., Bourdette, D., Chou, C.H., Hashim, G., Offner, H. & Vandenbark, A.A. (1991). Specificity of human T cell clones reactive to immunodominant epitopes of myelin basic protein. *Journal of Neuroscience Research*, **28**, 280–90.

Chou, Y.K., Morrison, W.J., Weinberg, A.D., Dedrick, R., Whitham, R., Bourdette, D.N., Hashim, G., Offner, H. & Vandenbark, A.A. (1994). Immunity to TCR peptides in multiple sclerosis. II. T cell recognition of V beta 5.2 and V beta 6.1 CDR2 peptides. *Journal of Immunology*, **152**, 2520–9.

Chou, Y.K., Vainiene, M., Whitham, R., Bourdette, D., Chou, C.H., Hashim, G., Offner, H. & Vandenbark, A.A. (1989). Response of human T lymphocyte lines to myelin basic protein: association of dominant epitopes with HLA class II restriction molecules. *Journal of Neuroscience Research*, **23**, 207–16.

Cohen, S.R., Herndon, R.M. & McKhann, G.M. (1976). Radioimmunoassay of myelin basic protein in spinal fluid. An index of active demyelination. *New England Journal of Medicine*, **295**, 1455–7.

Compston, A. (1988). The 150th anniversary of the first depiction of the lesions of multiple sclerosis. *Journal of Neurology, Neurosurgery and Psychiatry*, **51**, 1249–52.

Compston, D.A., Morgan, B.P., Campbell, A.K., Wilkins, P., Cole, G., Thomas, N.D. & Jasani, B. (1989). Immunocytochemical localization of the terminal complement complex in multiple sclerosis. *Neuropathology and Applied Neurobiology*, **15**, 307–16.

Compston, D.A., Vakarelis, B.N., Paul, E., McDonald, W.I., Batchelor, J.R. & Mims, C.A. (1986). Viral infection in patients with multiple sclerosis and HLA-DR matched controls. *Brain*, **109**, 325–44.

Cook, S.D., Devereux, C., Troiano, R., Hafstein, M.P., Zito, G., Hernandez, E., Lavenhar, M., Vidaver, R. & Dowling, P.C. (1986). Effect of total lymphoid irradiation in chronic progressive multiple sclerosis. *Lancet*, **1**, 1405–9.

Correale, J., Mix, E., Olsson, T., Kostulas, V., Fredrikson, S., Hojeberg, B. & Link, H. (1991). $CD5^+$ B cells and $CD4^-8^-$ T cells in neuroimmunological diseases. *Journal of Neuroimmunology*, **32**, 123–32.

Corrigan, E., Hutchinson, M. & Feighery, C. (1990). Fluctuations in T helper subpopulations in relapsing-remitting multiple sclerosis. *Acta Neurologica Scandinavica*, **81**, 443–7.

Coyle, P.K. & Procyk Dougherty, Z. (1984). Multiple sclerosis immune complexes: an analysis of component antigens and antibodies. *Annals of Neurology*, **16**, 660–7.

Crockard, A.D., McNeill, T.A., McKirgan, J. & Hawkins, S.A. (1988). Determination of activated lymphocytes in peripheral blood of patients with multiple sclerosis. *Journal of Neurology, Neurosurgery and Psychiatry*, **51**, 139–41.

Cruz, M., Olsson, T., Ernerudh, J., Hojeberg, B. & Link, H. (1987). Immunoblot detection of oligoclonal anti-myelin basic protein IgG antibodies in cerebrospinal fluid in multiple sclerosis. *Neurology*, **37**, 1515–19.

Cuzner, M.L., Hayes, G.M., Newcombe, J. & Woodroofe, M.N. (1988). The nature of inflammatory components during demyelination in multiple sclerosis. *Journal of Neuroimmunology*, **20**, 203–9.

Davie, C.A., Hawkins, C.P., Barker, G.J., Brennan, A., Tofts, P.S., Miller, D.H. & McDonald, W.I. (1993). Detection of myelin breakdown products by proton magnetic resonance spectroscopy. *Lancet*, **341**, 630–1.

Davie, C.A., Hawkins, C.P., Barker, G.J., Brennan, A., Tofts, P.S., Miller, D.H. & McDonald, W.I. (1994). Serial proton magnetic resonance spectroscopy in acute multiple sclerosis lesions. *Brain*, **117**, 49–58.

De Keyser, J. (1988). Autoimmunity in multiple sclerosis. *Neurology*, **38**, 371–4.

de Silva, S.M. & McFarland, H.F. (1991). Multiple sclerosis patients have reduced HLA class II-restricted cytotoxic responses specific for both measles and herpes virus. *Journal of Neuroimmunology*, **35**, 219–26.

Desquenne Clark, L., Esch, T.R., Otvos, L.J. & Heber Katz, E. (1991). T-cell receptor peptide immunization leads to enhanced and chronic experimental allergic encephalomyelitis. *Proceedings of the National Academy of Sciences USA*, **88**, 7219–23.

Dhib Jalbut, S., Lewis, K., Bradburn, E., McFarlin, D.E. & McFarland, H.F. (1990). Measles virus polypeptide-specific antibody profile in multiple sclerosis. *Neurology*, **40**, 430–5.

Doolittle, T., Myers, R., McDermott, T. & Hauser, S. (1990). Familial aggregation of autoimmune disease in multiplex multiple sclerosis kindreds. *Annals of Neurology*, **28**, 275–6.

Dore Duffy, P., Donaldson, J.O., Koff, T., Longo, M. & Perry, W. (1986). Prostaglandin release in multiple sclerosis: correlation with disease activity. *Neurology*, **36**, 1587–90.

Dore Duffy, P. & Donovan, C. (1991). Functional desensitization of monocytes from patients with multiple sclerosis due to prostaglandin E. *Clinical Immunology and Immunopathology*, **61**, 119–28.

Dore Duffy, P., Donovan, C. & Todd, R.F. (1992). Expression of monocyte activation antigen Mo3 on the surface of peripheral blood monocytes from patients with multiple sclerosis. *Neurology*, **42**, 1609–14.

Durelli, L., Cocito, D., Riccio, A., Barile, C., Bergamasco, B., Baggio, G.F., Perla, F., Delsedime, M., Gusmaroli, G. & Bergamini, L. (1986). High-dose intravenous methylprednisolone in the treatment of multiple sclerosis: clinical-immunologic correlations. *Neurology*, **36**, 238–43.

Ebers, G.C., Bulman, D.E., Sadovnick, A.D., Paty, D.W., Warren, S., Hader, W., Murray, T.J., Seland, T.P., Duquette, P., Grey, T., Nelson, R., Nicolle, M. & Brunet, D. (1986). A population-based study of multiple sclerosis in twins. *New England Journal of Medicine*, **315**, 1638–42.

Ehrlich, G.D., Glaser, J.B., Bryz Gornia, V., Maese, J., Waldmann, T.A., Poiesz, B.J., Greenberg, S.J. & the HTLV-MS Working Group (1991). Multiple sclerosis, retroviruses, and PCR. *Neurology*, **41**, 335–43.

Eoli, M., Ferrarini, M., Dufour, A., Heltaj, S., Bevilacqua, L., Comi, G., Cosi, V., Filippini, G., Martinelli, V., Milanese, C. *et al.* (1993). Presence of T-cell subset abnormalities in newly diagnosed cases of multiple sclerosis and relationship with short-term clinical activity. *Journal of Neurology*, **240**, 79–82.

Esiri, M.M. (1980). Multiple sclerosis: a quantitative and qualitative study of immunoglobulin-containing cells in the central nervous system. *Neuropathology and Applied Neurobiology*, **6**, 9–21.

Esiri, M.M. & Reading, M.C. (1987). Macrophage populations associated with multiple sclerosis plaques. *Neuropathology and Applied Neurobiology*, **13**, 451–65.

Felgenhauer, K., Schadlich, H.J., Nekic, M. & Ackermann, R. (1985). Cerebrospinal fluid virus antibodies. A diagnostic indicator for multiple sclerosis? *Journal of the Neurological Sciences*, **71**, 291–9.

Ferraro, A. & Jervis, G.A. (1940). Experimental disseminated encephalopathy in the monkey. *Archives of Neurology and Psychiatry*, **43**, 195–209.

Fesenmeier, J.T., Whitaker, J.N., Herman, P.K. & Walker, D.P. (1991). Cerebrospinal fluid levels of myelin basic protein-like material and soluble interleukin-2 receptor in multiple sclerosis. *Journal of Neuroimmunology*, **34**, 77–80.

Fog, T. & Bardram, M. (1953). Experimentel dissemineret encefalomyelitis cg iridocyclitis hos grise. *Nordisk Medicin*, **49**, 851–5.

Fredrikson, S., Baig, S. & Link, H. (1991). Immunoglobulin producing cells in bone marrow and blood of patients with multiple sclerosis and controls. *Journal of Neurology, Neurosurgery and Psychiatry*, **54**, 412–14.

Freedman, M.S., Buu, N.N., Ruijs, T.C., Williams, K. & Antel, J.P. (1992). Differential expression of heat shock proteins by human glial cells. *Journal of Neuroimmunology*, **41**, 231–8.

Freedman, M.S., Ruijs, T.C., Selin, L.K. & Antel, J.P. (1991). Peripheral blood gamma-delta T cells lyse fresh human brain-derived oligodendrocytes. *Annals of Neurology*, **30**, 794–800.

Frei, K., Fredrikson, S., Fontana, A. & Link, H. (1991). Interleukin-6 is elevated in plasma in multiple sclerosis. *Journal of Neuroimmunology*, **31**, 147–53.

Frequin, S.T., Barkhof, F., Lamers, K.J., Hommes, O.R. & Borm, G.F. (1992). CSF myelin basic protein, IgG and IgM levels in 101 MS patients before and after treatment with high-dose intravenous methylprednisolone. *Acta Neurologica Scandinavica*, **86**, 291–7.

Frick, E. (1989). Immunological studies of the pathogenesis of multiple sclerosis. Cell-mediated cytotoxicity by peripheral blood lymphocytes against basic protein of myelin, encephalitogenic peptide, cerebrosides and gangliosides. *Acta Neurologica Scandinavica*, **79**, 1–11.

Fugger, L., Sandberg Wollheim, M., Morling, N., Ryder, L.P. & Svejgaard, A. (1990). The germline repertoire of T-cell receptor beta chain genes in patients with relapsing/remitting multiple sclerosis or optic neuritis. *Immunogenetics*, **31**, 278–80.

Gallo, P., Piccinno, M., Pagni, S. & Tavolato, B. (1988). Interleukin-2 levels in serum and cerebrospinal fluid of multiple sclerosis patients. *Annals of Neurology*, **24**, 795–7.

Gallo, P., Piccinno, M.G., Pagni, S., Argentiero, V., Giometto, B., Bozza, F. & Tavolato, B. (1989*a*). Immune activation in multiple sclerosis: study of IL-2, sIL-2R, and gamma-IFN levels in serum and cerebrospinal fluid. *Journal of the Neurological Sciences*, **92**, 9–15.

Gallo, P., Piccinno, M.G., Tavolato, B. & Siden, A. (1991). A longitudinal study on IL-2, sIL-2R, IL-4 and IFN-gamma in multiple sclerosis CSF and serum. *Journal of the Neurological Sciences*, **101**, 227–32.

Gallo, P., Tavolato, B., Bergenbrant, S. & Siden, A. (1989*b*). Immunoglobulin light chain patterns in the cerebrospinal fluid. A study with special reference to the occurrence of free light chains in cerebrospinal fluid with and without oligoclonal immunoglobulin G. *Journal of the Neurological Sciences*, **94**, 241–53.

Gambi, D., Porrini, A.M., Giampietro, A. & Macor, S. (1991). CD21+ (B2 antigen+) cell decrement and CD4+CD29+ (helper-inducer) cell increment suggest an activation of cell immune reactivity in multiple sclerosis. *Journal of Neuroimmunology*, **33**, 97–102.

Gammon, G.A. & Dilworth, M.J. (1953). Effect of corticotropin on paralysis of experimental allergic encephalomyelitis. *Archives of Neurology and Psychiatry*, **69**, 649.

Geffard, M., Boullerne, A. & Brochet, B. (1993). Seric immune complexes in multiple sclerosis do not contain MBP epitopes. *Brain Research Bulletin*, **30**, 365–8.

Gerritse, K., Deen, C., Fasbender, M., Ravid, R., Boersma, W. & Claassen, E. (1994). The involvement of specific anti myelin basic protein antibody-forming cells in multiple sclerosis immunopathology. *Journal of Neuroimmunology*, **49**, 153–9.

Ghatak, N.R., Leshner, R.T., Price, A.C. & Felton, W.L. (1989). Remyelination in the human central nervous system. *Journal of Neuropathology and Experimental Neurology*, **48**, 507–18.

Giegerich, G., Pette, M., Meinl, E., Epplen, J.T., Wekerle, H. & Hinkkanen, A. (1992). Diversity of T cell receptor alpha and beta chain genes expressed by human T cells specific for similar myelin basic protein peptide/major histocompatibility complexes [published erratum appears in *Eur J Immunol* 1992 May;**22**(5):1331]. *European Journal of Immunology*, **22**, 753–8.

Godec, M.S., Asher, D.M., Murray, R.S., Shin, M.L., Greenham, L.W., Gibbs, C.J.J. & Gajdusek, D.C. (1992). Absence of measles, mumps, and rubella viral genomic sequences from multiple sclerosis brain tissue by polymerase chain reaction. *Annals of Neurology*, **32**, 401–4.

Goodman, A.D., Jacobson, S. & McFarland, H.F. (1989). Virus-specific cytotoxic T lymphocytes in multiple sclerosis: a normal mumps virus response adds support for a distinct impairment in the measles virus response. *Journal of Neuroimmunology*, **22**, 201–9.

Goswami, K.K., Randall, R.E., Lange, L.S. & Russell, W.C. (1987). Antibodies against the paramyxovirus SV5 in the cerebrospinal fluids of some multiple sclerosis patients. *Nature*, **327**, 244–7.

Graham, E.M., Francis, D.A., Sanders, M.D. & Rudge, P. (1989). Ocular inflammatory changes in established multiple sclerosis. *Journal of Neurology, Neurosurgery and Psychiatry*, **52**, 1360–3.

Grimaldi, L.M., Roos, R.P., Nalefski, E.A. & Arnason, B.G. (1985). Oligoclonal IgA bands in multiple sclerosis and subacute sclerosing panencephalitis. *Neurology*, **35**, 813–17.

Haegert, D.G. & Francis, G.S. (1992). Contribution of a single DQ beta chain residue to multiple sclerosis in French Canadians. *Human Immunology*, **34**, 85–90.

Hafler, D.A., Buchsbaum, M. & Weiner, H.L. (1985*a*). Decreased autologous mixed lymphocyte reaction in multiple sclerosis. *Journal of Neuroimmunology*, **9**, 339–47.

Hafler, D.A., Chofflon, M., Kurt Jones, E. & Weiner, H.L. (1991). Interleukin-1 corrects the defective autologous mixed lymphocyte response in multiple sclerosis. *Clinical Immunology and Immunopathology*, **58**, 115–25.

Hafler, D.A., Duby, A.D., Lee, S.J., Benjamin, D., Seidman, J.G. & Weiner, H.L. (1988*a*). Oligoclonal T lymphocytes in the cerebrospinal fluid of patients with multiple sclerosis [published erratum appears in *J Exp Med* 1988 Jul 1;**168**(1):459]. *Journal of Experimental Medicine*, **167**, 1313–22.

Hafler, D.A., Fox, D.A., Manning, M.E., Schlossman, S.F., Reinherz, E.L. & Weiner, H.L. (1985*b*). *In vivo* activated T lymphocytes in the peripheral blood and cerebrospinal fluid of patients with multiple sclerosis. *New England Journal of Medicine*, **312**, 1405–11.

Hafler, D.A., Ritz, J., Schlossman, S.F. & Weiner, H.L. (1988*b*). Anti-CD4 and anti-CD2 monoclonal antibody infusions in subjects with multiple sclerosis. Immunosuppressive effects and human anti-mouse responses. *Journal of Immunology*, **141**, 131–8.

Hafler, D.A. & Weiner, H.L. (1987). *In vivo* labeling of blood T cells: rapid traffic into cerebrospinal fluid in multiple sclerosis. *Annals of Neurology*, **22**, 89–93.

Halawa, I., Lolli, F. & Link, H. (1989). Terminal component of complement C9 in CSF and plasma of patients with MS and aseptic meningitis. *Acta Neurologica Scandinavica*, **80**, 130–5.

Hanefeld, F., Bauer, H.J., Christen, H.J., Kruse, B., Bruhn, H. & Frahm, J. (1991). Multiple sclerosis in childhood: report of 15 cases. *Brain and Development*, **13**, 410–16.

Hao, Q., Saida, T., Kawakami, H., Mine, H., Maruya, E., Inoko, H. & Saji, H. (1992). HLAs and genes in Japanese patients with multiple sclerosis: evidence for increased frequencies of HLA-Cw3, HLA-DR2, and HLA-DQB1*0602. *Human Immunology*, **35**, 116–24.

Hao, Q., Saida, T., Nishimura, M., Ozawa, K. & Saida, K. (1994). Failure to transfer multiple sclerosis into severe combined immunodeficiency mice by mononuclear cells from CSF of patients. *Neurology*, **44**, 163–5.

Harding, A.E., Sweeney, M.G., Miller, D.H., Mumford, C.J., Kellar Wood, H., Menard, D., McDonald, W.I. & Compston, D.A. (1992). Occurrence of a multiple sclerosis-like illness in women who have a Leber's hereditary optic neuropathy mitochondrial DNA mutation. *Brain*, **115**, 979–89.

Hartung, H.P., Hughes, R.A., Taylor, W.A., Heininger, K., Reiners, K. & Toyka, K.V. (1990). T cell activation in Guillain–Barré syndrome and in MS: elevated serum levels of soluble IL-2 receptors. *Neurology*, **40**, 215–18.

Hartung, H.P., Michels, M., Reiners, K., Seeldrayers, P., Archelos, J.J. & Toyka, K.V. (1993). Soluble ICAM-1 serum levels in multiple sclerosis and viral encephalitis. *Neurology*, **43**, 2331–5.

Hauser, S.L., Bhan, A.K., Gilles, F., Kemp, M., Kerr, C. & Weiner, H.L. (1986). Immunohistochemical analysis of the cellular infiltrate in multiple sclerosis lesions. *Annals of Neurology*, **19**, 578–87.

Hauser, S.L., Dawson, D.M., Lehrich, J.R., Beal, M.F., Kevy, S.V., Propper, R.D., Mills, J.A. & Weiner, H.L. (1983*a*). Intensive immunosuppression in progressive multiple sclerosis. A randomized, three-arm study of high-dose intravenous cyclophosphamide, plasma exchange, and ACTH. *New England Journal of Medicine*, **308**, 173–80.

Hauser, S.L., Doolittle, T.H., Lincoln, R., Brown, R.H. & Dinarello, C.A. (1990). Cytokine accumulations in CSF of multiple sclerosis patients: frequent detection of interleukin-1 and tumor necrosis factor but not interleukin-6. *Neurology*, **40**, 1735–9.

Hauser, S.L., Reinherz, E.L., Hoban, C.J., Schlossman, S.F. & Weiner, H.L. (1983*b*). CSF cells in multiple sclerosis: monoclonal antibody analysis and relationship to peripheral blood T-cell subsets. *Neurology*, **33**, 575–9.

Hayashi, T., Morimoto, C., Burks, J.S., Kerr, C. & Hauser, S.L. (1988). Dual-label immunocytochemistry of the active multiple sclerosis lesion: major histocompatibility complex and activation antigens. *Annals of Neurology*, **24**, 523–31.

Hayes, G.M., Woodroofe, M.N. & Cuzner, M.L. (1987). Microglia are the major cell type expressing MHC class II in human white matter. *Journal of the Neurological Sciences*, **80**, 25–37.

Hedlund, G., Sandberg Wollheim, M. & Sjogren, H.O. (1989). Increased proportion of $CD4^+CDw29^+CD45R^-UCHL\text{-}1^+$ lymphocytes in the cerebrospinal fluid of both multiple sclerosis patients and healthy individuals. *Cellular Immunology*, **118**, 406–12.

Henneberg, A., Mayle, D.M. & Kornhuber, H.H. (1991). Antibodies to brain tissue in sera of patients with chronic progressive multiple sclerosis. *Journal of Neuroimmunology*, **34**, 223–7.

Hillert, J. (1993). Immunoglobulin gamma constant gene region polymorphisms in multiple sclerosis. *Journal of Neuroimmunology*, **43**, 9–14.

Hillert, J., Gronning, M., Nyland, H., Link, H. & Olerup, O. (1992*a*). An immunogenetic heterogeneity in multiple sclerosis. *Journal of Neurology, Neurosurgery and Psychiatry*, **55**, 887–90.

Hillert, J., Kall, T., Vrethem, M., Fredrikson, S., Ohlson, M. & Olerup, O. (1994). The HLA-Dw2 haplotype segregates closely with multiple sclerosis in multiplex families. *Journal of Neuroimmunology*, **50**, 95–100.

Hillert, J., Leng, C. & Olerup, O. (1991). No association with germline T cell receptor beta-chain gene alleles or haplotypes in Swedish patients with multiple sclerosis. *Journal of Neuroimmunology*, **32**, 141–7.

Hillert, J., Leng, C. & Olerup, O. (1992*b*). T-cell receptor alpha chain germline gene polymorphisms in multiple sclerosis. *Neurology*, **42**, 80–4.

Hillert, J. & Olerup, O. (1993). HLA and MS. *Neurology*, **43**, 2426–7.

Hirsch, R.L. (1986). Defective autologous mixed lymphocyte reactivity in multiple sclerosis. *Clinical and Experimental Immunology*, **64**, 107–13.

Hofman, F.M., von Hanwehr, R.I., Dinarello, C.A., Mizel, S.B., Hinton, D. & Merrill, J.E. (1986). Immunoregulatory molecules and IL 2 receptors identified in multiple sclerosis brain. *Journal of Immunology*, **136**, 3239–45.

Hofman, F.M., Hinton, D.R., Johnson, K. & Merrill, J.E. (1989). Tumor necrosis factor identified in multiple sclerosis brain. *Journal of Experimental Medicine*, **170**, 607–12.

Hughes, P.J., Kirk, P.F. & Compston, D.A. (1989). Dual labelling of circulating CD8 cells in patients with multiple sclerosis. *Journal of Neurology, Neurosurgery and Psychiatry*, **52**, 118–21.

Hvas, J., Oksenberg, J.R., Fernando, R., Steinman, L. & Bernard, C.C. (1993). Gamma delta T cell receptor repertoire in brain lesions of patients with multiple sclerosis. *Journal of Neuroimmunology*, **46**, 225–34.

Ichioka, T., Uobe, K., Stoskopf, M., Kishimoto, Y., Tennekoon, G. & Tourtellotte, W.W. (1988). Anti-galactocerebroside antibodies in human cerebrospinal fluids determined by enzyme-linked immunosorbent assay (ELISA). *Neurochemical Research*, **13**, 203–7.

IFNB Multiple Sclerosis Study Group (1993). Interferon beta-1b is effective in relapsing-remitting multiple sclerosis. I. Clinical results of a multicenter, randomized, double-blind, placebo-controlled trial. *Neurology*, **43**, 655–61.

Ilonen, J., Surcel, H.M., Jagerroos, H., Nurmi, T. & Reunanen, M. (1990). T-lymphocyte subsets defined by double immunofluorescence in multiple sclerosis. *Acta Neurologica Scandinavica*, **81**, 128–30.

Imamura, K., Suzumura, A., Hayashi, F. & Marunouchi, T. (1993). Cytokine production by peripheral blood monocytes/macrophages in multiple sclerosis patients. *Acta Neurologica Scandinavica*, **87**, 281–5.

Ioppoli, C., Meucci, G., Mariotti, S., Martino, E., Lippi, A., Gironelli, L., Pinchera, A. & Muratorio, A. (1990). Circulating thyroid and gastric parietal cell autoantibodies in patients with multiple sclerosis. *Italian Journal of Neurological Sciences*, **11**, 31–6.

Jacobson, S., Flerlage, M.L. & McFarland, H.F. (1985). Impaired measles virus-specific cytotoxic T cell responses in multiple sclerosis. *Journal of Experimental Medicine*, **162**, 839–50.

Jaraquemada, D., Martin, R., Rosen Bronson, S., Flerlage, M., McFarland, H.F. & Long, E.O. (1990). HLA-DR2a is the dominant restriction molecule for the cytotoxic T cell response to myelin basic protein in DR2Dw2 individuals. *Journal of Immunology*, **145**, 2880–5.

Jersild, C., Fog, T., Hansen, G.S., Thomsen, M., Svejgaard, A. & Dupont, B. (1973). Histocompatibility determinants in multiple sclerosis, with special reference to clinical course. *Lancet*, **2**, 1221–5.

Johnson, D., Hafler, D.A., Fallis, R.J., Lees, M.B., Brady, R.O., Quarles, R.H. & Weiner, H.L. (1986). Cell-mediated immunity to myelin-associated glycoprotein, proteolipid protein, and myelin basic protein in multiple sclerosis. *Journal of Neuroimmunology*, **13**, 99–108.

Johnson, M.D., Lavin, P. & Whetsell, W.O.J. (1990). Fulminant monophasic multiple sclerosis, Marburg's type. *Journal of Neurology, Neurosurgery and Psychiatry*, **53**, 918–21.

Jones, R.E., Bourdette, D., Offner, H. & Vandenbark, A.A. (1992). The synthetic 87–99 peptide of myelin basic protein is encephalitogenic in Buffalo rats. *Journal of Neuroimmunology*, **37**, 203–12.

Karaszewski, J.W., Reder, A.T., Anlar, B. & Arnason, B.G. (1993). Increased high affinity beta-adrenergic receptor densities and cyclic AMP responses of CD8 cells in multiple sclerosis. *Journal of Neuroimmunology*, **43**, 1–7.

Karaszewski, J.W., Reder, A.T., Anlar, B., Kim, W.C. & Arnason, B.G. (1991). Increased lymphocyte beta-adrenergic receptor density in progressive multiple sclerosis is specific for the $CD8^+$, $CD28^-$ suppressor cell. *Annals of Neurology*, **30**, 42–7.

Karaszewski, J.W., Reder, A.T., Maselli, R., Brown, M. & Arnason, B.G. (1990). Sympathetic skin responses are decreased and lymphocyte beta-adrenergic receptors are increased in progressive multiple sclerosis. *Annals of Neurology*, **27**, 366–72.

Karkhanis, Y.D., Carlo, D.J., Brostoff, S.W. & Eylar, E.H. (1975). Allergic encephalomyelitis. Isolation of an encephalitogenic peptide active in the monkey. *Journal of Biological Chemistry*, **250**, 1718–22.

Kerlero de Rosbo, N., Milo, R., Lees, M.B., Burger, D., Bernard, C.C. & Ben Nun, A. (1993). Reactivity to myelin antigens in multiple sclerosis. Peripheral blood lymphocytes respond predominantly to myelin oligodendrocyte glycoprotein. *Journal of Clinical Investigation*, **92**, 2602–8.

Kermode, A.G., Thompson, A.J., Tofts, P., MacManus, D.G., Kendall, B.E., Kingsley, D.P., Moseley, I.F., Rudge, P. & McDonald, W.I. (1990). Breakdown of the blood–brain barrier precedes symptoms and other MRI signs of new lesions in multiple sclerosis. Pathogenetic and clinical implications. *Brain*, **113**, 1477–89.

Kesselring, J., Miller, D.H., MacManus, D.G., Johnson, G., Milligan, N.M., Scolding, N., Compston, D.A. & McDonald, W.I. (1989). Quantitative magnetic resonance imaging in multiple sclerosis: the effect of high dose intravenous methylprednisolone. *Journal of Neurology, Neurosurgery and Psychiatry*, **52**, 14–17.

Khan, M.A. & Kushner, I. (1979). Ankylosing spondylitis and multiple sclerosis: a possible association. *Arthritis and Rheumatism*, **22**, 784–6.

Kibler, R.F. (1965). Large dose corticosteroid therapy of experimental and human demyelinating diseases. *Annals of the New York Academy of Sciences*, **122**, 469–79.

Kiessling, W.R. & Pflughaupt, K.W. (1980). Antithyroid antibodies in multiple sclerosis. *Lancet*, **1**, 41.

Kittur, S.D., Kittur, D.S., Soncrant, T.T., Rapoport, S.I., Tourtellotte, W.W., Nagel, J.E. & Adler, W.H. (1990). Soluble interleukin-2 receptors in cerebrospinal fluid from individuals with various neurological disorders. *Annals of Neurology*, **28**, 168–73.

Konttinen, Y.T., Bergroth, V., Kinnunen, E., Nordstrom, D. & Kouri, T. (1987). Activated T lymphocytes in patients with multiple sclerosis in clinical remission. *Journal of the Neurological Sciences*, **81**, 133–9.

Koopmans, R.A., Li, D.K., Zhu, G., Allen, P.S., Penn, A. & Paty, D.W. (1993). Magnetic resonance spectroscopy of multiple sclerosis: *in-vivo* detection of myelin breakdown products. *Lancet*, **341**, 631–2.

Koprowski, H., DeFreitas, E.C., Harper, M.E., Sandberg Wollheim, M., Sheremata, W.A., Robert Guroff, M., Saxinger, C.W., Feinberg, M.B., Wong Staal, F. & Gallo, R.C. (1985). Multiple sclerosis and human T-cell lymphotropic retroviruses. *Nature*, **318**, 154–60.

Kotzin, B.L., Karuturi, S., Chou, Y.K., Lafferty, J., Forrester, J.M., Better, M., Nedwin, G.E., Offner, H. & Vandenbark, A.A. (1991). Preferential T-cell receptor beta-chain variable gene use in myelin basic protein-reactive T-cell clones from patients with multiple sclerosis. *Proceedings of the National Academy of Sciences USA*, **88**, 9161–5.

Lamers, K.J., Uitdehaag, B.M., Hommes, O.R., Doesburg, W., Wevers, R.A. & von Geel, W.J. (1988). The short-term effect of an immunosuppressive treatment on CSF myelin basic protein in chronic progressive multiple sclerosis. *Journal of Neurology, Neurosurgery and Psychiatry*, **51**, 1334–7.

Larsen, P.D., Bloomer, L.C. & Bray, P.F. (1985). Epstein–Barr nuclear antigen and viral capsid antigen antibody titers in multiple sclerosis. *Neurology*, **35**, 435–8.

Lassmann, H. (1983). *Comparative Neuropathology of Chronic Experimental Allergic Encephalomyelitis and Multiple Sclerosis*. Berlin: Springer-Verlag.

Lassmann, H., Budka, H. & Schnaberth, G. (1981). Inflammatory demyelinating polyradiculitis in a patient with multiple sclerosis. *Archives of Neurology*, **38**, 99–102.

Lassmann, H. & Wisniewski, H.M. (1979). Chronic relapsing experimental allergic encephalomyelitis: clinicopathological comparison with multiple sclerosis. *Archives of Neurology*, **36**, 490–7.

Lee, S.C., Moore, G.R., Golenwsky, G. & Raine, C.S. (1990). Multiple sclerosis: a role for astroglia in active demyelination suggested by class II MHC expression and ultrastructural study. *Journal of Neuropathology and Experimental Neurology*, **49**, 122–36.

Lee, S.C. & Raine, C.S. (1989). Multiple sclerosis: oligodendrocytes in active lesions do not express class II major histocompatibility complex molecules. *Journal of Neuroimmunology*, **25**, 261–6.

Lee, S.J., Wucherpfennig, K.W., Brod, S.A., Benjamin, D., Weiner, H.L. & Hafler, D.A. (1991). Common T-cell receptor V beta usage in oligoclonal T lymphocytes derived from cerebrospinal fluid and blood of patients with multiple sclerosis. *Annals of Neurology*, **29**, 33–40.

Liblau, R., Tournier Lasserve, E., Maciazek, J., Dumas, G., Siffert, O., Hashim, G. & Bach, M.A. (1991). T cell response to myelin basic protein epitopes in multiple sclerosis patients and healthy subjects. *European Journal of Immunology*, **21**, 1391–5.

Lightman, S., McDonald, W.I., Bird, A.C., Francis, D.A., Hoskins, A., Batchelor, J.R. & Halliday, A.M. (1987). Retinal venous sheathing in optic neuritis. Its significance for the pathogenesis of multiple sclerosis. *Brain*, **110**, 405–14.

Linington, C., Gunn, C.A. & Lassmann, H. (1990). Identification of an encephalitogenic determinant of myelin proteolipid protein for the rabbit. *Journal of Neuroimmunology*, **30**, 135–44.

Link, H. & Müller, R. (1971). Immunoglobulins in multiple sclerosis and infections of the nervous system. *Archives of Neurology*, **25**, 326–44.

Link, H., Sun, J.B., Wang, Z., Xu, Z., Love, A., Fredrikson, S. & Olsson, T. (1992). Virus-reactive and autoreactive T cells are accumulated in cerebrospinal fluid in multiple sclerosis. *Journal of Neuroimmunology*, **38**, 63–73.

Link, J., Fredrikson, S., Soderstrom, M., Olsson, T., Hojeberg, B., Ljungdahl, A. & Link, H. (1994*a*). Organ-specific autoantigens induce transforming growth factor-beta mRNA expression in mononuclear cells in multiple sclerosis and myasthenia gravis. *Annals of Neurology*, **35**, 197–203.

Link, J., Soderstrom, M., Ljungdahl, A., Hojeberg, B., Olsson, T., Xu, Z., Fredrikson, S., Wang, Z.Y. & Link, H. (1994*b*). Organ-specific autoantigens induce interferon-gamma and interleukin-4 mRNA expression in mononuclear cells in multiple sclerosis and myasthenia gravis. *Neurology*, **44**, 728–34.

Lisak, R.P. & Zweiman, B. (1977). *In vitro* cell-mediated immunity of cerebrospinal-fluid lymphocytes to myelin basic protein in primary demyelinating diseases. *New England Journal of Medicine*, **297**, 850–3.

Lolli, F., Halawa, I. & Link, H. (1989). Intrathecal synthesis of IgG, IgA, IgM and IgD in untreated multiple sclerosis and controls. *Acta Neurologica Scandinavica*, **80**, 238–47.

Losy, J., Mehta, P.D. & Wisniewski, H.M. (1990). Identification of IgG subclasses' oligoclonal bands in multiple sclerosis CSF. *Acta Neurologica Scandinavica*, **82**, 4–8.

Lynch, S.G., Rose, J.W., Petajan, J.H., Stauffer, D., Kamerath, C. & Leppert, M. (1991). Discordance of T-cell receptor beta-chain genes in familial multiple sclerosis. *Annals of Neurology*, **30**, 402–10.

Maimone, D., Gregory, S., Arnason, B.G. & Reder, A.T. (1991). Cytokine levels in the cerebrospinal fluid and serum of patients with multiple sclerosis. *Journal of Neuroimmunology*, **32**, 67–74.

Maimone, D. & Reder, A.T. (1991). Soluble CD8 levels in the CSF and serum of patients with multiple sclerosis. *Neurology*, **41**, 851–4.

Maimone, D., Reder, A.T. & Gregory, S. (1993). T cell lymphokine-induced secretion of cytokines by monocytes from patients with multiple sclerosis. *Cellular Immunology*, **146**, 96–106.

Marrosu, M.G. (1991). Decrease in memory (CDw29-high) cerebrospinal fluid cells from acute MS patients. *Acta Neurologica Scandinavica*, **84**, 487–490.

Martin, R., Howell, M.D., Jaraquemada, D., Flerlage, M., Richert, J., Brostoff, S., Long, E.O., McFarlin, D.E. & McFarland, H.F. (1991). A myelin basic protein peptide is recognized by cytotoxic T cells in the context of four HLA-DR types associated with multiple sclerosis. *Journal of Experimental Medicine*, **173**, 19–24.

Martin, R., Jaraquemada, D., Flerlage, M., Richert, J., Whitaker, J., Long, E.O., McFarlin, D.E. & McFarland, H.F. (1990). Fine specificity and HLA restriction of myelin basic protein-specific cytotoxic T cell lines from multiple sclerosis patients and healthy individuals. *Journal of Immunology*, **145**, 540–8.

Martin, R., Utz, U., Coligan, J.E., Richert, J.R., Flerlage, M., Robinson, E., Stone, R., Biddison, W.E., McFarlin, D.E. & McFarland, H.F. (1992). Diversity in fine specificity and T cell receptor usage of the human CD4+ cytotoxic T cell response specific for the immunodominant myelin basic protein peptide 87–106. *Journal of Immunology*, **148**, 1359–66.

Martin, R., Voskuhl, R., Flerlage, M., McFarlin, D.E. & McFarland, H.F. (1993). Myelin basic protein-specific T-cell responses in identical twins discordant or concordant for multiple sclerosis. *Annals of Neurology*, **34**, 524–35.

Martinez Naves, E., Victoria Gutierrez, M., Uria, D.F. & Lopez Larrea, C. (1993). The germline repertoire of T cell receptor beta-chain genes in multiple sclerosis patients from Spain. *Journal of Neuroimmunology*, **47**, 9–13.

Martino, G., Olsson, T., Fredrikson, S., Hojeberg, B., Kostulas, V., Grimaldi, L.M. & Link, H. (1991). Cells producing antibodies specific for myelin basic protein region 70–89 are predominant in cerebrospinal fluid from patients with multiple sclerosis. *European Journal of Immunology*, **21**, 2971–6.

Martyn, C.N., Cruddas, M. & Compston, D.A. (1993). Symptomatic Epstein–Barr virus infection and multiple sclerosis. *Journal of Neurology, Neurosurgery and Psychiatry*, **56**, 167–8.

Matsiota, P., Blancher, A., Doyon, B., Guilbert, B., Clanet, M., Kouvelas, E.D. & Avrameas, S. (1988). Comparative study of natural autoantibodies in the serum and cerebrospinal fluid of normal individuals and patients with multiple sclerosis and other neurological diseases. *Annales de l' Institut Pasteur Immunology*, **139**, 99–108.

Matsui, M., Mori, K.J. & Saida, T. (1990). Cellular immunoregulatory mechanisms in the central nervous system: characterization of noninflammatory and inflammatory cerebrospinal fluid lymphocytes. *Annals of Neurology*, **27**, 647–51.

Matsui, M., Mori, K.J., Saida, T., Akiguchi, I. & Kameyama, M. (1988). The imbalance in CSF T cell subsets in active multiple sclerosis. *Acta Neurologica Scandinavica*, **77**, 202–9.

McCallum, K., Esiri, M.M., Tourtellotte, W.W. & Booss, J. (1987). T cell subsets in multiple sclerosis. Gradients at plaque borders and differences in nonplaque regions. *Brain*, **110**, 1297–308.

McCombe, P.A., Chalk, J.B. & Pender, M.P. (1990). Familial occurrence of multiple sclerosis with thyroid disease and systemic lupus erythematosus. *Journal of the Neurological Sciences*, **97**, 163–71.

McCombe, P.A., Clark, P., Frith, J.A., Hammond, S.R., Stewart, G.J., Pollard, J.D. & McLeod, J.G. (1985). Alpha-1 antitrypsin phenotypes in demyelinating disease: an association between demyelinating disease and the allele PiM3. *Annals of Neurology*, **18**, 514–16.

McDonald, W.I. & Sears, T.A. (1970). The effects of experimental demyelination on conduction in the central nervous system. *Brain*, **93**, 583–98.

McGeer, P.L., Itagaki, S. & McGeer, E.G. (1988). Expression of the histocompatibility glycoprotein HLA-DR in neurological disease. *Acta Neuropathologica (Berlin)*, **76**, 550–7.

McLean, B.N., Luxton, R.W. & Thompson, E.J. (1990). A study of immunoglobulin G in the cerebrospinal fluid of 1007 patients with suspected neurological disease using isoelectric focusing and the Log IgG-Index. A comparison and diagnostic applications. *Brain*, **113**, 1269–89.

McLean, B.N. & Thompson, E.J. (1989). Antibodies against the paramyxovirus SV5 are not specific for cerebrospinal fluid from multiple sclerosis patients. *Journal of the Neurological Sciences*, **92**, 261–6.

Mehta, P.D., Patrick, B.A., Mehta, S.P. & Wisniewski, H.M. (1987). Specificity of oligoclonal IgG bands against myelin proteins in chronic relapsing EAE in guinea pigs. *Journal of Immunology*, **138**, 746–51.

Meisler, D.M., Tomsak, R.L., Khoury, S., Hanson, M.R., Schwab, I.R. & Ransohoff, R.M. (1989). Anterior uveitis and multiple sclerosis. *Cleveland Clinic Journal of Medicine*, **56**, 535–8.

Mendell, J.R., Kolkin, S., Kissel, J.T., Weiss, K.L., Chakeres, D.W. & Rammohan, K.W. (1987). Evidence for central nervous system demyelination in chronic inflammatory demyelinating polyradiculoneuropathy. *Neurology*, **37**, 1291–4.

Miller, D.H., Rudge, P., Johnson, G., Kendall, B.E., MacManus, D.G., Moseley, I.F., Barnes, D. & McDonald, W.I. (1988). Serial gadolinium enhanced magnetic resonance imaging in multiple sclerosis. *Brain*, **111**, 927–39.

Milligan, N.M., Newcombe, R. & Compston, D.A. (1987). A double-blind controlled trial of high dose methylprednisolone in patients with multiple sclerosis: 1. clinical effects. *Journal of Neurology, Neurosurgery and Psychiatry*, **50**, 511–16.

Minuk, G.Y. & Lewkonia, R.M. (1986). Possible familial association of multiple sclerosis and inflammatory bowel disease. *New England Journal of Medicine*, **314**, 586.

Mix, E., Olsson, T., Correale, J., Kostulas, V. & Link, H. (1990). $CD4^+$, $CD8^+$, and $CD4^-$ $CD8^-$ T cells in CSF and blood of patients with multiple sclerosis and tension headache. *Scandinavian Journal of Immunology*, **31**, 493–501.

Moller, J.R., Johnson, D., Brady, R.O., Tourtellotte, W.W. & Quarles, R.H. (1989). Antibodies to myelin-associated glycoprotein (MAG) in the cerebrospinal fluid of multiple sclerosis patients. *Journal of Neuroimmunology*, **22**, 55–61.

Morgan, B.P., Campbell, A.K. & Compston, D.A. (1984). Terminal component of complement (C9) in cerebrospinal fluid of patients with multiple sclerosis. *Lancet*, **2**, 251–4.

Morimoto, C., Hafler, D.A., Weiner, H.L., Letvin, N.L., Hagan, M., Daley, J. & Schlossman, S.F. (1987). Selective loss of the suppressor-inducer T-cell subset in progressive multiple sclerosis. Analysis with anti-2H4 monoclonal antibody. *New England Journal of Medicine*, **316**, 67–72.

Moyer, A.W., Jervis, G.A., Black, J., Koprowski, H. & Cox, H.R. (1950). Action of adrenocorticotropic hormone (ACTH) in experimental allergic encephalomyelitis of the guinea pig. *Proceedings of the Society for Experimental Biology and Medicine*, **75**, 387–90.

Multiple Sclerosis Study Group (1990). Efficacy and toxicity of cyclosporine in chronic progressive multiple sclerosis: a randomized, double-blinded, placebo-controlled clinical trial. *Annals of Neurology*, **27**, 591–605.

Munschauer, F.E., Stewart, C., Jacobs, L., Kaba, S., Ghorishi, Z., Greenberg, S.J. & Cookfair, D. (1993). Circulating CD3+ CD4+ CD8+ T lymphocytes in multiple sclerosis. *Journal of Clinical Immunology*, **13**, 113–18.

Murray, R.S., Brown, B., Brian, D. & Cabirac, G.F. (1992). Detection of coronavirus RNA and antigen in multiple sclerosis brain. *Annals of Neurology*, **31**, 525–33.

Nath, A. & Wolinsky, J.S. (1990). Antibody response to rubella virus structural proteins in multiple sclerosis. *Annals of Neurology*, **27**, 533–6.

Nishimura, M., Adachi, A., Maeda, M., Akiguchi, I., Ishimoto, A. & Kimura, J. (1990). Human T lymphotrophic virus type I may not be associated with multiple sclerosis in Japan. *Journal of Immunology*, **144**, 1684–8.

Noronha, A., Richman, D.P. & Arnason, B.G. (1985). Multiple sclerosis: activated cells in cerebrospinal fluid in acute exacerbations. *Annals of Neurology*, **18**, 722–5.

Noronha, A., Toscas, A. & Jensen, M.A. (1990). Interferon beta augments suppressor cell function in multiple sclerosis. *Annals of Neurology*, **27**, 207–10.

Noronha, A., Toscas, A. & Jensen, M.A. (1992). Contrasting effects of alpha, beta, and gamma interferons on nonspecific suppressor function in multiple sclerosis. *Annals of Neurology*, **31**, 103–6.

Noronha, A., Toscas, A. & Jensen, M.A. (1993). Interferon beta decreases T cell activation and interferon gamma production in multiple sclerosis. *Journal of Neuroimmunology*, **46**, 145–53.

Noronha, A.B.C., Richman, D.P. & Arnason, B.G. (1980). Detection of *in vivo* stimulated cerebrospinal-fluid lymphocytes by flow cytometry in patients with multiple sclerosis. *New England Journal of Medicine*, **303**, 713–17.

Norrby, E. (1978). Viral antibodies in multiple sclerosis. *Progress in Medical Virology*, **24**, 1–39.

O'Gorman, M.R., Aziz, T. & Oger, J. (1989). Chronic progressive multiple sclerosis: changes in phenotype and function of T helper subsets. *Journal of Neuroimmunology*, **24**, 163–8.

Offner, H., Hashim, G.A., Celnik, B., Galang, A., Li, X.B., Burns, F.R., Shen, N., Heber Katz, E. & Vandenbark, A.A. (1989). T cell determinants of myelin basic protein include a unique encephalitogenic I-E-restricted epitope for Lewis rats. *Journal of Experimental Medicine*, **170**, 355–67.

Ofosu Appiah, W., Mokhtarian, F., Miller, A. & Grob, D. (1991). Characterization of *in vivo*-activated T cell clones from peripheral blood of multiple sclerosis patients. *Clinical Immunology and Immunopathology*, **58**, 46–55.

Ohguro, H., Chiba, S., Igarashi, Y., Matsumoto, H., Akino, T. & Palczewski, K. (1993). Beta-arrestin and arrestin are recognized by autoantibodies in sera from multiple sclerosis patients. *Proceedings of the National Academy of Sciences USA*, **90**, 3241–5.

Oksenberg, J.R., Panzara, M.A., Begovich, A.B., Mitchell, D., Erlich, H.A., Murray, R.S., Shimonkevitz, R., Sherritt, M., Rothbard, J., Bernard, C.C. *et al.* (1993). Selection for T-cell receptor V beta-D beta-J beta gene rearrangements with specificity for a myelin basic protein peptide in brain lesions of multiple sclerosis. *Nature*, **362**, 68–70.

Oksenberg, J.R., Sherritt, M., Begovich, A.B., Erlich, H.A., Bernard, C.C., Cavalli Sforza, L.L. & Steinman, L. (1989). T-cell receptor V alpha and C alpha alleles associated with multiple sclerosis and myasthenia gravis. *Proceedings of the National Academy of Sciences USA*, **86**, 988–92.

Oksenberg, J.R., Stuart, S., Begovich, A.B., Bell, R.B., Erlich, H.A., Steinman, L. & Bernard, C.C. (1990). Limited heterogeneity of rearranged T-cell receptor V alpha transcripts in brains of multiple sclerosis patients [published erratum appears in *Nature* 1991 Sep 5;**353**(6339):94]. *Nature*, **345**, 344–6.

Olerup, O., Hillert, J., Fredrikson, S., Olsson, T., Kam Hansen, S., Moller, E., Carlsson, B. & Wallin, J. (1989). Primarily chronic progressive and relapsing/remitting multiple sclerosis: two immunogenetically distinct disease entities. *Proceedings of the National Academy of Sciences USA*, **86**, 7113–17.

Olsson, T., Baig, S., Hojeberg, B. & Link, H. (1990*a*). Antimyelin basic protein and antimyelin antibody-producing cells in multiple sclerosis. *Annals of Neurology*, **27**, 132–6.

Olsson, T., Sun, J., Hillert, J., Hojeberg, B., Ekre, H.P., Andersson, G., Olerup, O. & Link, H. (1992). Increased numbers of T cells recognizing multiple myelin basic protein epitopes in multiple sclerosis. *European Journal of Immunology*, **22**, 1083–7.

Olsson, T., Zhi, W.W., Hojeberg, B., Kostulas, V., Jiang, Y.P., Anderson, G., Ekre, H.P. & Link, H. (1990*b*). Autoreactive T lymphocytes in multiple sclerosis determined by antigen-induced secretion of interferon-gamma. *Journal of Clinical Investigation*, **86**, 981–5.

Ormerod, I.E., Miller, D.H., McDonald, W.I., du Boulay, E.P., Rudge, P., Kendall, B.E., Moseley, I.F., Johnson, G., Tofts, P.S., Halliday, A.M. *et al.* (1987). The role of NMR imaging in the assessment of multiple sclerosis and isolated neurological lesions. A quantitative study. *Brain*, **110**, 1579–616.

Ota, K., Matsui, M., Milford, E.L., Mackin, G.A., Weiner, H.L. & Hafler, D.A. (1990). T-cell recognition of an immunodominant myelin basic protein epitope in multiple sclerosis. *Nature*, **346**, 183–7.

Panitch, H.S., Hirsch, R.L., Haley, A.S. & Johnson, K.P. (1987*a*). Exacerbations of multiple sclerosis in patients treated with gamma interferon. *Lancet*, **1**, 893–5.

Panitch, H.S., Hirsch, R.L., Schindler, J. & Johnson, K.P. (1987*b*). Treatment of multiple sclerosis with gamma interferon: exacerbations associated with activation of the immune system. *Neurology*, **37**, 1097–102.

Paty, D.W., Li, D.K., the UBC MS/MRI Study Group & the IFNB Multiple Sclerosis Study Group (1993). Interferon beta-1b is effective in relapsing-remitting multiple sclerosis. II. MRI analysis results of a multicenter, randomized, double-blind, placebo-controlled trial. *Neurology*, **43**, 662–7.

Pelfrey, C.M., Trotter, J.L., Tranquill, L.R. & McFarland, H.F. (1993). Identification of a novel T cell epitope of human proteolipid protein (residues 40–60) recognized by proliferative and cytolytic CD4+ T cells from multiple sclerosis patients. *Journal of Neuroimmunology*, **46**, 33–42.

Pender, M.P. (1989). Recovery from acute experimental allergic encephalomyelitis in the Lewis rat: early restoration of nerve conduction and repair by Schwann cells and oligodendrocytes. *Brain*, **112**, 393–416.

Pender, M.P. (1991). Cyclosporine and multiple sclerosis. *Annals of Neurology*, **29**, 226.

Pender, M.P. (1992). Demyelinating diseases. In *Drug Therapy in Neurology*, ed. M.J. Eadie, pp. 513–23. Edinburgh: Churchill Livingstone.

Pender, M.P., Nguyen, K.B. & Willenborg, D.O. (1989). Demyelination and early remyelination in experimental allergic encephalomyelitis passively transferred with myelin basic protein-sensitized lymphocytes in the Lewis rat. *Journal of Neuroimmunology*, **25**, 125–42.

Pender, M.P., Stanley, G.P., Yoong, G. & Nguyen, K.B. (1990). The neuropathology of chronic relapsing experimental allergic encephalomyelitis induced in the Lewis rat by inoculation with whole spinal cord and treatment with cyclosporin A. *Acta Neuropathologica (Berlin)*, **80**, 172–83.

Peter, J.B., Boctor, F.N. & Tourtellotte, W.W. (1991). Serum and CSF levels of IL-2, sIL-2R, TNF-alpha, and IL-1 beta in chronic progressive multiple sclerosis: expected lack of clinical utility. *Neurology*, **41**, 121–3.

Pette, M., Fujita, K., Kitze, B., Whitaker, J.N., Albert, E., Kappos, L. & Wekerle, H. (1990*a*). Myelin basic protein-specific T lymphocyte lines from MS patients and healthy individuals. *Neurology*, **40**, 1770–6.

Pette, M., Fujita, K., Wilkinson, D., Altmann, D.M., Trowsdale, J., Giegerich, G., Hinkkanen, A., Epplen, J.T., Kappos, L. & Wekerle, H. (1990*b*). Myelin autoreactivity in multiple sclerosis: recognition of myelin basic protein in the context of HLA-DR2 products by T lymphocytes of multiple-sclerosis patients and healthy donors. *Proceedings of the National Academy of Sciences USA*, **87**, 7968–72.

Périer, O. & Grégoire, A. (1965). Electron microscopic features of multiple sclerosis lesions. *Brain*, **88**, 937–52.

Polman, C.H., Matthaei, I., De Groot, C.J., Koetsier, J.C., Sminia, T. & Dijkstra, C.D. (1988). Low-dose cyclosporin A induces relapsing remitting experimental allergic encephalomyelitis in the Lewis rat. *Journal of Neuroimmunology*, **17**, 209–16.

Pontecorvo, M.J., Levinson, J.D. & Roth, J.A. (1992). A patient with primary biliary cirrhosis and multiple sclerosis. *American Journal of Medicine*, **92**, 433–6.

Porrini, A.M., Gambi, D. & Malatesta, G. (1992). Memory and naive CD4+ lymphocytes in multiple sclerosis. *Journal of Neurology*, **239**, 437–40.

Porter, R. (1972). Uveitis in association with multiple sclerosis. *British Journal of Ophthalmology*, **56**, 478–81.

Poser, C.M., Paty, D.W., Scheinberg, L., McDonald, W.I., Davis, F.A., Ebers, G.C., Johnson, K.P., Sibley, W.A., Silberberg, D.H. & Tourtellotte, W.W. (1983). New diagnostic criteria for multiple sclerosis: guidelines for research protocols. *Annals of Neurology*, **13**, 227–31.

Prineas, J.W. (1985). The neuropathology of multiple sclerosis. In *Handbook of Clinical Neurology*, vol. 3 (47): *Demyelinating Diseases*, ed. P.J. Vinken, G.W. Bruyn & H.L. Klawans, pp. 213–57. Amsterdam: Elsevier Science Publishers.

Prineas, J.W., Barnard, R.O., Kwon, E.E., Sharer, L.R. & Cho, E.S. (1993*a*). Multiple sclerosis: remyelination of nascent lesions. *Annals of Neurology*, **33**, 137–51.

Prineas, J.W., Barnard, R.O., Revesz, T., Kwon, E.E., Sharer, L. & Cho, E.S. (1993*b*). Multiple sclerosis. Pathology of recurrent lesions. *Brain*, **116**, 681–93.

Prineas, J.W. & Graham, J.S. (1981). Multiple sclerosis: capping of surface immunoglobulin G on macrophages engaged in myelin breakdown. *Annals of Neurology*, **10**, 149–58.

Prineas, J.W., Kwon, E.E., Cho, E.-S. & Sharer, L.R. (1984). Continual breakdown and regeneration of myelin in progressive multiple sclerosis plaques. *Annals of the New York Academy of Sciences*, **436**, 11–32.

Prineas, J.W., Kwon, E.E., Goldenberg, P.Z., Ilyas, A.A., Quarles, R.H., Benjamins, J.A. & Sprinkle, T.J. (1989). Multiple sclerosis. Oligodendrocyte proliferation and differentiation in fresh lesions. *Laboratory Investigation*, **61**, 489–503.

Prineas, J.W. & Wright, R.G. (1978). Macrophages, lymphocytes, and plasma cells in the perivascular compartment in chronic multiple sclerosis. *Laboratory Investigation*, **38**, 409–21.

Procaccia, S., Lanzanova, D., Caputo, D., Ferrante, P., Papini, E., Gasparini, A., Colucci, A., Bianchi, M., Villa, P., Blasio, R. *et al.* (1988). Circulating immune complexes in serum and in cerebrospinal fluid of patients with multiple sclerosis. Characterization and correlation with the clinical course. *Acta Neurologica Scandinavica*, **77**, 373–81

Racke, M.K., Martin, R., McFarland, H. & Fritz, R.B. (1992). Copolymer-1-induced inhibition of antigen-specific T cell activation: interference with antigen presentation. *Journal of Neuroimmunology*, **37**, 75–84.

Rang, E.H., Brooke, B.N. & Hermon-Taylor, J. (1982). Association of ulcerative colitis with multiple sclerosis. *Lancet*, **2**, 555.

Ransohoff, R.M., Devajyothi, C., Estes, M.L., Babcock, G., Rudick, R.A., Frohman, E.M. & Barna, B.P. (1991). Interferon-beta specifically inhibits interferon-gamma-induced class II major histocompatibility complex gene transcription in a human astrocytoma cell line. *Journal of Neuroimmunology*, **33**, 103–12.

Rasminsky, M. (1973). The effects of temperature on conduction in demyelinated single nerve fibers. *Archives of Neurology*, **28**, 287–92.

Rasminsky, M. (1980). Ephaptic transmission between single nerve fibres in the spinal nerve roots of dystrophic mice. *Journal of Physiology*, **305**, 151–69.

Rauch, H.C., Montgomery, I.N., Hinman, C.L. & Harb, W. (1987). Experimental allergic encephalomyelitis in mice: presence of myelin basic protein in cerebrospinal fluid. *Journal of Neuroimmunology*, **15**, 73–83.

Reder, A.T., Arnason, B.G., Maimone, D. & Rohwer Nutter, D. (1991). The function of the CD2 protein is abnormal in multiple sclerosis. *Journal of Autoimmunity*, **4**, 479–91.

Richert, J.R., Robinson, E.D., Johnson, A.H., Bergman, C.A., Dragovic, L.J., Reinsmoen, N.L. & Hurley, C.K. (1991). Heterogeneity of the T-cell receptor beta gene rearrangements generated in myelin basic protein-specific T-cell clones isolated from a patient with multiple sclerosis. *Annals of Neurology*, **29**, 299–306.

Rose, A.S., Kuzma, J.W., Kurtzke, J.F., Namerow, N.S., Sibley, W.A., Tourtellotte, W.W., Dixon, W.J., Foley, J.M., Geschwind, N., MacKay, R.P. *et al.* (1970). Cooperative study in the evaluation of therapy in multiple sclerosis. ACTH vs. placebo – final report. *Neurology*, **20** (No. 5, Pt. 2), 1–59.

Rose, J., Gerken, S., Lynch, S., Pisani, P., Varvil, T., Otterud, B. & Leppert, M. (1993). Genetic susceptibility in familial multiple sclerosis not linked to the myelin basic protein gene. *Lancet*, **341**, 1179–81.

Rose, L.M., Ginsberg, A.H., Rothstein, T.L., Ledbetter, J.A. & Clark, E.A. (1985). Selective loss of a subset of T helper cells in active multiple sclerosis. *Proceedings of the National Academy of Sciences USA*, **82**, 7389–93.

Rose, L.M., Ginsberg, A.H., Rothstein, T.L., Ledbetter, J.A. & Clark, E.A. (1988). Fluctuations of CD4+ T-cell subsets in remitting-relapsing multiple sclerosis. *Annals of Neurology*, **24**, 192–9.

Rubin, M., Karpati, G. & Carpenter, S. (1987). Combined central and peripheral myelinopathy. *Neurology*, **37**, 1287–90.

Rudick, R.A., Carpenter, C.S., Cookfair, D.L., Tuohy, V.K. & Ransohoff, R.M. (1993). *In vitro* and *in vivo* inhibition of mitogen-driven T-cell activation by recombinant interferon beta. *Neurology*, **43**, 2080–7.

Sadovnick, A.D., Paty, D.W. & Yannakoulias, G. (1989). Concurrence of multiple sclerosis and inflammatory bowel disease. *New England Journal of Medicine*, **321**, 762–3.

Saeki, Y., Mima, T., Sakoda, S., Fujimura, H., Arita, N., Nomura, T. & Kishimoto, T. (1992). Transfer of multiple sclerosis into severe combined immunodeficiency mice by mononuclear cells from cerebrospinal fluid of the patients. *Proceedings of the National Academy of Sciences USA*, **89**, 6157–61.

Sakai, K., Zamvil, S.S., Mitchell, D.J., Lim, M., Rothbard, J.B. & Steinman, L. (1988). Characterization of a major encephalitogenic T cell epitope in SJL/J mice with synthetic oligopeptides of myelin basic protein. *Journal of Neuroimmunology*, **19**, 21–32.

Salmaggi, A., LaMantia, L., Milanese, C., Bianchi, G., Eoli, M., Campi, A. & Nespolo, A. (1989). CSF T-cell subsets in multiple sclerosis: relationship to cerebrospinal fluid myelin basic protein and clinical activity. *Journal of Neurology*, **236**, 336–9.

Salmi, A., Reunanen, M., Ilonen, J. & Panelius, M. (1983). Intrathecal antibody synthesis to virus antigens in multiple sclerosis. *Clinical and Experimental Immunology*, **52**, 241–9.

Salonen, R., Ilonen, J., Jagerroos, H., Syrjala, H., Nurmi, T. & Reunanen, M. (1989). Lymphocyte subsets in the cerebrospinal fluid in active multiple sclerosis. *Annals of Neurology*, **25**, 500–2.

Salvetti, M., Buttinelli, C., Ristori, G., Carbonari, M., Cherchi, M., Fiorelli, M., Grasso, M.G., Toma, L. & Pozzilli, C. (1992). T-lymphocyte reactivity to the recombinant mycobacterial 65- and 70-kDa heat shock proteins in multiple sclerosis. *Journal of Autoimmunity*, **5**, 691–702.

Sanders, M.E., Koski, C.L., Robbins, D., Shin, M.L., Frank, M.M. & Joiner, K.A. (1986). Activated terminal complement in cerebrospinal fluid in Guillain–Barré syndrome and multiple sclerosis. *Journal of Immunology*, **136**, 4456–9.

Saruhan Direskeneli, G., Weber, F., Meinl, E., Pette, M., Giegerich, G., Hinkkanen, A., Epplen, J.T., Hohlfeld, R. & Wekerle, H. (1993). Human T cell autoimmunity against myelin basic protein: CD4+ cells recognizing epitopes of the T cell receptor beta chain from a myelin basic protein-specific T cell clone. *European Journal of Immunology*, **23**, 530–6.

Satyanarayana, K., Chou, Y.K., Bourdette, D., Whitham, R., Hashim, G.A., Offner, H. & Vandenbark, A.A. (1993). Epitope specificity and V gene expression of cerebrospinal fluid T cells specific for intact versus cryptic epitopes of myelin basic protein. *Journal of Neuroimmunology*, **44**, 57–67.

Schadlich, H.J., Mohrmann, G., Nekic, M. & Felgenhauer, K. (1990). Intrathecal synthesis of virus antibodies: a diagnostic test for multiple sclerosis. *European Neurology*, **30**, 302–4.

Scolozzi, R., Boccafogli, A., Tola, M.R., Vicentini, L., Camerani, A., Degani, D., Granieri, E., Caniatti, L. & Paolino, E. (1992). T-cell phenotypic profiles in the cerebrospinal fluid and peripheral blood of multiple sclerosis patients. *Journal of the Neurological Sciences*, **108**, 93–8.

Seboun, E., Robinson, M.A., Doolittle, T.H., Ciulla, T.A., Kindt, T.J. & Hauser, S.L. (1989). A susceptibility locus for multiple sclerosis is linked to the T cell receptor β chain complex. *Cell*, **57**, 1095–100.

Selmaj, K., Brosnan, C.F. & Raine, C.S. (1991). Colocalization of lymphocytes bearing gamma delta T-cell receptor and heat shock protein hsp65+ oligodendrocytes in multiple sclerosis. *Proceedings of the National Academy of Sciences USA*, **88**, 6452–6.

Selmaj, K., Plater Zyberk, C., Rockett, K.A., Maini, R.N., Alam, R., Perkin, G.D. & Rose, F.C. (1986). Multiple sclerosis: increased expression of interleukin-2 receptors on lymphocytes. *Neurology*, **36**, 1392–5.

Serjeantson, S.W., Gao, X., Hawkins, B.R., Higgins, D.A. & Yu, Y.L. (1992). Novel HLA-DR2-related haplotypes in Hong Kong Chinese implicate the DQB1*0602 allele in susceptibility to multiple sclerosis. *European Journal of Immunogenetics*, **19**, 11–19.

Seyfert, S., Klapps, P., Meisel, C., Fischer, T. & Junghan, U. (1990). Multiple sclerosis and other immunologic diseases. *Acta Neurologica Scandinavica*, **81**, 37–42.

Sharief, M.K. & Hentges, R. (1991*a*). Importance of intrathecal synthesis of IgD in multiple sclerosis. A combined clinical, immunologic, and magnetic resonance imaging study. *Archives of Neurology*, **48**, 1076–9.

Sharief, M.K. & Hentges, R. (1991*b*). Association between tumor necrosis factor-alpha and disease progression in patients with multiple sclerosis. *New England Journal of Medicine*, **325**, 467–72.

Sharief, M.K., Hentges, R. & Thompson, E.J. (1991). The relationship of interleukin-2 and soluble interleukin-2 receptors to intrathecal immunoglobulin synthesis in patients with multiple sclerosis. *Journal of Neuroimmunology*, **32**, 43–51.

Sharief, M.K., Keir, G. & Thompson, E.J. (1990). Intrathecal synthesis of IgM in neurological diseases: a comparison between detection of oligoclonal bands and quantitative estimation. *Journal of the Neurological Sciences*, **96**, 131–42.

Sharief, M.K. & Thompson, E.J. (1991). Intrathecal immunoglobulin M synthesis in multiple sclerosis. Relationship with clinical and cerebrospinal fluid parameters. *Brain*, **114**, 181–95.

Sharief, M.K. & Thompson, E.J. (1993). Correlation of interleukin-2 and soluble interleukin-2 receptor with clinical activity of multiple sclerosis. *Journal of Neurology, Neurosurgery and Psychiatry*, **56**, 169–74.

Sherritt, M.A., Oksenberg, J., de Rosbo, N.K. & Bernard, C.C. (1992). Influence of HLA-DR2, HLA-DPw4, and T cell receptor alpha chain genes on the susceptibility to multiple sclerosis. *International Immunology*, **4**, 177–81.

Shimada, K., Koh, C.S. & Yanagisawa, N. (1993). [Detection of interleukin-6 in serum and cerebrospinal fluid of patients with neuroimmunological diseases]. *Arerugi. Japanese Journal of Allergology*, **42**, 934–40.

Shimonkevitz, R., Colburn, C., Burnham, J.A., Murray, R.S. & Kotzin, B.L. (1993). Clonal expansions of activated gamma/delta T cells in recent-onset multiple sclerosis. *Proceedings of the National Academy of Sciences USA*, **90**, 923–7.

Shirazian, D., Mokhtarian, F., Herzlich, B.C., Miller, A.E. & Grob, D. (1993). Presence of cross-reactive antibodies to HTLV-1 and absence of antigens in patients with multiple sclerosis. *Journal of Laboratory and Clinical Medicine*, **122**, 252–9.

Shoenfeld, Y., Ben Yehuda, O., Messinger, Y., Bentwitch, Z., Rauch, J., Isenberg, D.I. & Gadoth, N. (1988). Autoimmune diseases other than lupus share common anti-DNA idiotypes. *Immunology Letters*, **17**, 285–91.

Shrager, P. & Rubinstein, C.T. (1990). Optical measurement of conduction in single demyelinated axons. *Journal of General Physiology*, **95**, 867–90.

Sibley, W.A., Bamford, C.R. & Clark, K. (1985). Clinical viral infections and multiple sclerosis. *Lancet*, **1**, 1313–15.

Sindic, C.J. & Laterre, E.C. (1991). Oligoclonal free kappa and lambda bands in the cerebrospinal fluid of patients with multiple sclerosis and other neurological diseases. An immunoaffinity-mediated capillary blot study. *Journal of Neuroimmunology*, **33**, 63–72.

Sindic, C.J., Monteyne, P., Bigaignon, G. & Laterre, E.C. (1994). Polyclonal and oligoclonal IgA synthesis in the cerebrospinal fluid of neurological patients: an immunoaffinity-mediated capillary blot study. *Journal of Neuroimmunology*, **49**, 109–14.

Sloan, J.B., Berk, M.A., Gebel, H.M. & Fretzin, D.F. (1987). Multiple sclerosis and systemic lupus erythematosus: occurrence in two generations of the same family. *Archives of Internal Medicine*, **147**, 1317–20.

Smith, K.J., Blakemore, W.F. & McDonald, W.I. (1981). The restoration of conduction by central remyelination. *Brain*, **104**, 383–404.

Smith, K.J., Bostock, H. & Hall, S.M. (1982). Saltatory conduction precedes remyelination in axons demyelinated with lysophosphatidyl choline. *Journal of the Neurological Sciences*, **54**, 13–31.

Smith, K.J. & McDonald, W.I. (1982). Spontaneous and evoked electrical discharges from a central demyelinating lesion. *Journal of the Neurological Sciences*, **55**, 39–48.

Smith, M.E., Stone, L.A., Albert, P.S., Frank, J.A., Martin, R., Armstrong, M., Maloni, H., McFarlin, D.E. & McFarland, H.F. (1993). Clinical worsening in multiple sclerosis is associated with increased frequency and area of gadopentetate dimeglumine-enhancing magnetic resonance imaging lesions. *Annals of Neurology*, **33**, 480–9.

Sobel, R.A., Hafler, D.A., Castro, E.E., Morimoto, C. & Weiner, H.L. (1988). The 2H4 (CD45R) antigen is selectively decreased in multiple sclerosis lesions. *Journal of Immunology*, **140**, 2210–14.

Sobel, R.A., Mitchell, M.E. & Fondren, G. (1990). Intercellular adhesion molecule-1 (ICAM-1) in cellular immune reactions in the human central nervous system. *American Journal of Pathology*, **136**, 1309–16.

Soderstrom, M., Link, H., Sun, J.B., Fredrikson, S., Kostulas, V., Hojeberg, B., Li, B.L. & Olsson, T. (1993). T cells recognizing multiple peptides of myelin basic protein are found in blood and enriched in cerebrospinal fluid in optic neuritis and multiple sclerosis. *Scandinavian Journal of Immunology*, **37**, 355–68.

Sola, P., Merelli, E., Marasca, R., Poggi, M., Luppi, M., Montorsi, M. & Torelli, G. (1993). Human herpesvirus 6 and multiple sclerosis: survey of anti-HHV-6 antibodies by immunofluorescence analysis and of viral sequences by polymerase chain reaction. *Journal of Neurology, Neurosurgery and Psychiatry*, **56**, 917–19.

Somer, H., Muller, K. & Kinnunen, E. (1989). Myasthenia gravis associated with multiple sclerosis. Epidemiological survey and immunological findings. *Journal of the Neurological Sciences*, **89**, 37–48.

Stanley, G.P., McCombe, P.A. & Pender, M.P. (1992). Focal conduction block in the dorsal root ganglion in experimental allergic neuritis. *Annals of Neurology*, **31**, 27–33.

Stanley, G.P. & Pender, M.P. (1991). The pathophysiology of chronic relapsing experimental allergic encephalomyelitis in the Lewis rat. *Brain*, **114**, 1827–53.

Sumaya, C.V., Myers, L.W., Ellison, G.W. & Ench, Y. (1985). Increased prevalence and titer of Epstein–Barr virus antibodies in patients with multiple sclerosis. *Annals of Neurology*, **17**, 371–7.

Sun, D. (1992). Synthetic peptides representing sequence 39 to 59 of rat V beta 8 TCR fail to elicit regulatory T cells reactive with V beta 8 TCR on rat encephalitogenic T cells. *Cellular Immunology*, **141**, 200–10.

Sun, J., Link, H., Olsson, T., Xiao, B.G., Andersson, G., Ekre, H.P., Linington, C. & Diener, P. (1991). T and B cell responses to myelin-oligodendrocyte glycoprotein in multiple sclerosis. *Journal of Immunology*, **146**, 1490–5.

Sun, J.B., Olsson, T., Wang, W.Z., Xiao, B.G., Kostulas, V., Fredrikson, S., Ekre, H.P. & Link, H. (1991). Autoreactive T and B cells responding to myelin proteolipid protein in multiple sclerosis and controls. *European Journal of Immunology*, **21**, 1461–8.

Svenningsson, A., Hansson, G.K., Andersen, O., Andersson, R., Patarroyo, M. & Stemme, S. (1993). Adhesion molecule expression on cerebrospinal fluid T lymphocytes: evidence for common recruitment mechanisms in multiple sclerosis, aseptic meningitis, and normal controls. *Annals of Neurology*, **34**, 155–61.

Tanaka, Y., Tsukada, N., Koh, C.S. & Yanagisawa, N. (1987). Anti-endothelial cell antibodies and circulating immune complexes in the sera of patients with multiple sclerosis. *Journal of Neuroimmunology*, **17**, 49–59.

Teitelbaum, D., Aharoni, R., Sela, M. & Arnon, R. (1991). Cross-reactions and specificities of monoclonal antibodies against myelin basic protein and against the synthetic copolymer 1. *Proceedings of the National Academy of Sciences USA*, **88**, 9528–32.

Teitelbaum, D., Milo, R., Arnon, R. & Sela, M. (1992). Synthetic copolymer 1 inhibits human T-cell lines specific for myelin basic protein. *Proceedings of the National Academy of Sciences USA*, **89**, 137–41.

Thomas, P.K., Walker, R.W., Rudge, P., Morgan Hughes, J.A., King, R.H., Jacobs, J.M., Mills, K.R., Ormerod, I.E., Murray, N.M. & McDonald, W.I. (1987). Chronic demyelinating peripheral neuropathy associated with multifocal central nervous system demyelination. *Brain*, **110**, 53–76.

Thompson, A.J., Kennard, C., Swash, M., Summers, B., Yuill, G.M., Shepherd, D.I., Roche, S., Perkin, G.D., Loizou, L.A., Ferner, R. *et al.* (1989). Relative efficacy of intravenous methylprednisolone and ACTH in the treatment of acute relapse in MS. *Neurology*, **39**, 969–71.

Thompson, A.J., Kermode, A.G., Wicks, D., MacManus, D.G., Kendall, B.E., Kingsley, D.P. & McDonald, W.I. (1991). Major differences in the dynamics of primary and secondary progressive multiple sclerosis. *Annals of Neurology*, **29**, 53–62

Tienari, P.J., Wikstrom, J., Sajantila, A., Palo, J. & Peltonen, L. (1992). Genetic susceptibility to multiple sclerosis linked to myelin basic protein gene. *Lancet*. **340**, 987–91.

Tomasevic, L., Nikolic, J., Lukic, M. & Levic, Z. (1990). Circulating autoantibodies in multiple sclerosis. *Neurologija*, **39**, 157–61.

Tournier Lasserve, E., Lyoncaen, O., Roullet, E. & Bach, M.A. (1987). IL-2 receptor and HLA class II antigens on cerebrospinal fluid cells of patients with multiple sclerosis and other neurological diseases. *Clinical and Experimental Immunology*, **67**, 581–6.

Traugott, U. & Lebon, P. (1988). Interferon-gamma and Ia antigen are present on astrocytes in active chronic multiple sclerosis lesions. *Journal of the Neurological Sciences*, **84**, 257–64.

Traugott, U. & Raine, C.S. (1985). Multiple sclerosis. Evidence for antigen presentation *in situ* by endothelial cells and astrocytes. *Journal of the Neurological Sciences*, **69**, 365–70.

Traugott, U., Reinherz, E.L. & Raine, C.S. (1983*a*). Multiple sclerosis. Distribution of T cells,

T cell subsets and Ia-positive macrophages in lesions of different ages. *Journal of Neuro-immunology*, **4**, 201–21.

Traugott, U., Reinherz, E.L. & Raine, C.S. (1983*b*). Multiple sclerosis: distribution of T cell subsets within active chronic lesions. *Science*, **219**, 308–10.

Traugott, U., Scheinberg, L.C. & Raine, C.S. (1985). On the presence of Ia-positive endothelial cells and astrocytes in multiple sclerosis lesions and its relevance to antigen presentation. *Journal of Neuroimmunology*, **8**, 1–14.

Trostle, D.C., Helfrich, D. & Medsger, T.A. Jr (1986). Systemic sclerosis (scleroderma) and multiple sclerosis. *Arthritis and Rheumatism*, **29**, 124–7.

Trotter, J.L., Clifford, D.B., Anderson, C.B., van der Veen, R.C., Hicks, B.C. & Banks, G. (1988). Elevated serum interleukin-2 levels in chronic progressive multiple sclerosis. *New England Journal of Medicine*, **318**, 1206.

Trotter, J.L., Clifford, D.B., McInnis, J.E., Griffeth, R.C., Bruns, K.A., Perlmutter, M.S., Anderson, C.B., Collins, K.G., Banks, G. & Hicks, B.C. (1989). Correlation of immunological studies and disease progression in chronic progressive multiple sclerosis. *Annals of Neurology*, **25**, 172–8.

Trotter, J.L., Hickey, W.F., van der Veen, R.C. & Sulze, L. (1991). Peripheral blood mononuclear cells from multiple sclerosis patients recognize myelin proteolipid protein and selected peptides. *Journal of Neuroimmunology*, **33**, 55–62.

Trotter, J.L., van der Veen, R.C. & Clifford, D.B. (1990). Serial studies of serum interleukin-2 in chronic progressive multiple sclerosis patients: occurrence of 'bursts' and effect of cyclosporine. *Journal of Neuroimmunology*, **28**, 9–14.

Tsukada, N., Matsuda, M., Miyagi, K. & Yanagisawa, N. (1991). Soluble CD4 and CD8 in the peripheral blood of patients with multiple sclerosis and HTLV-1-associated myelopathy. *Journal of Neuroimmunology*, **35**, 285–93.

Tsukada, N., Miyagi, K., Matsuda, M. & Yanagisawa, N. (1993). Increased levels of circulating intercellular adhesion molecule-1 in multiple sclerosis and human T-lymphotropic virus type I-associated myelopathy. *Annals of Neurology*, **33**, 646–9.

Tuohy, V.K., Lu, Z.J., Sobel, R.A., Laursen, R.A. & Lees, M.B. (1988). A synthetic peptide from myelin proteolipid protein induces experimental allergic encephalomyelitis. *Journal of Immunology*, **141**, 1126–30.

Tuohy, V.K., Lu, Z., Sobel, R.A., Laursen, R.A. & Lees, M.B. (1989). Identification of an encephalitogenic determinant of myelin proteolipid protein for SJL mice. *Journal of Immunology*, **142**, 1523–7.

Utz, U., Biddison, W.E., McFarland, H.F., McFarlin, D.E., Flerlage, M. & Martin, R. (1993). Skewed T-cell receptor repertoire in genetically identical twins correlates with multiple sclerosis. *Nature*, **364**, 243–7.

Valli, A., Sette, A., Kappos, L., Oseroff, C., Sidney, J., Miescher, G., Hochberger, M., Albert, E.D. & Adorini, L. (1993). Binding of myelin basic protein peptides to human histocompatibility leukocyte antigen class II molecules and their recognition by T cells from multiple sclerosis patients. *Journal of Clinical Investigation*, **91**, 616–28.

Vandenbark, A.A., Chou, Y.K., Bourdette, D., Whitham, R., Chilgren, J., Chou, C.H., Konat, G., Hashim, G., Vainiene, M. & Offner, H. (1989). Human T lymphocyte response to myelin basic protein: selection of T lymphocyte lines from MBP-responsive donors. *Journal of Neuroscience Research*, **23**, 21–30.

Vogel, C., Paty, D.W. & Kibler, R.F. (1972). Treatment of experimental allergic encephalomyelitis in the rabbit. *Archives of Neurology*, **26**, 366–73.

Voskuhl, R.R., Martin, R. & McFarland, H.F. (1993*a*). A functional basis for the association of HLA class II genes and susceptibility to multiple sclerosis: cellular immune responses to myelin basic protein in a multiplex family. *Journal of Neuroimmunology*, **42**, 199–207.

Voskuhl, R.R., McFarlin, D.E., Tranquill, L.R., Deibler, G., Stone, R., Maloni, H. &

McFarland, H.F. (1993*b*). A novel candidate autoantigen in a multiplex family with multiple sclerosis: prevalence of T-lymphocytes specific for an MBP epitope unique to myelination. *Journal of Neuroimmunology*, **46**, 137–44.

Wajgt, A., Gorny, M., Szczechowski, L., Grzybowski, G. & Ochudlo, S. (1989). Effect of immunosuppressive therapy on humoral immune response in multiple sclerosis. *Acta Medica Polona*, **30**, 121–8.

Walsh, M.J. & Tourtellotte, W.W. (1986). Temporal invariance and clonal uniformity of brain and cerebrospinal IgG, IgA, and IgM in multiple sclerosis. *Journal of Experimental Medicine*, **163**, 41–53.

Walter, M.A., Gibson, W.T., Ebers, G.C. & Cox, D.W. (1991). Susceptibility to multiple sclerosis is associated with the proximal immunoglobulin heavy chain variable region. *Journal of Clinical Investigation*, **87**, 1266–73.

Warren, K.G. & Catz, I. (1993). Increased synthetic peptide specificity of tissue-CSF bound anti-MBP in multiple sclerosis. *Journal of Neuroimmunology*, **43**, 87–96.

Warren, K.G., Catz, I., Jeffrey, V.M. & Carroll, D.J. (1986). Effect of methylprednisolone on CSF IgG parameters, myelin basic protein and anti-myelin basic protein in multiple sclerosis exacerbations. *Canadian Journal of Neurological Sciences*, **13**, 25–30.

Warren, K.G., Catz, I., Johnson, E. & Mielke, B. (1994). Anti-myelin basic protein and anti-proteolipid protein specific forms of multiple sclerosis. *Annals of Neurology*, **35**, 280–9.

Washington, R., Burton, J., Todd, R.F., Newman, W., Dragovic, L. & Dore Duffy, P. (1994). Expression of immunologically relevant endothelial cell activation antigens on isolated central nervous system microvessels from patients with multiple sclerosis. *Annals of Neurology*, **35**, 89–97.

Waxman, S.G. (1993). Peripheral nerve abnormalities in multiple sclerosis. *Muscle and Nerve*, **16**, 1–5.

Waxman, S.G., Black, J.A., Kocsis, J.D. & Ritchie, J.M. (1989). Low density of sodium channels supports action potential conduction in axons of neonatal rat optic nerve. *Proceedings of the National Academy of Sciences USA*, **86**, 1406–10.

Weber, W.E. & Buurman, W.A. (1988). Myelin basic protein-specific CD4+ cytolytic T-lymphocyte clones isolated from multiple sclerosis patients. *Human Immunology*, **22**, 97–109.

Weiner, H.L., Mackin, G.A., Matsui, M., Orav, E.J., Khoury, S.J., Dawson, D.M. & Hafler, D.A. (1993). Double-blind pilot trial of oral tolerization with myelin antigens in multiple sclerosis. *Science*, **259**, 1321–4.

Weller, M., Stevens, A., Sommer, N., Melms, A., Dichgans, J. & Wietholter, H. (1991). Comparative analysis of cytokine patterns in immunological, infectious, and oncological neurological disorders. *Journal of the Neurological Sciences*, **104**, 215–21.

Wertman, E., Zilber, N. & Abramsky, O. (1992). An association between multiple sclerosis and type I diabetes mellitus. *Journal of Neurology*, **239**, 43–5.

Whitaker, J.N. (1977). Myelin encephalitogenic protein fragments in cerebrospinal fluid of persons with multiple sclerosis. *Neurology*, **27**, 911–20.

Whitaker, J.N. & Herman, P.K. (1988). Human myelin basic protein peptide 69–89: immunochemical features and use in immunoassays of cerebrospinal fluid. *Journal of Neuroimmunology*, **19**, 47–57.

Wilborn, F., Schmidt, C.A., Brinkmann, V., Jendroska, K., Oettle, H. & Siegert, W. (1994). A potential role for human herpesvirus type 6 in nervous system disease. *Journal of Neuroimmunology*, **49**, 213–14.

Woodroofe, M.N., Bellamy, A.S., Feldmann, M., Davison, A.N. & Cuzner, M.L. (1986). Immunocytochemical characterisation of the immune reaction in the central nervous system in multiple sclerosis. Possible role for microglia in lesion growth. *Journal of the Neurological Sciences*, **74**, 135–52.

Wucherpfennig, K.W., Newcombe, J., Li, H., Keddy, C., Cuzner, M.L. & Hafler, D.A. (1992*a*). T cell receptor V_α–V_β repertoire and cytokine gene expression in active multiple sclerosis lesions. *Journal of Experimental Medicine*, **175**, 993–1002.

Wucherpfennig, K.W., Newcombe, J., Li, H., Keddy, C., Cuzner, M.L. & Hafler, D.A. (1992*b*). Gamma delta T-cell receptor repertoire in acute multiple sclerosis lesions. *Proceedings of the National Academy of Sciences USA*, **89**, 4588–92.

Wucherpfennig, K.W., Ota, K., Endo, N., Seidman, J.G., Rosenzweig, A., Weiner, H.L. & Hafler, D.A. (1990). Shared human T cell receptor V beta usage to immunodominant regions of myelin basic protein. *Science*, **248**, 1016–19.

Wucherpfennig, K.W., Sette, A., Southwood, S., Oseroff, C., Matsui, M., Strominger, J.L. & Hafler, D.A. (1994). Structural requirements for binding of an immunodominant myelin basic protein peptide to DR2 isotypes and for its recognition by human T cell clones. *Journal of Experimental Medicine*, **179**, 279–90.

Xiao, B.G., Linington, C. & Link, H. (1991). Antibodies to myelin-oligodendrocyte glycoprotein in cerebrospinal fluid from patients with multiple sclerosis and controls. *Journal of Neuroimmunology*, **31**, 91–6.

Zaffaroni, M., Gallo, L., Ghezzi, A. & Cazzullo, C.L. (1991). CD4+ lymphocyte subsets in the cerebrospinal fluid of multiple sclerosis and non-inflammatory neurological diseases. *Journal of Neurology*, **238**, 209–11.

Zaffaroni, M., Rossini, S., Ghezzi, A., Parma, R. & Cazzullo, C.L. (1990). Decrease of CD4+CD45+ T-cells in chronic-progressive multiple sclerosis. *Journal of Neurology*, **237**, 1–4.

Zanetta, J.P., Warter, J.M., Kuchler, S., Marschal, P., Rumbach, L., Lehmann, S., Tranchant, C., Reeber, A. & Vincendon, G. (1990). Antibodies to cerebellar soluble lectin CSL in multiple sclerosis. *Lancet*, **335**, 1482–4.

Zhang, J., Chin, Y., Henderikx, P., Medaer, R., Chou, C.H. & Raus, J.C. (1991). Antibodies to myelin basic protein and measles virus in multiple sclerosis: precursor frequency analysis of the antibody producing B cells. *Autoimmunity*, **11**, 27–34.

Zhang, J., Chou, C.H., Hashim, G., Medaer, R. & Raus, J.C. (1990). Preferential peptide specificity and HLA restriction of myelin basic protein-specific T cell clones derived from MS patients. *Cellular Immunology*, **129**, 189–98.

Zhang, J., Markovic Plese, S., Lacet, B., Raus, J., Weiner, H.L. & Hafler, D.A. (1994). Increased frequency of interleukin 2-responsive T cells specific for myelin basic protein and proteolipid protein in peripheral blood and cerebrospinal fluid of patients with multiple sclerosis. *Journal of Experimental Medicine*, **179**, 973–84.

Zhang, J., Medaer, R., Hashim, G.A., Chin, Y., van den Berg Loonen, E. & Raus, J.C. (1992*a*). Myelin basic protein-specific T lymphocytes in multiple sclerosis and controls: precursor frequency, fine specificity, and cytotoxicity. *Annals of Neurology*, **32**, 330–8.

Zhang, J., Medaer, R., Stinissen, P., Hafler, D. & Raus, J. (1993). MHC-restricted depletion of human myelin basic protein-reactive T cells by T cell vaccination. *Science*, **261**, 1451–4.

Zhang, J., Schreurs, M., Medaer, R. & Raus, J.C. (1992*b*). Regulation of myelin basic protein-specific helper T cells in multiple sclerosis: generation of suppressor T cell lines. *Cellular Immunology*, **139**, 118–30.

Zhang, Y., Burger, D., Saruhan, G., Jeannet, M. & Steck, A.J. (1993). The T-lymphocyte response against myelin-associated glycoprotein and myelin basic protein in patients with multiple sclerosis. *Neurology*, **43**, 403–7.

Zoukos, Y., Leonard, J.P., Thomaides, T., Thompson, A.J. & Cuzner, M.L. (1992). beta-Adrenergic receptor density and function of peripheral blood mononuclear cells are increased in multiple sclerosis: a regulatory role for cortisol and interleukin-1. *Annals of Neurology*, **31**, 657–62.

–5–
Acute disseminated encephalomyelitis

MICHAEL P. PENDER

Introduction

Acute disseminated encephalomyelitis (ADEM) (post-infectious encephalomyelitis or post-vaccinal encephalomyelitis) is an acute inflammatory demyelinating disease of the central nervous system (CNS) (Johnson, Griffin & Gendelman, 1985). Typically it follows infection by a virus, but it may also follow infection by other agents or may complicate vaccination. Sometimes it occurs without any obvious triggering factors. The clinical manifestations are diverse and include presentation with acute transverse myelitis. Acute haemorrhagic leukoencephalitis is a rare and more severe form of ADEM with a high mortality and morbidity (Hurst, 1941; Johnson *et al.*, 1985). There is good evidence that ADEM and acute haemorrhagic leukoencephalitis are autoimmune diseases similar to acute experimental autoimmune encephalomyelitis (EAE) and hyperacute EAE, respectively.

Clinical features

Triggering factors

Viral infection

Typically ADEM follows a viral infection such as measles, chickenpox, rubella, mumps, influenza or Epstein–Barr virus infections (Johnson *et al.*, 1985). It may also follow upper respiratory tract infections of undetermined aetiology, *Mycoplasma pneumoniae* infection and bacterial infections (Johnson *et al.*, 1985). Prior to the eradication of smallpox and the discontinuation of smallpox vaccination, smallpox and vaccinia were also important triggers of ADEM. In regions of the world that do not have a successful measles vaccination programme, ADEM complicates about one in 1000 measles virus infections (Johnson *et al.*, 1984).

Rabies vaccine containing nervous tissue

'Neuroparalytic accidents' were noted to develop in some patients receiving the rabies vaccine which was introduced by Pasteur in 1885 and which contained rabbit spinal cord tissue. The pathological findings in patients dying of neuroparalytic accidents could be distinguished from those of rabies and consisted of perivascular inflammation and demyelination of the CNS, which are the characteristic features of ADEM (Bassoe & Grinker, 1930). Attempts to replicate this complication in experimental animals ultimately led to the development of the model, EAE (see Chapter 3). In countries still using rabies vaccine containing CNS tissue, the incidence of neurological complications is as high as 1:220 (Swaddiwudhipong *et al.*, 1987).

Other vaccines

ADEM may also be triggered by the administration of vaccines that do not contain nervous tissue, although the incidence is much lower than when vaccines containing nervous tissue are used. A wide variety of vaccines have been reported to trigger ADEM or acute transverse myelitis, including influenza, measles, rubella, pneumococcal, recombinant hepatitis B, and tetanus toxoid vaccines (Poser, Roman & Emery, 1978; Fenichel, 1982; de la Monte *et al.*, 1986; Herroelen, De Keyser & Ebinger, 1991; Topaloglu *et al.*, 1992; Read, Schapel & Pender, 1992).

Injection of nervous tissue other than in vaccines

Injection of preparations containing nervous tissue, as a form of alternative medicine, can trigger ADEM (Sotelo *et al.*, 1984; Goebel, Walther & Meuth, 1986).

General clinical features

The symptoms of ADEM complicating viral exanthems, such as measles, usually commence 4–8 days after the onset of the skin rash, but may occasionally precede the rash or develop as long as three weeks after the rash (Johnson *et al.*, 1984, 1985). In the case of ADEM complicating the administration of rabies vaccine containing CNS tissue, the symptoms of ADEM typically commence 6–17 days after the first injection, but may begin as early as one day or as late as nine weeks after the first injection (Swamy *et al.*, 1984; Hemachudha *et al.*, 1987*b*). When ADEM complicates immunization with vaccines not containing nervous tissue, the symptoms usually commence 1–15 days after vaccination, but may begin later (Fenichel, 1982).

The clinical features vary according to which region of the nervous system bears the brunt of the immune attack. Constitutional symptoms such as fever, myalgia and malaise commonly accompany all forms of ADEM. Encephalitis is manifested by headache, a decreased level of consciousness, which may progress to coma, epileptic seizures, neck stiffness, and focal cerebral dysfunction with hemiparesis or dysphasia. Acute transverse myelitis is manifested by paraparesis or quadriparesis with a bilateral sensory level and urinary and faecal retention. Encephalitis and acute transverse myelitis may occur together or separately. Unilateral or bilateral optic neuritis, cerebellar ataxia or brainstem dysfunction may also occur separately or in combination with clinical involvement of any of the other regions of the CNS.

Usually the clinical course is monophasic and there is spontaneous clinical improvement, although frequently there is a residual neurological deficit and occasionally the disease is fatal. Occasionally relapses of ADEM occur, without apparent further triggering factors, after infection (Walker & Gawler, 1989) or after immunization with rabies vaccine containing CNS tissue (Hemachudha *et al.*, 1987*b*). However, when relapses occur six months or longer after the infection, the diagnosis of multiple sclerosis (MS) rather than recurrent ADEM needs to be considered (Kesselring *et al.*, 1990).

Involvement of the peripheral nervous system

Clinical involvement of the peripheral nervous system (PNS), including the Guillain–Barré syndrome, may occur in association with ADEM following infection (Amit *et al.*, 1986, 1992), immunization with rabies vaccine containing CNS tissue (Swamy *et al.*, 1984; Hemachudha *et al.*, 1987*b*), immunization with other vaccines (Poser *et al.*, 1978; de la Monte *et al.*, 1986) or by injections of preparations of CNS tissue as a form of alternative medicine (Bohl *et al.*, 1989). Involvement of the PNS without clinical evidence of ADEM may also occur following these events. Interestingly, both the PNS and the CNS are affected in animals with acute EAE induced by inoculation with whole CNS tissue or purified myelin basic protein (MBP) (Pender, 1987; see also Chapter 3).

Diagnosis

The diagnosis of ADEM is based on the presence of the clinical features and precipitating factors mentioned above. Laboratory investigations and neuroimaging studies are also important in establishing the diagnosis. Examination of the cerebrospinal fluid (CSF) usually reveals a lymphocytic pleocytosis and often an elevated protein content (Johnson *et al.*, 1984;

Swamy *et al.*, 1984; Hemachudha *et al.*, 1987*b*). Oligoclonal immunoglobulin G (IgG) bands may also be present in the CSF in some patients (Kesselring *et al.*, 1990). Electroencephalography may often reveal diffuse slowing or occasionally paroxysmal discharges (Swamy *et al.*, 1984; Johnson *et al.*, 1985). Visual, auditory and somatosensory evoked potential studies may reveal evidence of subclinical involvement of the CNS, whereas electromyography and nerve conduction studies may demonstrate involvement of the PNS. Typically, magnetic resonance imaging (MRI) of the brain shows multifocal white matter lesions indistinguishable from those seen in MS (Dun *et al.*, 1986; Kesselring *et al.*, 1990). However, in some cases of ADEM there are patterns that are unusual in MS, such as extensive symmetrical abnormalities in the cerebral or cerebellar white matter or basal ganglia, or isolated thalamic involvement (Kesselring *et al.*, 1990; Hamed *et al.*, 1993). Occasionally MRI of the brain demonstrates a solitary lesion suggesting a neoplasm and necessitating a biopsy, which reveals the histological features of ADEM (Miller *et al.*, 1993; Hamed *et al.*, 1993). MRI of the spinal cord may reveal evidence of myelitis. In the case of suspected acute transverse myelitis, myelography or MRI is necessary to exclude spinal cord compression, which may produce a similar clinical picture. It is often difficult initially to determine whether an individual patient has ADEM or is experiencing the first attack of MS, particularly as episodes of MS can also be triggered by viral infection (Sibley, Bamford & Clark, 1985). In such cases long-term clinical follow-up is essential in establishing the correct diagnosis. Serial MRI studies may also be helpful (Kesselring *et al.*, 1990).

Acute haemorrhagic leukoencephalitis

The clinical course of acute haemorrhagic leukoencephalitis differs from that of typical ADEM in that the course is fulminant and there is a high mortality and morbidity (Hurst, 1941; Johnson *et al.*, 1985). The majority of patients die within five days of onset, and most survivors have severe neurological deficits. CSF examination reveals a predominance of polymorphonuclear leukocytes and an accumulation of erythrocytes. MRI of the brain may demonstrate the haemorrhagic lesions.

Neuropathology

Regardless of whether ADEM is triggered by viral infection, the injection of rabies vaccine containing CNS tissue, or the administration of other vaccines, the same histological changes occur. The typical neuropathological features are perivascular inflammation and primary demyelination of the CNS (Adams & Kubik, 1952; Calabresi & Powers, 1994). Usually the lesions are distributed widely throughout the CNS with involvement of the spinal cord, brainstem, cerebrum, cerebellum and sometimes the optic nerves. In some cases with the clinical features of acute myelitis, the lesions predominate or occur exclusively in the spinal cord. Generally the lesions are predominantly located in the white matter, although the grey matter is not spared. The inflammatory infiltrates consist predominantly of lymphocytes, plasma cells and macrophages, and are present in the Virchow–Robin space and perivascular parenchyma. Inflammation and primary demyelination are also found in the subpial and subependymal regions. Meningeal inflammation may occur. Immunocytochemical studies have shown that there is a loss of MBP and myelin-associated glycoprotein in the regions of perivenous demyelination, which has been interpreted as indicating that the immune attack is directed primarily at the myelin sheath rather than at the oligodendrocyte (Gendelman *et al.*, 1984). When the PNS is also involved the histological findings are similar to those in the CNS (Swamy *et al.*, 1984). The neuropathological findings of ADEM closely resemble those of acute EAE (see Chapter 3).

In acute haemorrhagic leukoencephalitis there is intense infiltration with polymorphonuclear leukocytes, necrosis and fibrin impregnation of small blood vessel walls, and perivascular haemorrhage, necrosis, fibrinous exudation and oedema (Hurst, 1941; Adams & Kubik, 1952; Ravkina *et al.*, 1979). These neuropathological features closely resemble those of hyperacute EAE (Levine & Wenk, 1965; Ravkina *et al.*, 1979; also see Chapter 3). Necrosis of small blood vessel walls and perivascular necrosis, haemorrhage and fibrin exudation may also occur in some lesions of otherwise typical ADEM, indicating the relationship between acute haemorrhagic leukoencephalitis and ADEM (Adams & Kubik, 1952).

Pathophysiology

It is likely that the neurological symptoms and signs of ADEM are mainly due to nerve conduction block due to primary demyelination, as in acute EAE (Pender, 1987; see also Chapter 3) and the early stages of MS (see Chapter 4). Neurological improvement is probably due to restoration of conduction by remyelination, as occurs during recovery from acute EAE (Pender, 1989). Residual neurological deficits are likely to reflect axonal loss.

Immunological findings in the peripheral blood

T cell reactivity to myelin basic protein

As MBP is encephalitogenic in experimental animals (see Chapter 3), reactivity to this protein has been studied in patients with ADEM. Increased proliferation of peripheral blood lymphocytes in response to MBP has been found in the majority of patients with post-infectious ADEM (Behan *et al.*, 1968; Lisak *et al.*, 1974; Lisak & Zweiman, 1977; Abramsky & Teitelbaum, 1977; Johnson *et al.*, 1984). The blood lymphocyte proliferative response to MBP in ADEM is considerably higher than that in patients with MS (Lisak *et al.*, 1974; Lisak & Zweiman, 1977) and returns to normal after clinical recovery (Lisak *et al.*, 1974). Increased proliferative reactivity to MBP has also been found in the peripheral blood lymphocytes of patients with post-infectious or idiopathic acute transverse myelitis (Abramsky & Teitelbaum, 1977). Johnson *et al.* (1984) found an increased proliferative response to MBP in the single patient they examined with ADEM complicating the administration of rabies vaccine containing CNS tissue, while Hemachudha *et al.* (1987*b*) found an increased proliferative response to purified CNS myelin in patients with this complication, but did not examine the reactivity to MBP. The peripheral blood lymphocyte reactivity to other myelin antigens such as myelin proteolipid protein, which is also encephalitogenic in experimental animals, has not yet been examined in ADEM.

Antibodies to MBP, cerebroside and gangliosides

Elevated serum anti-MBP antibody levels have been demonstrated in patients with CNS or PNS involvement, complicating immunization with rabies vaccine containing CNS tissue, but not in those with minor complications without neurological deficits or in patients with sporadic Guillain–Barré syndrome (Hemachudha *et al.*, 1987*a*, 1988). In addition, elevated serum antibodies against cerebroside and gangliosides were found in patients with major neurological complications of this vaccination; however, elevated anti-cerebroside antibodies were also present in those with no or minor complications (Hemachudha *et al.*, 1987*a*). Lisak *et al.* (1974) did not detect serum anti-MBP antibodies in patients with post-infectious ADEM.

Immunological findings in the CSF

Non-specific findings

As mentioned above, a lymphocytic pleocytosis is usually present in the CSF (Johnson *et al.*, 1984; Swamy *et al.*, 1984; Hemachudha *et al.*, 1987*b*). Oligoclonal IgG bands may also be present in the CSF in some patients (Kesselring *et al.*, 1990).

T cell reactivity to MBP

CSF lymphocytes in patients with ADEM exhibit an increased proliferative response to MBP, similar to that observed in active MS and significantly higher than in stable MS or other inflammatory neurological diseases (Lisak & Zweiman, 1977; Lisak, Zweiman & Whitaker, 1981). Hafler *et al.* (1987) found that five of nine $CD4^+$ T cell clones directly isolated from the CSF of a patient with post-infectious ADEM reacted to MBP, but none of 235 clones from the CSF of patients with MS showed such reactivity.

Antibodies to MBP and cerebroside

Hemachudha *et al.* (1987*a*) found elevated levels of anti-MBP and anti-cerebroside antibodies in the CSF of patients with CNS or PNS involvement, complicating immunization with rabies vaccine containing CNS tissue. By comparing the reactivity of the CSF with that of serum diluted to contain the same amount of total IgG, they demonstrated intrathecal synthesis of anti-MBP antibody in 36% and of anti-cerebroside antibody in 40% of patients with these complications.

MBP

Antigenic material that is cross-reactive with MBP can be detected by radioimmunoassay in the CSF of patients with active myelin destruction (Cohen, Herndon & McKhann, 1976; Whitaker, 1977; also see Chapter 4). Immunoreactive MBP is elevated in the CSF of some patients with ADEM following viral infection or immunization with rabies vaccine containing CNS tissue (Lisak *et al.*, 1981; Johnson *et al.*, 1984; Hemachudha *et al.*, 1987*b*).

Pathogenesis

As indicated above, there is convincing evidence of increased T cell reactivity to MBP in post-infectious ADEM. It is highly likely that T cells specific for MBP and/or other myelin antigens mediate the inflammatory demyelination, as is the case in acute EAE; however, the role of antibody to myelin antigens is unclear. The question arises of how viral or other infections lead to the expansion of the autoreactive T cells. In the case of ADEM following measles virus infection, viral invasion of the CNS is not necessary for such T cell expansion, as there is a lack of intrathecal synthesis of antibody against measles virus (Johnson *et al.*, 1984) and as immunocytochemical studies have shown an absence of viral antigen in the CNS of patients who have died with this complication (Gendelman *et al.*, 1984). One possible mechanism for the triggering of myelin-specific autoimmunity by a viral infection is that a viral epitope may evoke specific sensitization that cross-reacts with a homologous sequence in MBP or other myelin antigens.

This mechanism has been termed molecular mimicry. Computer searches have revealed sequence homologies between human myelin proteins and proteins of viruses known to infect humans (Jahnke, Fischer & Alvord, 1985). Experimental evidence supporting molecular mimicry as a mechanism for inducing autoimmunity has been provided by Fujinami & Oldstone (1985). By inoculating rabbits with a peptide of hepatitis B virus polymerase sharing sequence homology with an encephalitogenic region of MBP, they induced CNS inflammation together with antibody and lymphocyte proliferative responses to the viral peptide and MBP.

Although viral invasion of the CNS does not appear to be necessary for the expansion of MBP-specific T cells in ADEM following measles, studies in Lewis rats have shown that intracerebral inoculation with measles virus leads to increased proliferative responses of splenic lymphocytes to MBP (Liebert, Linington & ter Meulen, 1988). Furthermore, MBP-specific T cell lines, which do not cross-react with measles virus and which transfer EAE, can be isolated from the spleens of infected animals (Liebert *et al.*, 1988). A T-cell-mediated autoimmune reaction to MBP also develops in Lewis rats after intracerebral inoculation with the murine coronavirus JHM (Watanabe, Wege & ter Meulen, 1983). However, it is unclear whether direct viral invasion of the CNS has any role in the pathogenesis of ADEM in humans. Another postulated mechanism for the induction of autoimmunity by viral infection is that infection of lymphoid tissues may interfere with the immunoregulation of autoreactive cells (Johnson *et al.*, 1985).

In the case of ADEM following the administration of rabies vaccine containing CNS tissue, myelin-specific autoimmunity results from direct sensitization to myelin antigens in the vaccine. However, the genetic or other factors determining individual patient susceptibility to ADEM after rabies vaccination are unknown.

Therapy

Corticosteroid therapy is widely used in the treatment of ADEM, although there have been no controlled clinical trials demonstrating its efficacy. High-dose intravenous corticosteroid therapy followed by a gradually tapering course of oral corticosteroid treatment appears to be the most effective regimen (Dowling, Bosch & Cook, 1980). Intravenous cyclophosphamide therapy was found to be effective in patients with neurological complications of rabies vaccination not responding to corticosteroid therapy (Swamy *et al.*, 1984), although high-dose intravenous corticosteroid therapy was not used. Stricker, Miller & Kiprov (1992) observed that plasmapheresis appears to have a beneficial effect in ADEM. However, controlled studies will be required to determine the role of plasmapheresis and immunosuppressant therapy in the management of this condition. Supportive therapy, including the maintenance of electrolyte and fluid balance and adequate ventilation, is essential in the management of ADEM. Anti-epileptic drugs are required for epileptic seizures.

Conclusions

There is convincing evidence of increased T cell reactivity to MBP in patients with ADEM; however, studies are needed to determine whether there is also enhanced T cell reactivity to other myelin antigens such as proteolipid protein. It is highly likely that T cells specific for MBP and/or other myelin antigens mediate the inflammatory demyelination in ADEM, as is the case in acute EAE; however, the role of antibody to myelin antigens is unclear. The induction of anti-myelin autoimmunity by viral infection is not dependent on viral invasion of the CNS and may be due to the cross-reactivity of anti-viral immune responses with homologous amino acid sequences in MBP or other myelin antigens. Controlled clinical trials will be required to determine the optimal therapy in the management of patients with ADEM.

References

Abramsky, O. & Teitelbaum, D. (1977). The autoimmune features of acute transverse myelopathy. *Annals of Neurology*, **2**, 36–40.

Adams, R.D. & Kubik, C.S. (1952). The morbid anatomy of the demyelinative diseases. *American Journal of Medicine*, **12**, 510–46.

Amit, R., Glick, B., Itzchak, Y., Dgani, Y. & Meyeir, S. (1992). Acute severe combined demyelination. *Childs Nervous System*, **8**, 354–6.

Amit, R., Shapira, Y., Blank, A. & Aker, M. (1986). Acute, severe, central and peripheral nervous system combined demyelination. *Pediatric Neurology*, **2**, 47–50.

Bassoe, P. & Grinker, R.R. (1930). Human rabies and rabies vaccine encephalomyelitis. A clinicopathologic study. *Archives of Neurology and Psychiatry*, **23**, 1138–60.

Behan, P.O., Geschwind, N., Lamarche, J.B., Lisak, R.P. & Kies, M.W. (1968). Delayed hypersensitivity to encephalitogenic protein in disseminated encephalomyelitis. *Lancet*, **2**, 1009–12.

Bohl, J., Goebel, H.H., Potsch, L., Esinger, W., Walther, G., Mattern, R. & Merkel, K.H. (1989). [Complications following cell therapy]. *Zeitschrift für Rechtsmedizin*, **103**, 1–20.

Calabresi, P.A. & Powers, J.M. (1994). An ultrastructural analysis of human post-infectious (allergic) encephalomyelitis. *Acta Neuropathologica*, **87**, 541–4.

Cohen, S.R., Herndon, R.M. & McKhann, G.M. (1976). Radioimmunoassay of myelin basic protein in spinal fluid. An index of active demyelination. *New England Journal of Medicine*, **295**, 1455–7.

de la Monte, S.M., Ropper, A.H., Dickersin, G.R., Harris, N.L., Ferry, J.A. & Richardson, E.P.J. (1986). Relapsing central and peripheral demyelinating diseases. Unusual pathologic features. *Archives of Neurology*, **43**, 626–9.

Dowling, P.C., Bosch, V.V. & Cook, S.D. (1980). Possible beneficial effect of high-dose intravenous steroid therapy in acute demyelinating disease and transverse myelitis. *Neurology*, **30** (2), 33–6.

Dun, V., Bale, J.F.J., Zimmerman, R.A., Perdue, Z. & Bell, W.E. (1986). MRI in children with postinfectious disseminated encephalomyelitis. *Magnetic Resonance Imaging*, **4**, 25–32.

Fenichel, G.M. (1982). Neurological complications of immunization. *Annals of Neurology*, **12**, 119–28.

Fujinami, R.S. & Oldstone, M.B. (1985). Amino acid homology between the encephalitogenic site of myelin basic protein and virus: mechanism for autoimmunity. *Science*, **230**, 1043–5.

Gendelman, H.E., Wolinsky, J.S., Johnson, R.T., Pressman, N.J., Pezeshkpour, G.H. & Boisset, G.F. (1984). Measles encephalomyelitis: lack of evidence of viral invasion of the central nervous system and quantitative study of the nature of demyelination. *Annals of Neurology*, **15**, 353–60.

Goebel, H.H., Walther, G. & Meuth, M. (1986). Fresh cell therapy followed by fatal coma. *Journal of Neurology*, **233**, 242–7.

Hafler, D.A., Benjamin, D.S., Burks, J. & Weiner, H.L. (1987). Myelin basic protein and proteolipid protein reactivity of brain- and cerebrospinal fluid-derived T cell clones in multiple sclerosis and postinfectious encephalomyelitis. *Journal of Immunology*, **139**, 68–72.

Hamed, L.M., Silbiger, J., Guy, J., Mickle, J.P., Sibony, P., Cossari, A. & Andriola, M. (1993). Parainfectious optic neuritis and encephalomyelitis. A report of two cases with thalamic involvement. *Journal of Clinical Neuro-ophthalmology*, **13**, 18–23.

Hemachudha, T., Griffin, D.E., Chen, W.W. & Johnson, R.T. (1988). Immunologic studies of rabies vaccination-induced Guillain–Barré syndrome. *Neurology*, **38**, 375–8.

Hemachudha, T., Griffin, D.E., Giffels, J.J., Johnson, R.T., Moser, A.B. & Phanuphak, P. (1987*a*). Myelin basic protein as an encephalitogen in encephalomyelitis and polyneuritis following rabies vaccination. *New England Journal of Medicine*, **316**, 369–74.

Hemachudha, T., Phanuphak, P., Johnson, R.T., Griffin, D.E., Ratanavongsiri, J. & Siriprasomsup, W. (1987*b*). Neurologic complications of Semple-type rabies vaccine: clinical and immunologic studies. *Neurology*, **37**, 550–6.

Herroelen, L., De Keyser, J. & Ebinger, G. (1991). Central-nervous-system demyelination after immunisation with recombinant hepatitis B vaccine. *Lancet*, **338**, 1174–5.

Hurst, E.W. (1941). Acute haemorrhagic leucoencephalitis: a previously undefined entity. *Medical Journal of Australia*, **2**, 1–6.

Jahnke, U., Fischer, E.H. & Alvord, E.C. (1985). Sequence homology between certain viral proteins and proteins related to encephalomyelitis and neuritis. *Science*, **229**, 282–4.

Johnson, R.T., Griffin, D.E. & Gendelman, H.E. (1985). Postinfectious encephalomyelitis. *Seminars in Neurology*, **5**, 180–90.

Johnson, R.T., Griffin, D.E., Hirsch, R.L., Wolinsky, J.S., Roedenbeck, S., De Soriano, I.L. & Vaisberg, A. (1984). Measles encephalomyelitis – clinical and immunologic studies. *New England Journal of Medicine*, **310**, 137–41.

Kesselring, J., Miller, D.H., Robb, S.A., Kendall, B.E., Moseley, I.F., Kingsley, D., du Boulay, E.P. & McDonald, W.I. (1990). Acute disseminated encephalomyelitis. MRI findings and the distinction from multiple sclerosis. *Brain*, **113**, 291–302.

Levine, S. & Wenk, E.J. (1965). A hyperacute form of allergic encephalomyelitis. *American Journal of Pathology*, **47**, 61–88.

Liebert, U.G., Linington, C. & ter Meulen, V. (1988). Induction of autoimmune reactions to myelin basic protein in measles virus encephalitis in Lewis rats. *Journal of Neuroimmunology*, **17**, 103–18.

Lisak, R.P., Behan, P.O., Zweiman, B. & Shetty, T. (1974). Cell-mediated immunity to myelin basic protein in acute disseminated encephalomyelitis. *Neurology*, **24**, 560–4.

Lisak, R.P. & Zweiman, B. (1977). *In vitro* cell-mediated immunity of cerebrospinal-fluid lymphocytes to myelin basic protein in primary demyelinating diseases. *New England Journal of Medicine*, **297**, 850–3.

Lisak, R.P., Zweiman, B. & Whitaker, J.N. (1981). Spinal fluid basic protein immunoreactive material and spinal fluid lymphocyte reactivity to basic protein. *Neurology*, **31**, 180–2.

Miller, D.H., Scaravilli, F., Thomas, D.C., Harvey, P. & Hirsch, N.P. (1993). Acute disseminated encephalomyelitis presenting as a solitary brainstem mass. *Journal of Neurology, Neurosurgery and Psychiatry*, **56**, 920–2.

Pender, M.P. (1987). Demyelination and neurological signs in experimental allergic encephalomyelitis. *Journal of Neuroimmunology*, **15**, 11–24.

Pender, M.P. (1989). Recovery from acute experimental allergic encephalomyelitis in the Lewis rat: early restoration of nerve conduction and repair by Schwann cells and oligodendrocytes. *Brain*, **112**, 393–416.

Poser, C.M., Roman, G. & Emery, E.S. III (1978). Recurrent disseminated vasculomyelinopathy. *Archives of Neurology*, **35**, 166–70.

Ravkina, L., Harib, I., Manovitch, Z., Deconenko, E., Letchinskaja, E. & Papilova, E. (1979). Hyperacute experimental allergic encephalomyelitis in rhesus monkeys as a model of acute necrotizing hemorrhagic encephalomyelitis. *Journal of Neurology*, **221**, 113–25.

Read, S.J., Schapel, G.J. & Pender, M.P. (1992). Acute transverse myelitis after tetanus toxoid vaccination. *Lancet*, **339**, 1111–12.

Sibley, W.A., Bamford, C.R. & Clark, K. (1985). Clinical viral infections and multiple sclerosis. *Lancet*, **1**, 1313–15.

Sotelo, J., Enriquez, R.G., Najera, R. & Zermeno, F. (1984). Allergic encephalomyelitis associated with holistic medicine (implantation of porcine hypophysis). *Lancet*, **2**, 702.

Stricker, R.B., Miller, R.G. & Kiprov, D.D. (1992). Role of plasmapheresis in acute disseminated (postinfectious) encephalomyelitis. *Journal of Clinical Apheresis*, **7**, 173–9.

Swaddiwudhipong, W., Prayoonwiwat, N., Kunasol, P. & Choomkasien, P. (1987). A high incidence of neurological complications following Semple anti-rabies vaccine. *Southeast Asian Journal of Tropical Medicine and Public Health*, **18**, 526–31.

Swamy, H.S., Shankar, S.K., Chandra, P.S., Aroor, S.R., Krishna, A.S. & Perumal, V.G. (1984). Neurological complications due to beta-propiolactone (BPL)-inactivated antirabies vaccination: clinical, electrophysiological and therapeutic aspects. *Journal of the Neurological Sciences*, **63**, 111–28.

Topaloglu, H., Berker, M., Kansu, T., Saatci, U. & Renda, Y. (1992). Optic neuritis and myelitis after booster tetanus toxoid vaccination. *Lancet*, **339**, 178–9.

Walker, R.W. & Gawler, J. (1989). Serial cerebral CT abnormalities in relapsing acute disseminated encephalomyelitis. *Journal of Neurology, Neurosurgery and Psychiatry*, **52**, 1100–2.

Watanabe, R., Wege, H. & ter Meulen, V. (1983). Adoptive transfer of EAE-like lesions from rats with coronavirus-induced demyelinating encephalomyelitis. *Nature*, **305**, 150–3.

Whitaker, J.N. (1977). Myelin encephalitogenic protein fragments in cerebrospinal fluid of persons with multiple sclerosis. *Neurology*, **27**, 911–20.

–6–
The stiff-man syndrome

MICHAEL P. PENDER

Introduction

The stiff-man syndrome is a rare disorder of the central nervous system (CNS) characterized by progressive fluctuating rigidity and painful spasms of the body musculature. It was first described in 1956 by Moersch & Woltman, although they observed the first case of this condition much earlier, in 1924. Ironically, they nicknamed the disorder 'stiff-man syndrome' to 'associate it with a memorable and descriptive term that could not be taken by anyone to be final'. Recently, evidence has accumulated that the stiff-man syndrome is an autoimmune disease directed against neurones secreting the inhibitory neurotransmitter, gamma-aminobutyric acid (GABA) (Solimena *et al.*, 1990). The syndrome usually develops spontaneously and often occurs in association with other autoimmune diseases, particularly type I (insulin-dependent) diabetes mellitus. However, it may also occur as a paraneoplastic syndrome complicating remote malignancy.

Clinical features

General clinical features and diagnosis

The characteristic clinical picture is the insidious development of muscular tightness, stiffness and rigidity, initially involving the axial musculature (neck, paraspinal and abdominal muscles) and later spreading to affect proximal limb muscles (Moersch & Woltman, 1956; Gordon, Januszko & Kaufman, 1967; Lorish, Thorsteinsson & Howard, 1989). Mobility is restricted by the simultaneous contraction of agonist and antagonist muscles, so that the patient may be observed to walk or fall like 'a wooden man'. Paraspinal rigidity may result in low-back discomfort and a prominent lordosis, and involvement of the thoracic musculature may lead to exertional dyspnoea. The cranial muscles may also be affected, with resultant difficulty in smiling, swallowing and phonating (Gordon *et al.*, 1967).

Superimposed upon the persistent muscular rigidity there are painful muscle spasms, which may be precipitated by noise, a sudden jar, voluntary movement, passive stretching of the muscles, and occasionally by fear or apprehension (Moersch & Woltman, 1956; Gordon *et al.*, 1967; Lorish *et al.*, 1989). These spasms last for several minutes. Neurological examination may reveal the muscular rigidity and spasms and resultant restriction of mobility but the motor examination is otherwise normal. The deep tendon reflexes may be increased, but the plantar responses are flexor (Lorish *et al.*, 1989). Prior to the availability of effective treatment, many patients eventually became severely disabled and totally bedbound (Moersch & Woltman, 1956; Lorish *et al.*, 1989). Paroxysmal autonomic dysfunction leading to hyperpyrexia, diaphoresis, tachypnoea, tachycardia, pupillary dilatation, arterial hypertension and sudden unexpected death may complicate the clinical picture (Mitsumoto *et al.*, 1991).

Accurate clinical diagnosis of the stiff-man syndrome is important both for patient management (see below) and for research studies. Laboratory investigations are helpful in establishing the diagnosis. Electromyography reveals continuous motor unit activity 'at rest' without other abnormalities (Lorish *et al.*, 1989). In addition to routine electromyography, simultaneous video-electroencephalographic-surface electromyographic recordings may be useful in confirming the diagnosis (Armon *et al.*, 1990). Cerebrospinal fluid (CSF) examination may reveal a normal cell count or a pleocytosis and, in some patients, oligoclonal immunoglobulin G (IgG) bands which are not present in the serum (Solimena *et al.*, 1988, 1990; Folli *et al.*, 1993; Meinck *et al.*, 1994).

Association with epilepsy

Epilepsy occurs in about 10% of patients with the stiff-man syndrome (Martinelli *et al.*, 1978; Solimena *et al.*, 1990). As this percentage is considerably higher than the prevalence of epilepsy in the general population, the association is unlikely to be coincidental. Solimena *et al.* observed that epilepsy occurred only in patients with antibodies against GABA-ergic neurones (see below). As a defect in GABA-ergic neurotransmission has been implicated in the pathophysiology of epilepsy, it is possible that the epilepsy associated with the stiff-man syndrome may also have an autoimmune basis.

Association with other autoimmune diseases

Patients with the stiff-man syndrome have an increased incidence of organ-specific autoimmune diseases, particularly insulin-dependent diabetes mellitus, but also Graves' disease, hypothyroidism, pernicious anaemia and vitiligo (Solimena *et al.*, 1990; Grimaldi *et al.*, 1993). They also have a high incidence of organ-specific autoantibodies, namely those directed against islet cells, gastric parietal cells, thyroid microsomal fraction and thyroglobulin. The concurrence with other autoimmune diseases is seen in patients with autoantibodies against GABA-ergic neurones (see below), but not in those without such antibodies (Solimena *et al.*, 1990; Grimaldi *et al.*, 1993). This association supports the hypothesis that the stiff-man syndrome is also an autoimmune disease.

Association with malignancy

Occasionally the stiff-man syndrome occurs as a paraneoplastic syndrome complicating remote malignancy, such as breast carcinoma (Folli *et al.*, 1993), pharyngeal carcinoma (Masson *et al.*, 1987), colonic carcinoma (Piccolo & Cosi, 1989), small cell lung cancer (Bateman, Weller & Kennedy, 1990) and Hodgkin's disease (Ferrari *et al.*, 1990). It has also been observed in association with paraneoplastic limbic encephalitis (Masson *et al.*, 1987). The onset of the stiff-man syndrome may precede the detection of the associated malignancy.

Genetics

Class II HLA genes

The proportion of patients with the stiff-man syndrome who carry the HLA-DQB1*0201 allele (72%) is significantly higher than the proportion of controls who carry this allele (38%) (Pugliese *et al.*, 1993). This indicates that the stiff-man syndrome is associated with this allele, as are insulin-dependent diabetes mellitus and other autoimmune diseases. Interestingly, the diabetes-protective DQB1*0602 allele and other sequence-related DQB1*06 alleles, which are rarely found in insulin-dependent diabetes, occur with the same frequency as in controls. Diabetes is more frequent in patients with the stiff-man syndrome who lack a DQB1*06 allele than in those with such an allele, suggesting that the presence of the DQB1*0602 allele or other DQB1*06 alleles may protect against diabetes in patients with the stiff-man syndrome (Pugliese *et al.*, 1993).

Neuropathology

Perivascular lymphocytic accumulation has been observed in the spinal cord, brainstem and basal ganglia of patients with the stiff-man syndrome with or without associated malignancy (Masson *et al.*, 1987; Bateman *et al.*, 1990; Mitsumoto *et al.*, 1991; Meinck *et al.*, 1994).

Pathophysiology

In a detailed neurophysiological study on a patient with the stiff-man syndrome, Meinck, Ricker & Conrad (1984) found abnormal enhancement of exteroceptive reflexes, particularly those elicited from the skin, but no abnormalities of the monosynaptic reflex arc. Administration of clomipramine, which results in an excess of serotonin and noradrenaline at synapses, severely aggravated the clinical symptoms. In contrast, clonidine, which leads to an inhibition of noradrenaline release, and diazepam, which increases GABA-ergic activity, decreased both the muscular stiffness and abnormal exteroceptive reflexes. Meinck *et al.* proposed that the clinical manifestations are due to a disorder of descending brainstem pathways that exert a net inhibitory control on axial and limb girdle muscle tone as well as on exteroceptive reflex transmission.

Immunological findings in the peripheral blood

Antibodies against glutamic acid decarboxylase

In 1988, Solimena *et al.* reported that the serum and the CSF of a patient with the stiff-man syndrome, epilepsy and insulin-dependent diabetes mellitus intensely and specifically stained all grey-matter regions in frozen sections of the rat brain studied by light-microscopic immunocytochemistry. The staining pattern consisted primarily of small puncta that often outlined the profiles of perikarya and dendrites, suggesting a predominant localization of immunoreactivity in a major subpopulation of synapses, each of which would be represented by a punctum. Furthermore, in all brain regions the pattern of immunoreactivity corresponded with the distribution of GABA-ergic nerve terminals and with the staining pattern obtained with antibodies to glutamic acid decarboxylase (GAD), the enzyme responsible for the synthesis of GABA. Interestingly, the serum and the CSF of this patient also intensely and specifically stained pancreatic islet beta cells, which contain a high concentration of GAD and which are destroyed in insulin-dependent diabetes mellitus. Double immunofluorescence studies revealed that this staining was almost indistinguishable from that produced by antibodies against GAD. Using Western blotting, Solimena *et al.* demonstrated that the serum and CSF labelled a band (approximately 60 kDa) with an electrophoretic mobility corresponding to that of the band labelled by GAD antiserum. On the basis of these exciting observations they hypothesized that the stiff-man syndrome is an autoimmune disease directed against GABA-ergic neurones.

In a subsequent study, Solimena *et al.* (1990) found that 60% of patients with the stiff-man syndrome had serum antibodies against GABA-ergic neurones, with GAD being the principal autoantigen. Antibodies against GABA-ergic neurones were not found in patients with other neurological disorders. Solimena *et al.* observed that insulin-dependent diabetes mellitus occurred frequently in the patients with the stiff-man syndrome and anti-GAD antibodies. This observation led to the finding that the 64-kDa pancreatic islet beta cell antigen, which is a major target of autoantibodies in insulin-dependent diabetes, is GAD (Baekkeskov *et al.*, 1990). However, differences were observed between the anti-GAD antibodies associated with the stiff-man syndrome and those associated with insulin-dependent diabetes mellitus. The antibody titre is much higher in patients with the stiff-man syndrome. Furthermore, the anti-GAD antibodies of most patients with the stiff-man syndrome react with GAD in Western blots, whereas the anti-GAD antibodies of the majority of diabetic patients do not (Baekkeskov *et al.*, 1990; Bjork *et al.*, 1994). Differences in GAD reactivity between the stiff-man syndrome and insulin-dependent diabetes indicate that there are differences in antigen presentation to the immune system during the development of these diseases (Bjork *et al.*, 1994). This hypothesis is supported by the observation that GAD is the only islet cell antigen recognized by islet cell antibodies in patients with the stiff-man syndrome, whereas sera from newly diagnosed insulin-dependent diabetics recognize other islet cell antigens in addition to GAD (Richter *et al.*, 1993).

Both soluble and membrane forms of GAD contribute to the activity of GAD in the brain (Nathan *et al.*, 1994). There are two isoforms of soluble GAD, a 65-kDa form (GAD-65) and a 67-kDa form (GAD-67), which are the products of two different genes and differ substantially only at their N-terminal regions (Bu *et al.*, 1992). Both proteins are expressed in the brain, but their expression in pancreatic beta cells varies among species (Petersen *et al.*, 1993; Velloso *et al.*, 1993). In neurones GAD is concentrated around synaptic vesicles, and in pancreatic beta cells it is concentrated around synaptic-like microvesicles and in the region of the Golgi complex (Reetz *et al.*, 1991). By separately expressing the cloned genes for GAD-65 and GAD-67 in Chinese hamster ovary cells and COS cells, Solimena *et al.* (1993) studied the mechanism of the subcellular targeting of GAD. They found that GAD-67 had a diffuse cytoplasmic localization, whereas GAD-65 had a punctate distribution that was mainly concentrated in the area of the Golgi complex. A chimeric protein in which the 88 N-terminal amino acid residues of GAD-67 had been replaced by the 83 N-terminal amino acid residues of GAD-65 was targeted to the Golgi complex, indicating that the

N-terminal region of GAD-65 contains a targeting signal sufficient for directing the remaining portion of the molecule, highly similar in GAD-65 and GAD-67, to the Golgi complex-associated structures (Solimena *et al.*, 1993).

In patients with the stiff-man syndrome the anti-GAD antibodies recognize GAD-65 but not GAD-67 on Western blots (Butler *et al.*, 1993; Li *et al.*, 1994). Butler *et al.* (1993) found that these antibodies recognized a conformational epitope in the C-terminal region (amino acid residues 475–585) of GAD-65 and at least one epitope in the N-terminal domain of GAD-65 (amino acid residues 1–95). Li *et al.* (1994) found that the antibodies recognized linear epitopes at 354–368 and, in one patient, 390–403 of GAD-65. Interestingly, the 390–403 region includes the binding site of the GAD cofactor, pyridoxal 5′-phosphate, suggesting that some anti-GAD antibodies may block the active site. Antibodies reactive to the membrane form of GAD have been found in the sera of patients with insulin-dependent diabetes mellitus (Nathan *et al.*, 1994), but it is unknown whether the sera of patients with the stiff-man syndrome exhibit this reactivity. Because the membrane form of GAD is presumed to have exposed extracellular domains, Nathan *et al.* (1994) have suggested that it is more likely than the soluble form of GAD to be involved in the pathogenesis of insulin-dependent diabetes and the stiff-man syndrome.

Antibodies against amphiphysin

Folli *et al.* (1993) found that patients with the stiff-man syndrome and breast cancer had serum autoantibodies directed against a 128-kDa brain antigen but did not have anti-GAD antibodies. They did not detect antibodies against this 128-kDa antigen in the sera of patients with the stiff-man syndrome without cancer or in the sera of patients with cancer without the syndrome. Grimaldi *et al.* (1993) also found antibodies against a 125/130-kDa brain protein, but not against GAD, in one patient with the stiff-man syndrome and colon cancer and in another with the syndrome and Hodgkin's lymphoma. Folli *et al.* demonstrated that this antigen was concentrated at synapses and had a highly restricted distribution outside the nervous system: it was subsequently identified as amphiphysin (De Camilli *et al.*, 1993), a recently discovered synaptic vesicle-associated protein (Lichte *et al.*, 1992). Unlike GAD, which is expressed only by GABA-secreting neurones, amphiphysin is not restricted to these neurones (Lichte *et al.*, 1992; Folli *et al.*, 1993). Although amphiphysin has not been detected in breast cancer tissue (Folli *et al.*, 1993), the stiff-man syndrome associated with cancer and anti-amphiphysin antibodies has the characteristics of an autoimmune paraneoplastic neurological disorder (see Chapter 12). The detection of anti-amphiphysin antibodies in patients with the stiff-man syndrome is an indication to search for an occult cancer, particularly of the breast (Folli *et al.*, 1993).

Amphiphysin and GAD are similar in that they are both non-intrinsic membrane proteins that are concentrated in nerve terminals where they are associated with the cytoplasmic surface of synaptic vesicles. They are the only two known targets of CNS autoimmunity with this subcellular distribution, suggesting a link between autoimmunity directed against cytoplasmic proteins associated with synaptic vesicles and the stiff-man syndrome (De Camilli *et al.*, 1993).

Antibodies against other neuronal antigens

Some patients with the stiff-man syndrome have antibodies against GABA-ergic neurones that do not recognize GAD (Solimena *et al.*, 1990; Gorin *et al.*, 1990). Serum antibodies recognizing an 80-kDa neuronal antigen, but not GAD, have been detected in two patients with the stiff-man syndrome (Darnell *et al.*, 1993). Immunohistochemistry demonstrated neuronal binding identical to that reported with anti-GAD antibodies and both sera depleted GAD activity from brain extracts, suggesting that the 80-kDa antigen was either a different form of GAD or a protein that co-immunoprecipitates with GAD. Anti-GAD antibodies together with antibodies reacting with an additional neuronal antigen(s) have been found in some patients with the stiff-man syndrome (Richter *et al.*, 1993).

Immunological findings in the cerebrospinal fluid

Anti-GAD antibodies are present in the CSF of most, but not all, patients with the stiff-man syndrome and serum anti-GAD antibodies (Solimena *et al.*, 1990). The presence of oligoclonal IgG bands in the CSF but not the serum in some patients with the stiff-man syndrome indicates intrathecal antibody synthesis, but it has not been determined whether this intrathecal synthesis involves anti-GAD antibodies (Solimena *et al.*, 1988, 1990). Patients with the stiff-man syndrome, breast cancer and serum anti-amphiphysin antibodies also have anti-amphiphysin antibodies in the CSF (Folli *et al.*, 1993).

Mechanism by which the autoimmune process interferes with the function of the nervous system

The presence of anti-GAD antibodies or anti-amphiphysin antibodies in patients with the stiff-man syndrome suggests that this disorder results from an autoimmune process directed against these synaptic vesicle-associated antigens; however, it is not known whether the antibodies themselves are pathogenic. Furthermore, the possible role of anti-GAD or anti-amphiphysin T cells in the pathogenesis of the stiff-man syndrome has not yet been examined. T cells specific for GAD play an important role in the spontaneous development of insulin-dependent diabetes in the non-obese diabetic mouse (Kaufman *et al.*, 1993; Tisch *et al.*, 1993), and patients with insulin-dependent diabetes exhibit increased proliferation of peripheral blood T cells in the presence of GAD-67 (Honeyman, Cram & Harrison, 1993).

Therapy

Diazepam, which potentiates the effect of endogenously released GABA on GABA receptors, is the most effective drug in the treatment of the stiff-man syndrome (Lorish *et al.*, 1989). Other drugs which may sometimes be beneficial include oral baclofen, clonazepam and sodium valproate (Lorish *et al.*, 1989). Patients who lose their responsiveness to diazepam as the disease progresses can benefit from the intrathecal administration of baclofen, a GABA agonist, by a programmable drug pump (Penn & Mangieri, 1993). Paraspinal muscle injection of botulinum toxin A was found to be beneficial in one patient (Davis & Jabbari, 1993). With regard to immunotherapy, plasmapheresis is beneficial in some patients with the stiff-man syndrome (Vicari *et al.*, 1989; Brashear & Phillips, 1991) but not in others (Harding *et al.*, 1989), and corticosteroid therapy also has resulted in improvement in some, but not all, patients (Piccolo *et al.*, 1988; Vicari *et al.*, 1989; Harding *et al.*, 1989). Further studies will be required to determine the place of plasmapheresis and immunosuppressant therapy in the management of patients with the stiff-man syndrome.

Conclusions

The hypothesis that the stiff-man syndrome is an autoimmune disease of the CNS is supported by the following observations: the association with HLA-DQB1*0201; the presence of oligoclonal IgG bands in the CSF; the finding of perivascular lymphocytic infiltration in the CNS; the presence of anti-GAD antibodies and the association with organ-specific autoimmune disease in a significant proportion of patients; the presence of anti-amphiphysin antibodies and association with remote malignancy in some of the other patients with this syndrome; and the beneficial effect of plasmapheresis in some patients. However, further studies will be required to determine the role of these anti-neuronal antibodies and the role of specific T cells in the pathogenesis of the disorder, as well as to determine the place of immunotherapy in patient management. The availability of recombinant GAD and amphiphysin may allow the development of animal models to facilitate studies on the pathogenesis of the stiff-man syndrome.

References

Armon, C., McEvoy, K.M., Westmoreland, B.F. & McManis, P.G. (1990). Clinical neurophysiologic studies in stiff-man syndrome: use of simultaneous video-electroencephalographic-surface electromyographic recording. *Mayo Clinic Proceedings*, **65**, 960–7.

Baekkeskov, S., Aanstoot, H.J., Christgau, S., Reetz, A., Solimena, M., Cascalho, M., Folli, F., Richter Olesen, H., DeCamilli, P. & Camilli, P.D.D.C. (1990). Identification of the 64K autoantigen in insulin-dependent diabetes as the GABA-synthesizing enzyme glutamic acid decarboxylase [published erratum appears in *Nature* 1990 Oct 25; **347**(6295):782]. *Nature*, **347**, 151–6.

Bateman, D.E., Weller, R.O. & Kennedy, P. (1990). Stiffman syndrome: a rare paraneoplastic disorder? *Journal of Neurology, Neurosurgery and Psychiatry*, **53**, 695–6.

Bjork, E., Velloso, L.A., Kampe, O. & Karlsson, F.A. (1994). GAD autoantibodies in IDDM, stiff-man syndrome, and autoimmune polyendocrine syndrome type I recognize different epitopes. *Diabetes*, **43**, 161–5.

Brashear, H.R. & Phillips, L.H. (1991). Autoantibodies to GABAergic neurons and response to plasmapheresis in stiff-man syndrome. *Neurology*, **41**, 1588–92.

Bu, D.F., Erlander, M.G., Hitz, B.C., Tillakaratne, N.J., Kaufman, D.L., Wagner McPherson, C.B., Evans, G.A. & Tobin, A.J. (1992). Two human glutamate decarboxylases, 65-kDa GAD and 67-kDa GAD, are each encoded by a single gene. *Proceedings of the National Academy of Sciences USA*, **89**, 2115–19.

Butler, M.H., Solimena, M., Dirkx, R.J., Hayday, A. & De Camilli, P. (1993). Identification of a dominant epitope of glutamic acid decarboxylase (GAD-65) recognized by autoantibodies in stiff-man syndrome. *Journal of Experimental Medicine*, **178**, 2097–106.

Darnell, R.B., Victor, J., Rubin, M., Clouston, P. & Plum, F. (1993). A novel antineuronal antibody in stiff-man syndrome. *Neurology*, **43**, 114–20.

Davis, D. & Jabbari, B. (1993). Significant improvement of stiff-person syndrome after paraspinal injection of botulinum toxin A. *Movement Disorders*, **8**, 371–3.

De Camilli, P., Thomas, A., Cofiell, R., Folli, F., Lichte, B., Piccolo, G., Meinck, H.M., Austoni, M., Fassetta, G., Bottazzo, G. *et al.* (1993). The synaptic vesicle-associated protein amphiphysin is the 128-kD autoantigen of Stiff-Man syndrome with breast cancer. *Journal of Experimental Medicine*, **178**, 2219–23.

Ferrari, P., Federico, M., Grimaldi, L.M. & Silingardi, V. (1990). Stiff-man syndrome in a patient with Hodgkin's disease. An unusual paraneoplastic syndrome. *Haematologica*, **75**, 570–2.

Folli, F., Solimena, M., Cofiell, R., Austoni, M., Tallini, G., Fassetta, G., Bates, D., Cartlidge, N., Bottazzo, G.F., Piccolo, G. *et al.* (1993). Autoantibodies to a 128-kd synaptic protein in three women with the stiff-man syndrome and breast cancer. *New England Journal of Medicine*, **328**, 546–51.

Gordon, E.E., Januszko, D.M. & Kaufman, L. (1967). A critical survey of stiff-man syndrome. *American Journal of Medicine*, **42**, 582–99.

Gorin, F., Baldwin, B., Tait, R., Pathak, R., Seyal, M. & Mugnaini, E. (1990). Stiff-man syndrome: a GABAergic autoimmune disorder with autoantigenic heterogeneity. *Annals of Neurology*, **28**, 711–14.

Grimaldi, L.M., Martino, G., Braghi, S., Quattrini, A., Furlan, R., Bosi, E. & Comi, G. (1993). Heterogeneity of autoantibodies in stiff-man syndrome. *Annals of Neurology*, **34**, 57–64.

Harding, A.E., Thompson, P.D., Kocen, R.S., Batchelor, J.R., Davey, N. & Marsden, C.D. (1989). Plasma exchange and immunosuppression in the stiff man syndrome. *Lancet*, **2**, 915.

Honeyman, M.C., Cram, D.S. & Harrison, L.C. (1993). Glutamic acid decarboxylase 67-reactive T cells: a marker of insulin-dependent diabetes. *Journal of Experimental Medicine*, **177**, 535–40.

Kaufman, D.L., Clare Salzler, M., Tian, J., Forsthuber, T., Ting, G.S., Robinson, P., Atkinson, M.A., Sercarz, E.E., Tobin, A.J. & Lehmann, P.V. (1993). Spontaneous loss of T-cell tolerance to glutamic acid decarboxylase in murine insulin-dependent diabetes. *Nature*, **366**, 69–72.

Li, L., Hagopian, W.A., Brashear, H.R., Daniels, T. & Lernmark, A. (1994). Identification of autoantibody epitopes of glutamic acid decarboxylase in stiff-man syndrome patients. *Journal of Immunology*, **152**, 930–4.

Lichte, B., Veh, R.W., Meyer, H.E. & Kilimann, M.W. (1992). Amphiphysin, a novel protein associated with synaptic vesicles [published erratum appears in *EMBO J* 1992 Oct;**11**(10):3809]. *EMBO Journal*, **11**, 2521–30.

Lorish, T.R., Thorsteinsson, G. & Howard, F.M. (1989). Stiff-man syndrome updated. *Mayo Clinic Proceedings*, **64**, 629–36.

Martinelli, P., Pazzaglia, P., Montagna, P., Coccagna, G., Rizzuto, N., Simonati, S. & Lugaresi, E. (1978). Stiff-man syndrome associated with nocturnal myoclonus and epilepsy. *Journal of Neurology, Neurosurgery and Psychiatry*, **41**, 458–62.

Masson, C., Prier, S., Benoit, C., Henin, D., Massón, M. & Cambier, J. (1987). [Amnesia and stiff-man syndrome. Manifestations disclosing paraneoplastic encephalomyelitis]. *Annales de Medecine Interne (Paris)*, **138**, 502–5.

Meinck, H.-M., Ricker, K. & Conrad, B. (1984). The stiff-man syndrome: new pathophysiological aspects from abnormal exteroceptive reflexes and the response to clomipramine, clonidine, and tizanidine. *Journal of Neurology, Neurosurgery and Psychiatry*, **47**, 280–7.

Meinck, H.M., Ricker, K., Hulser, P.J., Schmid, E., Peiffer, J. & Solimena, M. (1994). Stiff man syndrome: clinical and laboratory findings in eight patients. *Journal of Neurology*, **241**, 157–66.

Mitsumoto, H., Schwartzman, M.J., Estes, M.L., Chou, S.M , La Franchise, E.F., De Camilli, P. & Solimena, M. (1991). Sudden death and paroxysmal autonomic dysfunction in stiff-man syndrome. *Journal of Neurology*, **238**, 91–6.

Moersch, F.P. & Woltman, H.W. (1956). Progressive fluctuating muscular rigidity and spasm ('stiff-man' syndrome): report of a case and some observations in 13 other cases. *Proceedings of the Staff Meetings of the Mayo Clinic*, **31**, 421–7.

Nathan, B., Bao, J., Hsu, C.C., Aguilar, P., Wu, R., Yarom, M., Kuo, C.Y. & Wu, J.Y. (1994). A membrane form of brain L-glutamate decarboxylase: identification, isolation, and its relation to insulin-dependent diabetes mellitus. *Proceedings of the National Academy of Sciences USA*, **91**, 242–6.

Penn, R.D. & Mangieri, E.A. (1993). Stiff-man syndrome treated with intrathecal baclofen. *Neurology*, **43**, 2412.

Petersen, J.S., Russel, S., Marshall, M.O., Kofod, H., Buschard, K., Cambon, N., Karlsen, A.E., Boel, E., Hagopian, W.A., Hejnaes, K.R. *et al.* (1993). Differential expression of glutamic acid decarboxylase in rat and human islets. *Diabetes*, **42**, 484–95.

Piccolo, G. & Cosi, V. (1989). Stiff-man syndrome, dysimmune disorder, and cancer. *Annals of Neurology*, **26**, 105.

Piccolo, G., Cosi, V., Zandrini, C. & Moglia, A. (1988). Steroid-responsive and dependent stiff-man syndrome: a clinical and electrophysiological study of two cases. *Italian Journal of Neurological Sciences*, **9**, 559–66.

Pugliese, A., Solimena, M., Awdeh, Z.L., Alper, C.A., Bugawan, T., Erlich, H.A., De Camilli, P. & Eisenbarth, G.S. (1993). Association of HLA-DQB1*0201 with stiff-man syndrome. *Journal of Clinical Endocrinology and Metabolism*, **77**, 1550–3.

Reetz, A., Solimena, M., Matteoli, M., Folli, F., Takei, K. & De Camilli, P. (1991). GABA and pancreatic beta-cells: colocalization of glutamic acid decarboxylase (GAD) and GABA with synaptic-like microvesicles suggests their role in GABA storage and secretion. *EMBO Journal*, **10**, 1275–84.

Richter, W., Seissler, J., Northemann, W., Wolfahrt, S., Meinck, H.M. & Scherbaum, W.A. (1993). Cytoplasmic islet cell antibodies recognize distinct islet antigens in IDDM but not in stiff man syndrome. *Diabetes*, **42**, 1642–8.

Solimena, M., Aggujaro, D., Muntzel, C., Dirkx, R., Butler, M., De Camilli, P. & Hayday, A. (1993). Association of GAD-65, but not of GAD-67, with the Golgi complex of transfected Chinese hamster ovary cells mediated by the N-terminal region. *Proceedings of the National Academy of Sciences USA*, **90**, 3073–7.

Solimena, M., Folli, F., Aparisi, R., Pozza, G. & De Camilli, P. (1990). Autoantibodies to GABA-ergic neurons and pancreatic beta cells in stiff-man syndrome. *New England Journal of Medicine*, **322**, 1555–60.

Solimena, M., Folli, F., Denis Donini, S., Comi, G.C., Pozza, G., De Camilli, P. & Vicari, A.M. (1988). Autoantibodies to glutamic acid decarboxylase in a patient with stiff-man syndrome, epilepsy, and type I diabetes mellitus. *New England Journal of Medicine*, **318**, 1012–20.

Tisch, R., Yang, X.D., Singer, S.M., Liblau, R.S., Fugger, L. & McDevitt, H.O. (1993). Immune response to glutamic acid decarboxylase correlates with insulitis in non-obese diabetic mice. *Nature*, **366**, 72–5.

Velloso, L.A., Kampe, O., Eizirik, D.L., Hallberg, A., Andersson, A. & Karlsson, F.A. (1993). Human autoantibodies react with glutamic acid decarboxylase antigen in human and rat but not in mouse pancreatic islets. *Diabetologia*, **36**, 39–46.

Vicari, A.M., Folli, F., Pozza, G., Comi, G.C., Comola, M., Canal, N., Besana, C., Borri, A., Tresoldi, M., Solimena, M. *et al.* (1989). Plasmapheresis in the treatment of stiff-man syndrome. *New England Journal of Medicine*, **320**, 1499.

–7– Experimental autoimmune neuritis

PAMELA A. McCOMBE

Introduction

Experimental allergic (autoimmune) neuritis (EAN) is an autoimmune disease that can be induced by the inoculation of susceptible animals with peripheral nervous system (PNS) antigens and adjuvants. In many respects, EAN is similar to experimental allergic (or autoimmune) encephalomyelitis (EAE). Indeed, studies of EAE paved the way for the development of EAN as a model of inflammatory demyelinating disease of the PNS (Waksman & Adams, 1955). In early studies of EAE, inflammation of the nerve roots was present, but always in combination with inflammation in the central nervous system (CNS) (Innes, 1951; Ferraro & Roizin, 1954). Lumsden (1949) inoculated animals with peripheral nerve, but produced a disease like EAE. Waksman & Adams (1955) deliberately set out to produce an animal model in which inflammation was confined to the PNS and achieved this by inoculating rabbits with peripheral nerve antigens and adjuvants. Acute EAN has subsequently been induced in rats (Smith, Forno & Hofmann, 1979), guinea pigs (Waksman & Adams, 1956; Hall, 1967), mice (Waksman & Adams, 1956; Dieperink *et al.*, 1991), chickens (Petek & Quaglio, 1967) and monkeys (Lumsden, 1949; Wisniewski *et al.*, 1974; Eylar *et al.*, 1982) and serves as a good model of the human disease, the Guillain–Barré syndrome (GBS). Chronic relapsing EAN has been produced in Lewis rats (Adam *et al.*, 1989; McCombe, van der Kreek & Pender, 1990), guinea pigs (Pollard, King & Thomas, 1975; Madrid, 1983), rabbits (Harvey *et al.*, 1987*a*) and monkeys (Wisniewski *et al.*, 1974) and serves as a model of the human disease, chronic inflammatory demyelinating polyradiculoneuropathy (CIDP).

Induction of EAN and susceptibility to EAN

Acute EAN

EAN was first produced by inoculation with homogenized peripheral nerve tissue. Studies were soon performed to identify which component of peripheral nerve tissue was the 'neuritogen'. One major component of peripheral nerve, and an attractive target antigen in a demyelinating disease, is myelin. Inoculation with purified PNS myelin causes EAN, with the severity of disease depending on the dose of myelin in the inoculum (Hahn *et al.*, 1988). The importance of myelin, rather than other antigens, in producing EAN was shown when it was found that inoculation with unmyelinated fibres did not cause EAN (Robinson, Allt & Evans, 1972). Later, inoculation with purified myelin P_2 protein was found to produce EAN (Kadlubowski & Hughes, 1979; Hughes & Powell, 1984; Taylor & Hughes, 1985). Passive transfer of T cells reactive with P_2 protein can also produce acute EAN (Linington *et al.*, 1984; Rostami *et al.*, 1985). The peptide epitope of P_2 that causes EAN in Lewis rats was reported to be residues 57–81: this is a peptide with an amphipathic helical structure typical of a T cell epitope (Olee, Powers & Brostoff, 1988; Olee *et al.*, 1989). Later the epitope was reported as residues 53–78 (Rostami *et al.*, 1990; Rostami & Gregorian, 1991) and more recently as residues 61–70 (Olee, Powell & Brostoff, 1990). Myelin P_0 protein can induce mild EAN in guinea pigs (Wood & Dawson, 1974): it can also produce EAN in Lewis rats when injected together with lysolecithin (Milner *et al.*, 1987). As outlined by Linington *et al.* (1992), P_0 is a glycoprotein member of the immunoglobulin supergene family and T cell lines reactive with P_0 protein can transfer disease. P_0 may become a target of the immune system because of cross-reactivity between P_0 and common viral antigens (Adelmann & Linington, 1992).

Other possible target antigens for the immune attack in EAN include glycolipids such as galactocerebroside and gangliosides which are components of myelin. Repeated inoculation of rabbits with galactocerebroside causes a disease similar to EAN (T. Saida *et al.*, 1979*b*, 1981). This appears to be a specific response to galactocerebroside. On the other hand, glucocerebroside and galactocerebroside can augment the demyelination of P_2-induced EAN (P_2-EAN), in a non-specific manner (Milner *et al.*, 1987). The role of gangliosides in EAN is complex. Some studies have found that gangliosides could enhance the demyelination in EAN induced by P_2 protein (Takeda, Ikuta & Nagai, 1980); others have found that gangliosides emulsified with complete Freund's adjuvant could themselves produce a disease like EAN (Mizisin *et al.*, 1987). In rabbits, repeated inoculation with gangliosides produced a 'ganglioside syndrome', which included weakness and peripheral nerve degeneration (Nagai *et al.*, 1976), and inoculation of gangliosides with influenza vaccine can produce a disease like EAN (Ziegler *et al.*, 1983). However, in rats, the inclusion of gangliosides in the inoculum reduced the severity of EAN (Ponzin *et al.*, 1991; Wietholter *et al.*, 1992).

Hyperacute EAN

Hyperacute EAE can be induced by the use of pertussis vaccine in the inoculum (Levine & Wenk, 1965). Wenk, Levine & Wallquist (1965) used pertussis vaccine mixed with aqueous homogenates of nerve and produced a hyperacute form of EAN, with perivascular polymorphonuclear leukocyte infiltration, in Lewis rats that had been adrenalectomized. Behan *et al.* (1971) produced hyperacute EAN in monkeys by inoculation with sciatic nerve, complete Freund's adjuvant and pertussis toxin. However, others have found that simultaneous inoculation with pertussis vaccine reduces the severity of EAN induced by inoculation of Lewis rats with guinea pig sciatic nerve (Ballon-Landa, Paterson & Dal Canto, 1978).

Chronic relapsing EAN

Chronic relapsing EAN has been developed as a model of the human disease CIDP. Some types of chronic relapsing EAN have evolved spontaneously from acute EAN, usually after the administration of larger than usual doses of antigen. Chronic relapsing EAN has been induced in rabbits by a multiportal inoculation of a large dose (500 mg) of purified bovine myelin (Harvey *et al.*, 1987*a*). In guinea pigs, inoculation with rabbit sciatic nerve produced a chronic course of EAN in a small proportion of animals (Pollard *et al.*, 1975). Juvenile guinea pigs develop a more chronic form of EAN than adult animals (Suzumura *et al.*, 1985). Monkeys inoculated with 60–70 mg of rabbit sciatic nerve myelin developed chronic demyelination (Wisniewski *et al.*, 1974). In Lewis rats, the pathological changes of chronic EAN have been reported to occur spontaneously (Adam *et al.*, 1989). Another approach has been the use of low doses of cyclosporin A, which is an immunosuppressive agent with complex actions. Chronic relapsing EAN has been induced in Lewis rats inoculated with bovine intradural myelin by treatment with low-dose cyclosporin A (McCombe *et al.*, 1990). Chronic EAN has not been reported after inoculation with purified myelin antigens. However, repeated transfer of P_2-specific T cell lines to Lewis rats has also been used to produce chronic relapsing EAN (Lassmann *et al.*, 1991).

Susceptibility to EAN

Genetic susceptibility

As discussed above, EAN can be induced in many different species. However, some strains of animal are resistant to the development of EAN (Steinman, Smith & Forno, 1981; Rostami, 1990). In general, strains that are susceptible to EAN are also susceptible to EAE and vice versa. For example, the Lewis rat is susceptible to EAN, but some rat strains, such as Brown Norway, are resistant (Hoffman *et al.*, 1980; Steinman *et al.*, 1981), the SJL mouse is susceptible to EAN but other strains of mouse are resistant (Taylor & Hughes, 1985; Rostami, 1990), and strain 13 guinea pigs are susceptible to EAN and EAE but strain 2 guinea pigs are resistant (Geczy *et al.*, 1984). Different approaches have been used to define the differences in susceptibility. P_2-reactive T cell lines can be produced from the lymph nodes of Brown Norway rats inoculated with P_2 and can produce EAN when injected into naive syngeneic recipients (Linington *et al.*, 1986). The failure of these cells to produce EAN in Brown Norway rats after active inoculation with neuritogen seems likely to be due to an *in vitro* regulatory mechanism. In Lewis rats, susceptibility to EAE, which has many similarities to EAN, has been linked to an autosomal dominant gene that is linked to the major histocompatibility region (Gasser *et al.*, 1973; Williams & Moore, 1973). Other studies have shown that EAN-resistant Brown Norway rats have fewer mast cells in the peripheral nerves than EAN-susceptible Lewis rats (Johnson, Yasui & Seeldrayers, 1991). In the guinea pig, susceptibility to EAN and EAE correlates with the induction of macrophage pro-coagulant activity (Geczy *et al.*, 1984). It seems likely that a number of inherited factors may influence susceptibility to EAN.

Influence of age

Immature rabbits (less than four weeks) are less susceptible to EAN than adult animals (Allt, Evans & Evans, 1971). Adam *et al.* (1989) found that juvenile Lewis rats (age four weeks) had milder disease than adult rats. However, juvenile guinea pigs had an increased incidence of relapsing EAN (Suzumura *et al.*, 1985). These findings could indicate that the immature immune system is either inefficient at causing disease, as in the case of rabbits and rats, or inefficient at regulating immune responses, as in the case of guinea pigs.

Clinical features

Acute EAN

Rabbits with EAN develop a flaccid weakness associated with splaying of the limbs and unsteadiness of hopping (Waksman & Adams, 1955). Lewis rats inoculated with peripheral nerve myelin develop ascending flaccid weakness (Smith *et al.*, 1979). Other signs of EAN in the Lewis rat include weight loss and sometimes ataxia (Hahn *et al.*, 1988; McCombe *et al.*, 1990; Rosen *et al.*, 1990*a*). The severity of disease is related to the dose of inoculated myelin (Hahn *et al.*, 1988). The neurological signs of acute EAN persist for several days and then the animal spontaneously recovers. About one-third of rats may have a single spontaneous recurrence of signs (McCombe *et al.*, 1990) and some may develop a chronic course of disease (Adam *et al.*, 1989). Disturbance of the autonomic nervous system can be detected in rats with EAN by analysis of R-R intervals (Solders *et al.*, 1985). Dieperink *et al.* (1991) found that SJL/J mice inoculated with peripheral nerve myelin developed pathological changes typical of EAN, but that the disease was subclinical.

Chronic relapsing EAN

Rats inoculated with peripheral nerve myelin and treated with low-dose cyclosporin A develop a relapsing course of disease, with recurrent episodes of weakness. After acute EAN, some rats may develop pathological changes of chronic EAN without clinical episodes (Adam *et al.*, 1989). Guinea pigs with chronic EAN may have a progressive (Madrid, 1983) or a relapsing (Pollard, King & Thomas, 1975) course of disease. Rabbits with chronic EAN may have either a relapsing or a progressive course of disease (Harvey *et al.*, 1987*a*).

Neuropathology

Acute EAN

Acute EAN is characterized histologically by infiltration of the nerve roots and peripheral nerves with macrophages and lymphocytes, and by primary demyelination. These changes are similar to those found in GBS (see Chapter 8). During the development of EAN, the endothelial cells of the venules become cuboidal, with loss of tight junctions between the cells, and leukocytes interact with the vessel wall and later migrate into the endoneurial compartment (Powell *et al.*, 1991). Physiological studies have shown that these changes occur in association with a breakdown of the blood–nerve barrier (Hahn, Feasby & Gilbert, 1985). In EAN, the nerve roots are more severely affected than the peripheral nerves: this may relate to the relative permeability of the blood–nerve barrier at the nerve roots and dorsal root ganglia (Olsson, 1968; Jacobs, Macfarlane & Cavanagh, 1976; Pettersson, Sharma & Olsson, 1990). Åström, Webster & Arnason (1968) studied the pathological findings in the early stages of EAN in rats and emphasized the role of lymphocytes. Asbury, Arnason & Adams (1969) strongly emphasized the role of the inflammation in the subsequent demyelination. Myelin is stripped away by macrophages (Hartung *et al.*, 1988*b*). Vesicular dissolution of myelin, although frequently reported, may be an artefact of fixation. Paranodal changes may be the first evidence of demyelination (Ballin & Thomas, 1969; Allt, 1975; Stevens *et al.*, 1989). Wisniewski & Bloom (1975) considered that demyelination of peripheral nerve by macrophages could occur as a non-specific event requiring only the presence of inflammatory cells in the vicinity of myelinated fibres. Later studies showed that such non-specific damage is uncommon and that demyelination of peripheral nerve requires specific sensitization to myelin antigens (Powell *et al.*, 1984). It is not clear what causes macrophages to attack myelin. Specific binding of macrophages to myelin could be mediated by anti-myelin antibodies. Alternatively, the presence of specific T cells near their target antigens may provide a sufficient stimulus to activate macrophages to damage myelin.

Axonal damage may also occur in EAN. Lampert (1969) noted that axonal damage in EAN occurred in regions of demyelination and concluded that this was a secondary phenomenon. The studies of Asbury *et al.* (1969) and Madrid & Wisniewski (1977) also suggested that axonal damage in EAN occurs in association with primary demyelination. King, Thomas & Pollard (1977) concluded that axonal damage in EAN was a bystander phenomenon. Axonal damage has also been reported in the autonomic nervous system in EAN. Tuck, Pollard & McLeod (1981) found axonal degeneration and loss of small unmyelinated fibres in the vagus and splanchnic nerves of rats with EAN. Kalimo *et al.* (1982) found inflammatory changes in regions with mostly unmyelinated fibres, which are regions where a primary attack on myelin is unlikely and where other antigens may be the target of the immune attack. On the other hand, some authors have demonstrated that autonomic dysfunction may be due to inflammation and demyelination in myelinated autonomic nerves (Morey *et al.*, 1985). Other observations on the pathology of EAN include that of Allt (1972), who found extravasated protein between the layers of the perineurium in EAN, and that of Martinez *et al.* (1977), who described activation of the Schwann cell enzymes NADH-diaphorase and acid phosphatase in nerves from guinea pigs with EAN. During recovery from EAN, there is remyelination of axons by Schwann cells. After recovery, these remyelinated fibres can be identified by the presence of inappropriately thin myelin sheaths.

Chronic relapsing EAN

There are fewer studies of chronic relapsing EAN than of acute EAN. Pathological studies have concentrated on the questions of whether there is evidence of repeated attacks of demyelination in chronic relapsing EAN and whether there is evidence of onion bulb formation, which is found in patients with CIDP (see Chapter 9). In chronic experimental EAN in rabbits, Sherwin (1966) found evidence of continuing demyelination and evidence of remyelination, whereas Harvey *et al.* (1987*a*) found active demyelination and well-developed onion bulbs at 12 months after initial inoculation. In guinea pigs with recurrent EAN produced by repeated inoculations, Pollard, King & Thomas (1975) found continuing demyelination and onion bulb formation. Wisniewski *et al.* (1974) also found ongoing demyelination in monkeys. In Lewis rats with clinical evidence of chronic relapsing EAN there is continuing demyelination and onion bulb formation and evidence of some axonal degeneration (McCombe, van der Kreek & Pender, 1992). In rats studied at a late stage after clinical recovery from acute EAN there may also be some onion bulb formation (Adam *et al.*, 1989). These pathological studies indicate that these models are pathologically similar to the human disease, CIDP.

Pathophysiology

Acute EAN

The pathophysiological findings in EAN are related to the pathological features of primary demyelination and sometimes axonal degeneration. Primary demyelination is demonstrated by conduction block or conduction slowing. Cragg & Thomas (1964) studied electrical conduction in sciatic nerves removed from guinea pigs with EAN induced by the methods of Waksman & Adams and found conduction block or severe slowing of nerve conduction. Hall (1967) studied conduction across the nerve roots of guinea pigs with EAN and demonstrated slowing of conduction velocity. Tuck, Antony & McLeod (1982) studied F waves in guinea pigs and rabbits with EAN: they found prolongation of the F-wave latencies in the presence of normal M waves in 14% of the guinea pigs and 7% of the rabbits. In a study on Lewis rats with EAN induced by inoculation with bovine intra-dural root myelin, conduction block was found in many fibres in the dorsal roots, whereas the conduction in the peripheral nerves was normal (Stanley, McCombe & Pender, 1992). Harvey & Pollard (1992*b*) demonstrated conduction block and conduction slowing in the peripheral nerves of Lewis rats with acute EAN. In Lewis rats with clinical signs of EAN induced by the passive transfer of P_2-specific T cell lines, there is evidence of conduction failure and conduction slowing of peripheral nerves (Heininger *et al.*, 1986; Wietholter *et al.*, 1988). These changes are consistent with demyelination being the cause of the neurological signs in EAN. In the demyelinated fibres in EAN there are alterations in the ion channels, such that slow K^+ conduction becomes more common than fast K^+ conduction (Schwarz *et al.*, 1991).

Chronic EAN

There are few electrophysiological studies of chronic EAN. Rabbits with chronic EAN, induced by inoculation with a high dose of antigen, were studied at six and 12 months after inoculation by Harvey *et al.* (1987*a*). The rabbits had severe prolongation of distal latencies and slowing of conduction velocities, typical of demyelination. There was also dispersion and reduction in amplitude of the compound muscle action potential.

Immunopathology of the nervous system lesions

Characteristics of the inflammatory infiltrate

Immunocytochemical techniques have confirmed the findings of conventional histology. Studies in the Lewis rat demonstrate that T cells and $CD4^+$ cells are present in the peripheral nerve during the course of acute EAN (Olsson *et al.*, 1983, 1984; Mizisin *et al.*, 1987; Ota, Irie & Takahashi, 1987).

MHC class II (Ia) expression and antigen presentation

Macrophages are MHC class II positive and contribute to the MHC class II antigen expression in the peripheral nerve in acute EAN. Macrophages in the nerves may also act as antigen-presenting cells. Schmidt *et al.* (1990) found no expression of MHC class II antigen on Schwann cells in acute EAN in Lewis rats, even though cultured Schwann cells can express MHC class II antigen after treatment with interferon-γ (IFN-γ) or exposure to activated T cells and can act as antigen-presenting cells *in vitro* (Wekerle *et al.*, 1986; Armati, Pollard & Gatenby, 1990; Tsai, Pollard & Armati, 1991). Stevens *et al.* (1989) have described a resident phagocytic cell that is not derived from Schwann cells, but that can transform into a macrophage. Such a cell would be a possible antigen-presenting cell in EAN.

Antibody and complement deposition

With immunostaining, antibody can be detected bound to peripheral nerves in EAN (Olsson *et al.*, 1983). Complement deposition on Schwann cells and myelin has also been detected in EAN (Stoll *et al.*, 1991). This complement deposition precedes demyelination and therefore may play a primary role in the production of demyelination.

Pathogenesis of EAN

Role of T cells

As already stated, T cells can be detected by immunocytochemistry in the endoneurium during acute EAN. T cells reactive with P_2 can be found in the peripheral blood of rats (Taylor & Hughes, 1988) and of rabbits with acute EAN (Nomura *et al.*, 1987). The important role of T cells in the pathogenesis of EAN is demonstrated by the ability of $CD4^+$ T cells reactive with P_2 to transfer EAN to naive recipients (Linington *et al.*, 1984; Rostami *et al.*, 1985) and the inability of T-cell-deficient rats to develop EAN (Brosnan *et al.*, 1987). The prevention of EAN by treatment with antibody to the $\alpha\beta$ TCR suggests that the neuritogenic cells are TCR $\alpha\beta^+$ (Jung *et al.*, 1992). It is generally accepted that the $CD4^+$ cells recruit macrophages, which cause demyelination and tissue damage. However, $CD4^+$ P_2-specific T cell lines capable of transferring EAN are cytotoxic to Schwann cells, in an MHC class II restricted manner (Argall *et al.*, 1992*a*, *b*). There are few studies on TCR usage by the cells that produce EAN. It has been reported that neuritogenic cells use the same Vα2 and Vβ8 chains as those used by myelin basic protein (MBP)-reactive encephalitogenic cells (Clark, Heber Katz & Rostami, 1992).

Role of antibody and humoral factors

Antibodies to myelin are present in the serum of rabbits with EAN induced by inoculation with myelin (Harvey *et al.*, 1987*b*). Antibodies to P_0 (Archelos *et al.*, 1993*b*) and P_2 can be detected in the serum in EAN (Hughes *et al.*, 1981). Furthermore, antibodies to galactocerebroside are present in the serum of rabbits with EAN induced by inoculation with emulsified PNS tissue (Saida *et al.*, 1977). *In vitro* studies show that EAN serum causes demyelination of CNS cultures (Saida, K. Saida & Silberberg, 1979*c*) or dorsal root ganglion cultures (Yonezawa, Ishihara & Matsuyama, 1968; Raine & Bornstein, 1979). *In vivo* studies of the possible function of antibodies and humoral factors have been carried out. Systemic injection of EAN serum alone does not transfer disease; however, systemic administration of EAN serum can cause local demyelination of nerves that have been treated with serotonin, which increases vascular permeability (Harvey & Pollard, 1992*a*). Intraneural injection of anti-galactocerebroside antibody causes demyelination of rat sciatic nerves (Saida *et al.*, 1979). Subsequent studies of intraneural injection or direct topical application of anti-galactocerebroside antibody showed that conduction block developed at the injection or application site within 1–2 h and that the conduction block was due to disruption of the paranodal structures rather than to a direct effect on conduction (Lafontaine *et al.*, 1982; Sumner *et al.*, 1982). The systemic administration of antibody to galactocerebroside enhanced the demyelination produced by the adoptive transfer of neuritogenic T cells (Hahn *et al.*, 1993). Intraneural injection of EAN serum also causes demyelination (T. Saida, *et al.*, 1978, 1979*a*; K. Saida *et al.* 1978) with the earliest changes being paranodal demyelination and later abnormalities being a recruitment of macrophages to the site of injection and subsequent demyelination. Other studies have shown that sera from rats inoculated with whole nerve or with P_2 cause demyelination if the sera have high titres of antibody to P_2 (Rosen, Brown & Rostami, 1990*b*). On the other hand, Hughes *et al.* (1985) found that rabbit antisera to P_2 did not cause significant demyelination after injection into rat nerve, although rabbit antisera to P_0 cause substantial demyelination.

Role of macrophages

While T cells are sufficient to transfer disease, macrophages are required for the development of EAN (Hartung *et al.*, 1988*b*; Heininger *et al.*, 1988). Macrophages could play a role as antigen-presenting cells or as effector cells that destroy myelin. Blockade of macrophages by silica (Tansey & Brosnan, 1982; Craggs, King & Thomas, 1984) reduces the severity of actively induced EAN. This was confirmed by the use of dichloromethylenediphosphothionate-containing liposomes which reduced the severity of passively transferred as well as actively transferred EAN (Jung *et al.*, 1993); this finding suggests that the macrophages are necessary in the effector phase of disease. Scavenging of oxygen free radicals, which are produced by macrophages, suppresses EAN (Hartung *et al.*, 1988*c*).

Role of mast cells

Mast cell numbers increase during the course of EAN (C.F. Brosnan *et al.*, 1985). Treatment with reserpine, which depletes vasoactive amines, such as those released by mast cells, protects animals against EAN (Brosnan & Tansey, 1984). Strains of rats and mice that are susceptible to EAN (and EAE) have greater numbers of mast cells than strains that are resistant (Johnson *et al.*, 1991). Johnson, Weiner & Seeldrayers (1988) showed that EAN serum contains IgE antibodies that can cause mast cell degranulation.

Role of cytokines

There is strong evidence for a role for IFN-γ in the evolution of EAN. Strigård *et al.* (1989*a*) showed that treatment of rats with antibody to IFN-γ after the onset of EAN shortened the course of disease, reduced MHC class II antigen expression and reduced the number of T cells within the nerves. They also showed that treatment with the same antibody from the day of immunization with myelin increased the duration of disease. A role for IFN-γ in the development of EAN was confirmed by Hartung *et al.* (1990) who showed that administration of IFN-γ enhances EAN. Immunocytochemical studies have shown that IFN-γ is produced by T cells and polymorphonuclear cells in the endoneurium during the course of EAN (Schmidt *et al.*, 1992). Tsai *et al.* (1991) showed that IFN-γ has the ability to induce MHC class II antigen expression on cultured Schwann cells. IFN-γ may also act on T cells. Treatment with antibody to IL-2 receptor (IL-2R) suppresses EAN (Hartung *et al.*, 1988*a*, 1989). Tumour necrosis factor-α (TNF-α) is present in macrophages in the peripheral nerves of rats with actively and passively induced EAN, and antibody to TNF-α ameliorates the disease (Stoll *et al.*, 1993*b*).

Cell adhesion molecules

Intercellular adhesion molecule-1 (ICAM-1) is expressed on macrophages and endothelial cells in EAN (Stoll *et al.*, 1993*a*) and antibody to ICAM-1 suppresses both actively and passively transferred EAN (Archelos *et al.*, 1993*a*), which suggests that ICAM-1 may be important in both the induction and effector stages of EAN. Lymphocyte function-associated molecule-1 (LFA-1) is a cell adhesion molecule that is a ligand for ICAM-1 and is expressed on lymphocytes. Antibodies to LFA-1 block actively induced but not passively transferred EAN (Archelos *et al.*, 1994), which suggests that this molecule is important in the induction stage of disease.

Role of complement

As discussed above, complement is present in peripheral nerve before the onset of demyelination in EAN. Treatment with cobra venom factor, which depletes the C3 component of complement, delays the onset and reduces the severity of pathological findings of actively induced EAN (Feasby *et al.*, 1987). The demyelinating activity that can be demonstrated by the intraneural injection of EAN serum is complement-dependent, as it can be destroyed by heating and restored by the addition of fresh serum from normal animals (T. Saida *et al.*, 1978; K. Saida, K. *et al.*, 1978). These findings suggest that complement plays a role in the pathogenesis of EAN.

Immunological findings in the peripheral blood

In general, these studies have been performed in acute EAN. Feasby *et al.* (1984) studied the numbers of $CD4^+$ and $CD8^+$ cells in the blood of Lewis rats with acute EAN and found no significant difference from normal controls. They found a small increase in the ratio of $CD4^+$ to $CD8^+$ cells on day 13 after inoculation: this was due to a slight decline in the number of

$CD8^+$ cells at this time. J.V. Brosnan *et al.* (1985) found that the number of $CD8^+$ cells in the blood declined during clinical disease. Yamashita *et al.* (1988) also found a small rise in the ratio of $CD4^+$ to $CD8^+$ cells in the blood of rats with EAN: this was due to a slight rise in the numbers of $CD4^+$ cells. Associated with the onset of disease they found an increase in the proliferative response of peripheral blood cells to myelin P_2 protein. In a subsequent study they found an increase in the number of MHC class II^+ and $CD25^+$ (IL-2R) T cells in the blood during the clinical phase of EAN (Hamaguchi *et al.*, 1991).

Immunoregulation

Tolerance to neuritogens

Animals that have recovered from actively induced acute EAN acquire tolerance to the antigen causing the attack of EAN. Guinea pigs that have recovered from EAN do not develop another episode of disease when reinjected with the same inoculum (Pollard *et al.*, 1975). Similarly, after recovery from acute EAN induced by inoculation with bovine dorsal roots (Brosnan *et al.*, 1984), myelin inoculation (McCombe *et al.*, 1990) or P_2 inoculation (Strigard *et al.*, 1989*b*), rats are resistant to the development of a further attack of disease after reinoculation with the same inoculum. This tolerance does not develop after passively transferred EAN, and repeated attacks of EAN can be produced by the repeated transfer of P_2-reactive T cell lines (Lassmann *et al.*, 1991).

Animals that are preimmunized with neuritogenic antigen in a form that does not cause EAN can be made tolerant to the antigen. Although pretreatment with bovine dorsal root tissue does not confer protection (Brosnan *et al.*, 1984), pretreatment with P_2 protein in incomplete Freund's adjuvant leads to resistance to induction of EAN by immunization with P_2 protein in adjuvant (Cunningham, Powers & Brostoff, 1983). Tolerance to neuritogenic antigen can also be induced by treatment with antigen-coupled splenocytes, and such tolerance is peptide-specific (Gregorian *et al.*, 1993). It has been shown that rats that are tolerized to neuritogenic peptide by this treatment retain the ability to produce a delayed-type hypersensitivity response to the peptide (Gregorian & Rostami, 1994).

Role of T cells in immunoregulation

T cells may have a role in the regulation of EAN. Treatment with antibody to CD5, which is a marker of T cells, can cause relapses in rats that have recovered from P_2-EAN and reverse the resistance to disease produced by pretreatment with P_2, suggesting that T cells play a role in the resistance to development of disease (Strigard *et al.*, 1989*b*). A T cell line obtained from cells of the cauda equina of rats with EAN was able to protect recipient rats against the development of EAN (Taylor & Hughes, 1988). Elimination of $CD8^+$ cells did not break this acquired tolerance, suggesting that $CD8^+$ cells play little role in the regulation of EAN (Strigard *et al.*, 1988*a*). Vaccination of rats with a P_2-stimulated T cell line did not prevent actively induced P_2-EAN (Jung *et al.*, 1991). However, the protective effect of antigen-coupled splenocytes was associated with a lack of T cells proliferating in response to the tolerizing peptide (Gregorian *et al.*, 1993).

Role of antibody in immunoregulation

Antibody appears to play a role in the regulation of EAE (MacPhee, Day & Mason, 1990). Antibody may also play a role in the downregulation of EAN. Lehrich & Arnason (1971) found that prior immunization of rats with peripheral nerve homogenized in saline prevented the development of EAN after immunization with peripheral nerve homogenized with adjuvant. They also found that serum from animals immunized with nerve in saline protected trigeminal ganglion cultures from damage by lymph node cells obtained from animals immunized with nerve in adjuvant. This protective effect might be mediated by antibody.

Chronic relapsing EAN: a failure of immmunoregulation?

As outlined above, rats that have recovered from acute EAN are resistant to reinduction of further episodes of disease by reinoculation with the same antigen. Chronic EAN has been produced by measures that might overcome immunoregulatory mechanisms, such as the use of a large dose of inoculum in rabbits (Harvey *et al.*, 1987*a*) or mild immunosuppression in Lewis rats (McCombe *et al.*, 1990).

Therapy

Studies of the treatment of EAN are important, because of the possible relevance to the treatment of GBS and CIDP, and because of the information that can be obtained about the possible pathogenesis of EAN.

Corticosteroids

High-dose methylprednisolone (50 mg/kg) treatment of Lewis rats after the onset of acute EAN resulted in reduction in the clinical severity of the disease and reduction in the degree of inflammation and demyelination (Watts, Taylor & Hughes, 1989). Similarly, high-dose (4 mg/kg) dexamethasone treatment after the onset of signs of acute EAN resulted in clinical and electrophysiological improvement (Heininger *et al.*, 1988). Intraperitoneal methylprednisolone (10 mg/kg) also improved the clinical status and the histological appearances in rats with EAN, whether given from the time of inoculation or after the onset of signs. Stevens *et al.* (1990) showed that short-term and long-term treatment of EAN with prednisolone reduced the severity of disease and did not cause relapses.

Cyclosporin A

Cyclosporin A is a fungal metabolite that inhibits T cell responses. Oral cyclosporin A given at a dose of 50 mg/kg suppresses acute EAN in guinea pigs and rats, whether given from the time of inoculation or after the onset of signs (King *et al.*, 1983). Animals treated from the time of inoculation develop EAN after treatment is stopped. Cyclosporin A also suppresses the development of EAN mediated by the passive transfer of P_2- specific T cell lines (Hartung *et al.*, 1987). Nakayasu *et al.* (1990) found that cyclosporin A treatment suppressed actively and passively induced EAN and that, whereas the actively inoculated rats developed disease after ceasing treatment, the rats that had received T cell infusions did not. These studies all used high doses of cyclosporin A. However, treatment with low doses of cyclosporin A failed to prevent disease, and led to chronic relapsing EAN (McCombe *et al.* 1990).

Plasma exchange or plasma infusion

The role of plasma exchange in EAN is of interest because of the success of plasma exchange in treating GBS and CIDP. Antony, Pollard & McLeod (1981) showed that plasmapheresis reduced the clinical disability, the dispersion of the compound muscle action potential and the histological abnormalities in rabbits with acute EAN. Gross *et al.* (1983) also studied the effects of plasma exchange on EAN in rabbits and found that the treated animals had less severe clinical and histological signs. The authors commented that the rapidity of the response to plasma exchange was 'probably too rapid to be due to remyelination' and suggested that plasma exchange may have removed a factor that blocks nerve conduction. However, Pender (1989) showed that, after spontaneous recovery from acute EAE, there is ensheathment and early remyelination of the nerve roots at a time when conduction is restored and clinical recovery occurs. Such early remyelination of the nerve roots could occur after plasma exchange in EAN and contribute to the clinical improvement. One possible explanation for the beneficial effects of plasmapheresis is that there is removal of a circulating factor, such as an antibody, which causes demyelination. Such factors have been demonstrated in EAN serum (T. Saida *et al.*, 1978; Pollard, Harrison & Gatenby, 1981). Harvey *et al.* (1988) performed plasma exchange on rabbits with EAN and showed that 55–60% of circulating anti-myelin antibody was removed at each exchange. They subsequently showed that immunoabsorption of the IgG fraction of EAN serum had a beneficial effect similar to that of plasmapheresis (Harvey, Schindhelm & Pollard, 1989*b*). However, the same group also showed that infusion of plasma could reduce the signs of EAN, and reduce the levels of anti-myelin antibodies (Harvey *et al.*, 1989*a*) and commented that such a reduction might be associated with anti-idiotypic antibodies.

Vaccination with T cells or anti-TCR therapy

In Lewis rats, antibodies to CD4, CD8, Ia antigen and T cells can reduce the severity of EAN when given shortly before the expected onset of signs (Strigard *et al.*, 1988*b*). The same study showed that antibody to CD5 reduces the severity of disease when given from the time of inoculation, but makes EAN worse when given shortly before the expected onset of signs. Treatment with antibody to the $\alpha\beta$TCR can prevent the development of EAN induced by transfer of P_2-reactive cells or can reduce the severity of EAN when given after the onset of signs (Jung *et al.*, 1992). In another study, antibodies to a pan-T-cell marker inhibited EAN, whereas antibody to CD8 worsened the disease (Holmdahl *et al.*, 1985). Vaccination with glutaraldehyde-fixed P_2-specific cells did not protect against EAN induced by inoculation with P_2 protein and adjuvants (Jung *et al.*, 1991).

Antagonism of cytokines

The role of IFN-γ in EAN is not yet clear. In a study of EAN induced in Lewis rats by inoculation with peripheral nerve myelin, Strigard *et al.* (1989*a*) found that antibody to IFN-γ shortened the duration of disease when given after the onset of symptoms, but increased the duration of disease when given from the time of inoculation. However, Hartung *et al.* (1990) found that antibody to IFN-γ suppressed EAN, and that IFN-γ enhanced disease.

Other agents

Treatment with the protease inhibitors ε-amino-caproic acid and pepstatin limited the rate of development of EAN (Schabet *et al.*, 1991). Treatment of rats with EAN with gangliosides reduced the severity of disease (Ledeen *et al.*, 1990; Oderfeld Nowak *et al.*, 1990). The ACTH analogue, Org 2766, which has no corticotrophic activity, protects against EAN, possibly by preventing axonal degeneration (Duckers, Verhaagen & Gispen, 1993).

Conclusions

EAN is an experimental inflammatory demyelinating polyradiculoneuropathy. The development of EAN as a model owes much to previous work on EAE. Although $CD4^+$ T lymphocytes are critical to the development of EAN, there is considerable evidence that specific antibodies may also play a role in the pathogenesis of EAN. Initial studies suggested that the myelin P_2 protein was the target antigen of EAN, but is now clear that immunity against the myelin P_0 protein can also lead to EAN. It seems most helpful to think of EAN as an immune-mediated primary demyelinating disease of the peripheral nervous system, where more than one antigen may be the target of the immune attack. Acute EAN is a good model of the human disease GBS, and chronic relapsing EAN is a good model of CIDP (see Chapters 8 and 9).

References

Adam, A.M., Atkinson, P.F., Hall, S.M., Hughes, R.A. & Taylor, W.A. (1989). Chronic experimental allergic neuritis in Lewis rats. *Neuropathology and Applied Neurobiology*, **15**, 249–64.

Adelmann, M. & Linington, C. (1992). Molecular mimicry and the autoimmune response to the peripheral nerve myelin PO glycoprotein. *Neurochemical Research*, **17**, 887–91.

Allt, G. (1972). Involvement of the perineurium in experimental allergic neuritis; electron microscopic observations. *Acta Neuropathologica*, **20**, 139–49.

Allt, G. (1975). The node of Ranvier in experimental allergic neuritis: an electron microscope study. *Journal of Neurocytology*, **4**, 63–76.

Allt, G., Evans, E.M. & Evans, D.H. (1971). The vulnerability of immature rabbits to experimental allergic neuritis: a light and electron microscope study. *Brain Research*, **29**, 271–91.

Antony, J.H., Pollard, J.D. & McLeod, J.G. (1981). Effects of plasmapheresis on the course of experimental allergic neuritis in rabbits. *Journal of Neurology, Neurosurgery and Psychiatry*, **44**, 1124–8.

Archelos, J.J., Maurer, M., Jung, S., Miyasaka, M., Tamatani, T., Toyka, K.V. & Hartung, H.P. (1994). Inhibition of experimental autoimmune neuritis by an antibody to the lymphocyte function-associated antigen-1. *Laboratory Investigation*, **70**, 667–75.

Archelos, J.J., Maurer, M., Jung, S., Toyka, K.V. & Hartung, H.P. (1993*a*). Suppression of experimental allergic neuritis by an antibody to the intercellular adhesion molecule ICAM-1. *Brain*, **116**, 1043–58.

Archelos, J.J., Roggenbuck, K., Schneider Schaulies, J., Toyka, K.V. & Hartung, H.P. (1993*b*). Detection and quantification of antibodies to the extracellular domain of P_0 during experimental allergic neuritis. *Journal of the Neurological Sciences*, **117**, 197–205.

Argall, K.G., Armati, P.J., Pollard, J.D. & Bonner, J. (1992*a*). Interactions between CD4$^+$ T-cells and rat Schwann cells *in vitro*. 2. Cytotoxic effects of P_2-specific CD4$^+$ T-cell lines on Lewis rat Schwann cells. *Journal of Neuroimmunology*, **40**, 19–29.

Argall, K.G., Armati, P.J., Pollard, J.D., Watson, E. & Bonner, J. (1992b). Interactions between CD4$^+$ T-cells and rat Schwann cells *in vitro*. 1. Antigen presentation by Lewis rat Schwann cells to P_2-specific CD4$^+$ T-cell lines. *Journal of Neuroimmunology*, **40**, 1–18.

Armati, P.J., Pollard, J.D. & Gatenby, P. (1990). Rat and human Schwann cells *in vitro* can synthesize and express MHC molecules. *Muscle and Nerve*, **13**, 106–16.

Asbury, A.K., Arnason, B.G. & Adams, R.D. (1969). The inflammatory lesion in idiopathic polyneuritis. Its role in pathogenesis. *Medicine*, **48**, 173–215.

Åström, K.E., Webster, H.D. & Arnason, B.G. (1968). The initial lesion in experimental allergic neuritis. A phase and electron microscopic study. *Journal of Experimental Medicine*, **128**, 469–95.

Ballin, R.H. & Thomas, P.K. (1969). Electron microscope observations on demyelination and remyelination in experimental allergic neuritis. I. Demyelination. *Journal of the Neurological Sciences*, **8**, 1–18.

Ballon-Landa, G.R., Paterson, P.Y. & Dal Canto, M.C. (1978). Experimental allergic neuritis in Lewis rat: altered pattern of disease induced by pertussis vaccine. *Clinical Immunology and Immunopathology*, **10**, 148–57.

Behan, P.O., Feldman, R.G., Hunt, R.D. & Behan, W.M. (1971). Hyperacute experimental allergic neuritis. *Research Communications in Chemical Pathology and Pharmacology*, **2**, 889–97.

Brosnan, C.F., Lyman, W.D., Tansey, F.A. & Carter, T.H. (1985). Quantitation of mast cells in experimental allergic neuritis. *Journal of Neuropathology and Experimental Neurology*, **44**, 196–203.

Brosnan, C.F. & Tansey, F.A. (1984). Delayed onset of experimental allergic neuritis in rats treated with reserpine. *Journal of Neuropathology and Experimental Neurology*, **43**, 84–93.

Brosnan, J.V., Craggs, R.I., King, R.H. & Thomas, P.K. (1984). Attempts to suppress experimental allergic neuritis in the rat by pretreatment with antigen. *Acta Neuropathologica*, **64**, 153–60.

Brosnan, J.V., Craggs, R.I., King, R.H. & Thomas, P.K. (1987). Reduced susceptibility of T cell-deficient rats to induction of experimental allergic neuritis. *Journal of Neuroimmunology*, **14**, 267–82.

Brosnan, J.V., Fellowes, R., Craggs, R.I., King, R.H., Bowley, T.J. & Thomas, P.K. (1985). Changes in lymphocyte subsets during the course of experimental allergic neuritis. *Brain*, **108**, 315–34.

Clark, L., Heber Katz, E. & Rostami, A. (1992). Shared T-cell receptor gene usage in experimental allergic neuritis and encephalomyelitis. *Annals of Neurology*, **31**, 587–92.

Cragg, B.G. & Thomas, P.K. (1964). Changes in nerve conduction in experimental allergic neuritis. *Journal of Neurology, Neurosurgery and Psychiatry*, **27**, 106–15.

Craggs, R.I., King, R.H. & Thomas, P.K. (1984). The effect of suppression of macrophage activity on the development of experimental allergic neuritis. *Acta Neuropathologica*, **62**, 316–23.

Cunningham, J.M., Powers, J.M. & Brostoff, S.W. (1983). Prevention of experimental allergic neuritis in the Lewis rat with bovine P_2 protein. *Brain Research*, **258**, 285–9.

Dieperink, M.E., O'Neill, A., Maselli, R. & Stefansson, K. (1991). Experimental allergic neuritis in the SJL/J mouse: dysfunction of peripheral nerve without clinical signs. *Journal of Neuroimmunology*, **35**, 247–59.

Duckers, H.J., Verhaagen, J. & Gispen, W.H. (1993). The neurotrophic analogue of ACTH(4–9), Org 2766, protects against experimental allergic neuritis. *Brain*, **116**, 1059–75.

Eylar, E.H., Toro Goyco, E., Kessler, M.J. & Szymanska, I. (1982). Induction of allergic neuritis in rhesus monkeys. *Journal of Neuroimmunology*, **3**, 91–8.

Feasby, T.E., Gilbert, J.J., Hahn, A.F. & Neilson, M. (1987). Complement depletion suppresses Lewis rat experimental allergic neuritis. *Brain Research*, **419**, 97–103.

Feasby, T.E., Mazaheri, R., Hahn, A.F., Gilbert, J.J., Stiller, C.R. & Keown, P.A. (1984). Circulating lymphocyte subpopulations in experimental allergic neuritis. *Journal of Neuroimmunology*, **6**, 209–14.

Ferraro, A. & Roizin, L. (1954). Neuropathologic variations in experimental allergic encephalomyelitis. *Journal of Neuropathology and Experimental Neurology*, **13**, 60–89.

Gasser, D.L., Newlin, C.M., Palm, J. & Gonatas, N.K. (1973). Genetic control of susceptibility to experimental allergic encephalomyelitis in rats. *Science*, **181**, 872–3.

Geczy, C.L., Roberts, I.M., Meyer, P. & Bernard, C.C.A. (1984). Susceptibility and resistance to experimental autoimmune encephalomyelitis and neuritis in the guinea pig correlate with the induction of procoagulant and anticoagulant activities. *Journal of Immunology*, **133**, 3026–36.

Gregorian, S.K., Clark, L., Heber Katz, E., Amento, E.P. & Rostami, A. (1993). Induction of peripheral tolerance with peptide-specific anergy in experimental autoimmune neuritis. *Cellular Immunology*, **150**, 298–310.

Gregorian, S.K. & Rostami, A. (1994). Delayed-type hypersensitivity response in experimental autoimmune neuritis treated with peptide-coupled spleen cells. *Journal of Neuroimmunology*, **51**, 69–75.

Gross, M.L., Craggs, R.I., King, R.H. & Thomas, P.K. (1983). The treatment of experimental allergic neuritis by plasma exchange. *Journal of the Neurological Sciences*, **61**, 149–60.

Hahn, A.F., Feasby, T.E. & Gilbert, J.J. (1985). Blood–nerve barrier studies in experimental allergic neuritis. *Acta Neuropathologica*, **68**, 101–9.

Hahn, A.F., Feasby, T.E., Steele, A., Lovgren, D.S. & Berry, J. (1988). Demyelination and axonal degeneration in Lewis rat experimental allergic neuritis depend on the myelin dosage. *Laboratory Investigation*, **59**, 115–25.

Hahn, A.F., Feasby, T.E., Wilkie, L. & Lovgren, D. (1993). Antigalactocerebroside antibody increases demyelination in adoptive transfer experimental allergic neuritis. *Muscle and Nerve*, **16**, 1174–80.

Hall, J.I. (1967). Studies on demyelinated peripheral nerves in guinea-pigs with experimental allergic neuritis. A histological and electrophysiological study. II. Electrophysiological observations. *Brain*, **90**, 313–32.

Hamaguchi, K., Ohno, R., Tsuji, T., Yamashita, T., Negishi, T., Nomura, K. & Hosokawa, T. (1991). Activated T lymphocyte subsets in experimental allergic neuritis. *Journal of Neuroimmunology*, **34**, 191–6.

Hartung, H.P., Schafer, B., Diamantstein, T., Fierz, W., Heininger, K. & Toyka, K.V. (1988*a*). Suppression of P2-T-cell line mediated experimental autoimmune neuritis by interleukin-2 receptor blockade. *Annals of the New York Academy of Sciences*, **540**, 563–5.

Hartung, H.P., Schafer, B., Diamantstein, T., Fierz, W., Heininger, K. & Toyka, K.V. (1989). Suppression of P2-T cell line-mediated experimental autoimmune neuritis by interleukin-2 receptor targeted monoclonal antibody ART 18. *Brain Research*, **489**, 120–28.

Hartung, H.P., Schafer, B., Fierz, W., Heininger, K. & Toyka, K.V. (1987). Ciclosporin A prevents P2 T cell line-mediated experimental autoimmune neuritis (AT-EAN) in rat. *Neuroscience Letters*, **83**, 195–200.

Hartung, H.P., Schafer, B., Heininger, K., Stoll, G. & Toyka, K.V. (1988*b*). The role of macrophages and eicosanoids in the pathogenesis of experimental allergic neuritis. Serial clinical, electrophysiological, biochemical and morphological observations. *Brain*, **111**, 1039–59.

Hartung, H.P., Schafer, B., Heininger, K. & Toyka, K.V. (1988*c*). Suppression of experimental autoimmune neuritis by the oxygen radical scavengers superoxide dismutase and catalase. *Annals of Neurology*, **23**, 453–60.

Hartung, H.P., Schafer, B., van der Meide, P.H., Fierz, W., Heininger, K. & Toyka, K.V. (1990). The role of interferon-gamma in the pathogenesis of experimental autoimmune disease of the peripheral nervous system. *Annals of Neurology*, **27**, 247–57.

Harvey, G.K. & Pollard, J.D. (1992*a*). Peripheral nervous system demyelination from systemic transfer of experimental allergic neuritis serum. *Journal of Neuroimmunology*, **41**, 159–66.

Harvey, G.K. & Pollard, J.D. (1992*b*). Patterns of conduction impairment in experimental allergic neuritis. An electrophysiological and histological study. *Journal of Neurology, Neurosurgery and Psychiatry*, **55**, 909–15.

Harvey, G.K., Pollard, J.D., Schindhelm, K. & Antony, J. (1987*a*). Chronic experimental allergic neuritis. An electrophysiological and histological study in the rabbit. *Journal of the Neurological Sciences*, **81**, 215–25.

Harvey, G.K., Pollard, J.D., Schindhelm, K. & McLeod, J.G. (1989*a*). Experimental allergic neuritis: effect of plasma infusions. *Clinical and Experimental Immunology*, **76**, 452–7.

Harvey, G.K., Schindhelm, K., Antony, J.H. & Pollard, J.D. (1987*b*). Linear response curves from an ELISA assay: measurement of anti-myelin IgG and IgM during experimental allergic neuritis. *Journal of Neuroscience Methods*, **21**, 81–90.

Harvey, G.K., Schindhelm, K., Antony, J.H. & Pollard, J.D. (1988). Membrane plasma exchange in experimental allergic neuritis: effect on antibody levels and clinical course. *Journal of the Neurological Sciences*, **88**, 207–18.

Harvey, G.K., Schindhelm, K. & Pollard, J.D. (1989*b*). IgG immunoadsorption in experimental allergic neuritis: effect on antibody levels and clinical course. *Journal of Neurology, Neurosurgery and Psychiatry*, **52**, 865–70.

Heininger, K., Schafer, B., Hartung, H.P., Fierz, W., Linington, C. & Toyka, K.V. (1988). The role of macrophages in experimental autoimmune neuritis induced by a P_2-specific T-cell line. *Annals of Neurology*, **23**, 326–31.

Heininger, K., Stoll, G., Linington, C., Toyka, K.V. & Wekerle, H. (1986). Conduction failure and nerve conduction slowing in experimental allergic neuritis induced by P_2-specific T-cell lines. *Annals of Neurology*, **19**, 44–9.

Hoffman, P.M., Powers, J.M., Weise, M.J. & Brostoff, S.W. (1980). Experimental allergic neuritis. I. Rat strain differences in the response to bovine myelin antigens. *Brain Research*, **195**, 355–62.

Holmdahl, R., Olsson, T., Moran, T. & Klareskog, L. (1985). *In vivo* treatment of rats with monoclonal anti-T-cell antibodies. Immunohistochemical and functional analysis in normal rats and in experimental allergic neuritis. *Scandinavian Journal of Immunology*, **22**, 157–69.

Hughes, R.A., Kadlubowski, M., Gray, I.A. & Leibowitz, S. (1981). Immune responses in experimental allergic neuritis. *Journal of Neurology, Neurosurgery and Psychiatry*, **44**, 565–9.

Hughes, R.A. & Powell, H.C. (1984). Experimental allergic neuritis: demyelination induced by P_2 alone and non-specific enhancement by cerebroside. *Journal of Neuropathology and Experimental Neurology*, **43**, 154–61.

Hughes, R.A.C., Powell, H.C., Braheny, S.L. & Brostoff, S. (1985). Endoneurial injection of antisera to myelin antigens. *Muscle and Nerve*, **8**, 516–22.

Innes, J.R.M. (1951). Experimental 'allergic' encephalitis: attempts to produce the disease in sheep and goats. *Journal of Comparative Pathology*, **61**, 241–50.

Jacobs, J.M., Macfarlane, R.M. & Cavanagh, J.B. (1976). Vascular leakage in the dorsal root ganglia of the rat, studies with horseradish peroxidase. *Journal of the Neurological Sciences*, **29**, 95–107.

Johnson, D., Weiner, H.L. & Seeldrayers, P.A. (1988). Role of mast cells in peripheral nervous system demyelination. *Annals of the New York Academy of Sciences*, **540**, 727–8.

Johnson, D., Yasui, D. & Seeldrayers, P. (1991). An analysis of mast cell frequency in the rodent nervous system: numbers vary between different strains and can be reconstituted in mast cell-deficient mice. *Journal of Neuropathology and Experimental Neurology*, **50**, 227–34.

Jung, S., Huitinga, I., Schmidt, B., Zielasek, J., Dijkstra, C.D., Toyka, K.V. & Hartung, H.P. (1993). Selective elimination of macrophages by dichlormethylene diphosphonate-containing liposomes suppresses experimental autoimmune neuritis. *Journal of the Neurological Sciences*, **119**, 195–202.

Jung, S., Kramer, S., Schluesener, H.J., Hunig, T., Toyka, K. & Hartung, H.P. (1992). Prevention and therapy of experimental autoimmune neuritis by an antibody against T cell receptors-alpha/beta. *Journal of Immunology*, **148**, 3768–75.

Jung, S., Schluesener, H.J., Toyka, K. & Hartung, H.P. (1991). T cell vaccination does not induce resistance to experimental autoimmune neuritis. *Journal of Neuroimmunology*, **35**, 1–11.

Kadlubowski, M. & Hughes, R.A. (1979). Identification of the neuritogen for experimental allergic neuritis. *Nature*, **277**, 140–1.

Kalimo, H., Molnar, G.K., Saksa, M. & Riekkinen, P.J. (1982). Involvement of autonomic nervous system in experimental allergic neuritis. A light- and electron-microscopic study. *Journal of Neuroimmunology*, **2**, 9–19.

King, R.H., Craggs, R.I., Gross, M.L., Tompkins, C. & Thomas, P.K. (1983). Suppression of experimental allergic neuritis by Cyclosporin-A. *Acta Neuropathologica*, **59**, 262–8.

King, R.H.M., Thomas, P.K. & Pollard, J.D. (1977). Axonal and dorsal root ganglion cell changes in experimental allergic neuritis. *Neuropathology and Applied Neurobiology*, **3**, 471–86.

Lafontaine, S., Rasminsky, M., Saida, T. & Sumner, A.J. (1982). Conduction block in rat myelinated fibres following acute exposure to anti-galactocerebroside serum. *Journal of Physiology*, **323**, 287–306.

Lampert, P.W. (1969). Mechanism of demyelination in experimental allergic neuritis. Electron microscopic studies. *Laboratory Investigation*, **20**, 127–38.

Lassmann, H., Fierz, W., Neuchrist, C. & Meyermann, R. (1991). Chronic relapsing experimental allergic neuritis induced by repeated transfer of P_2-protein reactive T cell lines. *Brain*, **114**, 429–42.

Ledeen, R.W., Oderfeld Nowak, B., Brosnan, C.F. & Cervone, A. (1990). Gangliosides offer partial protection in experimental allergic neuritis. *Annals of Neurology*, **27 (Supplement)**, S69-S74.

Lehrich, J.R. & Arnason, B.G. (1971). Suppression of experimental allergic neuritis in rats by prior immunization with nerve in saline. *Acta Neuropathologica*, **18**, 144–9.

Levine, S. & Wenk, E.J. (1965). A hyperacute form of allergic encephalomyelitis. *American Journal of Pathology*, **47**, 61–88.

Linington, C., Izumo, S., Suzuki, M., Uyemura, K., Meyermann, R. & Wekerle, H. (1984). A permanent rat T cell line that mediates experimental allergic neuritis in the Lewis rat *in vivo*. *Journal of Immunology*, **133**, 1946–50.

Linington, C., Lassmann, H., Ozawa, K., Kosin, S. & Mongan, L. (1992). Cell adhesion molecules of the immunoglobulin supergene family as tissue-specific autoantigens: induction of experimental allergic neuritis (EAN) by PO protein-specific T cell lines. *European Journal of Immunology*, **22**, 1813–17.

Linington, C., Mann, A., Izumo, S., Uyemura, K., Suzuki, M., Meyermann, R. & Wekerle, H. (1986). Induction of experimental allergic neuritis in the BN rat: P2 protein-specific T cells overcome resistance to actively induced disease. *Journal of Immunology*, **137**, 3826–31.

Lumsden, C.E. (1949). Experimental 'allergic' encephalomyelitis. *Brain*, **72**, 198–226.

MacPhee, I.A., Day, M.J. & Mason, D.W. (1990). The role of serum factors in the suppression of experimental allergic encephalomyelitis: evidence for immunoregulation by antibody to the encephalitogenic peptide. *Immunology*, **70**, 527–34.

Madrid, R.E. (1983). Chronic progressive and relapsing experimental allergic neuritis in guinea pigs. In *Clinical and Biological Aspects of Peripheral Nerve Diseases*, ed. L. Battistin, G.A. Hashim & A. Lajtha. pp. 265–76. New York: Alan R. Liss.

Madrid, R.E. & Wisniewski, H.M. (1977). Axonal degeneration in demyelinating disorders. *Journal of Neurocytology*, **6**, 103–17.

Martinez, A., Blanes, A., Ramon, C.J.S., De Ispizua, I. & Campo, C. (1977). Early changes in the Schwann cells in experimental allergic neuritis. *Journal of the Neurological Sciences*, **33**, 61–9.

McCombe, P.A., van der Kreek, S.A. & Pender, M.P. (1990). The effects of prophylactic cyclosporin A on experimental allergic neuritis (EAN) in the Lewis rat. Induction of relapsing EAN using low dose cyclosporin A. *Journal of Neuroimmunology*, **28**, 131–40.

McCombe, P.A., van der Kreek, S.A. & Pender, M.P. (1992). Neuropathological findings in chronic relapsing experimental allergic neuritis induced in the Lewis rat by inoculation with intradural root myelin and treatment with low dose cyclosporin A. *Neuropathology and Applied Neurobiology*, **18**, 171–87.

Milner, P., Lovelidge, C.A., Taylor, W.A. & Hughes, R.A. (1987). P_0 myelin protein produces experimental allergic neuritis in Lewis rats. *Journal of the Neurological Sciences*, **79**, 275–85.

Mizisin, A.P., Wiley, C.A., Hughes, R.A. & Powell, H.C. (1987). Peripheral nerve demyelination in rabbits after inoculation with Freund's complete adjuvant alone or in combination with lipid haptens. *Journal of Neuroimmunology*, **16**, 381–95.

Morey, M.K., Wiley, C.A., Hughes, R.A. & Powell, H.C. (1985). Autonomic nerves in experimental allergic neuritis in the rat. *Acta Neuropathologica*, **67**, 75–80.

Nagai, Y., Momoi, T., Saito, M., Mitsuzawa, E. & Ohtani, S. (1976). Ganglioside syndrome, a new autoimmune neurological disorder, experimentally induced with brain gangliosides. *Neuroscience Letters*, **2**, 107–11.

Nakayasu, H., Ota, K., Tanaka, H., Irie, H. & Takahashi, K. (1990). Suppression of actively induced and passively transferred experimental allergic neuritis by cyclosporin A. *Journal of Neuroimmunology*, **26**, 219–27.

Nomura, K., Hamaguchi, K., Ohno, R., Hosokawa, T., Negishi, T., Yamashita, T., Suzuki, M. & Uyemura, K. (1987). Cell-mediated immunity to bovine P2 protein and neuritogenic synthetic peptide in experimental allergic neuritis. *Journal of Neuroimmunology*, **15**, 25–35.

Oderfeld Nowak, B., Brosnan, C., Cervone, A., Oderfeld, J. & Ledeen, R.W. (1990). Gangliosides improve the outcome of experimental allergic neuritis (EAN). *Acta Neurobiologiae Experimentalis*, **50**, 495–504.

Olee, T., Powell, H.C. & Brostoff, S.W. (1990). New minimum length requirement for a T cell epitope for experimental allergic neuritis. *Journal of Neuroimmunology*, **27**, 187–90.

Olee, T., Powers, J.M. & Brostoff, S.W. (1988). A T cell epitope for experimental allergic neuritis. *Journal of Neuroimmunology*, **19**, 167–73.

Olee, T., Weise, M., Powers, J. & Brostoff, S. (1989). A T cell epitope for experimental allergic neuritis is an amphipathic alpha-helical structure. *Journal of Neuroimmunology*, **21**, 235–40.

Olsson, T., Holmdahl, R., Klareskog, L. & Forsum, U. (1983). Ia-expressing cells and T lymphocytes of different subsets in peripheral nerve tissue during experimental allergic neuritis in Lewis rats. *Scandinavian Journal of Immunology*, **18**, 339–43.

Olsson, T., Holmdahl, R., Klareskog, L., Forsum, U. & Kristensson, K. (1984). Dynamics of Ia-expressing cells and T lymphocytes of different subsets during experimental allergic neuritis in Lewis rats. *Journal of the Neurological Sciences*, **66**, 141–9.

Olsson, Y. (1968). Topographical differences in the vascular permeability of the peripheral nervous system. *Acta Neuropathologica*, **10**, 26–33.

Ota, K., Irie, H. & Takahashi, K. (1987). T cell subsets and Ia-positive cells in the sciatic nerve during the course of experimental allergic neuritis. *Journal of Neuroimmunology*, **13**, 283–92.

Pender, M.P. (1989). Recovery from acute experimental allergic encephalomyelitis in the Lewis rat. Early restoration of nerve conduction and repair by Schwann cells and oligodendrocytes. *Brain*, **112**, 393–416.

Petek, M. & Quaglio, G.L. (1967). Experimental allergic neuritis in the chicken. *Pathologica Veterinaria*, **4**, 464–76.

Pettersson, C.A.V., Sharma, H.S. & Olsson, Y. (1990). Vascular permeability of spinal nerve roots. A study in the rat with Evans blue and lanthanum as tracers. *Acta Neuropathologica*, **81**, 148–54.

Pollard, J.D., Harrison, B. & Gatenby, P. (1981). Serum-induced demyelination: an electrophysiological and histological study. *Clinical and Experimental Neurology*, **18**, 70–80.

Pollard, J.D., King, R.H. & Thomas, P.K. (1975). Recurrent experimental allergic neuritis. An electron microscope study. *Journal of the Neurological Sciences*, **24**, 365–83.

Ponzin, D., Menegus, A.M., Kirschner, G., Nunzi, M.G., Fiori, M.G. & Raine, C.S. (1991). Effects of gangliosides on the expression of autoimmune demyelination in the peripheral nervous system. *Annals of Neurology*, **30**, 678–85.

Powell, H.C., Braheny, S.L., Hughes, R.A.C. & Lampert, P.W. (1984). Antigen-specific demyelination and significance of the bystander effect in peripheral nerves. *American Journal of Pathology*, **114**, 443–53.

Powell, H.C., Myers, R.R., Mizisin, A.P., Olee, T. & Brostoff, S.W. (1991). Response of the axon and barrier endothelium to experimental allergic neuritis induced by autoreactive T cell lines. *Acta Neuropathologica*, **82**, 364–77.

Raine, C.S. & Bornstein, M.B. (1979). Experimental allergic neuritis. Ultrastructure of serum-induced myelin aberrations in peripheral nervous system cultures. *Laboratory Investigation*, **40**, 423–32.

Robinson, H.C., Allt, G. & Evans, D.H. (1972). A study of the capacity of myelinated and unmyelinated nerves to induce experimental allergic neuritis. *Acta Neuropathologica*, **21**, 99–108.

Rosen, J.L., Brown, M.J., Hickey, W.F. & Rostami, A. (1990*a*). Early myelin lesions in experimental allergic neuritis. *Muscle and Nerve*, **13**, 629–36.

Rosen, J.L., Brown, M.J. & Rostami, A. (1990*b*). Effect of experimental allergic neuritis serum on normal rat peripheral nerve. *Pathobiology*, **58**, 95–8.

Rostami, A. (1990). Comparative study of experimental autoimmune neuritis in SJL mice and Lewis rats. *Immunologic Research*, **9**, 314–19.

Rostami, A., Burns, J.B., Brown, M.J., Rosen, J., Zweiman, B., Lisak, R.P. & Pleasure, D.E. (1985). Transfer of experimental allergic neuritis with P_2-reactive T-cell lines. *Cellular Immunology*, **91**, 354–61.

Rostami, A. & Gregorian, S.K. (1991). Peptide 53–78 of myelin P_2 protein is a T cell epitope for the induction of experimental autoimmune neuritis. *Cellular Immunology*, **132**, 433–41.

Rostami, A., Gregorian, S.K., Brown, M.J. & Pleasure, D.E. (1990). Induction of severe experimental autoimmune neuritis with a synthetic peptide corresponding to the 53–78 amino acid sequence of the myelin P_2 protein. *Journal of Neuroimmunology*, **30**, 145–51.

Saida, K., Saida, T., Brown, M.J. & Silberberg, D.H. (1979). *In vivo* demyelination induced by intraneural injection of anti-galactocerebroside serum. *American Journal of Pathology*, **95**, 99–116.

Saida, K., Saida, T., Brown, M.J., Silberberg, D.H. & Asbury, A.K. (1978). Antiserum-mediated demyelination *in vivo*: a sequential study using intraneural injection of experimental allergic neuritis serum. *Laboratory Investigation*, **39**, 449–62.

Saida, T., Saida, K., Brown, M.J. & Silberberg, D.H. (1979*a*). Peripheral nerve demyelination induced by intraneural injection of experimental allergic encephalomyelitis serum. *Journal of Neuropathology and Experimental Neurology*, **38**, 498–518.

Saida, T., Saida, K., Dorfman, S.H., Silberberg, D.H., Sumner, A.J., Manning, M.C., Lisak, R.P. & Brown, M.J. (1979*b*). Experimental allergic neuritis induced by sensitization with galactocerebroside. *Science*, **204**, 1103–6.

Saida, T., Saida, K. & Silberberg, D.H. (1979*c*). Demyelination produced by experimental allergic neuritis serum and anti-galactocerebroside antiserum in CNS cultures. An ultrastructural study. *Acta Neuropathologica*, **48**, 19–25.

Saida, T., Saida, K., Silberberg, D.H. & Brown, M.J. (1978). Transfer of demyelination by intraneural injection of experimental allergic neuritis serum. *Nature*, **272**, 639–41.

Saida, T., Saida, K., Silberberg, D.H. & Brown, M.J. (1981). Experimental allergic neuritis induced by galactocerebroside. *Annals of Neurology*, **9 (Supplement)**, 87–101.

Saida, T., Silberberg, D.H., Fry, J.M. & Manning, M.C. (1977). Demyelinating anti-galactocerebroside antibodies in EAN and EAE. *Journal of Neuropathology and Experimental Neurology*, **36**, 627.

Schabet, M., Whitaker, J.N., Schott, K., Stevens, A., Zurn, A., Buhler, R. & Wietholter, H. (1991). The use of protease inhibitors in experimental allergic neuritis. *Journal of Neuroimmunology*, **31**, 265–72.

Schmidt, B., Stoll, G., Hartung, H.P., Heininger, K., Schafer, B. & Toyka, K.V. (1990). Macrophages but not Schwann cells express Ia antigen in experimental autoimmune neuritis. *Annals of Neurology*, **28**, 70–7.

Schmidt, B., Stoll, G., van der Meide, P., Jung, S. & Hartung, H.P. (1992). Transient cellular expression of γ-interferon in myelin-induced and T-cell line-mediated experimental autoimmune neuritis. *Brain*, **115**, 1633–46.

Schwarz, J.R., Corrette, B.J., Mann, K. & Wietholter, H. (1991). Changes of ionic channel distribution in myelinated nerve fibres from rats with experimental allergic neuritis. *Neuroscience Letters*, **122**, 205–9.

Sherwin, A.L. (1966). Chronic allergic neuropathy in the rabbit. *Archives of Neurology*, **15**, 289–93.

Smith, M.E., Forno, L.S. & Hofmann, W.W. (1979). Experimental allergic neuritis in the Lewis rat. *Journal of Neuropathology and Experimental Neurology*, **38**, 377–91.

Solders, G., Persson, A., Kristensson, K. & Hansson, S. (1985). Autonomic dysfunction in experimental allergic neuritis. *Acta Neurologica Scandinavica*, **72**, 18–25.

Stanley, G.P., McCombe, P.A. & Pender, M.P. (1992). Focal conduction block in the dorsal root ganglion in experimental allergic neuritis. *Annals of Neurology*, **31**, 27–33.

Steinman, L., Smith, M.E. & Forno, L.S. (1981). Genetic control of susceptibility to experimental allergic neuritis and the immune response to P_2 protein. *Neurology*, **31**, 950–4.

Stevens, A., Schabet, M., Schott, K. & Wietholter, H. (1989). Role of endoneural cells in experimental allergic neuritis and characterisation of a resident phagocytic cell. *Acta Neuropathologica*, **77**, 412–19.

Stevens, A., Schabet, M., Wietholter, H. & Schott, K. (1990). Prednisolone therapy of experimental allergic neuritis in Lewis rats does not induce relapsing or chronic disease. *Journal of Neuroimmunology*, **28**, 141–51.

Stoll, G., Jander, S., Jung, S., Archelos, J.J., Tamatani, T., Miyasaka, M., Toyka, K.V. & Hartung, H.P. (1993*a*). Macrophages and endothelial cells express intercellular adhesion molecule-1 in immune-mediated demyelination but not in Wallerian degeneration of the rat peripheral nervous system. *Laboratory Investigation*, **68**, 637–44.

Stoll, G., Jung, S., Jander, S., van der Meide, P. & Hartung, H.P. (1993b). Tumor necrosis factor-α in immune-mediated demyelination and Wallerian degeneration of the rat peripheral nervous system. *Journal of Neuroimmunology*, **45**, 175–82.

Stoll, G., Schmidt, B., Jander, S., Toyka, K.V. & Hartung, H.P. (1991). Presence of the terminal complement complex (C5b–9) precedes myelin degradation in immune-mediated demyelination of the rat peripheral nervous system. *Annals of Neurology*, **30**, 147–155.

Strigård, K., Holmdahl, R., van der Meide, P.H., Klareskog, L. & Olsson, T. (1989*a*). *In vivo* treatment of rats with monoclonal antibodies against gamma interferon: effects on experimental allergic neuritis. *Acta Neurologica Scandinavica*, **80**, 201–7.

Strigård, K., Larsson, P., Holmdahl, R., Klareskog, L. & Olsson, T. (1989*b*). *In vivo* monoclonal antibody treatment with Ox19 (anti-rat CD5) causes disease relapse and terminates P_2-induced immunospecific tolerance in experimental allergic neuritis. *Journal of Neuroimmunology*, **23**, 11–18.

Strigård, K., Olsson, T., Larsson, P., Holmdahl, R., Hojeberg, B. & Klareskog, L. (1988*a*). Elimination of $CD8^+$ T cells *in vivo* does not break induced immunospecific tolerance to experimental allergic neuritis in rats. *Scandinavian Journal of Immunology*, **28**, 325–30.

Strigard, K., Olsson, T., Larsson, P., Holmdahl, R. & Klareskog, L. (1988*b*). Modulation of experimental allergic neuritis in rats by *in vivo* treatment with monoclonal anti T cell antibodies. *Journal of the Neurological Sciences*, **83**, 283–91.

Sumner, A.J., Saida, K., Saida, T., Silberberg, D.H. & Asbury, A.K. (1982). Acute conduction block asociated with experimental antiserum-mediated demyelination of peripheral nerve. *Annals of Neurology*, **11**, 469–77.

Suzumura, A., Sobue, G., Sugimura, K., Matsuoka, Y. & Sobue, I. (1985). Chronic experimental allergic neuritis (EAN) in juvenile guinea pigs: immunological comparison with acute EAN in adult guinea pigs. *Acta Neurologica Scandinavica*, **71**, 364–72.

Takeda, S., Ikuta, F. & Nagai, Y. (1980). Neuropathological comparative studies on experimental allergic neuritis (EAN) induced in rabbits by P2 protein-ganglioside complexes. *Japanese Journal of Experimental Medicine*, **50**, 453–62.

Tansey, F.A. & Brosnan, C.F. (1982). Protection against experimental allergic neuritis with silica quartz dust. *Journal of Neuroimmunology*, **3**, 169–79.

Taylor, W.A. & Hughes, R.A. (1985). Experimental allergic neuritis induced in SJL mice by bovine P_2. *Journal of Neuroimmunology*, **8**, 153–7.

Taylor, W.A. & Hughes, R.A. (1988). Responsiveness to P_2 of blood- and cauda equina-derived lymphocytes in experimental allergic neuritis in the Lewis rat: preliminary characterisation of a P2-specific cauda equina-derived T cell line. *Journal of Neuroimmunology*, **19**, 279–89.

Tsai, C.P., Pollard, J.D. & Armati, P.J. (1991). Interferon-γ inhibition suppresses experimental allergic neuritis: modulation of major histocompatibility complex expression of Schwann cells *in vitro*. *Journal of Neuroimmunology*, **31**, 133–45.

Tuck, R.R., Antony, J.H. & McLeod, J.G. (1982). F-wave in experimental allergic neuritis. *Journal of the Neurological Sciences*, **56**, 173–84.

Tuck, R.R., Pollard, J.D. & McLeod, J.G. (1981). Autonomic neuropathy in experimental allergic neuritis: an electrophysiological and histological study. *Brain*, **104**, 187–208.

Waksman, B.H. & Adams, R.D. (1955). Allergic neuritis: an experimental disease of rabbits induced by the injection of peripheral nervous tissue and adjuvants. *Journal of Experimental Medicine*, **102**, 213–35.

Waksman, B.H. & Adams, R.D. (1956). A comparative study of experimental allergic neuritis in the rabbit, guinea pig, and mouse. *Journal of Neuropathology and Experimental Neurology*, **15**, 293–332.

Watts, P.M., Taylor, W.A. & Hughes, R.A. (1989). High-dose methylprednisolone suppresses experimental allergic neuritis in the Lewis rat. *Experimental Neurology*, **103**, 101–4.

Wekerle, H., Schwab, M., Linington, C. & Meyermann, R. (1986). Antigen presentation in the peripheral nervous system: Schwann cells present endogenous myelin autoantigens to lymphocytes. *European Journal of Immunology*, **16**, 1551–7.

Wenk, E.J., Levine, S. & Wallquist, J. (1965). Allergic neuritis: a hyperacute from. *Federation Proceedings*, **24**, 242 (Abstract).

Wietholter, H., Hulser, P.J., Linington, C., Meier, D.H. & Wessel, K. (1988). Electrophysiological follow up of experimental allergic neuritis mediated by a permanent T cell line in rats. *Journal of the Neurological Sciences*, **83**, 1–14.

Wietholter, H., Schabet, M., Stevens, A., Melms, A., Sommer, N. & Weller, M. (1992). Influence of gangliosides on experimental allergic neuritis. *Journal of Neuroimmunology*, **38**, 221–8.

Williams, R.M. & Moore, M.J. (1973). Linkage of susceptibility to experimental allergic encephalomyelitis to the major histocompatibility locus in the rat. *Journal of Experimental Medicine*, **138**, 775–83.

Wisniewski, H.M. & Bloom, B.R. (1975). Primary demyelination as a nonspecific consequence of a cell-mediated immune reaction. *Journal of Experimental Medicine*, **141**, 346–59.

Wisniewski, H.M., Brostoff, S.W., Carter, H. & Eylar, E.H. (1974). Recurrent experimental allergic polyganglioradiculoneuritis. Multiple demyelinating episodes in rhesus monkey sensitized with rabbit sciatic nerve myelin. *Archives of Neurology*, **30**, 347–58.

Wood, J.G. & Dawson, R.M.C. (1974). Some properties of a major structural glycoprotein of sciatic nerve. *Journal of Neurochemistry*, **22**, 627–30.

Yamashita, T., Negishi, T., Nomura, K., Hosokawa, T., Ohno, R. & Hamaguchi, K. (1988). Changes in T-cell subsets in experimental allergic neuritis. *Annals of the New York Academy of Sciences*, **540**, 720–2.

Yonezawa, T., Ishihara, Y. & Matsuyama, H. (1968). Studies on experimental allergic peripheral neuritis. (I) Demyelinating patterns studied *in vitro*. *Journal of Neuropathology and Experimental Neurology*, **27**, 453–63.

Ziegler, D.W., Gardner, J.J., Warfield, D.T. & Walls, H.H. (1983). Experimental allergic neuritis-like disease in rabbits after injection with influenza vaccines mixed with gangliosides and adjuvants. *Infection and Immunology*, **42**, 824–30.

–8–

The Guillain–Barré syndrome and acute dysautonomia

PAMELA A. McCOMBE

The Guillain–Barré syndrome

Introduction

Guillain, Barré & Strohl (1916) described a syndrome of ascending weakness, associated with loss of deep tendon reflexes and early recovery, in two soldiers. During the same period, others reported rather similar patients with acute febrile polyneuritis and acute infective polyneuritis (Holmes, 1917; Bradford, Bashford & Wilson, 1918). Earlier, Landry (1859) had described a patient who died in respiratory failure after developing ascending weakness. As noted by Cosnett (1987), Wardrop (1834) had also reported a patient with an episode of weakness with spontaneous recovery. In 1949, Haymaker & Kernohan analysed the published reports and established the modern use of the term 'the Guillain–Barré syndrome' (GBS). Histories of the syndrome have been written by Horowitz (1989), Wiederholt, Mulder & Lambert (1964) and Asbury (1990). Guillain (1936) also reviewed the syndrome in 1936, 20 years after his original description. GBS is also known as acute inflammatory demyelinating polyradiculoneuropathy, which is a term that reflects the pathological features of the disease. There is increasing evidence that GBS is an autoimmune disease: some of this evidence comes from the finding of similarities between GBS and experimental autoimmune encephalomyelitis (EAN) (see Chapter 7).

Clinical features

Clinical symptoms and signs

Guillain (1936) described the clinical features of the GBS. These were ascending weakness, associated with hypotonia and loss of tendon reflexes.

The onset is sometimes associated with pain or paraesthesiae. GBS is more common in males than females. The most common presenting symptom is weakness of the lower limbs (Wiederholt *et al.*, 1964; McFarland & Heller, 1966). Sensory symptoms may occur and ataxia may be a dominant clinical finding (Sobue *et al.*, 1983). Cranial nerve involvement, particularly facial weakness, may occur. Papilloedema is a recognized finding in GBS: it was present in 10% of the patients in one series (Pleasure, Lovelace & Duvoisin, 1968). However, papilloedema was found in only 1% of the patients reported by Winer, Hughes and Osmond (1988*d*). Autonomic disturbance is not infrequent, with signs including hypertension, hypotension, cardiac arrhythmias, sweating and flushing (Lichtenfeld, 1971); it may be the cause of death in patients with GBS.

Clinical variants of GBS

In some instances, acute sensory loss and areflexia develop without associated weakness. Asbury (1981) suggested that such syndromes could be described as GBS if characterized by rapid onset and good recovery, and electrophysiological evidence of demyelination. Patients with such syndromes are clearly similar to patients with acute sensory neuronopathy (Sterman, Schaumberg & Asbury, 1980), which has some clinical features in common with GBS but does not appear to be a demyelinating disease. The Miller Fisher syndrome of ataxia, areflexia and ophthalmoplegia is regarded as a variant of GBS, although central nervous system (CNS) lesions may be present (Shuaib & Becker, 1987; Berlit & Rakicky, 1992). Pure polyneuritis cranialis, which may include facial weakness and bulbar palsies, may be a variant of GBS (Shuaib & Becker, 1987; Polo *et al.*, 1992). Furthermore, acute brachial neuritis, which is associated with pain and weakness and wasting of the muscles about the shoulder girdle, may be a focal variant of GBS. Some patients with GBS develop severe weakness and wasting and are thought to have 'axonal GBS' (Feasby *et al.*, 1986, 1993), although this has not been completely accepted as a separate entity (see below for further discussion).

Diagnosis

Guillain (1936) stated that the cardinal features of the syndrome were cytoalbuminological dissociation in the cerebrospinal fluid (CSF) and a good prognosis. The diagnostic criteria proposed by Asbury (1981) are widely accepted and include progressive weakness of more than one limb and areflexia, with other features such as cranial nerve and autonomic involvement, recovery and absence of other causes of the neurological signs. While elevation of the CSF protein level is usually found in the GBS, it may not be found in the early stages of disease. Neurophysiological studies providing evidence of demyelination are helpful in the diagnosis of GBS (McLeod, 1981).

Clinical course and risk of recurrence

The diagnostic criteria for GBS include the cessation of progression of weakness by four weeks after onset (Asbury, 1981). Recent studies of the clinical course of GBS are confounded by the treatments that may have influenced the course of disease. Guillain (1936) emphasized that patients with GBS usually recovered. However, before the use of artificial ventilation, patients with GBS that caused respiratory weakness frequently died. Gilpin, Moersch & Kernohan (1936) described 20 GBS patients. Of these, two died, and many of the others had prolonged weakness. In the study of Wiederholt *et al.* (1964), six of 97 patients died, 38 of 47 untreated patients had made a complete recovery within one year, and 42 of 47 untreated patients had made a complete recovery within two years. In a study of 81 patients (Pleasure *et al.*, 1968), four patients died of respiratory insufficiency and, of 49 patients followed for more than two years, eight had marked distal weakness. Winer *et al.* (1988*d*) studied 100 patients, of whom ten underwent plasmapheresis and 14 received steroids, and found that 13 had died and 19 were still disabled after one year. The most common cause of death was cardiac arrest. The reported frequency of recurrence of GBS varies. In earlier large series the risk of recurrence was about 10% (Wiederholt *et al.*, 1964; Pleasure *et al.*, 1968), but a more recent study found that at one year of follow-up 3% of patients had experienced recurrence (Winer *et al.*, 1988*d*).

Association with CNS disease

CNS involvement may sometimes occur in GBS, and GBS may sometimes occur in acute disseminated encephalomyelitis (see Chapter 5). In the series of Loffel *et al.* (1977), 10% of 123 patients had clinical signs such as pyramidal tract involvement, suggesting CNS abnormality. More recently, a patient has been described who developed optic neuritis and widespread magnetic resonance imaging abnormalities while recovering from GBS (Nadkarni & Lisak, 1993). In the series of McFarland & Heller (1966), 23 of 100 patients had personality changes such as anxiety. In the series of de Jager & Sluiter (1991) 13 of 60 patients had agitation and confusion. Such changes as anxiety, agitation and confusion may be an indirect response to the illness rather than a direct component of GBS.

Association with other autoimmune diseases

Autoimmune diseases may occur in families, and it has been suggested that the tendency to develop autoimmunity is inherited as an autosomal dominant trait (Bias *et al.*, 1986). If GBS is an autoimmune disease, it might be expected that patients with GBS or their relatives would have an increased incidence of other autoimmune diseases. In one study (Korn Lubetzki & Abramsky, 1986) some GBS patients were reported to have systemic lupus erythematosus, thyroid disease, ulcerative colitis or rheumatoid arthritis.

Triggering factors

Some patients with GBS report a preceding event that may have precipitated the GBS (Winer *et al.*, 1988*c*; de Jager & Sluiter, 1991). Guillain (1936) wrote that he was convinced the disease was of infectious origin. One study (Leneman, 1966) found that 735 of 1100 GBS patients had a possible precipitating cause, of which 638 were infections. In contrast, a study in Finland found that only 10% of patients had an identifiable preceding event (Farkkila, Kinnunen & Weckstrom, 1991). Controlled studies are required to determine whether the events that appear to precipitate GBS occur more frequently in the GBS population than in the normal population. Many of the preceding events are infections, although physical events such as surgery are also reported.

Preceding infections

In the series of 100 GBS patients described by Winer *et al.* (1988*c*), 38% had respiratory infections compared to 12% of controls, and 17% had gastrointestinal infections compared to 3% of controls. Serological evidence of infection was found in 31% of patients. In the series of 61 GBS patients described by de Jager & Sluiter (1991), 33 (54%) had a history of a preceding infection. The infections that are commonly reported to precede GBS include cytomegalovirus (Mozes *et al.*, 1984; Winer *et al.*, 1988*c*; Boucquey *et al.*, 1991), Epstein–Barr virus (Grose *et al.*, 1975; Glaser, Brennan & Berlin, 1979), *Campylobacter jejuni* (Kaldor & Speed, 1984; Winer *et al.*, 1988*c*; Gruenewald *et al.*, 1991) and *Mycoplasma pneumoniae* (Boucquey *et al.*, 1991) infections. Malaria (Wijesundere, 1992), hepatitis B (Feutren *et al.*, 1983), herpes zoster infection (Ormerod & Cockerell, 1993) and herpes simplex infection (Gerken *et al.*, 1985) have also been reported to precede development of GBS. Infections may trigger GBS because of cross-reactivity (molecular mimicry) between infectious agents and peripheral nerve antigens: in the case of *Campylobacter jejuni*, there is cross-reactivity between bacterial polysaccharides and gangliosides in myelin (Yuki *et al.*, 1993*b*; Aspinall *et al.*, 1994).

Vaccinations and antiserum treatment

Polyneuritis typical of GBS can occur as a complication of rabies vaccines prepared from animal brains, particularly those prepared from suckling mouse brains (Appelbaum, Greenberg & Nelson, 1953; Cabrera, Griffin & Johnson, 1987; Hemachudha *et al.*, 1987, 1988). An acute self-limited polyneuritis occurs as a rare complication of smallpox vaccination (Winkelman, 1949). Leneman (1966) found that eight of 1100 GBS cases occurred in association with smallpox vaccination. GBS was recorded in many patients who received the 1976 A/New Jersey swine influenza vaccine (Schonberger *et al.*, 1979; Keenlyside *et al.*, 1980). Subsequent influenza vaccination programmes have not been associated with an increased incidence of GBS (Hurwitz *et al.*, 1981). Vaccines may induce GBS because of molecular mimicry between vaccine antigens and myelin antigens.

Serum sickness results from the formation of circulating immune complexes, and was a common sequel of treatment with antiserum. Neurological complications of serum sickness, including peripheral neuropathy, were reported in the years when antiserum was used more regularly in treatment. While some patients with serum sickness had acute brachial neuritis, others had more widespread peripheral nerve involvement, with weakness, loss of reflexes and good recovery (Kennedy, 1929; Allen, 1931; Robertson & Varmus, 1944; Miller & Stanton, 1954).

Surgery

GBS is also reported after surgery (Arnason & Asbury, 1968). Many different types of operation have been reported before the onset of GBS. Some have included possible disturbance of the nervous system and others have included cardiothoracic surgery (Hogan, Briggs & Oldershaw, 1992; Baldwin, Pierce & Frazier, 1992).

Pregnancy

There have been reports of GBS commencing during pregnancy (McFarland & Heller, 1966; Ahlberg & Ahlmark, 1978; D'Ambrosio & De Angelis, 1985), but it is not clear whether the incidence of GBS during pregnancy is greater than would be expected in non-pregnant women. Another question is whether patients with an episode of GBS commencing during pregnancy will suffer a relapse of GBS with subsequent pregnancies. There have been reports of patients suffering a first episode of GBS in pregnancy and subsequent episodes with later pregnancies (Ungley, 1933; Novak & Johnson, 1973; Jones & Berry, 1981).

Drug or therapeutic agents

GBS has been reported after streptokinase treatment (Barnes & Hughes, 1992), and in one report the patients had circulating anti-streptokinase antibodies and oligoclonal bands in the CSF that reacted with streptokinase (Kaiser *et al.*, 1993). Because anti-ganglioside antibodies are found in the serum of GBS patients (see below), there has been concern that ganglioside therapy might predispose to GBS. Latov, Koski & Walicke (1991) and Landi *et al.* (1993) reported patients who developed GBS after ganglioside therapy. However, other studies have not found an association between ganglioside therapy and GBS (Granieri *et al.*, 1991; Diez Tejedor, Gutierrez Rivas & Gil Peralta, 1993). Ala, Perfettu & Frey (1994) have reported two patients who developed an immune response to the ganglioside GM1 after its intramuscular injection, but who did not develop neurological signs.

Genetics

Familial GBS

GBS has occasionally been reported to occur in families. Saunders and Rake (1965) reported two elderly siblings who developed the GBS. MacGregor (1965) and Korn-Lubetzki *et al.* (1994) have reported the development of GBS in father and daughter.

Genetic typing

One study of Mexican patients with the GBS found an association with HLA-DR3 (Gorodezky *et al.*, 1983). An association of GBS with HLA-A3 and -B8 has also been reported. However, other studies have found no HLA associations (Adams *et al.*, 1977; Stewart *et al.*, 1978; Latovitzki *et al.*, 1979; Kaslow *et al.*, 1984; Winer *et al.*, 1988*a*; Hillert, Osterman & Olerup, 1991). Immunoglobulin allotypes have been associated with the development of GBS; there is evidence of an association of GBS with the Gm haplotype 1,2,17;21 (Feeney *et al.*, 1989). Alpha-1 antitrypsin alleles may also be associated with GBS: there is an association of GBS and other demyelinating diseases with the Pi type M3 (McCombe *et al.*, 1985). Both the alpha-1 antitrypsin genes and the Gm markers are located on chromosome 14.

Neuropathology

Pathological findings

The most important pathological findings in GBS are inflammation and primary demyelination (Prineas, 1981). These are similar to the findings in acute EAN (see Chapter 7). Asbury, Arnason & Adams (1969) emphasized the importance of the inflammatory cells in the pathology of GBS. Later studies have concentrated on the mechanism of myelin removal, which is predominantly by the stripping of myelin by macrophages (Prineas, 1981). The pathology of GBS has been most studied in biopsies of the sural nerve, which is a distal sensory nerve. Such studies do not give information about motor fibres or the more proximal components of the peripheral nervous system (PNS). Nevertheless, much information about GBS has come from sural nerve biopsy. Prineas (1972) described the electron microscope findings in biopsies of patients with GBS and emphasized that active primary demyelination by macrophages was a prominent finding. Stripping of the myelin sheath and vesicular dissolution was carried out by macrophages in the presence of lymphocytes. A detailed electron microscope study of 65 biopsies also showed macrophage invasion and myelin stripping (Brechenmacher *et al.*, 1987). Recently, Hall *et al.* (1992) have studied a motor nerve biopsy from a patient with severe GBS: they found subperineurial oedema, macrophage infiltration and prominent primary demyelination.

Autopsy studies of GBS are uncommon. Haymaker & Kernohan (1949) described 50 fatal cases and found oedema of the nerves and loss of myelin. Asbury *et al.* (1969) reported 19 autopsied cases and emphasized the role of the inflammatory cells in producing damage. Carpenter (1972) emphasized the prevalence of demyelination and the lack of axonal damage. A recent study of nine patients confirmed the main findings of myelin loss and inflammation of the PNS (Honavar *et al.*, 1991).

Mechanism of demyelination

The main mechanism of myelin removal in GBS is the invasion of the Schwann cell basement membrane by macrophages that remove the myelin by stripping and phagocytosis (Prineas, 1972; Brechenmacher *et al.*, 1987; Honavar *et al.*, 1991). Vesicular dissolution has an honoured history as another mechanism of myelin damage, but may be an artefact of fixation. As discussed in the chapter on EAN (Chapter 7), Wisniewski & Bloom (1975) considered that demyelination and damage by macrophages could occur as a non-specific event. However, later studies have showed that demyelination of peripheral nerve requires specific sensitization to myelin antigens (Powell *et al.*, 1984). Another possibility is that the Schwann cell is the primary target of damage in GBS and that myelin is removed because the Schwann cell no longer supports the myelin. There is little evidence to support this hypothesis. In most studies the Schwann cells appear morphologically normal (Carpenter, 1972; Brechenmacher *et al.*, 1987), although one study found that there was increased peripheral nerve acid phosphatase and proteinase activity: this may have been produced by Schwann cells (Arstila *et al.*, 1971).

Axonal GBS

In most studies of GBS, primary demyelination is the major finding, although some axonal damage occurs, as in the study of Prineas (1972). Some patients, with clinical features resembling GBS, have been found to have significant axonal damage as well as primary demyelination (Vallat *et al.*, 1990). Other patients with a clinical course typical of GBS have predominantly axonal damage, with electrically inexcitable nerves. It has been suggested that such patients have an acute axonal form of GBS (Feasby *et al.*, 1986). In such patients, axonal damage may occur with little inflammation (Feasby *et al.*, 1993). However, the existence of pure axonal GBS has been disputed and the issue is controversial (Fuller *et al.*, 1992; Cros & Triggs, 1994). It seems probable that more severe forms of GBS are associated with significant axonal degeneration. It also seems probable that an axonal form of GBS may exist. Patients with GBS following *Campylobacter jejuni* infection have a high incidence of axonal degeneration (Rees *et al.*, 1993) and the Chinese patients with 'acute motor axonal neuropathy' reported by McKhann *et al.* (1993) may have an axonal form of GBS.

Pathophysiology

Neurophysiological studies demonstrate abnormalities in the majority of GBS patients, with abnormalities being more frequent in the later stages of disease (McLeod, 1981). In a study of 113 patients with GBS, the most common findings were proximal conduction block (27%), proximal conduction block associated with distal abnormalities (27%) and generalized slowing (22%) (Ropper, Wijdicks & Shahani, 1990). It is probable that conduction block, rather than slowing of conduction, is the main cause of weakness and other neurological signs. One study detected peripheral nerve conduction abnormalities in 33 of 44 motor nerves in 44 patients (Olney & Aminoff, 1990). Phrenic nerve conduction may be abnormal in GBS (Gourie-Devi & Ganapathy, 1985). Studies of proximal PNS conduction, which assess conduction across nerve roots, show abnormalities in patients with GBS, including some patients with normal distal conduction velocities

(Kimura & Butzer, 1975; King & Ashby, 1976; Kimura, 1978; Olney & Aminoff, 1990). This is consistent with the pathological findings that demyelination and inflammation predominate in the nerve roots. The finding of electrically inexcitable nerves may represent either severe demyelination with conduction failure or axonal degeneration (Triggs *et al.*, 1992; Brown, Feasby & Hahn, 1993; Cros & Triggs, 1994). Although the existence of a pure axonal GBS is controversial, patients with severe forms of GBS often have evidence of axonal degeneration and denervation of muscles. This appears to contribute significantly to weakness and slowness of recovery.

Immunopathology of PNS lesions

Characteristics of the inflammatory infiltrate

The majority of cells infiltrating the nerves in GBS are macrophages, although T cells can also be demonstrated in some biopsies. The failure to demonstrate T cells in all biopsied nerves probably relates to the stage of disease, as T cells are likely to infiltrate the nerves early in disease. Using immunofluorescent techniques and rabbit antisera, Nyland, Matre & Mork (1981) found occasional T cells in the nerves of five GBS patients. Pollard, Baverstock & McLeod (1987) found occasional $CD4^+$ and $CD8^+$ T cells and many macrophages in sural nerves from two GBS patients. Hughes *et al.* (1992) also found that, whereas all of ten GBS patients had increased macrophages, only two of ten patients had increased lymphocytes in biopsied nerve. Others have also found T lymphocytes in the peripheral nerves of some GBS patients (Schroder *et al.*, 1988; Cornblath *et al.*, 1990). Honavar *et al.* (1991) identified lymphocytes with immunocytochemistry in a number of autopsy cases.

MHC class II antigen expression

There is increased MHC class II antigen expression in peripheral nerves in GBS. Much of this antigen expression occurs on macrophages. Whether Schwann cells express MHC class II antigen *in vivo* has been the subject of much study. Pollard *et al.* (1987) found MHC class II antigen on infiltrating cells and Schwann cells in nerves from GBS patients. Other studies confirmed MHC class II expression by Schwann cells in GBS, but also found such expression in non-inflammatory neuropathies (Mancardi *et al.*, 1988; Schroder *et al.*, 1988). However, in a study of neuropathies other than GBS, Atkinson *et al.* (1993) found no MHC class II antigen expression on Schwann cells.

Antibody and complement deposition

Studies have found complement deposition in the nerves of some GBS nerve biopsies (Luijten & Baart de la Faille Kuyper, 1972; Nyland *et al.*, 1981; Koski *et al.*, 1987; Hays, Lee & Latov, 1988). Complement is usually deposited in the tissues as part of immune complexes. In some patients with GBS in association with hepatitis B infection, immune complex deposition in small blood vessels in peripheral nerve has been demonstrated (Tsukada *et al.*, 1987).

Immunological findings in the peripheral blood

Non-specific findings

Lisak *et al.* (1985) found that the ratio of $CD4^+/CD8^+$ cells is disturbed in GBS, being elevated in some patients and decreased in others. In a study of 100 patients, Winer *et al.* (1988*b*) found that the number of circulating $CD8^+$ lymphocytes was reduced in the first week of disease. The proportion of circulating T cells bearing activation markers was increased in GBS compared to controls (Taylor & Hughes, 1989). GBS sera also had elevated levels of the adhesion molecule E-selectin compared to controls (Hartung *et al.*, 1994). Increased levels of soluble interleukin-2 receptor and interleukin-2 have been found in the blood of subjects with GBS (Hartung *et al.*, 1990, 1991; Bansil *et al.*, 1991). Serum levels of tumour necrosis factor α are elevated in GBS (Sharief, McLean & Thompson, 1993). Serum levels of neopterin are also elevated in GBS, probably reflecting immune activation (Bansil *et al.*, 1992). Koski *et al.* (1987) found evidence of complement activation in all of 19 GBS patients, but no controls. Kamolvarin *et al.* (1991) found raised serum C3c complement levels in four patients with GBS. However, Winer *et al.* (1988*b*) found that serum C3 and C4 complement levels were normal in 100 patients with GBS. Frampton *et al.* (1988) demonstrated that GBS patients had significantly higher levels of serum anti-cardiolipin antibody than did normal controls, and that the levels of anti-cardiolipin antibody correlated with severity of GBS.

Specific T cell responses

Early studies of T lymphocytes from the peripheral blood of patients with GBS indicated the presence of T cells reactive with peripheral nerve antigens. Knowles *et al.* (1969) demonstrated that peripheral blood lymphocytes from patients with GBS, but not from normal controls or patients with other neuropathies, were stimulated to proliferate by culture with peripheral nerve antigen. Behan *et al.* (1972) used macrophage migration inhibition to demonstrate that peripheral blood lymphocytes from GBS patients but not controls with other neurological diseases were sensitized to peripheral nerve antigens. Later studies have measured responses of lymphocytes to purified myelin antigens. Luijten *et al.* (1984) found that peripheral blood lymphocytes from GBS patients, but not normal controls, proliferated in response to P_2 protein. Taylor, Brostoff & Hughes (1991) confirmed that peripheral blood lymphocytes from two of four patients with early GBS, but no normal controls, showed proliferation to P_2 protein. Burns *et al.* (1986) isolated P_2- reactive cell lines from the peripheral blood of four normals and one patient with GBS. Khalili-Shirazi *et al.* (1992) showed that peripheral blood lymphocytes responded to P_2 and to P_0. Further detailed studies are required to assess the significance of P_0- and P_2-specific T lymphocytes in the blood of GBS patients. The consistent findings of increased numbers of myelin-specific T cells in GBS patients would provide circumstantial evidence that such cells play a role in the disease.

Specific antibody responses

Antibodies to myelin and purified myelin proteins

Using immunofluorescence, Tse *et al.* (1971) demonstrated that the sera of four of six GBS patients contained anti-myelin antibodies that bound to normal nerve. With the same technique, McCombe, Pollard & McLeod (1988) found 12 of 68 GBS patients, but no normals, had circulating anti-myelin antibodies. Hughes *et al.* (1984) found complement- fixing anti-nerve antibodies in two of 17 GBS patients. In a larger study Winer *et al.* (1988*b*) found complement-fixing anti-nerve antibodies in 7% of GBS patients and 1% of controls. Koski and colleagues (Koski, Humphrey & Shin, 1985; Koski, 1990) found a higher incidence of complement-fixing anti-myelin antibodies in GBS sera and showed that the levels of antibody were highest early in disease (Koski *et al.*, 1986). Vedeler, Matre & Nyland (1988), using an ELISA technique, found serum anti-myelin antibodies in 59% of GBS patients and 8% of normal blood donors. Using ELISA, Cruz *et al.* (1988) found serum anti-myelin antibodies in four of 14 (28%) GBS patients and 16% of blood donors. Other studies have investigated the presence in GBS sera of antibodies to purified myelin proteins. Quarles, Ilyas & Willison (1990) and Khalili Shirazi *et al.* (1993) found that some GBS patients had antibodies to P_2 and P_0. Other studies found little evidence of antibody to P_2 protein (Zweiman *et al.*, 1983; Winer *et al.*, 1988*b*). Lymphocytes from the peripheral blood of GBS patients include cells that secrete antibody to P_2 protein (Luijten *et al.*, 1984). Taken together, these studies suggest that only some GBS patients have evidence of circulating antibodies to myelin and its proteins.

Antibody to gangliosides and other glycolipids

Gangliosides are sialic-acid-containing glycosphingolipids, which are found in cell membranes and particularly in myelin. The gangliosides are named according to the number of sialic acid residues and the number of neutral sugar residues. The different gangliosides contain similar sugar residues and are structurally related, so that antibody directed against one ganglioside may react with a related ganglioside. Other non-sialic-acid-containing glycolipids, such as the sulphated glycolipids, are also found in myelin. The glycolipids contain antigenic determinants that are also found in the major myelin glycoproteins, which can also lead to cross-reactivity of antibodies against glycolipids and glycoproteins. Ilyas *et al.* (1988) found antibodies to gangliosides in five of 26 patients with GBS. These antibodies reacted with sialosyl paragloboside, GD1a, GD1b and GT1b gangliosides. Other studies have found that patients with GBS have antibodies to GM1 (Ilyas *et al.*, 1992; van den Berg *et al.*, 1992; Simone *et al.*, 1993; Willison & Kennedy, 1993). In GBS, antibodies to GM1 are found in patients with axonal damage and a poor prognosis (Kornberg *et al.*, 1994) and may identify patients with prior *Campylobacter* infection (Walsh *et al.*, 1991). Severe axonal GBS has also been associated with antibodies to GD1 (Yuki *et al.*, 1992). With immunostaining, GD1 has been demonstrated in dorsal root ganglia, sympathetic ganglia and paranodal regions of peripheral myelin (Kusunoki *et al.*, 1993). The Miller Fisher syndrome is associated with antibodies to the ganglioside GQ1b (Chiba *et al.*, 1992; Willison *et al.*, 1993; Yuki *et al.*, 1993*a*). Patients with ophthalmoplegia in association with typical GBS also have antibodies to GQ1b, while GBS patients without ophthalmoplegia do not have such antibodies (Chiba *et al.*, 1993). The antibody to GQ1b found in Miller Fisher syndrome also reacts with GT1a (Chiba *et al.*, 1993). The antibodies found in Miller Fisher syndrome may be biologically important, because, using a mouse phrenic-nerve diaphragm preparation, Roberts *et al.* (1994) found that serum from patients with Miller Fisher syndrome could block neurotransmitter release evoked by nerve stimulation (Roberts *et al.*, 1994). Willison and Veitch (1994) have analysed the IgG subclasses of anti-GQ1b antibodies in Miller Fisher patients and anti-GM1 antibodies in GBS patients: they found the antibodies to be of the IgG1 and IgG3 subclasses. They argued that such a pattern of responsiveness probably resulted from an immune response directed against a glycoprotein rather than against a glycolipid. They therefore suggested that the anti-ganglioside antibodies in

GBS and Miller Fisher syndrome result from cross-reactivity with a glycolipid target. Antibodies to sulphated glycolipids have also been found in GBS (Ilyas *et al.*, 1991; van den Berg *et al.*, 1993). Such antibodies are important, because these glycoplipids share antigenic determinants with myelin glycoproteins such as myelin-associated glycoprotein.

Antibodies to galactocerebroside can cause experimental demyelination (see Chapter 7), but do not appear to play a role in GBS. Rostami *et al.* (1987) found no elevations in anti-galactocerebroside antibody in GBS patients. Using a complement fixation assay, Winer *et al.* (1988*b*) found no evidence of anti-galactocerebroside antibodies in GBS sera, although they did find increased antibody responses to galactocerebroside with enzyme-linked assays.

Toxic and demyelinating factors in serum

Sera from GBS patients contain agents that are cytotoxic to rat Schwann cells (Sawant-Mane, Estep & Koski, 1994) and cause myelin destruction in tissue culture (Mithen *et al.*, 1992). Some GBS sera cause local demyelination, greater than that produced by control sera, when injected into rat sciatic nerve (Feasby, Hahn & Gilbert, 1982; Saida *et al.*, 1982; Harrison *et al.*, 1984). Other studies have found that GBS sera do not cause significant demyelination after intraneural injection (Low *et al.*, 1982; Winer *et al.*, 1988*b*; Oomes *et al.*, 1991). Roberts *et al.* (1994) have shown that serum from patients with the Miller Fisher syndrome, but not from normal controls or patients with other neurological diseases, blocks phrenic nerve conduction *in vitro* after local application.

Immunological findings in the CSF

The original description by Guillain, Barré and Strohl (1916) noted that the CSF albumin levels were elevated but that the cell count was not increased. Subsequent studies have confirmed that CSF protein levels are elevated in GBS. Much of the increased protein is due to entry from the blood, which is demonstrated by elevated CSF albumin and immunoglobulin levels. Detailed studies show that much of the antibody in the CSF is produced in the extrathecal compartment, although some intrathecal antibody production may also occur (Ryberg, 1984; Vedeler, Matre & Nyland, 1986). A factor present in the CSF of GBS patients can block Na^+ channels (Brinkmeier *et al.*, 1992). Activated complement components have been demonstrated in the CSF of GBS patients by Hartung *et al.* (1987).

Therapy

Corticosteroids

Early uncontrolled trials indicated that corticosteroids may lessen the duration of GBS (Jackson, Miller & Schapira, 1957). However, in a double-blind controlled trial, Hughes *et al.* (1978) found that treatment with oral prednisolone 60 mg/day did not shorten the duration of GBS, and was associated with more relapses than placebo treatment. A trial of high-dose intravenous methylprednisolone also failed to show any benefit (Guillain–Barré syndrome Steroid Trial Group, 1993).

Plasmapheresis

Some early reports of the benefit of plasma exchange in GBS (Valbonesi *et al.*, 1981) were followed by major controlled trials of this form of treatment. The GBS study group showed that plasma exchange was effective therapy when commenced within seven days of onset (The Guillain–Barré Syndrome Study Group, 1985). A large French study also showed that plasmapheresis was beneficial (French Cooperative Group on Plasma Exchange in Guillain–Barré syndrome, 1987, 1992) and that the benefit was equivalent in patients given albumin or fresh frozen plasma as replacement fluid. Relapses of GBS may occur if the course of plasmapheresis is too short (Osterman *et al.*, 1988).

Intravenous immunoglobulin

Treatment of GBS with high-dose intravenous immunoglobulin was attempted following the demonstration that plasmapheresis was successful. Two studies reported that high-dose intravenous immunoglobulin therapy was beneficial in GBS (van der Meche & Meulstee, 1988; Jackson, Godwin Austen & Whiteley, 1993). Another larger trial demonstrated that it was as effective as plasmapheresis in GBS (van der Meche & Schmitz, 1992). However, this study was criticized by Raphael *et al.* (1992), and others have found immunoglobulin therapy to be of less benefit (Castro & Ropper, 1993). One study found that more relapses occurred after immunoglobulin treatment than after plasmapheresis or no treatment (Irani *et al.*, 1993). Intravenous immunoglobulin therapy is likely to contain anti-idiotype antibodies that downregulate the immunological events in GBS, but may also modulate the activity of lymphocytes and adsorb complement (Hall, 1993; Thornton & Griggs, 1994).

Acute dysautonomia and experimental autonomic neuropathy

Acute dysautonomia

Autonomic dysfunction can occur as part of the GBS. It can also occur as an isolated clinical syndrome. Early descriptions of such a syndrome were given by Young *et al.* (1969) and Thomashefsky, Horwitz and Feingold (1972). Many more cases have been described (Hart & Kanter, 1990) and the syndrome can now be subdivided into acute cholinergic dysautonomia and acute pandysautonomia. In the syndrome of pandysautonomia described by Young *et al.* (1969), the patients had 'lethargy, decreased endurance, postural fainting, difficulty with vision, decreased potency, urinary difficulty, obstipation, and decrease of tears, saliva and sweat'. Appenzeller and Kornfeld (1973) described similar features. Adie's syndrome of tonic pupils and areflexia, which is an acquired and persistent disorder, might be a combined sensory and autonomic disturbance of similar aetiology (Adie, 1932; Rubenstein *et al.*, 1980). Acquired acute pandysautonomia has sometimes followed viral infections (Neville & Sladen, 1984), and has occurred in patients with autoimmune diseases (Gudesblatt *et al.*, 1985), and in association with malignancy. Acute cholinergic dysautonomia has been reported in a patient with low serum complement and anti-nuclear antibodies suggestive of an autoimmune process (Takayama *et al.*, 1987). In patients with acute pandysautonomia, sural nerve biopsies have been reported as showing axonal degeneration (Feldman *et al.*, 1991) or selective loss of small myelinated and unmyelinated fibres (Low *et al.*, 1983). In a man who had recovered from acute dysautonomia, there was an increase in the number of small unmyelinated nerve fibres, consistent with regeneration of these fibres (Appenzeller & Kornfeld, 1973).

The production of an animal model of acute autonomic neuropathy (see below) provides support for the concept that such neuropathies may have an immune pathogenesis. There are no detailed studies of the immunology of acute dysautonomia. However, a disorder confined to the autonomic nerves might occur after immune attack on antigens restricted to these nerves. The appearance of autonomic neuropathy with sensory neuropathy might suggest an immune attack on targets derived from neural crest tissue.

Experimental autonomic neuropathy

An animal model of experimental autonomic neuropathy (EAUN) can be produced by inoculation of rabbits with extracts of human sympathetic ganglia (Becker, Livett & Appenzeller, 1979). This model was first reported by Appenzeller, Arnason & Adams in 1965 and was produced before the first description by Young *et al.* (1969) of acute pandysautonomia in humans. In the rabbits inoculated with sympathetic ganglia, a deficiency in reflex vasodilatation was apparent within 6–14 days after inoculation and had disappeared when retesting was performed two months after inoculation (Appenzeller *et al.*, 1965; Becker *et al.*, 1979). Examination of the paravertebral ganglia from rabbits with EAUN revealed infiltration with lymphocytes and macrophages (Becker *et al.*, 1979). No active destruction of myelinated or unmyelinated fibres could be seen, but there was a reduction in the numbers of unmyelinated fibres during disease and evidence of regenerating fibres after recovery.

Conclusions

GBS is a dramatic illness that is now more readily treated and less likely to cause death than in previous years. There is evidence of immune activation in GBS and considerable support for the concept that GBS may be an autoimmune disease, possibly triggered by external factors such as infections or vaccinations. The cardinal pathological findings in GBS are inflammation and primary demyelination, although it is increasingly recognized that axonal degeneration may occur in GBS. There are important clinical variants of GBS such as the Miller Fisher syndrome; acute dysautonomia may be another variant of GBS. The primary target antigen in GBS is not known, and future studies are needed to determine whether there is a single important target or whether many different PNS antigens can be involved in the pathogenesis of GBS. It is also not clear whether there are several subgroups of GBS with possibly different pathogenic mechanisms. The response of GBS to plasmapheresis suggests that humoral factors are important in GBS, but analogy with experimental autoimmune neuritis suggests that T cells are also likely to be important.

References

Adams, D., Gibson, J.D., Thomas, P.K., Batchelor, J.R., Hughes, R.A., Kennedy, L., Festenstein, H. & Sachs, J. (1977). HLA antigens in Guillain–Barré syndrome. *Lancet*, **2**, 504–5.

Adie, W.J. (1932). Tonic pupils and absent tendon reflexes: a benign disorder sui generis; its complete and incomplete forms. *Brain*, **98**, 113.

Ahlberg, G. & Ahlmark, G. (1978). The Landry–Guillain–Barré syndrome and pregnancy. *Acta Obstetricia Gynecologica Scandinavica*, **57**, 377–80.

Ala, T.A., Perfettu, P.A. & Frey, W.H. (1994). Two cases of acute anti-GM1 antibody elevations in response to exogenous GM1 without neurological symptoms. *Journal of Neuroimmunology*, **53**, 109–13.

Allen, I.M. (1931). The neurological complications of serum treatment. With report of a case. *Lancet*, **2**, 1128–31.

Appelbaum, E., Greenberg, M. & Nelson, J. (1953). Neurological complications following antirabies vaccination. *Journal of the American Medical Association*, **151**, 188–91.

Appenzeller, O., Arnason, B.G. & Adams, R.D. (1965). Experimental autonomic neuropathy: an immunologically induced disorder of reflex vasomotor function. *Journal of Neurology, Neurosurgery and Psychiatry*, **28**, 510–15.

Appenzeller, O. & Kornfeld, M. (1973). Acute pandysautonomia. Clinical and morphological study. *Archives of Neurology*, **29**, 334–9.

Arnason, B.G. & Asbury, A.K. (1968). Idiopathic polyneuritis after surgery. *Archives of Neurology*, **18**, 500–7.

Arstila, A.U., Reikkinen, P.J., Rinne, U.K., Pelliniemi, T.T. & Nevalainen, T. (1971). Guillain–Barré syndrome. Neurochemical and ultrastructural study. *European Neurology*, **5**, 257–69.

Asbury, A.K. (1981). Diagnostic considerations in Guillain–Barré syndrome. *Annals of Neurology*, **9 (Supplement)**, 1–5.

Asbury, A.K. (1990). Guillain–Barré syndrome: historical aspects. *Annals of Neurology*, **27 (Supplement)**, S2–S6.

Asbury, A.K., Arnason, B.G. & Adams, R.D. (1969). The inflammatory lesion in idiopathic polyneuritis. Its role in pathogenesis. *Medicine*, **48**, 173–215.

Aspinall, G.O., McDonald, A.G., Pang, H., Kurjanczyk, L.A. & Penner, J.L. (1994). Lipopolysaccharides of *Campylobacter jejuni* serotype O:19: structures of core oligosaccharide regions from the serostrain and two bacterial isolates from patients with the Guillain–Barré syndrome. *Biochemistry*, **33**, 241–9.

Atkinson, P.F., Perry, M.E., Hall, S.M. & Hughes, R.A.C. (1993). Immunoelectronmicroscopical demonstration of major histocompatibility class II antigen: expression on endothelial and perivascular cells but not Schwann cells in human neuropathy. *Neuropathology and Applied Neurobiology*, **19**, 22–30.

Baldwin, R.T., Pierce, R.R. & Frazier, O.H. (1992). Guillain–Barré syndrome after heart transplantation. *Journal of Heart and Lung Transplantation*, **41**, 817–19.

Bansil, S., Mithen, F.A., Cook, S.D., Sheffet, A. & Rohowsky Kochan, C. (1991). Clinical correlation with serum-soluble interleukin-2 receptor levels in Guillain–Barré syndrome. *Neurology*, **41**, 1302–5.

Bansil, S., Mithen, F.A., Singhal, B.S., Cook, S.D. & Rohowsky Kochan, C. (1992). Elevated neopterin levels in Guillain–Barré syndrome. Further evidence of immune activation. *Archives of Neurology*, **49**, 1277–80.

Barnes, D. & Hughes, R.A. (1992). Guillain–Barré syndrome after treatment with streptokinase. *British Medical Journal*, **304**, 1225.

Becker, W., Livett, B.G. & Appenzeller, O. (1979). Experimental autonomic neuropathy: ultrastructure and immunohistochemical study of a disorder of reflex vasomotor function. *Journal of the Autonomic Nervous System*, **1**, 53–67.

Behan, P.O., Behan, W.M.H., Feldman, R.G. & Kies, M.W. (1972). Cell-mediated hypersensitivity to neural antigens. Occurrence in human patients and nonhuman primates with neurological diseases. *Archives of Neurology*, **27**, 145–52.

Berlit, P. & Rakicky, J. (1992). The Miller Fisher syndrome. Review of the literature. *Journal of Clinical Neuro-ophthalmology*, **12**, 57–63.

Bias, W.B., Reveille, J.D., Beaty, T.H., Meyers, D.A. & Arnett, F.C. (1986). Evidence that autoimmunity in man is a mendelian dominant trait. *American Journal of Human Genetics*, **39**, 584–602.

Boucquey, D., Sindic, C.J., Lamy, M., Delmee, M., Tomasi, J.P. & Laterre, E.C. (1991). Clinical and serological studies in a series of 45 patients with Guillain–Barré syndrome. *Journal of the Neurological Sciences*, **104**, 56–63.

Bradford, J.R., Bashford, E.F. & Wilson, J.A. (1918). Acute infective polyneuritis. *Quarterly Journal of Medicine*, **12**, 88–103.

Brechenmacher, C., Vital, C., Deminiere, C., Laurentjoye, L., Castaing, Y., Gbikpi Benissan, G., Cardinaud, J.P. & Favarel Garrigues, J.P. (1987). Guillain–Barré syndrome: an ultrastructural study of peripheral nerve in 65 patients. *Clinical Neuropathology*, **6**, 19–24.

Brinkmeier, H., Wollinsky, K.H., Hulser, P.J., Seewald, M.J., Mehrkens, H.H., Kornhuber, H.H. & Rudel, R. (1992). The acute paralysis in Guillain–Barré syndrome is related to a Na^+ channel blocking factor in the cerebrospinal fluid. *Pflugers Archiv European Journal of Physiology*, **421**, 552–7.

Brown, W.F., Feasby, T.E. & Hahn, A.F. (1993). Electrophysiological changes in the acute 'axonal' form of Guillain–Barré syndrome. *Muscle and Nerve*, **16**, 200–5.

Burns, J., Krasner, L.J., Rostami, A. & Pleasure, D. (1986). Isolation of P_2 protein-reactive T-cell lines from human blood. *Annals of Neurology*, **19**, 391–3.

Cabrera, J., Griffin, D.E. & Johnson, R.T. (1987). Unusual features of the Guillain–Barré syndrome after rabies vaccine prepared in suckling mouse brain. *Journal of the Neurological Sciences*, **81**, 239–45.

Carpenter, S. (1972). An ultrastructural study of an acute fatal case of the Guillain–Barré syndrome. *Journal of the Neurological Sciences*, **15**, 125–40.

Castro, L.H. & Ropper, A.H. (1993). Human immune globulin infusion in Guillain–Barré syndrome: worsening during and after treatment. *Neurology*, **43**, 1034–6.

Chiba, A., Kusunoki, S., Obata, H., Machinami, R. & Kanazawa, I. (1993). Serum anti-GQ1b IgG antibody is associated with ophthalmoplegia in Miller Fisher syndrome and Guillain–Barré syndrome: clinical and immunohistochemical studies. *Neurology*, **43**, 1911–17.

Chiba, A., Kusunoki, S., Shimizu, T. & Kanazawa, I. (1992). Serum IgG antibody to ganglioside GQ1b is a possible marker of Miller Fisher syndrome. *Annals of Neurology*, **31**, 677–9.

Cornblath, D.R., Griffin, D.E., Welch, D., Griffin, J.W. & McArthur, J.C. (1990). Quantitative analysis of endoneurial T-cells in human sural nerve biopsies. *Journal of Neuroimmunology*, **26**, 113–18.

Cosnett, J.E. (1987). Wardrop–Landry–Guillain–Barré–Strohl. *Lancet*, **1**, 861–2.

Cros, D. & Triggs, W.J. (1994). There are no neurophysiologic features characteristic of 'axonal' Guillain– Barré syndrome. *Muscle and Nerve*, **17**, 675–7.

Cruz, M., Ernerudh, J., Olsson, T., Hojeberg, B. & Link, H. (1988). Occurrence and isotype of antibodies against peripheral nerve myelin in serum from patients with peripheral neuropathy and healthy controls. *Journal of Neurology, Neurosurgery and Psychiatry*, **51**, 820–5.

D'Ambrosio, G. & De Angelis, G. (1985). Syndrome de Guillain–Barré au cours de la grossesse. *Revue Neurologique*, **141**, 33–7.

de Jager, A.E. & Sluiter, H.J. (1991). Clinical signs in severe Guillain–Barré syndrome: analysis of 63 patients. *Journal of the Neurological Sciences*, **104**, 143–50.

Diez Tejedor, E., Gutierrez Rivas, E. & Gil Peralta, A. (1993). Gangliosides and Guillain–Barré syndrome: the Spanish data. *Neuroepidemiology*, **12**, 251–6.

Farkkila, M., Kinnunen, E. & Weckstrom, P. (1991). Survey of Guillain–Barré syndrome in southern Finland. *Neuroepidemiology*, **10**, 236–41.

Feasby, T.E., Gilbert, J.J., Brown, W.F., Bolton, C.F., Hahn, A.F., Koopman, W.F. & Zochodne, D.W. (1986). An acute axonal form of Guillain–Barré polyneuropathy. *Brain*, **109**, 1115–26.

Feasby, T.E., Hahn, A.F., Brown, W.F., Bolton, C.F., Gilbert, J.J. & Koopman, W.J. (1993). Severe axonal degeneration in acute Guillain–Barré syndrome: evidence of two different mechanisms? *Journal of the Neurological Sciences*, **116**, 185–92.

Feasby, T.E., Hahn, A.F. & Gilbert, J.J. (1982). Passive transfer studies in Guillain–Barré polyneuropathy. *Neurology*, **32**, 1159–67.

Feeney, D.J., Pollard, J.D., McLeod, J.G., Stewart, G.J. & De Lange, G.G. (1989). Gm haplotypes in inflammatory demyelinating polyneuropathies. *Annals of Neurology*, **26**, 790–2.

Feldman, E.L., Bromberg, M.B., Blaivas, M. & Junck, L. (1991). Acute pandysautonomic neuropathy. *Neurology*, **41**, 746–8.

Feutren, G., Gerbal, J.L., Allinquant, B. & Schuller, E. (1983). Association of Guillain–Barré syndrome and B-virus hepatitis: simultaneous presence of anti-DS-DNA antibodies and HBs antigen in cerebrospinal-fluid. *Journal of Clinical and Laboratory Immunology*, **11**, 161–4.

Frampton, G., Winer, J.B., Cameron, J.S. & Hughes, R.A. (1988). Severe Guillain–Barré syndrome: an association with IgA anti-cardiolipin antibody in a series of 92 patients. *Journal of Neuroimmunology*, **19**, 133–9.

French Cooperative Group on Plasma Exchange in Guillain–Barré syndrome (1987). Efficiency of plasma exchange in Guillain–Barré syndrome: role of replacement fluids. *Annals of Neurology*, **22**, 753–61.

French Cooperative Group on Plasma Exchange in Guillain–Barré syndrome (1992). Plasma exchange in Guillain–Barré syndrome: one-year follow-up. *Annals of Neurology*, **32**, 94–7.

Fuller, G.N., Jacobs, J.M., Lewis, P.D. & Lane, R.J. (1992). Pseudoaxonal Guillain–Barré syndrome: severe demyelination mimicking axonopathy. A case with pupillary involvement. *Journal of Neurology, Neurosurgery and Psychiatry*, **55**, 1079–83.

Gerken, G., Trautmann, F., Kohler, H., Falke, D., Bohl, J., Nix, W. & Meyer zum Buschenfelde, K.H. (1985). Rare association of herpes simplex virus IgM-specific antibodies and Guillain–Barré syndrome successfully treated with plasma exchange and immunosuppression. *Klinische Wochenschrift*, **63**, 468–74.

Gilpin, S.F., Moersch, F.P. & Kernohan, J.W. (1936). Polyneuritis. A clinical and pathological study of a special group of cases frequently referred to as instances of neuronitis. *Archives of Neurology and Psychiatry*, **35**, 937–63.

Glaser, R., Brennan, R. & Berlin, C.M. (1979). Guillain–Barré syndrome associated with Epstein-Barr virus in a cytomegalovirus-negative patient. *Developmental Medicine and Child Neurology*, **21**, 787–90.

Gorodezky, C., Varela, B., Castro Escobar, L.E., Chavez Negrete, A., Escobar Gutierrez, A. & Martinez Mata, J. (1983). HLA-DR antigens in Mexican patients with Guillain–Barré syndrome. *Journal of Neuroimmunology*, **4**, 1–7.

Gourie-Devi, M. & Ganapathy, G.R. (1985). Phrenic nerve conduction time in Guillain–Barré syndrome. *Journal of Neurology, Neurosurgery and Psychiatry*, **48**, 245–9.

Granieri, E., Casetta, I., Govoni, V., Tola, M.R., Paolino, E. & Rocca, W.A. (1991). Ganglioside therapy and Guillain–Barré syndrome. A historical cohort study in Ferrara, Italy, fails to demonstrate an association. *Neuroepidemiology*, **10**, 161–9.

Grose, C., Henle, W., Henle, G. & Feorino, P.M. (1975). Primary Epstein–Barr-virus infections in acute neurologic diseases. *New England Journal of Medicine*, **292**, 392–5.

Gruenewald, R., Ropper, A.H., Lior, H., Chan, J., Lee, R. & Molinaro, V.S. (1991). Serologic evidence of *Campylobacter jejuni/coli* enteritis in patients with Guillain–Barré syndrome. *Archives of Neurology*, **48**, 1080–2.

Gudesblatt, M., Goodman, A.D., Rubenstein, A.E., Bender, A.N. & Choi, H.S. (1985). Autonomic neuropathy associated with autoimmune disease. *Neurology*, **35**, 261–4.

Guillain, G. (1936). Radiculoneuritis with acellular hyperalbuminosis of the cerebrospinal fluid. *Archives of Neurology and Psychiatry*, **36**, 975–90.

Guillain, G., Barré, J.A. & Strohl, A. (1916). Sur un syndrome de radiculonévrite avec hyperalbuminose du liquide cephalo-rachidien sans reaction cellulaire. Remarques sur les caractères cliniques et graphiques des réflexes tendineux. *Bulletin de la Société Médicale des Hôpitaux de Paris*, **40**, 1462–70.

Guillain–Barré syndrome Steroid Trial Group (1993). Double-blind trial of intravenous methylprednisolone in Guillain–Barré syndrome. *Lancet*, **341**, 586–90.

Hall, P.D. (1993). Immunomodulation with intravenous immunoglobulin. *Pharmacotherapy*, **13**, 564–73.

Hall, S.M., Hughes, R.A., Atkinson, P.F., McColl, I. & Gale, A. (1992). Motor nerve biopsy in severe Guillain–Barré syndrome. *Annals of Neurology*, **31**, 441–4.

Harrison, B.M., Hansen, L.A., Pollard, J.D. & McLeod, J.G. (1984). Demyelination induced by serum from patients with Guillain–Barré syndrome. *Annals of Neurology*, **15**, 163–70.

Hart, R.G. & Kanter, M.C. (1990). Acute autonomic neuropathy. Two cases and a clinical review. *Archives of Internal Medicine*, **150**, 2373–6.

Hartung, H.P., Hughes, R.A., Taylor, W.A., Heininger, K., Reiners, K. & Toyka, K.V. (1990). T cell activation in Guillain–Barré syndrome and in MS: elevated serum levels of soluble IL-2 receptors. *Neurology*, **40**, 215–18.

Hartung, H.P., Reiners, K., Michels, M., Hughes, R.A.C., Heidenreich, F., Zielasek, J., Enders, U. & Toyka, K.V. (1994). Serum levels of soluble E-selectin (ELAM-1) in immune-mediated neuropathies. *Neurology*, **44**, 1153–8.

Hartung, H.P., Reiners, K., Schmidt, B., Stoll, G. & Toyka, K.V. (1991). Serum interleukin-2 concentrations in Guillain–Barré syndrome and chronic idiopathic demyelinating polyradiculoneuropathy: comparison with other neurological diseases of presumed immunopathogenesis. *Annals of Neurology*, **30**, 48–53.

Hartung, H.P., Schwenke, C., Bitter Suermann, D. & Toyka, K.V. (1987). Guillain–Barré syndrome: activated complement components C3a and C5a in CSF. *Neurology*, **37**, 1006–9.

Haymaker, W. & Kernohan, J.W. (1949). The Landry–Guillain–Barré syndrome. A clinicopathological report of fifty fatal cases and a critique of the literature. *Medicine*, **28**, 59–141.

Hays, A.P., Lee, S.S.L. & Latov, N. (1988). Immune reactive C3d on the surface of myelin sheaths in neuropathy. *Journal of Neuroimmunology*, **18**, 231–44.

Hemachudha, T., Griffin, D.E., Chen, W.W. & Johnson, R.T. (1988). Immunologic studies of rabies vaccination-induced Guillain–Barré syndrome. *Neurology*, **38**, 375–8.

Hemachudha, T., Phanuphak, P., Johnson, R.T., Griffin, D.E., Ratanavongsiri, J. & Siriprasomsup, W. (1987). Neurological complications of Semple-type rabies vaccine: clinical and immunological studies. *Neurology*, **37**, 550–6.

Hillert, J., Osterman, P.O. & Olerup, O. (1991). No association with HLA-DR, -DQ or -DP alleles in Guillain–Barré syndrome. *Journal of Neuroimmunology*, **31**, 67–72.

Hogan, J.C., Briggs, T.P. & Oldershaw, P.J. (1992). Guillain–Barré syndrome following cardiopulmonary bypass. *International Journal of Cardiology*, **35**, 427–8.

Holmes, G. (1917). Acute febrile polyneuritis. *British Medical Journal*, **2**, 37–9.

Honavar, M., Tharakan, J.K., Hughes, R.A., Leibowitz, S. & Winer, J.B. (1991). A clinicopathological study of the Guillain–Barré syndrome. Nine cases and literature review. *Brain*, **114**, 1245–69.

Horowitz, S.H. (1989). The idiopathic polyradiculoneuropathies: a historical guide to an understanding of the clinical syndromes. *Acta Neurologica Scandinavica*, **80**, 369–86.

Hughes, R., Atkinson, P., Coates, P., Hall, S. & Leibowitz, S. (1992). Sural nerve biopsies in Guillain–Barré syndrome: axonal degeneration and macrophage-associated demyelination and absence of cytomegalovirus genome. *Muscle and Nerve*, **15**, 568–75.

Hughes, R.A., Gray, I.A., Gregson, N.A., Kadlubowski, M., Kennedy, M., Leibowitz, S. & Thompson, H. (1984). Immune responses to myelin antigens in Guillain–Barré syndrome. *Journal of Neuroimmunology*, **6**, 303–12.

Hughes, R.A.C., Newsom Davis, J., Perkin, G.D. & Pierce, J.M. (1978). Controlled trial of prednisolone in acute polyneuropathy. *Lancet*, **2**, 750–3.

Hurwitz, E.S., Schonberger, L.B., Nelson, D.B. & Holman, R.C. (1981). Guillain–Barré syndrome and the 1978–1979 influenza vaccine. *New England Journal of Medicine*, **304**, 1557–61.

Ilyas, A.A., Mithen, F.A., Chen, Z.W. & Cook, S.D. (1992). Anti-GM1 IgA antibodies in Guillain–Barré syndrome. *Journal of Neuroimmunology*, **36**, 69–76.

Ilyas, A.A., Mithen, F.A., Dalakas, M.C., Wargo, M., Chen, Z.W., Bielory, L. & Cook, S.D. (1991). Antibodies to sulfated glycolipids in Guillain–Barré syndrome. *Journal of the Neurological Sciences*, **105**, 108–17.

Ilyas, A.A., Willison, H.J., Quarles, R.H., Jungalwala, F.B., Cornblath, D.R., Trapp, B.D., Griffin, D.E., Griffin, J.W. & McKhann, G.M. (1988). Serum antibodies to gangliosides in Guillain–Barré syndrome. *Annals of Neurology*, **23**, 440–7.

Irani, D.N., Cornblath, D.R., Chaudhry, V., Borel, C. & Hanley, D.F. (1993). Relapse in Guillain–Barré syndrome after treatment with human immune globulin. *Neurology*, **43**, 872–5.

Jackson, M.C., Godwin Austen, R.B. & Whiteley, A.M. (1993). High-dose intravenous immunoglobulin in the treatment of Guillain–Barré syndrome: a preliminary open study. *Journal of Neurology*, **240**, 51–3.

Jackson, R.H., Miller, H. & Schapira, K. (1957). Polyradiculitis (Landry–Guillain–Barré syndrome). Treatment with cortisone and corticotrophin. *British Medical Journal*, **1**, 480–4.

Jones, M.W. & Berry, K. (1981). Chronic relapsing polyneuritis associated with pregnancy. *Annals of Neurology*, **9**, 413.

Kaiser, R., Kaufmann, R., Czygan, M., Lang, H. & Lucking, C.H. (1993). Guillain–Barré syndrome following streptokinase therapy. *Clinical Investigation*, **71**, 795–801.

Kaldor, J. & Speed, B.R. (1984). Guillain–Barré syndrome and *Campylobacter jejuni*: a serological study. *British Medical Journal*, **288**, 1867–70.

Kamolvarin, N., Hemachudha, T., Ongpipattanakul, B., Phanthumchinda, K. & Sueblinvong, T. (1991). Plasma C3c in immune-mediated neurological diseases: a preliminary report. *Acta Neurologica Scandinavica*, **83**, 382–7.

Kaslow, R.A., Sullivan Bolyai, J.Z., Hafkin, B., Schonberger, L.B., Kraus, L., Moore, M.J., Yunis, E. & Williams, R.M. (1984). HLA antigens in Guillain–Barré syndrome. *Neurology*, **34**, 240–2.

Keenlyside, R.A., Schonberger, L.B., Bregman, D.J. & Bolyai, J.Z. (1980). Fatal Guillain–Barré syndrome after the national influenza immunization program. *Neurology*, **30**, 929–33.

Kennedy, F. (1929). Certain nervous complications following the use of therapeutic and prophylactic sera. *American Journal of the Medical Sciences*, **177**, 555–9.

Khalili Shirazi, A., Atkinson, P., Gregson, N. & Hughes, R.A. (1993). Antibody responses to P_0 and P_2 myelin proteins in Guillain–Barré syndrome and chronic idiopathic demyelinating polyradiculoneuropathy. *Journal of Neuroimmunology*, **46**, 245–51.

Khalili Shirazi, A., Hughes, R.A., Brostoff, S.W., Linington, C. & Gregson, N. (1992). T cell responses to myelin proteins in Guillain–Barré syndrome. *Journal of the Neurological Sciences*, **111**, 200–3.

Kimura, J. (1978). Proximal versus distal slowing of motor nerve conduction velocity in the Guillain–Barré syndrome. *Annals of Neurology*, **3**, 344–50.

Kimura, J. & Butzer, J.F. (1975). F-wave conduction velocity in Guillain–Barré syndrome. Assessment of nerve segment between axilla and spinal cord *Archives of Neurology*, **32**, 524–9.

King, D. & Ashby, P. (1976). Conduction velocity in the proximal segments of a motor nerve in the Guillain–Barré syndrome. *Journal of Neurology, Neurosurgery and Psychiatry*, **39**, 538–44.

Knowles, M., Currie, S., Saunders, M., Walton, J.N. & Field, E.J. (1969). Lymphocyte transformation in the Guillain–Barré syndrome. *Lancet*, **2**, 1168–70.

Korn Lubetzki, I. & Abramsky, O. (1986). Acute and chronic demyelinating inflammatory polyradiculoneuropathy. Association with autoimmune diseases and lymphocyte response to human neuritogenic protein. *Archives of Neurology*, **43**, 604–8.

Korn-Lubetzki, I., Steiner, I., Brenner, T., Brautbar, C. & Argov, Z. (1994). Familial inflammatory demyelinating polyneuropathy: a Guillain–Barré syndrome variant without autoimmune predilection. *Journal of Neurology, Neurosurgery and Psychiatry*, **57**, 1008–16.

Kornberg, A.J., Pestronk, A., Bieser, K., Ho, T.W., McKhann, G.M., Wu, H.S. & Jiang, Z. (1994). The clinical correlates of high-titre IgG anti-GM1 antibodies. *Annals of Neurology*, **35**, 234–7.

Koski, C.L. (1990). Characterization of complement-fixing antibodies to peripheral nerve myelin in Guillain–Barré syndrome. *Annals of Neurology*, **27 Supplement**, S44-S47.

Koski, C.L., Gratz, E., Sutherland, J. & Mayer, R.F. (1986). Clinical correlation with anti-peripheral-nerve myelin antibodies in Guillain–Barré syndrome. *Annals of Neurology*, **19**, 573–7.

Koski, C.L., Humphrey, R. & Shin, M.L. (1985). Anti-peripheral myelin antibody in patients with demyelinating neuropathy: quantitative and kinetic determination of serum antibody by complement component 1 fixation. *Proceedings of the National Academy of Science of the United States of America*, **82**, 905–9.

Koski, C.L., Sanders, M.E., Swoveland, P.T., Lawley, T.J., Shin, M.L., Frank, M.M. & Joiner, K.A. (1987). Activation of terminal components of complement in patients with Guillain–Barré syndrome and other demyelinating neuropathies. *Journal of Clinical Investigation*, **80**, 1492–7.

Kusunoki, S., Chiba, A., Tai, T. & Kanazawa, I. (1993). Localization of GM1 and GD1b antigens in the human peripheral nervous system. *Muscle and Nerve*, **16**, 752–6.

Landi, G., D'Alessandro, R., Dossi, B.C., Ricci, S., Simone, I.L. & Ciccone, A. (1993). Guillain–Barré syndrome after exogenous gangliosides in Italy *British Medical Journal*, **307**, 1463–4.

Landry, O. (1859). Note sur la paralysie ascendante aigüe. *Gazette Hebdomaire de Médicine et de Chirurgie Paris*, **6**, 472–86.

Latov, N., Koski, C. & Walicke, P.A. (1991). Guillain–Barré syndrome and parenteral gangliosides. *Lancet*, **338**, 757.

Latovitzki, N., Suciu Foca, N., Penn, A.S., Olarte, M.R. & Chutorian, A.M. (1979). HLA typing and Guillain–Barré syndrome. *Neurology*, **29**, 743–5.

Leneman, F. (1966). The Guillain–Barré syndrome. *Archives of Internal Medicine*, **118**, 139–44.

Lichtenfeld, P. (1971). Autonomic dysfunction in the Guillain–Barré syndrome. *American Journal of Medicine*, **50**, 772–80.

Lisak, R.P., Zweiman, B., Guerrero, F. & Moskovitz, A.R. (1985). Circulating T-cell subsets in Guillain–Barré syndrome. *Journal of Neuroimmunology*, **8**, 93–101.

Loffel, N.B., Rossi, L.N., Mumenthaler, M., Lutschg, J. & Ludin, H.-P. (1977). The Landry–Guillain–Barré syndrome. Complications, prognosis and natural history in 123 cases. *Journal of the Neurological Sciences*, **33**, 71–9.

Low, P.A., Dyck, P.J., Lambert, E.H., Brimijoin, W.S., Trautmann, J.C., Malagelada, J.R., Fealey, R.D. & Barrett, D.M. (1983). Acute panautonomic neuropathy. *Annals of Neurology*, **13**, 412–17.

Low, P.A., Schmelzer, J., Dyck, P.J. & Kelly, J.J. Jr (1982). Endoneurial effects of sera from patients with acute inflammatory polyradiculoneuropathy: electrophysiologic studies on normal and demyelinated rat nerves. *Neurology*, **32**, 720–4.

Luijten, J.A. & Baart de la Faille Kuyper, E.H. (1972). The occurrence of IgM and complement factors along myelin sheaths of peripheral nerves. An immunohistochemical study of the Guillain–Barré syndrome. Preliminary communication. *Journal of the Neurological Sciences*, **15**, 219–24.

Luijten, J.A., De Jong, W.A., Demel, R.A., Heijnen, C.J. & Ballieux, R.E. (1984). Peripheral nerve P2 basic protein and the Guillain–Barré syndrome. *In vitro* demonstration of P2-specific antibody-secreting cells. *Journal of the Neurological Sciences*, **66**, 209–16.

MacGregor, G.A. (1965). Familial Guillain–Barré syndrome. *Lancet*, **2**, 1296.

Mancardi, G.L., Cadoni, A., Zicca, A., Schenone, A., Tabaton, M., De Martini, I. & Zaccheo, D. (1988). HLA-DR Schwann cell reactivity in peripheral neuropathies of different origins. *Neurology*, **38**, 848–51.

McCombe, P.A., Clark, P., Frith, J., Hammond, S., Stewart, G.J., Pollard, J.D. & McLeod, J.G. (1985). Alpha-1 antitrypsin phenotypes in demyelinating disease. An association between demyelinating disease and the allele PiM3. *Annals of Neurology*, **18**, 514–16.

McCombe, P.A., Pollard, J.D. & McLeod, J.G. (1988). Absence of antimyelin antibodies and serum demyelinating factors in most patients with chronic inflammatory demyelinating polyradiculoneuropathy. *Clinical and Experimental Neurology*, **25**, 53–60.

McFarland, R.H. & Heller, G.L. (1966). Guillain–Barré disease complex. A statement of diagnostic criteria and analysis of 100 cases. *Archives of Neurology*, **14**, 196–201.

McKhann, G.M., Cornblath, D.R., Griffin, J.W., Ho, T.W., Li, C.Y., Jiang, Z., Wu, H.S., Zhaori, G., Liu, Y., Jou, L.P. *et al.* (1993). Acute motor axonal neuropathy: a frequent cause of acute flaccid paralysis in China. *Annals of Neurology*, **33**, 333–42.

McLeod, J.G. (1981). Electrophysiological studies in the Guillain–Barré syndrome. *Annals of Neurology*, **9 (Supplement)**, 20–7.

Miller, H.G. & Stanton, J.B. (1954). Neurological sequelae of prophylactic inoculation. *Quarterly Journal of Medicine*, **23**, 1–27.

Mithen, F.A., Ilyas, A.A., Birchem, R. & Cook, S.D. (1992). Effects of Guillain–Barré sera containing antibodies against glycolipids in cultures of rat Schwann cells and sensory neurons. *Journal of the Neurological Sciences*, **112**, 223–32.

Mozes, B., Pines, A., Sayar, Y., Kaplinsky, N. & Frankl, O. (1984). Guillain–Barré syndrome associated with acute cytomegalovirus mononucleosis syndrome. *European Neurology*, **23**, 237–9.

Nadkarni, N. & Lisak, R.P. (1993). Guillain–Barré syndrome (GBS) with bilateral optic neuritis and central white matter disease. *Neurology*, **43**, 842–3.

Neville, B.G.R. & Sladen, G.E. (1984). Acute autonomic neuropathy following primary herpes simplex infection. *Journal of Neurology, Neurosurgery and Psychiatry*, **47**, 648–50.

Novak, D.J. & Johnson, K.P. (1973). Relapsing idiopathic polyneuritis during pregnancy. Immunological aspects and literature review. *Archives of Neurology*, **28**, 219–23.

Nyland, H., Matre, R. & Mork, S. (1981). Immunological characterization of sural nerve biopsies from patients with Guillain–Barré syndrome. *Annals of Neurology*, **9 (Supplement)**, 80–6.

Olney, R.K. & Aminoff, M.J. (1990). Electrodiagnostic features of the Guillain–Barré syndrome: the relative sensitivity of different techniques. *Neurology*, **40**, 471–5.

Oomes, P.G., van der Meche, F.G., Markus Silvis, L., Meulstee, J. & Kleyweg, R.P. (1991). *In vivo* effects of sera from Guillain–Barré subgroups: an electrophysiological and histological study on rat nerves. *Muscle and Nerve*, **14**, 1013–20.

Ormerod, I.E. & Cockerell, O.C. (1993). Guillain–Barré syndrome after herpes zoster infection: a report of 2 cases. *European Neurology*, **33**, 156–8.

Osterman, P.O., Fagius, J., Safwenberg, J. & Wikstrom, B. (1988). Early relapse of acute inflammatory polyradiculoneuropathy after successful treatment with plasma exchange. *Acta Neurologica Scandinavica*, **77**, 273–7.

Pleasure, D.E., Lovelace, R.E. & Duvoisin, R.C. (1968). The prognosis of acute polyradiculoneuritis. *Neurology*, **18**, 1143–8.

Pollard, J.D., Baverstock, J. & McLeod, J.G. (1987). Class II antigen expression and inflammatory cells in the Guillain–Barré syndrome. *Annals of Neurology*, **21**, 337–41.

Polo, A., Manganotti, P., Zanette, G. & De Grandis, D. (1992). Polyneuritis cranialis: clinical and electrophysiological findings. *Journal of Neurology, Neurosurgery and Psychiatry*, **55**, 398–400.

Powell, H.C., Braheny, S.L., Hughes, R.A.C. & Lampert, P.W. (1984). Antigen-specific demyelination and significance of the bystander effect in peripheral nerves. *American Journal of Pathology*, **114**, 443–53.

Prineas, J.W. (1972). Acute idiopathic polyneuritis. An electron microscope study. *Laboratory Investigation*, **26**, 133–47.

Prineas, J.W. (1981). Pathology of the Guillain–Barré syndrome. *Annals of Neurology*, **9 (Supplement)**, 6–19.

Quarles, R.H., Ilyas, A.A. & Willison, H.J. (1990). Antibodies to gangliosides and myelin proteins in Guillain–Barré syndrome. *Annals of Neurology*, **27 (Supplement)**, S48–S52.

Raphael, J.-C., Chastang, C., Chevret, S. & Gajdos, P. (1992). Intravenous immune globulin versus plasma exchange in Guillain–Barré syndrome. *New England Journal of Medicine*, **324**, 816.

Rees, J.H., Gregson, N.A., Griffiths, P.L. & Hughes, R.A. (1993). *Campylobacter jejuni* and Guillain–Barré syndrome. *Quarterly Journal of Medicine*, **86**, 623–34.

Roberts, M., Willison, H., Vincent, A. & Newsom Davis, J. (1994). Serum factor in Miller-Fisher variant of Guillain–Barré syndrome and neurotransmitter release. *Lancet*, **343**, 454–5.

Robertson, H.F. & Varmus, F. (1944). Report of a case of peripheral neuritis with hypertension following serum therapy. *The Military Surgeon*, **95**, 129–32.

Ropper, A.H., Wijdicks, E.F.M. & Shahani, B.T. (1990). Electrodiagnostic abnormalities in 113 consecutive patients with Guillain–Barré syndrome. *Archives of Neurology*, **47**, 881–7.

Rostami, A.M., Burns, J.B., Eccleston, P.A., Manning, M.C., Lisak, R.P. & Silberberg, D.H. (1987). Search for antibodies to galactocerebroside in the serum and cerebrospinal fluid in human demyelinating disorders. *Annals of Neurology*, **22**, 381–3.

Rubenstein, A.E., Yahr, M.D., Mytilineou, C., Sivak, M., Mindel, J. & Frontera, A.F. (1980). Orthostatic hypotension in the Holmes–Adie syndrome. *Mt Sinai Journal of Medicine*, **47**, 57–61.

Ryberg, B. (1984). Extra- and intrathecal production of antinerve and antibrain antibodies in Guillain–Barré syndrome: evaluation by an antibody index. *Neurology*, **34**, 1378–81.

Saida, T., Saida, K., Lisak, R.P., Brown, M.J., Silberberg, D.H. & Asbury, A.K. (1982). *In vivo* demyelinating activity of sera from patients with Guillain–Barré syndrome. *Annals of Neurology*, **11**, 69–75.

Saunders, M. & Rake, M. (1965). Familial Guillain–Barré syndrome. *Lancet*, **2**, 1106–7.

Sawant-Mane, S., Estep, A. & Koski, C.L. (1994). Antibody of patients with Guillain–Barré syndrome mediates complement-dependent cytolysis of rat Schwann cells: susceptibility to cytolysis reflects Schwann cell phenotype. *Journal of Neuroimmunology*, **49**, 145–52.

Schonberger, L.B., Bregman, D.J., Sullivan-Bolyai, J.Z., Keenlyside, R.A., Ziegler, D.W., Retailliau, H.F., Eddins, D.L. & Bryan, J.A. (1979). Guillain–Barré syndrome following vaccination in the national influenza immunization program, United States, 1976–1977. *American Journal of Epidemiology*, **110**, 105–23.

Schroder, H.D., Olsson, T., Solders, G., Kristensson, K. & Link, H. (1988). HLA-DR-expressing cells and T-lymphocytes in sural nerve biopsies. *Muscle and Nerve*, **11**, 864–70.

Sharief, M.K., McLean, B. & Thompson, E.J. (1993). Elevated serum levels of tumor necrosis factor-alpha in Guillain–Barré syndrome. *Annals of Neurology*, **33**, 591–6.

Shuaib, A. & Becker, W.J. (1987). Variants of Guillain–Barré syndrome: Miller Fisher syndrome, facial diplegia and multiple cranial nerve palsies. *Canadian Journal of Neurological Sciences*, **14**, 611–16.

Simone, I.L., Annunziata, P., Maimone, D., Liguori, M., Leante, R. & Livrea, P. (1993). Serum and CSF anti-GM1 antibodies in patients with Guillain–Barré syndrome and chronic inflammatory demyelinating polyneuropathy. *Journal of the Neurological Sciences*, **114**, 49–55.

Sobue, G., Senda, Y., Matsuoka, Y. & Sobue, I. (1983). Sensory ataxia. A residual disability of Guillain–Barré syndrome. *Archives of Neurology*, **40**, 86–9.

Sterman, A.B., Schaumberg, H.H. & Asbury, A.H. (1980). The acute sensory neuronopathy syndrome: a distinct clinical entity. *Annals of Neurology*, **7**, 354–8.

Stewart, G.J., Pollard, J.D., McLeod, J.G. & Wolnizer, C.M. (1978). HLA antigens in the Landry–Guillain–Barré syndrome and chronic relapsing polyneuritis. *Annals of Neurology*, **4**, 285–9.

Takayama, H., Kazahaya, Y., Kashihara, N., Kuroda, H., Miyawaki, S., Ota, Z. & Ogawa, N. (1987). A case of postganglionic cholinergic dysautonomia. *Journal of Neurology, Neurosurgery and Psychiatry*, **50**, 915–18.

Taylor, W.A., Brostoff, S.W. & Hughes, R.A. (1991). P_2 specific lymphocyte transformation in Guillain–Barré syndrome and chronic idiopathic demyelinating polyradiculoneuropathy. *Journal of the Neurological Sciences*, **104**, 52–5.

Taylor, W.A. & Hughes, R.A. (1989). T lymphocyte activation antigens in Guillain–Barré syndrome and chronic idiopathic demyelinating polyradiculoneuropathy. *Journal of Neuroimmunology*, **24**, 33–9.

The Guillain–Barré Syndrome Study Group (1985). Plasmapheresis and acute Guillain–Barré syndrome. *Neurology*, **35**, 1096–104.

Thomashefsky, A.J., Horwitz, S.J. & Feingold, M.H. (1972). Acute autonomic neuropathy. *Neurology*, **22**, 251–5.

Thornton, C.A. & Griggs, R.C. (1994). Plasma exchange and intravenous immunoglobulin treatment of neuromuscular disease. *Annals of Neurology*, **35**, 260–8.

Triggs, W.J., Cros, D., Gominak, S.C., Zuniga, G., Beric, A., Shahani, B.T., Ropper, A.H. & Roongta, S.M. (1992). Motor nerve inexcitability in Guillain–Barré syndrome. The spectrum of distal conduction block and axonal degeneration. *Brain*, **115**, 1291–302.

Tse, K.S., Arbesman, C.E., Tomasi, T.B. Jr & Tourville, D. (1971). Demonstration of antimyelin antibodies by immunofluorescence in Guillain–Barré syndrome. *Clinical and Experimental Immunology*, **8**, 881–7.

Tsukada, N., Koh, C.S., Inoue, A. & Yanagisawa, N. (1987). Demyelinating neuropathy associated with hepatitis B virus infection. Detection of immune complexes composed of hepatitis B virus surface antigen. *Journal of the Neurological Sciences*, **77**, 203–16.

Ungley, C.C. (1933). Recurrent polyneuritis in pregnancy and the puerperium affecting three members of a family. *Journal of Neurology and Psychopathology*, **14**, 15–26.

Valbonesi, M., Garelli, S., Mosconi, L., Zerbi, D. & Celano, I. (1981). Plasma exchange as a therapy for Guillain–Barré syndrome with immune complexes. *Vox Sanguinis*, **41**, 74–8.

Vallat, J.M., Hugon, J., Tabaraud, F., Leboutet, M.J., Chazot, F. & Dumas, M. (1990). Quatre cas de syndrome de Guillain–Barré avec lésions axonales. *Revue Neurologique*, **146**, 420–4.

van den Berg, L.H., Lankamp, C.L.A.M., de Jager, A.E., Notermans, N.C., Sodaar, P., Marrink, J., de Jong, H.J., Bar, P.R. & Wokke, J.H.J. (1993). Anti-sulphatide antibodies in peripheral neuropathy. *Journal of Neurology, Neurosurgery and Psychiatry*, **56**, 1164–8.

van den Berg, L.H., Marrink, J., de Jager, A.E., de Jong, H.J., van Imhoff, G.W., Latov, N. & Sadiq, S.A. (1992). Anti-GM1 antibodies in patients with Guillain–Barré syndrome. *Journal of Neurology, Neurosurgery and Psychiatry*, **55**, 8–11.

van der Meche, F.G. & Meulstee, J. (1988). Guillain–Barré syndrome: a model of random conduction block. *Journal of Neurology, Neurosurgery and Psychiatry*, **51**, 1158–63.

van der Meche, F.G. & Schmitz, P.I. (1992). A randomized trial comparing intravenous immune globulin and plasma exchange in Guillain–Barré syndrome. Dutch Guillain–Barré Study Group. *New England Journal of Medicine*, **326**, 1123–9.

Vedeler, C.A., Matre, R. & Nyland, H. (1986). Immunoglobulins in serum and cerebrospinal fluid from patients with acute Guillain–Barré syndrome. *Acta Neurologica Scandinavica*, **73**, 388–93.

Vedeler, C.A., Matre, R. & Nyland, H. (1988). Class and IgG subclass distribution of antibodies against peripheral nerve myelin in sera from patients with inflammatory demyelinating polyradiculoneuropathy. *Acta Neurologica Scandinavica*, **78**, 401–7.

Walsh, F.S., Cronin, M., Koblar, S., Doherty, P., Winer, J., Leon, A. & Hughes, R.A. (1991). Association between glycoconjugate antibodies and *Campylobacter* infection in patients with Guillain–Barré syndrome. *Journal of Neuroimmunology*, **34**, 43–51.

Wardrop, J. (1834). Clinical observations of various diseases. *Lancet*, **1**, 380–1.

Wiederholt, W.C., Mulder, D.W. & Lambert, E.H. (1964). The Landry–Guillain–Barré–Strohl syndrome or polyradiculoneuropathy: historical review, report on 97 patients, and present concepts. *Mayo Clinic Proceedings*, **39**, 427–51.

Wijesundere, A. (1992). Guillain–Barré syndrome in *Plasmodium falciparum* malaria. *Postgraduate Medical Journal*, **68**, 376–7.

Willison, H.J. & Kennedy, P.G. (1993). Gangliosides and bacterial toxins in Guillain–Barré syndrome. *Journal of Neuroimmunology*, **46**, 105–12.

Willison, H.J. & Veitch, J. (1994). Immunoglobulin subclass distribution and binding characteristics of anti-GQ1b antibodies in Miller-Fisher syndrome. *Journal of Neuroimmunology*, **50**, 159–65.

Willison, H.J., Veitch, J., Paterson, G. & Kennedy, P.G. (1993). Miller Fisher syndrome is associated with serum antibodies to GQ1b ganglioside. *Journal of Neurology, Neurosurgery and Psychiatry*, **56**, 204–6.

Winer, J.B., Briggs, D., Welsh, K. & Hughes, R.A. (1988*a*). HLA antigens in the Guillain–Barré syndrome. *Journal of Neuroimmunology*, **18**, 13–16.

Winer, J.B., Gray, I.A., Gregson, N.A., Hughes, R.A., Leibowitz, S., Shepherd, P., Taylor, W.A. & Yewdall, V. (1988*b*). A prospective study of acute idiopathic neuropathy. III. Immunological studies. *Journal of Neurology, Neurosurgery and Psychiatry*, **51**, 619–25.

Winer, J.B., Hughes, R.A.C., Anderson, M.J., Jones, D.M., Kangro, H. & Watkins, R.P.F. (1988*c*). A prospective study of acute idiopathic neuropathy. II. Antecedent events. *Journal of Neurology, Neurosurgery and Psychiatry*, **51**, 613–18.

Winer, J.B., Hughes, R.A.C. & Osmond, C. (1988*d*). A prospective study of acute idiopathic neuropathy. I. Clinical features and their prognostic value. *Journal of Neurology, Neurosurgery and Psychiatry*, **51**, 605–12.

Winkelman, N.W. (1949). Peripheral nerve and root disturbances following vaccination against smallpox. Study of five cases, review of literature and discussion of related entities. *Archives of Neurology and Psychiatry*, **62**, 421–38.

Wisniewski, H.M. & Bloom, B.R. (1975). Primary demyelination as a nonspecific consequence of a cell-mediated immune reaction. *Journal of Experimental Medicine*, **141**, 346–59.

Young, R.R., Asbury, A.K., Adams, R.D. & Corbett, J.L. (1969). Pure pan-dysautonomia with recovery. *Transactions of the American Neurological Association*, **94**, 355–7.

Yuki, N., Sato, S., Tsuji, S., Ohasawa, T. & Miyatake, T. (1993*a*). Frequent presence of anti-GQ1b antibody in Fisher's syndrome. *Neurology*, **43**, 414–17.

Yuki, N., Taki, T., Inagaki, F., Kasama, T., Takahashi, M., Saito, K., Handa, S. & Miyatake, T. (1993*b*). A bacterium lipopolysaccharide that elicits Guillain–Barré syndrome has a GM1 ganglioside-like structure. *Journal of Experimental Medicine*, **178**, 1771–5.

Yuki, N., Yoshino, H., Sato, S., Shinozawa, K. & Miyatake, T. (1992). Severe acute axonal form of Guillain–Barré syndrome associated with IgG anti-GD1a antibodies. *Muscle and Nerve*, **15**, 899–903.

Zweiman, B., Rostami, A., Lisak, R.P., Moskovitz, A.R. & Pleasure, D.E. (1983). Immune reactions to P2 protein in human inflammatory demyelinative neuropathies. *Neurology*, **33**, 234–7.

–9–
Chronic immune-mediated neuropathies

PAMELA A. McCOMBE

Chronic inflammatory demyelinating polyradiculoneuropathy

Introduction

Chronic inflammatory demyelinating polyradiculoneuropathy (CIDP) is the term used to describe chronic progressive and chronic relapsing polyneuropathies associated with inflammation and primary demyelination of the nerves and nerve roots. Austin (1958) gave an early description of recurrent polyneuropathies responsive to corticosteroid treatment. Such responsiveness to corticosteroids is a feature of CIDP. Austin regarded the case described by Targowla (1894) as the first description of relapsing polyneuropathy. Another early description was given by Hinman & Magee (1967): they highlighted the similarity of the chronic disease to the Guillain–Barré syndrome (GBS) and the elevation of cerebrospinal fluid (CSF) protein, which is another typical feature of CIDP. Thomas *et al.* (1969) and Prineas & McLeod (1976) highlighted the relapsing course of disease and described 'chronic relapsing polyneuritis'. Later the term 'chronic inflammatory polyradiculoneuropathy' was used by Dyck *et al.* (1975), who also included patients with a progressive course of disease. More recently, the term 'chronic inflammatory demyelinating polyradiculoneuropathy' has been accepted. This term is used for patients with relapsing and non-relapsing disease. It is difficult to make a distinction between patients with recurrent attacks of GBS and those with CIDP (Thomas *et al.*, 1969; McCombe, Pollard & McLeod, 1987*b*). Some authors have suggested that recurrences of GBS are distinguished from relapses of CIDP by rapidity of onset and completeness of recovery (Grand'Maison *et al.*, 1992). In this chapter, recurrent GBS is not differentiated from chronic relapsing CIDP.

Multifocal motor neuropathy and paraproteinaemic neuropathy are two syndromes that overlap with CIDP. Multifocal motor neuropathy is primarily a motor syndrome that may present with weakness and wasting. The relationship between CIDP and multifocal motor neuropathy remains to be clarified. Paraproteinaemic neuropathies have a variety of presentations. However, some patients who appear to have CIDP have a circulating paraprotein and it is not clear whether such patients should be classified as having CIDP (Vital *et al.*, 1991; Bromberg, Feldman & Albers, 1992).

Clinical features

Clinical symptoms and signs

Dyck *et al.* (1975) described a series of 53 patients with CIDP. They reported that the ratio of males to females was 2:1 and that the incidence was maximal in the fifth and sixth decades. Limb weakness was prominent but sensory symptoms were also common and cranial nerve involvement was present in about 10% of patients. Prineas & McLeod (1976) also found that males predominated in a series of patients with relapsing polyradiculoneuropathy. Oh (1978) described patients with weakness and a subacute onset. Some of these patients developed a relapsing course after corticosteroid treatment. McCombe, Pollard and McLeod (1987*b*) confirmed that CIDP has prominent motor symptoms, although some sensory impairment is usually present. Patients with CIDP may develop muscle wasting, especially in the later stages. Some patients who have the pathological features of CIDP affecting both motor and sensory nerves have the clinical features of a pure sensory neuropathy (Oh, Joy & Kuruoglu, 1992). Other reported clinical features of CIDP include tremor (Dyck *et al.*, 1975; Prineas & McLeod, 1976; Dalakas, Teravainen & Engel, 1984) and autonomic disturbance (Ingall, McLeod & Tamura, 1990). Austin (1958) described nerve hypertrophy in CIDP, but this has been less commonly reported in more recent surveys (Dyck *et al.*, 1975; Prineas & McLeod, 1976; McCombe *et al.*, 1987*b*).

Diagnosis

Diagnosis of CIDP requires evidence of a demyelinating neuropathy, which is often provided by neurophysiological studies, and inflammation, which is often provided by evidence of raised CSF protein. Further evidence of both inflammation and demyelination may be obtained from a nerve biopsy. Criteria for the strict diagnosis of CIDP have been produced (Barohn *et al.*, 1989; Ad Hoc Subcommittee of the American Academy of Neurology AIDS Task Force, 1991); these are particularly intended for use in research studies.

Association with other autoimmune diseases

If CIDP is an autoimmune disease, it might be expected to occur in association with other autoimmune diseases. CIDP has been reported in association with systemic lupus erythematosus (Rechthand *et al.*, 1984), rheumatoid arthritis (McCombe *et al.*, 1991*b*), thyroid disease and iritis (McCombe *et al.*, 1987*b*). CIDP has also been reported with glomerulonephritis (Witte & Burke, 1987; Kohli, Tandon & Kher, 1992).

Involvement of the central nervous system

Thomas *et al.* (1987) reported six patients with CIDP associated with CNS abnormalities resembling multiple sclerosis (MS). In a subsequent series, Ormerod *et al.* (1990) found that while six of 30 CIDP patients had clinical evidence of CNS involvement, 14 of 28 patients had abnormalities on magnetic resonance imaging (MRI). Other studies have found that MRI and evoked potential abnormalities are present in some patients with CIDP (Gigli *et al.*, 1989; Uncini *et al.*, 1991). However, some studies show that only a minority of CIDP patients have MRI evidence of CNS damage (Mendell *et al.*, 1987; Hawke, Hallinan & McLeod, 1990; Ohtake *et al.*, 1990; Feasby *et al.*, 1990). It is not clear whether CNS involvement in some patients with CIDP reflects the occurrence of CIDP together with another disease such as MS or whether CNS tissue can be damaged by the process causing CIDP. Patients with MS sometimes have abnormalities of the peripheral nervous system (PNS) (see Chapter 4).

Triggering factors

Infections and vaccinations

Both the onset of CIDP and relapses of CIDP may follow a precipitating event. Patients often report that initial symptoms of CIDP commence after an infection (McCombe *et al.*, 1987*b*). Relapses of CIDP may also follow infections such as hepatitis B (Inoue *et al.*, 1987) or vaccinations, for example with tetanus toxoid (Pollard & Selby, 1978). Exacerbation of disease after infection or vaccination may occur because of cross-reactivity of the infectious agent with PNS antigens (molecular mimicry).

Pregnancy and immunosuppression

There appears to be an increased risk of relapses of CIDP in the post-partum period (McCombe *et al.*, 1987*a*). Exacerbation of disease in the post-partum period may be associated with a decline in the immunosuppressive effects of pregnancy. CIDP has been reported to occur in other immunosuppressed patients such as those treated with FK506 (Wilson *et al.*, 1994). FK506 is related to cyclosporin A, which can be used to produce chronic relapsing experimental autoimmune neuritis, the animal model of CIDP (McCombe, van der Kreek & Pender, 1990).

Clinical course and follow-up studies

Patients with CIDP may develop severe weakness during relapses of disease. At follow-up, patients usually have continuing signs of neuropathy, but many are living independently (Dyck *et al.*, 1975; McCombe *et al.*, 1987*b*; Barohn *et al.*, 1989). However, some patients eventually develop severe unremitting weakness and wasting.

Genetics

Familial CIDP

If CIDP is an autoimmune disease, it might be expected that familial cases of CIDP would occur, because autoimmune diseases tend to run in families. However, in clinical neurology, the finding of demyelinating neuropathy in a family suggests a diagnosis of a genetic disorder such as hereditary motor and sensory neuropathy. Dyck *et al.* (1982*b*) described patients with corticosteroid-responsive demyelinating neuropathy who also had clinical features suggestive of hereditary motor and sensory neuropathy. It was thought that such patients might have inflammatory neuropathy superimposed on underlying genetic neuropathy. Further studies are needed to determine whether first-degree relatives of patients with CIDP have an increased incidence of CIDP and other autoimmune diseases.

Genetic typing

Feeney *et al.* (1990) found an increase in the frequencies of the linked antigens HLA-A3, -B7 and -DR2 in CIDP patients compared to controls, but this was not statistically significant. Van Doorn *et al.* (1991) found no HLA association in 52 patients with CIDP. The Gm (immunoglobulin allotype) allelic system has been associated with some autoimmune diseases such as myasthenia gravis. The frequency of the Gm haplotype 1,2,17:21 was slightly but not significantly increased in patients with CIDP (Feeney *et al.*, 1989). An increase in the frequency of the alpha-1 antitrypsin allele PiM3 has also been found in CIDP (McCombe *et al.*, 1985).

Neuropathology

Sural nerve biopsies

The pathology of CIDP is usually studied in peripheral nerve biopsies. Dyck *et al.* (1975) found that the abnormalities in CIDP include perivascular inflammation, mononuclear cell infiltration of the endoneurium, oedema of the endoneurium and the subperineurial space, and onion bulb formation. Prineas & McLeod (1976) reviewed biopsies from 23 patients with CIDP and found primary demyelination, onion bulb formation and active demyelination by macrophages. A study by Krendel *et al.* (1989) of 14 patients confirmed the presence of inflammatory cells and onion bulbs in some patients and demyelination in 50% of patients. Chou (1992) analysed onion bulbs in different types of neuropathies and found that those in CIDP are composed of Schwann cells, activated macrophages and a few fibroblasts. Ultrastructural studies of CIDP have shown that demyelination is produced by macrophages (Prineas, 1971; Prineas & McLeod, 1976). Other studies have shown that axonal degeneration (Dyck *et al.*, 1975; Pollard *et al.*, 1983; Julien *et al.*, 1989) and loss of small fibres (Gibbels & Kentenich, 1990; Ingall *et al.*, 1990) may occur in CIDP. It is not clear whether axonal damage occurs in patients with more severe disease, as is the case in EAN, or occurs in a subset of patients who may have a different disease process from that in patients with the predominantly demyelinating type of CIDP.

Autopsy studies

Autopsy studies are less common than nerve biopsy studies. Hyland and Russell (1930) reported the findings of an autopsied case and found nerve enlargement, demyelination, particularly of the nerve roots, and infiltration of the nerves with inflammatory cells. Harris & Newcombe (1929) had previously reported the presence of demyelination and onion bulb formation. Later, Thomas *et al.* (1969) described two autopsied cases, and found nerve swelling, loss of myelinated fibres and perivascular collections of lymphocytes.

Pathophysiology

The neurological deficit in CIDP is likely to be secondary to demyelination-induced nerve conduction block. However, axonal degeneration also occurs in CIDP and may play an important role in the production of persistent weakness and wasting (Pollard *et al.*, 1983). Nerve conduction studies are important in the diagnosis of CIDP and are used as evidence that primary demyelination is present. Bromberg (1991) has compared different means of assessing the presence of demyelination. Demyelination causes conduction slowing (detected as a reduction in the conduction velocity or as temporal dispersion of the compound muscle action potential) or conduction block, which causes a reduction in the amplitude of the compound muscle action potential on proximal stimulation when the amplitude is normal on distal stimulation. If the amplitude is low at all sites of stimulation, the underlying pathology may be either axonal degeneration or extensive demyelination, causing conduction failure. Biopsies of nerves with conduction block show evidence of demyelination (Feasby *et al.*, 1985). Many authors have found severe slowing of the motor nerve conduction in CIDP (Dyck *et al.*, 1975; Prineas & McLeod, 1976; Oh, 1978; Dalakas & Engel, 1981).

Immunopathology of the PNS lesions

Immunocytochemical staining of biopsies from six patients with CIDP showed infiltration of the endoneurium with macrophages and small numbers of $CD4^+$ and $CD8^+$ T cells (Pollard *et al.*, 1986). MHC class II antigen expression on Schwann cells in CIDP was described by Pollard *et al.* (1986) and later by Mitchell *et al.* (1991). However, subsequent studies have been unable to demonstrate MHC class II antigen expression on Schwann cells in CIDP (Atkinson *et al.*, 1993) or have found that Schwann cells can express MHC class II antigen in non-inflammatory conditions (Mitchell *et al.*, 1991) as well as in CIDP. Further studies are needed to clarify whether Schwann cell expression of MHC class II antigen is important in the pathogenesis of CIDP.

Using immunofluorescence, Dalakas & Engel (1980) found complement and antibody deposition in the small blood vessels in the nerves of seven patients with CIDP. With immunofluorescence, McCombe, Pollard & McLeod (1988) found that only one of 28 CIDP nerves had immunoglobulin bound to myelin sheaths. Complement deposition was found in the nerves of two of four CIDP patients examined by Hays, Lee & Latov (1988).

Immunological findings in the peripheral blood

Non-specific findings

Serum levels of interleukin-2 (IL-2) are elevated in CIDP, although not to the same extent as in GBS (Hartung *et al.*, 1991). In some CIDP patients there are elevated levels of soluble interleukin-2 receptor (IL-2R) (Hartung *et al.*, 1990). The elevations of serum IL-2 and soluble IL-2R indicate systemic T cell activation. This has been confirmed by a study showing that the numbers of circulating activated T cells in CIDP patients were increased (although not to the same extent as in GBS patients) (Taylor & Hughes, 1989). Serum complement (C3c) levels were elevated (Kamolvarin *et al.*, 1991) but serum IL-6 levels were not elevated in CIDP (Maimone *et al.*, 1993).

T cells

Taylor, Brostoff & Hughes (1991) found T cells responsive to myelin P_2 protein in the blood of some GBS patients, but not in CIDP patients. Lin *et al.* (1982) reported T cells responsive to P_2 protein in a patient with CIDP. A later study found that T cells responsive to P_2 or P_0 protein were present in six of 13 CIDP patients compared with four of 17 normal controls (Khalili Shirazi *et al.*, 1992).

Antibodies

The response to plasmapheresis (see below) suggested that antibody might play a role in the pathogenesis of CIDP as it does in myasthenia gravis, which also responds to plasma exchange. However, antibodies to peripheral nerve antigens have been difficult to demonstrate in the sera of patients with CIDP. Circulating antibodies to peripheral nerve (Nyland & Aarli, 1978), myelin (McCombe *et al.*, 1988), and P_2 and P_0 proteins (Khalili Shirazi *et al.*, 1993) have been found in only a minority of CIDP patients. Antibodies to Schwann cells and galactocerebroside were not present in the serum in CIDP patients (McCombe *et al.*, 1988). Occasional CIDP patients have circulating antibodies directed against the ganglioside GM1 (McCombe, Wilson & Prentice, 1992; Simone *et al.*, 1993). Circulating antibodies to neuroblastoma cells have also been reported in CIDP patients (van Doorn, Brand & Vermeulen, 1988). Antibodies to tubulin have been found in 57% of CIDP patients, 20% of GBS patients and 2% of controls (Connolly *et al.*, 1993). The role of antibodies in the pathogenesis of CIDP is not clear, as it has been shown that patients with other neuropathies such as Charcot–Marie–Tooth disease have anti-myelin antibodies, which probably arise as a response to tissue damage (Cruz *et al.*, 1988).

Toxic factors in the serum

Serum from patients with CIDP contains a factor that is cytotoxic to Schwann cells in culture (Armati & Pollard, 1987). CIDP serum does not usually cause demyelination in rat nerves after intraneural inoculation

(McCombe *et al.*, 1988). However, Heininger *et al.* (1984) demonstrated slowing of conduction velocities in monkey nerves after injection of CIDP serum.

Immunological findings in the cerebrospinal fluid

In CIDP there may be marked elevation of the CSF protein levels (Dyck *et al.*, 1975; McCombe *et al.*, 1987*b*). This elevation is usually associated with increases in both CSF albumin and immunoglobulin levels and indicates leakage of protein from the blood. However, there may also be intrathecal synthesis of immunoglobulin. Dalakas & Engel (1980) found monoclonal IgG bands in the CSF of 14 of 15 CIDP patients and McCombe *et al.* (1991*a*) found a monoclonal IgA band in the CSF of one patient with CIDP. Increased IL-6 levels were found in the CSF of 43% of CIDP patients (Maimone *et al.*, 1993).

Therapy

Corticosteroids

As already mentioned, the responsiveness to corticosteroids is a characteristic feature of CIDP. Controlled studies have confirmed that some CIDP patients respond to oral corticosteroids (Dyck *et al.*, 1982*a*). Some CIDP patients become dependent on these corticosteroids and experience relapses when the treatment is withdrawn ('pharmacorelapses') (Matthews, Howell & Hughes, 1970). The best response to corticosteroids occurs with shorter duration of disease, and rapid reduction in the dose is associated with relapses (Wertman, Argov & Abramsky, 1988).

Plasmapheresis

Early uncontrolled studies suggested that plasma exchange may be useful in CIDP (Server *et al.*, 1979; Gross & Thomas, 1981). Dyck *et al.* (1986) performed a double-blind trial and confirmed this benefit. Pollard *et al.* (1983) showed that patients with axonal degeneration respond poorly to plasma exchange.

Intravenous immunoglobulin

Intravenous immunoglobulin was used in CIDP because of the possibility that the benefits of plasma exchange might be due to the replacement fluid rather than the removal of plasma. Vermeulen *et al.* (1985) found that infusion of fresh frozen plasma was beneficial in CIDP. This was followed by reports of successful high-dose immunoglobulin therapy in adults (Faed *et al.*, 1989; Cornblath, Chaudry & Griffin, 1991*a*) and children (Vedanarayanan *et al.*, 1991). A double-blind placebo-controlled trial confirmed that high- dose immunoglobulin was effective in CIDP (van Doorn *et al.*, 1990*a*) and the investigators suggested that the benefits were due to anti-idiotype antibodies (van Doorn *et al.*, 1990*b*). However, a subsequent double-blind trial did not confirm the initial findings (Vermeulen *et al.*, 1993) and the authors suggested that a subgroup of CIDP patients may benefit from immunoglobulin therapy. One complication has been recurrent aseptic meningitis in a CIDP patient treated with intravenous immunoglobulin (Vera Ramirez, Charlet & Parry, 1992).

Other immunosuppressive agents

In uncontrolled trials, cyclosporin A was shown to be helpful in the management of patients with CIDP (Jongen *et al.*, 1988; Hodgkinson, Pollard & McLeod, 1990) and with CIDP associated with IgG paraproteinaemia (Waterston *et al.*, 1992). The chief side-effect was nephrotoxicity (Kolkin, Nahman & Mendell, 1987). Further studies are required to define the role of cyclosporin in therapy of CIDP. There are uncontrolled studies indicating that azathioprine may be helpful in CIDP (Palmer, 1966; Yuill, Swinburn & Liversedge, 1970; Walker, 1979; Pentland, 1980; Pentland, Adams & Mawdsley, 1982) and azathioprine is widely used as a steroid-sparing agent in CIDP. In a controlled trial, azathioprine was added to prednisone treatment, and shown to provide no additional benefit (Dyck *et al.*, 1985). Cyclophosphamide is not commonly used in the treatment of CIDP, although the successful use of oral cyclophosphamide has been reported (Prineas & McLeod, 1976) and intravenous cyclophosphamide is used in the treatment of patients with multifocal motor neuropathy (see below), which may be a variant of CIDP with prominent focal demyelination of motor nerves.

Multifocal motor neuropathy

Introduction

Multifocal motor neuropathy (MMN) is a recently described syndrome presenting with progressive weakness and wasting, evidence of mutifocal conduction block on careful neurophysiological testing and, often, with high titres of circulating antibodies to the ganglioside GM1 (Parry & Clarke, 1988). Patients with such a condition were described by Lewis *et al.* (1982), who suggested that this condition was a variant of CIDP. Other patients with MMN were described by Parry & Clarke (1988), who commented that the slowly progressive weakness resembled motor neurone disease. Other patients are described who have lower motor neurone weakness affecting the proximal or distal limb muscles and circulating anti-GM1 antibodies, but no evidence of multifocal conduction block: such patients do not have MMN (Pestronk *et al.*, 1990; Pestronk, 1991). It now seems likely that MMN may represent a variant of CIDP (Parry & Sumner, 1992). It is important to make the diagnosis, because aggressive therapy may be beneficial (see below).

Clinical features

Clinical symptoms and signs

Patients with MMN have progressive weakness and wasting of the limb muscles, and the deep tendon reflexes are reduced. The weakness may be asymmetrical. There may be wasting of the tongue (Kaji, Shibasaki & Kimura, 1992). Although patients with MMN usually have a pure motor neuropathy, sensory abnormalities are sometimes reported to be present (Lewis *et al.*, 1982; Parry & Clarke, 1988).

Diagnosis

The diagnosis of MMN depends on the demonstration of multifocal conduction block by neurophysiological techniques. Many neuropathies such as GBS and CIDP may have conduction block, but MMN requires the demonstration of block across a small segment. Patients with MMN are clinically similar to patients with progressive muscular atrophy, the lower motor neurone form of motor neurone disease (Lange *et al.*, 1992) and other lower motor neurone syndromes that are not associated with conduction block (Pestronk, 1991). Pestronk *et al.* (1990) found that a combination of electrophysiological and clinical findings defines MMN patients. Others experience more difficulty in separating MMN from other causes of lower motor neurone weakness and from demyelinating neuropathies such as CIDP. It would appear that clear evidence of multifocal conduction block is the most important diagnostic feature of MMN, although it must be noted that true conduction block can be difficult to distinguish from changes due to dispersion of the compound muscle action potential (Cornblath *et al.*, 1991*b*).

Neuropathology

A biopsy from the region of conduction block in a patient with MMN showed a perivascular area of scattered demyelination and small onion bulb formation (Kaji *et al.*, 1993). In other patients with MMN the sural nerve, a sensory nerve, was normal (Feldman *et al.*, 1991). IgM has been demonstrated at the nodes of Ranvier in the peripheral nerve of a patient with multifocal conduction block, anti-GM1 antibodies and motor neurone disease (Santoro *et al.*, 1990). Further studies of the pathology of the nerves in MMN are needed to define the features of this disease. It will be important to determine whether there is deposition of antibody on motor nerves and whether this is associated with morphological changes such paranodal damage or segmental demyelination and inflammation.

Immunological findings in the peripheral blood

Circulating antiganglioside antibodies

Anti-ganglioside antibodies are found in the sera of many patients with MMN, but are not specific for MMN. Circulating antibodies to gangliosides, including GM1, occur in the Guillain–Barré syndrome and CIDP (McCombe *et al.*, 1992; Heidenreich, Leifeld & Jovin, 1994), motor neurone disease and certain paraproteinaemic neuropathies (Pestronk *et al.*, 1990; Pestronk, 1991). There is considerable cross-reactivity between antibodies to gangliosides. In MMN the important target of anti-ganglioside antibodies is GM1, but there may be considerable heterogeneity of these antibodies (Baba *et al.*, 1989). The anti-GM1 antibodies react with the galactosyl-(β1–3)-*N*-acetyl-galactosamine epitope (Sadiq *et al.*, 1990; Lugaresi *et al.*, 1991). Kornberg & Pestronk (1994) have found that sera from patients with MMN are characterized by elevated levels of IgM antibodies to GM1 and a white matter antigen NP-9 and reduced levels of antibody to histone 3. Others have attempted to find the cellular target of the anti-GM1 antibodies. Anti-GM1 antibodies bind to motor neurones in the spinal cord but not to dorsal root ganglion cells (Lugaresi *et al.*, 1991; Corbo *et al.*, 1992). In addition, anti-GM1 antibodies bind to perineuronal networks and to the nodes of Ranvier (Nardelli *et al.*, 1994). Anti-GM1 antibodies bind to glycoproteins as well as gangliosides, suggesting that glycoproteins could also be the target of the antibodies (Lugaresi *et al.*, 1991). The B cells that secrete the anti-ganglioside antibodies are T cell dependent (Heidenreich *et al.*, 1994).

Experimental studies

Injection of serum containing anti-GM1 antibodies from a patient with multifocal conduction block led to deposition of IgM in rat nerve (Santoro *et al.*, 1990) and conduction block and demyelination at the site of the injection (Santoro *et al.*, 1992). A later study showed that such changes are produced by anti-GM1 serum from patients with MMN but not from patients with progressive muscular atrophy, the lower motor neurone form of motor neurone disease (Uncini *et al.*, 1993). Parry (1994) interprets this as indicating that factors other than anti-GM1 antibodies are responsible for the experimental demyelination. Kaji *et al.* (1994) have suggested that anti-GM1 antibodies impair remyelination and thus contribute to the continuation of conduction block.

Therapy

Patients with MMN fail to respond to corticosteroids or plasmapheresis and indeed may become worse after oral prednisolone therapy (Donaghy *et al.*, 1994). However, patients with MMN may improve after treatment with intravenous cyclophosphamide (Pestronk *et al.*, 1988; Feldman *et al.*, 1991). Because of the potential toxicity, this treatment should be reserved for patients with clear MMN, as patients with other lower motor neurone syndromes do not have a good response to cyclophosphamide (Pestronk *et al.*, 1990; Pestronk, 1991). Initial reports showed that some patients with MMN improved with high-dose intravenous immunoglobulin therapy (Kaji *et al.*, 1992; Chaudhry *et al.*, 1993; Nobile Orazio *et al.*, 1993; Donaghy *et al.*, 1994). A controlled trial has confirmed that patients with MMN, with anti-GM1 antibodies and conduction block, benefit from intravenous immunoglobulin (Azulay *et al.*, 1994). The apparent improvement after immunoglobulin infusion, but not after plasmapheresis, suggests that components of the infused immunoglobulin, such as anti-idiotypic antibodies, may be beneficial.

Neuropathies associated with paraproteinaemias

Introduction

Neuropathies are recognized complications of multiple myeloma, Waldenström's macroglobulinaemia and cryoglobulinaemia. Since the report of Forssman *et al.* (1973), neuropathies have also been recognized in patients with monoclonal gammopathy not associated with haematological disease (monoclonal gammopathies of unknown significance [MGUS]). The paraproteins associated with malignancy may not differ greatly from those of the MGUS. Kyle (1992) reported that 22% of patients with a benign gammopathy later developed evidence of conditions such as myeloma. At times, the neuropathy associated with a paraprotein may be due to physical disturbances such as ischaemia secondary to the intravascular precipitation of protein (Prior *et al.*, 1992). In other cases the paraprotein may be involved in the pathogenesis of the neuropathy through immunological means. In this section, the neuropathies associated with paraproteins will be discussed according to the subtype of immunoglobulin (IgG, IgM or IgA). The neuropathies associated with paraproteinaemias can also be classified on the basis of the underlying pathology in the nerve (demyelination or axonal damage) or according to the target antigen for the antibody. Patients with primary inflammatory neuropathies such as CIDP or GBS may also have a circulating monoclonal protein, or may develop the monoclonal band during the course of the illness. One study found little difference between CIDP patients with MGUS and CIDP patients without MGUS (Bromberg *et al.*, 1992). This could indicate that the monoclonal protein in CIDP is not of primary pathogenic significance, but is a response to the disease.

Incidence of neuropathy with MGUS

In about 10% of patients with undiagnosed neuropathy, monoclonal immunoglobulin bands can be demonstrated in the serum (Bosch & Smith, 1993). Kelly *et al.* (1981*b*) found that 2.5% of patients with neuropathy associated with systemic disease and 10% of patients with neuropathy unassociated with systemic disease had a circulating monoclonal immunoglobulin. From the other point of view, other studies found that 58–71% of patients with monoclonal gammopathy had evidence of neuropathy (Osby *et al.*, 1982; Vrethem *et al.*, 1993).

Clinical features

Neuropathies associated with IgM paraproteins

Neuropathy occurs in patients with Waldenström's macroglobulinaemia (Logothetis, Silverstein & Coe, 1960) and with cryoglobulinaemia. In 1973, neuropathy was reported in a patient with an IgM MGUS (Forssman *et al.*, 1973). Subsequent studies have shown that neuropathy occurs in 31% of IgM MGUS (Nobile Orazio *et al.*, 1992). Neuropathies associated with IgM

MGUS are well characterized and can be clinically separated from those associated with other types of MGUS (Gosselin, Kyle & Dyck, 1991). The clinical features vary according to the target of the IgM paraprotein. The neuropathy associated with an antibody to myelin-associated glycoprotein (MAG) is a chronic sensorimotor neuropathy, usually in later life (Smith *et al.*, 1983). Patients may have tremor and ataxia. Two patients reported by Sherman *et al.* (1983) had a syndrome of sensory neuropathy and epidermolysis in association with an IgM kappa antibody directed against chondroitin sulphate. Quattrini *et al.* (1991) also reported a patient with a sensory neuropathy and an IgM MGUS reactive with chondroitin sulphate. A patient reported by Yee *et al.* (1989) had a neuropathy with features of mononeuritis multiplex with an IgM antibody to chondroitin sulfate and to neural proteins. Other patients with IgM MGUS have motor neuropathy and conduction block and antibodies to GM1 (Sadiq *et al.*, 1990) and fall into the category of MMN (see above). Patients with MMN with an IgM paraprotein do not differ from those without a paraprotein.

Neuropathies associated with IgG paraproteins

Neuropathy can occur with myeloma (Kelly *et al.*, 1981*a*), often as a subclinical disorder (Walsh, 1971). Neuropathy also occurs in 6% of patients with IgG MGUS (Nobile Orazio *et al.*, 1992). A variety of clinical disorders have been described in the neuropathy accompanying IgG paraproteinaemia. For example, Nobile Orazio *et al.* (1992) found that the neuropathy associated with IgG MGUS had prominent motor involvement. Others (Read, Vanhegan & Matthews, 1978; Sewell *et al.*, 1981) have described patients with prominent weakness accompanied by sensory loss. Bleasel *et al.* (1993) and Contamin *et al.* (1976) described patients with IgG paraproteins and a relapsing–remitting course of a sensorimotor neuropathy.

Neuropathies associated with IgA paraproteins

A mixed sensorimotor neuropathy has been reported in IgA myeloma (Dhib-Jalbut & Liwnicz, 1986). Neuropathies associated with IgA MGUS are less common than those associated with IgG and IgM MGUS. In the series of Gosselin *et al.* (1991), only ten of 65 patients with MGUS and neuropathy had an IgA paraprotein. Simmons *et al.* (1993) reported that patients with IgA MGUS-associated neuropathy experienced painful paraesthesiae, with sensory loss and/or weakness. In two of the three patients described by Nemni *et al.* (1991), burning paraesthesiae were also a prominent feature. Bailey *et al.* (1986) described a patient with an IgA lambda protein and neuropathy with dysautonomia.

Pathophysiology

Neuropathies associated with IgM paraproteins

In one group of 23 patients with neuropathy associated with IgM MGUS, there was slowing of mean nerve conduction velocity and prolongation of the mean distal latency, suggestive of primary demyelination (Suarez & Kelly, 1993). However, within the group some patients had nerve conduction studies suggestive of axonal neuropathy. In anti-MAG neuropathy there is usually evidence of severe conduction slowing, indicating demyelination (Smith *et al.*, 1983). Suarez & Kelly (1993) found that the neurophysiological features of patients with IgM MGUS and anti-MAG antibody could not be distinguished from those with IgM MGUS without anti-MAG activity.

Neuropathies associated with IgG paraproteins

In a group of patients with neuropathy associated with IgG MGUS, there was no significant slowing of mean nerve conduction although electromyographic studies showed mild chronic denervation of the distal muscles of the lower limbs (Suarez & Kelly, 1993). In the study of Bleasel *et al.* (1993), four of five patients had marked slowing of conduction velocities, suggestive of demyelination.

Neuropathies associated with IgA paraproteins

Simmons *et al.* (1993) reported the electrophysiological findings of five patients with neuropathy associated with an IgA MGUS: there was no clear pattern of abnormality, with one patient having nerve conduction studies consistent with primary demyelination and the others having evidence of varying degrees of axonal degeneration. Hemachudha *et al.* (1989) reported a patient with an IgA paraprotein and serum anti-MAG antibody, who had slowing of motor nerve conduction.

Neuropathology

Neuropathies associated with IgM paraproteins

In many patients with IgM MGUS associated neuropathy, there is a widening of the myelin lamellae (Vital *et al.*, 1989). In anti-MAG neuropathy there is primary demyelination, without inflammation (Smith *et al.*,

1983) and widening of the myelin lamellae along the intraperiod line. IgM kappa paraproteins have also been described in patients with axonal polyneuropathy and antibody to chondroitin sulphate (Sherman *et al.*, 1983; Quattrini *et al.*, 1991). In one of these cases the antibody bound to Schmidt–Lanterman incisures (Quattrini *et al.*, 1991).

Neuropathies associated with IgG paraproteins

The pathological findings with IgG MGUS-associated neuropathy have included axonal degeneration (Nobile Orazio *et al.*, 1992), although some patients have had primary demyelination (Bleasel *et al.*, 1993).

Neuropathies associated with IgA paraproteins

Sural nerve biopsies from four patients with IgA MGUS-associated neuropathy were found to have a mixture of axonal degeneration and demyelination (Simmons *et al.*, 1993). In these nerves there was no evidence of the widening of the myelin lamellae that is found in some IgM paraprotein-associated neuropathies. Another study of sural nerves from three patients with IgA MGUS-associated neuropathy found axonal degeneration (Nemni *et al.*, 1991).

Immunopathology of the peripheral nerves

Little is known about the immunopathology of the peripheral nerves in neuropathies associated with paraproteinaemia. IgM is found bound to the myelin sheaths of peripheral nerve in anti-MAG neuropathy, and complement is also present (Hays *et al.*, 1988). McCombe *et al.* (1988) also found binding of IgM to myelin in three patients with IgM- kappa-associated neuropathy. Deposition of immunoglobulin and complement has been found in peripheral nerve from some patients with IgG MGUS-associated neuropathy (Sewell *et al.*, 1981; Bleasel *et al.*, 1993), but others have failed to find such immunoglobulin deposition (Read *et al.*, 1978; Nobile Orazio *et al.*, 1992).

IgA lambda was found in the peripheral nerve of a patient with osteosclerotic myeloma and peripheral neuropathy (Rousseau *et al.*, 1978). Simmons *et al.* (1993) did not find evidence of IgA bound to peripheral nerve in three patients with neuropathy associated with IgA MGUS. However, Bailey *et al.* (1986) found IgA and kappa light chains bound to the biopsied peripheral nerve of a patient with IgA kappa MGUS and neuropathy.

Immunological findings in the peripheral blood

Neuropathies associated with IgM paraproteins

The target antigen has been identified for a number of IgM paraproteins associated with neuropathy. The first target to be identified was MAG (Latov *et al.*, 1980; Braun, Frail & Latov, 1982). Anti-MAG antibodies appear to be directed against glycolipid determinants on the MAG molecule (Ilyas *et al.*, 1992; van den Berg *et al.*, 1993). Pestronk *et al.* (1994) have shown that Western blot analysis is the best method for identifying anti-MAG antibodies. Studies of the sequence of anti-MAG antibodies from different patients showed that all antibodies were members of the VH3 gene family (Ayadi *et al.*, 1992; Spatz *et al.*, 1992). Intraneural injection of serum from a patient with an IgM kappa MGUS and typical anti-MAG neuropathy did not cause disease in rats (Bosch *et al.*, 1982). However, injection of anti-MAG serum into cat sciatic nerve did cause demyelination (Hays *et al.*, 1987). Passive transfer of anti-MAG antiserum into chickens caused a demyelinating neuropathy (Tatum, 1993). In some patients with IgM MGUS-associated neuropathy, the paraproteins are directed against other targets including the gangliosides GM1 and GD1b (Daune *et al.*, 1992; Ilyas *et al.*, 1992) and sulphatides (van den Berg *et al.*, 1993). Chondroitin sulphate (Sherman *et al.*, 1983) may also be a target.

Neuropathies associated with IgG paraproteins and IgA paraproteins

No target antigen has been identified for the IgG monoclonal proteins. Bleasel *et al.* (1993) found that their patients with IgG paraprotein-associated neuropathy did not have elevated serum anti-myelin antibodies. Hemachudha *et al.* (1989) described a patient with neuropathy, IgA lambda MGUS and evidence of serum anti-MAG activity. Nemni *et al.* (1991) described three patients with IgA MGUS and neuropathy: these patients had circulating IgG, which reacted with a 66-kDa axonal protein and which stained axons. The IgA lambda paraprotein from a patient with sensorimotor neuropathy associated with myeloma bound to peripheral nerve from another subject and, by immunoblot analysis, reacted with three different molecular weight myelin components (Dhib-Jalbut & Liwnicz, 1986).

Therapy

Neuropathies associated with IgM paraproteins

Although there are no controlled studies of the use of corticosteroids in patients with IgM MGUS, corticosteroids are frequently used in association with other agents as treatment of such patients (Kelly *et al.*, 1988; Nobile-Orazio *et al.*, 1988). There are reports of patients who do not appear to benefit from corticosteroids and require other forms of treatment (Cook *et al.*, 1990). Plasmapheresis appears to be helpful in IgM neuropathy (Ernerudh *et al.*, 1986; Dyck *et al.*, 1991). Haas & Tatum (1988) found that removal of anti-MAG antibody by plasmapheresis was associated with clinical improvement. Cook *et al.* (1990) reported that two patients with neuropathy associated with an IgM monoclonal paraprotein, who had failed to respond to corticosteroid or immunosuppressive therapy, had rapid clinical improvement after treatment with high-dose intravenous immunoglobulin therapy. In anti-MAG neuropathy, immunosuppressive treatment with cytotoxic agents or plasmapheresis is beneficial in some patients (Kelly *et al.*, 1988; Haas & Tatum, 1988). Nobile-Orazio *et al.* (1988) found that two of five patients had clinical improvement and a decline in the levels of anti-MAG antibody after treatment with chlorambucil and prednisone.

Neuropathies associated with IgG paraproteins and IgA paraproteins

Corticosteroids may be helpful in neuropathy associated with IgG MGUS (Contamin *et al.*, 1976). Plasmapheresis is also of benefit in this neuropathy (Dyck *et al.*, 1991; Bleasel *et al.*, 1993). One patient with IgA MGUS and antibodies to MAG responded to prednisone treatment (Hemachudha *et al.*, 1989). Of the five patients with IgA MGUS reported by Simmons *et al.* (1993), three improved with prednisone or immunoglobulin therapy.

Conclusions

CIDP, MMN and the neuropathies associated with paraproteinaemia are important, because these conditions are potentially treatable. In these conditions T cells and antibodies are implicated, to varying degrees, in the pathogenesis. To some extent, the target antigens for the immune system have been identified. However, the pathogenic mechanisms are not yet fully established. Furthermore, the fundamental abnormality, presumably one of immunoregulation, that permits the development of these conditions is unknown. Future developments are likely to come from immunogenetic studies, studies of the mechanisms of tolerance to autoantigens and the effects of outside agents (such as microorganisms) in overcoming tolerance.

References

Ad Hoc Subcommittee of the American Academy of Neurology AIDS Task Force (1991). Research criteria for diagnosis of chronic inflammatory demyelinating polyneuropathy (CIDP). *Neurology*, **41**, 617–18.

Armati, P.J. & Pollard, J.D. (1987). Cytotoxic response of serum from patients with chronic inflammatory demyelinating polyradiculoneuropathy (CIDP) *Acta Neurologica Scandinavica*, **76**, 24–7.

Atkinson, P.F., Perry, M.E., Hall, S.M. & Hughes, R.A.C. (1993). Immunoelectronmicroscopical demonstration of major histocompatibility class II antigen: expression on endothelial and perivascular cells but not Schwann cells in human neuropathy. *Neuropathology and Applied Neurobiology*, **19**, 22–30.

Austin, J.H. (1958). Recurrent polyneuropathies and their corticosteroid treatment. With five-year observations of a placebo-controlled case treated with corticotrophin, cortisone, and prednisone. *Brain*, **81**, 11–192.

Ayadi, H., Mihaesco, E., Congy, N., Roy, J.-P., Gendron, M.-C., Laperriere, J., Prelli, J.-P., Frangione, B. & Brouet, J.-C. (1992). H chain V region sequences of three human monoclonal IgM with anti-myelin-associated glycoprotein activity. *Journal of Immunology*, **148**, 2812–16.

Azulay, J.P., Blin, O., Pouget, J., Boucraut, J., Bille-Turc, F., Carles, G. & Serratrice, G. (1994). Intravenous immunoglobulin treatment in patients with motor neuron syndromes associated with anti-GM1 antibodies. *Neurology*, **44**, 429–32.

Baba, H., Daune, G.C., Ilyas, A.A., Pestronk, A., Cornblath, D.R., Chaudhry, V., Griffin, J.W. & Quarles, R.H. (1989). Anti-GM1 ganglioside antibodies with differing fine specificities in patients with multifocal motor neuropathy. *Journal of Neuroimmunology*, **25**, 143–50.

Bailey, R.O., Ritaccio, A.L., Bishop, M.B. & Wu, A.Y. (1986). Benign monoclonal IgA kappa gammopathy associated with polyneuropathy and dysautonomia. *Acta Neurologica Scandinavica*, **73**, 574–80.

Barohn, R.J., Kissel, J.T., Warmolts, J.R. & Mendell, J.R. (1989). Chronic inflammatory demyelinating polyradiculoneuropathy. Clinical characteristics, course, and recommendations for diagnostic criteria. *Archives of Neurology*, **46**, 878–84.

Bleasel, A.F., Hawke, S.H.B., Pollard, J.D. & McLeod, J.G. (1993). IgG monoclonal paraproteinemia and peripheral neuropathy. *Journal of Neurology, Neurosurgery and Psychiatry*, **56**, 52–7.

Bosch, E.P., Ansbacher, L.E., Goeken, J.A. & Cancilla, P.A. (1982). Peripheral neuropathy associated with monoclonal gammopathy. Studies of intraneural injections of monoclonal immunoglobulin sera. *Journal of Neuropathology and Experimental Neurology*, **41**, 446–59.

Bosch, E.P. & Smith, B.E. (1993). Peripheral neuropathies associated with monoclonal proteins. *Medical Clinics of North America*, **77**, 125–39.

Braun, P.E., Frail, D.E. & Latov, N. (1982). Myelin-associated glycoprotein is the antigen for a monoclonal IgM in polyneuropathy. *Journal of Neurochemistry*, **39**, 1261–5.

Bromberg, M.B. (1991). Comparison of electrodiagnostic criteria for primary demyelination in chronic polyneuropathy. *Muscle and Nerve*, **14**, 968–76.

Bromberg, M.B., Feldman, E.L. & Albers, J.W. (1992). Chronic inflammatory demyelinating polyradiculoneuropathy: comparison of patients with and without an associated monoclonal gammopathy. *Neurology*, **42**, 1157–63.

Chaudhry, V., Corse, A.M., Cornblath, D.R., Kuncl, R.W., Drachman, D.B., Freimer, M.L., Miller, R.G. & Griffin, J.W. (1993). Multifocal motor neuropathy: response to human immune globulin. *Annals of Neurology*, **33**, 237–42.

Chou, S.M. (1992). Immunohistochemical and ultrastructural classification of peripheral neuropathies with onion-bulbs. *Clinical Neuropathology*, **11**, 109–14.

Connolly, A.M., Pestronk, A., Trotter, J.L., Feldman, E.L., Cornblath, D.R. & Olney, R.K. (1993). High-titer selective serum anti-beta-tubulin antibodies in chronic inflammatory demyelinating polyneuropathy. *Neurology*, **43**, 557–62.

Contamin, F., Singer, B., Mignot, B., Ecoffet, M. & Kazatchine, M. (1976). Polyneuropathy a rechutes, évoluant depuis 19 ans, associée a une gammapathie monoclonale IgG bénigne. Effet favorable de la corticothérapie. *Revue Neurologique*, **132**, 741–62.

Cook, D., Dalakas, M., Galdi, A., Biondi, D. & Porter, H. (1990). High-dose intravenous immunoglobulin in the treatment of demyelinating neuropathy associated with monoclonal gammopathy. *Neurology*, **40**, 212–14.

Corbo, M., Quattrini, A., Lugaresi, A., Santoro, M., Latov, N. & Hays, A.P. (1992). Patterns of reactivity of human anti-GM1 antibodies with spinal cord and motor neurons. *Annals of Neurology*, **32**, 487–93.

Cornblath, D.R., Chaudry, V. & Griffin, J.W. (1991*a*). Treatment of chronic inflammatory demyelinating polyneuropathy with intravenous immunoglobulin. *Annals of Neurology*, **30**, 104–6.

Cornblath, D.R., Sumner, A.J., Daube, J., Gilliatt, R.W., Brown, W.F., Parry, G.J., Albers, J.W., Miller, R.G. & Petajan, J. (1991*b*). Conduction block in clinical practice. *Muscle and Nerve*, **14**, 869–71.

Cruz, M., Ernerudh, J., Olsson, T., Hojeberg, B. & Link, H. (1988). Occurrence and isotype of antibodies against peripheral nerve myelin in serum from patients with peripheral neuropathy and healthy controls. *Journal of Neurology, Neurosurgery and Psychiatry*, **51**, 820–5.

Dalakas, M.C. & Engel, W.K. (1980). Immunoglobulin and complement deposits in nerves of patients with chronic relapsing polyneuropathy. *Archives of Neurology*, **37**, 637–40.

Dalakas, M.C. & Engel, W.K. (1981). Chronic relapsing (dysimmune) polyneuropathy: pathogenesis and treatment. *Annals of Neurology*, **9 (Supplement)**, 134–45.

Dalakas, M.C., Teravainen, H. & Engel, W.K. (1984). Tremor as a feature of chronic relapsing and dysglobulinemic polyneuropathies. Incidence and management. *Archives of Neurology*, **41**, 711–14.

Daune, G.C., Farrer, R.G., Dalakas, M.C. & Quarles, R.H. (1992). Sensory neuropathy associated with monoclonal immunoglobulin M to GD1b ganglioside. *Annals of Neurology*, **31**, 683–5.

Dhib-Jalbut, S. & Liwnicz, B.H. (1986). Binding of serum IgA of multiple myeloma to normal peripheral nerve. *Acta Neurologica Scandinavica*, **73**, 381–7.

Donaghy, M., Mills, K.R., Boniface, S.J., Simmons, J., Wright, I., Gregson, N. & Jacobs, J. (1994). Pure motor demyelinating neuropathy: deterioration after steroid treatment and improvement with intravenous immunoglobulin. *Journal of Neurology, Neurosurgery and Psychiatry*, **57**, 778–83.

Dyck, P.J., Daube, J., O'Brien, P., Pineda, A., Low, P.A., Windebank, A.J. & Swanson, C. (1986). Plasma exchange in chronic inflammatory demyelinating polyradiculoneuropathy. *New England Journal of Medicine*, **314**, 461–5.

Dyck, P.J., Lais, A.C., Ohta, M., Bastron, J.A., Okazaki, H. & Groover, R.V. (1975). Chronic inflammatory polyradiculoneuropathy. *Mayo Clinic Proceedings*, **50**, 621–37.

Dyck, P.J., Low, P.A., Windebank, A.J., Jaradeh, S.S., Gosselin, S., Bourque, P., Smith, B.E., Kratz, K.M., Karnes, J.L., Evans, B.A., Pineda, A.A., O'Brien, P.C. & Kyle, R.A. (1991). Plasma exchange in polyneuropathy associated with monoclonal gammopathy of undetermined significance. *New England Journal of Medicine*, **325**, 1482–5.

Dyck, P.J., O'Brien, P., Swanson, C., Low, P. & Daube, J. (1985). Combined azathioprine and prednisone in chronic inflammatory–demyelinating polyneuropathy. *Neurology*, **35**, 1173–6.

Dyck, P.J., O'Brien, P.C., Oviatt, K., Dinapoli, R.P., Daube, J.R., Bartleson, J.D., Mokri, B., Swift, T., Low, P.A. & Windebank, A.J. (1982*a*). Prednisone improves chronic inflammatory demyelinating polyradiculoneuropathy more than no treatment. *Annals of Neurology*, **11**, 136–41.

Dyck, P.J., Swanson, C.J., Low, P.A., Bartelson, J.D. & Lambert, E.H. (1982*b*). Prednisone-responsive hereditary motor and sensory neuropathy. *Mayo Clinic Proceedings*, **57**, 239–46.

Ernerudh, J., Brodtkorb, E., Olsson, T., Vedeler, C.A., Nyland, H. & Berlin, G. (1986). Peripheral neuropathy and monoclonal IgM with antibody activity against peripheral nerve myelin; effect of plasma exchange. *Journal of Neuroimmunology*, **11**, 171–8.

Faed, J.M., Day, B., Pollock, M., Taylor, P.K., Nukada, H. & Hammond-Tocke, G.D. (1989). High-dose intravenous human immunoglobulin in chronic inflammatory demyelinating polyneuropathy. *Neurology*, **39**, 422–5.

Feasby, T.E., Brown, W.F., Gilbert, J.J. & Hahn, A.F. (1985). The pathological basis of conduction block in human neuropathies. *Journal of Neurology, Neurosurgery and Psychiatry*, **48**, 239–44.

Feasby, T.E., Hahn, A.F., Koopman, W.J. & Lee, D.H. (1990) Central lesions in chronic inflammatory demyelinating polyneuropathy: an MRI study. *Neurology*, **40**, 476–8.

Feeney, D.J., Pollard, J.D., McLeod, J.G., Stewart, G.J. & De Lange, G.G. (1989). Gm haplotypes in inflammatory demyelinating polyneuropathies. *Annals of Neurology*, **26**, 790–2.

Feeney, D.J., Pollard, J.D., McLeod, J.G., Stewart, G.J. & Doran, T.J. (1990). HLA antigens in chronic inflammatory demyelinating polyneuropathy. *Journal of Neurology, Neurosurgery and Psychiatry*, **53**, 170–2.

Feldman, E.L., Bromberg, M.B., Albers, J.W. & Pestronk, A. (1991). Immunosuppressive treatment in multifocal motor neuropathy. *Annals of Neurology*, **30**, 397–401.

Forssman, O., Bjorkman, M.L., Hollender, A. & Englund, N.E. (1973). IgM-producing lymphocytes in peripheral nerves in a patient with benign monoclonal gammopathy. *Scandinavian Journal of Haematology*, **11**, 332–5.

Gibbels, E. & Kentenich, M. (1990). Unmyelinated fibers in sural nerve biopsies of chronic inflammatory demyelinating polyneuropathy. *Acta Neuropathologica*, **80**, 439–47.

Gigli, G.L., Carlesimo, A., Valente, M., Mazza, S., Di Trapani, G., Hernandez, R. & Tomassetti, P. (1989). Evoked potentials suggest cranial nerves and CNS involvement in chronic relapsing polyradiculoneuropathy. *European Neurology*, **29**, 145–9.

Gosselin, S., Kyle, R.A. & Dyck, P.J. (1991). Neuropathy associated with monoclonal gammopathies of undetermined significance. *Annals of Neurology*, **30**, 54–61.

Grand'Maison, F., Feasby, T.E., Hahn, A.F. & Koopman, W.J. (1992). Recurrent Guillain–Barré syndrome. Clinical and laboratory features. *Brain*, **115**, 1093–106.

Gross, M.L. & Thomas, P.K. (1981). The treatment of chronic relapsing and chronic progressive idiopathic inflammatory polyneuropathy by plasma exchange. *Journal of the Neurological Sciences*, **52**, 69–78.

Haas, D.C. & Tatum, A.H. (1988). Plasmapheresis alleviates neuropathy accompanying IgM anti-myelin-associated glycoprotein paraproteinemia. *Annals of Neurology*, **23**, 394–6.

Harris, W. & Newcomb, W.D. (1929). A case of relapsing interstitial hypertrophic polyneuritis. *Brain*, **52**, 108–16.

Hartung, H.-P., Hughes, R.A., Taylor, W.A., Heininger, K., Reiners, K. & Toyka, K.V. (1990). T cell activation in Guillain–Barré syndrome and in MS: elevated serum levels of soluble IL-2 receptors. *Neurology*, **40**, 215–18.

Hartung, H.-P., Reiners, K., Schmidt, B., Stoll, G. & Toyka, K.V. (1991). Serum interleukin-2 concentrations in Guillain–Barré syndrome and chronic idiopathic demyelinating polyradiculoneuropathy: comparison with other neurological diseases of presumed immunopathogenesis. *Annals of Neurology*, **30**, 48–53.

Hawke, S.H., Hallinan, J.M. & McLeod, J.G. (1990). Cranial magnetic resonance imaging in chronic demyelinating polyneuropathy. *Journal of Neurology, Neurosurgery and Psychiatry*, **53**, 794–6.

Hays, A.P., Latov, N., Takatsu, M. & Sherman, W.H. (1987). Experimental demylination of nerve induced by serum of patients with neuropathy and an anti-MAG IgM M-protein. *Neurology*, **372**, 242–56.

Hays, A.P., Lee, S.S.L. & Latov, N. (1988). Immune reactive C3d on the surface of myelin sheaths in neuropathy. *Journal of Neuroimmunology*, **18**, 231–44.

Heidenreich, F., Leifeld, L. & Jovin, T. (1994). T cell-dependent activity of ganglioside GM1-specific B cells in Guillain–Barré syndrome and multifocal motor neuropathy *in vitro*. *Journal of Neuroimmunology*, **49**, 97–108.

Heininger, K., Liebert, U.G., Toyka, K.V., Haneveld, F.T., Schwendemann, G., Kolb-Bachofen, V., Ross, H.-G., Cleveland, S., Besinger, U.A., Gibbels, E. & Wechsler, W. (1984). Chronic inflammatory polyneuropathy. Reduction of nerve conduction velocities in monkeys by systemic passive transfer of immunoglobulin G. *Journal of the Neurological Sciences*, **66**, 1–14.

Hemachudha, T., Phanuphak, P., Phanthumichinda, K. & Kasempinolporn, S. (1989). Proximal motor neuropathy, IgA paraproteinemia and anti-myelin-associated glycoprotein activity. *Postgraduate Medical Journal*, **65**, 662–4.

Hinman, R.C. & Magee, K.R. (1967). Guillain–Barré syndrome with slow progressive onset and persistent elevation of spinal fluid protein. *Annals of Internal Medicine*, **67**, 1007–12.

Hodgkinson, S.J., Pollard, J.D. & McLeod, J.G. (1990). Cyclosporin A in the treatment of chronic demyelinating polyradiculoneuropathy. *Journal of Neurology, Neurosurgery and Psychiatry*, **53**, 327–30.

Hyland, H.H. & Russell, W.R. (1930). Chronic progressive polyneuritis with report of a fatal case. *Brain*, **53**, 278–89.

Ilyas, A.A., Cook, S.D., Dalakas, M.C. & Mithen, F.A. (1992). Anti-MAG IgM paraproteins from some patients with polyneuropathy associated with IgM paraproteinemia also react with sulfatide. *Journal of Neuroimmunology*, **37**, 85–92.

Ingall, T.J., McLeod, J.G. & Tamura, N. (1990). Autonomic function and unmyelinated fibers in chronic inflammatory demyelinating polyradiculoneuropathy. *Muscle and Nerve*, **13**, 70–6.

Inoue, A., Tsukada, N., Koh, C.S. & Yanagisawa, N. (1987). Chronic relapsing demyelinating polyneuropathy associated with hapatitis B infection. *Neurology*, **37**, 1663–6.

Jongen, P.J., Joosten, E.M., Berden, J.H. & Gabreels Festen, A.A. (1988). Cyclosporine therapy in chronic inflammatory demyelinating polyradiculoneuropathy – a preliminary report of clinical results in two patients. *Transplantation Proceedings*, **20**, 329–32.

Julien, J., Vital, C., Lagueny, A., Ferrer, X. & Brechenmacher, C. (1989). Chronic relapsing idiopathic polyneuropathy with primary axonal lesions. *Journal of Neurology, Neurosurgery and Psychiatry*, **52**, 871–5.

Kaji, R., Hirota, N., Oka, N., Kohara, N., Watanabe, T., Nishio, T. & Kimura, J. (1994). Anti-GM1 antibodies and impaired blood–nerve barrier may interfere with remyelination in multifocal motor neuropathy. *Muscle and Nerve*, **17**, 108–10.

Kaji, R., Oka, N., Tsuji, T., Mezaki, T., Nishio, T., Akiguchi, I. & Kimura, J. (1993). Pathological findings at the site of conduction block in multifocal motor neuropathy. *Annals of Neurology*, **33**, 152–8.

Kaji, R., Shibasaki, H. & Kimura, J. (1992). Multifocal demyelinating motor neuropathy: cranial nerve involvement and immunoglobulin therapy. *Neurology*, **42**, 506–9.

Kamolvarin, N., Hemachudha, T., Ongpipattanakul, B., Phanthumchinda, K. & Sueblinvong, T. (1991). Plasma C3c in immune-mediated neurological diseases: a preliminary report. *Acta Neurologica Scandinavica*, **83**, 382–7.

Kelly, J.J., Adelman, L.S., Berkman, E. & Bhan, I. (1988). Polyneuropathies associated with IgM monoclonal gammopathies. *Archives of Neurology*, **45**, 1355–9.

Kelly, J.J., Kyle, R.A., Miles, J.M., O'Brien, P.C. & Dyck, P.J. (1981*a*). The spectrum of peripheral neuropathy in myeloma. *Neurology*, **31**, 24–31.

Kelly, J.J., Kyle, R.A., O'Brien, P.C. & Dyck, P.J. (1981*b*). Prevalence of monoclonal protein in peripheral neuropathy. *Neurology*, **31**, 1480–9.

Khalili Shirazi, A., Atkinson, P., Gregson, N. & Hughes, R.A. (1993). Antibody responses to P_0 and P_2 myelin proteins in Guillain–Barré syndrome and chronic idiopathic demyelinating polyradiculoneuropathy. *Journal of Neuroimmunology*, **46**, 245–51.

Khalili Shirazi, A., Hughes, R.A., Brostoff, S.W., Linington, C. & Gregson, N. (1992). T cell responses to myelin proteins in Guillain–Barré syndrome. *Journal of the Neurological Sciences*, **111**, 200–3.

Kohli, A., Tandon, P. & Kher, V. (1992). Chronic inflammatory demyelinating polyradiculoneuropathy with membranous glomerulonephritis: report of one case. *Clinical Neurology and Neurosurgery*, **94**, 31–3.

Kolkin, S., Nahman, N.S.J. & Mendell, J.R. (1987). Chronic nephrotoxicity complicating cyclosporine treatment of chronic inflammatory demyelinating polyradiculoneuropathy. *Neurology*, **37**, 147–9.

Kornberg, A.J. & Pestronk, A. (1994). The clinical and diagnostic role of anti-GM1 antibody testing. *Muscle and Nerve*, **17**, 100–4.

Krendel, D.A., Parks, H.P., Anthony, D.C., St.Clair, M.B. & Graham, D.G. (1989). Sural nerve biopsy in chronic inflammatory demyelinating polyradiculoneuropathy. *Muscle and Nerve*, **12**, 252–64.

Kyle, R.A. (1992). Current concepts on monoclonal gammopathies. *Australian and New Zealand Journal of Medicine*, **22**, 291–302.

Lange, D.J., Trojaborg, W., Latov, N., Hays, A.P., Younger, D.S., Uncini, A., Blake, D.M., Hirano, M., Burns, S.M., Lovelace, R.E. *et al.* (1992). Multifocal motor neuropathy with conduction block: is it a distinct clinical entity? *Neurology*, **42**, 497–505.

Latov, N., Sherman, W.H., Nemni, R., Galassi, G., Shyong, J.S., Penn, A.S., Chess, L., Olarte, M.R., Rowland, L.P. & Osserman, E.F. (1980). Plasma-cell dyscrasia and peripheral neuropathy with a monoclonal antibody to peripheral-nerve myelin. *New England Journal of Medicine*, **303**, 618–21.

Lewis, R.A., Sumner, A.J., Brown, M.J. & Asbury, A.K. (1982). Multifocal demyelinating neuropathy with persistent conduction block. *Neurology*, **32**, 958–64.

Lin, J.T., Rowe, V., Brostoff, S.W. & Abdou, N.I. (1982). Lymphocyte studies in a patient with chronic polyradiculoneuropathy. *Neurology*, **32**, 1127–32.

Logothetis, J., Silverstein, P. & Coe, J. (1960). Neurologic aspects of Waldenström's macroglobulinemia. *Archives of Neurology*, **3**, 564–73.

Lugaresi, A., Corbo, M., Thomas, F.P., Miyatani, N., Ariga, T., Yu, R.K., Hays, A.P. & Latov, N. (1991). Identification of glycoconjugates which are targets for anti-Gal(β1–3)GalNAc autoantibodies in spinal motor neurones. *Journal of Neuroimmunology*, **34**, 69–76.

Maimone, D., Annunziata, P., Simone, I.L., Livrea, P. & Guazzi, G.C. (1993). Interleukin-6 levels in the cerebrospinal fluid and serum of patients with Guillain–Barré syndrome and chronic inflammatory demyelinating polyradiculoneuropathy. *Journal of Neuroimmunology*, **47**, 55–61.

Matthews, W.B., Howell, D.A. & Hughes, R.C. (1970). Relapsing corticosteroid-dependent polyneuritis. *Journal of Neurology, Neurosurgery and Psychiatry*, **33**, 330–7.

McCombe, P.A., Brown, N.N., Barr, A.E. & Parkin, L. (1991*a*). Monoclonal immunoglobulin bands in the cerebrospinal fluid. *Australian and New Zealand Journal of Medicine*, **21**, 227–9.

McCombe, P.A., Clark, P., Frith, J., Hammond, S., Stewart, G.J., Pollard, J.D. & McLeod, J.G. (1985). Alpha-1 antitrypsin phenotypes in demyelinating disease. An association between demyelinating disease and the allele PiM3. *Annals of Neurology*, **18**, 514–16.

McCombe, P.A., Klestov, A.C., Tannenberg, A.E., Chalk, J.B. & Pender, M.P. (1991*b*). Sensorimotor peripheral neuropathy in rheumatoid arthritis. *Clinical and Experimental Neurology*, **28**, 146–53.

McCombe, P.A., McManis, P.G., Frith, J.A., Pollard, J.D. & McLeod, J.G. (1987*a*). Chronic inflammatory demyelinating polyradiculoneuropathy associated with pregnancy. *Annals of Neurology*, **21**, 102–4.

McCombe, P.A., Pollard, J.D. & McLeod, J.G. (1987*b*). Chronic inflammatory demyelinating polyradiculoneuropathy. A clinical and electrophysiological study of 92 cases. *Brain*, **110**, 1617–30.

McCombe, P.A., Pollard, J.D. & McLeod, J.G. (1988). Absence of antimyelin antibodies and serum demyelinating factors in most patients with chronic inflammatory demyelinating polyradiculoneuropathy. *Clinical and Experimental Neurology*, **25**, 53–60.

McCombe, P.A., van der Kreek, S.A. & Pender, M.P. (1990). The effects of prophylactic cyclosporin A on experimental allergic neuritis (EAN) in the Lewis rat. Induction of relapsing EAN using low dose cyclosporin A. *Journal of Neuroimmunology*, **28**, 131–40.

McCombe, P.A., Wilson, R. & Prentice, R.L. (1992). Antiganglioside antibodies in peripheral neuropathy. *Clinical and Experimental Neurology*, **29**, 182–8.

Mendell, J.R., Kolkin, S., Kissel, J.T., Weiss, K.L., Chakeres, D.W. & Rammohan, K.W. (1987). Evidence for central nervous system demyelination in chronic inflammatory demyelinating polyradiculoneuropathy. *Neurology*, **37**, 1291–4.

Mitchell, G.W., Williams, G.S., Bosch, E.P. & Hart, M.N. (1991). Class II antigen expression in peripheral neuropathies. *Journal of the Neurological Sciences*, **102**, 170–6.

Nardelli, E., Anzini, P., Moretto, G., Rizutto, N. & Steck, A.J. (1994). Pattern of nervous tissue immunostaining by human anti-glycolipid antibodies. *Journal of the Neurological Sciences*, **122**, 220–7.

Nemni, R., Mamoli, A., Fazio, R., Camerlingo, M., Quattrini, A., Lorenzetti, I., Comola, M., Galardi, G. & Canal, N. (1991). Polyneuropathy associated with IgA monoclonal gammopathy: a hypothesis of its pathogenesis. *Acta Neuropathologica*, **81**, 371–6.

Nobile Orazio, E., Barbieri, S., Baldini, L., Marmiroli, P., Carpo, M., Premoselli, S., Manfredini, E. & Scarlato, G. (1992). Peripheral neuropathy in monoclonal gammopathy of undetermined significance: prevalence and immunopathogenetic studies. *Acta Neurologica Scandinavica*, **85**, 383–90.

Nobile Orazio, E., Meucci, N., Barbieri, S., Carpo, M. & Scarlato, G. (1993). High-dose intravenous immunoglobulin therapy in multifocal motor neuropathy. *Neurology*, **43**, 537–44.

Nobile-Orazio, E., Baldini, L., Barbieri, S., Marmiroli, P., Spagnol, G., Francomano, E. & Scarlato, G. (1988). Treatment of patients with neuropathy and anti-MAG IgM M-proteins. *Annals of Neurology*, **24**, 93–7.

Nyland, H. & Aarli, J.A. (1978). Guillain–Barré syndrome: demonstration of antibodies to peripheral nerve tissue. *Acta Neurologica Scandinavica*, **58**, 35–43.

Oh, S.J. (1978). Subacute demyelinating polyneuropathy responding to corticosteroid treatment. *Archives of Neurology*, **35**, 509–16.

Oh, S.J., Joy, J.L. & Kuruoglu, R. (1992). 'Chronic sensory demyelinating neuropathy': chronic inflammatory demyelinating polyneuropathy presenting as a pure sensory neuropathy. *Journal of Neurology, Neurosurgery and Psychiatry*, **55**, 677–80.

Ohtake, T., Komori, T., Hirose, K. & Tanabe, H. (1990). CNS involvement in Japanese patients with chronic inflammatory demyelinating polyradiculoneuropathy. *Acta Neurologica Scandinavica*, **81**, 108–12.

Ormerod, I.E.C., Waddy, H.M., Kermode, A.G., Murray, N.M.F. & Thomas, P.K. (1990). Involvement of the central nervous system in chronic inflammatory demyelinating polyradiculoneuropathy: a clinical electrophysiological and magnetic resonance study. *Journal of Neurology, Neurosurgery and Psychiatry*, **53**, 789–93.

Osby, E., Noring, L., Hast, R., Kjellin, K.G., Knuttson, E. & Siden, A. (1982). Benign monoclonal gammopathy and peripheral neuropathy. *British Journal of Haematology*, **51**, 531–9.

Palmer, K.N.V. (1966). Polyradiculoneuropathy treated with cytotoxic drugs. *Lancet*, **1**, 265.

Parry, G.J. (1994). Antiganglioside antibodies do not necessarily play a role in multifocal motor neuropathy. *Muscle and Nerve*, **17**, 97–9.

Parry, G.J. & Clarke, S. (1988). Multifocal acquired demyelinating neuropathy masquerading as motor neurone disease. *Muscle and Nerve*, **11**, 103–7.

Parry, G.J. & Sumner, A.J. (1992). Multifocal motor neuropathy. *Neurologic Clinics*, **10**, 671–84.

Pentland, B. (1980). Azathioprine in chronic relapsing polyneuropathy. *Postgraduate Medical Journal*, **56**, 734–5.

Pentland, B., Adams, G.G.W. & Mawdsley, C. (1982). Chronic idiopathic polyneuropathy treated with azathioprine. *Journal of Neurology, Neurosurgery and Psychiatry*, **45**, 866–9.

Pestronk, A. (1991). Invited review: motor neuropathies, motor neuron disorders, and antiglycolipid antibodies. *Muscle and Nerve*, **14**, 927–36.

Pestronk, A., Bieser, K., Choksi, R., Whitton, A., Kornberg, A.J., Goldstein, J.M. & Yee, W-C. (1994). Anti-MAG antibodies: major effects of antigen purity and antibody cross-reactivity on ELISA results and clinical correlation. *Neurology*, **44**, 1131–7.

Pestronk, A., Chaudhry, V., Feldman, E.L., Griffin, J.W., Cornblath, D.R., Denys, E.H., Glasberg, M., Kuncl, R.W., Olney, R.K. & Yee, W.C. (1990). Lower motor neuron syndromes defined by patterns of weakness, nerve conduction abnormalities, and high titers of antiglycolipid antibodies. *Annals of Neurology*, **27**, 316–26.

Pestronk, A., Cornblath, D.R., Ilyas, A.A., Baba, H., Quarles, R.H., Griffin, J.W., Alderson, K. & Adams, R.N. (1988). A treatable multifocal motor neuropathy with antibodies to GM1 ganglioside. *Annals of Neurology*, **24**, 73–8.

Pollard, J.D., McCombe, P.A., Baverstock, J., Gatenby, P.A. & McLeod, J.G. (1986). Class II antigen expression and T lymphocyte subsets in chronic inflammatory demyelinating polyneuropathy. *Journal of Neuroimmunology*, **13**, 123–34.

Pollard, J.D., McLeod, J.G., Gatenby, P. & Kronenberg, H. (1983). Prediction of response to plasma exchange in chronic relapsing polyneuropathy. *Journal of the Neurological Sciences*, **58**, 269–87.

Pollard, J.D. & Selby, G. (1978). Relapsing neuropathy due to tetanus toxoid. *Journal of the Neurological Sciences*, **37**, 113–25.

Prineas, J.W. (1971). Demyelination and remyelination in recurrent idiopathic polyneuropathy. *Acta Neuropathologica*, **18**, 34–57.

Prineas, J.W. & McLeod, J.G. (1976). Chronic relapsing polyneuritis. *Journal of the Neurological Sciences*, **27**, 427–58.

Prior, R., Schober, R., Scharffetter, K. & Wechsler, W. (1992). Occlusive microangiopathy by immunoglobulin (IgM-kappa) precipitation: pathogenetic relevance in paraneoplastic cryoglobulinemic neuropathy. *Acta Neuropathologica*, **83**, 423–6.

Quattrini, A., Nemni, R., Fazio, R., Iannaccone, S., Lorenzetti, I., Grassi, F. & Canal, N. (1991). Axonal neuropathy in a patient with monoclonal IgM kappa reactive with Schmidt–Lanterman incisures. *Journal of Neuroimmunology*, **33**, 73–9.

Read, D.J., Vanhegan, R.I. & Matthews, W.B. (1978). Peripheral neuropathy and benign IgG paraproteinemia. *Journal of Neurology, Neurosurgery and Psychiatry*, **41**, 215–19.

Rechthand, E., Cornblath, D.R., Stern, B.J. & Meyerhoff, J.O. (1984). Chronic demyelinating polyneuropathy in systemic lupus erythematosus. *Neurology*, **34**, 1375–7.

Rousseau, J.J., Franck, G., Grisar, T., Reznik, M., Heynen, G. & Salmon, J. (1978). Osteosclerotic myeloma with polyneuropathy and ectopic secretion of calcitonin. *European Journal of Cancer*, **14**, 133–40.

Sadiq, S.A., Thomas, F.P., Kilidireas, K., Portopsaltis, S., Hays, A.P., Lee, K.-W., Romas, S.N., Kumar, N., van den Berg, L., Santoro, M. *et al.* (1990). The spectrum of neurological disease associated with anti-GM1 antibodies. *Neurology*, **40**, 1067–72.

Santoro, M., Thomas, F.P., Fink, M.E., Lange, D.J., Uncini, A., Wadia, N.H., Latov, N. & Hays, A.P. (1990). IgM deposits at nodes of Ranvier in a patient with amyotrophic lateral sclerosis, anti-GM1 antibodies, and multifocal motor conduction block. *Annals of Neurology*, **28**, 373–7.

Santoro, M., Uncini, A., Corbo, M., Staugaitis, S.M., Thomas, F.P., Hays, A.P. & Latov, N. (1992). Experimental conduction block induced by serum from a patient with anti-GM1 antibodies. *Annals of Neurology*, **385**, 390.

Server, A.C., Lefkowith, J., Braine, H. & McKhann, G.M. (1979). Treatment of chronic relapsing inflammatory polyradiculoneuropathy by plasma exchange. *Annals of Neurology*, **6**, 258–61.

Sewell, H.F., Matthews, J.B., Gooch, E., Millac, P., Willox, A., Stern, M.A. & Walker, F. (1981). Autoantibody to nerve tissue in a patient with a peripheral neuropathy and an IgG paraprotein. *Journal of Clinical Pathology*, **34**, 1163–6.

Sherman, W.H., Latov, N., Hays, A.P., Takatsu, M., Nemni, R., Galassi, G. & Osserman, E.F. (1983). Monoclonal IgM kappa antibody precipitating with chondroitin sulfate C from patients with axonal polyneuropathy and epidermolysis. *Neurology*, **33**, 192–201.

Simmons, Z., Bromberg, M.B., Feldman, E.L. & Blaivas, M. (1993). Polyneuropathy associated with IgA monoclonal gammopathy of undetermined significance. *Muscle and Nerve*, **16**, 77–83.

Simone, I.L., Annunziata, P., Maimone, D., Liguori, M., Leante, R. & Livrea, P. (1993). Serum and CSF anti-GM1 antibodies in patients with Guillain–Barré syndrome and chronic inflammatory demyelinating polyneuropathy. *Journal of the Neurological Sciences*, **114**, 49–55.

Smith, I.S., Kahn, S.N., Lacey, B.W., King, R.H.M., Eames, R.A., Whybrew, D.J. & Thomas, P.K. (1983). Chronic demyelinating neuropathy associated with benign IgM paraproteinemia. *Brain*, **106**, 169–95.

Spatz, L.A., Williams, M., Brender, B., Desai, R. & Latov, N. (1992). DNA sequence analysis and comparison of the variable heavy and light chain regions of two IgM, monoclonal, anti-myelin associated glycoprotein antibodies. *Journal of Neuroimmunology*, **36**, 29–39.

Suarez, G.A. & Kelly, J.J. (1993). Polyneuropathy associated with monoclonal gammopathy of undetermined significance: further evidence that IgM-MGUS neuropathies are different than IgG-MGUS. *Neurology*, **43**, 1304–8.

Targowla, J. (1894). Polynévrite récidivante, envahissement des nerfs craniens et diplegie faciale. *Revue Neurologique*, **2**, 465–72.

Tatum, A.H. (1993). Experimental paraprotein neuropathy, demyelination by passive transfer of human IgM anti-myelin-associated glycoprotein. *Annals of Neurology*, **33**, 502–6.

Taylor, W.A., Brostoff, S.W. & Hughes, R.A. (1991). P_2 specific lymphocyte transformation in Guillain–Barré syndrome and chronic idiopathic demyelinating polyradiculoneuropathy. *Journal of the Neurological Sciences*, **104**, 52–5.

Taylor, W.A. & Hughes, R.A. (1989). T lymphocyte activation antigens in Guillain–Barré syndrome and chronic idiopathic demyelinating polyradiculoneuropathy. *Journal of Neuroimmunology*, **24**, 33–9.

Thomas, P.K., Lascelles, R.G., Hallpike, J.F. & Hewer, R.L. (1969). Recurrent and chronic relapsing Guillain–Barré polyneuritis. *Brain*, **92**, 589–606.

Thomas, P.K., Walker, R.W.H., Rudge, P., Morgan-Hughes, J.A., King, R.H.M., Jacobs, J.M., Mills, K.R., Ormerod, I.E.C., Murray, N.M.F. & McDonald, W.I. (1987). Chronic demyelinating peripheral neuropathy associated with multifocal central nervous system demyelination. *Brain*, **110**, 53–76.

Uncini, A., Gallucci, M., Lugaresi, A., Porrini, A.M., Onofrj, M. & Gambi, D. (1991). CNS involvement in chronic inflammatory demyelinating polyneuropathy: an electrophysiological and MRI study. *Electromyography and Clinical Neurophysiology*, **31**, 365–71.

Uncini, A., Santoro, M., Corbo, M., Lugaresi, A. & Latov, N. (1993). Conduction abnormalities induced by sera of patients with multifocal motor neuropathy and anti-GM1 antibodies. *Muscle and Nerve*, **16**, 610–15.

van den Berg, L.H., Lankamp, C.L.A.M., de Jager, A.E., Notermans, N.C., Sodaar, P., Marrink, J., de Jong, H.J., Bar, P.R. & Wokke, J.H.J. (1993). Anti-sulphatide antibodies in peripheral neuropathy. *Journal of Neurology, Neurosurgery and Psychiatry*, **56**, 1164–8.

van Doorn, P.A., Brand, A., Strengers, P.F.W., Meulstee, J. & Vermeulen, M. (1990*a*). High-dose intravenous immunoglobulin treatment in chronic inflammatory demyelinating polyneuropathy: a double-blind, placebo-controlled, crossover study. *Neurology*, **40**, 209–12.

van Doorn, P.A., Brand, A. & Vermeulen, M. (1988). Anti-neuroblastoma cell line antibodies in inflammatory demyelinating polyneuropathy: inhibition *in vitro* and *in vivo* by IV immunoglobulin. *Neurology*, **38**, 1592–5.

van Doorn, P.A., Rossi, F., Brand, A., van Lint, M., Vermeulen, M. & Kazatchkine, M.D. (1990*b*). On the mechanism of high-dose intravenous immunoglobulin treatment of patients with chronic inflammatory demyelinating polyneuropathy. *Journal of Neuroimmunology*, **29**, 57–64.

van Doorn, P.A., Schreuder, G.M.T., Vermeulen, M., d'Amaro, J. & Brand, A. (1991). HLA antigens in patients with chronic inflammatory demyelinating polyneuropathy. *Journal of Neuroimmunology*, **32**, 133–9.

Vedanarayanan, V., Kandt, R.S., Lewis, D.V. & DeLong, G.R. (1991). Chronic inflammatory demyelinating polyradiculoneuropathy of childhood: treatment with high-dose intravenous immunoglobulin. *Neurology*, **41**, 828–30.

Vera Ramirez, M., Charlet, M. & Parry, G.J. (1992). Recurrent aseptic meningitis complicating intravenous immunoglobulin therapy for chronic inflammatory demyelinating polyradiculoneuropathy. *Neurology*, **42**, 1636–7.

Vermeulen, M., van der Meche, F.G.A., Speelman, J.D., Weber, A. & Busch, H.F.M. (1985). Plasma and gamma-globulin infusion in chronic inflammatory polyneuropathy. *Journal of the Neurological Sciences*, **70**, 317–26.

Vermeulen, M., van Doorn, P.A., Brand, A., Strengers, P.F., Jennekens, F.G. & Busch, H.F. (1993). Intravenous immunoglobulin treatment in patients with chronic inflammatory demyelinating polyneuropathy: a double blind, placebo controlled study. *Journal of Neurology, Neurosurgery and Psychiatry*, **56**, 36–9.

Vital, A., Latinville, D., Aupy, M., Dumas, P. & Vital, C. (1991). Inflammatory demyelinating lesions in two patients with IgM monoclonal gammopathy and polyneuropathy. *Neuropathology and Applied Neurobiology*, **17**, 415–20.

Vital, A., Vital, C., Julien, J., Baquey, A. & Steck, A.J. (1989). Polyneuropathy associated with IgM monoclonal gammopathy. Immunological and pathological study in 31 patients. *Acta Neuropathologica*, **79**, 160–7.

Vrethem, M., Cruz, M., Wen Xin, H., Malm, C., Holmgren, H. & Ernerudh, J. (1993). Clinical, neurophysiological and immunological evidence of polyneuropathy in patients with monoclonal gammopathies. *Journal of the Neurological Sciences*, **114**, 193–9.

Walker, G.L. (1979). Progressive polyradiculoneuropathy: treatment with azathioprine. *Australian and New Zealand Journal of Medicine*, **9**, 184–7.

Walsh, J.C. (1971). The neuropathy of multiple myeloma. An electrophysiological and histological study. *Archives of Neurology*, **25**, 404–14.

Waterston, J.A., Brown, M.M., Ingram, D.A. & Swash, M. (1992). Cyclosporin A therapy in paraprotein-associated neuropathy. *Muscle and Nerve*, **15**, 445–8.

Wertman, E., Argov, Z. & Abramsky, O. (1988). Chronic inflammatory demyelinating polyradiculoneuropathy: features and prognostic factors with corticosteroid therapy. *European Neurology*, **28**, 199–204.

Wilson, J.R., Conwit, R.A., Eidelman, B.H., Starzl, T. & Abu-Elmagd, K. (1994). Sensorimotor neuropathy resembling CIDP in patients receiving FK506. *Muscle and Nerve*, **17**, 528–32.

Witte, A.S. & Burke, J.F. (1987). Membranous glomerulonephritis associated with chronic progressive demyelinating neuropathy. *Neurology*, **37**, 342–5.

Yee, W.C., Hahn, A.F., Hearn, S.A. & Rupar, A.R. (1989). Neuropathy in IgM lambda paraproteinemia. Immunoreactivity to neuronal proteins and chondroitin sulfate. *Acta Neuropathologica*, **78**, 57–64.

Yuill, G.M., Swinburn, W.R. & Liversedge, L.A. (1970). Treatment of polyneuropathy with azathioprine. *Lancet*, **2**, 854–6.

–10–
Autoimmune diseases of the neuromuscular junction and other disorders of the motor unit

PAMELA A. McCOMBE

Myasthenia gravis

Introduction

As discussed by Drachman (1981), a patient with the features of myasthenia gravis (MG) was recorded by Willis in 1672. A full description of the disease was given in 1900 by Campbell & Bramwell, who described the clinical features, mentioning that the weakness frequently started with ptosis and diplopia. The concept that MG was an autoimmune disease was suggested by Simpson (1960), because MG was often associated with other autoimmune diseases. Nastuk, Plescia & Osserman (1960) also suggested an autoimmune pathogenesis for MG, on the basis of alterations in serum complement levels. The finding that injection of purified acetylcholine receptor (AChR) into rabbits caused an autoimmune disease similar to MG (Patrick & Lindstrom, 1973) was further evidence that MG has an immune aetiology. Most patients with MG have elevated levels of circulating antibodies to the AChR (Lindstrom *et al.*, 1976*c*), although some patients do not (seronegative MG) (Birmanns *et al.*,1991). Seronegative MG (Birmanns *et al.*, 1991; Lu *et al.*, 1993) and MG induced by exposure to penicillamine (Heidenreich, Vincent & Newsom-Davis, 1988) also appear to have an autoimmune aetiology.

Clinical features

General clinical features

MG is a relatively uncommon disease. Kurtzke (1978) suggested that the prevalence of MG is about 4 per 100 000. In a study of MG in Finland,

Hokkanen (1969) suggested that the true prevalence is probably 5–7.5 per 100 000. The chief clinical features of MG are weakness and abnormal fatiguability. Symptoms and signs of MG usually commence in the extraocular muscles. There is no impairment of sensation. In a series of 282 patients reviewed by Osserman *et al.* (1958), 57% of patients presented with ptosis, 78% of all patients eventually developed ptosis and 55% of patients eventually developed generalized weakness. Other symptoms included oculomotor disorders such as diplopia, dysarthria, dysphagia and weakness of the face, trunk and limbs. Oh & Kuruoglu (1992) reported that 12 of 314 patients with MG presented with limb weakness. Osserman *et al.* (1958) devised a clinical classification of MG, using the location and severity of weakness. The first category was localized MG, the second was generalized MG and the other categories included an acute fulminating form, a late severe form and a category with muscle atrophy. Patients with MG with anti-AChR antibodies can also be classified into three groups: those with thymoma (type A), those with early onset without thymoma (type B) and those without thymoma with late onset (type C) (Compston *et al.*, 1980). Neonatal MG is a transient syndrome that occurs in the offspring of myasthenic mothers and is due to the transfer of anti-AChR antibodies to the foetus (Plauché, 1994).

Some patients with the clinical features of MG are seronegative for anti-AChR antibodies (Lindstrom *et al.*, 1976*c*; Marchiori *et al.*, 1989). Birmans *et al.* (1991) reported that, of 12 patients with seronegative MG, seven had generalized muscle weakness and five had weakness confined to ocular and bulbar muscles. Evoli *et al.* (1989) found that patients with generalized seronegative MG were more frequently male and more often had mild disease than did patients with seropositive MG.

Abnormalities of the thymus

The thymus is frequently abnormal in MG. A minority of patients have a thymic tumour (Palmisani *et al.*, 1993) while the remainder have evidence of thymic hyperplasia or sometimes thymic atrophy. Patients with thymoma have more severe disease than non-thymoma patients and show less response to thymectomy (Palmisani *et al.*, 1993).

Association with other autoimmune diseases

The association of MG with recognized autoimmune diseases led Simpson (1960) to propose that MG was itself an autoimmune disease. Some patients with MG have other muscle diseases such as dermatomyositis (Vasilescu *et al.*, 1978). Other diseases associated with MG include autoimmune thyroid disease, systemic lupus erythematosus, primary Sjögren's syndrome and scleroderma (Bhalla *et al.*, 1993), which are mostly found in patients with MG without thymoma (Aarli, Gilhus & Matre, 1992). In general, MG patients with thymoma do not have an increased incidence of non-muscle autoimmune diseases (Aarli *et al.*, 1992), although they may have evidence of red cell aplasia.

Precipitating factors

Campbell & Bramwell (1900) mentioned that symptoms often commence after an infection and Edgeworth (1930) described the onset of her symptoms after an infection. In the series of Osserman *et al.* (1958) some patients associated the onset of MG with preceding infections, but the authors found this was not of statistical significance. Increased anti-virus antibody titres have not been detected in the sera of patients with MG (Klavinskis *et al.*, 1985). Plauché (1994) has reported that women with MG may have exacerbations or remissions of disease during pregnancy. He also reported that one-third of women experience exacerbations of MG in the postpartum period.

Diagnosis

Patients with MG usually have oculomotor weakness and sometimes more generalized weakness. Clinical examination may reveal abnormal fatiguability of muscles and an increase in strength after administration of edrophonium (Tensilon®). The neurophysiological findings characteristic of MG are a reduction of the amplitude of the compound muscle action potential on repetitive nerve stimulation and increased jitter with single fibre electromyography. Most patients with MG have circulating anti-AChR antibodies. Computerized tomography of the thorax should be performed to exclude a thymoma.

Genetics

Familial myasthenia gravis

Inherited congenital and infantile forms of myasthenia do not have an autoimmune basis. Namba *et al.* (1971*a*) described familial autoimmune MG where many of the patients had elevated levels of autoantibodies in the serum. Pirskanen (1977) found that 19 of 264 patients had familial MG, and that other autoimmune diseases were common in patients and family members. Electrophysiological abnormalities and anti-AChR antibodies may be found in asymptomatic relatives of patients with MG (Pirskanen *et al.*, 1981; Pascuzzi *et al.*, 1987). Bergoffen, Zmijewski & Fischbeck (1994) reported a family from a consanguineous marriage where five of ten siblings had autoimmune MG. They showed that the MHC genes, the AChR β subunit genes and the T cell receptor genes were not involved in the inheritance of this form of MG.

Twin studies

MG has been reported to occur in both members of pairs of monozygotic twins (Osborne & Simcock, 1966; Murphy & Murphy, 1986), which suggests that genetic factors are involved. Others have reported MG occurring in only one member of pairs of monozygotic and dizygotic twins (Alter & Talbert, 1960; Motoki *et al.*, 1966; Namba *et al.*, 1971*b*). In a large study of the familial incidence of MG, Pirskanen (1977) found no concordance of MG in twins. A larger study comparing the concordance of MG in monozygotic and dizygotic twins would help to determine the importance of genetic factors in MG.

HLA typing and Gm typing

Many studies have shown that MG is influenced by HLA type, which can predispose to the development of disease or can confer protection. Dawkins *et al.* (1987) found an association of generalized MG with HLA A1, B8 and DR3. Further studies showed a strong association with HLA DR3 in women and in patients with early age of onset of MG (Compston *et al.*, 1980; Vieira *et al.*, 1993). Vieira *et al.* (1993) found that patients with thymoma-associated MG had an association with DQB1.0604 and that DR1 was a protective allele in females. Penicillamine-induced MG is associated with HLA DR1 (Delamere *et al.*, 1983). The HLA DR associations may reflect linkage of the HLA DR genes with other markers in the HLA region. Dawkins and colleagues have pioneered studies that show that MG is associated with the ancestral haplotype 8.1, which contains regions other than HLA markers. It appears that a region between HLA B and tumour necrosis factor (TNF) contains the important gene (Degli Esposti *et al.*, 1992*a*). The BAT (B-associated transcript) gene is in this region and the BAT1 B allele is correlated with the presence of MG (Degli Esposti, Leelayuwat & Dawkins, 1992*b*). The PERB6 gene is located between BAT and HLA B and may also be a useful probe of this area (Marshall *et al.*, 1994). There is also an association of MG with immunoglobulin allotypes (Gm typing) (Gilhus *et al.*, 1990). This has been confirmed with molecular techniques (Demaine *et al.*, 1992).

Pathology

Pathology of the neuromuscular junction and muscle

Engel (1980) described the pathology of the muscle in MG: in myasthenic muscles, there is degeneration of the postsynaptic regions of the motor endplate, with widening of the clefts and debris in the synaptic space, but the presynaptic regions show normal synaptic vesicles. There is deficiency of the AChR at MG endplates. There is no inflammation at the motor endplates, but collections of inflammatory cells (lymphorrhages) are sometimes found around blood vessels in muscle (Russell, 1953) or in the muscle parenchyma (Oosterhuis & Bethlem, 1973).

Pathology of the thymus

The thymus is frequently abnormal in MG. Bell (1917) reported that there was thymic enlargement, either tumour or hyperplasia, in nearly half the patients with MG. Castelman & Norris (1949) found that ten of 35 patients with MG had thymic tumours and the remainder had microscopic abnormalities of the thymic medulla. One study of 115 MG patients showed that 13% had a thymoma (Berrih Aknin *et al.*, 1987) and another study showed that 30 of 42 patients with seropositive MG had an abnormal thymus (Degli Esposti *et al.*, 1992*a*). In patients with seropositive MG without thymoma and with a younger age of onset, the thymus frequently shows hyperplasia, characterized by the presence of increased numbers of germinal centres (Levine & Rosai, 1978). Germinal centres in the thymus in MG are similar to those in lymph nodes and contain B cells (Staber, Fink & Sack, 1975). Patients without thymoma and with a later age of onset of MG have thymic atrophy rather than hyperplasia (Compston *et al.*, 1980; Bhalla *et al.*, 1993). Patients with seronegative MG have fewer thymic abnormalities than those with seropositive MG: in one study, six of eight seronegative patients had a normal thymus (Verma & Oger, 1992). In another study of seronegative MG, lymph-node-like areas were found in the thymic medulla, but there were fewer germinal centres and less Ig production (per B cell) than in seropositive MG (Willcox *et al.*, 1991). Thymomas are tumours of thymic epithelial cells (Levine & Rosai, 1978; Fukai *et al.*, 1992; Kornstein, 1992). Thymomas can be classified according to the tumour morphology and associated lymphocyte infiltration (Lewis *et al.*, 1987), or according to the type of epithelium in the tumour (Fukai *et al.*, 1992).

Pathophysiology

A decrement of the amplitude of the compound muscle action potential following repetitive nerve stimulation is a cardinal finding in MG and explains the abnormal fatiguability. Harvey & Masland (1941*a*) described a quantitative method of recording motor activity, and showed that curarization caused a decline in amplitude with repeated stimulation. They then showed a similar defect in MG (Harvey & Masland, 1941*b*). Today, repetitive stimulation is a useful diagnostic tool in MG. The other main abnormality in MG is the finding, described by Elmqvist *et al.* (1964) using intracellular recordings, that the amplitude of miniature endplate potentials (mepps), which are produced by the spontaneous release of ACh, is reduced. This reduction is related to deficiency of the AChR on the postsynaptic junction.

Immunopathology

Immunopathology of the neuromuscular junction

Fambrough, Drachman & Satyamurti (1973) showed that the number of AChRs was decreased in MG. Antibody complexes and complement are present at the endplates (Engel, Lambert & Howard, 1977; Sahashi *et al.*, 1980). *In vitro*, antibody to AChR produces a decrease in the number of AChRs (Reiness & Weinberg, 1978; Stanley & Drachman, 1978) and can do so in the absence of complement (Heinemann, Merlie & Lindstrom, 1978). Turnover of AChR by endocytosis is a physiological process, but in MG the rate of turnover is increased. This may be due to enhanced degradation of AChRs that have been cross-linked by antibody and/or damage to AChRs by antibody together with complement (Drachman *et al.*, 1980).

Immunopathology of the thymus

Presence of AChR in the thymus

The thymus is usually morphologically abnormal in MG (see above) and appears to play a primary role in the pathogenesis of MG. Because the AChR is the target of the immune attack in MG, there has been considerable interest in whether the AChR is expressed in the thymus, and by what cells. Kirchner *et al.* (1988) demonstrated AChR antigens in myasthenic and non-myasthenic tumour-free thymuses and also in thymic tumours. In non-thymomatous thymuses, the AChR expression was on myoid cells. Schluep *et al.* (1987) found AChR expression but not MHC class II expression on myoid cells in normal and myasthenic thymuses, and found that the cells expressing AChR were not near germinal centres. Analysis of expression of mRNA of the different AChR subunits showed that myoid cells from the non-neoplastic thymus of myasthenic patients express AChR (Geuder *et al.*, 1992*b*). A similar study found expression of AChR subunits in non-myasthenic thymic tumours and hyperplastic thymic tissue from myasthenic patients (Kaminski *et al.*, 1994). In MG-associated thymomas, epithelial cells have been shown by immunohistochemistry to contain proteins with epitopes in common with the AChR (Kirchner *et al.*, 1988). Marx *et al.* (1989, 1990) have characterized a 153–kDa protein containing such epitopes in tissue from thymomas. Geuder *et al.* (1992*a*) showed that, in MG-associated thymomas, genomic DNA encoding the AChR is present but is not transcribed. However, they also showed that RNA in thymomas contains sequences homologous to the AChR α subunit which could lead to the production of proteins with AChR epitopes.

Presence of lymphocytes specific for AChR in the thymus

Armstrong, Nowak & Falk (1973) found that phytohaemagglutinin-stimulated thymocytes from MG patients but not from normal controls were cytotoxic to foetal muscle. T cells specific for the AChR can be isolated from the thymus of patients with MG (Melms *et al.*, 1988). B lymphoid lines can be cultured from MG thymuses, but not from control thymuses (Vilquin *et al.*, 1993). Antibody to AChR can be produced *in vitro* by thymic cells (Fujii *et al.*, 1984, 1985*a*) and a B cell line secreting antibody to AChR was produced from the thymus of a patient with MG (Kamo *et al.*, 1982). Transplantation of thymic tissue from myasthenic thymuses to SCID mice results in production of AChR antibodies in the recipients.

Immunological findings in the peripheral blood

Antibodies

Antibodies in seropositive MG

Between 67 and 87% of patients with MG have circulating antibodies to the AChR (Lindstrom *et al.*, 1976*c*; Marchiori *et al.*, 1989), which is a transmembrane protein containing four subunits arranged in a pentamer $\alpha 2\beta\gamma\delta$ (Changeux, Devillers-Thiery & Chemouilli, 1984). The AChR has both T and B cell epitopes (Manfredi *et al.*, 1992*a*,*b*). In MG, the majority of anti-

AChR antibodies are directed against the α subunit (Tzartos *et al.*, 1991*a*); the part of the AChR that is the target of antibodies is known as the main immunogenic region (MIR) (Tzartos *et al.*, 1991*b*). Most anti-AChR antibodies are IgG, although some are IgM or IgA (Hofstad *et al.*, 1992). Antibodies from the one patient can be heterogeneous in their fine specificity and ability to transfer disease, and levels of anti-AChR antibodies do not always correlate with disease activity (Tindall, 1981; Cardona *et al.*, 1994). Cells from the thymus and lymph nodes (Fujii *et al.*, 1985*a*), from the peripheral blood (Yi, Pirskanen & Lefvert, 1993) and possibly from the bone marrow (Fujii *et al.*, 1985*b*) are capable of producing antibody to AChR. Passive transfer of human MG serum to mice causes a disease resembling MG (Toyka *et al.*, 1975). Patients with penicillamine-induced MG also have circulating antibodies to AChR (Morel *et al.*, 1991). In mice it has been found that penicillamine administration causes elevation of the level of anti-AChR antibodies (Bever & Asofsky, 1991).

Antibodies to striated muscle (striational autoantibodies) are present in the sera of some patients with MG, particularly those with thymoma (Sano & Lennon, 1993). Some antibodies to AChR are cross-reactive with muscle proteins such as troponin (Osborn *et al.*, 1992) and myosin (Mohan, Barohn & Krolick, 1992). In MG, other antibodies have been reported to react with titin (Williams *et al.*, 1992). Antibodies to ryanodine, a calcium release channel in sarcoplasmic reticulum, are found in about 50% of patients with MG and thymoma (Mygland *et al.*, 1992, 1994). MG sera also contain antibodies to a presynaptic membrane protein that binds bungarotoxin and may be a presynaptic receptor (Lu *et al.*, 1991). Furthermore, antibodies to the β-adrenergic receptor have also been described in MG (Eng *et al.*, 1992) and antibodies to thymic epithelial cells are found in MG patients with thymic hyperplasia (Safar *et al.*, 1991).

Antibodies in seronegative MG

About 15% of patients do not have detectable levels of circulating AChR antibodies. Such 'seronegative' patients probably also have an autoimmune disorder (Birmanns *et al.*, 1991). In these patients, cells can be found that secrete antibody against both the AChR and against the presynaptic membrane protein (Lu *et al.*, 1993). An IgM antibody that inhibits sodium flux through the AChR has also been reported in seronegative MG (Yamamoto *et al.*, 1991).

T cells

While antibody alone can transfer MG (Toyka *et al.*, 1975), the production of antibody to AChR is dependent on T cells. Abramsky *et al.* (1975) found that peripheral blood lymphocytes from patients with MG were stimulated to transform by AChR. Subsequent studies have found that AChR-reactive T cells are present in the blood of MG patients (Newsom-Davis *et al.*, 1989; Protti *et al.*, 1990; Ahlberg *et al.*, 1992; Link *et al.*, 1992; Sun *et al.*, 1992; Yi *et al.*, 1993) and also in healthy subjects (Salvetti *et al.*, 1991). In MG, the circulating AChR-specific cells are sensitive to low concentrations of interleukin-2 (IL-2), suggesting that these cells are activated *in vivo* (Cohen Kaminsky *et al.*, 1989*a*,*b*). T cells from different subjects with MG react with different regions of the main extracellular part of the α chain of the AChR (Oshima *et al.*, 1990). Cultured AChR-stimulated T cells can produce IL-2, interferon-γ (IFN-γ) and interleukin-4 (IL-4), although these cytokines may be produced by different subsets of cells (Yi *et al.*, 1994). AChR-specific T cells can proliferate in the presence of MHC class II antigen-positive muscle cell lines (Baggi *et al.*, 1993).

Non-specific findings

Elevated levels of soluble IL-2 receptor (IL-2R) are found in the serum of some of MG patients. Levels of soluble IL-2R correlate with severity of disease and decline after thymectomy (Cohen Kaminsky *et al.*, 1992; Confalonieri *et al.*, 1993). Levels of TNF and IFN-γ are not elevated in the serum of MG patients (Confalonieri *et al.*, 1993). Some workers find increased numbers of $CD5^+$ B cells, which are thought to have a role in autoimmunity, in the peripheral blood of MG patients (Ragheb & Lisak, 1992). However, others find the numbers of circulating $CD5^+$ B cells to be the same in MG patients as in normal controls (Yi *et al.*, 1992).

Immunoregulation

Anti-idiotype antibodies directed against anti-AChR antibodies appear to have a role in the regulation of MG (Lefvert, Holm & Pirskanen, 1987; Lefvert & Holm, 1987; Souroujon & Fuchs, 1987). T cells that are stimulated by anti-AChR antibodies and by anti-idiotype antibodies against the anti-AChR antibodies are also found in MG; such T cells may participate in a regulatory network (Yi, Ahlberg & Lefvert, 1992). It is thought that $CD8^+$ T cells may play a downregulatory role, because removal of $CD8^+$ T cells facilitates the *in vitro* detection of $CD4^+$ T cells reactive with the AChR (Manfredi *et al.*, 1992*b*).

Therapy

Early treatments for MG included strychnine, arsenic and thyroid extract (Simon, 1935). Edgeworth (1930) reported the beneficial effects of ephedrine on her own MG, and suggested that the stimulant properties were beneficial. Today, symptomatic treatment is based on the use of acetylcholinesterase inhibitors, which increase the levels of AChR available at the neuromuscular junction. Modern treatment also aims to interrupt the underlying immunological process.

Thymectomy

Blalock *et al.* (1941), aware that many patients with MG had thymic abnormalities, reported that thymectomy was helpful in MG. Simpson (1958) concluded that thymectomy is beneficial in MG patients with and without thymoma. Thymectomy has been useful as primary therapy of MG (Olanow *et al.*, 1987) and also in combination with immunosuppressive agents (Lindberg *et al.*, 1992). The best responses to thymectomy are found in patients with early onset of disease and with thymic hyperplasia, but patients with late onset have less benefit (Olanow *et al.*, 1987). Evoli *et al.* (1988) showed that thymectomy is of no benefit for patients with ocular MG, and that MG patients with thymoma show less improvement after thymectomy than non-thymoma patients. Some studies have shown that serum anti-AChR antibodies decrease after thymectomy (Kuks *et al.*, 1991*b*). However, others have found that such a decrease may not occur and is not required for the thymectomy to be helpful (Olanow *et al.*, 1987). Possible adverse effects might occur if thymectomy produced a deficiency of T cells. Melms *et al.* (1993) found no significant change in the phenotype of T cells in the peripheral blood of patients after thymectomy. However, there are reports of other autoimmune diseases such as systemic lupus erythematosus developing after thymectomy (Kennes *et al.*, 1978; Alarcon Segovia *et al.*, 1963). Interestingly, MG has also been reported to develop after the removal of a thymoma (Hassel *et al.*, 1992).

Corticosteroids

Corticosteroids are widely used in the treatment of MG. Early studies reported the benefit of the use of anterior pituitary extract (Simon, 1935). The use of corticotrophin was pioneered by Torda & Wolff (1951). Short-term treatment (Osserman & Genkins, 1966) and repeated courses of corticotrophin (Grob & Namba, 1966) were shown to be of benefit, although patients often experienced temporary worsening of symptoms after the commencement of treatment. Brunner, Namba and Grob (1972) found that high-dose intramuscular methylprednisolone therapy was of similar benefit to adrenocorticotrophic hormone (ACTH). Kjaer (1971) found that oral prednisone was also of benefit, but that relapses followed its withdrawal. Later studies have concentrated on the long-term use of oral corticosteroids and have confirmed that this treatment is of benefit. MG patients may have increasing weakness in the early stages of corticosteroid treatment (Pascuzzi, Coslett & Johns, 1984; Sghirlanzoni *et al.*, 1984; Evoli *et al.*, 1992). Some authors have advocated the gradual introduction of oral corticosteroids in an attempt to prevent deterioration after commencing treatment (Seybold & Drachman, 1974). In the long term, alternate day therapy appears to be satisfactory (Warmolts & Engel, 1972). The percentage of patients responding to corticosteroids in these studies ranged from 72 to 82%. Patients with thymoma are less responsive to corticosteroids than non-thymoma patients (Evoli *et al.*, 1992).

Azathioprine

Azathioprine appears to be of benefit in MG, either alone or in combination with corticosteroids (Kuks, Djojoatmodjo & Oosterhuis, 1991*a*). In one study of 99 patients, 38% showed marked improvement and 33% showed some improvement (Matell, 1987). Factors that were predictive of a response to azathioprine included a later age of onset, the presence of anti-AChR antibodies, HLA B8 negativity and male gender. A recent trial has suggested that azathioprine may be more beneficial than prednisone (Myasthenia Gravis Clinical Study Group, 1993). There have been reports of reactivation of clinical disease after ceasing azathioprine (Hohlfeld *et al.*, 1985). The long-term adverse effects of azathioprine treatment include an increased risk of developing lymphoma or other malignancies (Kuks *et al.*, 1991*a*).

Plasmapheresis

Bergstrom *et al.* (1973) showed that thoracic duct drainage was beneficial in MG, and that patients became worse when their own cell-free lymph was reinfused. The first report of the use of plasmapheresis in MG showed that this form of treatment was beneficial in two patients with acquired MG but was of no benefit in a patient with congenital MG (Pinching, Peters & Newsom-Davis, 1976). Subsequent authors confirmed the benefits of short courses of plasma exchange. Others showed chronic long-term plasma exchange could be used in MG (Rodnitzky & Bosch, 1984). The mechanism of action of plasma exchange seems likely to be the removal of anti-AChR antibodies. However, there is often a rebound effect, with levels of antibody to AChR rising after plasmapheresis. This is a general effect, as other antibody levels also rise. Such an increase in antibody levels after plasmapheresis may result from the removal of anti-idiotypic antibodies. The increase in antibody levels can be prevented by azathioprine (Nasca *et al.*, 1990). Patients with myasthenic crisis have been reported who failed to respond to immunoglobulin therapy but who responded to plasmapheresis (Stricker *et al.*, 1993). Plasma exchange requires the use of albumin or plasma as replacement fluid. The use of an immunoabsorbent column may reduce the need for replacement fluid (Ichikawa *et al.*, 1993; Sawada *et al.*, 1993).

Intravenous immunoglobulin

High-dose intravenous immunoglobulin therapy is of benefit in patients with MG (Fateh-Moghadam *et al.*, 1984; Gajdos *et al.*, 1984; Ippoliti *et al.*, 1984). An uncontrolled trial showed that more than half of 37 patients improved with a five-day course of this therapy (Cosi *et al.*, 1991). The mechanism of action is not clear, but may involve the transfer of anti-idiotypic antibodies that bind to anti-AChR antibodies (Liblau *et al.*, 1991). Aseptic meningitis has been reported as a complication of this form of therapy (Ellis, Swenson & Bajorek, 1994).

Cyclosporin A

Tindall *et al.* (1987) have shown that cyclosporin A is of benefit in patients with late-onset MG and also in patients with severe corticosteroid-dependent MG (Tindall *et al.*, 1993). Nephrotoxicity is the main adverse effect.

Other measures

Anti-AChR antibodies mediate the loss of AChR from the motor endplate, and the production of these antibodies is dependent on $CD4^+$ T cells. Treatment of one patient with a monoclonal antibody to CD4 produced several months of improvement (Ahlberg *et al.*, 1993). A novel approach, which may become applicable to the treatment of MG, is the use of 3-deazaadenosine to prevent the breakdown of AChR (Kuncl *et al.*, 1993). In the future it may become possible to downregulate the autoimmune attack on the AChR in a more specific manner. Some of the experimental therapies being used in experimental autoimmune myasthenia gravis (see below) may become applicable to MG.

Experimental autoimmune (allergic) myasthenia gravis

Introduction

Experimental autoimmune myasthenia gravis (EAMG) was first induced by Patrick and Lindstrom in attempt to make antibodies to the AChR (Patrick & Lindstrom, 1973; Lindstrom, 1980). EAMG has been produced in rabbits (Patrick & Lindstrom, 1973; Heilbron *et al.*, 1976), rats (Seybold *et al.*, 1976), guinea pigs (Seybold *et al.*, 1976), mice (Fuchs *et al.*, 1976) and monkeys (Tarrab-Hazdai *et al.*, 1975*b*). Acute EAMG is a self-limited disease with considerable inflammation at the motor endplate. Chronic EAMG, induced in rats, is a good model of human MG.

Induction

The AChR is a transmembrane glycoprotein containing four subunits (Changeux *et al.*, 1984). The α-subunits appear to be the antigen involved in EAMG. EAMG can be actively induced by direct inoculation with AChR, or components of the AChR and adjuvants. EAMG can also be induced by the passive transfer of antibody (Lindstrom *et al.*, 1976*b*) or lymph node cells (Tarrab-Hazdai *et al.*, 1975*a*) from animals with EAMG. Another model of MG can be induced by the transfer of human myasthenic thymic tissue to SCID mice (Schonbeck *et al.*, 1992).

Actively induced EAMG

Recombinant AChR α-subunit induces chronic EAMG when inoculated with adjuvants into Lewis rats (Lennon *et al.*, 1991). Age influences the susceptibility to EAMG. Graus *et al.* (1993) showed that rats aged 10–12 weeks developed clinical and pathological features of EAMG after immunization with AChR, whereas rats aged 120–130 weeks developed no clinical signs of EAMG. Lennon, Lindstrom and Seybold (1975) showed that rats recover from acute EAMG by day 11–15 after inoculation, but from day 26–35 develop a second progressive phase of weakness. The same study found that guinea pigs with EAMG also develop relapses after the first episode of weakness and have progressive weakness from day 42 after inoculation.

Passively transferred EAMG

EAMG can be induced by the passive transfer to naive animals of antibody from patients with MG (Toyka *et al.*, 1975) and from animals inoculated with AChR (Lindstrom *et al.*, 1976*b*). In strain 13 guinea pigs, EAMG can be transferred to naive animals by lymph node cells obtained from animals inoculated with AChR (Tarrab-Hazdai *et al.*, 1975*a*).

EAMG induced by transfer of thymic tissue

Goldstein & Whittingham (1966) found that four of 15 animals immunized with thymus in complete Freund's adjuvant developed electrophysiological evidence of impaired neuromuscular transmission. This effect was abolished by thymectomy. Schonbeck *et al.* (1992) have shown that transplantation of tissue from human MG thymuses into SCID mice resulted in the production of antibodies to AChR.

Susceptibility to EAMG

Mice of different strains vary in susceptibility to EAMG and this is linked to the MHC loci (Fuchs *et al.*, 1976; Berman & Patrick, 1980; Christadoss *et al.*, 1981). Susceptibility is not linked to the ability to produce antibody to AChR (Berman & Patrick, 1980). The T cell repertoire may be important in susceptibility to EAMG. Lewis rats, which are susceptible to EAMG, have T cells reactive with sequence 100–116 of the α-subunit of the AChR, but Wistar Furth rats, which are resistant, do not (Zoda & Krolick, 1993). In mice, the epitope recognized by AChR-reactive T cells varies with MHC type (Bellone *et al.*, 1991*a*). A mutation that confers resistance to EAMG causes a deficiency of T cells responsive to the AChR epitopes recognized by the T cells of susceptible mice (Bellone *et al.*, 1991*b*). Mice that are deficient in the C5 complement component are resistant to EAMG (Christadoss, 1988).

Clinical features

Actively induced EAMG

The rabbits that developed EAMG after inoculation with AChR by Patrick & Lindstrom (1973) developed acute severe weakness. Monkeys also developed acute severe weakness (Tarrab-Hazdai *et al.*, 1975*b*). In rats immunized with AChR with pertussis vaccine, an acute phase of weakness occurred 8–11 days after inoculation; on day 28–30 after inoculation a chronic phase of disease commenced, with progressive weakness that sometimes led to death (Lennon *et al.*, 1975; Lindstrom *et al.*, 1976*a*). In guinea pigs, the clinical course was similarly prolonged (Lennon *et al.*,

1975). Mice inoculated twice, at an interval of nine weeks, with AChR developed weight loss, fatigue, hypoactivity and paralysis of the limbs (Fuchs *et al.*, 1976). Severely affected animals died, whereas other animals had a transient illness.

Passively induced EAMG

Lindstrom *et al.* (1976*b*) found that rats became weak within 12 h of a single intravenous injection of antibody to AChR. The weakness became maximal by 48–60 h and started to improve by 72 h, although some weakness persisted for seven days. The weakness was associated with weight loss. In strain 13 guinea pigs, signs of generalized weakness commenced 7–14 days after injection with sensitized lymph node cells and lasted for 3–4 days (Tarrab-Hazdai *et al.*, 1975*a*).

Pathology

Pathology of muscle

In rabbits with EAMG, the light-microscopic appearances of skeletal muscle are normal. However, electron microscopy shows dense material in the synaptic clefts and increased folding of the synaptic membranes (Heilbron *et al.*, 1976). In rats, in the acute phase of EAMG, there is infiltration of the motor endplates with mononuclear cells and destruction of the postsynaptic regions (Engel *et al.*, 1976; Lennon *et al.*, 1978). This is associated with a reduction in the amount of AChR that can be obtained from the muscle (Lindstrom *et al.*, 1976*a*). In the chronic phase of disease there is less inflammation of the muscles, although there is ultrastructural evidence of immune complex deposition on, and destruction of, the junctional folds (Engel *et al.*, 1976; Sahashi *et al.*, 1978).

Pathology of thymus

In actively and passively induced EAMG, the thymus is essentially normal, and shows none of the changes seen in the thymus in human MG (Meinl, Klinkert & Wekerle, 1991). This suggests that the changes seen in human MG are primary and are not a response to the disease.

Pathophysiology

In EAMG there are changes in the miniature endplate potentials similar to those in MG (Lambert, Lindstrom & Lennon, 1976; Lindstrom *et al.*,

1976*a*). There is also a decremental response of the compound muscle action potential to repetitive nerve stimulation (Patrick & Lindstrom, 1973; Lennon *et al.*, 1975), similar to that found in human MG.

Pathogenesis and immunoregulation

B cell response

The B cell response and antibody production play a central role in the pathogenesis of EAMG. Passive transfer of antibodies to the AChR can cause EAMG in recipient animals (Lindstrom *et al.*, 1976*b*; Tzartos *et al.*, 1987). After immunization with AChR in complete Freund's adjuvant, there is an increase in the numbers of B cells producing antibodies directed against all subunits of the AChR (Wang *et al.*, 1993*a*).

T cell response

In EAMG, the antibody production by B cells is dependent on T cell help (Fujii & Lindstrom, 1988*a*,*b*). Clones of AChR-specific T cells from Lewis rats with EAMG were all $CD4^{+}CD8^{-}$ and helped antibody production by AChR-primed lymph node B cells (Fujii & Lindstrom, 1988*b*). In Lewis rats the epitope recognized by cloned AChR-specific T cells was found to be the residue [Tyr100]α100–116 (Fujii & Lindstrom, 1988*a*). Other rat strains recognize different epitopes. In EAMG-susceptible C57BL/6 mice, the T cell receptor usage by T cells responsive to AChR is restricted (Infante *et al.*, 1992).

Macrophages

MHC class II-positive macrophages accumulate at the motor endplate in EAMG (Engel *et al.*, 1976). Kinoshita *et al.* (1988) showed that silica injection, which inhibits macrophage function, prolonged survival in EAMG, and reduced the accumulation of macrophages at the motor endplates. They suggested that the macrophages invading the endplates act as antigen-presenting cells for the induction of the chronic phase of disease.

Complement

Complement has a role in the development of EAMG. It can be demonstrated at the motor endplate in EAMG (Sahashi *et al.*, 1978) as well as in MG (Sahashi *et al.*, 1980). Removal of complement by cobra venom factor

(Lennon *et al.*, 1978) or by antibody (Biesecker & Gomez, 1989) inhibits acute EAMG in rats. Mice that are deficient in C5 are resistant to EAMG (Christadoss, 1988).

Immunoregulation

By using cyclosporin A, McIntosh & Drachman (1986) isolated suppressor T cells, specific for AChR, from rats with EAMG. These cells suppressed the *in vitro* production of anti-AChR antibody by lymphocytes from rats with EAMG and may play a role in regulating the disease.

Therapy

Non-specific agents

Terbutaline, a β-2 adrenergic agonist, suppresses passively transferred EAMG (Chelmicka Schorr *et al.*, 1993). Alpha-foetoprotein confers some protection against EAMG induced in mice by the transfer of human myasthenic immunoglobulin (Buschman *et al.*, 1987). Cyclosporin A prevents the development of EAMG when administered at the time of sensitization, and suppresses EAMG when administered after clinical onset (Drachman *et al.*, 1985). Antibody to complement reduces weakness, and prevents the loss of AChR and macrophage accumulation in muscle in passively transferred EAMG (Biesecker & Gomez, 1989).

Specific immunotherapy

A number of experimental therapies have been used to produce tolerance to AChR and to treat EAMG. In one study, treatment with anti-idiotypic antibodies directed against anti-AChR antibodies did not suppress disease (Verschuuren *et al.*, 1991) but in another, such antibodies provided some protection (Souroujon, Pachner & Fuchs, 1986). Oral administration of AChR to Lewis rats prior to immunization with AChR and adjuvants prevented the development of EAMG (Wang *et al.*, 1993*b*). Mice can be rendered resistant to the development of EAMG by tolerization with the main myasthenogenic region of the α-subunit of the AChR by injection of a synthetic peptide conjugated to monomethylpolyethylene glycol (Atassi *et al.*, 1992). Treatment of rats with established EAMG with AChR conjugated to the toxin gelonin also suppressed the disease (Urbatsch *et al.*, 1993). In Lewis rats, vaccination with AChR-specific T cells does not suppress actively induced EAMG and may increase the magnitude of the antibody response (Kahn, McIntosh & Drachman, 1990). However, treatment of

Lewis rats with AChR-coupled spleen cells can suppress both T cell and antibody responses to AChR inoculation (McIntosh & Drachman, 1992). Incubation of AChR-specific T cells with fixed AChR-coupled B cells also reduces the proliferative response of these T cells to AChR *in vitro* (Reim *et al.*, 1992).

The Lambert–Eaton myasthenic syndrome

Introduction

In 1957, Eaton & Lambert described six patients with a disorder that resembled MG but that could be distinguished from it by the effects of repetitive nerve stimulation. Some of these patients had intrathoracic neoplasms, and it was suggested that the neurological syndrome may have been related to the malignancy. This clinical syndrome is now known as the Lambert–Eaton myasthenic syndrome (LEMS). LEMS is most commonly found in association with small cell carcinoma of the lung (O'Neill, Murray & Newsom-Davis, 1988; Chalk *et al.*, 1990), but may also occur with other malignancies (O'Neill *et al.*, 1988; Sutton *et al.*, 1988). LEMS can also develop in patients without evidence of malignancy (O'Neill *et al.*, 1988; Gutmann & Phillips, 1992). Non-paraneoplastic LEMS may occur together with other autoimmune diseases (Gutmann *et al.*, 1972; O'Neill *et al.*, 1988). It now is clear that LEMS, with or without associated malignancy, is an autoimmune disease. Ultrastructural studies have shown that there is a reduction in the number of large intramembrane particles in presynaptic membrane active zones of motor nerve terminals (Fukunaga *et al.*, 1982). These particles are thought to represent voltage-gated calcium channels, which appear to be the target antigen of the immune attack in LEMS. The weakness in LEMS is due to reduced release of ACh.

Clinical features

Clinical features and genetic associations

As with MG, weakness and abnormal fatiguability occur in LEMS. A distinguishing feature of LEMS is that muscle strength characteristically increases after sustained contraction. For example, ptosis may improve after sustained upgaze (Breen *et al.*, 1991). In the series of O'Neill *et al.* (1988), 70% of patients had weakness of the muscles supplied by cranial nerves, 100% had lower limb weakness and 78% had upper limb weakness.

Respiratory muscle weakness may also occur (Laroche *et al.*, 1989) and may be the presenting problem (Barr *et al.*, 1993; Beydoun, 1994). Typically, the deep tendon reflexes are depressed, but increase after sustained maximal voluntary muscle contraction (O'Neill *et al.*, 1988). There is no sensory involvement. Cholinergic autonomic dysfunction, resulting in dry mouth, impotence and constipation (O'Neill *et al.*, 1988), is described in LEMS. The occurrence of such symptoms suggests that the defect in ACh release may not be confined to the neuromuscular junction (Rubenstein, Horowitz & Bender, 1979). There is an association of LEMS with the genetic markers HLA B8 and the Gm allele Glm2 (Willcox *et al.*, 1985). The diagnosis of LEMS is made by electrophysiological testing and requires the finding of an increase in the amplitude of the compound muscle action potential after sustained contraction or after repetitive stimulation at 20 Hz.

Association with malignancy

The malignancy most commonly associated with LEMS is small cell carcinoma of the lung (Eaton & Lambert, 1957; O'Neill *et al.*, 1988; Chalk *et al.*, 1990). The prevalence of LEMS among patients with this carcinoma is about 3% (Elrington *et al.*, 1991). LEMS may also occur with other malignancies (Lauritzen *et al.*, 1980; O'Neill *et al.*, 1988; Sutton *et al.*, 1988; Morrow *et al.*, 1988). LEMS may coexist with other paraneoplastic neurological syndromes, for example subacute cerebellar degeneration (Blumenfeld *et al.*, 1991). LEMS may present before the diagnosis of malignancy, but in patients with LEMS for longer than five years, it is unlikely that a malignancy will become apparent (O'Neill *et al.*, 1988).

Association with other autoimmune disease

LEMS has been reported in association with other autoimmune diseases such as thyroid disease, vitiligo and pernicious anaemia (Gutmann *et al.*, 1972; O'Neill *et al.*, 1988).

Pathology

The morphological changes in LEMS are found at the neuromuscular junction (Fukuhara *et al.*, 1972) and in particular at the active zones on the presynaptic membrane. Using freeze–fracture techniques, Fukunaga *et al.* (1982) have shown that there is a reduction in the numbers of active zones and active zone particles and an aggregation of these particles into clusters. There are no studies of antibody at the neuromuscular junction in patients with LEMS. However, when LEMS serum is transferred to mice, IgG is bound to the active zones of the presynaptic membrane and may cause cross-linking of the active zone particles (Fukuoka *et al.*, 1987*b*).

Pathophysiology

Lambert and Elmqvist (Elmqvist & Lambert, 1968; Lambert and Elmqvist, 1971) studied the intercostal muscle of patients with LEMS. They showed that miniature endplate potentials (mepps) were normal and that the endplate potentials were reduced. These findings indicated that there was reduced release of ACh from nerve terminals on stimulation. The release of ACh increased with repetitive stimulation, with guanidine treatment and with increasing calcium concentrations. This accounts for the weakness in LEMS and the improvement with increasing effort. Schwartz and Stahlberg (1975) used single fibre electromyography to demonstrate jitter and blocking in the muscle of a patient with LEMS. They showed that these abnormalities, which indicate insecurity of neuromuscular transmission, declined when the frequency of discharge of the potentials occurred at higher rates.

Immunological findings in the peripheral blood

Antibodies

LEMS sera contain antibodies that bind to voltage gated calcium channels (VGCCs); such antibodies are not present in patients with other neurological diseases, but are occasionally found in patients with rheumatoid arthritis or systemic lupus erythematosus (Leys *et al.*, 1991; Hewett & Atchison, 1992*a*). VGCCs are composed of a number of subunits. There are four types of VGCC (L-type, N-type, P-type and T-type) which are identified by the agent that blocks the channel (Mori *et al.*, 1993). The N-type calcium channel is present on neurones, is blocked by ω-conotoxin and is involved in the release of ACh from nerve terminals (Hong, Tsuji & Chang, 1992). Antibodies in LEMS bind to ω-conotoxin-labelled calcium channel complexes (Leys *et al.*, 1991; Lang *et al.*, 1993). Some antibodies associated with LEMS may also bind to the protein, synaptotagmin, which is associated with VGCCs (Leveque *et al.*, 1992). LEMS sera may also contain antibodies to L-type and P-type channels (Lang *et al.*, 1993). Rosenfeld *et al.* (1993) have cloned a target antigen that is homologous with the β subunit of calcium channels and that was recognized by three of seven LEMS sera but none of 34 controls. Binding of antibodies to VGCCs appears to lead to morphological changes of the active zone particles at the nerve terminals (Leys *et al.*,

1991; Hewett & Atchison, 1992*a*,*b*). Immunoglobulin from patients with LEMS reduces the release of ACh in mice (Lambert & Lennon, 1988), probably by action of the antibody on presynaptic VGCCs (Kim & Neher, 1988; Lang, Newsom-Davis & Wray, 1988; Hewett & Atchison, 1992*a*). Studies of the transfer of LEMS IgG to mice show that IgG binds to the active zone particles and probably causes cross-linking (Fukuoka *et al.*, 1987*a*,*b*) (see below). Serum from a LEMS patient also inhibited calcium channels on a small cell carcinoma line (Roberts *et al.*, 1985). This finding suggests that, in paraneoplastic LEMS, the autoimmune response arises because of cross-reactivity between antigens on the carcinoma cells and antigens at the neuromuscular junction.

Therapy

The agent 3,4-diaminopyridine, which blocks potassium channels (Kirsch & Narahashi, 1978) and enhances neuromuscular transmission, provides symptomatic relief to patients with LEMS (Lundh, Nilsson & Rosen, 1984). Guanidine, which also enhances neuromuscular transmission, can improve weakness in LEMS, but has been associated with toxic effects including interstitial nephritis and bone marrow suppression (Joong & Kim, 1973; Cherington, 1976). In LEMS associated with malignancy, treatment of the malignancy results in improvement of the neurological syndrome (Berglund *et al.*, 1982; Sutton *et al.*, 1988; Chalk *et al.*, 1990). Long-term treatment with oral prednisone improves muscle strength in LEMS (Streib & Rothner, 1981). Plasma exchange combined with immunosuppression is also useful in LEMS (Dau & Denys, 1982; Newsom-Davis & Murray, 1984). High-dose intravenous immunoglobulin therapy has been reported to be of benefit in LEMS (Bird, 1992).

Animal model of LEMS

Inoculation of Lewis rats with cholinergic synaptosomes in complete Freund's adjuvant causes a presynaptic defect of neuromuscular transmission similar to that found in LEMS (Chapman *et al.*, 1990). Serum from patients with LEMS can transfer to mice the electrophysiological abnormalities of LEMS (Lang *et al.*, 1981, 1983, 1984). Mice with this form of passively transferred LEMS have abnormalities of the presynaptic membranes that are similar to those found in human LEMS (Fukunaga *et al.*, 1982, 1983; Fukuoka *et al.*, 1987*a*). IgG can be detected at the active zones of the presynaptic membranes and probably causes cross-linking of the active zone particles (Fukuoka *et al.*, 1987*b*).

Isaacs' syndrome

Introduction

Isaacs' syndrome is a disorder characterized by muscle cramps and weakness and myokymia. It was described by Isaacs (1961), in a report of two patients with muscle weakness and continuous muscle fibre activity. Denny-Brown & Foley (1948) had previously described a similar patient as having undulating myokymia. Newsom-Davis & Mills (1993) have suggested that Isaacs' syndrome is of autoimmune origin and have suggested the use of the term 'acquired neuromyotonia'. Jamieson & Katirji (1994) have recently reviewed a group of patients with 'idiopathic generalized myokymia' – many of these appear to have Isaacs' syndrome.

Clinical features and muscle pathology

Isaacs' syndrome is characterised by spontaneous muscle fibre activity (myokymia) associated with muscle cramps (neuromyotonia) and sometimes weakness (Newsom-Davis & Mills, 1993). Although most cases probably arise spontaneously, acquired neuromyotonia has been reported in association with small cell lung cancer (Partanen *et al.*, 1980), after penicillamine treatment (Reeback *et al.*, 1979) and in association with the Guillain–Barré syndrome (Vasilescu, Alexianu & Dan, 1984). Halbach, Homberg & Freund (1987) have reported patients with acquired neuromyotonia in association with thymoma. The EMG findings include spontaneous muscle discharges, typically fibrillations, fasciculations and myotonic activity (Newsom-Davis & Mills, 1993). Muscle biopsies from the two patients reported by Isaacs (1961) displayed some variation in fibre size, but no other abnormalities. The patient reported by Nagashima *et al.* (1985) had evidence of IgA deposition at motor endplates.

Immunological findings in the peripheral blood and cerebrospinal fluid

Nagashima *et al.* (1985) described a patient with Isaacs' syndrome who had circulating immune complexes. Sinha *et al.* (1991) found that serum from a patient with Isaacs' syndrome enhanced resistance to tubocurarine at the neuromuscular junction *in vitro*. They suggested that this was due to effects of an antibody directed against potassium channels, which have been shown by Bostock & Baker (1988) to be present on human motor axons. Newsom-

Davis & Mills (1993) reported that three of five patients with Isaacs' syndrome had oligoclonal bands in the cerebrospinal fluid. These findings suggest that Isaacs' syndrome is associated with activation of the immune system and may be mediated by antibody to potassium channels.

Therapy

Symptomatic treatment with carbamazepine or phenytoin may be helpful in Isaacs' syndrome. Newsom-Davis & Mills (1993) have reported improvement after plasmapheresis. It might be expected that high-dose immunoglobulin therapy would also be useful, but it has been reported that one patient became worse after such treatment (Ishii *et al.*, 1994). One of the patients described by Halbach *et al.* (1987) improved after thymectomy.

Amyotrophic lateral sclerosis

Introduction

Amyotrophic lateral sclerosis (ALS) was the term used by Charcot in his initial description of this condition (see Bonduelle, 1975). The term 'motor neurone disease' (MND) is used synonymously with ALS. ALS is a progressive disorder, which presents with weakness and wasting of the muscles in association with spasticity and increased deep tendon reflexes, typical of upper motor neurone lesions. Degeneration of the lower motor neurones without upper motor neurone involvement also occurs: such patients were first described by Aran (see Norris, 1975), and are now regarded as having progressive muscular atrophy, a subgroup of ALS. The primary pathology in these conditions is loss of motor neurones. Many workers have tried to determine the cause of ALS and recently there has been interest in a possible role for the immune system. Clearly, some forms of ALS, such as the familial form and the form found on Guam, are not of autoimmune aetiology. Other possible non-immune aetiologies for ALS include excitotoxicity, which may be related to impaired glutamate uptake (Rothstein, Martin & Kuncl, 1992) and deficiency in neurotrophic factors (Masu *et al.*, 1993). The main evidence for an immune basis for ALS is the development of autoimmune animal models and the finding of antibodies to calcium channels and the ganglioside GM1 in many patients with ALS. The question that needs to be addressed is whether ALS in some patients is immune-mediated. The present chapter will review the immune abnormalities found in ALS.

Clinical features

General clinical features

The predominant clinical feature of ALS is weakness. The weakness is associated with the lower motor neurone signs of wasting and fasciculations of the muscles. It may also be associated with upper motor neurone signs such as an increase in the deep tendon reflexes. There is no sensory loss. Variable involvement of the upper and lower motor neurones allows the subdivision of ALS into categories such as progressive muscular atrophy, progressive bulbar palsy, primary lateral sclerosis and progressive pseudobulbar palsy.

Recently there has been considerable interest in the condition multifocal motor neuropathy (see Chapter 9), which has clinical features in common with progressive muscular atrophy and which can be distinguished by the finding of multifocal conduction block. Some authors have defined other lower motor neurone syndromes where there is evidence of peripheral degeneration of motor neurones and no evidence of conduction block (Pestronk *et al.*, 1990; Pestronk, 1991). Clearly, there is considerable overlap between such syndromes and progressive muscular atrophy.

Diagnosis

There is no single diagnostic test for ALS and the clinical features may not be fully developed at onset. Electromyography is useful in demonstrating fasciculations and denervation. Nerve conduction studies are important in distinguishing the lower motor neurone forms of ALS from motor neuropathies such as multifocal motor neuropathy with conduction block (Parry & Clarke, 1988). The diagnosis of these conditions requires careful study for conduction block, which must be distinguished from temporal dispersion on the one hand and from amplitude reduction due to axonal degeneration on the other.

Genetics

Familial MND

About 5–10% of ALS is familial and in these patients the disease is not autoimmune. Mulder *et al.* (1986) described 72 families with a total of 329 affected members. Familial ALS is associated with mutations in the gene for superoxide dismutase (Rosen, 1993; Rosen *et al.*, 1993) and patients with familial ALS but not sporadic ALS have reduced activity of red blood cell superoxide dismutase (Robberecht *et al.*, 1994).

HLA associations

Non-familial ALS has been associated with HLA A3 (Antel *et al.*, 1976; Kott *et al.*, 1979), with HLA A2 and A28 (Behan, Durward & Dick, 1976), with HLA B35 (Bartfeld *et al.*, 1982) and with HLA B40 (Kott *et al.*, 1979). Other studies have failed to find significant associations with HLA A and B loci (Pedersen *et al.*, 1977) or with HLA D loci (Woo *et al.*, 1986). However, if a subset of patients with ALS have an autoimmune disease, then studies of the entire group would not be expected to show an immunogenetic association.

Neuropathology

The pathological changes in ALS are slight and chiefly comprise degeneration of motor neurones and the major descending fibre pathways. The mechanism of cell death is not known; it would be of interest to know whether motor neurones in ALS die by the process of apoptosis (programmed cell death), which can be produced by growth factor deprivation and by cytotoxic T cells. Munoz *et al.* (1988) found an accumulation of phosphorylated neurofilaments in the perikarya of anterior horn cells in ALS. Others have confirmed changes in the cytoskeleton in lower motor neurones, and occasionally in upper motor neurones in ALS (Murayama, Bouldin & Suzuki, 1992). Heterotopic neurones have been found in the spinal cord of seven patients with ALS (Kozlowski *et al.*, 1989) which could indicate a developmental disorder that predisposes to ALS. As would be expected, in the peripheral nerves of patients with ALS there is a reduction in the number of myelinated fibres (Rosales *et al.*, 1988).

Immunopathology of the nervous system lesions

Immunocytochemistry has allowed the detection of infiltrating T cells in the central nervous system in ALS (Troost *et al.*, 1989; Lampson, Kushner & Sobel, 1990; Troost, van den Oord & Vianney de Jong, 1990; Kawamata *et al.*, 1992; Engelhardt, Tajti & Appel, 1993). Reactive microglia have also been detected (Kawamata *et al.*, 1992; Engelhardt *et al.*, 1993), but this is a non-specific finding. Troost *et al.* (1989; 1990) found lymphocytes in the spinal cord, with $CD8^+$ cells outnumbering $CD4^+$ cells. Others have also found small numbers of T cells in the spinal cord (Lampson *et al.*, 1990;

Kawamata *et al.*, 1992), but the importance of these cells in the pathogenesis of ALS is by no means clear. Lampson *et al.*, (1990) found no expression of MHC antigens on motor neurones in ALS or in controls, although in ALS there was MHC class I and II antigen expression on macrophages in areas of degeneration. J.I. Engelhardt & Appel (1990) found immunoglobulin deposition on motor neurones in the spinal cord and motor cortex from patients with ALS, but not from normal controls. They found no deposition on astrocytes, although an earlier study had found antibodies on astrocytes in the spinal cord in ALS and also complement deposition (Donnenfeld, Kascsak & Bartfeld, 1984). Immunoglobulin deposition in spinal motor neurones has been found in experimental animal models of ALS (Engelhardt, Appel & Killian, 1989) (see below).

Immunological findings in the peripheral blood and cerebrospinal fluid

Antibody

Antibody to calcium channels

Antibody to L-type calcium channels, which are present in all excitable tissues, are found in the sera of patients with ALS (Delbono *et al.*, 1991*a*,*b*; Rowland, 1992; Engel, 1993; Wierzbicki, 1993; Mori *et al.*, 1993) and are reactive with the $\alpha 1$ subunit (Kimura *et al.*, 1994). Such antibodies may be responsible for the changes in calcium current produced *in vitro* in skeletal muscle fibres by ALS immunoglobulins (Delbono *et al.*, 1991*a*,*b*). ALS immunoglobulins can enhance neurotransmitter release from the presynaptic membrane (Uchitel *et al.*, 1988) and after passive transfer cause increased neurotransmitter release at neuromuscular junctions of recipient mice (Appel *et al.*, 1991; Uchitel *et al.*, 1992). Cell death by apoptosis is often preceded by changes in intracellular calcium levels; possibly alterations in calcium channels could lead to the death of target cells. ALS immunoglobulins cause death, by a mechanism that is dependent on extracellular calcium, of a motor neurone/neuroblastoma hybrid cell line *in vitro* (Smith *et al.*, 1994).

Anti-GM1 antibodies

Pestronk *et al.* (1989) have found elevated levels of antibodies to GM1 in patients with ALS. Others have confirmed that a small percentage of patients with upper motor neurone forms of ALS have elevated serum anti-GM1 titres, but that anti-GM1 antibodies are present in higher titres in patients with motor nerve conduction block than with ALS (Salazar Grueso *et al.*, 1990; Sanders *et al.*, 1993). The anti-GM1 antibodies found in ALS sera show greater binding to GM1 incorporated into liposomes than do such antibodies from other patients (Li & Pestronk, 1991). In the cerebrospinal fluid a pattern of anti-ganglioside antibody reactivity has been found that appears to be specific for ALS: in 35 ALS patients there were elevated IgM antibodies to all the mono-, di- and trisialogangliosides tested but no antibodies to asialogangliosides (Stevens, Weller & Wietholter, 1993).

Other antibodies

Some have found antibody to components of foetal but not adult muscle (Ordonez & Sotelo, 1989). In a patient with paraneoplastic ALS, a monoclonal antibody reactive with cytoskeletal proteins was present in the serum (Hays *et al.*, 1990). The vulnerability of neurones in ALS has been related to the presence of antibodies to acetyl cholinesterase in ALS sera (Conradi & Ronnevi, 1993). ALS sera are toxic to erythrocytes (Conradi & Ronnevi, 1985).

Monoclonal immunoglobulin bands

Monoclonal immunoglobulin bands are reported in the serum of some patients with ALS. Duarte *et al.* (1991) found that up to 60% of ALS patients had such paraproteins, which were usually IgG or IgM. An IgG kappa paraprotein from a patient with ALS failed to inhibit sprouting of mouse nerve terminals (Donaghy & Duchen, 1986). An IgA paraprotein has also been reported in ALS (Hays *et al.*, 1990).

Complement and immune complexes

Elevation of serum C4 complement levels (Apostolski *et al.*, 1991) and cerebrospinal fluid C4d complement levels (Tsuboi & Yamada, 1994) has been reported in patients with ALS. Oldstone *et al.* (1976) reported that circulating immune complexes were present in ALS sera.

Therapy

No successful treatment has been found for ALS. Because of the possibility that ALS may have an autoimmune aetiology, many forms of immunosuppression have been tried, all without success. However, Drachman & Kuncl (1989), in their review of a possible autoimmune aetiology for ALS, suggest that more powerful and specific immunosuppressants, or a longer course of treatment, may be required. Because ALS is characterized by the permanent loss of motor neurones, it is unlikely that any form of treatment will lead to clinical improvement, but it is possible that treatment may halt progression of disease.

Plasmapheresis and immunosuppressive therapy

Neither plasmapheresis alone (Olarte *et al.*, 1980) nor plasmapheresis combined with azathioprine is of benefit in ALS (Kelemen *et al.*, 1983). Therapy with high-dose intravenous cyclophosphamide does not alter the course of the disease (Brown *et al.*, 1986). A trial of total lymphoid irradiation also failed to benefit patients with ALS (Drachman *et al.*, 1994). The authors of this study argued that this was evidence against a role of the immune system in the pathogenesis of ALS. However, if a subgroup of patients with ALS have an autoimmune disorder, then a trial may not show beneficial results for the whole group.

Protecting neurones from death

Flunarazine, which is a calcium channel blocker, protects motor neurones from cell death after growth factor deprivation (Rich & Hollowell, 1990). This may be of relevance if ALS is caused by growth factor deprivation. It may also be important because of the possible role of calcium channel abnormalities in causing cell death in ALS (see above). Another calcium channel blocker, nifedipine, protects against excitotoxins (Weiss *et al.*, 1990), which have been implicated in ALS. There has also been recent interest in the possible use of ciliary neurotrophic factor (CNTF), which arrests apoptosis in certain motor neurones (Wewetzer *et al.*, 1990), and which might protect motor neurones from death caused by growth factor deprivation.

Autoimmune animal models of ALS

There are animal models of motor neurone disease that do not have an immunological basis (Sillevis Smitt & de Jong, 1989). The present section deals only with the autoimmune models of ALS (Smith *et al.*, 1993). Experimental autoimmune motor neurone disease (EAMND) can be induced by inoculation with bovine motor neurones (Gilpin, Moersch & Kernohan, 1936; Engelhardt *et al.*, 1989) isolated by centrifugation (Engelhardt *et al.*, 1985) and is characterized by weight loss, loss of muscle tone and weakness. Experimental autoimmune grey matter disease (EAGMD) can be produced by the inoculation of guinea pigs with bovine ventral horn homogenate and is characterized by decreased tone of the abdomen and weakness and decreased tone in the hind legs (Engelhardt, Appel & Killian, 1990). EAGMD is more severe than EAMND. Cyclophosphamide treatment prevents EAGMD (Tajti, Stefani & Appel, 1991).

In EAMND there is degeneration of the lower motor neurones in the spinal cord and brainstem with neuronophagia. The muscles of the hindlimbs show evidence of denervation (Engelhardt *et al.*, 1989). In EAGMD there is a loss of motor neurones and scattered inflammatory foci in the spinal cord (Engelhardt *et al.*, 1990). In EAMND the inoculated animals develop high titres of circulating IgG antibody to motor neurones (Engelhardt *et al.*, 1989). In both EAGMD and EAMND, IgG can be demonstrated within motor neurones and at motor endplates (Engelhardt *et al.*, 1989, 1990). Serum from animals with EAMND and EAGMD binds to motor neurones with immunocytochemical staining and is transported to these neurones following limb injection (J. Engelhardt & Appel, 1990). Passive transfer of EAGMD and EAMND sera to mice causes increased miniature endplate potentials, indicating increased quantal release of ACh from neuromuscular junctions (Appel *et al.*, 1991).

Conclusions

The conditions in this chapter are similar in two ways. Firstly, all are disorders of motor function. Secondly, in all disorders there is evidence that an antibody-mediated autoimmune process may be occurring: this evidence is very strong in MG, LEMS and the respective animal models, is circumstantial in Isaacs' syndrome and is less convincing in ALS. Evidence that an autoimmune process is occurring has led to successful immunosuppressive treatment in MG and LEMS and is likely to lead to more specific and successful treatments in the future.

References

Aarli, J.A., Gilhus, N.E. & Matre, R. (1992). Myasthenia gravis with thymoma is not associated with an increased incidence of non-muscle autoimmune disorders. *Autoimmunity*, **11**, 159–62.

Abramsky, O., Aharonov, A., Webb, C. & Fuchs, S. (1975). Cellular immune response to acetylcholine receptor receptor-rich fraction, in patients with myasthenia gravis. *Clinical and Experimental Immunology*, **19**, 11–16.

Ahlberg, R., Yi, Q., Eng, H., Pirskanen, R. & Lefvert, A.K. (1992). T-cell epitopes on the human acetylcholine receptor alpha-subunit residues 10–84 in myasthenia gravis. *Scandinavian Journal of Immunology*, **36**, 435–42.

Ahlberg, R., Yi, Q., Pirskanen, R., Matell, G., Swerup, C., Rieber, P., Riethmuller, G., Holm, G. & Lefvert, A.K. (1993). Clinical improvement of myasthenia gravis by treatment with a chimeric anti-CD4 monoclonal antibody. *Annals of the New York Academy of Sciences*, **681**, 552–5.

Alarcon Segovia, D., Galbraith, R.F., Maldonado, J.E. & Howard, F.M. (1963). Systemic lupus erythematosus following thymectomy for myasthenia gravis. *Lancet*, **2**, 662–5.

Alter, M. & Talbert, R. (1960). Myasthenia gravis in one monozygotic twin. *Neurology*, **10**, 793–8.

Antel, J.P., Arnason, B.G., Fuller, T.C. & Lehrich, J.R. (1976). Histocompatibility typing in amyotrophic lateral sclerosis. *Archives of Neurology*, **33**, 423–5.

Apostolski, S., Nikolic, J., Bugarski Prokopljevic, C., Miletic, V., Pavlovic, S. & Filipovic, S. (1991). Serum and CSF immunological findings in ALS. *Acta Neurologica Scandinavica*, **83**, 96–8.

Appel, S.H., Engelhardt, J.I., Garcia, J. & Stefani, E. (1991). Immunoglobulins from animal models of motor neuron disease and from human amyotrophic lateral sclerosis patients passively transfer physiological abnormalities to the neuromuscular junction. *Proceedings of the National Academy of Science of the United States of America*, **88**, 647–51.

Armstrong, R.M., Nowak, R.M. & Falk, R.E. (1973). Thymic lymphocyte function in myasthenia gravis. *Neurology*, **23**, 1078–83.

Atassi, M.Z., Ruan, K.H., Jinnai, K., Oshima, M. & Ashizawa, T. (1992). Epitope-specific suppression of antibody response in experimental autoimmune myasthenia gravis by a monomethoxypolyethylene glycol conjugate of a myasthenogenic synthetic peptide. *Proceedings of the National Academy of Science of the United States of America*, **89**, 5852–6.

Baggi, F., Nicolle, M., Vincent, A., Matsuo, H., Willcox, N. & Newsom-Davis, J. (1993). Presentation of endogenous acetylcholine receptor epitope by an MHC class-II transfected human muscle cell line to a specific $CD4^+$ T cell clone from a myasthenia gravis patient. *Journal of Neuroimmunology*, **46**, 57–66.

Barr, C.W., Claussen, G., Thomas, D., Fesenmeier, J.T., Pearlman, R.L. & Oh, S.J. (1993). Primary respiratory failure as the presenting symptom in Lambert–Eaton myasthenic syndrome. *Muscle and Nerve*, **16**, 712–15.

Bartfeld, H., Pollack, M.S., Cunningham Rundles, S. & Donnenfeld, H. (1982). HLA frequencies in amyotrophic lateral sclerosis. *Archives of Neurology*, **39**, 270–1.

Behan, P.O., Durward, W.F. & Dick, H. (1976). Histocompatibility antigens associated with motor-neurone disease. *Lancet*, **2**, 803.

Bell, E.T. (1917). Tumors of the thymus in myasthenia gravis. *Journal of Nervous and Mental Disease*, **45**, 130–43.

Bellone, M., Ostlie, N., Lei, S. & Conti Tronconi, B.M. (1991*a*). Experimental myasthenia gravis in congenic mice. Sequence mapping and H-2 restriction of T helper epitopes on the alpha subunits of *Torpedo californica* and murine acetylcholine receptors. *European Journal of Immunology*, **21**, 2303–10.

Bellone, M., Ostlie, N., Lei, S.J., Wu, X.D. & Conti Tronconi, B.M. (1991*b*). The $I\text{-}A^{bm12}$ mutation, which confers resistance to experimental myasthenia gravis, drastically affects the epitope repertoire of murine $CD4^+$ cells sensitized to nicotinic acetylcholine receptor. *Journal of Immunology*, **147**, 1484–91.

Berglund, S., Eriksson, M., von Eyben, F.E., Hellekant, C. & Mattsson, W. (1982). Remission by chemotherapy of the Eaton–Lambert myasthenic syndrome in a patient with small cell bronchogenic carcinoma. *Acta Medica Scandinavica*, **212**, 429–32.

Bergoffen, J., Zmijewski, C.M. & Fischbeck, K.H. (1994). Familial autoimmune myasthenia gravis. *Neurology*, **44**, 551–4.

Bergstrom, K., Franksson, C., Matell, G. & von Reiss, G. (1973). The effect of thoracic duct lymph drainage in myasthenia gravis. *European Neurology*, **9**, 157–67.

Berman, P.W. & Patrick, J. (1980). Linkage between the frequency of muscular weakness and the loci that regulate immune responsiveness in murine experimental myasthenia gravis. *Journal of Experimental Medicine*, **152**, 507–20.

Berrih Aknin, S., Morel, E., Raimond, F., Safar, D., Gaud, C., Binet, J.P., Levasseur, P. & Bach, J.F. (1987). The role of the thymus in myasthenia gravis: immunohistological and immunological studies in 115 cases. *Annals of the New York Academy of Sciences*, **505**, 50–70.

Bever, C.T.J. & Asofsky, R. (1991). Augmented IgG anti-acetylcholine receptor response following chronic penicillamine administration. *Journal of Neuroimmunology*, **35**, 131–7.

Beydoun, S.R. (1994). Delayed diagnosis of Lambert–Eaton myasthenic syndrome in a patient presenting with recurrent refractory respiratory failure. *Muscle and Nerve*, **17**, 689–90.

Bhalla, R., Swedler, W.I., Lazarevic, M.B., Ajmani, H.S. & Skosey, J.L. (1993). Myasthenia gravis and scleroderma. *Journal of Rheumatology*, **20**, 1409–10.

Biesecker, G. & Gomez, C.M. (1989). Inhibition of acute passive transfer experimental autoimmune myasthenia gravis with Fab antibody to complement C6. *Journal of Immunology*, **142**, 2654–9.

Bird, S.J. (1992). Clinical and electrophysiologic improvement in Lambert–Eaton syndrome with intravenous immunoglobulin therapy. *Neurology*, **42**, 1422–3.

Birmanns, B., Brenner, T., Abramsky, O. & Steiner, I. (1991). Seronegative myasthenia gravis: clinical features, response to therapy and synthesis of acetylcholine receptor antibodies *in vitro*. *Journal of the Neurological Sciences*, **102**, 184–9.

Blalock, A., Harvey, A.M., Ford, F.R. & Lilienthal, J.L. (1941). The treatment of myasthenia gravis by removal of the thymus gland. *Journal of the American Medical Association*, **117**, 1529–33.

Blumenfeld, A.M., Recht, L.D., Chad, D.A., DeGirolami, U., Griffin, T. & Jaeckle, K.A. (1991). Coexistence of Lambert–Eaton myasthenic syndrome and subacute cerebellar degeneration: differential effects of treatment. *Neurology*, **41**, 1682–85.

Bonduelle, M. (1975). Amyotrophic lateral sclerosis. In *Handbook of Clinical Neurology*, volume 22, *Systemic Disorders and Atrophies*, Part II, ed. P.J. Vinken & G.W. Bruyn, pp. 281–338. Amsterdam: North-Holland.

Bostock, H. & Baker, M. (1988). Evidence for two types of potassium channel in human motor axons *in vivo*. *Brain Research*, **462**, 354–8.

Breen, L.A., Gutmann, L., Brick, J.F. & Riggs, J.R. (1991). Paradoxical lid elevation with sustained upgaze: a sign of Lambert–Eaton syndrome. *Muscle and Nerve*, **14**, 863–6.

Brown, R.H., Hauser, S.L., Harrington, H. & Weiner, H.L. (1986). Failure of immunosuppression with a ten- to 14-day course of high-dose intravenous cyclophosphamide to alter the progression of amyotrophic lateral sclerosis. *Archives of Neurology*, **43**, 383–4.

Brunner, N.G., Namba, T. & Grob, D. (1972). Corticosteroids in management of severe, generalized myasthenia gravis. Effectiveness and comparison with corticotrophin therapy. *Neurology*, **22**, 603–10.

Buschman, E., van Oers, N., Katz, M. & Murgita, R.A. (1987). Experimental myasthenia gravis induced in mice by passive transfer of human myasthenic immunoglobulin. Evidence for an ameliorating effect by alpha-fetoprotein. *Journal of Neuroimmunology*, **13**, 315–30.

Campbell, H. & Bramwell, E. (1900). Myasthenia gravis. *Brain*, **23**, 277–336.

Cardona, A., Garchon, H.J., Vernet-der-Garabedian, B., Morel, E., Gajdos, P. & Bach, J.F. (1994). Human IgG monoclonal antibodies against muscle acetylcholine receptor: direct evidence for clonal heterogeneity of the antiself humoral response in myasthenia gravis. *Journal of Neuroimmunology*, **53**, 9–16.

Castleman, B. & Norris, E.H. (1949). The pathology of the thymus in myasthenia gravis. A study of 35 cases. *Medicine*, **28**, 27–58.

Chalk, C.H., Murray, N.M., Newsom-Davis, J., O'Neill, J.H. & Spiro, S.G. (1990). Response of the Lambert–Eaton myasthenic syndrome to treatment of associated small-cell lung carcinoma. *Neurology*, **40**, 1552–6.

Changeux, J.-P., Devillers-Thiery, A. & Chemouilli, P. (1984). Acetylcholine receptor: an allosteric protein. *Science*, **225**, 1335–45.

Chapman, J., Rabinowitz, R., Korczyn, A.D. & Michaelson, D.M. (1990). Rats immunized with cholinergic synaptosomes: a model for Lambert–Eaton syndrome. *Muscle and Nerve*, **13**, 726–33.

Chelmicka Schorr, E., Wollmann, R.L., Kwasniewski, M.N., Kim, D.H. & Dupont, B.L. (1993). The beta 2-adrenergic agonist terbutaline suppresses acute passive transfer experimental autoimmune myasthenia gravis (EAMG). *International Journal of Immunopharmacology*, **15**, 19–24.

Cherington, M. (1976). Guanidine and germine in Eaton–Lambert syndrome. *Neurology*, **26**, 944–6.

Christadoss, P. (1988). C5 gene influences the development of murine myasthenia gravis. *Journal of Immunology*, **140**, 2589–92.

Christadoss, P., Lennon, V.A., Krco, C.J., Lambert, E.H. & David, C.S. (1981). Genetic control of autoimmunity to acethylcholine receptors: role of Ia molecules. *Annals of the New York Academy of Sciences*, **377**, 258–77.

Cohen Kaminsky, S., Gaud, C., Morel, E. & Berrih Aknin, S. (1989*a*). High recombinant interleukin-2 sensitivity of peripheral blood lymphocytes from patients with myasthenia gravis: correlations with clinical parameters. *Journal of Autoimmunity*, **2**, 241–58.

Cohen Kaminsky, S., Jacques, Y., Aime, C., Safar, D., Morel, E. & Berrih Aknin, S. (1992). Follow-up of soluble interleukin-2 receptor levels after thymectomy in patients with myasthenia gravis. *Clinical Immunology and Immunopathology*, **62**, 190–8.

Cohen Kaminsky, S., Levasseur, P., Binet, J.P. & Berrih Aknin, S. (1989*b*). Evidence of enhanced recombinant interleukin-2 sensitivity in thymic lymphocytes from patients with myasthenia gravis: possible role in autoimmune pathogenesis. *Journal of Neuroimmunology*, **24**, 75–85.

Compston, D.A.S., Vincent, A., Newsom-Davis, J. & Batchelor, J.R. (1980). Clinical, pathological, HLA antigen and immunological evidence for disease heterogeneity in myasthenia gravis. *Brain*, **103**, 579–601.

Confalonieri, P., Antozzi, C., Cornelio, F., Simoncini, O. & Mantegazza, R. (1993). Immune activation in myasthenia gravis: soluble interleukin-2 receptor, interferon-γ and tumor necrosis factor-α levels in patients' serum. *Journal of Neuroimmunology*, **48**, 33–6.

Conradi, S. & Ronnevi, L.O. (1985). Cytotoxic activity in the plasma of amyotrophic lateral sclerosis (ALS) patients against normal erythrocytes. Quantitative determinations. *Journal of the Neurological Sciences*, **68**, 135–45.

Conradi, S. & Ronnevi, L.O. (1993). Selective vulnerability of alpha motor neurons in ALS: relation to autoantibodies toward acetylcholinesterase (AChE) in ALS patients. *Brain Research Bulletin*, **30**, 369–71.

Cosi, V., Lombardi, M., Piccolo, G. & Erbetta, A. (1991). Treatment of myasthenia gravis with high-dose intravenous immunoglobulin. *Acta Neurologica Scandinavica*, **84**, 81–4.

Dau, P.C. & Denys, E.H. (1982). Plasmapheresis and immunosuppressive drug therapy in the Eaton–Lambert syndrome. *Annals of Neurology*, **11**, 570–5.

Dawkins, R.L., Kay, P.H., Garlepp, M.J. & Christiansen, F.T. (1987). Immunogenetics of spontaneous, drug-induced, and experimental myasthenia gravis. *Annals of the New York Academy of Sciences*, **505**, 398–406.

Degli Esposti, M.A., Andreas, A., Christiansen, F.T., Schalke, B., Albert, E. & Dawkins, R.L. (1992*a*). An approach to the localization of the susceptibility genes for generalized myasthenia gravis by mapping recombinant ancestral haplotypes. *Immunogenetics*, **35**, 355–64.

Degli Esposti, M.A., Leelayuwat, C. & Dawkins, R.L. (1992*b*). Ancestral haplotypes carry haplotypic and haplospecific polymorphisms of BAT1: possible relevance to autoimmune disease. *European Journal of Immunogenetics*, **19**, 121–7.

Delamere, J.P., Jobson, S., Mackintosh, L.P., Wells, L. & Walton, K.W. (1983). Penicillamine-induced myasthenia in rheumatoid arthritis: its clinical and genetic features. *Annals of the Rheumatic Diseases*, **42**, 500–4.

Delbono, O., Garcia, J., Appel, S.H. & Stefani, E. (1991*a*). Calcium current and charge movement of mammalian muscle: action of amyotrophic lateral sclerosis immunoglobulins. *Journal of Physiology*, **444**, 723–42.

Delbono, O., Garcia, J., Appel, S.H. & Stefani, E. (1991*b*). IgG from amyotrophic lateral sclerosis affects tubular calcium channels of skeletal muscle. *American Journal of Physiology*, **260**, C1347–C1351.

Demaine, A., Willcox, N., Janer, M., Welsh, K. & Newsom-Davis, J. (1992). Immunoglobulin heavy chain gene associations in myasthenia gravis: new evidence for disease heterogeneity. *Journal of Neurology*, **239**, 53–6.

Denny-Brown, D. & Foley, J.M. (1948). Myokymia and the benign fasciculations of muscular cramps. *Transactions of the Association of American Physicians*, **61**, 88–96.

Donaghy, M. & Duchen, L.W. (1986). Sera from patients with motor neuron disease and associated paraproteinaemia fail to inhibit experimentally induced sprouting of motor nerve terminals. *Journal of Neurology, Neurosurgery and Psychiatry*, **49**, 817–19.

Donnenfeld, H., Kascsak, R.J. & Bartfeld, H. (1984). Deposits of IgG and C3 in the spinal cord and motor cortex of ALS patients. *Journal of Neuroimmunology*, **6**, 51–7.

Drachman, D.B. (1981). The biology of myasthenia gravis. *Annual Review of Neuroscience*, **4**, 195–225.

Drachman, D.B., Adams, R.N., McIntosh, K. & Pestronk, A. (1985). Treatment of experimental myasthenia gravis with cyclosporin A. *Clinical Immunology and Immunopathology*, **34**, 174–88.

Drachman, D.B., Adams, R.H., Stanley, E.F. & Pestronk, A. (1980). Mechanisms of acetylcholine receptor loss in myasthenia gravis. *Journal of Neurology, Neurosurgery and Psychiatry*, **43**, 601–10.

Drachman, D.B., Chaudry, V., Cornblath, D., Kubcl, R.W., Pestronk, A., Clawson, L., Mellits, E.D., Quaskey, S., Quinn, T., Calkins, A. & Order, S. (1994). Trial of immunosuppression in amyotrophic latreal sclerosis using total lymphoid irradiation. *Annals of Neurology*, **35**, 142–50.

Drachman, D.B. & Kuncl, R.W. (1989). Amyotrophic lateral sclerosis: an unconventional autoimmune disease? *Annals of Neurology*, **26**, 269–74.

Duarte, F., Binet, S., Lacomblez, L., Bouche, P., Preud'homme, J.L. & Meininger, V. (1991). Quantitative analysis of monoclonal immunoglobulins in serum of patients with amyotrophic lateral sclerosis. *Journal of the Neurological Sciences*, **104**, 88–91.

Eaton, L.M. & Lambert, E.H. (1957). Electromyography and electric stimulation of nerves in diseases of motor unit. Observations on myasthenic syndrome associated with malignant tumors. *Journal of the American Medical Association*, **163**, 1117–24.

Edgeworth, H. (1930). A report on the use of ephedrine in a case of myasthenia gravis. *Journal of the American Medical Association*, **94**, 1136.

Ellis, R.J., Swenson, M.R. & Bajorek, J. (1994). Aseptic meningitis as a complication of intravenous immunoglobulin therapy for myasthenia gravis. *Muscle and Nerve*, **17**, 683–4.

Elmqvist, D., Hofmann, W.W., Kugelberg, J. & Quastel, D.M.J. (1964). An electrophysiological investigation of neuromuscular transmission in myasthenia gravis. *Journal of Physiology*, **174**, 417–34.

Elmqvist, D. & Lambert, E.H. (1968). Detailed analysis of neuromuscular transmission in a patient with the myasthenic syndrome sometimes associated with bronchogenic carcinoma. *Mayo Clinic Proceedings*, **43**, 689–713.

Elrington, G.M., Murray, N.M., Spiro, S.G. & Newsom-Davis, J. (1991). Neurological paraneoplastic syndromes in patients with small cell lung cancer. A prospective survey of 150 patients. *Journal of Neurology, Neurosurgery and Psychiatry*, **54**, 764–7.

Eng, H., Magnusson, Y., Matell, G., Lefvert, A.K., Saponja, R. & Hoebeke, J. (1992). Beta 2-adrenergic receptor antibodies in myasthenia gravis. *Journal of Autoimmunity*, **5**, 213–27.

Engel, A.G. (1980). Morphologic and immunopathological findings in myasthenia gravis and in congenital myasthenic syndromes. *Journal of Neurology, Neurosurgery and Psychiatry*, **43**, 577–89.

Engel, A.G., Lambert, E.H. & Howard, F.M. (1977). Immune complexes (IgG and C3) at the motor end-plate in myasthenia gravis. Ultrastructural and light microscopic localization and electrophysiologic correlations. *Mayo Clinic Proceedings*, **52**, 267–80.

Engel, A.G., Tsujihata, M., Lindstrom, J.M. & Lennon, V.A. (1976). The motor end plate in myasthenia gravis and in experimental autoimmune myasthenia gravis. A quantitative ultrastructural study. *Annals of the New York Academy of Sciences*, **274**, 60–79.

Engel, W.K. (1993). Antibodies to L-type calcium channels in amyotrophic lateral sclerosis. *New England Journal of Medicine*, **328**, 1356–7.

Engelhardt, J. & Appel, S.H. (1990). Motor neuron reactivity of sera from animals with autoimmune models of motor neuron destruction. *Journal of the Neurological Sciences*, **96**, 333–52.

Engelhardt, J., Joo, F., Pakaski, M. & Kasa, P. (1985). An improved method for the bulk isolation of spinal motor neurones. *Journal of Neuroscience Methods*, **15**, 219–27.

Engelhardt, J.I. & Appel, S.H. (1990). IgG reactivity in the spinal cord and motor cortex in amyotrophic lateral sclerosis. *Archives of Neurology*, **47**, 1210–16.

Engelhardt, J.I., Appel, S.H. & Killian, J.M. (1989). Experimental autoimmune motorneuron disease. *Annals of Neurology*, **26**, 368–76.

Engelhardt, J.I., Appel, S.H. & Killian, J.M. (1990). Motor neurone destruction in guinea pigs immunized with bovine spinal cord ventral horn homogenate: experimental autoimmune gray matter disease. *Journal of Neuroimmunology*, **27**, 21–31.

Engelhardt, J.I., Tajti, J. & Appel, S.H. (1993). Lymphocytic infiltrates in the spinal cord in amyotrophic lateral sclerosis. *Archives of Neurology*, **50**, 30–6.

Evoli, A., Bartoccioni, E., Batocchi, A.P., Scuderi, F. & Tonali, P. (1989). Anti-AChR-negative myasthenia gravis: clinical and immunological features. *Clinical and Investigative Medicine*, **12**, 104–9.

Evoli, A., Batocchi, A.P., Palmisani, M.T., Lo Monaco, M. & Tonali, P. (1992). Long-term results of corticosteroid therapy in patients with myasthenia gravis. *European Neurology*, **32**, 37–43.

Evoli, A., Batocchi, A.P., Provenzano, C., Ricci, E. & Tonali, P. (1988). Thymectomy in the treatment of myasthenia gravis: report of 247 patients. *Journal of Neurology*, **235**, 272–6.

Fambrough, D.M., Drachman, D.B. & Satyamurti, S. (1973). Neuromuscular junction in myasthenia gravis: decreased acetylcholine receptors. *Science*, **182**, 293–5.

Fateh-Moghadam, A., Wick, M., Besinger, U. & Geursen, R.G. (1984). High-dose intravenous gammaglobulin for myasthenia gravis. *Lancet*, **1**, 848–9.

Fuchs, S., Nevo, D., Tarrab-Hazdai, R. & Yaar, I. (1976). Strain differences in the autoimmune response of mice to acetylcholine receptors. *Nature*, **263**, 329–30.

Fujii, Y. & Lindstrom, J. (1988*a*). Specificity of the T cell immune response to acetylcholine receptor in experimental autoimmune myasthenia gravis. Response to subunits and synthetic peptides. *Journal of Immunology*, **140**, 1830–7.

Fujii, Y. & Lindstrom, J. (1988*b*). Regulation of antibody production by helper T cell clones in experimental autoimmune myasthenia gravis. *Journal of Immunology*, **141**, 3361–9.

Fujii, Y., Monden, Y., Hashimoto, J., Nakahara, K. & Kawashima, Y. (1985*a*). Acetylcholine receptor antibody-producing cells in thymus and lymph nodes in myasthenia gravis. *Clinical Immunology and Immunopathology*, **34**, 141–6.

Fujii, Y., Monden, Y., Hashimoto, J., Nakahara, K. & Kawashima, Y. (1985*b*). Acetylcholine receptor antibody production by bone marrow cells in a patient with myasthenia gravis. *Neurology*, **35**, 577–9.

Fujii, Y., Monden, Y., Nakahara, K., Hashimoto, J. & Kawashima, Y. (1984). Antibody to acetylcholine receptor in myasthenia gravis: production by lymphocytes from thymus or thymoma. *Neurology*, **34**, 1182–6.

Fukai, I., Masaoka, A., Hashimoto, T., Yamakawa, Y., Mizuno, T., Tanamura, O., Hirokawa, K. & Ueda, R. (1992). An immunohistologic study of the epithelial components of 81 cases of thymoma. *Cancer*, **69**, 2463–8.

Fukuhara, N., Takamori, M., Gutmann, L. & Chou, S.M. (1972). Eaton–Lambert syndrome. Ultrastructural study of the motor end-plates. *Archives of Neurology*, **27**, 67–78.

Fukunaga, H., Engel, A.G., Lang, B., Newsom-Davis, J. & Vincent, A. (1983). Passive transfer of Lambert–Eaton myasthenic syndrome with IgG from man to mouse depletes the presynaptic membrane active zones. *Proceedings of the National Academy of Science of the United States of America*, **80**, 7636–40.

Fukunaga, H., Engel, A.G., Osame, M. & Lambert, E.H. (1982). Paucity and disorganization of presynaptic membrane active zones in the Lambert–Eaton myasthenic syndrome. *Muscle and Nerve*, **5**, 686–97.

Fukuoka, T., Engel, A.G., Lang, B., Newsom-Davis, J., Prior, C. & Wray, D.W. (1987*a*). Lambert-Eaton myasthenic syndrome: I. Early morphological effects of IgG on the presynaptic membrane active zones. *Annals of Neurology*, **22**, 193–9.

Fukuoka, T., Engel, A.G., Lang, B., Newsom-Davis, J. & Vincent, A. (1987*b*). Lambert–Eaton myasthenic syndrome: II. Immunoelectron microscopy localization of IgG at the mouse motor end-plate. *Annals of Neurology*, **22**, 200–11.

Gajdos, P., Outin, H., Elkharrat, D., Brunel, D., de Rohan-Chabot, P., Raphael, J.C., Goulon, M., Goulon-Goeau, C. & Morel, E. (1984). High-dose intravenous gammaglobulin for myasthenia gravis. *Lancet*, **1**, 406–7.

Geuder, K.I., Marx, A., Witzemann, V., Schalke, B., Kirchner, T. & Muller Hermelink, H.K. (1992*a*). Genomic organization and lack of transcription of the nicotinic acetylcholine receptor subunit genes in myasthenia gravis-associated thymoma. *Laboratory Investigation*, **66**, 452–8.

Geuder, K.I., Marx, A., Witzemann, V., Schalke, B., Toyka, K., Kirchner, T. & Muller Hermelink, H.K. (1992*b*). Pathogenetic significance of fetal-type acetylcholine receptors on thymic myoid cells in myasthenia gravis. *Developmental Immunology*, **2**, 69–75.

Gilhus, N.E., Pandey, J.P., Gaarder, P.I. & Aarli, J.A. (1990). Immunoglobulin allotypes in myasthenia gravis patients with a thymoma. *Journal of Autoimmunity*, **3**, 299–305.

Gilpin, S.F., Moersch, F.P. & Kernohan, J.W. (1936). Polyneuritis. A clinical and pathological study of a special group of cases frequently referred to as instances of neuronitis. *Archives of Neurology and Psychiatry*, **35**, 937–63.

Goldstein, G. & Whittingham, S. (1966). Experimental autoimmune thymitis. An animal model of human myasthenia gravis. *Lancet*, **2**, 315–18.

Graus, Y.M., Verschuuren, J.J., Spaans, F., Jennekens, F., van Breda Vriesman, P.J. & De Baets, M.H. (1993). Age-related resistance to experimental autoimmune myasthenia gravis in rats. *Journal of Immunology*, **150**, 4093–103.

Grob, D. & Namba, T. (1966). Corticotrophin in generalized myasthenia gravis. *Journal of the American Medical Association*, **198**, 703–7.

Gutmann, L., Crosby, T.W., Takamori, M. & Martin, J.D. (1972). The Eaton–Lambert syndrome and autoimmune disorders. *American Journal of Medicine*, **53**, 354–6.

Gutmann, L. & Phillips, L.H. (1992). Trends in the association of Lambert–Eaton myasthenic syndrome with carcinoma. *Neurology*, **42**, 848–50.

Halbach, M., Hömberg, V. & Freund, H.J. (1987). Neuromuscular, autonomic and central cholinergic hyperactivity associated with thymoma and acetylcholine receptor-binding antibody. *Journal of Neurology*, **234**, 433–6.

Harvey, A.M. & Masland, R.L. (1941*a*). A method for the study of neuromuscular transmission in human subjects. *Bulletin of the Johns Hopkins Hospital*, **68**, 81–93.

Harvey, A.M. & Masland, R.L. (1941*b*). The electromyogram in myasthenia gravis. *Bulletin of the Johns Hopkins Hospital*, **69**, 1–13.

Hassel, B., Gilhus, N.E., Aarli, J.A. & Skogen, O.R. (1992). Fulminant myasthenia gravis and polymyositis after thymectomy for thymoma. *Acta Neurologica Scandinavica*, **85**, 63–5.

Hays, A.P., Roxas, A., Sadiq, S.A., Vallejos, H., D'Agati, V., Thomas, F.P., Torres, R., Sherman, W.H., Bailey Braxton, D., Hays, A.G. *et al.* (1990). A monoclonal IgA in a patient with amyotrophic lateral sclerosis reacts with neurofilaments and surface antigen on neuroblastoma cells. *Journal of Neuropathology and Experimental Neurology*, **49**, 383–98.

Heidenreich, F., Vincent, A. & Newsom-Davis, J. (1988). Differences in fine specificity of anti-acetylcholine receptor antibodies between subgroups of spontaneous myasthenia gravis of recent onset, and of penicillamine induced myasthenia. *Autoimmunity*, **2**, 31–7.

Heilbron, E., Mattsson, C., Thornell, L.-E., Sjostrom, M., Stalberg, E., Hilton-Brown, P. & Elmqvist, D. (1976). Experimental myasthenia in rabbits: biochemical, electrophysiological, and morphological aspects. *Annals of the New York Academy of Sciences*, **274**, 337–53.

Heinemann, S., Merlie, J. & Lindstrom, J. (1978). Modulation of acetylcholine receptor in rat diaphragm by anti-receptor sera. *Nature*, **274**, 65–8.

Hewett, S.J. & Atchison, W.D. (1992*a*). Specificity of Lambert–Eaton myasthenic syndrome immunoglobulin for nerve terminal calcium channels. *Brain Research*, **599**, 324–32.

Hewett, S.J. & Atchison, W.D. (1992*b*). Disruption of synaptosomal calcium channel function by Lambert–Eaton myasthenic immunoglobulin is serum-dependent. *Brain Research*, **599**, 317–23.

Hofstad, H., Ulvestad, E., Gilhus, N.E., Matre, R. & Aarli, J.A. (1992). Myasthenia gravis muscle antibodies examined by ELISA: IgG and IgM antibodies characterize different patient subgroups. *Acta Neurologica Scandinavica*, **85**, 233–8.

Hohlfeld, R., Toyka, K.V., Besinger, U.A., Gerhold, B. & Heininger, K. (1985). Myasthenia gravis: reactivation of clinical disease and of autoimmune factors after discontinuation of long-term azathioprine. *Annals of Neurology*, **17**, 238–42.

Hokkanen, E. (1969). Epidemiology of myasthenia gravis in Finland. *Journal of the Neurological Sciences*, **9**, 463–478.

Hong, S.J., Tsuji, K. & Chang, C.C. (1992). Inhibition by neosurugatoxin and omega-conotoxin of acetylcholine release and muscle and neuronal nicotinic receptors in mouse neuromuscular junction. *Neuroscience*, **48**, 727–35.

Ichikawa, M., Koh, C.S., Hata, Y., Tohyama, M., Tsuno, T. & Komiyama, A. (1993). Immunoadsorption plasmapheresis for severe generalised myasthenia gravis. *Archives of Disease in Childhood*, **69**, 236–8.

Infante, A.J., Levcovitz, H., Gordon, V., Wall, K.A., Thompson, P.A. & Krolick, K.A. (1992). Preferential use of a T cell receptor V beta gene by acetylcholine receptor reactive T cells from myasthenia gravis-susceptible mice. *Journal of Immunology*, **148**, 3385–90.

Ippoliti, G., Cosi, V., Piccolo, G., Lombardi, M. & Mantegaz, R. (1984). High-dose intravenous gammaglobulin for myasthenia gravis. *Lancet*, **2**, 809.

Isaacs, H. (1961). A syndrome of continuous muscle-fibre activity. *Journal of Neurology, Neurosurgery and Psychiatry*, **24**, 319–25.

Ishii, A., Hayashi, A., Ohkoshi, N., Oguni, E., Maeda, M., Ueda, Y., Ishii, K., Arasaki, K., Mizusawa, H. & Shoji, S. (1994). Clinical evaluation of plasma exchange and high dose intravenous immunoglobulin in a patient with Isaacs' syndrome. *Journal of Neurology, Neurosurgery and Psychiatry*, **57**, 840–2.

Jamieson, P.W. & Katirji, M.B. (1994). Idiopathic generalized myokymia. *Muscle and Nerve*, **17**, 42–51.

Joong, S. & Kim, K.W. (1973). Guanidine hydrochloride in the Eaton–Lambert syndrome. Electrophysiological improvement. *Neurology*, **23**, 1084–90.

Kahn, C.R., McIntosh, K.R. & Drachman, D.B. (1990). T-cell vaccination in experimental myasthenia gravis: a double-edged sword. *Journal of Autoimmunity*, **3**, 659–69.

Kaminski, H.J., Fenstermaker, R.A., Abdul Karim, F.W., Clayman, J. & Ruff, R.L. (1994). Acetylcholine receptor subunit gene expression in thymic tissue. *Muscle and Nerve*, **16**, 1332–7.

Kamo, I., Furukawa, S., Tada, A., Mano, Y., Iwasaki, Y., Furuse, T., Ito, N., Hayashi, K. & Satoyoshi, E. (1982). Monoclonal antibody to acetylcholine receptor: cell line established from thymus of patient with myasthenia gravis. *Science*, **215**, 995–7.

Kawamata, T., Akiyama, H., Yamada, T. & McGeer, P.L. (1992). Immunologic reactions in amyotrophic lateral sclerosis brain and spinal cord tissue. *American Journal of Pathology*, **140**, 691–707.

Kelemen, J., Hedlund, W., Orlin, J.B., Berkman, E.M. & Munsat, T.L. (1983). Plasmapheresis with immunosuppression in amyotrophic lateral sclerosis. *Archives of Neurology*, **40**, 752–3.

Kennes, B., Delespesse, G., Vandenbossche, J.L. & Sternon, J. (1978). Systemic lupus erythematosus triggered by adult thymectomy in myasthenia gravis patient: report of a case. *Acta Clinica Belgica*, **33**, 110–15.

Kim, Y.I. & Neher, E. (1988). IgG from patients with Lambert–Eaton syndrome blocks voltage-dependent calcium channels. *Science*, **239**, 405–8.

Kimura, F., Smith, R.G., Delbono, O., Nyormoi, O., Schneider, T., Nastainczyk, W., Hofmann, F., Stefani, E. & Appel, S.H. (1994). Amyotrophic lateral sclerosis patient antibodies label Ca_{2+} channel $\alpha 1$ subunit. *Annals of Neurology*, **35**, 164–71.

Kinoshita, I., Nakamura, T., Satoh, A., Matsuo, H., Seto, M., Tomita, I., Tsujihata, M. & Nagataki, S. (1988). Role of the macrophage in the pathogenesis of experimental autoimmune myasthenia gravis. *Journal of the Neurological Sciences*, **87**, 49–59.

Kirchner, T., Tzartos, S., Hoppe, F., Schalke, B., Wekerle, H. & Muller Hermelink, H.K. (1988). Pathogenesis of myasthenia gravis. Acetylcholine receptor-related antigenic determinants in tumor-free thymuses and thymic epithelial tumors. *American Journal of Pathology*, **130**, 268–80.

Kirsch, G.E. & Narahashi, T. (1978). 3,4-diaminopyridine. A potent new potassium channel blocker. *Biophysical Journal*, **22**, 507–12.

Kjaer, M. (1971). Myasthenia gravis and myasthenic syndromes treated with prednisone. *Acta Neurologica Scandinavica*, **47**, 464–74.

Klavinskis, L.S., Willcox, N., Oxford, J.S. & Newsom-Davis, J. (1985). Antivirus antibodies in myasthenia gravis. *Neurology*, **35**, 1381–4.

Kornstein, M.J. (1992). Controversies regarding the pathology of thymomas. *Pathology Annual*, **27 Part 2**, 1–15.

Kott, E., Livni, E., Zamir, R. & Kuritzky, A. (1979). Cell-mediated immunity to polio and HLA antigens in amyotrophic lateral sclerosis. *Neurology*, **29**, 1040–4.

Kozlowski, M.A., Williams, C., Hinton, D.R. & Miller, C.A. (1989). Heterotopic neurons in spinal cord of patients with ALS. *Neurology*, **39**, 644–8.

Kuks, J.B., Djojoatmodjo, S. & Oosterhuis, H.J. (1991*a*). Azathioprine in myasthenia gravis: observations in 41 patients and a review of literature. *Neuromuscular Disorders*, **1**, 423–31.

Kuks, J.B., Oosterhuis, H.J., Limburg, P.C. & The, T.H. (1991*b*). Anti-acetylcholine receptor antibodies decrease after thymectomy in patients with myasthenia gravis. Clinical correlations. *Journal of Autoimmunity*, **4**, 197–211.

Kuncl, R.W., Drachman, D.B., Adams, R. & Lehar, M. (1993). 3-Deazaadenosine: a therapeutic strategy for myasthenia gravis by decreasing the endocytosis of acetylcholine receptors. *Journal of Pharmacology and Experimental Therapy*, **267**, 582–9.

Kurtzke, J.F. (1978). Epidemiology of myasthenia gravis. In *Neurological Epidemiology: Principles and Clinical Applications*, ed. B.S. Schoenberg, pp. 545–66. New York: Raven Press.

Lambert, E.H. & Elmqvist, D. (1971). Quantal components of end-plate potentials in the myasthenic syndrome. *Annals of the New York Academy of Sciences*, **183**, 183–99.

Lambert, E.H. & Lennon, V.A. (1988). Selected IgG rapidly induces Lambert–Eaton myasthenic syndrome in mice: complement independence and EMG abnormalities. *Muscle and Nerve*, **11**, 1133–45.

Lambert, E.H., Lindstrom, J.M. & Lennon, V.A. (1976). End-plate potentials in experimental autoimmune myasthenia gravis in rats. *Annals of the New York Academy of Sciences*, **274**, 300–18.

Lampson, L.A., Kushner, P.D. & Sobel, R.A. (1990). Major histocompatibility complex antigen expression in the affected tissues in amyotrophic lateral sclerosis. *Annals of Neurology*, **28**, 365–72.

Lang, B., Johnston, I., Leys, K., Elrington, G., Marqueze, B., Leveque, C., Martin-Moutot, N., Seagar, M., Hoshino, T., Takahashi, M., Sugimori, M., Cherskey, B.D., Llinas, R. & Newsom-Davis, J. (1993). Antibody specificities in the Lambert–Eaton myasthenic syndrome. *Annals of the New York Academy of Sciences*, **681**, 382–93.

Lang, B., Molenaar, P.C., Newsom-Davis, J. & Vincent, A. (1984). Passive transfer of Lambert–Eaton myasthenic syndrome in mice: decreased rates of resting and evoked release of acetylcholine from skeletal muscle. *Journal of Neurochemistry*, **42**, 658–62.

Lang, B., Newsom-Davis, J., Prior, C. & Wray, D. (1983). Antibodies to motor nerve terminals: an electrophysiological study of a human myasthenic syndrome transferred to mouse. *Journal of Physiology*, **344**, 335–45.

Lang, B., Newsom-Davis, J. & Wray, D.W. (1988). The effect of Lambert–Eaton myasthenic syndrome antibody on slow action potentials in mouse cardiac ventricle. *Proceedings of the Royal Society of London. Series B Biological Sciences*, **235**, 103–10.

Lang, B., Newsom-Davis, J., Wray, D., Vincent, A. & Murray, N. (1981). Autoimmune aetiology for myasthenic (Eaton–Lambert) syndrome. *Lancet*, **2**, 224–6.

Laroche, C.M., Mier, A.K., Spiro, S.G., Newsom-Davis, J., Moxham, J. & Green, M. (1989). Respiratory muscle weakness in the Lambert–Eaton myasthenic syndrome. *Thorax*, **44**, 913–18.

Lauritzen, M., Smith, T., Fischer Hansen, B., Sparup, J. & Olesen, J. (1980). Eaton–Lambert syndrome and malignant thymoma. *Neurology*, **30**, 634–8.

Lefvert, A.K. & Holm, G. (1987). Idiotypic network in myasthenia gravis demonstrated by human monoclonal B-cell lines. *Scandinavian Journal of Immunology*, **26**, 573–8.

Lefvert, A.K., Holm, G. & Pirskanen, R. (1987). Autoantiidiotypic antibodies in myasthenia gravis. *Annals of the New York Academy of Sciences*, **505**, 133–54.

Lennon, V.A., Lambert, E.H., Leiby, K.R., Okarma, T.B. & Talib, S. (1991). Recombinant human acetylcholine receptor α-subunit induces chronic experimental autoimmune myasthenia gravis. *Journal of Immunology*, **146**, 2245–8.

Lennon, V.A., Lindstrom, J.M. & Seybold, M.E. (1975). Experimental autoimmune myasthenia: a model of myasthenia gravis in rats and guinea pigs. *Journal of Experimental Medicine*, **141**, 1365–75.

Lennon, V.A., Seybold, M.E., Lindstrom, J.M., Cochrane, C. & Ulevitch, R. (1978). Role of complement in the pathogenesis of experimental autoimmune myasthenia gravis. *Journal of Experimental Medicine*, **147**, 973–83.

Leveque, C., Hoshino, T., David, P., Shoji Kasai, Y., Leys, K., Omori, A., Lang, B., el Far, O., Sato, K., Martin Moutot, N. *et al.* (1992). The synaptic vesicle protein synaptotagmin associates with calcium channels and is a putative Lambert–Eaton myasthenic syndrome antigen. *Proceedings of the National Academy of Science of the United States of America*, **89**, 3625–9.

Levine, G.D. & Rosai, J. (1978). Thymic hyperplasia: a review of current concepts. *Human Pathology*, **9**, 495–515.

Lewis, J.E., Wick, M.R., Scheithauer, B.W., Bernatz, P.E. & Taylor, W.F. (1987). Thymoma. A clinicopathological review. *Cancer*, **60**, 2727–43.

Leys, K., Lang, B., Johnston, I. & Newsom-Davis, J. (1991). Calcium channel autoantibodies in the Lambert–Eaton myasthenic syndrome. *Annals of Neurology*, **29**, 307–14.

Li, F. & Pestronk, A. (1991). Autoantibodies to GM1 ganglioside: different reactivity to GM1-liposomes in amyotrophic lateral sclerosis and lower motor neuron disorders. *Journal of the Neurological Sciences*, **104**, 209–14.

Liblau, R., Gajdos, P., Bustarret, F.A., el Habib, R., Bach, J.F. & Morel, E. (1991). Intravenous gamma-globulin in myasthenia gravis: interaction with anti-acetylcholine receptor autoantibodies. *Journal of Clinical Immunology*, **11**, 128–31.

Lindberg, C., Andersen, O., Larsson, S. & Oden, A. (1992). Remission rate after thymectomy in myasthenia gravis when the bias of immunosuppressive therapy is eliminated. *Acta Neurologica Scandinavica*, **86**, 323–8.

Lindstrom, J. (1980). Experimental autoimmune myasthenia gravis. *Journal of Neurology, Neurosurgery and Psychiatry*, **43**, 568–76.

Lindstrom, J.M., Einarson, B.L., Lennon, V.A. & Seybold, M.E. (1976*a*). Pathological mechanisms in experimental autoimmune myasthenia gravis. I Immunogenicity of syngeneic muscle acetylcholine receptor and quantitative extraction of receptor and antibody-receptor complexes from muscles of rats with experimental autoimmune myasthenia gravis. *Journal of Experimental Medicine*, **144**, 726–38.

Lindstrom, J.M., Engel, A.G., Seybold, M.E., Lennon, V.A. & Lambert, E.H. (1976*b*). Pathological mechanisms in experimental autoimmune myasthenia gravis. II. Passive transfer of experimental autoimmune myasthenia gravis in rats with anti-acetylcholine receptor antibodies. *Journal of Experimental Medicine*, **144**, 739–53.

Lindstrom, J.M., Seybold, M.E., Lennon, V.A., Whittingham, S. & Duane, D.D. (1976*c*). Antibody to acetylcholine receptor in myasthenia gravis. Prevalence, clinical correlates, and diagnostic value. *Neurology*, **26**, 1054–9.

Link, H., Xu, Z.Y., Melms, A., Kalbacher, H., Sun, J.B., Wang, Z.Y., Fredrikson, S. & Olsson, T. (1992). The T-cell repertoire in myasthenia gravis involves multiple cholinergic receptor epitopes. *Scandinavian Journal of Immunology*, **36**, 405–14.

Lu, C.Z., Link, H., Mo, X.A., Xiao, B.G., Zhang, Y.L. & Qin, Z (1991). Anti-presynaptic membrane receptor antibodies in myasthenia gravis. *Journal of the Neurological Sciences*, **102**, 39–45.

Lu, C.Z., Lu, L., Hao, Z.S., Xia, D.G., Qain, J. & Arnason, B.G. (1993). Antibody-secreting cells to acetylcholine receptor and to presynaptic membrane receptor in seronegative myasthenia gravis. *Journal of Neuroimmunology*, **43**, 145–9.

Lundh, H., Nilsson, O. & Rosen, I. (1984). Treatment of Lambert–Eaton syndrome: 3,4-diaminopyridine and pyridostigmine. *Neurology*, **34**, 1324–30.

Manfredi, A.A., Protti, M.P., Bellone, M., Moiola, L. & Conti Tronconi, B.M. (1992*a*). Molecular anatomy of an autoantigen: T and B epitopes on the nicotinic acetylcholine receptor in myasthenia gravis. *Journal of Laboratory and Clinical Medicine*, **120**, 13–21.

Manfredi, A.A., Protti, M.P., Wu, X.D., Howard, J.F.J. & Conti Tronconi, B.M. (1992*b*). $CD4^+$ T-epitope repertoire on the human acetylcholine receptor alpha subunit in severe myasthenia gravis: a study with synthetic peptides. *Neurology*, **42**, 1092–100.

Marchiori, P.E., dos Reis, M., Quevedo, M.E., Scaff, M., Cossermelli, W., Assis, J.L. & de Oliveira, R.M. (1989). Acetylcholine receptor antibody in myasthenia gravis. *Acta Neurologica Scandinavica*, **80**, 387–9.

Marshall, B., Leelayuwat, C., Abraham, L.J., Pinelli, M. & Dawkins, R.L. (1994). Large transcripts and sequence from a polymorphic 170 kb MHC region implicated in susceptibility to autoimmune disease. *Immunogenetics*, **39**, 15–20.

Marx, A., O'Connor, R., Geuder, K.I., Hoppe, F., Schalke, B., Tzartos, S., Kalies, I., Kirchner, T. & Muller-Hermelink, H.K. (1990). Characterization of a protein with an acetylcholine receptor epitope from myasthenia gravis-associated thymomas. *Laboratory Investigation*, **62**, 279–86.

Marx, A., O'Connor, R., Tzartos, S., Kalies, I., Kirchner, T. & Muller Hermelink, H.K. (1989). Acetylcholine receptor epitope in proteins of myasthenia gravis-associated thymomas and non-thymic tissues. *Thymus*, **14**, 171–8.

Masu, Y., Wolf, E., Holtmann, B., Sendtner, M., Brem, G. & Thoenen, H. (1993). Disruption of the CNTF gene results in motor neuron degeneration. *Nature*, **365**, 27–32.

Matell, G. (1987). Immunosuppressive drugs: azathioprine in the treatment of myasthenia gravis. *Annals of the New York Academy of Sciences*, **505**, 588–94.

McIntosh, K.R. & Drachman, D.B. (1986). Induction of suppressor cells specific for AChR in experimental autoimmune myasthenia gravis. *Science*, **232**, 401–3.

McIntosh, K.R. & Drachman, D.B. (1992). Tolerance to acetylcholine receptor induced by AChR-coupled syngeneic cells. *Journal of Neuroimmunology*, **38**, 75–84.

Meinl, E., Klinkert, W.E. & Wekerle, H. (1991). The thymus in myasthenia gravis. Changes typical for the human disease are absent in experimental autoimmune myasthenia gravis of the Lewis rat. *American Journal of Pathology*, **139**, 995–1008.

Melms, A., Malcherek, G., Gern, U., Sommer, N., Weissert, R., Wietholter, H. & Buhring, H.J. (1993). Thymectomy and azathioprine have no effect on the phenotype of CD4 T lymphocyte subsets in myasthenia gravis. *Journal of Neurology, Neurosurgery and Psychiatry*, **56**, 46–51.

Melms, A., Schalke, B.C.G., Kirchner, T., Muller-Hermelink, H.K., Albert, E. & Wekerle, H. (1988). Thymus in myasthenia gravis. Isolation of T-lymphocyte lines specific for the nicotinic acetylcholine receptor from the thymuses of myasthenic patients. *Journal of Clinical Investigation*, **81**, 902–8.

Mohan, S., Barohn, R.J. & Krolick, K.A. (1992). Unexpected cross-reactivity between myosin and a main immunogenic region (MIR) of the acetylcholine receptor by antisera obtained from myasthenia gravis patients. *Clinical Immunology and Immunopathology*, **64**, 218–26.

Morel, E., Feuillet Fieux, M.N., Vernet der Garabedian, B., Raimond, F., D'Anglejan, J., Bataille, R., Sany, J. & Bach, J.F. (1991). Autoantibodies in D-penicillamine-induced myasthenia gravis: a comparison with idiopathic myasthenia and rheumatoid arthritis. *Clinical Immunology and Immunopathology*, **58**, 318–30.

Mori, Y., Niidome, T., Fujita, Y., Mynlieff, M., Dirksen, R.T., Beam, K.G., Iwabe, N., Miyata, T., Furutama, D., Furuichi, T. & Mikoshiba, K. (1993). Molecular diversity of voltage-dependent calcium channels. *Annals of the New York Academy of Sciences*, **707**, 87–108.

Morrow, J.D., Manian, F.A., Clinton, M.E. & Stein, R.S. (1988). Eaton–Lambert syndrome in a patient with acute T cell lymphocytic leukemia. *Southern Medical Journal*, **81**, 1578–9.

Motoki, R., Harada, M., Chiba, A. & Honda, K. (1966). A case of myasthenia gravis in identical twin brothers. *International Surgery*, **45**, 674–7.

Mulder, D.W., Kurland, L.T., Offord, K.P. & Beard, M.C. (1986). Familial adult motor neuron disease: amyotrophic lateral sclerosis. *Neurology*, **36**, 511–17.

Munoz, D.G., Greene, C., Perl, D.P. & Selkoe, D.J. (1988). Accumulation of phosphorylated neurofilaments in anterior horn motoneurons of amyotrophic lateral sclerosis patients. *Journal of Neuropathology and Experimental Neurology*, **47**, 9–18

Murayama, S., Bouldin, T.W. & Suzuki, K. (1992). Immunocytochemical and ultrastructural studies of upper motor neurons in amyotrophic lateral sclerosis. *Acta Neuropathologica*, **83**, 518–24.

Murphy, J. & Murphy, S.F. (1986). Myasthenia gravis in identical twins. *Neurology*, **36**, 78–80.

Myasthenia Gravis Clinical Study Group (1993). A randomised clinical trial comparing prednisone and azathioprine in myasthenia gravis. Results of the second interim analysis. *Journal of Neurology, Neurosurgery and Psychiatry*, **56**, 1157–63.

Mygland, A., Aarli, J.A., Matre, R. & Gilhus, N.E. (1994). Ryanodine receptor antibodies realted to severity of thymoma associated myasthenia gravis. *Journal of Neurology, Neurosurgery and Psychiatry*, **57**, 843–6.

Mygland, A., Tysnes, O.B., Matre, R., Volpe, P., Aarli, J.A. & Gilhus, N.E. (1992). Ryanodine receptor autoantibodies in myasthenia gravis patients with a thymoma. *Annals of Neurology*, **32**, 589–91.

Nagashima, T., Kamegai, M., Hirose, K., Yamada, K., Uono, M., Tsubaki, T. & Nagashima, K. (1985). Creatine kinase (CK)-linked IgA in Isaacs' syndrome. An immune complex disease? *Journal of the Neurological Sciences*, **67**, 269–76.

Namba, T., Brunner, N.G., Brown, S.D., Muguruma, M. & Grob, D. (1971*a*). Familial myasthenia gravis. Report of 27 patients in 12 families and review of 164 patients in 73 families. *Archives of Neurology*, **25**, 49–60.

Namba, T., Shapiro, M.S., Bruner, N.G. & Grob, D. (1971*b*). Myasthenia gravis occurring in twins. *Journal of Neurology, Neurosurgery and Psychiatry*, **34**, 531–4.

Nasca, T.J., Muder, R.R., Thomas, D.B., Schrecker, J.C. & Ruben, F.L. (1990). Antibody response to pneumococcal polysaccharide vaccine in myasthenia gravis: effect of therapeutic plasmapheresis. *Journal of Clinical Apheresis*, **5**, 133–9.

Nastuk, W.L., Plescia, O.J. & Osserman, K.E. (1960). Changes in serum complement activity in patients with myasthenia gravis. *Proceedings of the Society for Experimental Biology and Medicine*, **105**, 177–84.

Newsom-Davis, J., Harcourt, G., Sommer, N., Beeson, D., Willcox, N. & Rothbard, J.B. (1989). T-cell reactivity in myasthenia gravis. *Journal of Autoimmunity*, **2 (Supplement)**, 101–8.

Newsom-Davis, J. & Mills, K.R. (1993). Immunological associations of acquired neuromyotonia (Isaacs' syndrome). Report of five cases and literature review *Brain*, **116**, 453–69.

Newsom-Davis, J. & Murray, N.M. (1984). Plasma exchange and immunosuppressive drug treatment in the Lambert–Eaton myasthenic syndrome. *Neurology*, **34**, 480–5.

Norris, F.H. (1975). Adult spinal motor neuron disease. Progressive muscular atrophy (Aran's disease) in relation to amyotrophic lateral sclerosis. In *Handbook of Clinical Neurology*, Volume 22. *Systemic Disorders and Atrophies*, Part II, ed. P.J. Vinken & G.W. Bruyn, pp. 1–56. Amsterdam: North-Holland.

O'Neill, J.H., Murray, N.M.F. & Newsom-Davis, J. (1988). The Lambert–Eaton myasthenic syndrome. A review of 50 cases. *Brain*, **111**, 577–96.

Oh, S.J. & Kuruoglu, R. (1992). Chronic limb-girdle myasthenia gravis. *Neurology*, **42**, 1153–6.

Olanow, C.W., Wechsler, A.S., Sirotkin, M., Sjajich, J. & Roses, A.D. (1987). Thymectomy as primary therapy in myasthenia gravis. *Annals of the New York Academy of Sciences*, **505**, 595–606.

Olarte, M., Schoenfeldt, R.S., McKiernan, G. & Rowland, L.P. (1980). Plasmapheresis in amyotrophic lateral sclerosis. *Annals of Neurology*, **8**, 644–5.

Oldstone, M.B., Wilson, C.B., Perrin, L.H. & Norris, F.H. Jr (1976). Evidence for immune-complex formation in patients with amyotrophic lateral sclerosis. *Lancet*, **2**, 169–72.

Oosterhuis, H.J. & Bethlem, J. (1973). Neurogenic muscle involvement in myasthenia gravis. A clinical and histopathological study. *Journal of Neurology, Neurosurgery and Psychiatry*, **36**, 244–54.

Ordonez, G. & Sotelo, J. (1989). Antibodies against fetal muscle proteins in serum from patients with amyotrophic lateral sclerosis. *Neurology*, **39**, 683–6.

Osborn, M., Marx, A., Kirchner, T., Tzartos, S.J., Plessman, U. & Weber, K. (1992). A shared epitope in the acetylcholine receptor-alpha subunit and fast troponin I of skeletal muscle. Is it important for myasthenia gravis? *American Journal of Pathology*, **140**, 1215–23.

Osborne, D. & Simcock, J. (1966). Myasthenia gravis in identical twins. *British Medical Journal*, **1**, 1025–6.

Oshima, M., Ashizawa, T., Pollack, M.S. & Atassi, M.Z. (1990). Autoimmune T cell recognition of human acetylcholine receptor: the sites of T cell recognition in myasthenia gravis on the extracellular part of the alpha subunit. *European Journal of Immunology*, **20**, 2563–9.

Osserman, K.E. & Genkins, G. (1966). Studies in myasthenia gravis. Short-term massive corticotrophin therapy. *Journal of the American Medical Association*, **198**, 699–702.

Osserman, K.E., Kornfeld, P., Cohen, E., Genkins, G., Mendelow, H., Goldberg, H., Windsley, H. & Kaplan, L.I. (1958). Studies in myasthenia gravis. Review of two hundred eighty-two cases at The Mount Sinai Hospital, New York City. *Annals of Internal Medicine*, **102**, 72–81.

Palmisani, M.T., Evoli, A., Batocchi, A.P., Provenzano, C. & Tonali, P. (1993). Myasthenia gravis associated with thymoma: clinical characteristics and long-term outcome. *European Neurology*, **34**, 78–82.

Parry, G.J. & Clarke, S. (1988). Multifocal acquired demyelinating neuropathy masquerading as motor neurone disease. *Muscle and Nerve*, **11**, 103–7.

Partanen, V.S.J., Soininen, H., Saksa, M. & Riekkinen, P. (1980). Electromyography and nerve conduction findings in a patient with neuromyotonia, normocalcemic tetany and small-cell lung cancer. *Acta Neurologica Scandinavica*, **61**, 216–26.

Pascuzzi, R.M., Coslett, H.B. & Johns, T.R. (1984). Long-term corticosteroid treatment of myasthenia gravis: report of 116 patients. *Annals of Neurology*, **15**, 291–8.

Pascuzzi, R.M., Phillips, L.H., Johns, T.R. & Lennon, V.A. (1987). The prevalence of electrophysiological and immunological abnormalities in asymptomatic relatives of patients with myasthenia gravis. *Annals of the New York Academy of Sciences*, **505**, 407–15.

Patrick, J. & Lindstrom, J.L. (1973). Autoimmune response to acetylcholine receptor. *Science*, **180**, 871–2.

Pedersen, L., Platz, P., Jersild, C. & Thomsen, M. (1977). HLA (SD and LD) in patients with amyotrophic lateral sclerosis (ALS). *Journal of the Neurological Sciences*, **31**, 313–18.

Pestronk, A. (1991). Invited review: motor neuropathies, motor neuron disorders, and antiglycolipid antibodies. *Muscle and Nerve*, **14**, 927–36.

Pestronk, A., Adams, R.N., Cornblath, D., Kuncl, R.W., Drachman, D.B. & Clawson, L. (1989). Patterns of serum IgM antibodies to GM1 and GD1a gangliosides in amyotrophic lateral sclerosis. *Annals of Neurology*, **25**, 98–102.

Pestronk, A., Chaudhry, V., Feldman, E.L., Griffin, J.W., Cornblath, D.R., Denys, E.H., Glasberg, M., Kuncl, R.W., Olney, R.K. & Yee, W.C. (1990). Lower motor neuron syndromes defined by patterns of weakness, nerve conduction abnormalities, and high titers of antiglycolipid antibodies. *Annals of Neurology*, **27**, 316–26.

Pinching, A.J., Peters, D.K. & Newsom-Davis, J. (1976). Remission of myasthenia gravis following plasma-exchange. *Lancet*, **2**, 1373–6.

Pirskanen, R. (1977). Genetic aspects in myasthenia gravis. A family study of 264 Finnish patients. *Acta Neurologica Scandinavica*, **56**, 365–88.

Pirskanen, R., Bergstrom, K., Hammarstrom, L., Knutsson, E., Lefvert, A.K., Matell, G., Nilsson, B.Y. & Smith, C.I.E. (1981). Neuromuscular safety margin: genetical, immunological and electrophysiological determinants in relatives of myasthenia gravis patients: a preliminary report. *Annals of the New York Academy of Sciences*, **377**, 605–12.

Plauché, W.C. (1994). Myasthenia gravis in mothers and their newborns. *Clinical Obstetrics and Gynaecology*, **34**, 82–99.

Protti, M.P., Manfredi, A.A., Straub, C., Wu, X.D., Howard, J.F. Jr & Conti Tronconi, B.M. (1990). Use of synthetic peptides to establish anti-human acetylcholine receptor $CD4^+$ cell lines from myasthenia gravis patients. *Journal of Immunology*, **144**, 1711–20.

Ragheb, S. & Lisak, R.P. (1992). Effect of clinical status and treatment on the frequency of $CD5^+$ B cells in patients with myasthenia gravis. *Neurology*, **42**, 1076–80.

Reeback, J., Benton, S., Swash, M. & Schwartz, M.S. (1979). Penicillamine-induced neuromyotonia. *British Medical Journal*, **1**, 1464–5.

Reim, J., McIntosh, K., Martin, S. & Drachman, D.B. (1992). Specific immunotherapeutic strategy for myasthenia gravis: targeted antigen-presenting cells. *Journal of Neuroimmunology*, **41**, 61–70.

Reiness, C.G. & Weinberg, C.B. (1978). Antibody to acetylcholine receptor increases degradation of junctional and extrajunctional receptors in adult muscle. *Nature*, **274**, 68–70.

Rich, K.M. & Hollowell, J.P. (1990). Flunarizine protects neurons from death after axotomy or NGF deprivation. *Science*, **248**, 1419–21.

Robberecht, W., Sapp, P., Viaene, M.K., Rosen, D., McKenna Yasek, D., Haines, J., Horvitz, R., Theys, P. & Brown, R.J. (1994). Cu/Zn superoxide dismutase activity in familial and sporadic amyotrophic lateral sclerosis. *Journal of Neurochemistry*, **62**, 384–7.

Roberts, A., Perera, S., Lang, B., Vincent, A. & Newsom-Davis, J. (1985). Paraneoplastic myasthenic syndrome IgG inhibits $^{45}Ca^{2+}$ flux in a human small cell carcinoma line. *Nature*, **317**, 737–9.

Rodnitzky, R.L. & Bosch, E.P. (1984). Chronic long-interval plasma exchange in myasthenia gravis. *Archives of Neurology*, **41**, 715–17.

Rosales, R.L., Osmame, M., Madriaga, E.P., Navarro, J.C. & Igata, A. (1988). Morphometry of intramuscular nerves in amyotrophic lateral sclerosis. *Muscle and Nerve*, **11**, 223–6.

Rosen, D.R. (1993). Mutations in Cu/Zn superoxide dismutase gene are associated with familial amyotrophic lateral sclerosis. *Nature*, **364**, 362.

Rosen, D.R., Siddique, T., Patterson, D., Figlewicz, D.A., Sapp, P., Hentati, A., Donaldson, D., Goto, J., O'Regan, J.P., Deng, H.X. *et al.* (1993). Mutations in Cu/Zn superoxide dismutase gene are associated with familial amyotrophic lateral sclerosis. *Nature*, **362**, 59–62.

Rosenfeld, M.R., Wong, E., Dalmau, J., Manley, G., Posner, J.B., Sher, E. & Furneaux, H.M. (1993). Cloning and characterization of a Lambert–Eaton myasthenic syndrome antigen. *Annals of Neurology*, **33**, 113–20.

Rothstein, J.D., Martin, L.J. & Kuncl, R.W. (1992). Decreased glutamate transport by the brain and spinal cord in amyotrophic lateral sclerosis. *New England Journal of Medicine*, **326**, 1464–8.

Rowland, L.P. (1992). Amyotrophic lateral sclerosis and autoimmunity. *New England Journal of Medicine*, **327**, 1752–3.

Rubenstein, A.E., Horowitz, S.H. & Bender, A.N. (1979). Cholinergic dysautonomia and Eaton–Lambert syndrome. *Neurology*, **29**, 720–3.

Russell, D.S. (1953). Histological changes in the striped muscles in myasthenia gravis. *Journal of Pathology and Bacteriology*, **65**, 279–94.

Safar, D., Aime, C., Cohen Kaminsky, S. & Berrih Aknin, S. (1991). Antibodies to thymic epithelial cells in myasthenia gravis. *Journal of Neuroimmunology*, **35**, 101–10.

Sahashi, K., Engel, A.G., Lambert, E.H. & Howard, F.M. (1980). Ultrastructural localization of the terminal and lytic ninth complement component (C9) at the motor end-plate in myasthenia gravis. *Journal of Neuropathology and Experimental Neurology*, **39**, 160–72.

Sahashi, K., Engel, A.G., Lambert, E.H. & Lennon, V.A. (1978). Ultrastructural localization of immune complexes (IgG and C3) at the end-plate in experimental myasthenia gravis. *Journal of Neuropathology and Experimental Neurology*, **37**, 212–23.

Salazar Grueso, E.F., Routbort, M.J., Martin, J., Dawson, G. & Roos, R.P. (1990). Polyclonal IgM anti-GM1 ganglioside antibody in patients with motor neuron disease and variants. *Annals of Neurology*, **27**, 558–63.

Salvetti, M., Jung, S., Chang, S.-F., Will, H., Schalke, B.C.G. & Wekerle, H. (1991). Acetylcholine receptor-specific T-lymphocyte clones in the normal human immune repertoire: target epitopes, HLA restriction, and membrane properties. *Annals of Neurology*, **29**, 508–16.

Sanders, K.A., Rowland, L.P., Murphy, P.L., Younger, D.S., Latov, N., Sherman, W.H., Pesce, M. & Lange, D.J. (1993). Motor neuron diseases and amyotrophic lateral sclerosis: GM1 antibodies and paraproteinemia. *Neurology*, **43**, 418–20.

Sano, M. & Lennon, V.A. (1993). Enzyme immunoassay of anti-human acetylcholine receptor autoantibodies in patients with myasthenia gravis reveals correlation with striational autoantibodies. *Neurology*, **43**, 573–8.

Sawada, K., Malchesky, P.S., Koo, A.P. & Mitsumoto, H. (1993). Myasthenia gravis therapy: immunoadsorbent may eliminate need for plasma products. *Cleveland Clinic Journal of Medicine*, **60**, 60–4.

Schluep, M., Willcox, N., Vincent, A., Dhoot, G.K. & Newsom-Davis, J. (1987). Acetylcholine receptors in human thymic myoid cells *in situ*: an immunohistological study. *Annals of Neurology*, **22**, 212–22.

Schonbeck, S., Padberg, F., Hohlfeld, R. & Wekerle, H. (1992). Transplantation of thymic autoimmune microenvironment to severe combined immunodeficiency mice. A new model of myasthenia gravis. *Journal of Clinical Investigation*, **90**, 245–50.

Schwartz, M.S. & Stahlberg, E. (1975). Myasthenic syndrome studied with single fibre electromyography. *Archives of Neurology*, **32**, 815–17.

Seybold, M.E. & Drachman, D.B. (1974). Gradually increasing doses of prednisone in myasthenia gravis. Reducing the hazards of treatment. *New England Journal of Medicine*, **290**, 81–4.

Seybold, M.E., Lambert, E.H., Lennon, V.A. & Lindstrom, J.M. (1976). Experimental autoimmune myasthenia: clinical, neurophysiologic, and pharmacologic aspects. *Annals of the New York Academy of Sciences*, **274**, 275–82.

Sghirlanzoni, A., Peluchetti, D., Mantegazza, R., Fiacchino, F. & Ferdinando, C. (1984). Myasthenia gravis: prolonged treatment with steroids. *Neurology*, **34**, 170–4.

Sillevis Smitt, P.A.E. & de Jong, J.M.B.V. (1989). Animal models of amyotrophic lateral sclerosis and the spinal muscular atrophies. *Journal of the Neurological Sciences*, **91**, 231–58.

Simon, H.E. (1935). Myasthenia gravis. Effect of treatment with anterior pituitary extract: preliminary report. *Journal of the American Medical Association*, **104**, 2065–6.

Simpson, J.A. (1958). An evaluation of thymectomy in myasthenia gravis. *Brain*, **81**, 112–44.

Simpson, J.A. (1960). Myasthenia gravis: a new hypothesis. *Scottish Medical Journal*, **5**, 419–36.

Sinha, S., Newsom-Davis, J., Mills, K., Byrne, N., Lang, B. & Vincent, A. (1991). Autoimmune aetiology for acquired neuromyotonia (Isaacs' syndrome). *Lancet*, **338**, 75–7.

Smith, R.G., Alexianu, M.E., Crawford, G., Nyormoi, O., Stefani, E. & Appel, S.H. (1994). Cytotoxicity of immunoglobulins from amyotrophic lateral sclerosis patients on a hybrid motoneuron cell line. *Proceedings of the National Academy of Science of the United States of America*, **91**, 3393–7.

Smith, R.G., Engelhardt, J.I., Tajti, J. & Appel, S.H. (1993). Experimental immune-mediated motor neuron diseases: models for human ALS. *Brain Research Bulletin*, **30**, 373–80.

Souroujon, M.C. & Fuchs, S. (1987). Antiidiotypic antibodies in the regulation of experimental autoimmune myasthenia gravis. *Annals of the New York Academy of Sciences*, **505**, 676–82.

Souroujon, M.C., Pachner, A.R. & Fuchs, S. (1986). The treatment of passively transferred experimental myasthenia with anti-idiotypic antibodies. *Neurology*, **36**, 622–5.

Staber, F.G., Fink, U. & Sack, W. (1975). B lymphocytes in the thymus of patients with myasthenia gravis. *New England Journal of Medicine*, **292**, 1032–3.

Stanley, E.F. & Drachman, D.B. (1978). Effect of myasthenic immunoglobulin on acetylcholine receptors of intact mammalian neuromuscular junctions. *Science*, **200**, 1285–7.

Stevens, A., Weller, M. & Wietholter, H. (1993). A characteristic ganglioside antibody pattern in the CSF of patients with amyotrophic lateral sclerosis. *Journal of Neurology, Neurosurgery and Psychiatry*, **56**, 361–4.

Streib, E.W. & Rothner, A.D. (1981). Eaton–Lambert myasthenic syndrome: long-term treatment of three patients with prednisone. *Annals of Neurology*, **10**, 448–53.

Stricker, R.B., Kwiatkowska, B.J., Habis, J.A. & Kiprov, D.D. (1993). Myasthenic crisis. Response to plasmapheresis following failure of intravenous gamma-globulin. *Archives of Neurology*, **50**, 837–40.

Sun, J.B., Harcourt, G., Wang, Z.Y., Hawke, S., Olsson, T., Fredrikson, S. & Link, H. (1992). T cell responses to human recombinant acetylcholine receptor-alpha subunit in myasthenia gravis and controls. *European Journal of Immunology*, **22**, 1553–9.

Sutton, G.P., Siemers, E., Stehman, F.B. & Ehrlich, C.E. (1988). Eaton–Lambert syndrome as a harbinger of recurrent small-cell carcinoma of the cervix with improvement after combination chemotherapy. *Obstetrics and Gynaecology*, **72**, 516–8.

Tajti, J., Stefani, E. & Appel, S.H. (1991). Cyclophosphamide alters the clinical and pathological expression of experimental autoimmune gray matter disease. *Journal of Neuroimmunology*, **34**, 143–51.

Tarrab-Hazdai, R., Ahronov, A., Abramsky, O., Yaar, I. & Fuchs, S. (1975*a*). Passive transfer of experimental autoimmune myasthenia by lymph node cells in inbred guinea pigs. *Journal of Experimental Medicine*, **142**, 785–9.

Tarrab-Hazdai, R., Ahronov, A., Silman, I. & Fuchs, S. (1975*b*). Experimental autoimmune myasthenia induced in monkeys by purified acetyl choline receptor. *Nature*, **256**, 128–30.

Tindall, R.S. (1981). Humoral immunity in myasthenia gravis: biochemical characterization of acquired antireceptor antibodies and clinical correlations. *Annals of Neurology*, **10**, 437–47.

Tindall, R.S., Phillips, J.T., Rollins, J.A., Wells, L. & Hall, K. (1993). A clinical therapeutic trial of cyclosporine in myasthenia gravis. *Annals of the New York Academy of Sciences*, **681**, 539–51.

Tindall, R.S., Rollins, J.A., Phillips, J.T., Greenlee, R.G., Wells, L. & Belenduik, G. (1987). Preliminary results of a double-blind, randomized, placebo-controlled trial of cyclosporin in myasthenia gravis. *New England Journal of Medicine*, **316**, 719–24.

Torda, C. & Wolff, H.G. (1951). Effects of administration of the adrenocorticotropic hormone (ACTH) on patients with myasthenia gravis. *Archives of Neurology and Psychiatry*, **66**, 163–70.

Toyka, K.V., Drachman, D.B., Pestronk, A. & Kao, I. (1975). Myasthenia gravis: passive transfer from man to mouse. *Science*, **190**, 397–9.

Troost, D., van den Oord, J.J., de Jong, J.M. & Swaab, D.F. (1989). Lymphocytic infiltration in the spinal cord of patients with amyotrophic lateral sclerosis. *Clinical Neuropathology*, **8**, 289–94.

Troost, D., van den Oord, J.J. & Vianney de Jong, J.M. (1990). Immunohistochemical characterization of the inflammatory infiltrate in amyotrophic lateral sclerosis. *Neuropathology and Applied Neurobiology*, **16**, 401–10.

Tsuboi, Y. & Yamada, T. (1994). Increased concentration of C4d complement protein in CSF in amyotrophic lateral sclerosis. *Journal of Neurology, Neurosurgery and Psychiatry*, **57**, 859–61.

Tzartos, S., Hochschwender, S., Vasquez, P. & Lindstrom, J. (1987). Passive transfer of experimental autoimmune myasthenia gravis by monoclonal antibodies to the main immunogenic region of the acetylcholine receptor. *Journal of Neuroimmunology*, **15**, 185–94.

Tzartos, S.J., Barkas, T., Cung, M.T., Kordossi, A., Loutrari, H., Marraud, M., Papadouli, I., Sakarellos, C., Sophianos, D. & Tsikaris, V. (1991*a*). The main immunogenic region of the acetylcholine receptor. Structure and role in myasthenia gravis. *Autoimmunity*, **8**, 259–70.

Tzartos, S.J., Cung, M.T., Demange, P., Loutrari, H., Mamalaki, A., Marraud, M., Papadouli, I., Sakarellos, C. & Tsikaris, V. (1991*b*). The main immunogenic region (MIR) of the nicotinic acetylcholine receptor and the anti-MIR antibodies. *Molecular Neurobiology*, **5**, 1–29.

Uchitel, O.D., Appel, S.H., Crawford, F. & Sczcupak, L. (1988). Immunoglobulins from amyotrophic lateral sclerosis patients enhance spontaneous transmitter release from motor-nerve terminals. *Proceedings of the National Academy of Science of the United States of America*, **85**, 7371–4.

Uchitel, O.D., Scornik, F., Protti, D.A., Fumberg, C.G., Alvarez, V. & Appel, S.H. (1992). Long-term neuromuscular dysfunction produced by passive transfer of amyotrophic lateral sclerosis immunoglobulins. *Neurology*, **42**, 2175–80.

Urbatsch, I.L., Sterz, R.K., Peper, K. & Trommer, W.E. (1993). Antigen-specific therapy of experimental myasthenia gravis with acetylcholine receptor-gelonin conjugates *in vivo*. *European Journal of Immunology*, **23**, 776–9.

Vasilescu, C., Alexianu, M. & Dan, A. (1984). Muscle hypertrophy and a syndrome of continuous motor unit activity in prednisone-responsive Guillain–Barré syndrome. *Journal of Neurology*, **231**, 276–9.

Vasilescu, C., Bucur, G., Petrovici, A. & Florescu, A. (1978). Myasthenia in patients with dermatomyositis. Clinical, electrophysiological and ultrastructural studies. *Journal of the Neurological Sciences*, **38**, 129–44.

Verma, P.K. & Oger, J.J. (1992). Seronegative generalized myasthenia gravis: low frequency of thymic
pathology. *Neurology*, **42**, 586–9.

Verschuuren, J.J., Graus, Y.M., van Breda Vriesman, P.J., Tzartos, S. & De Baets, M.H. (1991). *In vivo* effects of neonatal administration of antiidiotype antibodies on experimental autoimmune myasthenia gravis. *Autoimmunity*, **10**, 173–9.

Vieira, M.L., Caillat-Zucman, S., Gajdos, P., Cohen-Kaminsky, S., Casteur, A. & Bach, J.-F. (1993). Identification by genomic typing of non-DR3 HLA class II genes associated with myasthenia gravis. *Journal of Neuroimmunology*, **47**, 115–22.

Vilquin, J.T., Braun, S., Labouret, P., Tranchant, C., Hartmann, D., Lombard, Y., Goetz, J., Urlacher, A., Wihlm, J.M., Warter, J.M. *et al.* (1993). Establishment and characterization of B-like lymphoblastoid cell lines by long-term culture of primary explants from human myasthenic thymus. *Thymus*, **21**, 25–42.

Wang, Z.-Y., Link, H., Qiao, J., Olsson, T. & Huang, W.-X. (1993*a*). B cell autoimmunity to acetylcholine receptor and its subunits in Lewis rats over the course of experimental autoimmune myasthenia gravis. *Journal of Neuroimmunology*, **45**, 103–12.

Wang, Z.Y., Qiao, J., Melms, A. & Link, H. (1993*b*). T cell reactivity to acetylcholine receptor in rats orally tolerized against experimental autoimmune myasthenia gravis. *Cellular Immunology*, **152**, 394–404.

Warmolts, J.R. & Engel, W.K. (1972). Benefit from alternate-day prednisone in myasthenia gravis. *New England Journal of Medicine*, **286**, 17–20.

Weiss, J.H., Hartley, D.M., Koh, J. & Choi, D.W. (1990). The calcium channel blocker nifedipine attenuates slow excitatory amino acid neurotoxicity. *Science*, **247**, 1474–7.

Wewetzer, K., MacDonald, J.R., Collins, F. & Unsicker, K. (1990). CNTF rescues motor-neurons from ontogenetic cell death *in-vivo* but not *in-vitro*. *NeuroReport*, **1**, 203–6.

Wierzbicki, A.S. (1993). Antibodies to L-type calcium channels in amyotrophic lateral sclerosis. *New England Journal of Medicine*, **328**, 1355–6.

Willcox, N., Demaine, A.G., Newsom-Davis, J., Welsh, K.I., Robb, S.A. & Spiro, S.G. (1985). Increased frequency of IgG heavy chain marker Glm(2) and of HLA-B8 in Lambert–Eaton myasthenic syndrome with and without associated lung carcinoma. *Human Immunology*, **14**, 29–36.

Willcox, N., Schluep, M., Ritter, M.A. & Newsom-Davis, J. (1991). The thymus in seronegative myasthenia gravis patients. *Journal of Neurology*, **238**, 256–61.

Williams, C.L., Hay, J.E., Huiatt, T.W. & Lennon, V.A. (1992). Paraneoplastic IgG striational autoantibodies produced by clonal thymic B cells and in serum of patients with myasthenia gravis and thymoma react with titin. *Laboratory Investigation*, **66**, 331–6.

Woo, E., Nightingale, S., Dick, D.J., Walls, T.J., French, J.M. & Bates, D. (1986). A study of histocompatibility antigens in patients with motor neuron disease in the northern region of England. *Journal of Neurology, Neurosurgery and Psychiatry*, **49**, 435–7.

Yamamoto, T., Vincent, A., Ciulla, T.A., Lang, B., Johnston, I. & Newsom-Davis, J. (1991). Seronegative myasthenia gravis: a plasma factor inhibiting agonist-induced acetylcholine receptor function copurifies with IgM. *Annals of Neurology*, **30**, 550–7.

Yi, Q., Ahlberg, R. & Lefvert, A.K. (1992). T cells with specificity for idiotypic determinants on human monoclonal autoantibodies in myasthenia gravis. *Research in Immunology*, **143**, 149–56.

Yi, Q., Ahlberg, R., Pirskanen, R. & Lefvert, A.K. (1992). Levels of $CD5^+$ B lymphocytes do not differ between patients with myasthenia gravis and healthy individuals. *Neurology*, **42**, 1081–4.

Yi, Q., Ahlberg, R., Pirskanen, R. & Lefvert, A.K. (1994). Acetylcholine receptor-reactive T cells in myasthenia gravis: evidence for the involvement of different subpopulations of T helper cells. *Journal of Neuroimmunology*, **50**, 177–86.

Yi, Q., Pirskanen, R. & Lefvert, A.K. (1993). Human muscle acetylcholine receptor reactive T and B lymphocytes in the peripheral blood of patients with myasthenia gravis. *Journal of Neuroimmunology*, **42**, 215–22.

Zoda, T.E. & Krolick, K.A. (1993). Antigen presentation and T cell specificity repertoire in determining responsiveness to an epitope important in experimental autoimmune myasthenia gravis. *Journal of Neuroimmunology*, **43**, 131–8.

–11–
Inflammatory myopathies and experimental autoimmune myositis

PAMELA A. McCOMBE

Idiopathic inflammatory myopathy (myositis)

Introduction

Inflammatory myopathies have been recognized for many years (see Marinacci, 1965); an early review was written by Steiner (1903). The inflammatory myopathies include primary inflammatory muscle diseases and inflammatory muscle diseases in association with other autoimmune diseases (the overlap syndromes) or with malignancy. Bohan and colleagues (Bohan & Peter, 1975*a*,*b*; Bohan *et al.*, 1977) established diagnostic criteria for myositis. They divided patients with myositis into five categories: polymyositis, dermatomyositis, polymyositis or dermatomyositis associated with malignancy, childhood polymyositis or dermatomyositis, and polymyositis or dermatomyositis associated with connective tissue disorder (overlap group). Inclusion body myositis is another inflammatory myopathy that is now regarded as a distinct entity, separate from polymyositis (Yunis & Samaha, 1971; Lotz *et al.*, 1989). As outlined by Dalakas (1992*a*), the clinical and pathological features of polymyositis, dermatomyositis and inclusion body myositis remain constant whether or not these diseases are ...sociated with malignancy or with connective tissue diseases. With the ...ption of inclusion body myositis, which at present is of unknown ...gy, it seems likely that these conditions have an autoimmune basis.

...tures

... of adults. It usually develops subacutely, presenting ...kness and later producing widespread weakness of the limb muscles and sometimes the bulbar muscles (Dalakas, 1992*a*). Muscle pain and tenderness are usually present, but are not severe. Clinical examination reveals muscle weakness and decreased deep tendon reflexes. Some patients with polymyositis have interstitial lung disease (Targoff *et al.*, 1989; Lohr *et al.*, 1993) and some patients have cardiac muscle involvement (Behan, Behan & Gairns, 1987*b*). There is elevation of the serum creatine kinase levels. Diagnosis is made on the basis of electromyography (see below) and muscle biopsy. Patients with polymyositis in association with other connective tissue diseases are described as having overlap syndromes (see below).

Dermatomyositis

Patients with dermatomyositis have muscle weakness in association with skin changes characterized by a heliotrope rash on the upper eyelids, a red rash on the face and upper trunk and erythema of the knuckles (Dalakas, 1992*b*). These skin changes may precede the development of muscle weakness. Dermatomyositis in children has clinical and pathological features that differ from those of dermatomyositis in adults (Banker & Victor, 1966; Bohan & Peter, 1975*a*; Pachman & Cooke, 1980; Crowe *et al.*, 1982). In particular, there is evidence of systemic involvement in the childhood form.

Inclusion body myositis

Inclusion body myositis was named by Yunis & Samaha (1971), although earlier studies had noted cellular inclusions in the muscles of some patients with chronic polymyositis (Adams, Kakulas & Samaha, 1965; Chou, 1967). Inclusion body myositis is a chronic disease, more common in males, with a mean age of onset of 63 years. Patients with inclusion body myositis usually have symmetrical weakness of proximal and distal limb muscles (Ringel *et al.*, 1987). Other studies have confirmed the slight male predominance and the older age of onset in inclusion body myositis compared to other forms of myositis (Lotz *et al.*, 1989; Beyenburg, Zierz & Jerusalem, 1993). Dysphagia occurs in some patients with inclusion body myositis (Ringel *et al.*, 1987; Wintzen *et al.*, 1988; Lotz *et al.*, 1989) and may be the presenting complaint (Riminton *et al.*, 1993). In the series reported by Lindberg *et al.* (1994), five of 18 patients with inclusion body myositis had immunoglobulin deficiency.

Focal myositis

Focal myositis was reported by Heffner, Armbrustmacher & Earle (1977), who described a localized soft tissue swelling that had the histological appearances of lymphocytic infiltration of the muscle with patchy muscle fibre necrosis. Focal myositis may also have an autoimmune basis. Focal or localized myositis has been reported to affect the extraocular muscles (ocular myositis) (Shah *et al.*, 1992) and the temporalis muscle (Naumann *et al.*, 1993) or one limb (Lederman *et al.*, 1984).

Overlap syndromes

Overlap syndromes are found in patients where features of polymyositis occur with non-organ-specific connective tissue diseases. Bohan *et al.* (1977) considered that patients with overlap syndromes should fulfil strict diagnostic criteria for both myositis and one other connective tissue disease. Using this definition, he found that 21% of 153 patients with myositis had overlap syndromes. Patients in the overlap group have polymyositis more frequently than dermatomyositis. The diseases frequently associated with myositis are scleroderma, systemic lupus erythematosus, rheumatoid arthritis and primary Sjögren's syndrome. Inclusion body myositis has recently been reported in association with rheumatoid arthritis (Soden *et al.*, 1994).

Association with organ-specific autoimmune disease

Myositis can also occur with organ-specific autoimmune diseases such as primary biliary cirrhosis (Milosevic & Adams, 1990), myasthenia gravis (Bohan *et al.*, 1977) and Crohn's disease (Leibowitz *et al.*, 1994).

Association with malignancy

Polymyositis and especially dermatomyositis may occur in association with malignancy such as ovarian cancer (Cherin *et al.*, 1993; Whitmore, Rosenshein & Provost, 1994) and colon carcinoma (Gluck *et al.*, 1993).

Magnetic resonance imaging and spectroscopy

Magnetic resonance imaging can detect areas of abnormality on the T_2 weighted scans in polymyositis/dermatomyositis, and magnetic resonance spectroscopy shows metabolic abnormalities (Park *et al.*, 1994). The magnetic resonance abnormalities resolve with treatment (Chapman *et al.*, 1994). Magnetic resonance imaging has been used to guide muscle biopsy of patients with myositis (Pitt *et al.*, 1993).

Genetics

Familial myositis

The familial occurrence of polymyositis has been reported (Garcia de la Torre, Ramirez Casillas & Hernandez Vazquez, 1991) In one family a child had fatal dermatomyositis and the father had adult-onset polymyositis (Lewkonia & Buxton, 1973). First-degree relatives of patients with polymyositis or dermatomyositis have evidence of elevated serum anti-nuclear antibodies (Valentini *et al.*, 1991). Familial inclusion body myositis, transmitted as an autosomal dominant condition, has been described (Neville *et al.*, 1992). Deletions of mitochondrial DNA have also been described in inclusion body myositis (Oldfors *et al.*, 1993).

Genetic typing

Juvenile dermatomyositis is associated with HLA B8 and HLA DR3 (Friedman *et al.*, 1983; Pachman, 1986; Robb *et al.*, 1987; Garlepp, 1993), whereas adult polymyositis is associated with HLA B8 (Behan, Behan & Dick, 1978), HLA B14 (Cumming *et al.*, 1977) which may cross-react with HLA B8, and with HLA DR3 (Garlepp, 1993). Myositis with circulating anti-Jo antibodies (see below) is closely linked with HLA DRw52 (Goldstein *et al.*, 1990). Robb *et al.* (1987) found that juvenile dermatomyositis was strongly associated with null alleles of C4, which is a major histocompatibility complex (MHC) class III gene. Patients with C4 null alleles may have decreased clearance of immune complexes which may predispose to the development of the vasculitis found in juvenile dermatomyositis (Banker & Victor, 1966; Kissel, Mendell & Rammohan, 1986). Moulds *et al.* (1990) found there was no association of adult myositis with the C4 null alleles.

Pathology

Polymyositis

Muscle biopsies show evidence of inflammation and necrosis of muscle fibres, with macrophage ingestion of damaged fibres. The inflammatory infiltrates and necrotic fibres are scattered diffusely in the fascicles (Dalakas, 1992*b*).

Dermatomyositis

As in polymyositis, in dermatomyositis there is muscle inflammation and necrosis. The inflammation is predominantly perivascular or in the interfascicular septae, and the muscles show clear perifascicular atrophy (Dalakas, 1992*b*). There is also evidence of microangiopathy of small intramuscular blood vessels (Emslie Smith & Engel, 1990). In the childhood form of dermatomyositis, which has been called 'systemic angiopathy', there is evidence of widespread vasculitis (Banker & Victor, 1966).

Inclusion body myositis

Inclusion body myositis is associated with inflammation of the muscles, but the cardinal histological feature is the presence of rimmed vacuoles with a clear centre and a basophilic, granular edge which, at electron microscopy, are a collection of vacuoles containing debris and filaments (Ringel *et al.*, 1987). These vacuoles may be derived from lysosomes and contain amyloid precursor protein (Mendell *et al.*, 1991; Villanova *et al.*, 1993), ubiquitin (Askanas *et al.*, 1992), α-chymotrypsin (Bilak, Askanas & Engel, 1993) and prion protein (Askanas *et al.*, 1993). Another feature that distinguishes inclusion body myositis from polymyositis is that muscle fibre hypertrophy occurs in the former (Verma *et al.*, 1992). The finding of inclusion bodies suggests that inclusion body myositis may have an infectious aetiology rather than an autoimmune aetiology.

Pathophysiology

Electromyography is used to demonstrate the presence of muscle damage in myositis. In polymyositis, the motor unit action potentials are of low amplitude and short duration, with an increased number of phases (Buchthal & Pinelli, 1953; Richardson, 1956; Streib, Wilbourn & Mitsumoto, 1979). This appears to represent loss of muscle fibres from the motor unit. Spontaneous electrical activity also occurs (Henriksson & Stalberg, 1978; Streib *et al.*, 1979) and may arise from isolated denervated segments of muscle produced by the patchy muscle fibre necrosis. Marinacci (1965) emphasized that in polymyositis there may be positive sharp waves and high-frequency discharges, indicating muscle irritability.

Immunopathology of the muscle lesions

Characteristics of the inflammatory infiltrate

Behan *et al.* (1987*a*) found many T cells and macrophages in the muscles of patients with inflammatory myopathy. Lemoine *et al.* (1986) found that the predominant inflammatory cells in polymyositis were $CD8^+$ cells and macrophages. Giorno & Ringel (1986) also found lymphocytes and macrophages in polymyositis and inclusion body myositis. Arahata and Engel (Engel & Arahata, 1984, 1986; Arahata & Engel, 1986, 1988*a*) described the inflammatory infiltrate in inflammatory myopathies, emphasized the role of $CD8^+$ cells and showed that these $CD8^+$ cells had the characteristics of cytotoxic cells (Arahata & Engel, 1988*b*). The protein, granzyme, which is a product of cytotoxic lymphocytes, may be involved in the degradation of muscle fibres (Nakamura *et al.*, 1993). B cells and $CD4^+$ T cells are not a prominent feature of the inflammatory infiltrate in polymyositis, but B cells may be present in dermatomyositis (Arahata & Engel, 1984; Behan *et al.*, 1987*a*). Beyenburg *et al.* (1993) also showed that the majority of T cells in inclusion body myositis were $CD8^+$. The $\alpha\beta$ T cell receptor genes used by the infiltrating lymphocytes have been analysed by O'Hanlon *et al.* (1994), who found that in polymyositis the majority of cells used the $V\alpha1$ or $V\beta6$ genes, whereas in dermatomyositis there was no restriction of gene usage. One patient with polymyositis was found to have inflammation of the muscle with $\gamma\delta$ T cells (Hohlfeld *et al.*, 1991; Hohlfeld & Engel, 1992).

MHC antigen expression

$CD8^+$ T cells are the prominent cell found in the muscle in polymyositis and inclusion body myositis. Such cells would be expected to interact with MHC class I antigen-positive structures. MHC class I antigen is not expressed on normal muscle fibres, but is expressed on the sarcolemma in polymyositis and inclusion body myositis in areas of inflammation (Isenberg *et al.*, 1986; Emslie Smith, Arahata & Engel, 1989; Bartoccioni *et al.*, 1994). In dermatomyositis, MHC class I antigen is expressed on perifascicular fibres (Karpati, Pouliot & Carpenter, 1988; Emslie Smith *et al.*, 1989). Isenberg *et al.* (1986) found that MHC class I expression was present in regions of cytokine production, but others have been unable to confirm this (Emslie Smith *et al.*, 1989). Some infiltrating T cells in myositis are MHC class II antigen-positive (Giorno *et al.*, 1984; Engel & Arahata, 1986) as are macrophages. MHC class II antigen is sometimes observed on muscle fibres in areas of inflammation in polymyositis and dermatomyositis (Zuk & Fletcher, 1988; Bartoccioni *et al.*, 1994).

Studies of T cells derived from muscle

Rosenschein *et al.* (1987) derived $CD4^+$ and $CD8^+$ T cell lines from the muscle of a patient with dermatomyositis. These lines exhibited non-HLA-restricted responses to human muscle antigen. Hohlfeld & Engel (1991) established T cell lines from the muscles of patients with polymyositis, inclusion body myositis and dermatomyositis. These were a mixture of $CD4^+$ and $CD8^+$ cells, some of which were cytotoxic to cultured myotubes.

Role of complement

Whitaker & Engel (1972) found deposition of complement and immunoglobulin in the walls of blood vessels of muscle in patients with myositis, especially childhood myositis. Morgan *et al.* (1984) found evidence of the complement membrane attack complex on the muscle fibres of patients with myositis. Kissel *et al.* (1986) found deposition of the complement membrane attack complex on the small vessels of five of 19 patients with adult dermatomyositis and ten of 12 patients with childhood dermatomyositis. C3 complement deposition on vascular endothelium appears to have an important role in the production of vascular damage in childhood polymyositis and dermatomyositis (Crowe *et al.*, 1982).

Role of cytokines and adhesion molecules

Immunostaining has demonstrated the presence of interferons α, β and γ at the site of inflammation in polymyositis (Isenberg *et al.*, 1986). Intercellular adhesion molecule-1 (ICAM-1)-positive fibres have been found in regions of inflammation in myositis, but many of these were regenerating fibres (Bartoccioni *et al.*, 1994).

Immunological findings in the peripheral blood

Non-specific findings

Patients with myositis have increased numbers of activated T cells, detected by expression of interleukin-2 receptors (IL-2R) and late activation markers, in the peripheral blood compared to controls (Miller *et al.*, 1990). Levels of interleukin-2 (IL-2), soluble IL-2R and interleukin-1α (IL-1α) (Wolf & Baethge, 1990) and soluble CD8 (Tokano *et al.*, 1993) are elevated in the blood in myositis; these changes indicate T cell activation.

Specific T cell abnormalities

Currie *et al.* (1971) found that lymphocytes from the blood of patients with polymyositis showed a higher proliferative response to muscle antigens than did lymphocytes from patients with other diseases, and were cytotoxic towards muscle cultures, whereas lymphocytes from patients with other diseases such as muscular dystrophy were not. Dawkins & Mastaglia (1973) found that lymphocytes from patients with active polymyositis were cytotoxic to muscle cells, whereas lymphocytes from patients with inactive disease were not. Others have confirmed the finding of lymphocytes that are cytotoxic towards muscle in the blood of patients with myositis (Esiri, Maclennan & Hazleman, 1973; Haas & Arnason, 1974).

Antibodies

Autoantibodies are frequently found in the sera of patients with myositis. Reichlin & Arnett (1984) found that 89% of patients had evidence of either antibody to calf thymus extract (demonstrated by immunoprecipitation) or antibody against HEp2 cells (demonstrated by immunofluorescence). The immunofluorescent staining was nuclear, nucleolar and cytoplasmic. The targets of many of the autoantibodies in myositis sera have been characterized (Targoff, 1992, 1993). Patients may have anti-nuclear antibodies, antibodies directed against synthetases and other myositis-specific targets and antibodies to muscle proteins. Some of these antibodies are associated with clinical subsets of patients with myositis. Love *et al.* (1991) have proposed an alternative classification of patients with myositis, using the presence of different antibodies (see below) to define the groups. It is not clear whether these antibodies, which are directed against intracellular antigens, play a role in the pathogenesis of myositis.

Antinuclear antibodies

Antinuclear antibodies are frequently found in high titres in patients with myositis, especially those with overlap syndromes or features of other connective tissue diseases. The antibodies that are commonly found are anti-rRNP, anti-Sm, anti-Ro and anti-La. The presence of the anti-Ro antibody may correlate with cardiac involvement (Behan *et al.*, 1987*b*). Antibodies to the Ku antigen (Mimori & Hardin, 1986) are usually present in patients with the polymyositis/scleroderma overlap syndrome (Mimori *et al.*, 1990) but are occasionally found in other autoimmune diseases (Yaneva & Arnett, 1989). In the polymyositis/scleroderma overlap syndrome there are also antibodies to a nucleolar particle named PM-Scl (Reimer *et al.*,

1986; Alderuccio, Chan & Tan, 1991). Others have described antibodies to a 56-kDa nuclear protein in patients with polymyositis or dermatomyositis (Arad Dann *et al.*, 1989). This antibody was found in 12 of 17 patients in one study (Ehrenstein, Snaith & Isenberg, 1992). One novel anti-nuclear antibody found in myositis is an antibody to nuclear pore complexes (Dagenais, Bibor Hardy & Senecal, 1988).

Antibodies to cytoplasmic components

'Myositis-specific antibodies' (MSA) are found in about one-third of patients with myositis (Love *et al.*, 1991; Targoff, 1993). Many of these antibodies react with tRNA synthetases (Arad Dann *et al.*, 1987; Bernstein & Mathews, 1987; Bunn & Mathews, 1987*a*). In polymyositis associated with interstitial lung disease anti-synthetase antibodies are characteristically present (Hochberg *et al.*, 1984; Saito *et al.*, 1989; Targoff *et al.*, 1989, 1992; Marguerie *et al.*, 1990). The Jo-1 antigen, which was the first of these to be characterized, is histidyl tRNA-synthase (Matthews & Bernstein, 1983; Walker & Jeffrey, 1987; Biswas *et al.*, 1987; Fahoum & Yang, 1987). Anti-Jo-1 antibodies recognize a variety of different epitopes on the histidyl tRNA-synthetase molecule (Ramsden *et al.*, 1989) and are found in idiopathic polymyositis (Shi, Tsui & Rubin, 1991) with an incidence ranging from one of 25 patients (Ehrenstein *et al.*, 1992) to nine of 32 patients (Yoshida *et al.*, 1983). Antibodies directed against other synthetases are also found in patients with polymyositis. Antibodies have been described against alanine tRNA and alanine tRNA-synthetase (PL-12) (Bunn, Bernstein & Mathews, 1986; Bunn & Mathews, 1987*a*,*b*; Targoff & Arnett, 1990) as well as threonyl-tRNA synthetase (PL-7) (Matthews *et al.*, 1984; Dang, Tan & Traugh, 1988) and the tRNA synthetases for isoleucine (OJ) and glycine (EJ) (Targoff, 1990). Antibodies to cytoplasmic components other than the synthetases have also been reported in the sera of patients with myositis. Antibody to signal recognition particle (SRP) was detected in sera from 13 of 265 patients with polymyositis and is a marker of patients who do not develop lung disease (Targoff, Johnson & Miller, 1990). Antibody to the Mi-2 antigen is present in the sera of patients with dermatomyositis (Targoff & Reichlin, 1985). Other myositis-related antibodies, which are less common, are the anti-Fer, anti-Mas and anti-KJ antibodies (Targoff, 1992, 1993). Antibodies to muscle contractile proteins are reported in patients with idiopathic myositis (Koga *et al.*, 1987) and also in a patient with paraneoplastic polymyositis (Ueyama, Kumamoto & Araki, 1992). Anti-myoglobin antibodies were found in 11 patients with polymyositis and no patients with connective tissue diseases (Nishikai & Homma, 1972).

Immunoregulation

The autologous mixed lymphocyte reaction, which assesses the proliferation of T lymphocytes in the presence of inactivated autologous non-T mononuclear cells, is impaired in patients with myositis (Laffon, Alcocer-Varela & Alarcon-Segovia, 1983; Ransohoff & Dustoor, 1983). Such impairment is found in other autoimmune diseases such as systemic lupus erythematosus and multiple sclerosis (see Chapter 4). It has been suggested that impairment of this reaction may reflect impaired self-recognition and immunoregulation. Peripheral blood lymphocytes from adults with polymyositis also have impaired proliferative responses to T cell mitogens, compared to those from controls (Cambridge *et al.*, 1989). Peripheral blood lymphocytes from children with dermatomyositis have increased immunoglobulin production compared to controls (Cambridge *et al.*, 1989). Gonzalez-Amaro, Alcocer-Varela & Alarcon-Segovia (1987) found that natural killer cell activity was reduced in patients with active myositis.

Therapy

In the cases reviewed by Steiner (1903), 17 of 28 patients had a fatal outcome. With modern treatment, myositis is not usually fatal. In the patients reviewed by Ehrenstein, Snaith & Isenberg (1992), three of 25 had a fatal outcome, although many had continuing weakness despite extensive treatment.

Corticosteroids

Although there are no controlled trials of the use of corticosteroids, oral prednisone is the first line of treatment of polymyositis and dermatomyositis (Dalakas, 1992*b*). In a large survey of the predictors of response to prednisone therapy, it was found that patients with anti-synthetase antibodies had a poorer response than those without such antibodies (Joffe *et al.*, 1993). Inclusion body myositis responds poorly to corticosteroid therapy (Ringel *et al.*, 1987; Joffe *et al.*, 1993).

Other immunosuppressive agents

In patients with dermatomyositis or polymyositis who fail to respond or who become resistant to prednisone, azathioprine or methotrexate may be used (Dalakas, 1992*b*). Patients with inclusion body myositis do not appear to benefit from azathioprine (Beyenburg *et al.*, 1993; Soueidan & Dalakas, 1993). In polymyositis and dermatomyositis, cyclophosphamide has been found to be beneficial by some workers (Bombardieri *et al.*, 1989; De Vita & Fossaluzza, 1992), but not by others (Cronin *et al.*, 1989).

Plasmapheresis and intravenous immunoglobulin

A controlled trial of plasmapheresis and leukapheresis in polymyositis and dermatomyositis failed to show any greater benefit than sham plasmapheresis (Miller *et al.*, 1992). High-dose intravenous immunoglobulin therapy was beneficial in some patients with polymyositis and dermatomyositis who failed to respond to other treatment (Cherin *et al.*, 1990; Jann *et al.*, 1992; Collet *et al.*, 1994). A controlled trial of high-dose intravenous immunoglobulin has shown clear benefits in dermatomyositis (Dalakas *et al.*, 1993). A trial of this therapy in four patients with inclusion body myositis showed some improvement in muscle strength (Soueidan & Dalakas, 1993).

Experimental autoimmune myositis

Introduction

Experimental autoimmune myositis (EAM) has been developed as a model of the human inflammatory myopathies. The successful production of this model is evidence that these human disorders have an autoimmune aetiology. Dawkins (1965) produced EAM by the inoculation of guinea pigs with a mixture of muscle tissue and Freund's adjuvant. Previously, Pearson (1956) and Tal & Liban (1962) had reported muscle abnormalities in rats, rabbits and guinea pigs inoculated with muscle and adjuvants, but the work of Dawkins gave a clear description of the production of inflammation and damage of muscles. EAM has subsequently been induced in rats (Morgan, Peter & Newbould, 1971), SJL/J mice (Rosenberg, Ringel & Kotzin, 1987) and guinea pigs (Webb, 1970*a*). In general, EAM is a good model of inflammatory myopathy and in the future may be useful in the testing of possible treatments for the human diseases.

Induction

Actively induced EAM

EAM was first induced in guinea pigs and rats by inoculation with homogenized muscle tissue and adjuvants (Dawkins, 1965; Webb, 1970*b*; Morgan *et* *al.*, 1971). Later studies have tried to define the component of muscle tissue that is the target antigen. Manghani *et al.* (1974) found that the myofibrillar fraction of muscle was able to produce EAM. Further studies in the guinea pig found that the myosin B component of muscle was the most efficient antigen and showed that strain 13 guinea pigs were more susceptible than Hartley guinea pigs (Matsubara & Takamori, 1987*a*). EAM has also been produced in SJL/J mice by injection of muscle homogenate and complete Freund's adjuvant (Rosenberg *et al.*, 1987) or purified myosin B fraction and adjuvants (Matsubara, Shima & Takamori, 1993). SJL/J mice, which are susceptible to EAM, express a different C3 complement allele from other mice, which are resistant to EAM (Lynch *et al.*, 1993).

Passively transferred EAM

Lymphoid cells from rats with EAM produced by immunization with muscle antigens can transfer disease to normal recipients (Morgan *et al.*, 1971; Esiri & MacLennan, 1974). Another model of EAM was produced by the transfer from SJL/J and BALB/c mice of splenocytes that had been cultured in the presence of syngeneic myotubes: transfer of these cells resulted in inflammatory myopathy in SJL/J but not in BALB/c mice (Hart *et al.*, 1987).

Matsubara *et al.* (1993) reported that when IgG from SJL/J mice with histological evidence of EAM induced by immunization with myosin B fraction was injected into normal mice, the recipient mice also developed histological evidence of EAM. This is the first report of the passive transfer of EAM by antibody and, if confirmed, will provide evidence of the pathogenic role of antibody in this disease.

Clinical features

In early studies in rats, EAM was recognized by pathological rather than clinical features (Morgan *et al.*, 1971). Esiri & MacLennan (1974) could not find evidence of muscle weakness in rats with EAM. In SJL/J mice with EAM recognized by pathological abnormalities, there was no apparent clinical abnormality (Rosenberg *et al.*, 1987). In a recent study where muscle power was specifically assessed, Matsubara *et al.* (1993) found no weakness in SJL/J mice with EAM. Similarly in guinea pigs with EAM, no weakness was reported (Whitaker, 1982). The lack of apparent weakness is likely to be due to difficulties in assessing power in these animals.

Pathology and pathogenesis

Pathology of the muscles

In strain 13 guinea pigs with EAM, there is degeneration of muscle fibres and infiltration of the muscle with lymphocytes and macrophages (Matsubara & Takamori, 1987*a*,*b*). In rats with EAM, there was focal myositis, with necrosis, phagocytosis of muscle fibres and infiltration of the muscle by inflammatory cells (Morgan *et al.*, 1971).

Antibodies

In the sera of animals with EAM, circulating antibodies to striated muscle can be detected by indirect immunofluorescence (Dawkins, Eghtedari & Holborow, 1971; Rosenberg *et al.*, 1987) or by enzyme-linked immunosorbent assay (ELISA) (Rosenberg *et al.*, 1987). Antibody deposition can be demonstrated in the inflamed muscle (Rosenberg *et al.*, 1987; Matsubara *et al.*, 1993). With immunoblotting it has been shown that antibody from guinea pigs with EAM reacts with heavy and light chains of myosin, actin, troponin and other muscle proteins (Matsubara & Takamori, 1987*b*).

T cell responses

Early studies showed that lymphocytes from animals with EAM undergo transformation in the presence of muscle antigens (Currie, 1971; Esiri & Maclennan, 1975). Kakulas (1966) found that lymphocytes from rats inoculated with muscle tissue are able to destroy muscle cultures. Splenocytes from rats that have been immunized with muscle and complete Freund's adjuvant undergo transformation in response to muscle antigens (Esiri & Maclennan, 1975) and splenocytes activated by culture with muscle antigens can transfer disease (Hart *et al.*, 1987).

Role of complement

Complement is deposited on the surface of muscle fibres in EAM in SJL/J mice. Depletion of complement inhibited the transfer of disease by IgG from mice with EAM (Matsubara *et al.*, 1993).

Immunoregulation

Dawkins (1965) found that guinea pigs given weekly injections of homogenized muscle and adjuvant had a single episode of disease, which then declined in severity and was not reactivated by further injections. This is similar to the findings in experimental autoimmune encephalomyelitis and experimental autoimmune neuritis, where, after recovery from disease, animals become resistant to the induction of further episodes of disease by reinoculation. Antibody to muscle antigens was present in guinea pigs injected weekly for up to 94 weeks (Dawkins *et al.*, 1971) and Dawkins (1975) has suggested that antibody to muscle components may inhibit disease.

Conclusions

The evidence suggests that polymyositis is an autoimmune disease mediated by cytotoxic T cells. Dermatomyositis is associated with microangiopathy. A large number of antibodies are found in the serum of patients with these conditions and may also have a role in pathogenesis. Inclusion body myositis is associated with inflammation of the muscles and has some clinical features in common with polymyositis, but the role of autoimmunity is less clear. Animal models of polymyositis have been developed and may play a role in the elucidation of the human diseases. In the future, it will be important to obtain further information about the possible target antigens of these diseases, so that the possibility of specific immunotherapy can be explored. Further studies of the role of immunoregulation of these specific immune responses will aid our understanding of how these diseases develop and may also provide possible future treatments.

References

Adams, R.D., Kakulas, B.A. & Samaha, F.A. (1965). A myopathy with cellular inclusions. *Transactions of the American Neurological Association*, **90**, 213–16.

Alderuccio, F., Chan, E.K. & Tan, E.M. (1991). Molecular characterization of an autoantigen of PM-Scl in the polymyositis/scleroderma overlap syndrome: a unique and complete human cDNA encoding an apparent 75-kD acidic protein of the nucleolar complex. *Journal of Experimental Medicine*, **173**, 941–52.

Arad Dann, H., Isenberg, D., Ovadia, E., Shoenfeld, Y., Sperling, J. & Sperling, R. (1989). Autoantibodies against a nuclear 56 kDa protein: a marker for inflammatory muscle disease. *Journal of Autoimmunity*, **2**, 877–88.

Arad Dann, H., Isenberg, D.A., Shoenfeld, Y., Offen, D., Sperling, J. & Sperling, R. (1987). Autoantibodies against a specific nuclear RNP protein in sera of patients with autoimmune rheumatic diseases associated with myositis. *Journal of Immunology*, **138**, 2463–8.

Arahata, K. & Engel, A.G. (1984). Monoclonal antibody analysis of mononuclear cells in myopathies. I: quantitation of subsets according to diagnosis and sites of accumulation and demonstration and counts of muscle fibres invaded by T cells. *Annals of Neurology*, **16**, 193–208.

Arahata, K. & Engel, A.G. (1986). Monoclonal antibody analysis of mononuclear cells in myopathies. III: Immunoelectron microscopy aspects of cell-mediated muscle fiber injury. *Annals of Neurology*, **19**, 112–25.

Arahata, K. & Engel, A.G. (1988*a*). Monoclonal antibody analysis of mononuclear cells in myopathies. IV: Cell-mediated cytotoxicity and muscle fiber necrosis. *Annals of Neurology*, **23**, 168–73.

Arahata, K. & Engel, A.G. (1988*b*). Monoclonal antibody analysis of mononuclear cells in myopathies. V: Identification and quantitation of $T8^+$ cytotoxic and $T8^+$ suppressor cells. *Annals of Neurology*, **23**, 493–9.

Askanas, V., Bilak, M., Engel, W.K., Alvarez, R.B., Tome, F. & Leclerc, A. (1993). Prion protein is abnormally accumulated in inclusion-body myositis. *Neuroreport*, **5**, 25–8.

Askanas, V., Serdaroglu, P., Engel, W.K. & Alvarez, R.B. (1992). Immunocytochemical localization of ubiquitin in inclusion body myositis allows its light-microscopic distinction from polymyositis. *Neurology*, **42**, 460–1.

Banker, B.Q. & Victor, M. (1966). Dermatomyositis (systemic angiopathy) of childhood. *Medicine*, **45**, 261–89.

Bartoccioni, E., Gallucci, S., Scuderi, F., Ricci, E., Servidei, S., Broccolini, A. & Tonali, P. (1994). MHC class I, MHC class II and intercellular adhesion molecule-1 (ICAM-1) expression in inflammatory myopathies. *Clinical and Experimental Immunology*, **95**, 166–72.

Behan, W.H., Behan, P.O. & Dick, H.A. (1978). HLA B8 in polymyositis. *New England Journal of Medicine*, **298**, 1260–1.

Behan, W.M., Behan, P.O., Durward, W.F. & McQueen, A. (1987*a*). The inflammatory process in polymyositis: monoclonal antibody analysis of muscle and peripheral blood immunoregulatory lymphocytes. *Journal of Neurology, Neurosurgery and Psychiatry*, **50**, 1468–74.

Behan, W.M., Behan, P.O. & Gairns, J. (1987*b*). Cardiac damage in polymyositis associated with antibodies to tissue ribonucleoproteins. *British Heart Journal*, **57**, 176–80.

Bernstein, R.M. & Mathews, M.B. (1987). Autoantibodies to intracellular antigens, with particular reference to transfer RNA and related proteins in myositis. *Journal of Rheumatology*, **14 (Supplement 13)**, 83–8.

Beyenburg, S., Zierz, S. & Jerusalem, F. (1993). Inclusion body myositis: clinical and histopathological features of 36 patients. *Clinical Investigation*, **71**, 351–61.

Bilak, M., Askanas, V. & Engel, W.K. (1993). Strong immunoreactivity of alpha 1-antichymotrypsin co-localizes with beta-amyloid protein and ubiquitin in vacuolated muscle fibers of inclusion-body myositis. *Acta Neuropathologica*, **85**, 378–82.

Biswas, T., Miller, F.W., Takagaki, Y. & Plotz, P.H. (1987). An enzyme-linked immunosorbent assay for the detection and quantitation of anti-Jo-1 antibody in human serum. *Journal of Immunological Methods*, **98**, 243–8.

Bohan, A. & Peter, J.B. (1975*a*). Polymyositis and dermatomyositis (first of two parts). *New England Journal of Medicine*, **292**, 344–7.

Bohan, A. & Peter, J.B. (1975*b*). Polymyositis and dermatomyositis (second of two parts). *New England Journal of Medicine*, **292**, 403–7.

Bohan, A., Peter, J.B., Bowman, R.L. & Pearson, C.M. (1977). A computer-assisted analysis of 153 patients with polymyositis and dermatomyositis. *Medicine*, **56**, 255–86.

Bombardieri, S., Hughes, G.V.R., Neri, R., Del Bravo, P. & Del Bono, L. (1989). Cyclophosphamide in severe polymyositis. *Lancet*, **1**, 1138–9.

Buchthal, F. & Pinelli, P. (1953). Muscle action potentials in polymyositis. *Neurology*, **3**, 424–36.

Bunn, C.C., Bernstein, R.M. & Mathews, M.B. (1986). Autoantibodies against alanyl-tRNA synthetase and tRNAAla coexist and are associated with myositis. *Journal of Experimental Medicine*, **163**, 1281–91.

Bunn, C.C. & Mathews, M.B. (1987*a*). Two human tRNA(Ala) families are recognized by autoantibodies in polymyositis sera. *Molecular Biology and Medicine*, **4**, 21–36.

Bunn, C.C. & Mathews, M.B. (1987*b*). Autoreactive epitope defined as the anticodon region of alanine transfer RNA. *Science*, **238**, 1116–19.

Cambridge, G., Faith, A., Saunders, C. & Dubowitz, V. (1989). A comparative study of *in vitro* proliferative responses to mitogens and immunoglobulin production in patients with inflammatory muscle disease. *Clinical and Experimental Rheumatology*, **7**, 27–33.

Chapman, S., Southwood, T.R., Fowler, J. & Ryder, C.A. (1994). Rapid changes in magnetic resonance imaging of muscle during the treatment of juvenile dermatomyositis. *British Journal of Rheumatology*, **33**, 184–6.

Cherin, P., Herson, S., Wechsler, R., Bletry, O., Degennes, C., Piette, J.C., Ziza, J.M. & Godeau, P. (1990). Intravenous immunoglobulin for polymyositis and dermatomyositis. *Lancet*, **336**, 116.

Cherin, P., Piette, J.C., Herson, S., Bletry, O., Wechsler, B., Frances, C. & Godeau, P. (1993). Dermatomyositis and ovarian cancer: a report of 7 cases and literature review. *Journal of Rheumatology*, **20**, 1897–9.

Chou, S.-M. (1967). Myxovirus-like structures in a case of human chronic polymyositis. *Science*, **158**, 1453–5.

Collet, E., Dalac, S., Maerens, B., Courtois, J.M., Izac, M. & Lambert, D. (1994). Juvenile dermatomyositis: treatment with intravenous gammaglobulin. *British Journal of Dermatology*, **130**, 231–4.

Cronin, M.E., Miller, F.W., Hicks, J.E., Dalakas, M. & Plotz, P.H. (1989). The failure of intravenous cyclophosphamide therapy in refractory idiopathic inflammatory myopathy. *Journal of Rheumatology*, **16**, 1225–8.

Crowe, W.E., Bove, K.E., Levinson, J.E. & Hilton, P.K. (1982). Clinical and pathological implications of histopathology in childhood dermatomyositis. *Arthritis and Rheumatism*, **25**, 126–39.

Cumming, W.J.K., Hudgson, P., Lattimer, D., Sussman, M. & Wilcox, C.B. (1977). HLA and serum complement in polymyositis. *Lancet*, **2**, 978–9.

Currie, S. (1971). Experimental myositis: the *in-vivo* and *in-vitro* activity of lymph-node cells. *Journal of Pathology*, **105**, 169–85.

Currie, S., Saunders, M., Knowles, M. & Brown, A.E. (1971). Immunological aspects of polymyositis. The *in vitro* activity of lymphocytes on incubation with muscle antigen and muscle cultures. *Quarterly Journal of Medicine*, **40**, 63–84.

Dagenais, A., Bibor Hardy, V. & Senecal, J.L. (1988). A novel autoantibody causing a peripheral fluorescent antinuclear antibody pattern is specific for nuclear pore complexes. *Arthritis and Rheumatism*, **31**, 1322–7.

Dalakas, M.C. (1992*a*). Inflammatory myopathies. In *Handbook of Clinical Neurology*, volume 18, *Myopathies*, ed. L.P. Rowland & S. DiMauro, pp. 369–90. Amsterdam: Elsevier Science Publishers.

Dalakas, M.C. (1992*b*). Clinical, immunopathologic, and therapeutic considerations of inflammatory myopathies. *Clinical Neuropharmacology*, **15**, 327–51.

Dalakas, M.C., Illa, I., Dambrosia, J.M., Soueidan, S.A., Stein, D.P., Otero, C., Dinsmore, S.T. & McCrosky, S. (1993). A controlled trial of high-dose intravenous immune globulin infusions as treatment for dermatomyositis. *New England Journal of Medicine*, **329**, 1993–2000.

Dang, C.V., Tan, E.M. & Traugh, J.A. (1988). Myositis autoantibody reactivity and catalytic function of threonyl-tRNA synthetase. *FASEB Journal*, **2**, 2376–9.

Dawkins, R.L. (1965). Experimental myositis associated with hypersensitivity to muscle. *Journal of Pathology and Bacteriology*, **90**, 619–25.

Dawkins, R.L. (1975). Experimental autoallergic myositis, polymyositis and myasthenia gravis. Autoimmune muscle disease associated with immunodeficiency and neoplasia. *Clinical and Experimental Immunology*, **21**, 185–201.

Dawkins, R.L., Eghtedari, A. & Holborow, E.J. (1971). Antibodies to skeletal muscle demonstrated by immunofluorescence in experimental autoallergic myositis. *Clinical and Experimental Immunology*, **9**, 329–37.

Dawkins, R.L. & Mastaglia, F.L. (1973). Cell-mediated cytotoxicity to muscle in polymyositis. Effect of immunosuppression. *New England Journal of Medicine*, **288**, 434–8.

De Vita, S. & Fossaluzza, V. (1992). Treatment of idiopathic inflammatory myopathies with cyclophosphamide pulses: clinical experience and a review of the literature. *Acta Neurologica Belgica*, **92**, 215–27.

Ehrenstein, M.R., Snaith, M.L. & Isenberg, D.A. (1992). Idiopathic myositis: a rheumatological view. *Annals of the Rheumatic Diseases*, **51**, 41–4.

Emslie Smith, A.M., Arahata, K. & Engel, A.G. (1989). Major histocompatibility complex class I antigen expression, immunolocalization of interferon subtypes, and T cell-mediated cytotoxicity in myopathies. *Human Pathology*, **20**, 224–31.

Emslie Smith, A.M. & Engel, A.G. (1990). Microvascular changes in early and advanced dermatomyositis: a quantitative study. *Annals of Neurology*, **27**, 343–56.

Engel, A.G. & Arahata, K. (1984). Monoclonal antibody analysis of mononuclear cells in myopathies. II: Phenotypes of autoinvasive cells in polymyositis and inclusion body myositis. *Annals of Neurology*, **16**, 209–15.

Engel, A.G. & Arahata, K. (1986). Mononuclear cells in myopathies: quantitation of functionally distinct subsets, recognition of antigen-specific cell-mediated cytotoxicity in some diseases, and implications for the pathogenesis of the different inflammatory myopathies. *Human Pathology*, **17**, 704–21.

Esiri, M.M. & Maclennan, I.C. (1975). Experimental myositis in rats. II. The sensitivity of spleen cells to syngeneic muscle antigen. *Clinical and Experimental Immunology*, **19**, 513–20.

Esiri, M.M., Maclennan, I.C. & Hazleman, B.L. (1973). Lymphocyte sensitivity to skeletal muscle in patients with polymyositis and other disorders. *Clinical and Experimental Immunology*, **14**, 25–35.

Esiri, M.M. & MacLennan, I.C.M. (1974). Experimental myositis in rats. I Histological and creatine phoshphokinase changes and passive transfer to normal syngeneic rats. *Clinical and Experimental Immunology*, **17**, 139–50.

Fahoum, S.K. & Yang, D.C. (1987). Purification of mammalian histidyl-tRNA synthetase and its interaction with myositis-specific anti-Jo-1 antibodies. *Biochemistry*, **26**, 5871–7.

Friedman, J.M., Pachman, L.M., Maryjowski, M.L., Radvany, R.M., Crowe, W.E., Hanson, V., Levinson, J.E. & Spencer, C.H. (1983). Immunogenetic studies of juvenile dermatomyositis: HLA-DR antigen frequencies. *Arthritis and Rheumatism*, **26**, 214–16.

Garcia de la Torre, I., Ramirez Casillas, A. & Hernandez Vazquez, L. (1991). Acute familial myositis with a common autoimmune response. *Arthritis and Rheumatism*, **34**, 744–50.

Garlepp, M.J. (1993). Immunogenetics of inflammatory myopathies. *Baillière's Clinical Neurology*, **2**, 579–97.

Giorno, R., Barden, M.T., Kohler, P.F. & Ringel, S.P. (1984). Immunohistochemical characterization of the mononuclear cells infiltrating muscle of patients with inflammatory and noninflammatory myopathies. *Clinical Immunology and Immunopathology*, **30**, 405–12.

Giorno, R. & Ringel, S.P. (1986). Analysis of macrophages, activated cells and T cell subsets in inflammatory myopathies using monoclonal antibodies. *Pathology and Immunopathology Research*, **5**, 491–9.

Gluck, Z., Kutsherowsky, M., Abraham, Z. & Galper, I. (1993). Dermatomyositis, carcinoma of colon and meningioma in the same patient. *Journal of Dermatology*, **20**, 719–22.

Goldstein, R., Duvic, M., Targoff, I.N., Reichlin, M., McMenemy, A.M., Reveille, J.D., Warner, N.B., Pollack, M.S. & Arnett, F.C. (1990). HLA-D region genes associated with autoantibody responses to histidyl-transfer RNA synthetase (Jo-1) and other translation-related factors in myositis. *Arthritis and Rheumatism*, **33**, 1240–8.

Gonzalez-Amaro, R., Alcocer-Varela, J. & Alarcon-Segovia, D. (1987). Natural killer cell activity in dermatomyositis-polymyositis. *Journal of Rheumatology*, **14**, 307–10.

Haas, D.C. & Arnason, B.G.W. (1974). Cell-mediated immunity in polymyositis. Creatine phosphokinase release from muscle cultures. *Archives of Neurology*, **31**, 192–6.

Hart, M.N., Linthicum, D.S., Waldschmidt, M.M., Tassell, S.K., Schelper, R.L. & Robinson, R.A. (1987). Experimental autoimmune inflammatory myopathy. *Journal of Neuropathology and Experimental Neurology*, **46**, 511–21.

Heffner, R.R., Armbrustmacher, V.W. & Earle, K.M. (1977). Focal myositis. *Cancer*, **40**, 301–6.

Henriksson, K.G. & Stalberg, E. (1978). The terminal innervation pattern in polymyositis: a histochemical and SFEMG study. *Muscle and Nerve*, **1**, 3–13.

Hochberg, M.C., Feldman, D., Stevens, M.B., Arnett, F.C. & Reichlin, M. (1984). Antibody to Jo-1 in polymyositis/dermatomyositis: association with interstitial pulmonary disease. *Journal of Rheumatology*, **11**, 663–5.

Hohlfeld, R. & Engel, A.G. (1991). Coculture with autologous myotubes of cytotoxic T cells isolated from muscle in inflammatory myopathies. *Annals of Neurology*, **29**, 498–507.

Hohlfeld, R. & Engel, A.G. (1992). The role of gamma-delta T lymphocytes in inflammatory muscle disease. *Chemical Immunology*, **53**, 75–85.

Hohlfeld, R., Engel, A.G., Ii, K. & Harper, M.C. (1991). Polymyositis mediated by T lymphocytes that express the gamma/delta receptor. *New England Journal of Medicine*, **324**, 877–81.

Isenberg, D.A., Rowe, D., Shearer, M., Novick, D. & Beverley, P.C. (1985). Localization of interferons and interleukin 2 in polymyositis and muscular dystrophy. *Clinical and Experimental Immunology*, **63**, 450–8.

Jann, S., Beretta, S., Moggio, M., Adobbati, L. & Pellegrini, G. (1992). High-dose intravenous human immunoglobulin in polymyositis resistant to treatment. *Journal of Neurology, Neurosurgery and Psychiatry*, **55**, 60–2.

Joffe, M.M., Love, L.A., Leff, R.L., Fraser, D.D., Targoff, I.N., Hicks, J.E., Plotz, P.H. & Miller, F.W. (1993). Drug therapy of the idiopathic inflammatory myopathies: predictors of response to prednisone, azathioprine, and methotrexate and a comparison of their efficacy. *American Journal of Medicine*, **94**, 379–87.

Kakulas, B.A. (1966). Destruction of differentiated muscle cultures by sensitised lymphoid cells. *Journal of Pathology and Bacteriology*, **91**, 495–503.

Karpati, G., Pouliot, Y. & Carpenter, S. (1988). Expression of immunoreactive major histocompatibility complex products in human skeletal muscles. *Annals of Neurology*, **23**, 64–72.

Kissel, J.T., Mendell, J.R. & Rammohan, K.W. (1986). Microvascular deposition of complement membrane attack complex in dermatomyositis. *New England Journal of Medicine*, **314**, 329–34.

Koga, K., Abe, S., Hashimoto, H. & Yamaguchi, M. (1987). Western-blotting method for detecting antibodies against human muscle contractile proteins in myositis. *Journal of Immunological Methods*, **105**, 15–21.

Laffon, A., Alcocer-Varela, J. & Alarcon-Segovia, D. (1983). Differences in the kinetics of the autologous mixed lymphocyte reaction between the various connective tissue diseases. *Rheumatology International*, **3**, 117–28.

Lederman, R.J., Salanga, V.D., Wilbourn, A.J., Hanson, M.R. & Dudley, A.W. (1984). Focal inflammatory myopathy. *Muscle and Nerve*, **7**, 142–6.

Leibowitz, G., Eliakim, R., Amir, G. & Rachmilewitz, D. (1994). Dermatomyositis associated with Crohn's disease. *Journal of Clinical Gastroenterology*, **18**, 48–52.

Lemoine, N.R., Ryan, J.F., Cox, E.L., Mayston, V., Revell, P.A. & Swash, M. (1986). Immunohistochemical analysis of mononuclear cell subsets in inflammatory and non-inflammatory myopathies. *Journal of Clinical Pathology*, **39**, 271–4.

Lewkonia, R.M. & Buxton, P.H. (1973). Myositis in father and daughter. *Journal of Neurology, Neurosurgery and Psychiatry*, **36**, 820–5.

Lindberg, C., Persson, L.I., Bjorkander, J. & Oldfors, A. (1994). Inclusion body myositis: clinical, morphological, physiological and laboratory findings in 18 cases. *Acta Neurologica Scandinavica*, **89**, 123–31.

Lohr, H.F., Bocher, W.O., Hermann, E., Muller Quernheim, J., Schwickert, H., Meyer zum Buschenfelde, K.H. & Gerken, G. (1993). Interstitial alveolitis as early manifestation of anti-Jo-1 positive polymyositis. *Zeitschrift fur Rheumatologie*, **52**, 307–11.

Lotz, B.P., Engel, A.G., Nishino, H., Stevens, J.C. & Litchy, W.J. (1989). Inclusion body myositis. Observations in 40 patients. *Brain*, **112**, 727–47.

Love, L.A., Leff, R.L., Fraser, D.D., Targoff, I.N., Dalakas, M., Plotz, P.H. & Miller, F.W. (1991). A new approach to the classification of idiopathic inflammatory myopathy: myositis-specific autoantibodies define useful homogeneous patient groups. *Medicine*, **70**, 360–74.

Lynch, D.M., Kay, P.H., Papadimitriou, J.M. & Grounds, M.D. (1993). Studies on the structure of complement C3 and the stability of C3 derived phagocytic ligands C3b/iC3b in SJL/J and BALB/c mice. *European Journal of Immunogenetics*, **20**, 1–9.

Manghani, D., Partridge, T.A. & Sloper, J.C. (1974). The role of myofibrillar fraction of skeletal muscle in the production of experimental polymyositis. *Journal of the Neurological Sciences*, **23**, 489–503.

Marguerie, C., Bunn, C.C., Beynon, H.L., Bernstein, R.M., Hughes, J.M., So, A.K. & Walport, M.J. (1990). Polymyositis, pulmonary fibrosis and autoantibodies to aminoacyl-tRNA synthetase enzymes. *Quarterly Journal of Medicine*, **77**, 1019–38.

Marinacci, A.A. (1965). Electromyography in the diagnosis of polymyositis. *Electromyography*, **5**, 255–68.

Matsubara, S., Shima, T. & Takamori, M. (1993). Experimental allergic myositis in SJL/J mice immunized with rabbit myosin B fraction: immunohistochemical analysis and transfer. *Acta Neuropathologica*, **85**, 138–44.

Matsubara, S. & Takamori, M. (1987*a*). Experimental allergic myositis: strain 13 guinea pig immunised with rabbit myosin B fraction. *Acta Neuropathologica*, **74**, 158–62.

Matsubara, S. & Takamori, M. (1987*b*). Experimental allergic myositis: ultrastructural, histochemical, immunological and immunohistochemical studies. *Acta Neuropathologica*, **74**, 151–7.

Matthews, M.B. & Bernstein, R.M. (1983). Myositis autoantibody inhibits histidyl-tRNA synthetase: a model for autoimmunity. *Nature*, **304**, 177–9.

Matthews, M.B., Reichlin, M., Hughes, G.V.R. & Bernstein, R.M. (1984). Anti-threonyl-tRNA synthetase, a second myositis-related autoantibody. *Journal of Experimental Medicine*, **160**, 420–34.

Mendell, J.R., Sahenk, Z., Gales, T. & Paul, L. (1991). Amyloid filaments in inclusion body myositis. Novel findings provide insight into nature of filaments. *Archives of Neurology*, **48**, 1229–34.

Miller, F.W., Leitman, S.F., Cronin, M.E., Hicks, J.E., Leff, R.L., Wesley, R., Fraser, D.D., Dalakas, M. & Plotz, P.H. (1992). Controlled trial of plasma exchange and leukapheresis in polymyositis and dermatomyositis. *New England Journal of Medicine*, **326**, 1380–4.

Miller, F.W., Love, L.A., Barbieri, S.A., Balow, J.E. & Plotz, P.H. (1990). Lymphocyte activation markers in idiopathic myositis: changes with disease activity and differences among clinical and autoantibody subgroups. *Clinical and Experimental Immunology*, **81**, 373–9.

Milosevic, M. & Adams, P. (1990). Primary biliary cirrhosis and polymyositis. *Journal of Clinical Gastroenterology*, **12**, 332–5.

Mimori, T. & Hardin, J.A. (1986). Mechanism of interaction between Ku protein and DNA. *Journal of Biological Chemistry*, **261**, 10375–9.

Mimori, T., Ohosone, Y., Hama, N., Suwa, A., Akizuki, M., Homma, M., Griffith, A.J. & Hardin, J.A. (1990). Isolation and characterization of cDNA encoding the 80-kDa subunit protein of the human autoantigen Ku (p70/p80) recognized by autoantibodies from patients with scleroderma-polymyositis overlap syndrome. *Proceedings of the National Academy of Science of the United States of America*, **87**, 1777–81.

Morgan, B.P., Sewry, C.A., Siddle, K., Luzio, J.P. & Campbell, A.K. (1984). Immunolocalization of complement component C9 on necrotic and non-necrotic muscle fibres in myositis using monoclonal antibodies: a primary role of complement in autoimmune cell damage. *Immunology*, **52**, 181–8.

Morgan, G., Peter, J.B. & Newbould, B.B. (1971). Experimental allergic myositis in rats. *Arthritis and Rheumatism*, **14**, 599–609.

Moulds, J.M., Rolih, C., Goldstein, R., Whittington, K.F., Warner, N.B., Targoff, I.N., Reichlin, M. & Arnett, F.C. (1990). C4 null genes in American whites and blacks with myositis. *Journal of Rheumatology*, **17**, 331–4.

Nakamura, K., Arahata, K., Ishiura, S., Osame, M. & Sugita, H. (1993). Degradative activity of granzyme A on skeletal muscle proteins *in vitro*: a possible molecular mechanism for muscle fiber damage in polymyositis. *Neuromuscular Disorders*, **3**, 303–10.

Naumann, M., Toyka, K.V., Goebel, H.H., Hofmann, E. & Reichmann, H. (1993). Focal myositis of the temporal muscle. *Muscle and Nerve*, **16**, 1374–6.

Neville, H.E., Baumbach, L.L., Ringel, S.P., Russo, L.S.J., Sujansky, E. & Garcia, C.A. (1992). Familial inclusion body myositis: evidence for autosomal dominant inheritance. *Neurology*, **42**, 897–902.

Nishikai, M. & Homma, M. (1972). Anti-myoglobin antibody in polymyositis. *Lancet*, **2**, 1205–6.

O'Hanlon, T.P., Dalakas, M.C., Plotz, P.H. & Miller, F.W. (1994). Predominant TCR-alpha beta variable and joining gene expression by muscle-infiltrating lymphocytes in the idiopathic inflammatory myopathies. *Journal of Immunology*, **152**, 2569–76.

Oldfors, A., Larsson, N.G., Lindberg, C. & Holme, E. (1993). Mitochondrial DNA deletions in inclusion body myositis. *Brain*, **116**, 325–36.

Pachman, L.M. (1986). Juvenile dermatomyositis. *Pediatric Clinics of North America*, **33**, 1097–117.

Pachman, L.M. & Cooke, N. (1980). Juvenile dermatomyositis: a clinical and immunologic study. *Journal of Pediatrics*, **96**, 226–34.

Park, J.H., Vital, T.L., Ryder, N.M., Hernanz Schulman, M., Partain, C.L., Price, R.R. & Olsen, N.J. (1994). Magnetic resonance imaging and P-31 magnetic resonance spectroscopy provide unique quantitative data useful in the longitudinal management of patients with dermatomyositis. *Arthritis and Rheumatism*, **37**, 736–46.

Pearson, C. (1956). Development of arthritis, periarthritis and periostitis in rats given adjuvants. *Proceedings of the Society for Experimental Biology and Medicine*, **91**, 95–101.

Pitt, A.M., Fleckenstein, J.L., Greenlee, R.G.J., Burns, D.K., Bryan, W.W. & Haller, R. (1993). MRI-guided biopsy in inflammatory myopathy: initial results. *Magnetic Resonance Imaging*, **11**, 1093–9.

Ramsden, D.A., Chen, J., Miller, F.W., Misener, V., Bernstein, R.M., Siminovitch, K.A. & Tsui, F.W. (1989). Epitope mapping of the cloned human autoantigen, histidyl-tRNA synthetase. Analysis of the myositis-associated anti-Jo-1 autoimmune response. *Journal of Immunology*, **143**, 2267–72.

Ransohoff, R.M. & Dustoor, M.M. (1983). Impaired autologous mixed lymphocyte reaction with normal concanavalin A-induced suppression in adult polymyositis/dermatomyositis. *Clinical and Experimental Immunology*, **53**, 67–75.

Reichlin, M. & Arnett, F.C. Jr (1984). Multiplicity of antibodies in myositis sera. *Arthritis and Rheumatism*, **27**, 1150–6.

Reimer, G., Scheer, U., Peters, J.M. & Tan, E.M. (1986). Immunolocalization and partial characterization of a nucleolar autoantigen (PM-Scl) associated with polymyositis/scleroderma overlap syndromes. *Journal of Immunology*, **137**, 3802–8.

Richardson, A.T. (1956). Clinical and electromyographic aspects of polymyositis. *Proceedings of the Royal Society of Medicine*, **49**, 111–14.

Riminton, D.S., Chambers, S.T., Parkin, P.J., Pollock, M. & Donaldson, I.M. (1993). Inclusion body myositis presenting solely as dysphagia. *Neurology*, **43**, 1241–3.

Ringel, S.P., Kenny, C.E., Neville, H.E., Giorno, R. & Carry, M.R. (1987). Spectrum of inclusion body myositis. *Archives of Neurology*, **44**, 1154–7.

Robb, S.A., Fielder, A.H.L., Saunders, C.E., Davey, N.J., Burley, M.W., Lord, D.H., Batchelor, J.R. & Dubowitz, V. (1987). C4 complement allotypes in juvenile dermatomyositis. *Human Immunology*, **22**, 31–8.

Rosenberg, N.L., Ringel, S.P. & Kotzin, B.L. (1987). Experimental autoimmune myositis in SJL/J mice. *Clinical and Experimental Immunology*, **68**, 117–29.

Rosenschein, U., Radnay, J., Shoham, D., Shainberg, A., Klajman, A. & Rozenszajn, L.A. (1987). Human muscle-derived, tissue specific, myocytotoxic T cell lines in dermatomyositis. *Clinical and Experimental Immunology*, **67**, 309–18.

Saito, E., Yoshimoto, Y., Oshima, H., Yoshida, H. & Kinoshita, M. (1989). Fluorescent antibodies in polymyositis using cultured human skin fibroblasts: granular perinuclear cytoplasmic staining pattern by sera from patients with polymyositis and pulmonary fibrosis. *Journal of Rheumatology*, **16**, 47–54.

Shah, S.S., Lowder, C.Y., Schmitt, M.A., Wilke, W.S., Kosmorsky, G.S. & Meisler, D.M. (1992). Low-dose methotrexate therapy for ocular inflammatory disease. *Ophthalmology*, **99**, 1419–23.

Shi, M.H., Tsui, F.W. & Rubin, L.A. (1991). Cellular localization of the target structures recognized by the anti-Jo-1 antibody: immunofluorescence studies on cultured human myoblasts. *Journal of Rheumatology*, **18**, 252–8.

Soden, M., Boundy, K., Burrow, D., Blumbergs, P. & Ahern, M. (1994). Inclusion body myositis in association with rheumatoid arthritis. *Journal of Rheumatology*, **21**, 344–6.

Soueidan, S.A. & Dalakas, M.C. (1993). Treatment of inclusion-body myositis with high-dose immunoglobulin. *Neurology*, **34**, 876–9.

Steiner, W.R. (1903). Dermatomyositis, with report of a case which presented with a rare muscle anomaly but once described in man. *Journal of Experimental Medicine*, **6**, 407–42.

Streib, E.W., Wilbourn, A.J. & Mitsumoto, H. (1979). Spontaneous electrical muscle fiber activity in polymyositis and dermatomyositis. *Muscle and Nerve*, **2**, 14–18.

Tal, C. & Liban, E. (1962). Experimental production of muscular dystrophy-like lesions in rabbits and guinea pigs by an auto-immune process. *British Journal of Experimental Pathology*, **43**, 525–9.

Targoff, I.N. (1990). Autoantibodies to aminoacyl-transfer RNA synthetases for isoleucine and glycine. Two additional synthetases are antigenic in myositis. *Journal of Immunology*, **144**, 1737–43.

Targoff, I.N. (1992). Autoantibodies in polymyositis. *Rheumatic Diseases Clinics of North America*, **18**, 455–82.

Targoff, I.N. (1993). Humoral immunity in polymyositis/dermatomyositis. *Journal of Investigative Dermatology*, **100**, 116S–123S.

Targoff, I.N. & Arnett, F.C. (1990). Clinical manifestations in patients with antibody to PL-12 antigen (alanyl-tRNA synthetase). *American Journal of Medicine*, **88**, 241–51.

Targoff, I.N., Arnett, F.C., Berman, L., O'Brien, C. & Reichlin, M. (1989). Anti-KJ: a new antibody associated with the syndrome of polymyositis and interstitial lung disease. *Journal of Clinical Investigation*, **84**, 162–72.

Targoff, I.N., Johnson, A.E. & Miller, F.W. (1990). Antibody to signal recognition particle in polymyositis. *Arthritis and Rheumatism*, **33**, 1361–70.

Targoff, I.N. & Reichlin, M. (1985). The association between Mi-2 antibodies and dermatomyositis. *Arthritis and Rheumatism*, **28**, 796–803.

Targoff, I.N., Trieu, E.P., Plotz, P.H. & Miller, F.W. (1992). Antibodies to glycyl-transfer RNA synthetase in patients with myositis and interstitial lung disease. *Arthritis and Rheumatism*, **35**, 821–30.

Tokano, Y., Obara, T., Hashimoto, H., Okumura, K. & Hirose, S. (1993). Soluble CD4, CD8 in patients with polymyositis/dermatomyositis. *Clinical Rheumatology*, **12**, 368–74.

Ueyama, H., Kumamoto, T. & Araki, S. (1992). Circulating autoantibody to muscle protein in a patient with paraneoplastic myositis and colon cancer. *European Neurology*, **32**, 281–4.

Valentini, G., Improta, R.D., Resse, M., Migliaresi, S., Minucci, P.B., Tirri, R., Farzati, B. & Tirri, G. (1991). Antinuclear antibodies in first-degree relatives of patients with polymyositis-dermatomyositis: analysis of the relationship with HLA haplotypes. *British Journal of Rheumatology*, **30**, 429–32.

Verma, A., Bradley, W.G., Soule, N.W., Pendlebury, W.W., Kelly, J., Adelman, L.S., Chou, S.M., Karpati, G. & Brenner, J.F. (1992). Quantitative morphometric study of muscle in inclusion body myositis. *Journal of the Neurological Sciences*, **112**, 192–8.

Villanova, M., Kawai, M., Lubke, U., Oh, S.J., Perry, G., Six, J., Ceuterick, C., Martin, J.J. & Cras, P. (1993). Rimmed vacuoles of inclusion body myositis and oculopharyngeal muscular dystrophy contain amyloid precursor protein and lysosomal markers. *Brain Research*, **603**, 343–7.

Walker, E.J. & Jeffrey, P.D. (1987). Purification of bovine liver histidyl-tRNA synthetase, the Jo-1 antigen of polymyositis: size of the whole enzyme and its characteristic proteolytic fragments. *Biological Chemistry Hoppe-Seyler*, **368**, 531–7.

Webb, J.N. (1970*a*). Experimental immune myositis in guinea pigs. *Journal of the Reticuloendothelial Society*, **7**, 305–16.

Webb, J.N. (1970*b*). *In vitro* transformation of lymphocytes in experimental immune myositis. *Journal of the Reticuloendothelial Society*, **7**, 445–52.

Whitaker, J.N. (1982). Inflammatory myopathy: a review of etiologic and pathogenetic factors. *Muscle and Nerve*, **5**, 573–92.

Whitaker, J.N. & Engel, W.K. (1972). Vascular deposits of immunoglobulin and complement in idiopathic inflammatory myopathy. *New England Journal of Medicine*, **286**, 333–8.

Whitmore, S.E., Rosenshein, N.B. & Provost, T.T. (1994). Ovarian cancer in patients with dermatomyositis. *Medicine*, **73**, 153–60.

Wintzen, A.R., Bots, G.T., de Bakker, H.M., Hulshof, J.H. & Padberg, G.W. (1988). Dysphagia in inclusion body myositis. *Journal of Neurology, Neurosurgery and Psychiatry*, **51**, 1542–5.

Wolf, R.E. & Baethge, B.A. (1990). Interleukin-1 alpha, interleukin-2, and soluble interleukin-2 receptors in polymyositis. *Arthritis and Rheumatism*, **33**, 1007–14.

Yaneva, M. & Arnett, F.C. (1989). Antibodies against Ku protein in sera from patients with autoimmune diseases. *Clinical and Experimental Immunology*, **76**, 366–72.

Yoshida, S., Akizuki, M., Mimori, T., Yamagata, H., Inada, S. & Homma, M. (1983). The precipitating antibody to an acidic nuclear protein antigen, the Jo-1, in connective tissue diseases. *Arthritis and Rheumatism*, **26**, 604–11.

Yunis, E.J. & Samaha, F.J. (1971). Inclusion body myositis. *Laboratory Investigation*, **25**, 240–8.

Zuk, J.A. & Fletcher, A. (1988). Skeletal muscle expression of class II histocompatibility antigens (HLA-DR) in polymyositis and other muscle disorders with an inflammatory infiltrate. *Journal of Clinical Pathology*, **41**, 410–14.

–12–
Paraneoplastic neurological disorders

MICHAEL P. PENDER

Introduction

Paraneoplastic neurological disorders are diseases of the nervous system that occur as a remote effect of malignant neoplasms and that are not due to infiltration of the nervous system by neoplastic tissue. These disorders have been described in association with a wide variety of neoplasms, with the lung, ovary and breast being common sites of origin. There is increasing evidence that paraneoplastic neurological disorders are due to an autoimmune attack on specific regions of the nervous system triggered by the aberrant expression of neuronal antigens by the neoplasm (Posner, 1992). Many regions of the nervous system can be involved, either in isolation or in combination, and this involvement determines the clinical features. The following paraneoplastic neurological syndromes have been described: subacute sensory neuronopathy (Denny-Brown, 1948), the Lambert–Eaton myasthenic syndrome (Eaton & Lambert, 1957), subacute cerebellar degeneration (Brain & Wilkinson, 1965), paraneoplastic motor neurone disease (Brain, Croft & Wilkinson, 1965; Henson, Hoffman & Urich, 1965), brainstem encephalitis (Henson *et al.*, 1965), limbic encephalitis (Corsellis, Goldberg & Norton, 1968), opsoclonus and myoclonus (Brandt *et al.*, 1974), the visual paraneoplastic syndrome (Grunwald *et al.*, 1987), dysautonomia (Veilleux, Bernier & Lamarche, 1990), the stiff-man syndrome (Ferrari *et al.*, 1990; Folli *et al.*, 1993) and cochleovestibular dysfunction (Gulya, 1993). At least some of these syndromes can occur on an autoimmune basis in the absence of any detectable neoplasm. As the Lambert–Eaton myasthenic syndrome and the stiff-man syndrome commonly occur in the absence of an associated neoplasm, they are dealt with in separate specific chapters (Chapters 10 and 6, respectively).

Clinical features

Because of the diversity of clinical syndromes, the clinical features of the paraneoplastic neurological disorders will be discussed separately for each syndrome.

Subacute sensory neuronopathy

This disorder is most commonly seen in association with small cell carcinoma of the lung, but may also occur with a wide variety of other neoplasms, including breast cancer (Horwich *et al.*, 1977; Chalk *et al.*, 1992). The incidence of subacute sensory neuronopathy in small cell lung cancer is about 1% (Elrington *et al.*, 1991). A similar disorder can develop in association with primary Sjögren's syndrome (Malinow *et al.*, 1986; Griffin *et al.*, 1990; see Chapter 13) or may occur in the absence of any detectable associated disease (Kaufman, Hopkins & Hurwitz, 1981). Paraneoplastic subacute sensory neuronopathy may become manifest before or after the diagnosis of the associated neoplasm. Typically the syndrome comprises the subacute onset of pain, paraesthesiae, dysaesthesiae and numbness in the limbs commencing distally and spreading proximally and sometimes involving the trunk and face (Denny-Brown, 1948; Horwich *et al.*, 1977; Chalk *et al.*, 1992). Physical examination reveals loss of light touch, pain and temperature sensation, and severe impairment of joint position sense and vibration sense. Sensory ataxia and areflexia are also characteristic features. Strength is preserved. In one series, about half of the patients had associated autonomic, cerebellar or cerebral abnormalities (Chalk *et al.*, 1992). Electrophysiological studies are useful in confirming the selective sensory involvement. Examination of the cerebrospinal fluid (CSF) usually reveals an elevated protein level and sometimes a mononuclear pleocytosis (Horwich *et al.*, 1977).

Subacute cerebellar degeneration

Subacute cerebellar degeneration is most commonly seen in association with small cell carcinoma of the lung, gynaecological cancers (especially of the ovary or breast) and Hodgkin's disease (Brain & Wilkinson, 1965; Hammack *et al.*, 1992), but may also occur with other malignancies, including carcinoma of the colon (Tsukamoto *et al.*, 1993). When it occurs in Hodgkin's disease, it is more common in men and has a younger age of onset than when associated with other malignancies (Hammack *et al.*, 1992). Paraneoplastic subacute cerebellar degeneration may become clinically evident either before or after detection of the malignancy. The typical clinical pattern is the subacute evolution (over weeks to months) of truncal and limb ataxia and dysarthria (Brain & Wilkinson, 1965; Hammack *et al.*, 1992). The ataxia can become so severe that the patient has difficulty sitting up in bed. Nystagmus, particularly downbeat nystagmus, may occur, but is often absent. Subacute cerebellar degeneration is often accompanied by evidence of involvement of other regions of the nervous system (Brain & Wilkinson, 1965). Examination of the CSF often reveals an elevated protein level and a lymphocytic pleocytosis (Peterson *et al.*, 1992). Computerized tomography or magnetic resonance imaging may reveal cerebellar atrophy, particularly in the later stages (Peterson *et al.*, 1992). Although spontaneous improvement may occur (Hammack *et al.*, 1992), the disorder is usually irreversible.

Paraneoplastic motor neurone disease

A lower motor neurone syndrome with or without upper motor neurone involvement may occur in association with malignancy, particularly that of the lung (Brain *et al.*, 1965; Dhib Jalbut & Liwnicz, 1986). This paraneoplastic disorder may also be accompanied by clinical evidence of involvement of other regions of the nervous system (Henson *et al.*, 1965), but when it occurs in the absence of such involvement it resembles idiopathic motor neurone disease. There is evidence that the latter may sometimes have an autoimmune basis (see Chapter 10).

Brainstem encephalitis

Paraneoplastic brainstem encephalitis occurs particularly in association with lung cancer and manifests itself in ophthalmoplegia, bulbar palsy, vertigo and nystagmus (Henson *et al.*, 1965). It may also be accompanied by clinical involvement of other regions of the nervous system. Baloh *et al.* (1993) have recently reported a novel brainstem syndrome occurring in patients with prostatic carcinoma and consisting of a loss of voluntary horizontal saccadic eye movements and severe persistent muscle spasms of the face, jaw and pharynx together with mild unsteadiness of gait.

Limbic encephalitis

Limbic encephalitis occurs particularly in conjunction with small cell carcinoma of the lung (Brierley *et al.*, 1960; Corsellis *et al.*, 1968; Bakheit, Kennedy & Behan, 1990), but also with other tumours, such as thymoma (McArdle & Millingen, 1988; Ingenito *et al.*, 1990), carcinoma of the testis (Burton *et al.*, 1988) and carcinoma of the colon (Tsukamoto *et al.*, 1993). Characteristically, the disorder is manifested by the onset over several months of a marked disturbance of affect, such as severe anxiety or depression, and of a selective impairment of recent memory (Corsellis *et al.*, 1968; Bakheit *et al.*, 1990). Hallucinations and epilepsy may also occur. The clinical picture may resemble that of schizophrenia (Frommer *et al.*, 1993). Clinical involvement of other regions of the nervous system may accompany the picture of limbic encephalitis (Tsukamoto *et al.*, 1993). Examination of the CSF often reveals a mononuclear pleocytosis and an elevated protein level, while electroencephalography may demonstrate paroxysmal activity and/or slow waves over one or both temporal lobes (Corsellis *et al.*, 1968). On magnetic resonance imaging there may be abnormal high-signal intensity in the medial temporal lobes on T_2-weighted scans followed by the development of temporal lobe atrophy on T_1-weighted scans (Dirr *et al.*, 1990; Kodama *et al.*, 1991).

Opsoclonus and myoclonus

A syndrome of opsoclonus ('dancing eyes'), truncal and limb myoclonus, and ataxia may occur in children with neuroblastoma (Brandt *et al.*, 1974), and in adults with cancer, particularly small cell carcinoma of the lung (Anderson *et al.*, 1988*a*). Opsoclonus is defined as the occurrence of involuntary, arrhythmic, large-amplitude, multidirectional, conjugate saccadic eye movements without an intersaccadic interval. The syndrome is characterized by the acute onset of vertigo, nausea, vomiting, opsoclonus, truncal and limb myoclonus, truncal and (to a lesser extent) limb ataxia, and encephalopathy (Brandt *et al.*, 1974; Anderson *et al.*, 1988*a*). The truncal ataxia often becomes so severe that the patient is unable to stand or sit without support. The encephalopathy is manifested by apathy, lethargy and confusion, and may progress to stupor or coma. Unlike most other paraneoplastic neurological syndromes, the course is often remitting and relapsing (Anderson *et al.*, 1988*a*). CSF examination may reveal a lymphocytic pleocytosis, a mild elevation of the protein level, and the presence of oligoclonal immunoglobulin (Ig) bands. Electro-oculography allows accurate definition of the involuntary eye movements. Patients with this syndrome differ clinically from those with the more common paraneoplastic cerebellar degeneration by the predominance of truncal over limb ataxia, the presence of opsoclonus and myoclonus, the absence of severe dysarthria and a tendency for remission (Anderson *et al.*, 1988*a*). A similar opsoclonus–myoclonus syndrome can occur in children without detectable neuroblastoma (Kinsbourne, 1962) and can occur in adults without malignancy as an acute self-limited disorder following a respiratory or gastrointestinal infection (Baringer, Sweeney & Winkler, 1968).

Other paraneoplastic neurological syndromes

The Lambert–Eaton myasthenic syndrome, which can occur in association with small cell carcinoma of the lung (Eaton & Lambert, 1957), and the stiff-man syndrome, which can occur with Hodgkin's disease (Ferrari *et al.*, 1990) and breast cancer (Folli *et al.*, 1993), are discussed in detail in Chapters 10 and 6, respectively. Other paraneoplastic neurological syndromes include: the visual paraneoplastic syndrome, which occurs in association with small cell carcinoma of the lung and results in binocular visual loss (Grunwald *et al.*, 1987); cochleovestibular dysfunction, which has been observed accompanying other paraneoplastic neurological syndromes (Gulya, 1993); and dysautonomia manifested by orthostatic hypotension, abnormal pupillary reflexes, hyperhidrosis, urinary retention, constipation, impotence, cardiac arrhythmias, hypothermia and sleep apnoea (Veilleux *et al.*, 1990; Dalmau *et al.*, 1992*b*). Posterior uveitis may also occur in association with paraneoplastic neurological involvement (Antoine *et al.*, 1993). A severe impairment of gastrointestinal motility with intestinal pseudo-obstruction, gastroparesis and oesophageal dysmotility can occur in patients with small cell lung cancer with or without other autonomic dysfunction (Chinn & Schuffler, 1988; Sodhi *et al.*, 1989; Lennon *et al.*, 1991). Turner *et al.* (1993) found subclinical cardiovascular autonomic dysfunction in 80% of patients with Hodgkin's disease or non-Hodgkin's lymphoma at the time of presentation, and suggested that this was due to a paraneoplastic syndrome.

Neuropathology

The typical neuropathological features of the paraneoplastic neurological disorders are neuronal loss, neuronal pyknosis, neuronophagia, microglial nodules (or nodules of Nageotte in the dorsal root ganglia), meningeal lymphocytic infiltration, perivascular lymphocytic cuffing, parenchymal infiltration with lymphocytes and macrophages, and astrocytic gliosis (Denny-Brown, 1948; Henson *et al.*, 1965; Brain & Wilkinson, 1965; Corsellis *et al.*, 1968; Horwich *et al.*, 1977). The distribution of these changes varies with the clinical syndrome. Thus, the dorsal root ganglion is the main site in subacute sensory neuronopathy (Denny-Brown, 1948; Horwich *et al.*, 1977); the cerebellar Purkinje cell layer in subacute cerebellar degeneration (Brain & Wilkinson, 1965); the anterior horn cells of the spinal cord in paraneoplastic motor neurone syndromes (Henson *et al.*, 1965; Brain *et al.*, 1965); the lower brainstem nuclei in brainstem encephalitis (Henson *et al.*, 1965; Baloh *et al.*, 1993); the limbic grey matter (hippocampal formation, amygdaloid nucleus, and the cingulate and orbital cortex) in limbic encephalitis (Corsellis *et al.*, 1968); and the retinal ganglion cell layer in the visual paraneoplastic syndrome (Grunwald *et al.*, 1987). The paravertebral sympathetic ganglia, brainstem grey matter and spinal cord are among the sites of involvement in dysautonomia (Veilleux *et al.*, 1990; Dalmau *et al.*, 1992*b*). In intestinal pseudo-obstruction and gastroparesis the pathological changes are found in the myenteric plexus (Chinn & Schuffler, 1988; Chu *et al.*, 1993). The neuropathological basis of the opsoclonus–myoclonus syndrome is unknown (Anderson *et al.*, 1988*a*). Involvement of the limbic grey matter, the lower brainstem nuclei, the anterior horn cells of the spinal cord and the dorsal root ganglia often occur together in various combinations (Henson *et al.*, 1965); these combinations are often referred to as 'paraneoplastic encephalomyelitis'.

Immunopathology of the lesions in the nervous system

Characteristics of the inflammatory infiltrate in the nervous system

Immunohistochemical studies in patients with paraneoplastic encephalomyelitis and sensory neuronopathy have shown that the perivascular inflammatory infiltrates are composed mainly of B cells and $CD4^+$ T cells with some $CD8^+$ T cells and macrophages, while the interstitial inflammatory infiltrates consist predominantly of $CD8^+CD11b^-$ (reportedly cytotoxic) T cells, although $CD4^+$ T cells, macrophages and occasional B cells are also present (Graus *et al.*, 1990; Yoshioka *et al.*, 1992; Jean *et al.*, 1994). Neurones do not express class I or class II major histocompatibility complex (MHC) antigens, although satellite cells in the dorsal root ganglia express HLA-DR in both patients and controls (Graus *et al.*, 1990; Yoshioka *et al.*, 1992). By incubating tissue sections with biotinylated HuD neuronal antigen (see below), Szabo *et al.* (1991) have demonstrated HuD-reactive B lymphocytes in the brain of a patient with a paraneoplastic neurological disorder. Interestingly, a predominance of $CD8^+$ T cells has also been observed in the dorsal root ganglion inflammatory infiltrate of a patient with subacute sensory neuronopathy due to primary Sjögren's syndrome (Griffin *et al.*, 1990), suggesting that a similar mechanism may be responsible for the neuronal destruction in this syndrome and in the paraneoplastic one.

Localization of antibody in the nervous system

IgG bound to neurones has been demonstrated *in situ* in patients with paraneoplastic neurological disorders and with circulating anti-Hu antibodies (Graus *et al.*, 1990; Brashear *et al.*, 1991; Dalmau *et al.*, 1991). Dalmau *et al.* (1991) found that the amount of anti-Hu IgG relative to total IgG was higher in some areas of the brain than in the serum and CSF. The anti-Hu IgG within the nervous system is predominantly of the IgG1 isotype and to a lesser extent of the IgG2 and IgG3 isotypes (Jean *et al.*, 1994). There is also a minor degree of complement deposition within the nervous system parenchyma (Jean *et al.*, 1994). Binding of Ig to neurones *in situ* has been demonstrated in patients with small cell lung cancer and circulating anti-neuronal antibodies in the absence of clinical evidence of a paraneoplastic neurological disorder, but not in cancer patients without circulating anti-neuronal antibodies (Drlicek *et al.*, 1992). Immune deposits have also been found in the retina of a patient with the visual paraneoplastic syndrome (Grunwald *et al.*, 1987).

Immunological findings in the peripheral blood

Anti-neuronal antibodies can be demonstrated in the sera of patients with paraneoplastic neurological disorders. Different antibodies have been defined according to their specificities and will be discussed separately below. The antibodies have been called 'anti-Yo', 'anti-Hu' and 'anti-Ri' after the first two letters of the last names of patients with the respective antibodies.

Antibodies against Purkinje cell cytoplasm (anti-Yo antibodies)

Antibodies against Purkinje cell cytoplasm (anti-Yo antibodies) are present in the sera of patients with subacute cerebellar degeneration and gynaecological cancer (mainly ovarian and breast) but not in normal healthy controls or patients with other paraneoplastic neurological disorders or other neurological diseases (Greenlee & Brashear, 1983; Jaeckle *et al.*, 1985; Peterson *et al.*, 1992). Generally, they are not present in patients with subacute cerebellar degeneration associated with other malignancies. These antibodies are also present in some patients with gynaecological cancer without clinical evidence of cerebellar degeneration, although they are absent in the majority of such patients (Greenlee & Brashear, 1983; Brashear *et al.*, 1989). Therefore, serum anti-Yo antibodies are a specific marker for gynaecological cancer (Peterson *et al.*, 1992). Their presence in patients with cerebellar dysfunction should prompt a careful search for such an underlying malignancy.

Western blot analysis of purified Purkinje neurones has shown that the autoantibodies recognize at least two proteins: a major antigen of 62 kDa (CDR 62, cerebellar degeneration-related 62-kDa protein) and a minor antigen of 34 kDa (CDR 34) (Cunningham *et al.*, 1986). The gene encoding CDR 34 has been isolated and characterized and found to reside on the X chromosome (Dropcho *et al.*, 1987; Furneaux *et al.*, 1989; Chen *et al.*, 1990). It is uniquely expressed in Purkinje cells of the cerebellum and has also been detected in tumour tissue from a patient with paraneoplastic cerebellar degeneration (Furneaux *et al.*, 1989). Screening of a human expression library has also resulted in the isolation of cDNA clones encoding the major CDR 62 antigen (Fathallah Shaykh *et al.*, 1991). Sequence analysis revealed the presence of leucine-zipper and zinc-fingers motifs in the predicted open reading frame, suggesting that the CDR 62 protein plays a role in the regulation of gene expression. In contrast to the minor antigen CDR 34, the recombinant CDR 62 antigen is highly reactive with anti-Yo sera and provides the basis for a simple diagnostic enzyme-linked immunosorbent assay for the presence of anti-Yo antibodies (Fathallah Shaykh *et al.*, 1991). Interestingly, H.M. Furneaux *et al.* (1990) have found that the CDR 62 protein is expressed by gynaecological tumours from patients with paraneoplastic cerebellar degeneration but not by gynaecological tumours from patients without this neurological complication. They hypothesize that paraneoplastic cerebellar degeneration is a result of an immunological response directed against the Purkinje cell but provoked by the tumour-induced expression of the Yo antigen.

An antibody specifically reacting against Purkinje cell cytoplasm, but in a different, more diffuse pattern than that obtained with anti-Yo antibodies, has been found in the sera of some patients with paraneoplastic cerebellar degeneration and Hodgkin's disease, but Western blotting has not identified a discrete Purkinje cell antigen (Hammack *et al.*, 1992). Furthermore, non-anti-Yo antibodies reacting with Purkinje cell cytoplasm and recognizing 62-kDa or 110-kDa neuronal antigens have been detected in the sera of men with subacute sensory neuronopathy without tumours (Nemni *et al.*, 1993).

Antibodies against neuronal nuclei (anti-Hu antibodies)

Antibodies specifically reactive against neuronal nuclei, but not the nuclei of most other cells, (anti-Hu antibodies) are present in the sera of patients with subacute sensory neuronopathy, or paraneoplastic encephalomyelitis (including limbic encephalitis, motor neurone dysfunction, cerebellar dysfunction, brainstem encephalitis and dysautonomia) and small cell lung cancer (Graus, Cordon-Cardo & Posner, 1985; Dick *et al.*, 1988; Anderson *et al.*, 1988*b*; Moll *et al.*, 1990; Dalmau *et al.*, 1990, 1992*b*; Lennon *et al.*, 1991). They are predominantly of the IgG1 isotype and to a lesser extent of the IgG2 and IgG3 isotypes (Jean *et al.*, 1994). The antibodies are also present, although at lower titre, in the sera of a minority of patients with small cell lung cancer without clinical evidence of a paraneoplastic neurological disorder. They are not present in normal healthy individuals. Furthermore, they are not usually present in cases of subacute sensory neuronopathy associated with other cancers or occurring without malignancy (Anderson *et al.*, 1988*b*) although they can be detected in some patients with primary Sjögren's syndrome with or without sensory neuronopathy (Moll *et al.*, 1993). With the latter exception, the anti-Hu antibody is a specific marker for the paraneoplastic syndromes associated with small cell lung cancer; its detection in a patient not known to have cancer should prompt a careful search for this malignancy.

The antibodies stain predominantly the neuronal nuclei, with sparing of the nucleoli, and with weaker staining of the neuronal cytoplasm. Western blot analysis of nuclear extracts of human and rat brain has revealed that the antibodies react with a closely arranged set of protein bands of 35–40 kDa (Graus *et al.*, 1986; Dalmau *et al.*, 1990). Using immunohistochemistry or Western blot analysis, Dalmau *et al.* (1992*a*) studied the expression of the Hu antigen in normal human tissues and in tumours of different histological types. They found that in normal tissues the Hu antigen was restricted to neurones (including those of the myenteric plexus), adrenal chromaffin cells and ganglion cells of the bronchus. With regard to tumours, the antigen was present in all small cell lung cancers, but not other lung cancers; it was not present in most other cancers, except for neuroendocrine-related cancers, especially neuroblastoma. Given that all small cell lung cancers express the Hu antigen, it is unclear why only a minority of patients with this cancer develop anti-Hu antibodies.

By screening a phage lambda cerebellar expression library, Szabo *et al.* (1991) have isolated a recombinant neuronal antigen (HuD) that is recognized by anti-Hu antibodies and that can be used to provide an unambiguous assay for these antibodies. In normal tissues, HuD mRNA is uniquely expressed in the nervous system. The HuD antigen is homologous to the *Drosophila* proteins Elav (embryonic lethal abnormal vision) and couch potato, which are essential RNA-binding proteins expressed early during neuronal development (Szabo *et al.*, 1991; Bellen *et al.*, 1992). In view of this homology it is likely that HuD plays a role in neurone-specific RNA processing. Sakai *et al.* (1994) have isolated a hippocampal 38-kDa antigen (PLE21) that is also recognized by anti-Hu antibodies. This protein contains RNA recognition motifs and is highly homologous to the HuC antigen isolated by Szabo *et al.* (1991).

Anti-Ri antibodies

Patients with opsoclonus, ataxia and breast cancer have serum antibodies specifically directed against neuronal nuclei (Luque *et al.*, 1991). Histochemically these antibodies appear identical to anti-Hu antibodies, but

Western blot analysis with cerebral cortex neuronal extracts reveals that the protein antigens have a different molecular mass (55 kDa and 80 kDa) than the antigens recognized by anti-Hu antibodies (35–40 kDa) (Luque *et al.*, 1991). Serum anti-Ri antibodies are not present in normal individuals. Generally they are not detected in patients with breast cancer without opsoclonus, although they have been found in some patients with breast cancer and ataxia in the absence of opsoclonus (Luque *et al.*, 1991; Escudero *et al.*, 1993). Furthermore, these antibodies have not been detected in the sera of patients with paraneoplastic opsoclonus associated with small cell lung cancer or neuroblastoma. While they are generally absent in patients with non-paraneoplastic opsoclonus (Luque *et al.*, 1991), they have been detected in a patient with steroid-responsive opsoclonus–myoclonus in the absence of tumour (Dropcho, Kline & Riser, 1993). Anti-Ri antibodies react with the tumours of patients with the respective antibodies and opsoclonus, but do not react with the breast cancers of those without anti-Ri antibodies (Luque *et al.*, 1991). Therefore, the situation in anti-Ri paraneoplastic opsoclonus is similar to that in anti-Yo paraneoplastic cerebellar degeneration, where the antigen is present only in the tumours of those patients who develop the antibody response. It is different from the situation with anti-Hu antibodies and from the paraneoplastic Lambert–Eaton myasthenic syndrome, where the antigen appears to be present in all small cell lung cancers but where only a small proportion of patients mount an antibody response.

Immunological findings in the cerebrospinal fluid

Furneaux, Reich & Posner (1990) quantified the activity of anti-Yo and anti-Hu antibodies in simultaneously obtained samples of serum and CSF of patients with paraneoplastic neurological disorders. In the majority of patients the autoantibody activity per milligram of total IgG was substantially greater in the CSF than in the serum, indicating intrathecal production of these autoantibodies in the paraneoplastic syndromes. Plasmapheresis reduced the level of antibody in the serum without affecting that in the CSF in five of six patients. In patients with the anti-Ri paraneoplastic syndrome there is also evidence of intrathecal production of the anti-Ri antibodies (Luque *et al.*, 1991).

Mechanism of neuronal destruction and/or dysfunction

It is likely that the anti-neuronal antibodies that are present in the serum, CSF and nervous tissue in the paraneoplastic disorders play a role in the neuronal destruction that is characteristic of these disorders; however, this has not yet been definitely established. Greenlee, Parks & Jaeckle (1993) found that anti-Hu antibodies from patients with paraneoplastic disorders produced specific lysis of rat cerebellar granule neurones *in vitro* in the presence of complement, as compared with controls using normal serum or heat-inactivated complement. More prolonged incubation of cultures with anti-Hu antibodies without complement also resulted in specific lysis, whereas incubation with normal serum or serum from neurologically normal patients with small cell lung cancer did not. These results indicate that anti-Hu antibodies may cause neuronal destruction in the absence of lymphocytes. On the other hand, attempts to transfer the neurological disorder by injecting anti-Hu antibodies into experimental animals have so far been unsuccessful (Dick *et al.*, 1988; Szabo *et al.*, 1991). Repeated intraventricular injections of anti-Yo IgG from a patient with paraneoplastic cerebellar degeneration into guinea pigs have failed to produce either clinical or histological evidence of cerebellar disease, despite the presence of IgG in the Purkinje cell cytoplasm of the recipients (Graus *et al.*, 1991).

The $CD8^+$ lymphocytes infiltrating the nervous system (Graus *et al.*, 1990; Yoshioka *et al.*, 1992) may also contribute to the neuronal elimination by acting as cytotoxic T cells. However, as neurones do not express class I MHC antigens (Graus *et al.*, 1990; Yoshioka *et al.*, 1992), it is difficult to explain how $CD8^+$ cytotoxic T cells, which recognize antigen in the context of these MHC antigens, could specifically interact with the neurones. An alternative explanation is that some of the infiltrating $CD8^+$ cells represent natural killer cells which might be targeted by their Fc receptors to antibody-binding neurones. Natural killer cells have been shown to mediate the destruction of sympathetic neurones in the superior cervical ganglia of rats treated with guanethidine (Hickey *et al.*, 1992). However, Jean *et al.* (1994) did not find natural killer cells in the inflammatory infiltrates of patients with paraneoplastic encephalomyelitis.

While neuronal death is the cause of the clinical deficit in most of the paraneoplastic disorders, antibody-mediated dysfunction without neuronal death may be responsible for the manifestations of reversible central nervous system syndromes, for example opsoclonus–myoclonus, as in the case of the Lambert–Eaton myasthenic syndrome (see Chapter 10). The availability of recombinant neuronal antigens such as Yo and Hu may allow the production of animal models that will facilitate studies on the pathogenesis of the paraneoplastic neurological disorders.

Effect of the immune response on the tumour

Altman & Baehner (1976) observed that children with coincident opsoclonus–myoclonus and neuroblastoma had a much better prognosis for survival than those without opsoclonus–myoclonus. They acknowledged that this might be partly explained by earlier tumour detection in the former group, because of the striking neurological symptomatology. However, as five of the seven patients with opsoclonus–myoclonus and advanced malignancy also exhibited long-term survival, they suggested that an immune response might be responsible for controlling the growth and spread of the tumour, as well as being responsible for the neurological syndrome. This hypothesis has been supported by the observation that patients with small cell lung cancer who have low-titre anti-Hu antibodies and no paraneoplastic neurological syndrome are more likely to have their tumour limited to the chest than patients without anti-Hu antibodies (Dalmau *et al.*, 1990). Despite the fact that the presence of anti-Hu antibody appears to protect against death from the tumour, the median survival of patients with the associated paraneoplastic syndrome is similar to that of small cell lung cancer patients without the syndrome, because of the severity of the neurological disorder (Dalmau *et al.*, 1992*b*). Interestingly, spontaneous tumour regression can occur in patients with small cell lung carcinoma, paraneoplastic neurological disease and anti-neuronal antibodies (Darnell & DeAngelis, 1993). This raises the possibility that the absence of identifiable tumour in some patients with 'paraneoplastic' neurological syndromes may be explained by immune-mediated elimination of the tumour cells. Anti-Hu IgG and anti-Hu B lymphocytes have been demonstrated in the tumour as well as in the brain in patients with paraneoplastic neurological disorders (Dalmau *et al.*, 1991; Szabo *et al.*, 1991).

Therapy

In general, the clinical deficits in patients with the paraneoplastic neurological syndromes with underlying neuronal loss are irreversible, whereas syndromes without demonstrable neuronal loss such as paraneoplastic opsoclonus–myoclonus may spontaneously remit. In some instances of limbic encephalitis, clinical improvement has occurred following antineoplastic therapy or surgical removal of the tumour (Burton *et al.*, 1988; Kaniecki & Morris, 1993; Tsukamoto *et al.*, 1993), indicating either that neuronal loss was not responsible for the clinical manifestations or that any neuronal loss had been compensated for, perhaps by axonal sprouting. In some patients with paraneoplastic sensory neuronopathy, treatment of the neoplasm may halt progression of the neuronopathy but neurological improvement does not occur and most patients continue to worsen even when the tumour responds well to therapy (Chalk *et al.*, 1992).

With the exception of the paraneoplastic Lambert–Eaton myasthenic syndrome (see Chapter 10), the paraneoplastic neurological disorders do not respond to plasmapheresis, corticosteroid or other immunosuppressant therapy (Peterson *et al.*, 1992; Hammack *et al.*, 1992; Dalmau *et al.*, 1992*b*). Given the underlying neuronal loss, the most that could be expected from such therapy would be prevention of progression. By inhibiting the immune response against the tumour, immunosuppressive treatment may also allow the tumour to progress unless it is controlled by other therapy.

Conclusions

The hypothesis that paraneoplastic neurological syndromes are due to an autoimmune attack on the nervous system triggered by the aberrant expression of neuronal antigens by the neoplasm is supported by the following observations: lymphocytic pleocytosis in the CSF; lymphocytic infiltrate in the nervous system; circulating anti-neuronal antibodies that also react with the underlying tumour; intrathecal synthesis and localization of these autoantibodies in nervous tissue parenchyma; and (in one study) the lytic effect of anti-neuronal antibodies on neurones *in vitro*. Further studies are needed to determine the relative roles of T cells and antibodies in the pathogenesis of these disorders. At least some, and perhaps all, of these syndromes may occur on an autoimmune basis in the absence of any triggering neoplasm. Studies on the pathogenesis of the paraneoplastic neurological disorders may shed light on the pathogenesis of the corresponding non-paraneoplastic disorders. The availability of recombinant neuronal antigens should allow the development of animal models that will facilitate these studies.

References

Altman, A.J. & Baehner, R.L. (1976). Favorable prognosis for survival in children with coincident opso-myoclonus and neuroblastoma. *Cancer*, **37**, 846–52.

Anderson, N.E., Budde Steffen, C., Rosenblum, M.K., Graus, F., Ford, D., Synek, B.J. & Posner, J.B. (1988*a*). Opsoclonus, myoclonus, ataxia, and encephalopathy in adults with cancer: a distinct paraneoplastic syndrome. *Medicine Baltimore*, **67**, 100–9.

Anderson, N.E., Rosenblum, M.K., Graus, F., Wiley, R.G. & Posner, J.B. (1988*b*). Autoantibodies in paraneoplastic syndromes associated with small-cell lung cancer. *Neurology*, **38**, 1391–8.

Antoine, J.C., Honnorat, J., Vocanson, C., Koenig, F., Aguera, M., Belin, M.F. & Michel, D. (1993). Posterior uveitis, paraneoplastic encephalomyelitis and auto-antibodies reacting with developmental protein of brain and retina. *Journal of the Neurological Sciences*, **117**, 215–23.

Bakheit, A.M., Kennedy, P.G. & Behan, P.O. (1990). Paraneoplastic limbic encephalitis: clinico-pathological correlations. *Journal of Neurology, Neurosurgery and Psychiatry*, **53**, 1084–8.

Baloh, R.W., DeRossett, S.E., Cloughesy, T.F., Kuncl, R.W., Miller, N.R., Merrill, J. & Posner, J.B. (1993). Novel brainstem syndrome associated with prostate carcinoma. *Neurology*, **43**, 2591–6.

Baringer, J.R., Sweeney, V.P. & Winkler, G.F. (1968). An acute syndrome of ocular oscillations and truncal myoclonus. *Brain*, **91**, 473–80.

Bellen, H.J., Kooyer, S., D'Evelyn, D. & Pearlman, J. (1992). The *Drosophila* couch potato protein is expressed in nuclei of peripheral neuronal precursors and shows homology to RNA-binding proteins. *Genes and Development*, **6**, 2125–36.

Brain, L., Croft, P.B. & Wilkinson, M. (1965). Motor neurone disease as a manifestation of neoplasm (with a note on the course of classical motor neurone disease). *Brain*, **88**, 479–500.

Brain, L. & Wilkinson, M. (1965). Subacute cerebellar degeneration associated with neoplasms. *Brain*, **88**, 465–78.

Brandt, S., Carlsen, N., Glenting, P. & Helweg-Larsen, J. (1974). Encephalopathia myoclonica infantilis (Kinsbourne) and neuroblastoma in children. A report of three cases. *Developmental Medicine and Child Neurology*, **16**, 286–94.

Brashear, H.R., Caccamo, D.V., Heck, A. & Keeney, P.M. (1991). Localization of antibody in the central nervous system of a patient with paraneoplastic encephalomyeloneuritis. *Neurology*, **41**, 1583–7.

Brashear, H.R., Greenlee, J.E., Jaeckle, K.A. & Rose, J.W. (1989). Anticerebellar antibodies in neurologically normal patients with ovarian neoplasms. *Neurology*, **39**, 1605–9.

Brierley, J.B., Corsellis, J.A.N., Hierons, R. & Nevin, S. (1960). Subacute encephalitis of later adult life. Mainly affecting the limbic areas. *Brain*, **83**, 357–68.

Burton, G.V., Bullard, D.E., Walther, P.J. & Burger, P.C. (1988). Paraneoplastic limbic encephalopathy with testicular carcinoma. A reversible neurologic syndrome. *Cancer*, **62**, 2248–51.

Chalk, C.H., Windebank, A.J., Kimmel, D.W. & McManis, P.G. (1992). The distinctive clinical features of paraneoplastic sensory neuronopathy. *Canadian Journal of Neurological Sciences*, **19**, 346–51.

Chen, Y.T., Rettig, W.J., Yenamandra, A.K., Kozak, C.A., Chaganti, R.S., Posner, J.B. & Old, L.J. (1990). Cerebellar degeneration-related antigen: a highly conserved neuroectodermal marker mapped to chromosomes X in human and mouse. *Proceedings of the National Academy of Sciences USA*, **87**, 3077–81.

Chinn, J.S. & Schuffler, M.D. (1988). Paraneoplastic visceral neuropathy as a cause of severe gastrointestinal motor dysfunction. *Gastroenterology*, **95**, 1279–86.

Chu, G., Wilson, P.C., Carter, C.D., Lennon, V.A. & Roberts Thomson, I.C. (1993). Intestinal pseudo-obstruction, type 1 anti-neuronal nuclear antibodies and small-cell carcinoma of the lung. *Journal of Gastroenterology and Hepatology*, **8**, 604–6.

Corsellis, J.A.N., Goldberg, G.J. & Norton, A.R. (1968). 'Limbic encephalitis' and its association with carcinoma. *Brain*, **91**, 481–96.

Cunningham, J., Graus, F., Anderson, N. & Posner, J.B. (1986). Partial characterization of the Purkinje cell antigens in paraneoplastic cerebellar degeneration. *Neurology*, **36**, 1163–8.

Dalmau, J., Furneaux, H.M., Cordon Cardo, C. & Posner, J.B. (1992*a*). The expression of the Hu (paraneoplastic encephalomyelitis/sensory neuronopathy) antigen in human normal and tumor tissues. *American Journal of Pathology*, **141**, 881–6.

Dalmau, J., Furneaux, H.M., Gralla, R.J., Kris, M.G. & Posner, J.B. (1990). Detection of the anti-Hu antibody in the serum of patients with small cell lung cancer – a quantitative western blot analysis. *Annals of Neurology*, **27**, 544–52.

Dalmau, J., Furneaux, H.M., Rosenblum, M.K., Graus, F. & Posner, J.B. (1991). Detection of the anti-Hu antibody in specific regions of the nervous system and tumor from patients with paraneoplastic encephalomyelitis/sensory neuronopathy. *Neurology*, **41**, 1757–64.

Dalmau, J., Graus, F., Rosenblum, M.K. & Posner, J.B. (1992*b*). Anti-Hu-associated paraneoplastic encephalomyelitis/sensory neuronopathy. A clinical study of 71 patients. *Medicine Baltimore*, **71**, 59–72.

Darnell, R.B. & DeAngelis, L.M. (1993). Regression of small-cell lung carcinoma in patients with paraneoplastic neuronal antibodies. *Lancet*, **341**, 21–2.

Denny-Brown, D. (1948). Primary sensory neuropathy with muscular changes associated with carcinoma. *Journal of Neurology, Neurosurgery and Psychiatry*, **11**, 73–87.

Dhib Jalbut, S. & Liwnicz, B.H. (1986). Immunocytochemical binding of serum IgG from a patient with oat cell tumor and paraneoplastic motoneuron disease to normal human cerebral cortex and molecular layer of the cerebellum. *Acta Neuropathologica (Berlin)*, **69**, 96–102.

Dick, D.J., Harris, J.B., Falkous, G., Foster, J.B. & Xuereb, J.H. (1988). Neuronal anti-nuclear antibody in paraneoplastic sensory neuronopathy. *Journal of the Neurological Sciences*, **85**, 1–8.

Dirr, L.Y., Elster, A.D., Donofrio, P.D. & Smith, M. (1990). Evolution of brain MRI abnormalities in limbic encephalitis. *Neurology*, **40**, 1304–6.

Drlicek, M., Liszka, U., Jellinger, K., Mohn Staudner, A., Lintner, F. & Grisold, W. (1992). Circulating antineuronal antibodies reach neurons *in vivo*: an autopsy study. *Journal of Neurology*, **239**, 407–10.

Dropcho, E.J., Chen, Y.T., Posner, J.B. & Old, L.J. (1987). Cloning of a brain protein identified by autoantibodies from a patient with paraneoplastic cerebellar degeneration. *Proceedings of the National Academy of Sciences USA*, **84**, 4552–6.

Dropcho, E.J., Kline, L.B. & Riser, J. (1993). Antineuronal (anti-Ri) antibodies in a patient with steroid-responsive opsoclonus-myoclonus. *Neurology*, **43**, 207–11.

Eaton, L.M. & Lambert, E.H. (1957). Electromyography and electric stimulation of nerves in diseases of motor unit. Observations on myasthenic syndrome associated with malignant tumors. *Journal of the American Medical Association*, **163**, 1117–24.

Elrington, G.M., Murray, N.M., Spiro, S.G. & Newsom Davis, J. (1991). Neurological paraneoplastic syndromes in patients with small cell lung cancer. A prospective survey of 150 patients. *Journal of Neurology, Neurosurgery and Psychiatry*, **54**, 764–7.

Escudero, D., Barnadas, A., Codina, M., Fueyo, J. & Graus, F. (1993). Anti-Ri-associated paraneoplastic neurologic disorder without opsoclonus in a patient with breast cancer. *Neurology*, **43**, 1605–6.

Fathallah Shaykh, H., Wolf, S., Wong, E., Posner, J.B. & Furneaux, H.M. (1991). Cloning of a leucine-zipper protein recognized by the sera of patients with antibody-associated paraneoplastic cerebellar degeneration. *Proceedings of the National Academy of Sciences USA*, **88**, 3451–4.

Ferrari, P., Federico, M., Grimaldi, L.M. & Silingardi, V. (1990). Stiff-man syndrome in a patient with Hodgkin's disease. An unusual paraneoplastic syndrome. *Haematologica*, **75**, 570–2.

Folli, F., Solimena, M., Cofiell, R., Austoni, M., Tallini, G., Fassetta, G., Bates, D., Cartlidge, N., Bottazzo, G.F., Piccolo, G. *et al.* (1993). Autoantibodies to a 128-kd synaptic protein in three women with the stiff-man syndrome and breast cancer. *New England Journal of Medicine*, **328**, 546–51.

Frommer, J., Haass, A., Bergmann, M., Gullotta, F. & Schimrigk, K. (1993). [Schizophreniform psychosis in paraneoplastic limbic encephalitis]. *Nervenarzt*, **64**, 328–30.

Furneaux, H.F., Reich, L. & Posner, J.B. (1990). Autoantibody synthesis in the central nervous system of patients with paraneoplastic syndromes. *Neurology*, **40**, 1085–91.

Furneaux, H.M., Dropcho, E.J., Barbut, D., Chen, Y.T., Rosenblum, M.K., Old, L.J. & Posner, J.B. (1989). Characterization of a cDNA encoding a 34-kDa Purkinje neuron protein recognized by sera from patients with paraneoplastic cerebellar degeneration. *Proceedings of the National Academy of Sciences USA*, **86**, 2873–7.

Furneaux, H.M., Rosenblum, M.K., Dalmau, J., Wong, E., Woodruff, P., Graus, F. & Posner, J.B. (1990). Selective expression of Purkinje-cell antigens in tumor tissue from patients with paraneoplastic cerebellar degeneration. *New England Journal of Medicine*, **322**, 1844–51.

Graus, F., Cordon-Cardo, C. & Posner, J.B. (1985). Neuronal antinuclear antibody in sensory neuronopathy from lung cancer. *Neurology*, **35**, 538–43.

Graus, F., Elkon, K.B., Cordon Cardo, C. & Posner, J.B. (1986). Sensory neuronopathy and small cell lung cancer. Antineuronal antibody that also reacts with the tumor. *American Journal of Medicine*, **80**, 45–52.

Graus, F., Illa, I., Agusti, M., Ribalta, T., Cruz Sanchez, F. & Juarez, C. (1991). Effect of intraventricular injection of an anti-Purkinje cell antibody (anti-Yo) in a guinea pig model. *Journal of the Neurological Sciences*, **106**, 82–7.

Graus, F., Ribalta, T., Campo, E., Monforte, R., Urbano, A. & Rozman, C. (1990). Immunohistochemical analysis of the immune reaction in the nervous system in paraneoplastic encephalomyelitis. *Neurology*, **40**, 219–22.

Greenlee, J.E. & Brashear, H.R. (1983). Antibodies to cerebellar Purkinje cells in patients with paraneoplastic cerebellar degeneration and ovarian carcinoma. *Annals of Neurology*, **14**, 609–13.

Greenlee, J.E., Parks, T.N. & Jaeckle, K.A. (1993). Type IIa ('anti-Hu') antineuronal antibodies produce destruction of rat cerebellar granule neurons *in vitro*. *Neurology*, **43**, 2049–54.

Griffin, J.W., Cornblath, D.R., Alexander, E., Campbell, J., Low, P.A., Bird, S. & Feldman, E.L. (1990). Ataxic sensory neuropathy and dorsal root ganglionitis associated with Sjögren's syndrome. *Annals of Neurology*, **27**, 304–15.

Grunwald, G.B., Kornguth, S.E., Towfighi, J., Sassani, J., Simmonds, M.A., Housman, C.M. & Papadopoulos, N. (1987). Autoimmune basis for visual paraneoplastic syndrome in patients with small cell lung carcinoma. Retinal immune deposits and ablation of retinal ganglion cells. *Cancer*, **60**, 780–6.

Gulya, A.J. (1993). Neurologic paraneoplastic syndromes with neurotologic manifestations. *Laryngoscope*, **103**, 754–61.

Hammack, J., Kotanides, H., Rosenblum, M.K. & Posner, J.B. (1992). Paraneoplastic cerebellar degeneration. II. Clinical and immunologic findings in 21 patients with Hodgkin's disease. *Neurology*, **42**, 1938–43.

Henson, R.A., Hoffman, H.L. & Urich, H. (1965). Encephalomyelitis with carcinoma. *Brain*, **88**, 449–64.

Hickey, W.F., Ueno, K., Hiserodt, J.C. & Schmidt, R.E. (1992). Exogenously-induced, natural killer cell-mediated neuronal killing: a novel pathogenetic mechanism. *Journal of Experimental Medicine*, **176**, 811–17.

Horwich, M.S., Cho, L., Porro, R.S. & Posner, J.B. (1977). Subacute sensory neuropathy: a remote effect of carcinoma. *Annals of Neurology*, **2**, 7–19.

Ingenito, G.G., Berger, J.R., David, N.J. & Norenberg, M.D. (1990). Limbic encephalitis associated with thymoma. *Neurology*, **40**, 382.

Jaeckle, K.A., Graus, F., Houghton, A., Cardon-Cardo, C., Nielsen, S.L. & Posner, J.B. (1985). Autoimmune response of patients with paraneoplastic cerebellar degeneration to a Purkinje cell cytoplasmic protein antigen. *Annals of Neurology*, **18**, 592–600.

Jean, W.C., Dalmau, J., Ho, A. & Posner, J.B. (1994). Analysis of the IgG subclass distribution and inflammatory infiltrates in patients with anti-Hu-associated paraneoplastic encephalomyelitis. *Neurology*, **44**, 140–7.

Kaniecki, R. & Morris, J.C. (1993). Reversible paraneoplastic limbic encephalitis. *Neurology*, **43**, 2418–19.

Kaufman, M.D., Hopkins, L.C. & Hurwitz, B.J. (1981). Progressive sensory neuropathy in patients without carcinoma: a disorder with distinctive clinical and electrophysiological findings. *Annals of Neurology*, **9**, 237–42.

Kinsbourne, M. (1962). Myoclonic encephalopathy of infants. *Journal of Neurology, Neurosurgery and Psychiatry*, **25**, 271–6.

Kodama, T., Numaguchi, Y., Gellad, F.E., Dwyer, B.A. & Kristt, D.A. (1991). Magnetic resonance imaging of limbic encephalitis. *Neuroradiology*, **33**, 520–3.

Lennon, V.A., Sas, D.F., Busk, M.F., Scheithauer, B., Malagelada, J.R., Camilleri, M. & Miller, L.J. (1991). Enteric neuronal autoantibodies in pseudoobstruction with small-cell lung carcinoma. *Gastroenterology*, **100**, 137–42.

Luque, F.A., Furneaux, H.M., Ferziger, R., Rosenblum, M.K., Wray, S.H., Schold, S.C.J., Glantz, M.J., Jaeckle, K.A., Biran, H., Lesser, M. *et al.* (1991). Anti-Ri: an antibody associated with paraneoplastic opsoclonus and breast cancer. *Annals of Neurology*, **29**, 241–51.

Malinow, K., Yannakakis, G.D., Glusman, S.M., Edlow, D.W., Griffin, J., Pestronk, A., Powell, D.L., Ramsey-Goldman, R., Eidelman, B.H., Medsger, T.A.Jr & Alexander, E.L. (1986). Subacute sensory neuronopathy secondary to dorsal root ganglionitis in primary Sjögren's syndrome. *Annals of Neurology*, **20**, 535–7.

McArdle, J.P. & Millingen, K.S. (1988). Limbic encephalitis associated with malignant thymoma. *Pathology*, **20**, 292–5.

Moll, J.W., Henzen Logmans, S.C., Splinter, T.A., van der Burg, M.E. & Vecht, C.J. (1990). Diagnostic value of anti-neuronal antibodies for paraneoplastic disorders of the nervous system. *Journal of Neurology, Neurosurgery and Psychiatry*, **53**, 940–3.

Moll, J.W., Markusse, H.M., Pijnenburg, J.J., Vecht, C.J. & Henzen Logmans, S.C. (1993). Antineuronal antibodies in patients with neurologic complications of primary Sjögren's syndrome. *Neurology*, **43**, 2574–81.

Nemni, R., Camerlingo, M., Fazio, R., Casto, L., Quattrini, A., Mamoli, D., Lorenzetti, I., Canal, N. & Mamoli, A. (1993). Serum antibodies to Purkinje cells and dorsal root ganglia neurons in sensory neuronopathy without malignancy. *Annals of Neurology*, **34**, 848–54.

Peterson, K., Rosenblum, M.K., Kotanides, H. & Posner, J.B. (1992). Paraneoplastic cerebellar degeneration. I. A clinical analysis of 55 anti-Yo antibody-positive patients. *Neurology*, **42**, 1931–7.

Posner, J.B. (1992). Pathogenesis of central nervous system paraneoplastic syndromes. *Revue Neurologique (Paris)*, **148**, 502–12.

Sakai, K., Gofuku, M., Kitagawa, Y., Ogasawara, T., Hirose, G., Yamazaki, M., Koh, C.S., Yanagisawa, N. & Steinman, L. (1994). A hippocampal protein associated with paraneoplastic neurologic syndrome and small cell lung carcinoma. *Biochemical and Biophysical Research Communications*, **199**, 1200–8.

Sodhi, N., Camilleri, M., Camoriano, J.K., Low, P.A., Fealey, R.D. & Perry, M.C. (1989). Autonomic function and motility in intestinal pseudoobstruction caused by paraneoplastic syndrome. *Digestive Diseases and Sciences*, **34**, 1937–42.

Szabo, A., Dalmau, J., Manley, G., Rosenfeld, M., Wong, E., Henson, J., Posner, J.B. & Furneaux, H.M. (1991). HuD, a paraneoplastic encephalomyelitis antigen, contains RNA-binding domains and is homologous to Elav and Sex-lethal. *Cell*, **67**, 325–33.

Tsukamoto, T., Mochizuki, R., Mochizuki, H., Noguchi, M., Kayama, H., Hiwatashi, M. & Yamamoto, T. (1993). Paraneoplastic cerebellar degeneration and limbic encephalitis in a patient with adenocarcinoma of the colon. *Journal of Neurology, Neurosurgery and Psychiatry*, **56**, 713–16.

Turner, M.L., Boland, O.M., Parker, A.C. & Ewing, D.J (1993). Subclinical autonomic dysfunction in patients with Hodgkin's disease and non-Hodgkin's lymphoma. *British Journal of Haematology*, **84**, 623–6.

Veilleux, M., Bernier, J.P. & Lamarche, J.B. (1990). Paraneoplastic encephalomyelitis and subacute dysautonomia due to an occult atypical carcinoid tumour of the lung. *Canadian Journal of Neurological Sciences*, **17**, 324–8.

Yoshioka, A., Ueda, Y., Sakai, K., Negami, T. & Hirose, G. (1992). [Immunohistochemical studies of paraneoplastic subacute sensory neuropathy – an analysis of antineuronal antibody and infiltrated lymphocytes]. *Rinsho Shinkeigaku. Clinical Neurology (Tokyo)*, **32**, 397–404.

–13–
Neurological complications of connective tissue diseases and vasculitis

PAMELA A. McCOMBE

Connective tissue diseases such as systemic lupus erythematosus can have neurological manifestations. Furthermore, systemic vasculitides can result in neurological disease (Sigal, 1987; Moore, 1989*b*) and some vasculitides are restricted to the nervous system (Dyck *et al.*, 1987; Moore, 1989*a*; Crane, Kerr & Spiera, 1991). There are three possible means by which connective tissue diseases and vasculitides could be associated with neurological disorders. Firstly, the neurological complications of these conditions could be due to ischaemia secondary to vascular occlusion. Secondly, neurological complications could be due to a specific immune response directed against antigens in the parenchyma of the nervous system. Thirdly, neurological disturbance could result from a separate autoimmune neurological disorder occurring in an individual predisposed to autoimmune disease. This chapter reviews central nervous system (CNS) and peripheral nervous system (PNS) manifestations of connective tissue diseases and vasculitides, but does not attempt a comprehensive review of these systemic disorders.

Clinical features

Systemic lupus erythematosus

The neurological manifestations of systemic lupus erythematosus (SLE) are manifold (Johnson & Richardson, 1968; Feinglass *et al.*, 1976; Futrell, Schultz & Millikan, 1992). There are strict criteria for the diagnosis of SLE (Tan *et al.*, 1982) and these include the presence of neurological signs. In some patients, neurological symptoms and signs are the first manifestation of SLE (Tola *et al.*, 1992). SLE is associated with a wide range of neuropsychiatric abnormalities including psychosis and cognitive impairment (Feinglass *et al.*, 1976). In one series, 21% of SLE patients had cognitive impairment (Hanly *et al.*, 1992*a*). SLE can also be associated with encephalomyelitis, which sometimes has clinical and radiological features similar to those of multiple sclerosis (MS) (Penn & Rowan, 1968; Pender & Chalk, 1989; Tola *et al.*, 1992). In the PNS, SLE can occur in association with a chronic sensorimotor neuropathy (McCombe *et al.*, 1987). SLE can also occur in association with syndromes typical of the Guillain–Barré syndrome (Chaudhuri *et al.*, 1989) and chronic inflammatory demyelinating polyradiculoneuropathy (Rechthand *et al.*, 1984; Sindern *et al.*, 1991), although it is not clear whether this is an association of different diseases or whether these syndromes are a direct complication of SLE. SLE may occur in association with myositis (see Chapter 11), myasthenia gravis (Ben Chetrit *et al.*, 1990) and the Lambert–Eaton myasthenic syndrome (Bromberg, Albers & McCune, 1989). Modern imaging techniques have led to significant advances in the understanding of the CNS manifestations of connective tissue diseases. Magnetic resonance imaging (MRI) of the brain has demonstrated increased signal intensity in the periventricular regions in some patients with neuropsychiatric features of SLE (Stimmler, Coletti & Quismorio, 1993; Baum *et al.*, 1993). Single photon emission computerized tomography (SPECT) studies have found areas of reduced cerebral blood flow in patients with CNS complications of SLE (Emmi *et al.*, 1993). Positron emission tomography (PET) has shown deficiencies in cerebral glucose metabolism in patients with cognitive defects and SLE (Carbotte *et al.*, 1992).

Primary Sjögren's syndrome

Sjögren's syndrome (sicca syndrome) was named after Henrik Sjögren (see Mutlu & Scully, 1993). Sjögren's syndrome is characterized by dry eyes (xerophthalmia), dry mouth (xerostomia), lacrimal and salivary gland enlargement and punctate keratitis. The diagnosis of Sjögren's syndrome rests on the finding of xerophthalmia confirmed by a Schirmer's test and a lip biopsy showing lymphocytic infiltration of the salivary glands (Greenspan *et al.*, 1974). Sjögren's syndrome can be a primary disorder or may be secondary to other diseases such as rheumatoid arthritis. Patients with primary Sjögren's syndrome often have extraglandular involvement and in particular may have disease of the CNS or PNS. CNS disturbances, such as seizures, encephalopathy, cognitive impairment and focal deficits have been reported to occur in up to 25% of patients with primary Sjögren's syndrome (Alexander *et al.*, 1986*a*; Alexander, 1986; Spezialetti *et al.*, 1993) and often occur in patients with widespread cutaneous vasculitis (Alexander & Provost, 1987). However, others have found that the incidence of CNS abnormalities is much lower (Binder, Snaith & Isenberg, 1988; Mellgren *et al.*, 1989; Andonopoulos *et al.*, 1990). It has been reported that CNS involvement in primary Sjögren's syndrome can lead to widespread neurological abnormalities that mimic multiple sclerosis (Alexander *et al.*, 1986*b*). MRI has been reported to show patchy cerebral lesions in patients with CNS complications of primary Sjögren's syndrome (Alexander *et al.*, 1988*a*). However, others have found little evidence of MRI abnormalities in primary Sjögren's syndrome (Manthorpe, Manthorpe & Sjoberg, 1992). There is less controversy about the involvement of the PNS in primary Sjögren's syndrome. PNS involvement is frequently present (Mellgren *et al.*, 1989; Andonopoulos *et al.*, 1990; Mauch *et al.*, 1994) and includes trigeminal sensory neuropathy (Kaltreider & Talal, 1969), peripheral sensorimotor neuropathy, subacute sensory neuronopathy resembling that which occurs as a paraneoplastic syndrome (Graus *et al.*, 1988; Griffin *et al.*, 1990; McCombe *et al.*, 1992) and mononeuritis multiplex (Kaplan *et al.*, 1990).

Rheumatoid arthritis

Rheumatoid arthritis (RA) is a destructive arthritis associated with the presence in the serum of rheumatoid factor. In RA, the spinal cord and peripheral nerves may be subjected to physical compression secondary to disease of the cervical spine or disorders such as carpal tunnel syndrome. Peripheral neuropathy is frequently present and includes mild sensory or sensorimotor neuropathies as well as more severe sensorimotor neuropathies in association with vasculitis (Good *et al.*, 1965; Chamberlain & Bruckner, 1970). Patients with RA may also develop chronic inflammatory demyelinating polyradiculoneuropathy, although it is not clear whether this represents the simultaneous development of two conditions or whether RA can more directly cause the development of a demyelinating neuropathy (McCombe *et al.*, 1991). CNS abnormalities such as confusional states, seizures and focal neurological signs have occasionally been reported in RA (Skowronski & Gatter, 1974; Ramos & Mandybur, 1975; Gupta & Ehrlich, 1976; Kim, 1980).

Isolated angiitis of the CNS or PNS

Primary angiitis of the CNS

Vasculitis confined to the intracranial cerebral circulation was first described as granulomatous angiitis of the nervous system. More recently the terms 'isolated angiitis of the nervous system' (Moore, 1989*a*; Crane *et al.*, 1991) or 'primary angiitis of the CNS' (Calabrese *et al.*, 1992) have been adopted. Calabrese *et al.* (1992) reported that the symptoms of this condition included headache (62%), weakness (55%), cognitive impairment (51%) and impaired consciousness (29%). Other symptoms include seizures, cerebral haemorrhage and spinal cord disease. Diagnosis requires proof of vasculitis by cerebral angiography or biopsy.

Non-systemic vasculitic neuropathy

Dyck *et al.* (1987) have described peripheral neuropathy associated with vasculitis that, on clinical testing, was confined to the PNS, and remained confined to the PNS after lengthy follow-up. Most of their patients exhibited mononeuritis multiplex, while others had asymmetrical or symmetrical polyneuropathy. Torvik & Berntzen (1968) reported patients with vasculitis affecting nerves and muscles but without visceral involvement. Kissel *et al.* (1985) reported that four of 16 patients with necrotizing vasculitic neuropathy had no systemic involvement.

Other vasculitides

Other generalized vasculitides such as polyarteritis nodosa and Wegener's granulomatosus can cause neurological abnormalities. Mononeuritis multiplex is frequently associated with vasculitis (Cohen Tervaert & Kallenberg, 1993). Giant cell arteritis is a large vessel vasculitis that is restricted to the aortic arch and its branches and that can cause headache, loss of vision and occasionally cognitive impairment (Caselli & Hunder, 1993). Giant cell arteritis is diagnosed by elevation of the erythrocyte sedimentation rate and abnormalities on superficial temporal artery biopsy and is treated with corticosteroids. Behçet's disease, which may be an autoimmune vasculitis, can have relapsing and remitting neurological manifestations (Allen, 1993). In Behçet's disease MRI brain scans may show widespread white matter abnormalities and evidence of intracranial venous thrombosis (Morrissey *et al.*, 1993; Wechsler *et al.*, 1993). The cerebrospinal fluid (CSF) protein may be elevated (Hatzinikolaou *et al.*, 1993). Eales' disease is a vasculitis of the retina that can be associated with more widespread neurological involvement (Katz *et al.*, 1991).

Neuropathology

Systemic lupus erythematosus

Ischaemia secondary to vasculitis is one possible cause of the neurological disturbance in cerebral SLE, and is likely to be due to vascular changes affecting small blood vessels. Hanly, Walsh & Sangalang (1992*b*) found small-vessel damage and cerebral microinfarcts in the brain of patients with SLE. Others have found small-vessel hyalinization and platelet deposition in the walls of blood vessels (Ellison *et al.*, 1993). In a post-mortem study, Johnson & Richardson (1968) found destructive and proliferative changes of the small blood vessels of the brain of patients with neurological manifestations of SLE. They found no evidence of vasculitis of larger vessels. Devinsky, Petito and Alonso (1988) also found that there was no evidence of large-vessel vasculitis in patients with neurological complications of SLE. Immune complexes have been found in the choroid plexus of patients with confusional states associated with SLE (Atkins *et al.*, 1972). Sural nerve biopsies from patients with sensorimotor neuropathy associated with SLE showed axonal degeneration with little evidence of abnormalities of blood vessels (McCombe *et al.*, 1987), although this is not conclusive, because of the sampling problems of peripheral nerve biopsy.

Sjögren's syndrome

In the CNS in primary Sjögren's syndrome there may be vasculitis often associated with meningitis (Alexander, 1992). Aseptic meningitis without vasculitis has also been reported (Gerraty, McKelvie & Byrne, 1993), as has venous sinus thrombosis (Urban, Jabbari & Robles, 1994). In patients with subacute sensory neuronopathy associated with primary Sjögren's syndrome there is lymphocytic infiltration of the dorsal root ganglia (Griffin *et al.*, 1990). Peripheral nerve biopsies may show evidence of axonal degeneration and vasculitis (Peyronnard *et al.*, 1982; Mellgren *et al.*, 1989), although some studies have found little evidence of vasculitis (Gemignani *et al.*, 1994). One study of peripheral nerve from a patient with sensory neuronopathy and primary Sjögren's syndrome did not demonstrate antibody bound to peripheral nerve (Graus *et al.*, 1988), although such deposition would not be expected if the pathology was confined to the dorsal root ganglia.

Rheumatoid arthritis

Beckett & Dinn (1972) found that in sural nerves from RA patients with clinically mild neuropathy there was segmental demyelination and no vascular damage. They found that nerves from patients with more severe neuropathy showed evidence of vascular damage and axonal degeneration. Conn, McDuffie & Dyck (1972) found immunoglobulin deposition in the wall of a neural blood vessel in a patient with vasculitic neuropathy and RA, but there was no such deposition in the nerves of patients with chronic neuropathy associated with RA. In one patient studied by van Lis & Jennekens (1977) there was inflammation of the epineural arterioles and deposition of immunoglobulin. In the brains of patients with CNS manifestations of RA there may be severe necrotizing vasculitis, the presence of rheumatoid nodules, meningeal involvement or choroid plexus involvement (Ramos & Mandybur, 1975; Kim, 1980; Kim & Collins, 1981). IgM deposits have been found in the choroid plexus in one patient with RA and organic brain syndrome (Gupta & Ehrlich, 1976). Clearly, further clinicopathological correlation is needed to define the neurological complications of RA.

Isolated angiitis of the CNS and PNS

In primary angiitis of the CNS there is inflammation of the small veins and arterioles, with prominent involvement of the leptomeninges (Calabrese *et al.*, 1992). The infiltrate is usually granulomatous. In non-systemic vasculitic neuropathy, the pathological features are those of an ischaemic neuropathy associated with necrotizing vasculitis affecting small arterioles (Dyck *et al.*, 1987).

Immunological findings in the peripheral blood and cerebrospinal fluid

Systemic lupus erythematosus

SLE is characterized by the presence of increased levels of serum antinuclear antibodies (Warner, 1994). Anti-cardiolipin antibodies may be increased in the serum and CSF of patients with CNS manifestations of SLE (Lolli *et al.*, 1991) and are associated with ischaemia and thrombotic CNS disease (Brey, Gharavi & Lockshin, 1993). Increased levels of antibodies to brain antigens are also found in SLE (Klein, Richter & Berg, 1991; Hanly, Hong & White, 1993; Khin & Hoffman, 1993; Teh *et al.*, 1993). Correlation between the presence of anti-neuronal antibodies and cognitive impairment has been reported (Denburg, Carbotte & Denburg, 1987). It has been suggested that antibodies to synaptosomal particles may contribute to neurological complications of SLE (Hanly *et al.*, 1993). Such antibodies react with a 50-kDa membrane protein (Hanson *et al.*, 1992). SLE sera also contain antibodies reactive with ribosomal P proteins (Bonfa *et al.*, 1987). The anti-P antibodies react with a 38-kDa membrane protein (Koren *et al.*, 1992). Antibodies to a cytoskeletal protein L-fimbrin are present in the sera of patients with SLE and correlate with CNS complications (De Mendonca Neto *et al.*, 1992). CSF examination in patients with neurological complications of SLE may reveal intrathecal antibody synthesis (Hirohata & Miyamoto, 1986), intrathecal synthesis of the fourth component of complement (Jongen *et al.*, 1990) or elevated levels of interleukin-6 (Hirohata & Miyamoto, 1990).

Primary Sjögren's syndrome

Primary Sjögren's syndrome patients with circulating anti-Ro antibodies have a higher incidence of serious CNS disease than those without these antibodies (Alexander, 1992; Alexander *et al.*, 1994). Spezialetti *et al.* (1993) found that patients with CNS manifestations do not have increased levels of serum anti-ribosomal P proteins or anti-neuronal antibodies. However, Moll *et al.* (1993) have shown that some patients with neurological complications of primary Sjögren's syndrome have anti-neuronal antibodies including the anti-Hu antibodies found in patients with paraneoplastic syndromes (see Chapter 12). In the CSF in patients with neurological disease associated with primary Sjögren's syndrome, there are increased immunoglobulin levels and the presence of oligoclonal bands (Alexander *et al.*, 1986*a*; Vrethem *et al.*, 1990). Activated complement can be detected in the serum and CSF of patients with CNS disease associated with primary Sjögren's syndrome (Sanders *et al.*, 1987; Alexander *et al.*, 1988*b*).

Rheumatoid arthritis

Reduced levels of CSF complement have been reported in a patient with a confusional state associated with RA (Kim, 1980).

Isolated angiitis of the nervous system

There is no evidence of any immunological abnormality specific for primary angiitis of the CNS. It might be expected that primary angiitis of the CNS would be associated with inflammation directed against antigens specific for CNS blood vessel antigens. One antigen that is found on CNS endothelium but not other endothelium is HT7 (Unger *et al.*, 1993), which is also known as neurothelin or basigin (Seulberger, Unger & Risau, 1992) and which is a member of the immunoglobulin superfamily (Miyauchi, Masuzawa & Muramatsu, 1991; Seulberger *et al.*, 1991; Kasinrerk *et al.*, 1992). Similarly, it can be postulated that isolated angiitis of the PNS might be associated with an immune attack directed against antigens that are unique to vessels of the PNS.

Other vasculitides

The finding of elevated levels of serum anti-neutrophil cytoplasmic antibodies is an important part of the diagnosis of the systemic vasculitides (Kallenberg, Mulder & Tervaert, 1992; Geffriaud Ricouard *et al.*, 1993; Warner, 1994), but these antibodies are not likely to have a direct involvement in the development of neurological complications. In Behçet's disease, elevated serum anti-cardiolipin antibodies have been found (al Dalaan *et al.*, 1993). Elevated levels of anti-endothelial antibodies have also been reported in Behçet's disease (Aydintug *et al.*, 1993).

Pathogenesis

There is considerable evidence that ischaemia plays a major role in the neurological complications of connective tissue diseases and vasculitis. The consequences of ischaemia have been studied by Nukada & Dyck (1987), who showed that occlusion of small blood vessels in peripheral nerves causes axonal degeneration, with secondary demyelination. This is likely to be the case throughout the nervous system. It has also been suggested that vasculitis can lead to non-specific primary demyelination (vasculomyelinopathy) (Reik, 1980). In some of the neurological complications of these disorders, there is inflammatory cell infiltration of the parenchyma of the nervous system and circulating antibodies specific for nervous system antigens. These findings indicate a direct immune attack on the parenchyma of the nervous system. Furthermore, as susceptibility to autoimmunity appears to be inherited as an autosomal dominant trait (Bias *et al.*, 1986), patients with a connective tissue disease such as SLE may simultaneously have another autoimmune disease such as myasthenia gravis, chronic inflammatory demyelinating polyradiculoneuropathy or multiple sclerosis.

Systemic lupus erythematosus

Recent evidence from PET scanning (Stimmler *et al.*, 1993) strongly suggests that ischaemia and its metabolic consequences are important in producing the CNS complications of SLE. This is likely to be due to inflammation and obstruction of small blood vessels. There is also a considerable body of evidence supporting a role for antineuronal antibodies (see above), but the proof that these antibodies are pathogenic, namely passive transfer of disease to experimental animals, is not available.

Animal models of SLE

In the animal models of SLE there is evidence of vasculitis and anti-brain antibodies. In NZB/W F_1 mice, there is immune complex deposition in the brain capillaries and lymphoid cell infiltration of the subarachnoid regions and around blood vessels (Rudick & Eskin, 1983). Studies of MRL/lpr mice demonstrate infiltration of the CNS with $CD4^+$ T cells (Vogelweid *et al.*,

1991). Anti-brain antibodies are produced in the mice, which develop SLE-like syndromes (Narendran & Hoffman, 1989).

Sjögren's syndrome

Some of the neurological manifestations of primary Sjögren's syndrome are likely to be secondary to vasculitis. In sensory neuronopathy complicating primary Sjögren's syndrome there is inflammation of dorsal root ganglia and circulating anti-neuronal antibodies (including anti-Hu antibodies), indicating a specific immune attack on neural antigens. Models of Sjögren's syndrome have been developed in mice (Sato & Sullivan, 1994; Yeoman & Franklin, 1994), but have not yet been used to study the nervous system.

Other conditions

In rheumatoid arthritis, primary angiitis of the CNS, non-systemic vasculitic neuropathy and the other vasculitides discussed in this chapter there is strong evidence that ischaemia due to vasculitis is the primary cause of the neurological disturbance.

Therapy

Systemic lupus erythematosus

Since the report of Dubois *et al.* (1974), high doses of corticosteroids have been the main form of treatment in CNS lupus. Intravenous cyclophosphamide therapy is also of benefit in patients with CNS manifestations of SLE (Boumpas *et al.*, 1991).

Primary Sjögren's syndrome

Alexander (1992) has suggested that corticosteroids and other immunosuppressive agents may improve the neurological status of patients with CNS disease due to primary Sjögren's syndrome. Primary Sjögren's syndrome may produce a dementia that responds to corticosteroid treatment (Caselli *et al.*, 1991; Kawashima, Shindo & Kohno, 1993). Peripheral neuropathy or sensory neuronopathy in association with primary Sjögren's syndrome may stabilize or improve with immunosuppressive therapy (Caselli *et al.*, 1991; McCombe *et al.*, 1992).

Rheumatoid arthritis

Patients with neuropsychiatric abnormalities attributed to RA have responded to treatment with corticosteroids (Skowronski & Gatter, 1974; Gupta & Ehrlich, 1976).

Isolated angiitis of the nervous system

Patients with primary angiitis of the CNS were initially thought to have a poor prognosis. However, in the series of Calabrese *et al.* (1992) more than half of the patients who were diagnosed in life made a complete recovery, often after treatment with corticosteroids or other immunosuppressants. Moore (1989*a*) and Crane *et al.*, (1991) also suggested that aggressive treatment with corticosteroids and immunosuppressants was helpful. Dyck *et al.* (1987) reported that prednisone appeared to arrest the course of disease in some patients with non-systemic vasculitic neuropathy.

Other conditions

The systemic vasculitides are usually treated rather aggressively with immunosuppressive agents, which may lead to improvement of the neurological complications (Cohen *et al.*, 1993).

Conclusions

Connective tissue diseases and vasculitides are often complicated by involvement of the CNS and/or the PNS. Ischaemia associated with vasculitis is likely to be a common cause of this complication, but further studies of the exact mechanisms of ischaemia and its effects are required. There is also evidence that some neurological complications are due to a specific immune attack on antigens in the parenchyma of the nervous system, for example in the subacute sensory neuronopathy of primary Sjögren's syndrome. Further studies are required to determine the relative roles of anti-neuronal T cells and antibodies in the pathogenesis of these conditions. Understanding of the neurological complications of these diseases would be aided by the development of further animal models which would permit experimental studies. The most appropriate treatment of these conditions is not yet known and further study is required, because the types of treatment that appear likely to be helpful include potentially harmful immunosuppressive agents.

References

al Dalaan, A.N., al Ballaa, S.R., al Janadi, M.A., Bohlega, S. & Bahabri, S. (1993). Association of anti-cardiolipin antibodies with vascular thrombosis and neurological manifestation of Behçets disease. *Clinical Rheumatology*, **12**, 28–30.

Alexander, E. (1992). Central nervous system disease in Sjögren's syndrome. New insights into immunopathogenesis. *Rheumatic Diseases Clinics of North America*, **18**, 637–72.

Alexander, E. & Provost, T.T. (1987). Sjögren's syndrome. Association of cutaneous vasculitis with central nervous system disease. *Archives of Dermatology*, **123**, 801–10.

Alexander, E.L. (1986). Central nervous system (CNS) manifestations of primary Sjögren's syndrome: an overview. *Scandinavian Journal of Rheumatology*, **61**, 161–5.

Alexander, E.L., Beall, S.S., Gordon, B., Selnes, O.A., Yannakakis, G.D., Patronas, N., Provost, T.T. & McFarland, H.F. (1988*a*). Magnetic resonance imaging of cerebral lesions in patients with the Sjögren syndrome. *Annals of Internal Medicine*, **108**, 815–23.

Alexander, E.L., Lijewski, J.E., Jerdan, M.S. & Alexander, G.E. (1986*a*). Evidence of an immunopathogenic basis for central nervous system disease in primary Sjögren's syndrome. *Arthritis and Rheumatism*, **29**, 1223–31.

Alexander, E.L., Malinow, K., Lejewski, J.E., Jerdan, M.S., Provost, T.T. & Alexander, G.E. (1986*b*). Primary Sjögren's syndrome with central nervous system disease mimicking multiple sclerosis. *Annals of Internal Medicine*, **104**, 323–30.

Alexander, E.L., Provost, T.T., Sanders, M.E., Frank, M.M. & Joiner, K.A. (1988*b*). Serum complement activation in central nervous system disease in Sjögren's syndrome. *American Journal of Medicine*, **85**, 513–18.

Alexander, E.L., Ranzenbach, M.R., Kumar, A.J., Kozachuk, W.E., Rosenbaum, A.E., Patronas, N., Harley, J.B. & Reichlin, M. (1994). Anti-Ro(SS-A) autoantibodies in central nervous system disease associated with Sjögren's syndrome (CNS-SS): clinical, neuroimaging, and angiographic correlates. *Neurology*, **44**, 899–908.

Allen, N.B. (1993). Miscellaneous vasculitic syndromes including Behçet's disease and central nervous system vasculitis. *Current Opinion in Rheumatology*, **5**, 51–6.

Andonopoulos, A.P., Lagos, G., Drosos, A.A. & Moutsopoulos, H.M. (1990). The spectrum of neurological involvement in Sjögren's syndrome. *British Journal of Rheumatology*, **29**, 21–3.

Atkins, C.J., Kondon, J.J., Quismorio, F.P. & Friou, G.J. (1972). The choroid plexus in systemic lupus erythematosus. *Annals of Internal Medicine*, **76**, 65–72.

Aydintug, A.O., Tokgoz, G., D'Cruz, D.P., Gurler, A., Cervera, R., Duzgun, N., Atmaca, L.S., Khamashta, M.A. & Hughes, G.V.R. (1993). Antibodies to endothelial cells in patients with Behçet's disease. *Clinical Immunology and Immunopathology*, **67**, 157–62.

Baum, K.A., Hopf, U., Nehrig, C., Stover, M. & Schorner, W. (1993). Systemic lupus erythematosus: neuropsychiatric signs and symptoms related to cerebral MRI findings. *Clinical Neurology and Neurosurgery*, **95**, 29–34.

Beckett, V.L. & Dinn, J.J. (1972). Segmental demyelination in rheumatoid arthritis. *Quarterly Journal of Medicine*, **41**, 71–80.

Ben Chetrit, E., Pollack, A., Flusser, D. & Rubinow, A. (1990). Coexistence of systemic lupus erythematosus and myasthenia gravis: two distinct populations of anti-DNA and anti-acetylcholine receptor antibodies. *Clinical and Experimental Rheumatology*, **8**, 71–4.

Bias, W.B., Reveille, J.D., Beaty, T.H., Meyers, D.A. & Arnett, F.C. (1986). Evidence that autoimmunity in man is a mendelian dominant trait. *American Journal of Human Genetics*, **39**, 584–602.

Binder, A., Snaith, M.L. & Isenberg, D. (1988). Sjögren's syndrome: a study of its neurological complications. *British Journal of Rheumatology*, **27**, 275–80.

Bonfa, E., Golombek, S.J., Kaufman, L.D., Skelly, S., Weissbach, H., Brot, N. & Elkon, K.B. (1987). Association between lupus psychosis and anti-ribosomal P protein antibodies. *New England Journal of Medicine*, **317**, 265–71.

Boumpas, D.T., Yamada, H., Patronas, N.J., Scott, D., Klippel, J.H. & Balow, J.E. (1991). Pulse cyclophosphamide for severe neuropsychiatric lupus. *Quarterly Journal of Medicine*, **81**, 975–84.

Brey, R.L., Gharavi, A.E. & Lockshin, M.D. (1993). Neurologic complications of antiphospholipid antibodies. *Rheumatic Diseases Clinics of North America*, **19**, 833–50.

Bromberg, M.B., Albers, J.W. & McCune, W.J. (1989). Transient Lambert–Eaton myasthenic syndrome associated with systemic lupus erythematosus. *Muscle and Nerve*, **12**, 15–19.

Calabrese, L.H., Furlan, A.J., Gragg, L.A. & Ropos, T.J. (1992). Primary angiitis of the central nervous system: disgnostic criteria and clinical approach. *Cleveland Clinic Journal of Medicine*, **59**, 293–306.

Carbotte, R.M., Denburg, S.D., Denburg, J.A., Nahmias, C. & Garnett, E.S. (1992). Fluctuating cognitive abnormalities and cerebral glucose metabolism in neuropsychiatric systemic lupus erythematosus. *Journal of Neurology, Neurosurgery and Psychiatry*, **55**, 1054–9.

Caselli, R.J. & Hunder, G.G. (1993). Neurological aspects of giant cell (temporal) arteritis. *Rheumatic Diseases Clinics of North America*, **19**, 941–53.

Caselli, R.J., Scheithauer, B.W., Bowles, C.A., Trenerry, M.R., Meyer, F.B., Smigielski, J.S. & Rodriguez, M. (1991). The treatable dementia of Sjögren's syndrome. *Annals of Neurology*, **30**, 98–101.

Chamberlain, M.A. & Bruckner, F.E. (1970). Rheumatoid neuropathy. Clinical and electrophysiological features. *Annals of the Rheumatic Diseases*, **29**, 609–16.

Chaudhuri, K.R., Taylor, I.K., Niven, R.M. & Abbott, R.J. (1989). A case of systemic lupus erythematosus presenting as Guillain–Barré syndrome. *British Journal of Rheumatology*, **28**, 440–2.

Cohen Tervaert, J.W. & Kallenberg, C. (1993). Neurological manifestations of systemic vasculitides. *Rheumatic Diseases Clinics of North America*, **19**, 913–40.

Conn, D.L., McDuffie, F.C. & Dyck, P.J. (1972). Immunopathologic study of sural nerves in rheumatoid arthritis. *Arthritis and Rheumatism*, **15**, 135–43.

Crane, R., Kerr, L.D. & Spiera, H. (1991). Clinical analysis of isolated angiitis of the central nervous system. *Archives of Internal Medicine*, **151**, 2290–4.

De Mendonca Neto, E.C., Kumar, A., Shadick, N.A., Michon, A.M., Matsudaira, P., Eaton, R.B., Kumar, P. & Schur, P.H. (1992). Antibodies to T- and L-isoforms of the cytoskeletal protein, fimbrin, in patients with systemic lupus erythematosus. *Journal of Clinical Investigation*, **90**, 1037–42.

Denburg, J.A., Carbotte, R.M. & Denburg, S.D. (1987). Neuronal antibodies and cognitive function in systemic lupus erythematosus. *Neurology*, **37**, 464–7.

Devinsky, O., Petito, C.K. & Alonso, D.R. (1988). Clinical and neuropathological findings in systemic lupus erythematosus: the role of vasculitis, heart emboli, and thrombotic thrombocytopenic purpura. *Annals of Neurology*, **23**, 380–4.

Dubois, E.L., Wierzchowiecki, M., Cox, M.B. & Weiner, J.M. (1974). Duration and death in systemic lupus erythematosus. An analysis of 249 cases. *Journal of the American Medical Association*, **227**, 1399–402.

Dyck, P.J., Benstead, T.J., Conn, D.L., Stevens, J.C., Windebank, A.J. & Low, P.A. (1987). Nonsystemic vasculitic neuropathy. *Brain*, **110**, 843–54.

Ellison, D., Gatter, K., Heryet, A. & Esiri, M. (1993). Intramural platelet deposition in cerebral vasculopathy of systemic lupus erythematosus. *Journal of Clinical Pathology*, **46**, 37–40.

Emmi, L., Bramati, M., De Cristofaro, M.T., Mascalchi, M., Dal Pozzo, G., Marconi, G.P., Massai, G. & Passaleva, A. (1993). MRI and SPECT investigations of the CNS in SLE patients. *Clinical and Experimental Rheumatology*, **11**, 13–20.

Feinglass, E.J., Arnett, F.C., Dorsch, C.A., Zizic, M. & Stevens, M.B. (1976). Neuropsychiatric manifestations of systemic lupus erythematosus: diagnosis, clinical spectrum, and relationship to other features of the disease. *Medicine*, **55**, 323–39.

Futrell, N., Schultz, L.R. & Millikan, C. (1992). Central nervous system disease in patients with systemic lupus erythematosus. *Neurology*, **42**, 1649–57.

Geffriaud Ricouard, C., Noel, L.H., Chauveau, D., Houhou, S., Grunfeld, J.P. & Lesavre, P. (1993). Clinical significance of ANCA in 98 patients. *Advances in Experimental Medicine and Biology*, **336**, 273–9.

Gemignani, F., Marbibi, A., Pavesi, G., Di Vittorio, S., Manganelli, P., Cenacchi, G. & Mancia, D. (1994). Peripheral neuropathy associated with primary Sjögren's syndrome. *Journal of Neurology, Neurosurgery and Psychiatry*, **57**, 983–6.

Gerraty, R.P., McKelvie, P.A. & Byrne, E. (1993). Aseptic meningoencephalitis in primary Sjögren's syndrome. Response to plasmapheresis and absence of CNS vasculitis at autopsy. *Acta Neurologica Scandinavica*, **88**, 309–11.

Good, A.E., Christopher, R.P., Koepke, G.H., Bender, L.F & Tarter, M.E. (1965). Peripheral neuropathy associated with rheumatoid arthritis. A clinical and electrodiagnostic study of 70 consecutive rheumatoid arthritis patients. *Annals of Internal Medicine*, **63**, 87–99.

Graus, F., Pou, A., Kanterewicz, E. & Anderson, N.E. (1988). Sensory neuronopathy and Sjögren's syndrome: clinical and immunologic study of two patients. *Neurology*, **38**, 1637–9.

Greenspan, J.S., Daniels, T.E., Talal, N. & Sylvester, R.A. (1974). The histopathology of Sjögren's syndrome in labial salivary gland biopsies. *Oral Surgery, Oral Medicine, Oral Pathology*, **37**, 217–29.

Griffin, J.W., Cornblath, D.R., Alexander, E., Campbell, J., Low, P.A., Bird, S. & Feldman, E.L. (1990). Ataxic sensory neuropathy and dorsal root ganglionitis associated with Sjögren's syndrome. *Annals of Neurology*, **27**, 304–15.

Gupta, V.P. & Ehrlich, G.E. (1976). Organic brain syndrome in rheumatoid arthritis following corticosteroid withdrawal. *Arthritis and Rheumatism*, **19**, 1333–8.

Hanly, J.G., Fisk, J.D., Sherwood, G., Jones, E., Jones, J.V. & Eastwood, B. (1992*a*). Cognitive impairment in patients with systemic lupus erythematosus. *Journal of Rheumatology*, **19**, 562–7.

Hanly, J.G., Hong, C. & White, T.D. (1993). Brain synaptosomal antibodies in systemic lupus erythematosus. *Lupus*, **2**, 35–45.

Hanly, J.G., Walsh, N.M. & Sangalang, V. (1992*b*). Brain pathology in systemic lupus erythematosus. *Journal of Rheumatology*, **19**, 732–41.

Hanson, V.G., Horowitz, M., Rosenbluth, D., Spiera, H. & Puszkin, S. (1992). Systemic lupus erythematosus patients with central nervous system involvement show autoantibodies to a 50-kD neuronal membrane protein. *Journal of Experimental Medicine*, **176**, 565–73.

Hatzinikolaou, P., Vaiopoulos, G., Mavropoulos, S., Avdelidis, D., Stamatelos, G. & Kaklamanis, P. (1993). Adamantiadis–Behçet's syndrome: central nervous system involvement. *Acta Neurologica Scandinavica*, **87**, 290–3.

Hirohata, S. & Miyamoto, T. (1986). Increased intrathecal immunoglobulin synthesis of both kappa and lambda types in patients with systemic lupus erythematosus and central nervous system involvement. *Journal of Rheumatology*, **13**, 715–21.

Hirohata, S. & Miyamoto, T. (1990). Elevated levels of interleukin-6 in cerebrospinal fluid from patients with systemic lupus erythematosus and central nervous system involvement. *Arthritis and Rheumatism*, **33**, 644–9.

Johnson, R.T. & Richardson, E.P. (1968). The neurological manifestations of systemic lupus erythematosus. A clinico-pathological study of 24 cases and a review of the literature. *Medicine*, **47**, 337–69.

Jongen, P.J.H., Boerbooms, A.M.T., Lamers, K.J.B., Raes, B.C.M. & Vierwinden, G. (1990). Diffuse CNS involvement in systemic lupus erythematosus: intrathecal synthesis of the 4th component of complement. *Neurology*, **40**, 1593–6.

Kallenberg, C.G., Mulder, A.H. & Tervaert, J.W. (1992). Antineutrophil cytoplasmic antibodies: a still-growing class of autoantibodies in inflammatory disorders. *American Journal of Medicine*, **93**, 675–82.

Kaltreider, H.B. & Talal, N. (1969). The neuropathy of Sjögren's syndrome: trigeminal nerve involvement. *Annals of Internal Medicine*, **70**, 751–62.

Kaplan, J.G., Rosenberg, R., Reinitz, E., Buchbinder, S. & Schaumburg, H.H. (1990). Peripheral neuropathy in Sjögren's syndrome. *Muscle and Nerve*, **13**, 570–9.

Kasinrerk, W., Fiebiger, E., Stefanova, I., Baumruker, T., Knapp, W. & Stockinger, H. (1992). Human leukocyte activation antigen M6, a member of the Ig superfamily, is the species homologue of rat OX-47, mouse basigin, and chicken HT7 molecule. *Journal of Immunology*, **149**, 847–54.

Katz, B., Wheeler, D., Weinreb, R.N. & Swenson, M.R. (1991). Eales' disease with central nervous system infarction. *Annals of Ophthalmology*, **23**, 460–3.

Kawashima, N., Shindo, R. & Kohno, M. (1993). Primary Sjögren's syndrome with subcortical dementia. *Internal Medicine*, **32**, 561–4.

Khin, N.A. & Hoffman, S.A. (1993). Brain reactive monoclonal auto-antibodies: production and characterization. *Journal of Neuroimmunology*, **44**, 137–48.

Kim, R.C. (1980). Rheumatoid disease with encephalopathy. *Annals of Neurology*, **7**, 86–91.

Kim, R.C. & Collins, G.H. (1981). The neuropathology of rheumatoid disease. *Human Pathology*, **12**, 5–15.

Kissel, J.T., Slivka, A.P., Warmolts, J.R. & Mendell, J.R. (1985). The clinical spectrum of necrotizing angiopathy of the peripheral nervous system. *Annals of Neurology*, **18**, 251–7.

Klein, R., Richter, C. & Berg, P.A. (1991). Antibodies against central nervous system tissue (anti-CNS) detected by ELISA and western blotting: marker antibodies for neuropsychiatric manifestations in connective tissue diseases. *Autoimmunity*, **10**, 133–44.

Koren, E., Reichlin, M.W., Koscec, M., Fugate, R.D. & Reichlin, M. (1992). Autoantibodies to the ribosomal P proteins react with a plasma membrane-related target on human cells. *Journal of Clinical Investigation*, **89**, 1236–41.

Lolli, F., Mata, S., Baruffi, M.C. & Amaducci, L. (1991). Cerebrospinal fluid anti-cardiolipin antibodies in neurological diseases. *Clinical Immunology and Immunopathology*, **59**, 314–21.

Manthorpe, R., Manthorpe, T. & Sjoberg, S. (1992). Magnetic resonance imaging of the brain in patients with primary Sjögren's syndrome. *Scandinavian Journal of Rheumatology*, **21**, 148–9.

Mauch, E., Volk, C., Kratzsch, G., Krapf, H., Kornhuber, H.H., Laufen, H. & Hummel, K.J. (1994). Neurological and neuropsychiatric dysfunction in primary Sjögren's syndrome. *Acta Neurologica Scandinavica*, **89**, 31–5.

McCombe, P.A., Klestov, A.C., Tannenberg, A.E., Chalk, J.B. & Pender, M.P. (1991). Sensorimotor peripheral neuropathy in rheumatoid arthritis. *Clinical and Experimental Neurology*, **28**, 146–53.

McCombe, P.A., McLeod, J.G., Pollard, J.D., Guo, Y.P. & Ingall, T.J. (1987). Peripheral sensorimotor and autonomic neuropathy associated with systemic lupus erythematosus. Clinical, pathological and immunological features. *Brain*, **110**, 533–49.

McCombe, P.A., Sheean, G.L., McLaughlin, D.B. & Pender, M.P. (1992). Vestibular and ventilatory dysfunction in sensory and autonomic neuropathy associated with primary Sjögren's syndrome. *Journal of Neurology, Neurosurgery and Psychiatry*, **55**, 1211–12.

Mellgren, S.I., Conn, D.L., Stevens, J.C. & Dyck, P.J. (1989). Peripheral neuropathy in primary Sjögren's syndrome. *Neurology*, **39**, 390–4.

Miyauchi, T., Masuzawa, Y. & Muramatsu, T. (1991). The basigin group of the immunoglobulin superfamily: complete conservation of a segment in and around transmembrane domains of human and mouse basigin and chicken HT7 antigen. *Journal of Biochemistry (Tokyo)*, **110**, 770–4.

Moll, J.W., Markusse, H.M., Pijnenburg, J.J., Vecht, C.J. & Henzen Logmans, S.C. (1993). Antineuronal antibodies in patients with neurologic complications of primary Sjögren's syndrome. *Neurology*, **43**, 2574–81.

Moore, P.M. (1989*a*). Diagnosis and management of isolated angiitis of the central nervous system. *Neurology*, **39**, 167–73.

Moore, P.M. (1989*b*). Immune mechanisms in the primary and secondary vasculitices. *Journal of the Neurological Sciences*, **93**, 129–45.

Morrissey, S.P., Miller, D.H., Hermaszewski, R., Rudge, P., MacManus, D.G., Kendall, B. & McDonald, W.I. (1993). Magnetic resonance imaging of the central nervous system in Behçet's disease. *European Neurology*, **33**, 287–93.

Mutlu, S. & Scully, C. (1993). The person behind the eponym: Henrik Sjögren (1899–1986). *Journal of Oral Pathology and Medicine*, **22**, 439.

Narendran, A. & Hoffman, S.A. (1989). Characterization of brain-reactive autoantibodies in murine models of systemic lupus erythematosus. *Journal of Neuroimmunology*, **24**, 113–23.

Nukada, H. & Dyck, P.J. (1987). Acute ischemia causes axonal stasis, swelling, attenuation, and secondary demyelination. *Annals of Neurology*, **22**, 311–18.

Pender, M.P. & Chalk, J.B. (1989). Connective tissue disease mimicking multiple sclerosis. *Australian and New Zealand Journal of Medicine*, **19**, 469–72.

Penn, A.S. & Rowan, A.J. (1968). Myelopathy in systemic lupus erythematosus. *Archives of Neurology*, **18**, 337–49.

Peyronnard, J.M., Charron, L., Beaudet, F. & Couture, F. (1982). Vasculitic neuropathy in rheumatoid disease and Sjögrens's syndrome. *Neurology*, **32**, 839–45.

Ramos, M. & Mandybur, T.I. (1975). Cerebral vasculitis in rheumatoid arthritis. *Archives of Neurology*, **32**, 271–5.

Rechthand, E., Cornblath, D.R., Stern, B.J. & Meyerhoff, J.O. (1984). Chronic demyelinating polyneuropathy in systemic lupus erythematosus. *Neurology*, **34**, 1375–7.

Reik, L. (1980). Disseminated vasculomyelinopathy: an immune complex disease. *Annals of Neurology*, **7**, 291–6.

Rudick, R.A. & Eskin, T.A. (1983). Neuropathological features of a lupus-like disorder in autoimmune mice. *Annals of Neurology*, **14**, 325–32.

Sanders, M.E., Alexander, E.L., Koski, C.L., Frank, M.M. & Joiner, K.A. (1987). Detection of activated terminal complement (C5b–9) in cerebrospinal fluid from patients with central nervous system involvement of primary Sjögren's syndrome or systemic lupus erythematosus. *Journal of Immunology*, **138**, 2095–9.

Sato, E.H. & Sullivan, D.A. (1994). Comparative influence of steroid hormones and immunosuppressive agents on autoimmune expression in lacrimal glands of a female mouse model of Sjögren's syndrome. *Investigative Ophthalmology and Visual Science*, **35**, 2632–42.

Seulberger, H., Unger, C., Albrecht, U. & Risau, W. (1991). The inducible blood–brain barrier endothelium-specific antigen HT7, a novel immunoglobulin-like membrane glycoprotein. *Annals of the New York Academy of Sciences*, **633**, 611–14.

Seulberger, H., Unger, C.M. & Risau, W. (1992). HT7, Neurothelin, Basigin, gp42 and OX-47 – many names for one developmentally regulated immuno-globulin-like surface glycoprotein on blood–brain barrier endothelium, epithelial tissue barriers and neurons. *Neuroscience Letters*, **140**, 93–7.

Sigal, L.H. (1987). The neurological presentation of vasculitic and rheumatological syndromes. *Medicine*, **66**, 157–79.

Sindern, E., Stark, E., Haas, J. & Steck, A.J. (1991). Serum antibodies to GM1 and GM3-gangliosides in systemic lupus erythematosus with chronic inflammatory demyelinating polyradiculoneuropathy. *Acta Neurologica Scandinavica*, **83**, 399–402.

Skowronski, T. & Gatter, R.A. (1974). Cerebral vasculitis associated with rheumatoid disease. *Journal of Rheumatology*, **1**, 473–5.

Spezialetti, R., Bluestein, H.G., Peter, J.B. & Alexander, E.L. (1993). Neuropsychiatric disease in Sjögren's syndrome: anti-ribosomal P and anti-neuronal antibodies. *American Journal of Medicine*, **95**, 153–60.

Stimmler, M.M., Coletti, P.M. & Quismorio, F.P.J. (1993). Magnetic resonance imaging of the brain in neuropsychiatric systemic lupus erythematosus. *Seminars in Arthritis and Rheumatism*, **22**, 335–49.

Tan, E.M., Cohen, A.S., Freis, J.M., Masi, A.T., McShane, D.J., Rothfield, N.F., Schaller, J.G., Talal, N. & Winchester, R.J. (1982). The 1982 revised criteria for the classification of systemic lupus erythematosus. *Arthritis and Rheumatism*, **25**, 1271–7.

Teh, L.S., Hay, E.M., Amos, N., Black, D., Huddy, A., Creed, F., Bernstein, R.M., Holt, P.J. & Williams, B.D. (1993). Anti-P antibodies are associated with psychiatric and focal cerebral disorders in patients with systemic lupus erythematosus. *British Journal of Rheumatology*, **32**, 287–90.

Tola, M.R., Granieri, E., Caniatti, L., Paolino, E., Monetti, C., Dovigo, L., Scolozzi, R., De Bastiani, P. & Carreras, M. (1992). Systemic lupus erythematosus presenting with neurological disorders. *Journal of Neurology*, **239**, 61–4.

Torvik, A. & Berntzen, A.E. (1968). Necrotizing vasculitis without visceral involvement. *Acta Medica Scandinavica*, **184**, 69–77.

Unger, C.M., Seulberger, H., Breier, G., Albrecht, U., Achen, M.G. & Risau, W. (1993). Expression of the HT7 gene in blood–brain barrier. *Advances in Experimental Medicine and Biology*, **331**, 211–15.

Urban, E., Jabbari, B. & Robles, H. (1994). Concurrent cerebral venous sinus thrombosis and myeloradiculopathy in Sjögren's syndrome. *Neurology*, **44**, 554–6.

van Lis, J.M.J. & Jennekens, F.G.I. (1977). Immunofluorescence studies in a case of rheumatoid neuropathy. *Journal of the Neurological Sciences*, **33**, 313–21.

Vogelweid, C.M., Johnson, G.C., Besch Williford, C.L., Basler, J. & Walker, S.E. (1991). Inflammatory central nervous system disease in lupus-prone MRL/lpr mice: comparative histologic and immunohistochemical findings. *Journal of Neuroimmunology*, **35**, 89–99.

Vrethem, M., Ernerudh, J., Lindstrom, F. & Skogh, T. (1990). Immunoglobulins within the central nervous system in primary Sjögren's syndrome. *Journal of the Neurological Sciences*, **100**, 186–92.

Warner, N.B. (1994). Serologic tests for connective tissue diseases and the primary vasculitides. *Dermatology Clinics*, **12**, 161–73.

Wechsler, B., Dell'Isola, B., Vidailhet, M., Dormont, D., Piette, J.C., Bletry, O. & Godeau, P. (1993). MRI in 31 patients with Behçet's disease and neurological involvement: prospective study with clinical correlation. *Journal of Neurology, Neurosurgery and Psychiatry*, **56**, 793–8.

Yeoman, C.M. & Franklin, C.D. (1994). The treatment of Sjögren's disease in NZB/NZW F1 hybrid mice with azathioprine: a two-stage study. *Clinical and Experimental Rheumatology*, **12**, 49–53.

Index

For EU product safety concerns, contact us at Calle de José Abascal, 56–1°,
28003 Madrid, Spain or eugpsr@cambridge.org.

www.ingramcontent.com/pod-product-compliance
Lightning Source LLC
LaVergne TN
LVHW101456200926
848483LV00001B/142

* 9 7 8 0 5 2 1 4 6 1 1 3 9 *

SURVIVING THE LONG WARS

CREATIVE REBELLION AT THE ENDS OF EMPIRE

Bridge Books - bridge-books.org

CONTRIBUTORS

MAITHAM ALHARBI
BASSIM AL SHAKER
HIPÓLITO ARRIAGA III
ANDREA ASSAF
KEVIN BASL
DOROTHY BURGE
MIRIDITH CAMPBELL
JUNE CARPENTER
BRUCE CARTER
BRITTNEY CHANTELE
MAHWISH CHISHTY
ELEXA DAWSON
JOSE DEVERA
MELISSA DOUD
ROXANNE DUNBAR-ORTIZ
SABBA ELAHI
GILBERT KILLS PRETTY ENEMY III
RODNEY EWING
ALI EYAL
DARRELL WAYNE FAIR
SARAH FARAHAT
FRONTLINE ARTS
CHITRA GANESH
MARIAM GHANI
FREDERICK GOKLIZ
GOODW.Y.N.
HOCK E AYE VI EDGAR HEAP OF BIRDS
GINA HERRERA
AARON HUGHES
TOM JONES
RAJKAMAL KAHLON
RONAK K. KAPADIA
RUTH KANEKO
SHAYMAA KHALIL
LALEH KHALILI
ERIKA RENEE LAND
TERRAN LAST GUN
JOSEPH LEFTHAND
NATHAN LEWIS
MONTY LITTLE
HANAA MALALLAH
KYLE T. MAYS
HECTOR RENÉ MEMBREÑO-CANALES
DUNYA MIKHAIL
JAMES PAKOOTAS
CHRIS PAPPAN
ERIC PEREZ
YVETTE M. PINO
THERESE QUINN
ISRA RAHMAN
MICHAEL RAKOWITZ
JUNAID RANA
GREGORY RICK
MERANDA ROBERTS
JOSEPH RUNNING CRANE
SADA
RIJIN SAHAKIAN
GERALD SHEFFIELD
CARLOS SIRAH
HUSSEIN SMKO
STARLA THOMPSON
ANTHONY TORRES
DWAYNE WILCOX
YIRAN ZHANG
AMBER ZORA

SURVIVING THE LONG WARS

CREATIVE REBELLION AT THE ENDS OF EMPIRE

edited by

AARON HUGHES

RONAK K. KAPADIA

THERESE QUINN

MERANDA ROBERTS

AMBER ZORA

Land Acknowledgment

We honor and acknowledge the original peoples of the Chicagoland area, where the *Surviving the Long Wars* project is based—the Three Fires Confederacy: the Potawatomi, Odawa, and Ojibwe Nations, as well as other Tribal Nations that know this area as their ancestral homelands, including the Menominee, Ho-Chunk, Myaamia, Peoria, and Sac and Fox and their descendants. Today, this land is home to one of the largest urban Native American communities in the United States. This acknowledgment is not merely a rhetorical gesture, but a call to action. It serves as the foundation for any critique of violence, imperialism, militarism, and warfare presented here. To acknowledge is to act. We urge everyone to consider the multitude of ways to transform awareness into meaningful support for Indigenous peoples and communities—locally, nationally, and globally.

for the survivors and descendants of the long wars, including those war resisters creating art to upend US militarism at home and abroad

contents

All works are courtesy of the artist unless otherwise noted.

introduction

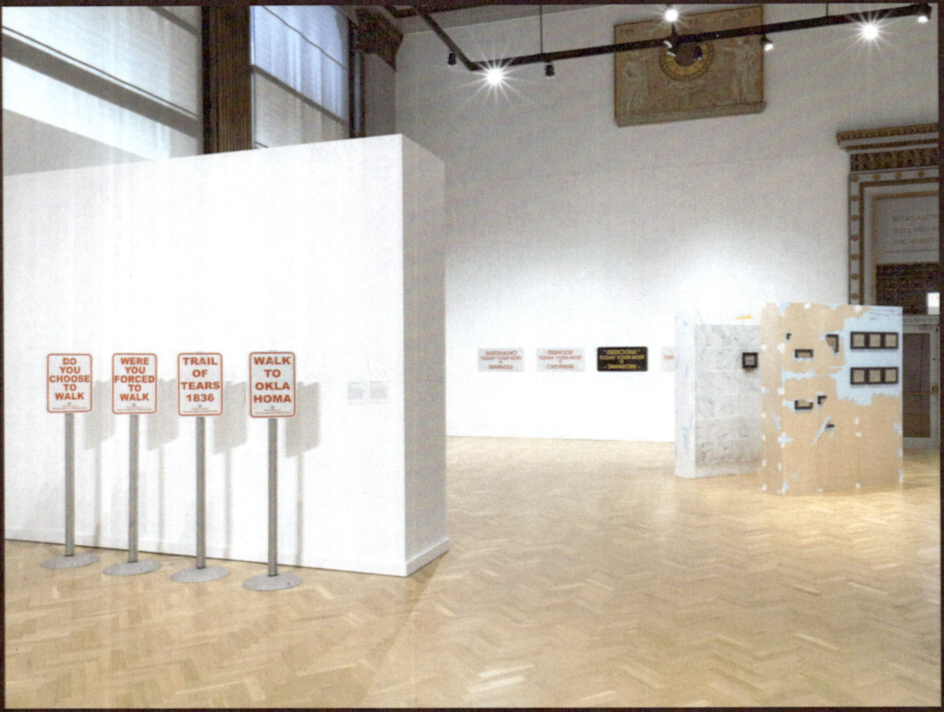

Work featured in *Reckon and Reimagine* at the Chicago Cultural Center

left: **HOCK E AYE VI EDGAR HEAP OF BIRDS**
Trail of Tears
see also: pp. 83, 96

center background: ***Native Host for Oklahoma***
see also: p. 276

right background: **ALI EYAL**
An indefinite appearance or two walls and
see also: pp. 113, 120–22

Introduction

SURVIVING THE LONG WARS EDITORIAL COLLECTIVE

Surviving the Long Wars is a testament to the power of creativity in our collective struggle against endless war and militarism. This book uncovers the multiple, overlapping histories that shape our understanding of warfare, as well as the alternative visions of peace, healing, and justice generated by diverse communities impacted by war. By weaving together a variety of voices and perspectives, we illuminate the profound connections between the two most protracted military conflicts in US history: the "American Indian Wars" of the eighteenth and nineteenth centuries and the twenty-first century's "Global War on Terror" (GWOT).[1] Despite their separation in time and space, these twin "long wars" share common military strategies, ideological justifications, and devastating impacts on marginalized communities. This book reframes these conflicts as part of a continuous thread of US imperialism spanning centuries.

Confronting this violent record, *Surviving the Long Wars* reveals a legacy of resistance and creative rebellion. Drawing inspiration from Indigenous responses to the "Indian Wars" and artists from the Greater Middle East and South Asia defying the "GWOT," this book explores the deep entanglements between these traditions and the experiences of contemporary Black, Indigenous, and People of Color (BIPOC) veterans.[2] These connections propose a complex coalition rooted in shared struggle, forging transformative parallels between those most targeted by and recruited into the machinery of state violence. Such alliances, akin to spiritual interventions or poetic insurrections, challenge the monolithic logic of imperialism, disrupt the binaries of oppressed and oppressor, and advocate for solidarity across differences in the pursuit of collective liberation.

At its core, this book argues that art is not merely a reflection of dissent but a powerful catalyst for building intersectional movements. Abolitionist art-making plays a pivotal role in opposing militarism and ending wars, channeling centuries of rebellious creativity from those most impacted by US imperialism. *Surviving the Long Wars* urges artists, activists, and scholars to unite in the pursuit of peace and justice, positioning art-making at the heart of an internationalist, demilitarized vision. This project embodies the spirit of BIPOC liberation, advocating for a future shaped by solidarity and "freedom dreams."[3]

Imperial Echoes and Creative Rebellion

Tracing the roots of US militarism from the "Indian Wars" to the "GWOT," this book underscores the importance of a comparative, relational, and transnational lens to forge solidarity against ongoing US state violence.[4] Building on a significant shift in comparative American and ethnic studies toward the postcolonial study of the US, this book investigates the intimacies between creative defiance at "home" and artistic insurgencies "abroad."[5] This approach unearths how settler-colonial histories—marked by land theft, Native genocide, African chattel slavery, and Asian exploitation—are integral to the genealogy of the US military and its sprawling architecture of social control.[6]

The term "long wars," originally coined by Secretary of Defense Donald H. Rumsfeld, is repurposed here to examine the US as a nation perpetually at war, exposing the unbroken lineage of military escalation and territorial acquisition that defines its past and present.[7] This framework allows us to juxtapose the eighteenth- and nineteenth-century "Indian Wars" with the twenty-first-century "GWOT," highlighting a continuous genealogy of US settler-colonial invasion, occupation, and genocide against Indigenous peoples.[8] Native and Black resistance to this oppressive security order has long inspired contemporary global movements against militarism and securitization. By revealing points of convergence and potential alliances between the twin "long wars," we underscore the urgency of forging dynamic coalitions to dismantle these violent systems and connect the brutal impacts of past conflicts to current struggles.

The echoes of US militarism reverberate through time. The "GWOT" is not an isolated conflict but a continuation of the expansionist logic that drove the "Indian Wars," once framed as the "taming of the frontier." This connection was made explicit by the George W. Bush Administration's Office of Legal Counsel, which traced a direct line from the 9/11 attacks to the "Indian Wars." The Barack Obama Administration further reinforced this link when it codenamed the operation to kill Osama Bin Laden "Geronimo," invoking the Apache resistance leader.[9] Such decisions reflect a deeply ingrained imperial mindset that views every frontier as a counterinsurgent battlefield, every Indigenous life as expendable.[10]

In *The Transit of Empire*, Chickasaw scholar Jodi Byrd considers how racialization and colonization have worked in tandem to dispossess entire peoples—enslaving, excluding, removing, and killing them in the name of progress and capitalism.[11] Recognizing these militarized residues of late-nineteenth- and early-twentieth-century settler colonialism is crucial for contemporary anti-war artists and the wider anti-imperialist, abolitionist struggle. The military strategies once, and arguably still, used to crush Native American resistance have been repurposed for modern counterinsurgency, targeting BIPOC communities both domestically and internationally.[12] Historically, the US has conscripted those it seeks to control—such as Native scouts, Iraqi Police, and the Afghan National Army—into its war machinery, turning them into reluctant agents complicit in colonial operations. This legacy demands a critical reckoning with the past to effectively challenge current cycles of militarized oppression and to forge dynamic coalitions to dismantle these violent systems.

A Rising Veteran Art Movement

Amid these seemingly endless wars, a radical praxis of anti-colonial resistance endures, shaping the landscape like an underground river that surfaces in the fierce creativity of contemporary BIPOC artists, including veterans. Drawing on traditions of creative dissent, these artists transform pain into power, challenge stereotypes, disrupt political narratives, and reclaim stories distorted by militarized cultural norms. This artistic uprising is about more than survival; it's about solidarity and forging connections across time and space.[13] Effective solidarity-building requires meeting people where they are and understanding both the commonalities and differences in their struggles. This process, though challenging, is central to our project, especially in addressing the heterogeneity within racialized and Indigenous communities. By linking past struggles with present movements, our work envisions a future where liberation from the long wars is not just a dream but a reality.

As this book details, resistance is a central theme across both conflicts, showcasing the agency, resilience, and sacrifices of affected communities. Indigenous protest to US expansion, whether through armed struggle, diplomacy, or aesthetic revolt, resonates with contemporary opposition to the "GWOT." These acts of insurgency, pursued at considerable personal and communal cost, challenge the devastating effects of US imperialism and militarism. *Surviving the Long Wars* explores these insurgent responses, focusing on how veterans and artists from Indigenous, Black, Latinx, Asian, Middle Eastern, and South Asian communities not only critique the intertwined histories of warfare but also offer a roadmap for future opposition, grounded in solidarity and the courage to confront oppressive systems.[14]

The Veteran Art Movement, rooted in legacies of creative rebellion, draws from veterans' involvement in international art movements—from DADA to Black Arts—and their indispensable contributions to anti-war, civil rights, abolition, and decolonization struggles.[15] For example, artists like T.C. Cannon (Kiowa and Caddo) and Rick Bartow (Mad River Band of the Wiyot), both Vietnam veterans, established an "insurgent aesthetics" that continues to inspire subsequent generations of Indigenous veteran artists featured in the Triennial, such as Monty Little (Diné) and Ruth Kaneko (Kanaka Wahine).[16] These contemporary artists build on the art activism of movement leaders like Dennis Banks (Chippewa), who, after serving in the US Air Force, co-founded the American Indian Movement in 1968. This lineage of creative organizing is extensively chronicled in movement newspapers—from the Mohawk Nation's *Akwesasne Notes* to Vietnam Veterans Against the War's *Winter Soldier*. It continues through actions like the 2016 veteran mobilizations in support of Water Protectors defending their lands against the Dakota Access Pipeline at Standing Rock.[17]

In the Black Arts Movement, famed writer Amiri Baraka, a former US Air Force gunner, bridged the gap between military service and radical art activism. This practice is deeply rooted in the Civil Rights Movement, where veterans like World War II hero and NAACP organizer Medgar Evers and the Black Panther Party's Minister of Defense Elmer "Geronimo" Pratt—who earned two Purple Hearts in Vietnam—played pivotal roles. These veterans navigated their commitment to radical activism, often at great personal cost, confronting the sense of betrayal and trespass associated with speaking out, demanding justice, and confronting racist, militarized norms. This spirit of radical Black creativity continues with Triennial artists like Rodney Ewing, whose collage prints *Pathfinder (Harriet Tubman)* (2021) and *Come the Mean Times* (2022) fuse art with activism. Gregory Rick's artist book *Black and Native Victories* (2017) and GOODW.Y.N.'s poem "It's Not All Dead" further extend this political legacy, demonstrating the power of art to challenge injustice. Similarly, Triennial artists Yvette M. Pino and Eric Perez channel the spirit of veteran artist Rupert García and the Chicano Art Movement. The Royal Chicano Air Force, co-founded by veteran artist José Montoya, remains a central collective in this field, demonstrating the enduring impact of veteran-led art movements on the broader landscape of creative rebellion across the long twentieth century. Together, these artists represent a lasting thread, demonstrating how veterans have consistently repurposed their lived experiences to challenge oppression and imagine alternative futures. The Veteran Art Movement, steeped in this rich history of radical art activism, continues to connect generations and communities, affirming art's indomitable power as a force for social change and collective liberation.[18]

The 2023 Veteran Art Triennial, Summit, and Scholarly Series

The 2023 Veteran Art Triennial in Chicago was a landmark event, redefining how we engage with the complex connections, contradictions, and solidarities within the expressive cultures of impacted communities.[19] Commemorating the twentieth anniversary of the US-led invasion of Iraq, the Triennial showcased the work of over fifty BIPOC artists who delivered powerful and urgent artistic responses to the profound consequences of war. Chicago art critic Lori Waxman, writing in *Hyperallergic*, lauded the exhibitions' bold focus on war-themed art from a diverse array of directly impacted communities, setting it apart from traditional, often patriotic, veteran art exhibitions. The Triennial stands out for its innovative curation and broad inclusion of voices, extending beyond conventional depictions of service members' experiences to foster an international arts dialogue.[20]

This powerful convergence of artists, scholars, students, and community leaders ignited an engagement with the relational histories and lived experiences of US military conflicts, spotlighting resistance to settler colonialism and white supremacy. The Triennial seamlessly integrated into Chicago's vibrant art scene, which has long been a crucible for groundbreaking exhibitions like *A Proximity of Consciousness* (2014), *The Long Term* (2018), *Do Not Resist* (2018), *Original Warrior* (2018), *Remaking the Exceptional* (2022), and the 2019 Veteran Art Triennial, *On War & Survival*. This rich cultural landscape builds on pioneering artist-run initiatives such as the Monster Roster, AfriCOBRA, Vietnam Veterans Art Group, and AREA Chicago, while contemporary projects like Justseeds, the #LetUsBreathe Collective, the PO Box Collective, and Walls Turned Sideways continue to drive a revolutionary arts discourse.

The Triennial and Summit served as a dynamic platform for dialogue, action, and reflection, bridging the intimate realities of the long wars with broader anti-war currents. The events celebrated the resilience and "survivance" of BIPOC communities, a concept eloquently articulated by Anishinaabe critic Gerald Vizenor.[21] With support from a National Endowment for the Humanities grant, Veteran Fellows—including Gina Herrera (Tesuque Pueblo), Monty Little (Diné), Eric Perez, Gerald Sheffield, Natasha Erskine, and Anthony Torres—led curated discussions on themes of intimacy, resilience, and solidarity.[22] These conversations resonated deeply with Indigenous scholar Jarrett Martineau's insight that "acts of creation are entwined with movements toward freedom."[23] The four-day Summit, which launched the Triennial, embodied a spirit of dissent, survivance, and healing, a spirit captured by storyteller James Pakootas (Confederate Tribes of Colville) in his reflection, "As we heal, our ancestors heal." This powerful sentiment framed the project from the outset and remains central to this book. The culminating program of the Summit, a closing circle and Iraq War Memorial Activation, provided a space for veterans, artists, students, and scholars to reflect, demonstrating how collaborative projects rooted in reciprocal care and driven by the collective agency of BIPOC communities offer a potent lens for advancing healing, justice, and solidarity.[24]

Anchoring the Triennial and Summit was a major scholarly seminar series at the University of Illinois Chicago (UIC) during the 2022–23 academic year.[25] Featuring prominent thinkers such as Roxanne Dunbar-Ortiz, Kyle T. Mays, Harsha Walia, Laleh Khalili, Nick Estes, Kelly Hayes, and Tiffany King, the series explored critical concepts across Indigenous Studies, Black Studies, Critical Ethnic Studies, Middle Eastern Studies, and Gender Studies. The free, livestreamed, and archived seminars cultivated a community of inquiry and action, exploring comparative and relational histories that laid the intellectual groundwork for the Triennial and Summit. *Surviving the Long Wars* captures the transformative energy and impact of these multi-sited public humanities programs, celebrating the art-making and movement-building that emerged. By documenting these collective efforts, this book deepens our understanding of how imperial warfare shapes diverse communities and serves as a blueprint for future resistance. It invites readers to forge new alliances and actively engage in ongoing struggles for justice and liberation.

Chicago as a Site of Resistance and Social-Justice-Informed Curation

Chicago emerges as a critical site of organizing and strategy within this book, renowned for its deep roots in overlapping social movements and art activism.[26] This book not only addresses the erasure of Indigenous history but also highlights Chicago's crucial role in global Indigenous struggles, aligning with the mission of the Center for Native Futures (CfNF), the only all-Native artist-led arts nonprofit in Zhegagoynak ("Chicago" in Potawatomi). The city, home to vibrant African, Black, Muslim, Middle Eastern, Arab, and South Asian communities, is also at the forefront of organizing against the apparatus of the "GWOT" and its repressive domestic surveillance. Additionally, Chicago's longstanding tradition of creative anti-war veteran activism by groups including Vietnam Veterans Against the War, Iraq Veterans Against the War, About Face: Veterans Against the War, and the emerging Veteran Art Movement, positions the city as an epicenter of twenty-first-century creative rebellion against the long wars.

Art plays a transformative role within these organizations. Building on Chicago's culture of creative activism, *Surviving the Long Wars* draws further inspiration from social museology, which advocates for leveraging standard museum practices—collecting, exhibiting, and programming—for popular education and social justice.[27] This approach is reflected in notable, movement-based cultural initiatives that have shaped resistance and solidarity from at least the 1970s to the present, including Brazil's *favela* museums, the People's Archive of Police Violence in Cleveland, UC Santa Cruz's Visualizing Abolition, and Decolonize This Place, among others.[28] These public initiatives serve as a touchstone for our approach, reflecting a commitment to transformative, community-centered art-making.

This project further aims to strengthen our connections with Native and Indigenous artists, educators, and activists, including veterans. It highlights how intersectional approaches to critical race and Indigenous thought—along with advancements in critical ethnic studies, transnational American studies, feminist and queer studies, disability studies, and Middle Eastern and South Asian studies—offer a nuanced analysis of racial capitalism, settler colonialism, warfare, and empire. We hope this book will serve as a model and template for future collaborative projects among artists, educators, organizers, and students, offering deep insights into the histories of Native uprisings and race-radical resistance to war and militarism.

Our Editorial Collective

The editorial collective behind *Surviving the Long Wars* comprises a diverse ensemble of scholars, artists, educators, and activists, united by a fierce commitment to queer feminist abolitionist anti-colonial politics and a spirit of experimentation. Each member brings a unique perspective to our collective effort. Meranda Roberts, a citizen of the Yerington Paiute tribe and Chicana, employs Indigenous methodologies to challenge and decolonize public representations of Native American histories, art, and cultures. Therese Quinn, a teacher, writer, and cultural worker, actively engages in queer and feminist anti-authoritarian, anti-capitalist formations and directs the justice-centered Museum and Exhibition Studies (MUSE) Program at UIC. Ronak K. Kapadia, a queer South Asian diasporic scholar in Gender and Women's Studies (GWS) at UIC, critically examines the carceral geographies of late modern warfare and the diasporas of South and Southwest Asia, illuminating the intersections of race, war, aesthetics, and US empire. Artist and anti-war veteran Amber Zora critiques militarism and imperialism through her solo and collaborative creative projects, drawing on her experiences joining the military at nineteen. Aaron Hughes, an artist, organizer, curator, and anti-war veteran, was radicalized by his deployment to Kuwait and Iraq in 2003. He has since dedicated himself to creating meaning out of personal and collective traumas and critiques militarism through art and activism, with projects like the emerging Veteran Art Movement.[29] Together, these distinct voices ensure that our collective is deeply rooted in a multiplicity of experiences and perspectives.

Our collective's diverse backgrounds in race, indigeneity, sexuality, gender, ability, region, employment status, and past military service infuse our work with a spectrum of viewpoints. We approach these differences with a keen awareness of power dynamics. Inspired by the Veteran Art Movement—which critically examines veterans' roles in US military interventions and occupations—we are committed to confronting these tensions directly. We acknowledge the cycles of harm perpetuated by militarism and state violence and are committed to actively engaging with critical feedback regarding the ethics of collaborating with veterans, especially at UIC, where many students come from the Global Majorities directly affected by US imperialism. This feedback compels us to continually reflect on our responsibilities and the impact of our partnerships and educational initiatives.

Abolition feminism teaches us that people are not defined solely by their worst actions and that everyone has the power to change.[30] This perspective enables us to address the complexities of working with anti-war veteran artists—recognizing the harm they have perpetuated, the harm they and their families have endured, and the broader cycles of violence embedded in our collective histories and daily lives. For war resisters, the stakes are particularly high: they must confront their past actions while actively opposing the militarized systems that once shaped their lives, often at significant personal cost. By rejecting imperialism and standing in solidarity with those most impacted, these veterans challenge the very institutions that seek to define them, risking alienation and further marginalization. Yet, it is through this very act of defiance that they harness the power to reclaim their narratives and advance broader movements for justice.

We aim to foster a dialogue that not only embraces these contradictions but uses them as a foundation for dismantling the military-industrial complex. Through creative rebellion and a steadfast commitment to transformative justice, we work towards a future where cycles of violence are not only acknowledged but systematically dismantled, paving the way for a more peaceful and just world.

Conclusion: A Call to Action

Surviving the Long Wars transcends the conventional exhibition catalog; it is a clarion call to bridge differences, reject imperialism, and envision a future shaped by peace and justice. By centering the lived experiences and radical creativity of those most impacted by US imperialism, this book highlights the transformative power of art to inspire, heal, and unite communities in their ongoing fight against war and militarism. For veteran artists, this requires shifting from alliances based solely on military experiences to coalitions rooted in solidarity with other targeted and impacted communities.

In Chicago, we urge cultural institutions to draw inspiration from our approach, leveraging their collective platforms and resources to confront uncomfortable truths, particularly in collaboration with Indigenous partners. The city's founding is deeply intertwined with the "Indian Wars" and the forced removal of several Indigenous nations, including the Ojibwe, Potawatomi, Odawa, Menominee, Myaamia, and Ho-Chunk. It is crucial for these institutions to recognize this legacy and support these Nations in their efforts to reclaim their sovereignty.[31] Ultimately, this book highlights the worldmaking power of art in intersectional movement building and its indispensable role in imagining abolitionist futures. We invite you to join us in this call to action—to engage, reflect, and act in solidarity towards dismantling systemic violence and working for a more just and equitable world.

NOTES

1. The "American Indian Wars" were a series of violent conflicts from the 1500s to the early 1900s, marked by land theft, forced relocations, and efforts to eradicate Indigenous cultures. In contrast, the "Global War on Terror," launched after the September 11, 2001, attacks, represents a contemporary phase of US military engagement in the Middle East, South Asia, and Africa marked by invasions, occupations, and counter-terrorism operations and perpetuating violence and destabilization in these regions.

2. The term "BIPOC" (Black, Indigenous, and People of Color) originated in Canada in the early 2010s to emphasize the distinct experiences of Black and Indigenous people under white supremacy and colonialism while also suggesting potential coalitions among racialized communities and people of the Global Majorities. See Sandra E. Garcia, "Where Did BIPOC Come From?," *New York Times*, June 17, 2020, https://www.nytimes.com/article/what-is-bipoc.html.

3. In studying art for social change, we draw inspiration from works such as Robin D.G. Kelley, *Freedom Dreams* (2003); Avery F. Gordon, *Ghostly Matters* (2008); Claudia Rankine, *Citizen: An American Lyric* (2014); Kellie Jones, *South of Pico* (2017); Alice Kim et al., *The Long Term* (2018); Jennifer Ponce de León, *Another Aesthetics Is Possible* (2021); Amber Ginsburg et al., *Remaking the Exceptional* (2022); Daphne Brooks, *Liner Notes for the Revolution* (2023); and others by, for instance, Angela Davis, Augusto Boal, Nicole Fleetwood, Kellie Jones, Lisa Lowe, Daphne Brooks, and Diana Taylor.

4. Our project's comparative and relational framework is inspired by interdisciplinary works such as Ann Stoler, *Haunted By Empire* (2006); Roderick Ferguson and Grace Hong, *Strange Affinities* (2011); Lisa Lowe, *The Intimacies of Four Continents* (2015); Gayatri Gopinath, *Unruly Visions* (2018); Tiffany King et al., *Otherwise Worlds* (2020); and Juliana Hu Pegues, *Space-Time Colonialism* (2021).

5. This reorientation in fields like American Studies challenges the denial of empire and positions imperialism as central to US national identity. Since Amy Kaplan and Donald E. Pease's *Cultures of United States Imperialism* (1993), scholars have rejected the myth of "American exceptionalism" and adopted a "post-exceptionalist" approach, integrating postcolonial tools to place the US within broader hemispheric and global frameworks. This New Americanist project, which builds on earlier critiques by figures like W. E. B. Du Bois, has reshaped the field and informs contemporary studies of US race, war, and empire including this work.

6. For more on the settler ideology underlying the founding of the Americas, see Ned Blackhawk, *The Rediscovery of America: Native Peoples and the Unmaking of US History* (2023).

7. See "Quadrennial Defense Review Report," February 6, 2006. http://archive.defense.gov/pubs/pdfs/QDR20060203.pdf. See also Andrew Bacevich, *The Long War: A New History of US National Security Policy Since World War II* (2007) and Nikhil Pal Singh, *Race and America's Long War* (2019).

8. For a range of perspectives on the concept of settler colonialism, which originated in Native and Indigenous studies and has since shaped fields like anthropology, geography, and American studies, see Frantz Fanon, *The Wretched of the Earth* (1961); Edward Said, "Zionism from the Standpoint of Its Victims" (1979); Sherene H. Razack, *Race, Space, and the Law* (2002); Patrick Wolfe, "Settler Colonialism and the Elimination of the Native" (2006); Alyosha Goldstein and Alex Lubin, "Settler Colonialism" (*South Atlantic Quarterly*, vol. 107, 2008); Lorenzo Veracini, *Settler Colonialism* (2010); Scott Lauria Morgensen, *Spaces between Us* (2011); Alyosha Goldstein, *Formations of United States Colonialism* (2014); Audra Simpson, *Mohawk Interruptus* (2014); Audra Simpson and Andrea Smith, *Theorizing Native Studies* (2014); Dana M. Olwan, "On Assumptive Solidarities in Comparative Settler Colonialisms" (2015); and Kēhaulani Kauanui, "'A Structure, Not an Event'" (2016).

9. For insights on the intersections of imperialism, visual culture, and racialization, see Keith P. Feldman, "Empire's Verticality: The Af/Pak Frontier, Visual Culture, and Racialization from Above," *Comparative American Studies* 9, no. 4 (2011): 325–41; and Anne McClintock, "Imperial Ghosting and National Tragedy: Revenants from Hiroshima and Indian Country in the War on Terror," *PMLA* 129, no. 4 (2014): 819–29. For Native studies critiques of the US (settler) state's long history, see Luana Ross, *Inventing the Savage* (1998); Ned Blackhawk, *Violence over the Land* (2008); Setsu Shigematsu and Keith Camacho, *Militarized Currents* (2010); Roxanne Dunbar-Ortiz, *An Indigenous People's History of the United States* (2014); Iyko Day, *Alien Capital* (2016); Heidi Kiiwetinepinesiik Stark, "Criminal Empire" (2016); Kelly Lytle Hernández, *City of Inmates* (2017); and Dean Saranillio, *Unsustainable Empire* (2018).

10. Key texts offering critical perspectives on US counterinsurgency include Eqbal Ahmad, "Counterinsurgency" (1971); Paul A. Kramer, *The Blood of Government* (2006); Roberto J. González, *American Counterinsurgency* (2009); Alfred W. McCoy, *Policing America's Empire* (2009); Network of Concerned Anthropologists, *Counter-Counterinsurgency Manual* (2009); Joseph Masco, "'Sensitive but Unclassified'" (2010); Nicholas Mirzoeff, *The Right to Look* (2011); Laleh Khalili, *Time in the Shadows* (2012); Paul Amar, *Security Archipelago* (2013); Nerissa Balce, *Body Parts of Empire* (2016); Jordan Camp, *Incarcerating the Crisis* (2016); Ronak K. Kapadia, *Insurgent Aesthetics* (2019); and Stuart Schrader, *Badges without Borders* (2019).

11. Jodi A. Byrd, *The Transit of Empire: Indigenous Critiques of Colonialism* (2011). On the problem of narrating synchronous histories of racialization and colonization, see Lisa Lowe, *The Intimacies of Four Continents* (2015): 10–11.

12. On the intersections of US imperial warfare and racialization abroad, see Timothy Mitchell, *Rule of Experts* (2002); Jodi Kim, *Ends of Empire* (2004); Paul A. Kramer, *The Blood of Government* (2006); Jasbir Puar, *Terrorist Assemblages* (2007); Robert Vitalis, *America's Kingdom* (2007); Moon-Ho Jung, *Coolies and Cane* (2008); Junaid Rana, *Terrifying Muslims* (2011); Laleh Khalili, *Time in the Shadows* (2012); and Lisa Lowe, *The Intimacies of Four Continents* (2015). For the role of race in the domestic US context, see Nayan Shah, *Contagious Divides* (2001); Robert O. Self, *American Babylon* (2003); Mae Ngai, *Impossible Subjects* (2004); Ruth Wilson Gilmore, *Golden Gulag* (2007); Daniel HoSang, *Racial Propositions* (2010); Chandan Reddy, *Freedom with Violence* (2011); Nadine Naber, *Arab America* (2012); Andrew Friedman, *Covert Capital* (2013); Maria Josefina Saldaña-Portillo, *Indian Given* (2016); and Walter Johnson, *River of Dark Dreams* (2017).

13. On solidarity politics, see Antonio Gramsci, *Prison Notebooks* (1929); Paulo Freire, *Pedagogy of the Oppressed* (1968); Sara Ahmed, *Living a Feminist Life* (2017); Keeanga-Yamahtta Taylor, *How We Get Free* (2017); Dean Spade, *Mutual Aid* (2020); Mariame Kaba and Kelly Hayes, *Let This Radicalize You* (2023); and Leah Hunt-Hendrix and Astra Taylor, *Solidarity* (2024).

14. Our approach in *Surviving the Long Wars* is shaped by our co-editor Ronak K. Kapadia's *Insurgent Aesthetics: Security and the Queer Life of the Forever War* (2019). Kapadia's analysis of contemporary art from Arab, Muslim, and South Asian diasporic artists provides essential intellectual grounding for the emerging Veteran Art Movement. His work examines how these art responses critique the expansion of US militarism in the Greater Middle East and its impact on gendered, racialized state violence, framing the post-9/11 era as a new phase in the long durée of US settler colonialism.

15. The emerging Veteran Art Movement (eVAM) grew out of the activism of Iraq Veterans Against the War (IVAW), as chronicled by Nan Levinson in *War is Not a Game* (2014) and in the Justseeds print portfolio *Celebrate People's History: Iraq Veterans Against the War* (2014). eVAM draws inspiration from Vietnam Veterans Against the War (VVAW), as documented by Richard Stacewicz in *Winter Soldiers* (1997) and Andrew E. Hunt in *The Turning* (1999), and from the Vietnam Veteran Art Group, featured in *Vietnam Reflexes and Reflections* (1998). It builds on the legacy of veterans working in international art movements, including DADA, Surrealism, Fluxus, the Monster Roster, the Black Arts Movement, the Chicano Art Movement, and the Royal Chicano Air Force. For more, see the eVAM website and related blog posts on the 2019 Triennial & Summit.

16. Anne Bolen, "An Art Revolution: T.C. Cannon Shows Native Life at The Edge Of America" (*American Indian*, Spring 2019 / Vol. 20 No. 1) discusses the internal conflict T.C. Cannon faced as an Indigenous veteran, reflected in his painting *Soldiers* (1970). Monty Little similarly explores his military experience as an Indigenous veteran in an interview with Larry Abbott, "The Art of Erasure & A Conversation with Monty Little" (*War, Literature & the Arts*, Vol. 31, 2019).

17. Louise Siddons considers the graphics, frequently distributed by the Liberation News Services, shared between the Red Power and Black Power movements, in "Red Power in the Black Panther: Radical Imagination and Intersectional Resistance at Wounded Knee" (*American Art*, summer 2021). Our work is also influenced by *Signal: A Journal of International Political Graphics and Culture*, the Interference Archive in New York City, and the Center for the Study of Political Graphics.

18. Building on legendary Monster Roster artist and World War II veteran Leon Golub's involvement in the 1980s campaign "Artists Call Against US Intervention in Central America," eVAM artists in 2020 joined Iraqi artists in calling for MoMA to divest from war profiteers and arms manufacturers (see the spring 2020 issue of VVAW's *The Veteran*). In 2023/2024, they also supported the global ceasefire campaign in response to the genocide in Gaza and Palestine.

19. For an archive of 2023 Veteran Art Triennial exhibitions, see https://www.survivingthelongwars.online/triennial. For the Summit, see https://www.survivingthelongwars.online/summit.

20. Lori Waxman, "Art by Survivors of America's Long Wars," *Hyperallergic*, May 7, 2023, https://hyperallergic.com/819534/art-by-survivors-of-americas-wars/.

21. Gerald Robert Vizenor, *Survivance: Narratives of Native Presence* (University of Nebraska Press, 2008).

22. In 2022, our team received a National Endowment for the Humanities (NEH) Dialogues on the Experiences of War grant to fund *Surviving the Long Wars: Visualizing Parallels Between the US "Indian Wars" and the "Global War on Terror."* This project integrated academic study, curatorial research, and a seminar series, culminating in veteran-led forums at the second National Veteran Art Triennial & Summit in Chicago in March 2023. This grant followed a 2019 project that offered a two-semester course at the University of Illinois Chicago, which included a workshop preparing veteran artists and curators to lead discussions on wars from World War I to the present at the National Veterans Art Museum's inaugural Triennial & Summit in Chicago.

23. Jarrett Martineau, nêhiyaw (Plains Cree) and Denesųłiné from Frog Lake Cree Nation, Alberta, discusses Indigenous art, resurgence, and decolonization in his PhD dissertation, "Creative Combat: Indigenous Art, Resurgence, and Decolonization" (University of Victoria, 2015): 3.

24. On the ideas of relational care and curatorial ethics, see Nicole R. Fleetwood, *Marking Time: Art in the Age of Mass Incarceration* (2020); and Laura Kina et al., "A&Q: Curation as Decolonial Practice" (*Verge: Studies in Global Asias* 8, no. 2, 2022): 46-64. On healing justice, see Cara Page and Erica Woodland, *Healing Justice Lineages: Dreaming at the Crossroads of Liberation, Collective Care, and Safety* (2023).

25. For the digital archive of the *STLW* virtual scholarly seminar series, visit https://www.survivingthelongwars.online/scholarlyseries. This series was supported by the University of Illinois Chicago (UIC) Institute for the Humanities Innovation Grant, UIC Award for Creative Activity, UIC Program in Museum and Exhibition Studies, UIC Program in Gender and Women's Studies, UIC Disability Cultural Center, Chicago Cultural Center, Hyde Park Art Center, Newberry Library, DEMIL Art Fund, and a National Endowment for the Humanities Dialogues on the Experience of War grant.

26. In Chicago this history is highlighted by influential groups such as BYP100, Let Us Breathe Collective, Black Lives Matter Chicago, We Charge Genocide, Chicago Torture Justice Memorials, Justseeds Artists' Cooperative, Prison + Neighborhood Arts/Education Project, Dissenters, Students for Justice in Palestine, REAL Youth Initiative, Organized Communities Against Deportation, Chi-Nations Youth Council, Southwest Youth Collaborative, Assata's Daughters, Chicago Alliance Against Racist and Political Repression, Little Village Environmental Justice Organization, Lifted Voices, Black and Pink, among many others.

27. For more on this history and framework, see the International Movement for a New Museology: https://www.minom-icom.net.

28. See also The Visitors of Color Project, #MuseumsAreNotNeutral, #MuseumWorkersSpeak, #MASSAction (Museums as Sites of Social Action), #MuseumsRespondToFerguson, MOTHA (the Museum of Trans Hirstory & Art), the Natural History Museum ("A Museum for the Movement"), P.A.I.N. (Prescription Addict on Intervention Now), and Alice Procter's Uncomfortable Art Tours at six British museums.

29. Kevin Basl, Aaron Hughes, Anthony Torres, and Amber Zora, working with fellow veteran artists, including Jesse Albrecht, Hipólito Arriaga III, Drew Cameron, Rodney Ewing, Alicia Dietz, Eric Garcia, GOODW.Y.N., Edgar Gonzalez-Baeza, Gina Herrera, Ash Kyrie, David Keefe, Jessica Putnam-Phillips, Nathan Lewis, Monty Little, Eric Perez, Yvette M. Pino, Gerald Sheffield, Carlos Sirah, Ehren Tool, and Eli Wright have played key roles in cultivating the emerging Veteran Art Movement (eVAM). This decentralized network of veterans and service members is committed to using creative practices to transform themselves, and US society as a whole, as they grapple with the ongoing realities of endless war, militarism, and dehumanization. For more on eVAM, see https://www.veteran-art-movement.net/.

30. Angela Y. Davis, Gina Dent, Erica R. Meiners, and Beth E. Richie, *Abolition. Feminism. Now.* (Haymarket Books, 2022).

31. This recognition is urgent given that Chicago's monuments perpetuate a romanticized and distorted portrayal of Native Peoples, erasing the true experiences and stewardship of the land and waterways. The stars on the city's flag, meant to symbolize settler "resilience," overlook the tragic truth of Indigenous removal and genocide. Despite being home to one of the largest urban Native American communities in the US, Chicago has yet to fully recognize or engage with these communities in meaningful ways. It is time for change

section one

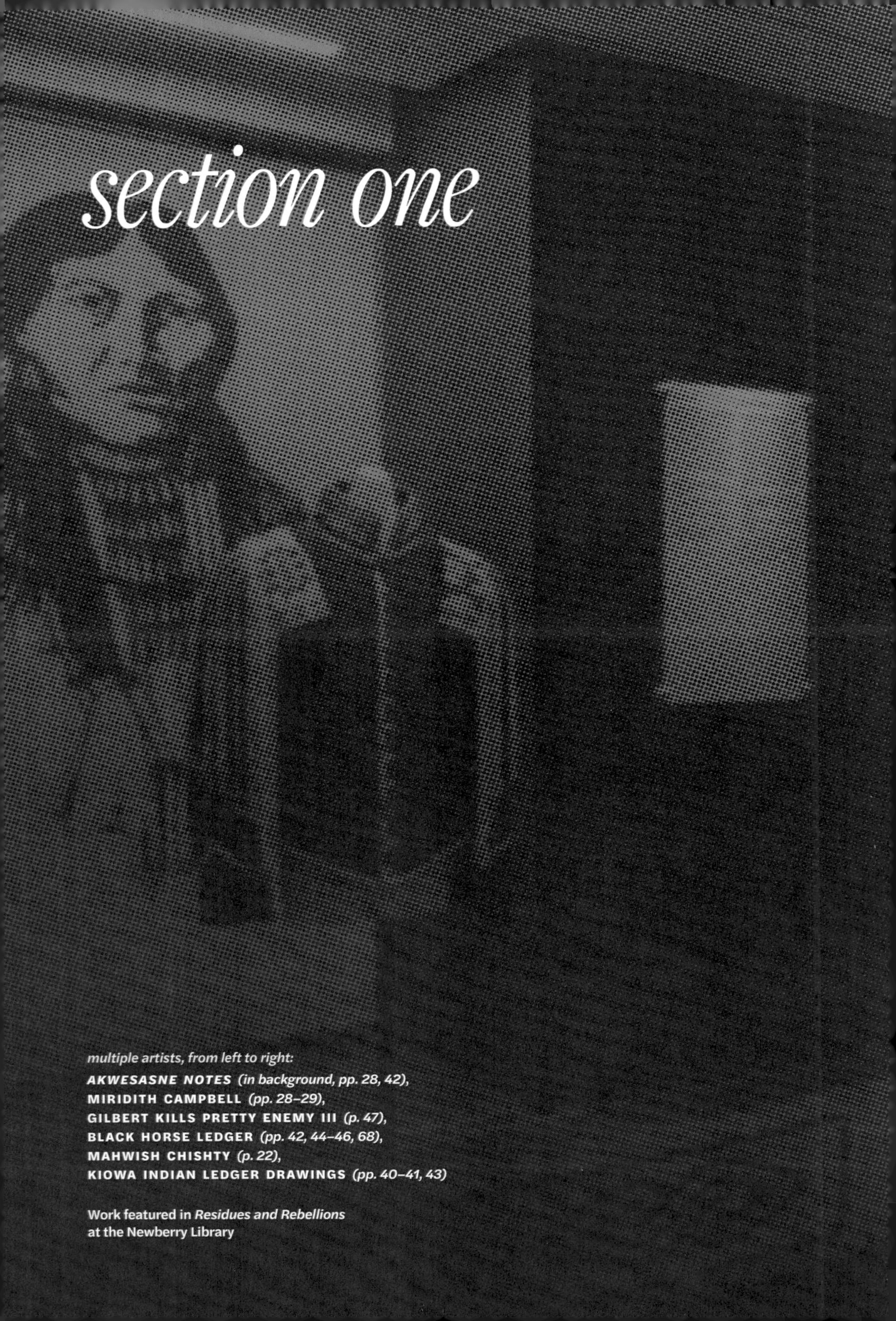

multiple artists, from left to right:
AKWESASNE NOTES *(in background, pp. 28, 42),*
MIRIDITH CAMPBELL *(pp. 28–29),*
GILBERT KILLS PRETTY ENEMY III *(p. 47),*
BLACK HORSE LEDGER *(pp. 42, 44–46, 68),*
MAHWISH CHISHTY *(p. 22),*
KIOWA INDIAN LEDGER DRAWINGS *(pp. 40–41, 43)*

Work featured in *Residues and Rebellions* at the Newberry Library

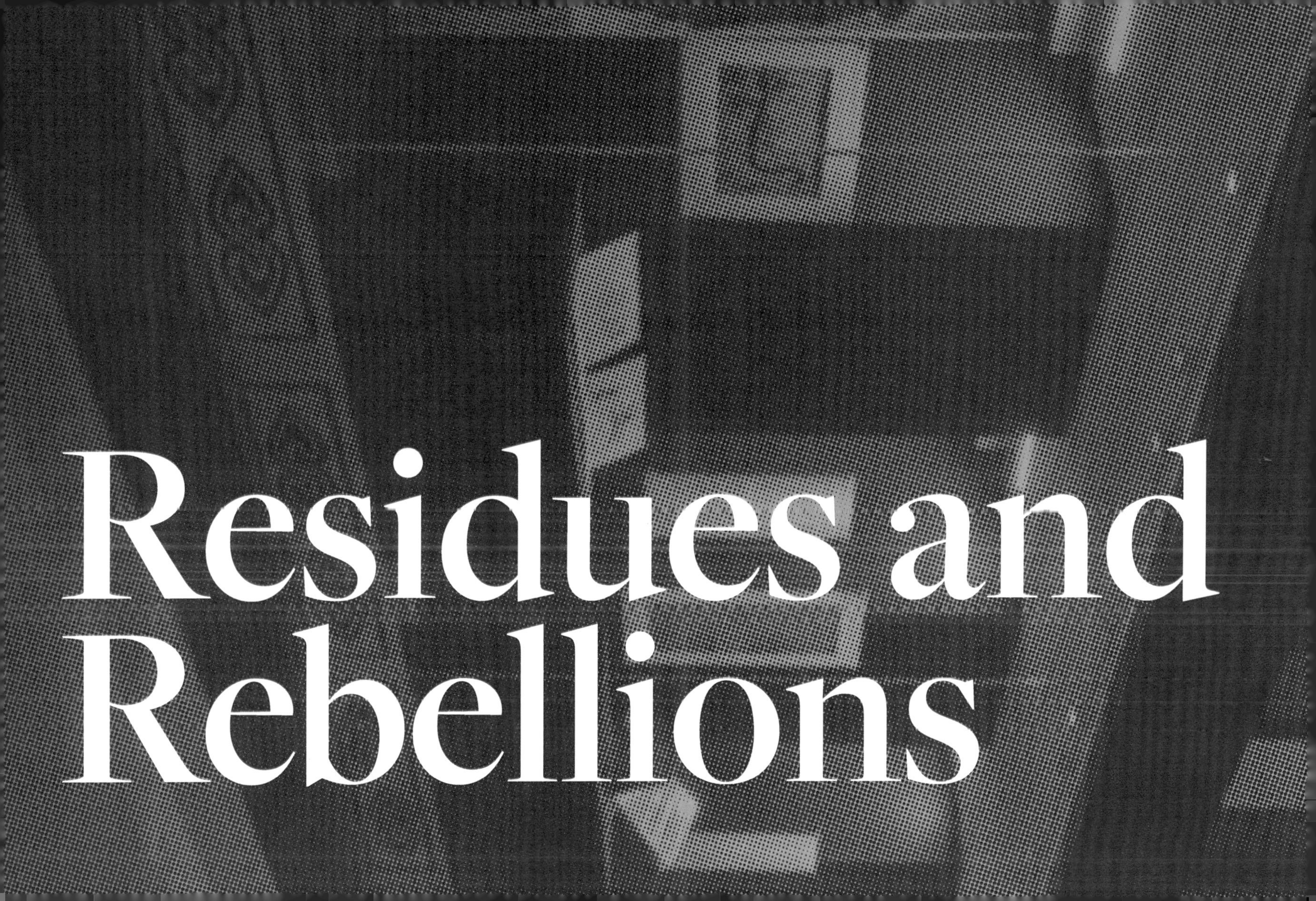

Residues and Rebellions

Residues and Rebellions

The War on Terror is literally just an extension of the Indian Wars. [...] We can go back to any modern war that the United States has fought and trace its tactics and how it characterizes the enemy to its approach to "the Indian."
—Nick Estes, "Red Planet" (*The New Inquiry*, 2019)

The enduring traces of people's efforts to confront the pain and ferocity of endless war lie within elders' stories, inherited traditions, repurposed uniforms, old sketchbooks, yellowed newspapers, and at times, contemporary conceptual artworks. When these efforts are juxtaposed, they resonate across histories and geographies, forming a chorus of perpetual creative rebellion.

This section, titled *Residues and Rebellions* after the Triennial exhibition at the Newberry Library (February 28–May 26, 2023), features artworks by Miridith Campbell (Kiowa), Mahwish Chishty, Gilbert Kills Pretty Enemy III (Standing Rock Sioux), Rodney Ewing, Darrell Wayne Fair, Frederick Gokliz (San Carlos Apache), Terran Last Gun (Piikani), and Monty Little (Diné). These artworks are presented alongside broadsides from the newspapers *Akwesasne Notes*, *Winter Soldier*, and *The Black Panther*, as well as selections from the Newberry's Edward E. Ayer Indigenous Studies collection, including the Black Horse Ledger and the Kiowa ledger drawings.

Spanning from the 1870s to the present, these works navigate and respond to the intertwined violence of the "American Indian Wars" and the "Global War on Terror." By drawing parallels between military strategies that profile, target, and devastate BIPOC communities and the persistent anti-colonial resistance that counters these forces, the relationships forged within these works propose uncommon alliances that serve as a foundation for solidarity.

The artworks are accompanied by original essays from American historian Roxanne Dunbar-Ortiz and Native/Chicana curator and writer Meranda Roberts, as well as poetry by veteran artist Erika R. Land.

In her essay "Why Is the United States the Most Militaristic State in History?," Roxanne Dunbar-Ortiz argues that US militarism is deeply rooted in the nation's founding as a fiscal-military state, designed to conquer the continent through settler militias, who were promised land in exchange for their participation in the frontier wars. This military culture, stemming from British-colonial "savage war" tactics and later enshrined in the US Constitution's Second Amendment, has persisted through continuous counterinsurgency operations both domestically and internationally, shaping the nation's identity and political mythology. This violent legacy elicits the insurgent aesthetic responses embodied in the exhibited artworks, from the Black Horse Ledger to *For Those Who Have No Voice* by Gilbert Kills Pretty Enemy III, and *MQ-9/3* by Mahwish Chishty.

Meranda Roberts's essay "Unlikely Rebellions, Reckonings, and Refusals," a reflection on the Triennial exhibitions and performances, is grounded in her personal experience as an Indigenous scholar and activist. In her review, Roberts considers how the exhibited artists actively refuse to let the long wars silence or shame them. She argues that through continuous and courageous creation, these artists demand that we bear witness to their joy, pain, and grief. This act of creation pierces the isolation perpetuated by the traumas of settler colonialism, fostering a shared experience of seeing and being seen.

Like Roberts, this section bears witness to the ceaseless manifestations of creative rebellion against the void of unrelenting war.

The Devil Will Always Find Work / "Watch Us Survive"

ERIKA RENEE LAND

Adapted from a spoken word poem performed at the STLW *Summit, in response to Rodney Ewing's artwork* Pathfinder (Harriet Tubman); *see p. 32.*

The devil went to war with Africa,
And African people were
Pillaged,
Captured,
Renamed,
Sold,
Transported,

Uprooted and Replanted
oceans away.

Through it all
Their spirits said,
"Watch us survive."

It's my job to mend and bring color
To the broken shadows of life.

When I think about surviving
the long wars
I think of the aftermath.
Paths taken to survive during and
after a war.
I think about how important
it is to shine a light on pathfinders,
not profiteers.

It's our job to keep their stories alive.
BECAUSE
The devil will always find work.
CENSORSHIP
WAR
REPRESSION
GENOCIDE
COLONIALISM
IMPERIALISM
7 DEADLY SINS

When I think about surviving
the long wars
I think of the aftermath.
Paths taken to survive during
and after a war.
I think about how important it is
to shine a light on pathfinders,
not profiteers.

When I look at Rodney Ewing's
work *Pathfinder*
I think about my ancestors,
And the paths they took to survive,
And the Pathfinders that led
the way.
I see Harriet Tubman as a telescopic
guide with a telescopic eye,
Measuring paths and slopes with
only her mind.

I hypothesize
She was able to commit
the shapes of trees
And walking paths to memory
flawlessly.

I imagine her vision ebbing
and flowing
As she calculated distances,
pensively looking for the devil.
Slave owners and their dogs.
City henchmen and their wives.
Tom, Dick and Harry, who lied
when they said they were on her side.

Harriet had to navigate hundreds of
people trying to take her life.

I think about
How mentally stable she was
or was not
navigating those railroad lines.

History doesn't always provide
the full story.

When I think about surviving
the long wars.
I think of the aftermath.
Paths taken to survive during
and after a war.
I think about how important it is
to shine a light on pathfinders.

The Devil Will Always Find Work.

HARRIET TUBMAN sang,
"Watch us survive."

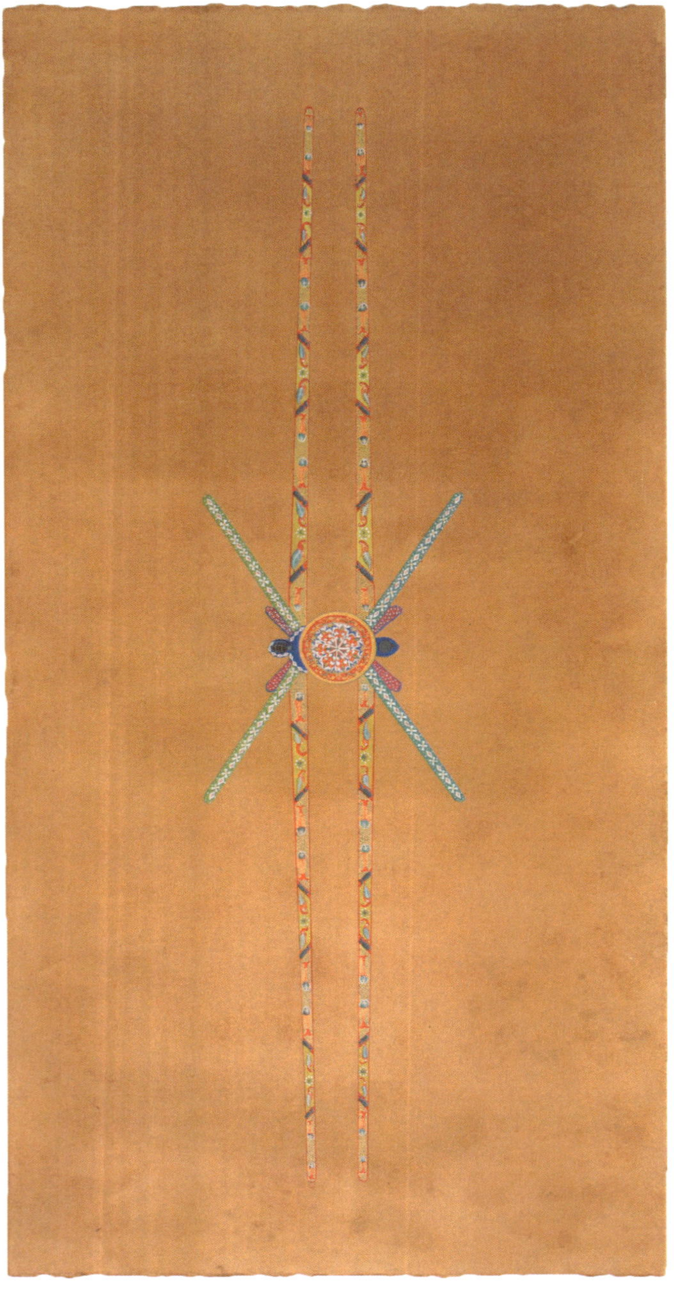

MAHWISH CHISHTY

(b. 1980)
this page: ***MQ-9/3***, 2013
Gouache and tea stain
on paper

opposite page: ***MQ-9/5***, 2013
Gouache and tea stain
on paper

In *MQ-9/5*, two eyes look back at the viewer from the center of the silhouette of a General Atomics MQ-9 Reaper. Each work in Mahwish Chishty's *Drone Art* series starts with a silhouette of an unmanned aerial vehicle (drone), on which she paints colorful symbols influenced by the Pakistani folk tradition of "truck art." Chishty utilizes the shape of these often unseen military vehicles to emphasize their presence and juxtapose the terror they produce with representations of beauty.

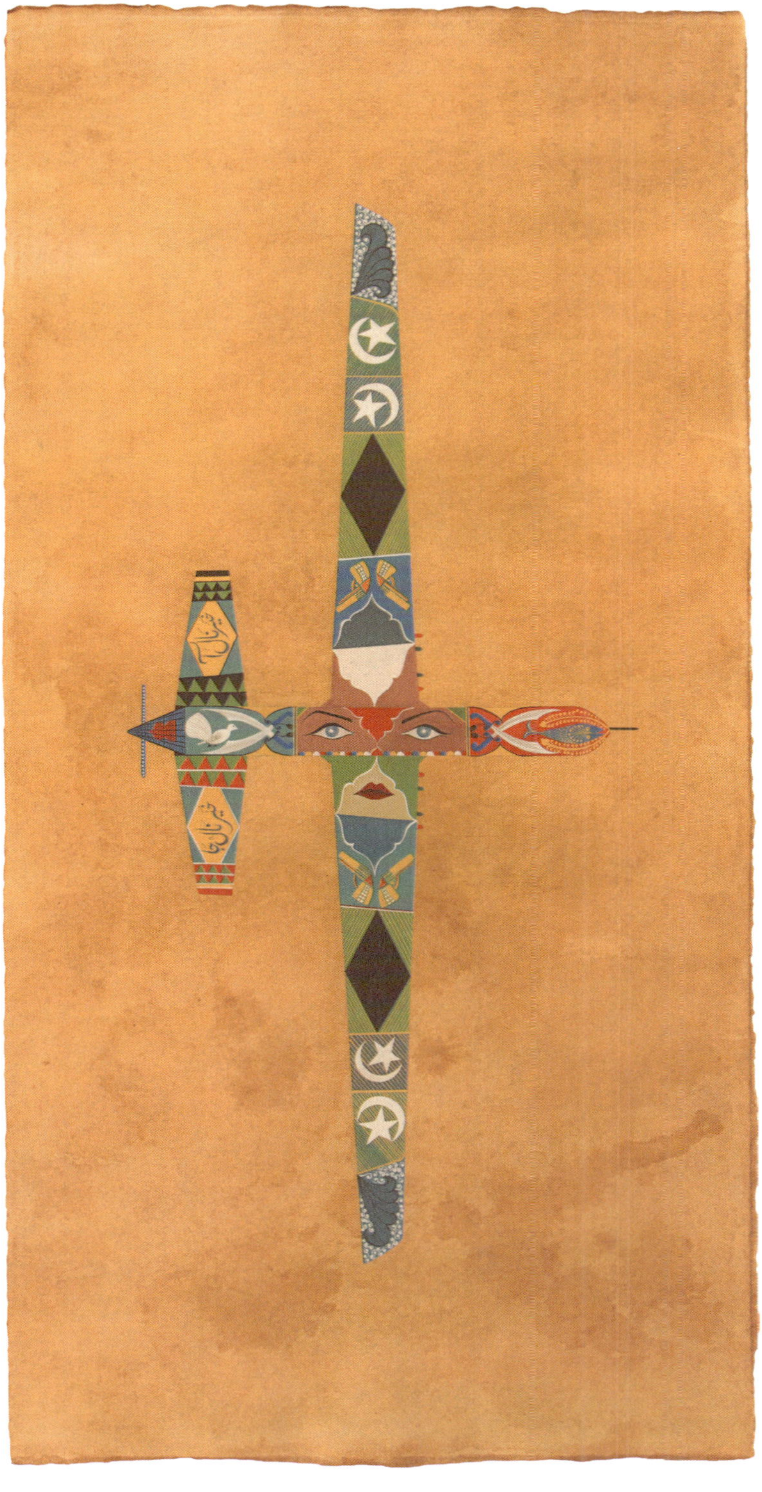

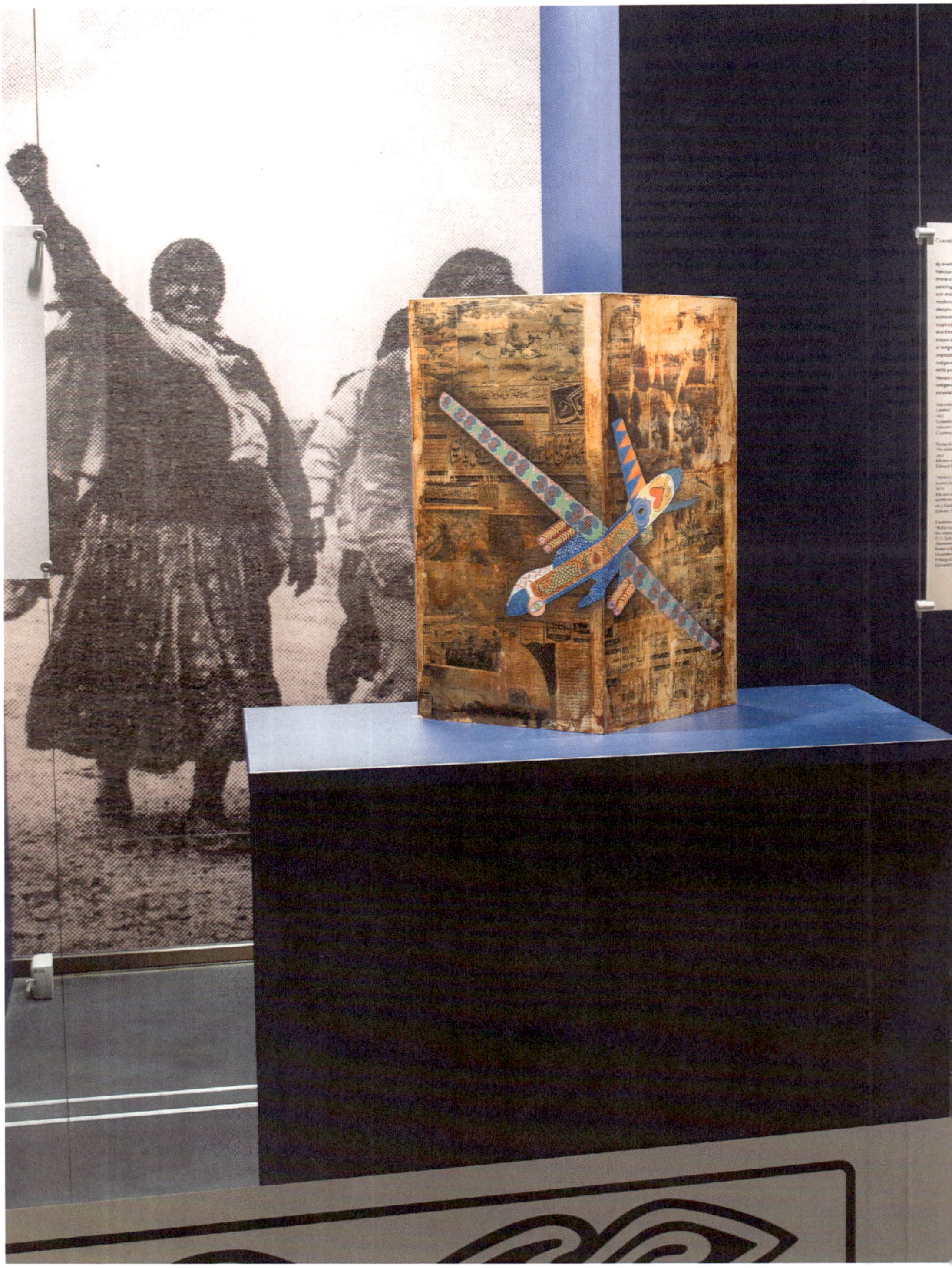

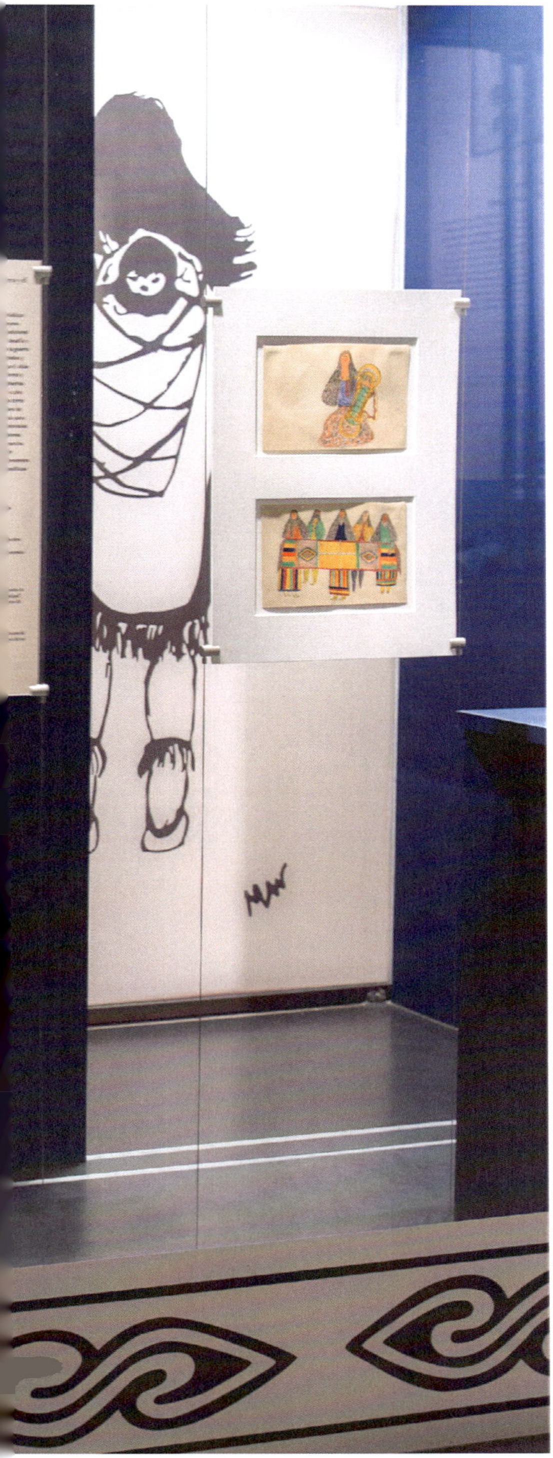

from left to right:

AKWESASNE NOTES
Unattributed photograph with caption, "Roberta Blackgoat of Big Mountain is one of the organizers of the march in support of Navajo JUA (Joint Use Area) residents"
Rooseveltown, NY: Mohawk Nation, December 1979
Enlarged digital reproduction
Courtesy of the Edward E. Ayer Collection

MAHWISH CHISHTY *(b. 1980)*
Untitled, 2013
Gouache, tea stain, and photo transfers on Masonite

By overlaying photo-transfers of Pakistani newspaper articles about US drone attacks with traditional miniature painting, Mahwish Chishty challenges and makes visible the cruel reality of modern warfare with ornate and colorful designs.

AKWESASNE NOTES
Illustration of a person carrying a cradleboard attributed with the initials "MW"
Rooseveltown, NY: Mohawk Nation, July/August 1970
Enlarged digital reproduction
Courtesy of the Edward E. Ayer Collection

FREDERICK GOKLIZ *(San Carlos Apache, 1863–1904) [US Army veteran and prisoner of war]*
top: ***Woman and baby in cradleboard***, ca. 1894–1899
bottom: ***Group presents blanket***, ca. 1894–1899
Ink and watercolor on paper
Courtesy of the Edward E. Ayer Collection

Miridith Campbell describes the importance of toy cradleboards to highlight how children learn "to love, take care and uphold their responsibilities as society members." The importance of the cradleboard and passing on generational knowledge is reflected in the brightly hued drawings of maternal and community care by Frederick Gokliz, made when he was paradoxically both imprisoned by the US—as an enemy POW—and serving in the US Army. Similar themes are evident in the illustration from *Akwesasne Notes*, a newspaper published by the Mohawk Nation from 1969 to 1996. Collectively, these works highlight resistance and "survivance" through maintaining community traditions.

see next spread

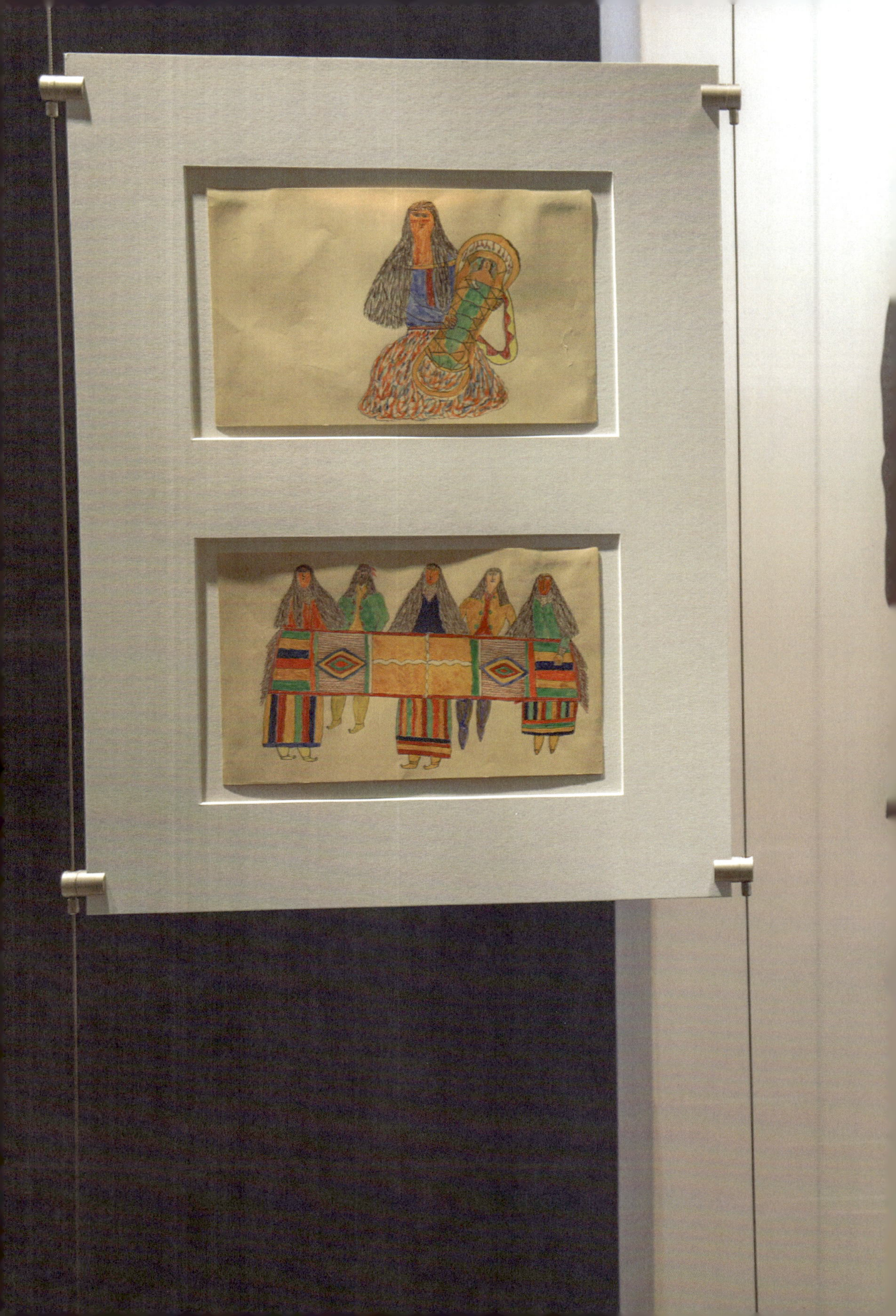

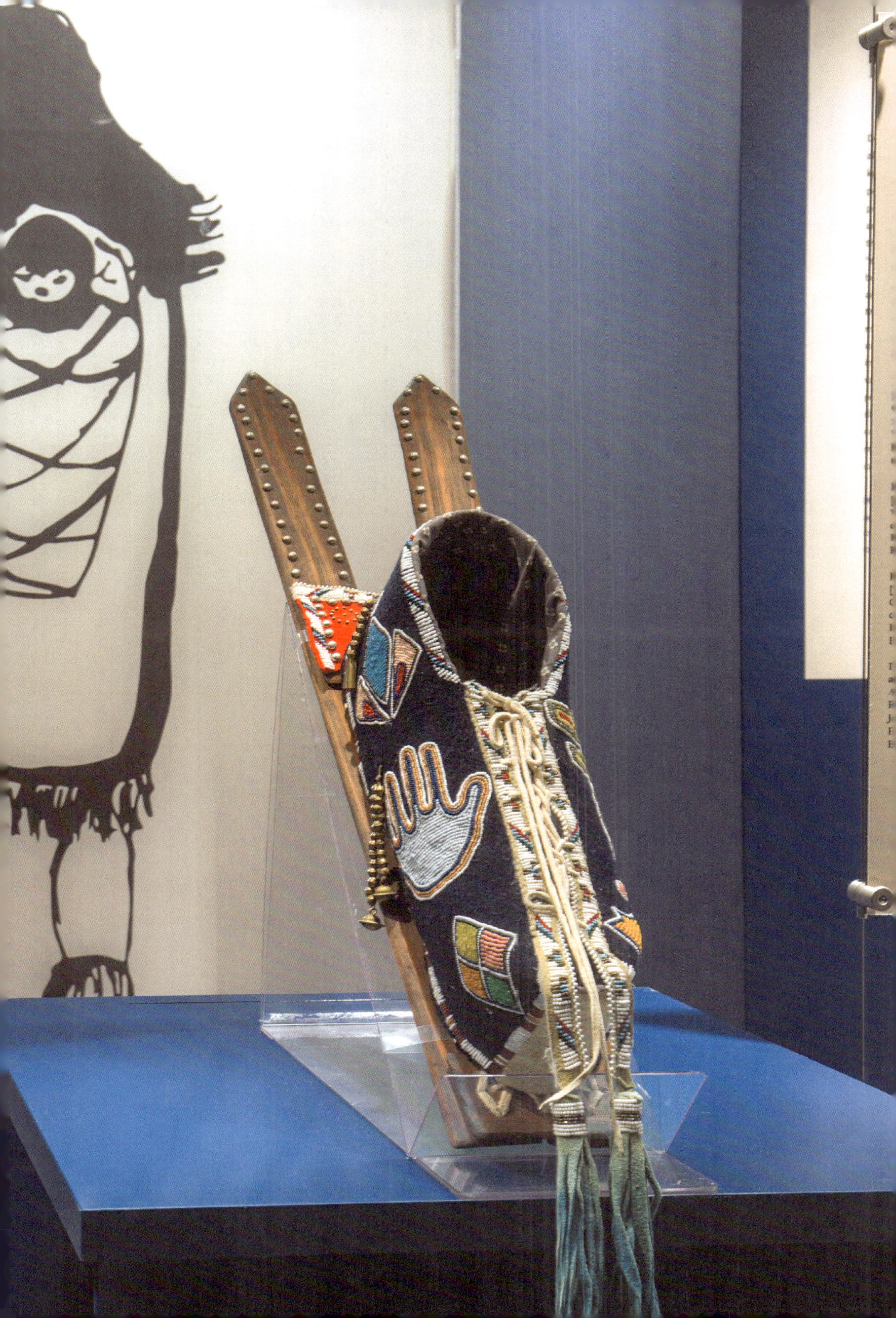

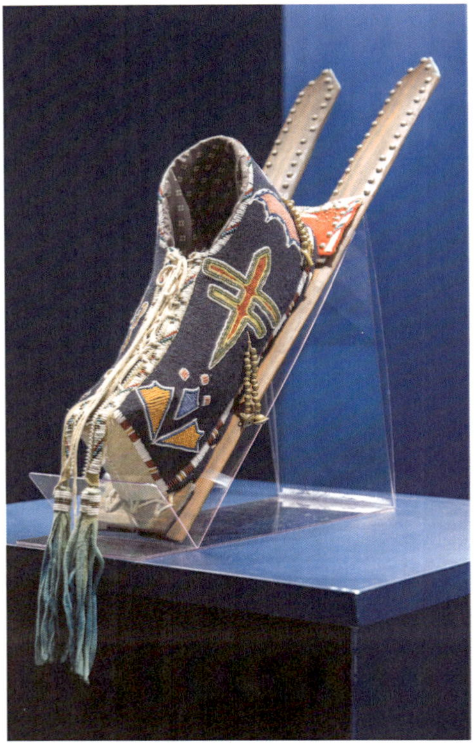

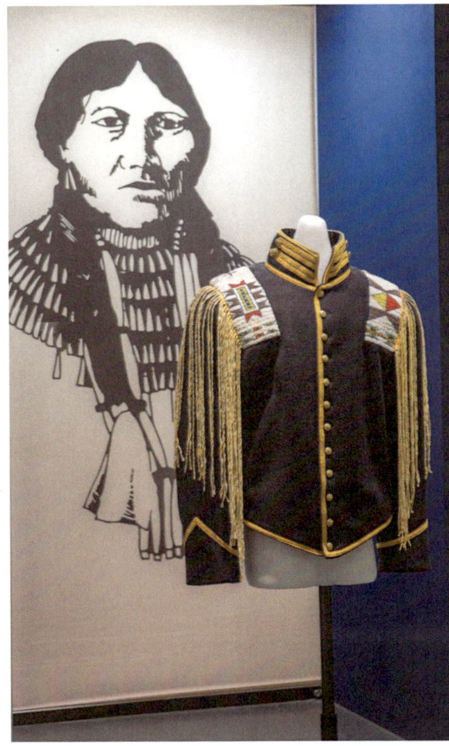

MIRIDITH CAMPBELL *(Kiowa, b. 1966)*
[US Marine Corps, Army, and Navy veteran]
left photo: ***Cradleboard***, 1998
Wood, leather, rawhide, brass tacks, wool, seed beads, and buckskin

right photo, background: ***AKWESASNE NOTES***
Unattributed illustration of an Indigenous person
Rooseveltown, NY: Mohawk Nation, April 1974
Enlarged digital reproduction
Courtesy of the Edward E. Ayer Collection

right photo, foreground: **MIRIDITH CAMPBELL**
Counting Coup, 2002
US cavalry coat, seed beads, and buckskin

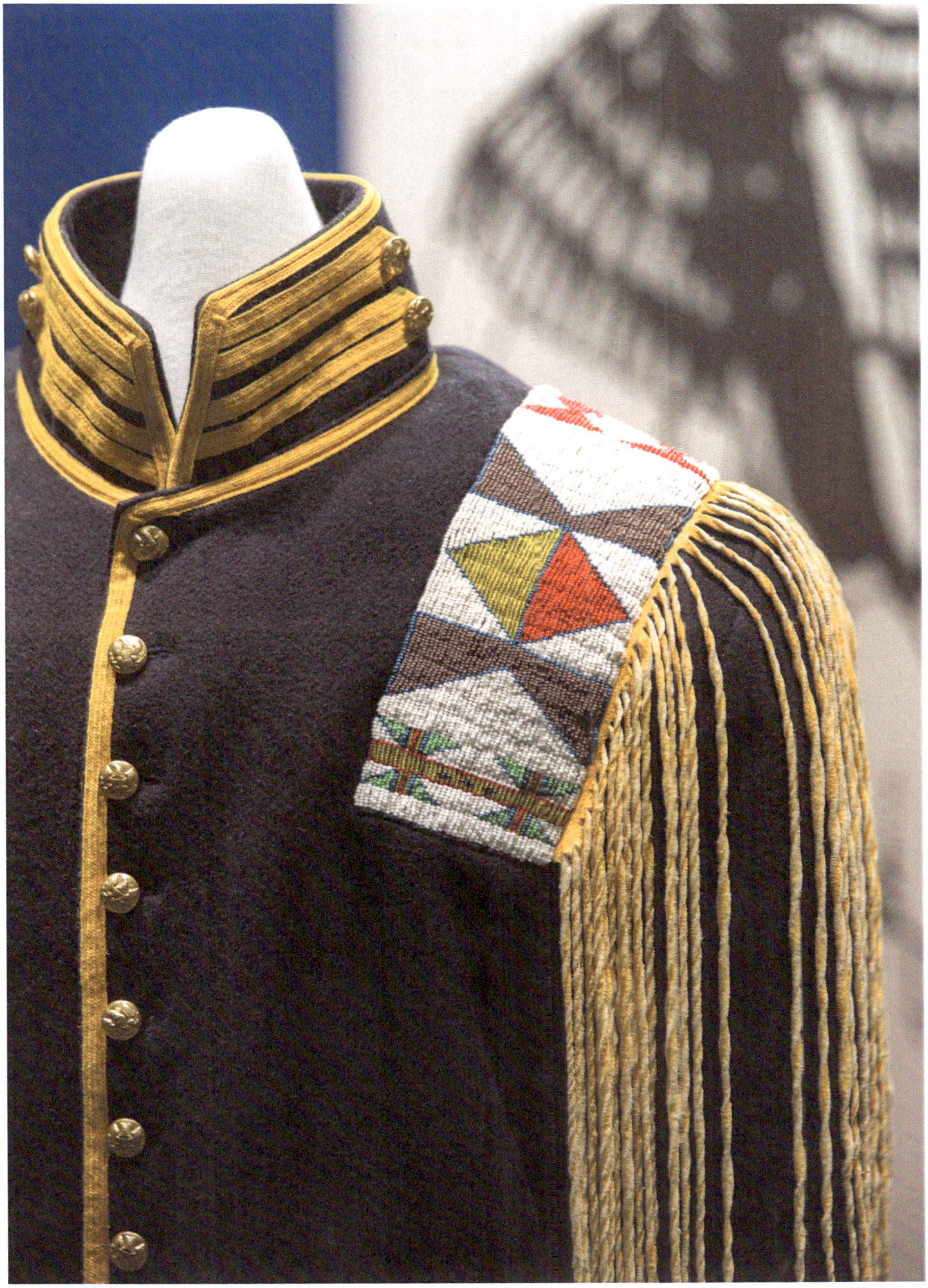

"Counting coup" refers to the Indigenous practice of counting successful touches, or strikes, a warrior makes against a foe during battle. Such acts of bravery also include confiscating and repurposing enemy property. For *Counting Coup*, Miridith Campbell appropriated a Civil War-era US cavalry coat and adorned it with Kiowa-style beadwork. She described the work as representing a "spoil of war."

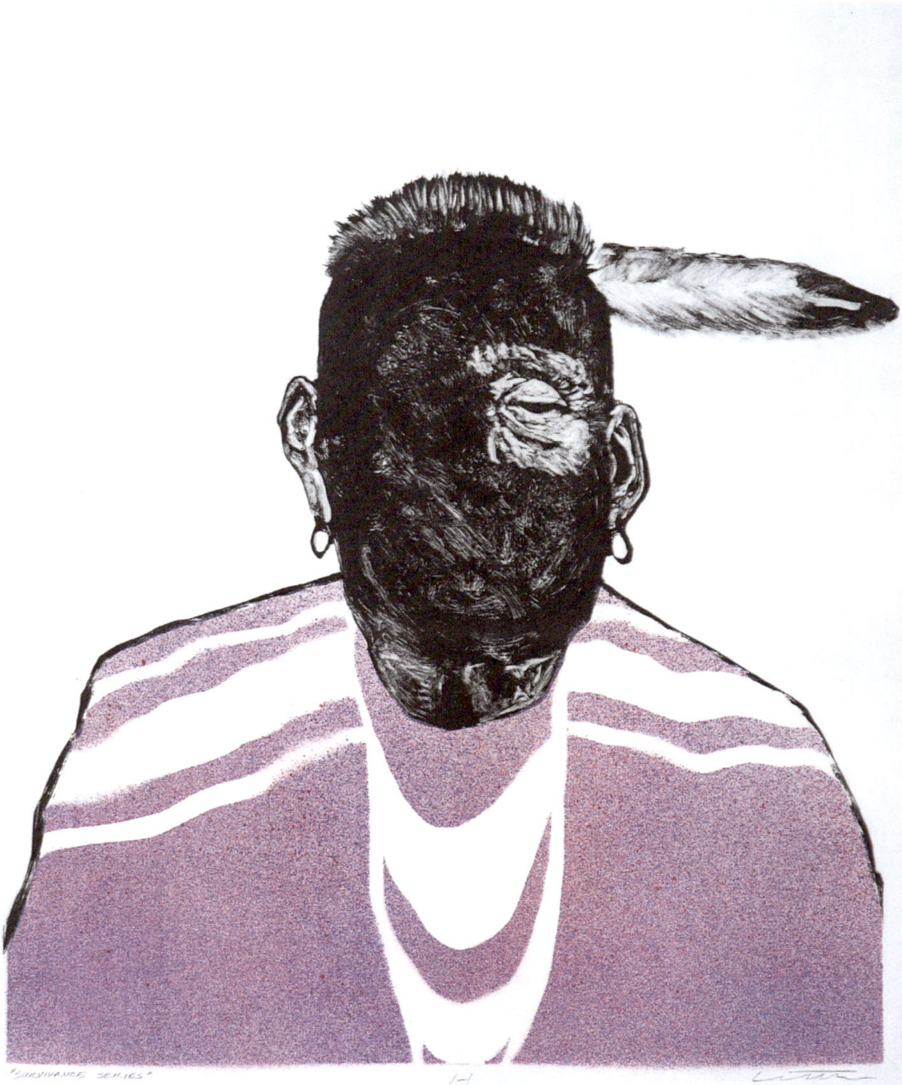

MONTY LITTLE *(Diné, b. 1983)*
[US Marine Corps veteran]
Survivance, 14, 2022–23
Monoprint on BFK Rives cotton paper

Coined by Anishinaabe author Gerald Vizenor, "survivance" refers to the continuation, presence, resistance, and survival of Indigenous peoples. Survivance becomes visible throughout Indigenous creative practices. In the ongoing *Survivance* monoprint series by Monty Little, subjects look back defiantly at the viewer, renouncing dominance, tragedy, and victimization. Their gaze is meant to show an active sense of presence and the continuance of Indigenous stories.

see detail on p. 54

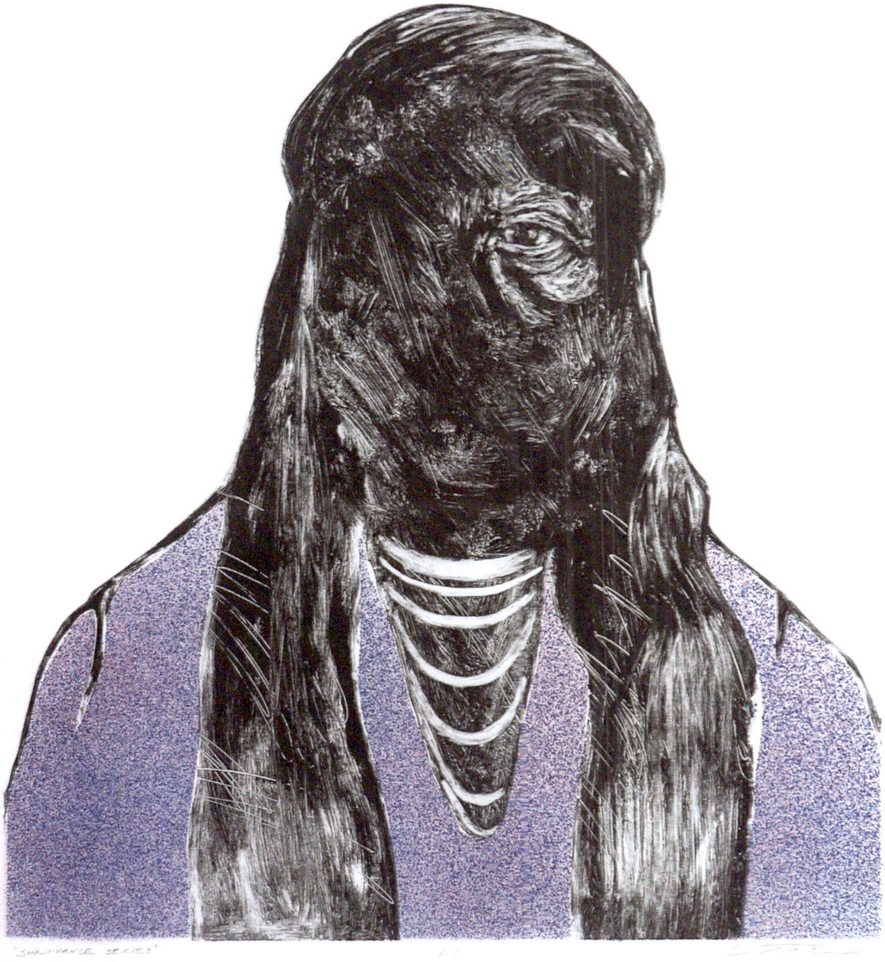

Survivance, 15, 2022–23
Monoprint on BFK Rives cotton paper

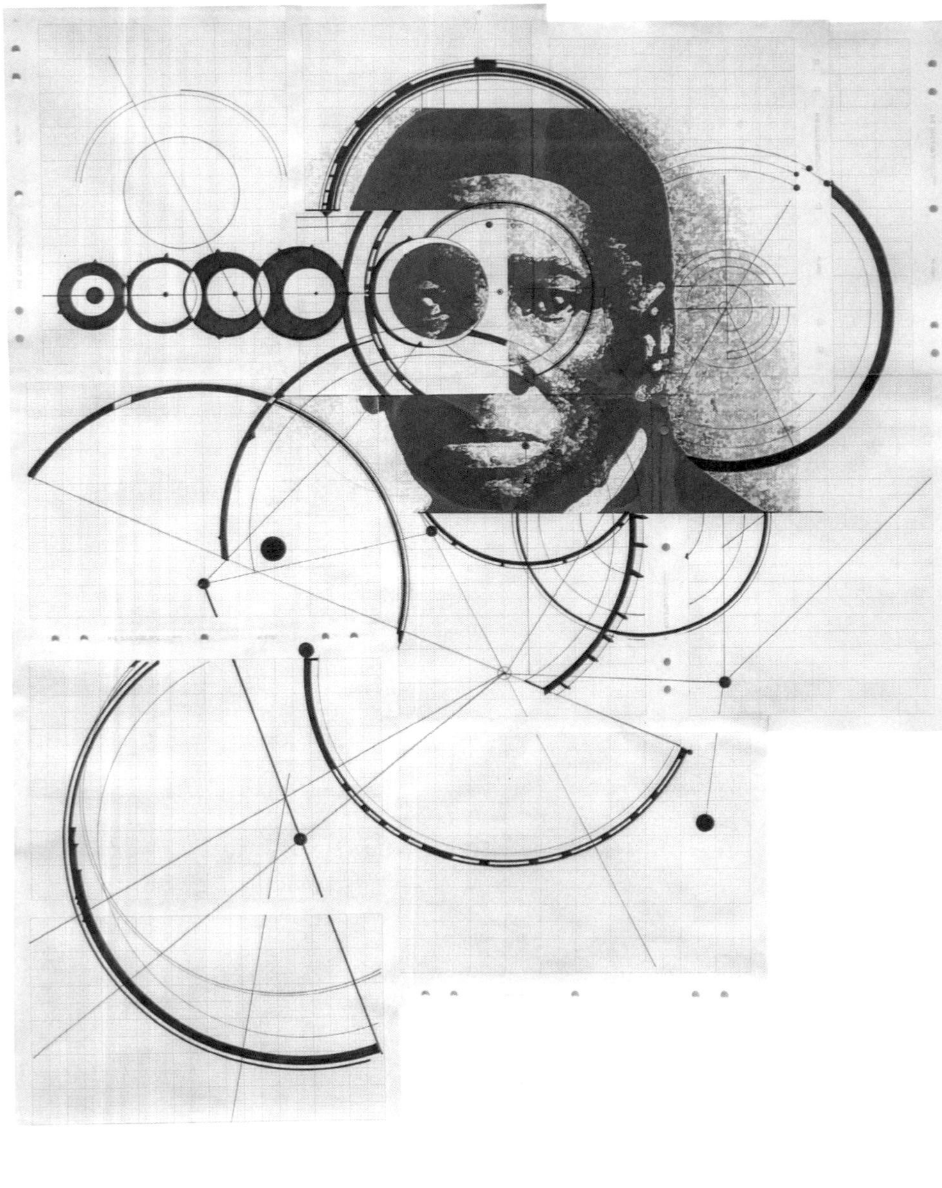

RODNEY EWING *(b. 1964) [US Army veteran]*
Pathfinder (Harriet Tubman), 2021
Hand-colored silkscreen on graph paper
Courtesy of the artist and Rena Bransten Gallery

The Devil Finds Work series by Rodney Ewing documents the history of the Black Body navigating hostile physical, social, and psychological spaces.

In *Conductor* and *Pathfinder*, Ewing uses ledger paper, a tool of colonial control that was co-opted by Indigenous artists to create works of cultural resistance during the "American Indian Wars." He portrays Harriet Tubman and William Still, two conductors on the Underground Railroad who helped hundreds of enslaved people escape to freedom in the nineteenth century.

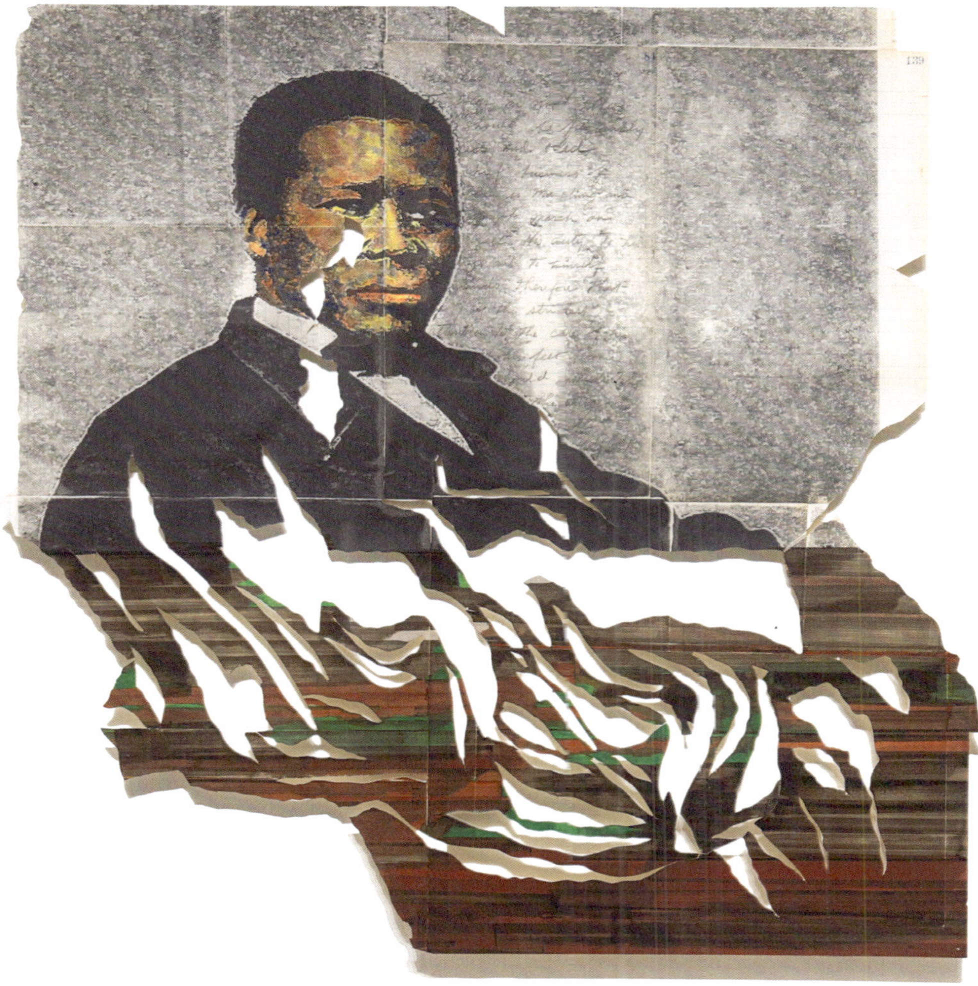

RODNEY EWING *(b. 1964) [US Army veteran]*
Conductor (William Still), 2021
Hand-colored silkscreen on ledger paper
Courtesy of the artist and Rena Bransten Gallery

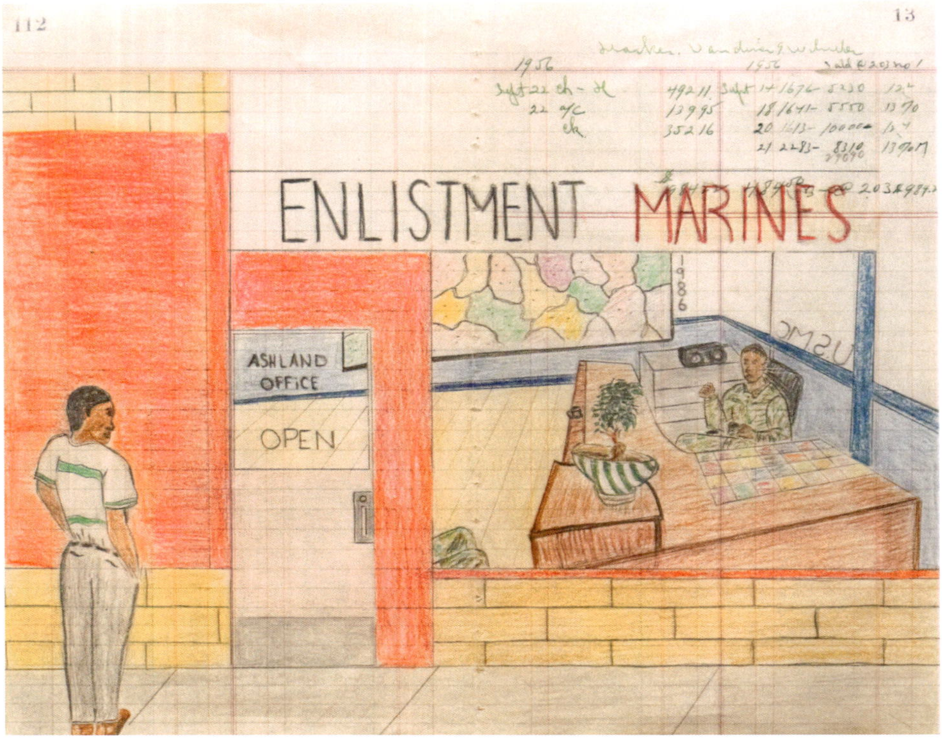

DARRELL WAYNE FAIR *(b. 1967)*
[US Marine Corps veteran]
Enlistment, 2022
Pencil and colored pencil on ledger paper
Courtesy of the artist and Prison + Neighborhood Arts/Education Project

see detail on p. 68

Inspired by nineteenth-century ledger art made by Indigenous prisoners of war, Darrell Wayne Fair uses ledger paper to document his life—from joining the military as a teenager, to his arrest and torture at a Chicago police station, to his time in prison. Through these lived experiences, Fair draws connections between mass incarceration, militarism, and colonialism.

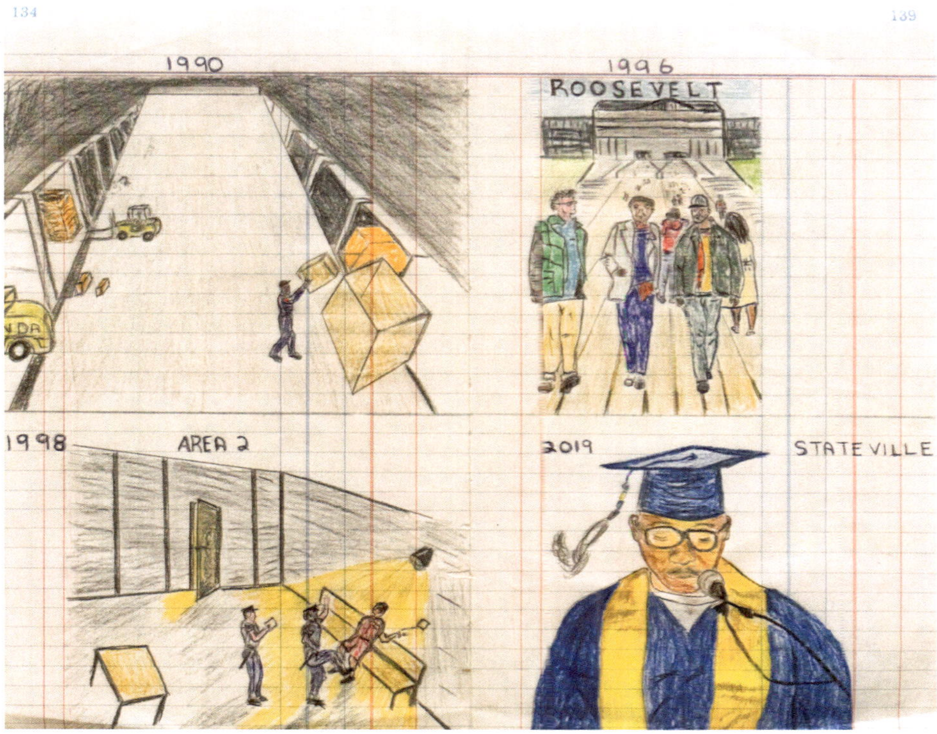

Panel Documentary, 2022
Pencil and colored pencil on ledger paper
Courtesy of the artist and Prison + Neighborhood Arts/Education Project

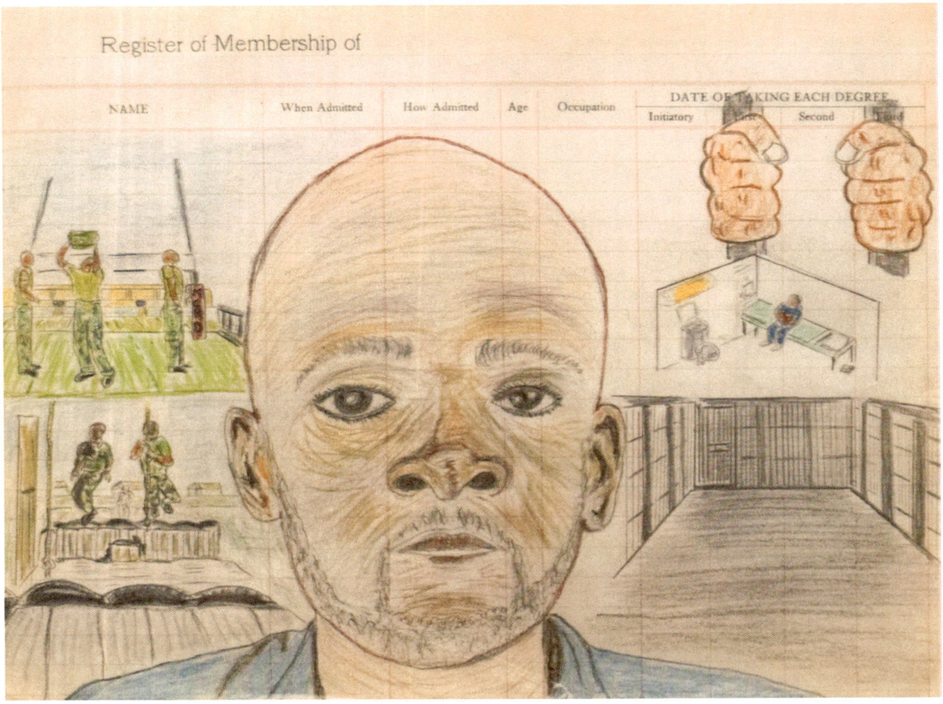

DARRELL WAYNE FAIR *(b. 1967)*
[US Marine Corps veteran]
Self Portrait, 2022
Pencil, colored pencil, acrylic paint, and ink on ledger paper

Courtesy of the artist and Prison + Neighborhood Arts/Education Project

see detail on p. 317

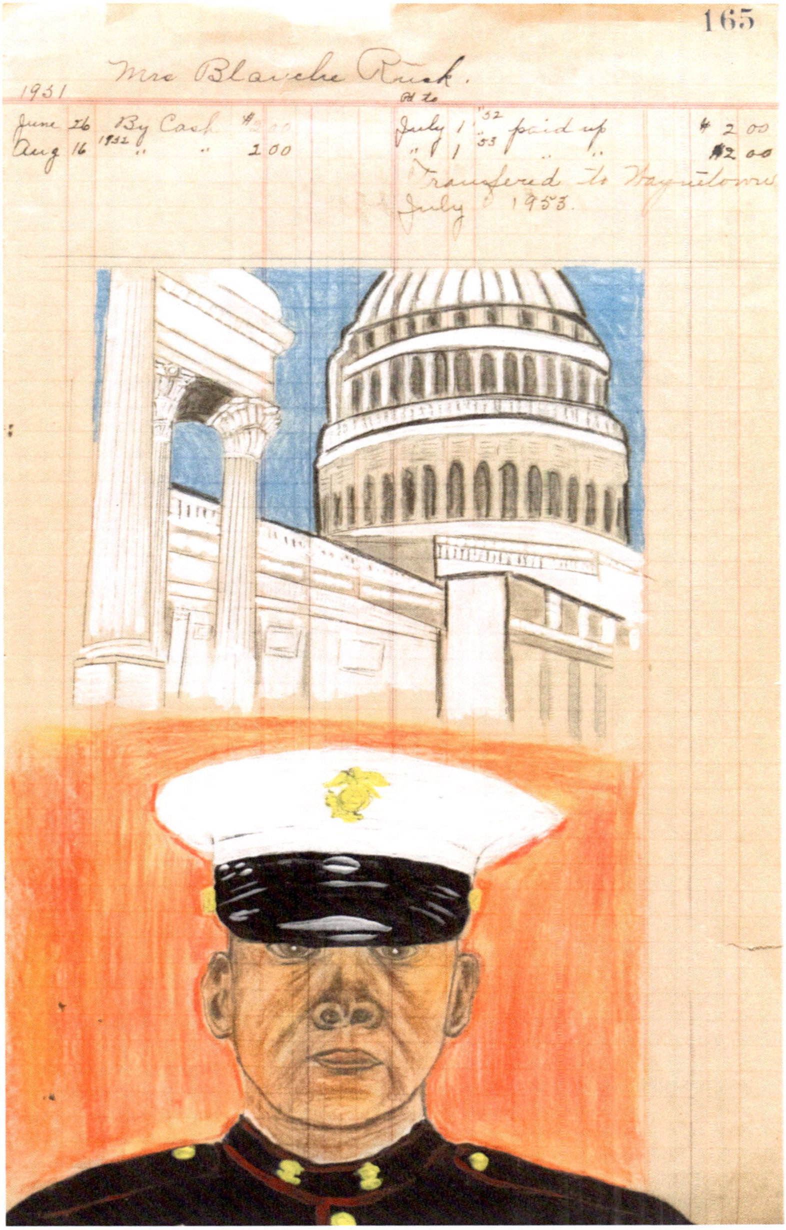

The Facade, 2022
Pencil and colored pencil on ledger paper
Courtesy of the artist and Prison + Neighborhood Arts/Education Project

In a reflection on his art, Fair notes, "Our government as well as uniformed service members . . . present this polished facade but many layers exist beneath both."

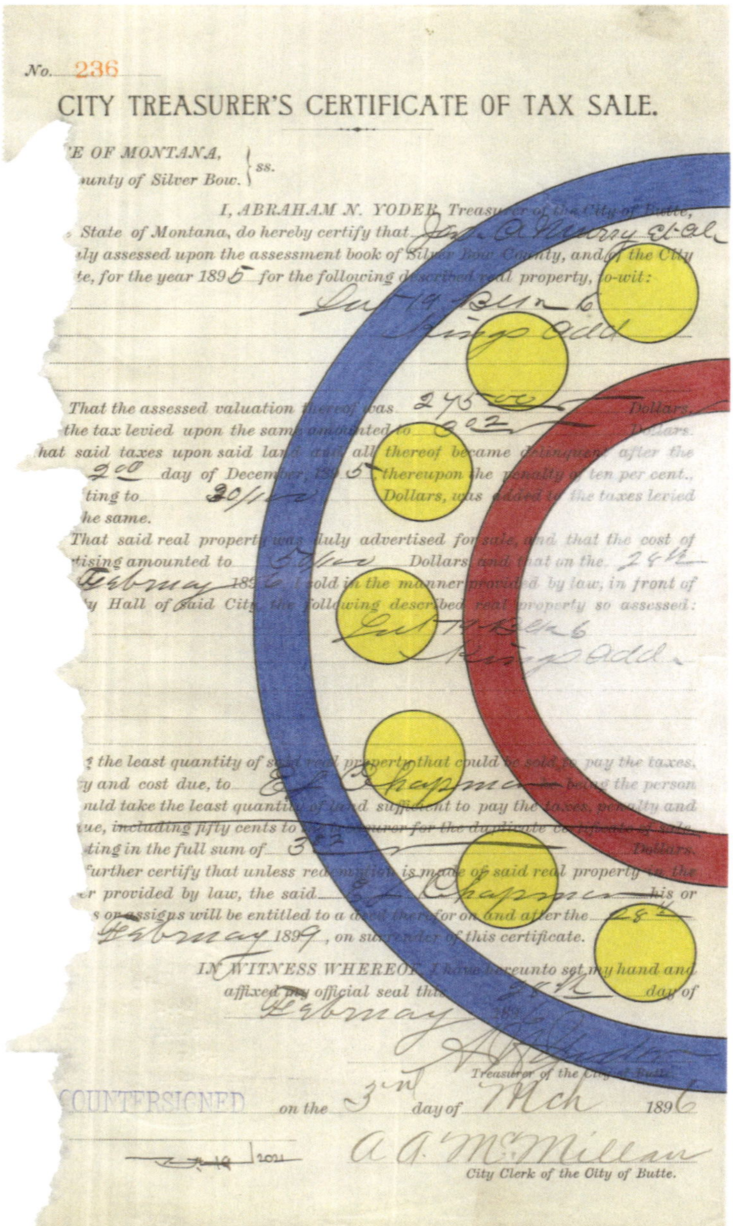

TERRAN LAST GUN *(Piikani, b. 1989)*
above: ***The ancient people of the West live on***, 2021
Ink and colored pencil on found paper
Courtesy of the Edward E. Ayer Collection

opposite page: ***10,000 journeys around the sun with moon***, 2021
Ink and colored pencil on a "City Treasurer's certificate of tax sale," dated in Butte, Montana, on March 3, 1896
Courtesy of the Edward E. Ayer Collection

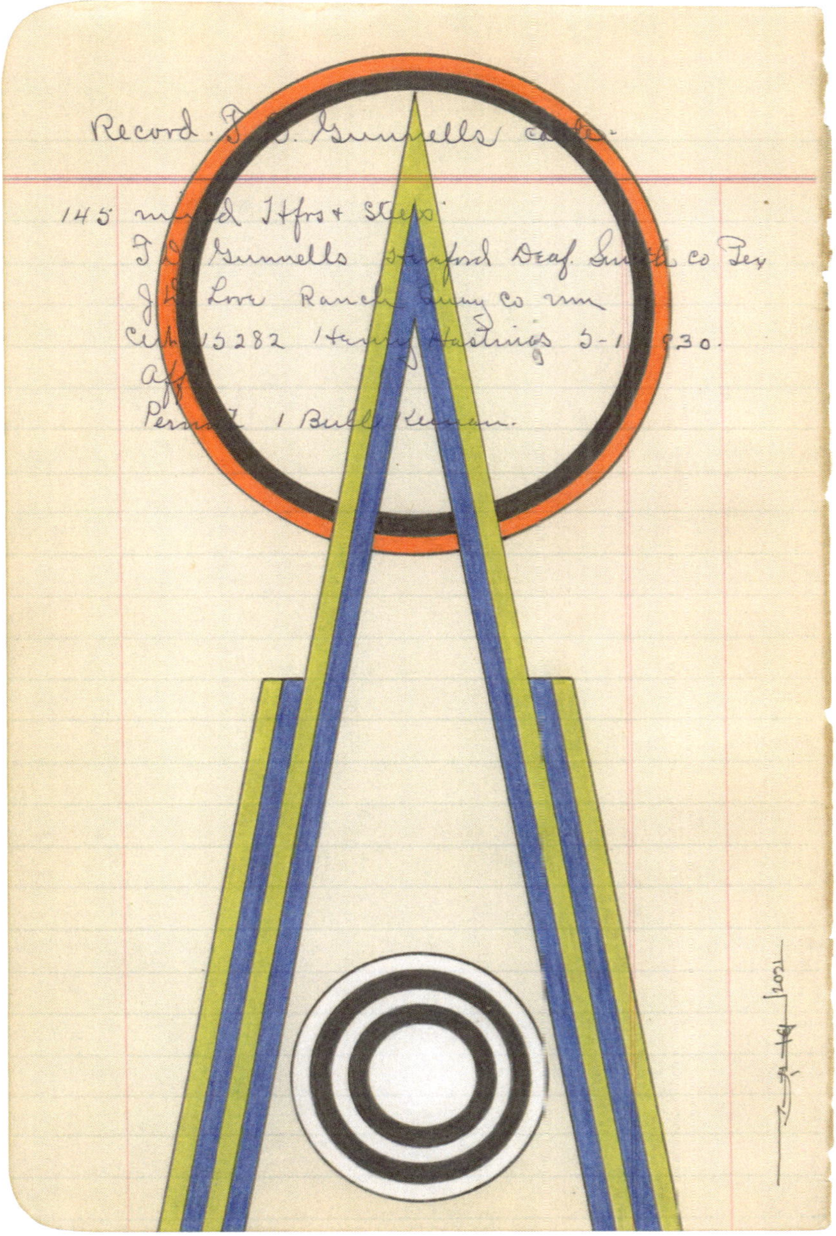

Terran Last Gun places explorations of color, form, and nature in images of Piikani, or Blackfoot, painted lodges (commonly known as "tipis") against the backdrop of ledger paper to interrupt the colonial implications of the paper and center Indigenous worldviews.

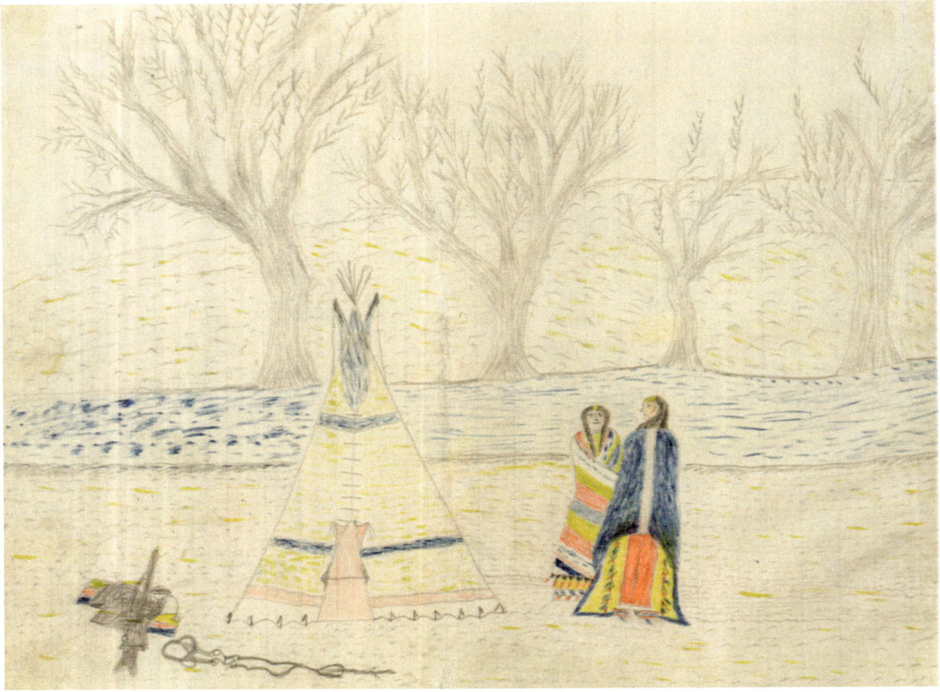

KIOWA INDIAN LEDGER DRAWINGS
ca. 1880–1890
Colored pencil on ledger paper
Courtesy of the Edward E. Ayer Collection

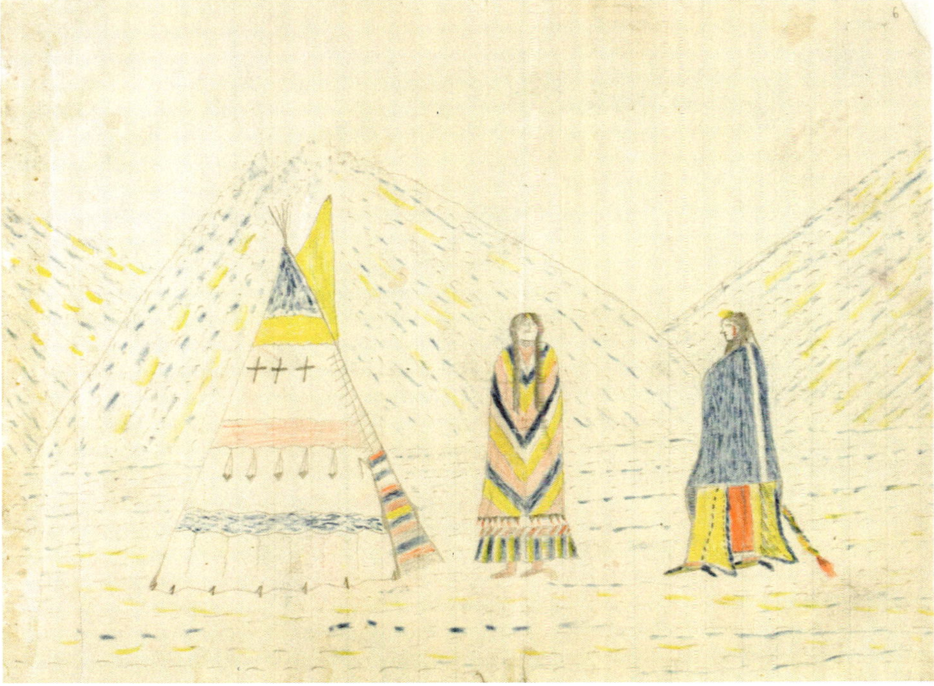

Ledger art is part of the long tradition of Indigenous people chronicling their lives both despite and in response to settler colonialism. A series of Kiowa ledger drawings on blank sheets of blue-ruled paper includes illustrations of family life, as well as scenes of hunting, courtship, and battles with US soldiers. Parallel colorful patterns appear in the bright ornamentation used in Mahwish Chishty's *Drone Art* series (pp. 22–23, 174–75), Terran Last Gun's ledger drawings (pp. 38–39), and Miridth Campbell's bead work (pp. 27–29, 71, 88–91, 250, 319). Each of these artists draws from their respective creative traditions to repurpose military technology as a means of returning the colonial gaze

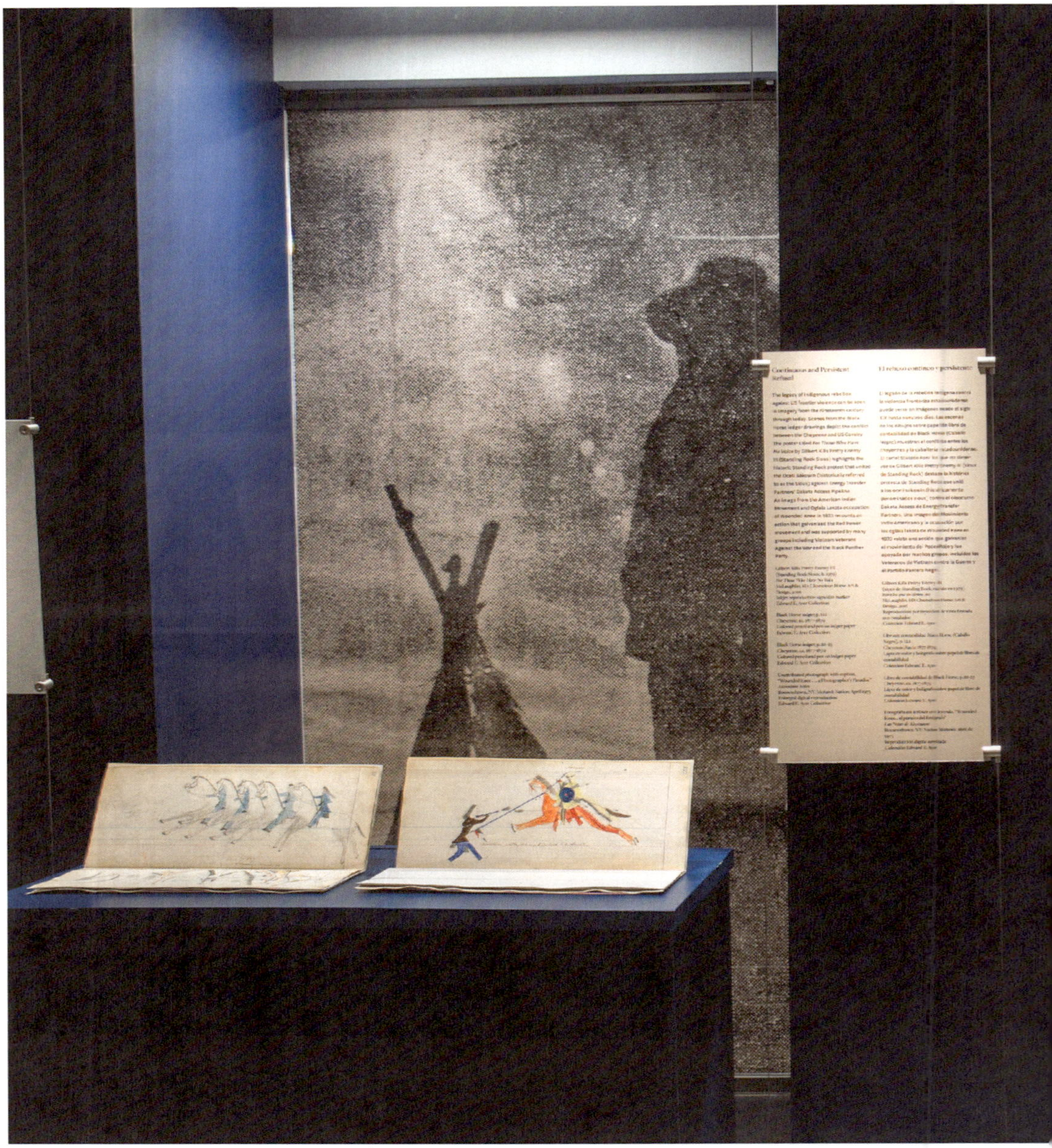

foreground: **BLACK HORSE LEDGER**
left: ***pp. 22–23 and*** *right:* ***p. 122***
see also: pp. 44–46, 68

background: ***AKWESASNE NOTES***
Unattributed photograph with caption,
"Wounded Knee . . . a Photographer's Paradise"
Rooseveltown, NY: Mohawk Nation, April 1973
Enlarged digital reproduction
Courtesy of the Edward E. Ayer Collection

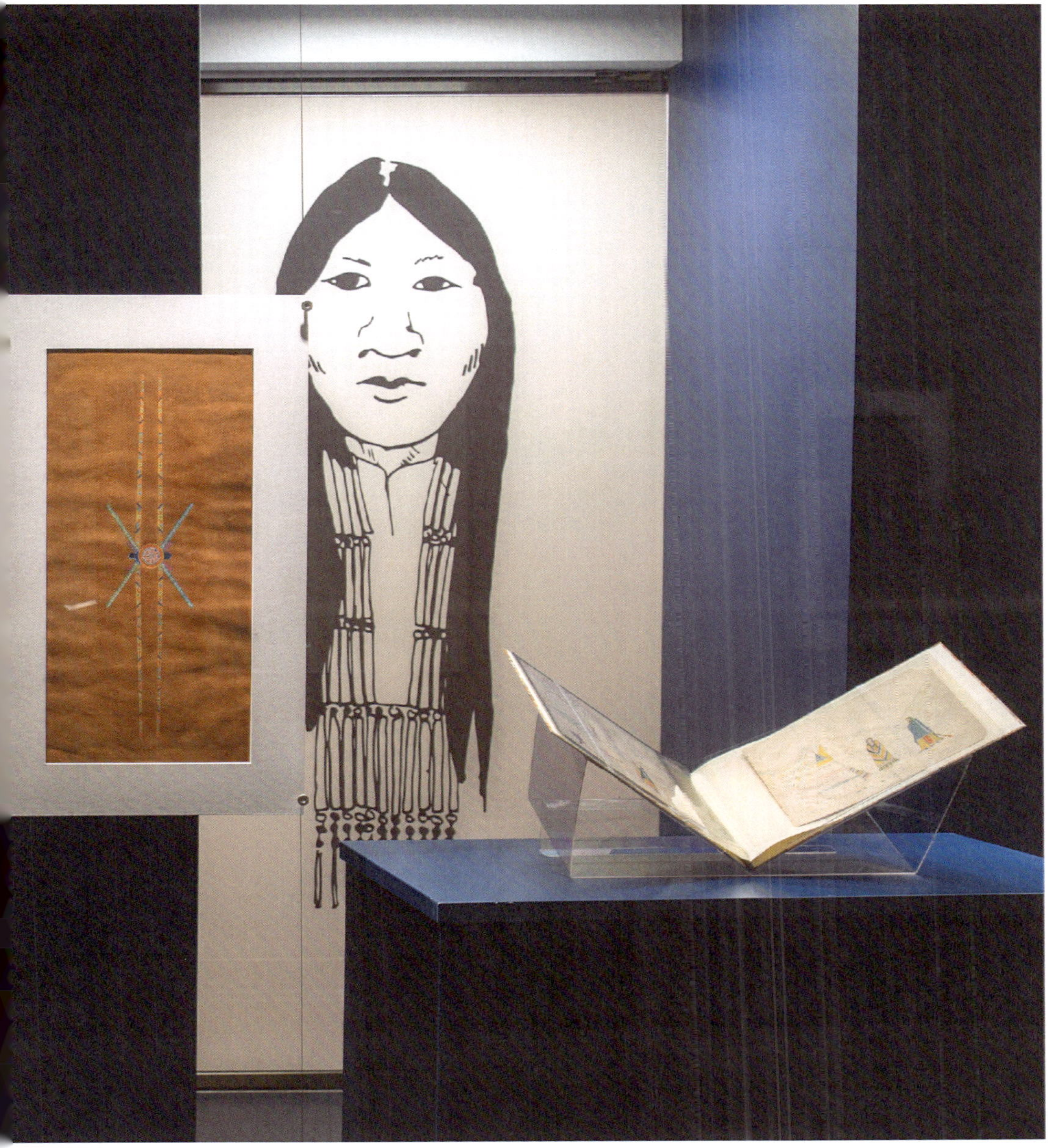

left foreground: **MAHWISH CHISHTY**
MQ-9/3 - *see also: p. 22*

right foreground: **KIOWA INDIAN LEDGER DRAWINGS** - *see also: pp. 40–41*

background: ***AKWESASNE NOTES***
Unattributed illustration of an Indigenous person
Rooseveltown, NY: Mohawk Nation, early autumn 1975
Enlarged digital reproduction
Courtesy of the Edward E. Ayer Collection

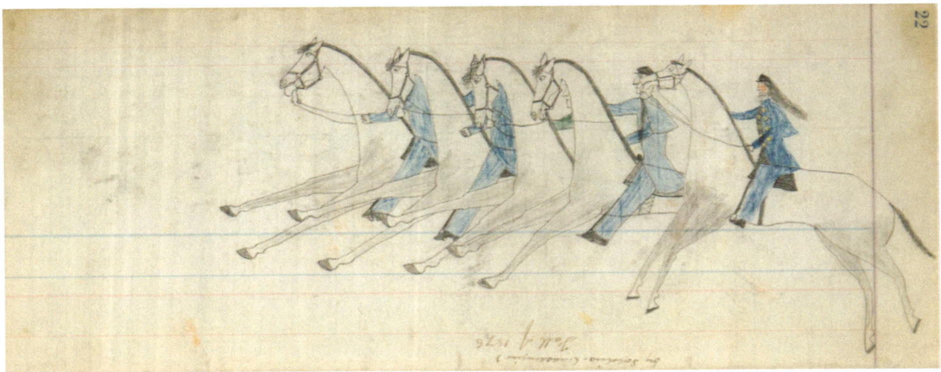

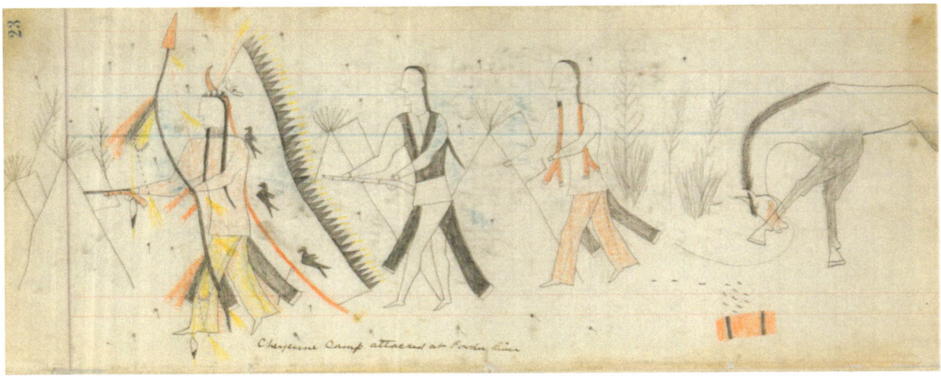

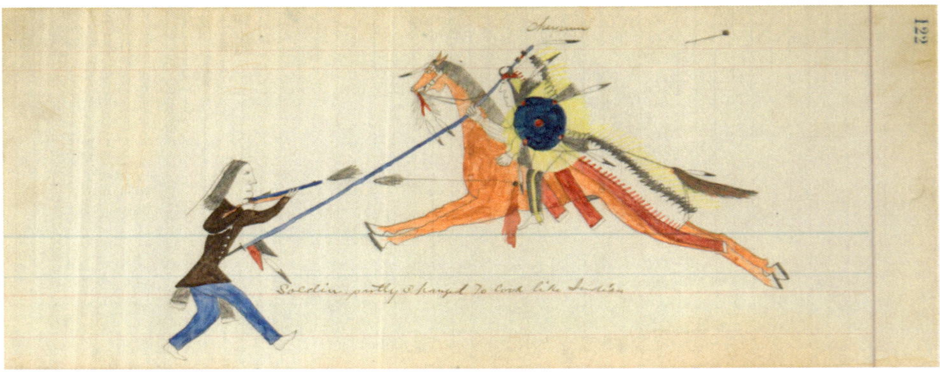

BLACK HORSE LEDGER
from top to bottom: ***p. 22, p. 23, p. 122***
Cheyenne, ca. 1877–1879
Colored pencil and pen on ledger paper
Courtesy of the Edward E. Ayer Collection

Scenes from the Black Horse ledger drawings depict the conflict between the Cheyenne and US Cavalry.

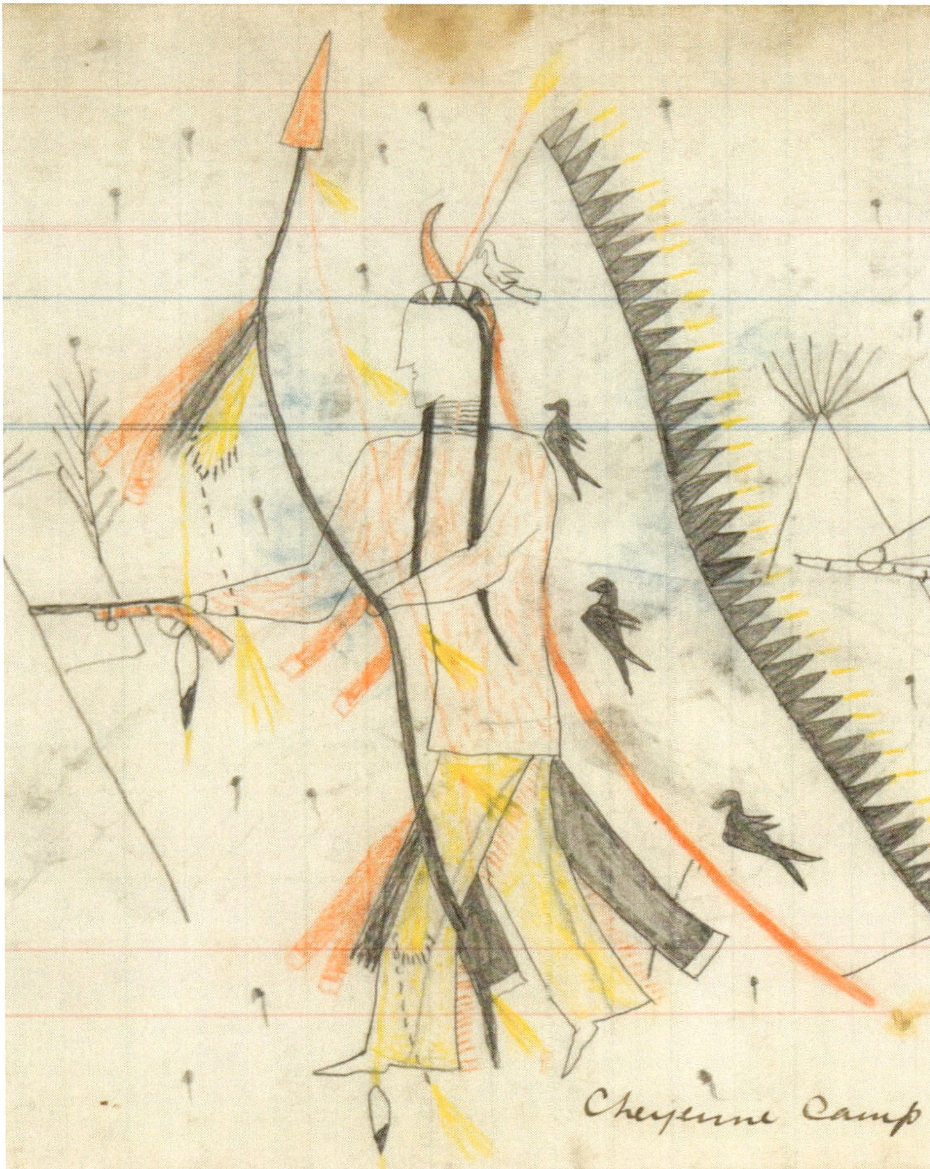

BLACK HORSE LEDGER
p. 23 (detail)

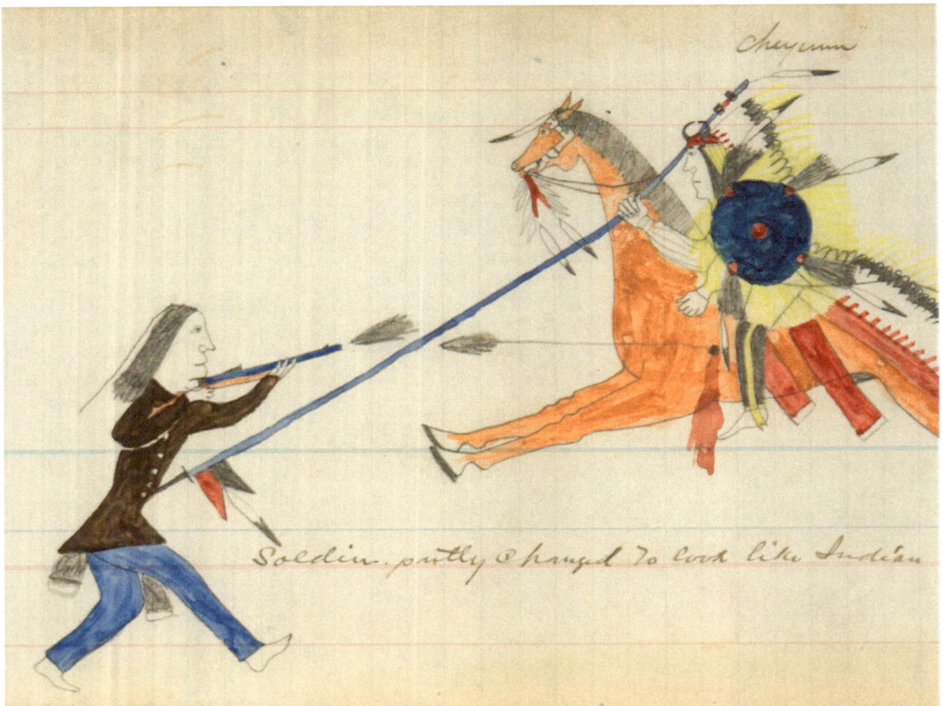

BLACK HORSE LEDGER
p. 122 (detail) - *see previous spread*

opposite page: **GILBERT KILLS PRETTY ENEMY III** *(Standing Rock Sioux, b. 1979)*
For Those Who Have No Voice
McLaughlin, South Dakota: Chameleon Horse Art & Design, 2016
Inkjet reproduction signed in marker
Courtesy of the Edward E. Ayer Collection

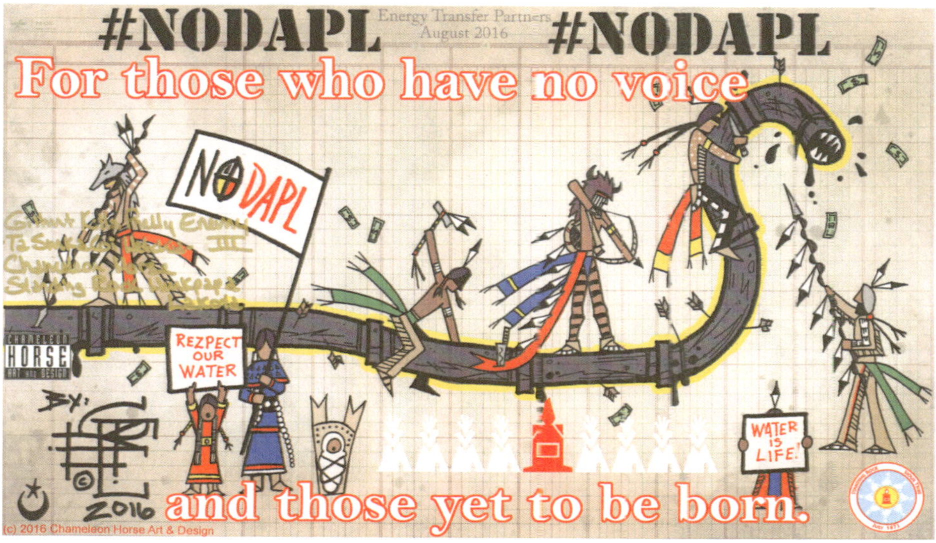
#NODAPL
Energy Transfer Partners
August 2016
#NODAPL
For those who have no voice
NO DAPL
REZPECT OUR WATER
WATER IS LIFE!
By:
2016
and those yet to be born.
(c) 2016 Chameleon Horse Art & Design

The legacy of Indigenous rebellion against US frontier violence can be seen in imagery from the nineteenth century through today. The poster titled *For Those Who Have No Voice* by Gilbert Kills Pretty Enemy III highlights the historic Standing Rock protest that united the Great Sioux Nation, or the Oceti Sakowin (Seven Council Fires), against Energy Transfer Partners' Dakota Access Pipeline.

The Standing Rock mobilization resonates with the historic 1973 American Indian Movement and Oglala Lakota occupation of Wounded Knee, an event that galvanized the Red Power Movement. The Wounded Knee occupation was supported by many activist groups, including Vietnam Veterans Against the War and the Black Panther Party, both of whom covered the direct action in their newspapers. Images of the action printed in *Akwesasne Notes* (see pp. 49–50) were also featured in *The Black Panther* (see p. 53) and *Winter Soldier* (see p. 52).

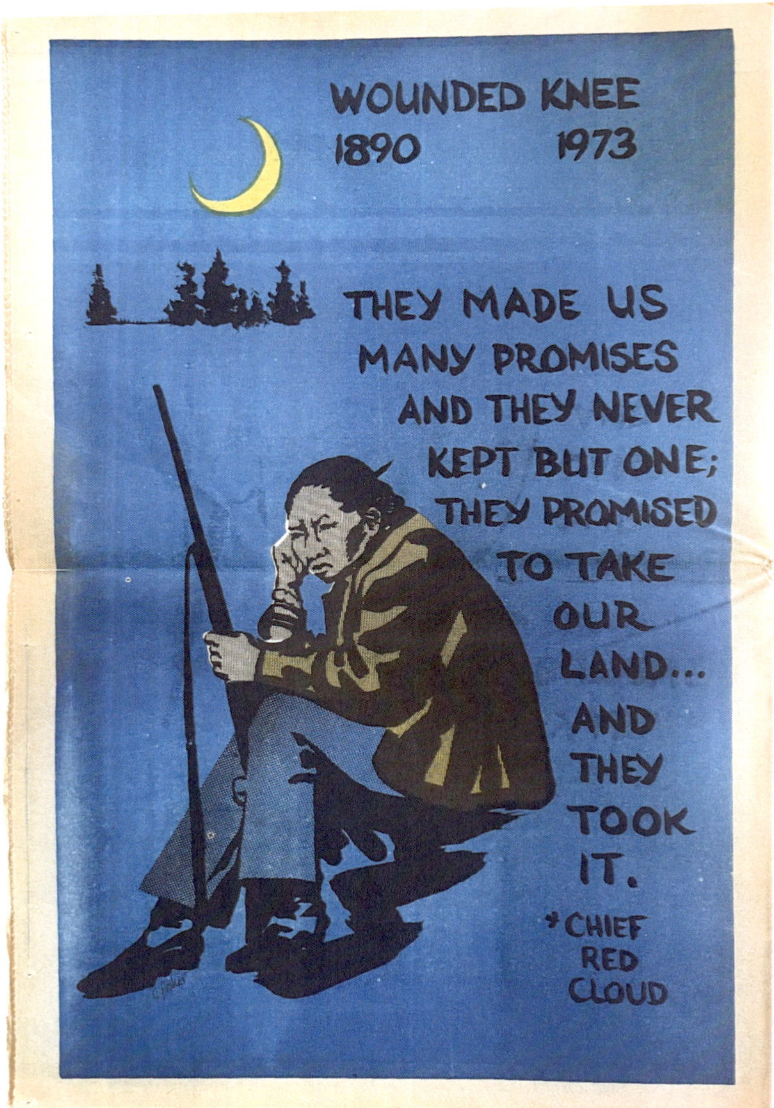
WOUNDED KNEE
1890 1973
THEY MADE US
MANY PROMISES
AND THEY NEVER
KEPT BUT ONE;
THEY PROMISED
TO TAKE
OUR
LAND...
AND
THEY
TOOK
IT.
*CHIEF
RED
CLOUD

above and opposite page, left:

VIETNAM VETERANS AGAINST THE WAR AND CAROL FISHER

Winter Soldier illustration with heading "Wounded Knee 1800–1973"

Chicago, IL: Vietnam Veterans Against the War, May 1973

Offset lithograph on paper

Courtesy of Vietnam Veterans Against the War

Unlikely coalitions become visible in the shared iconography of publications from different people's movements and groups, including *Akwesasne Notes* from the Mohawk Nation, *Winter Soldier* from Vietnam Veterans Against the War, and *The Black Panther* from the Black Panther Party.

The seated figure in the enlarged photograph of the Wounded Knee occupation in *Akwesasne Notes* is mirrored in the broadside illustration from *Winter Soldier*.

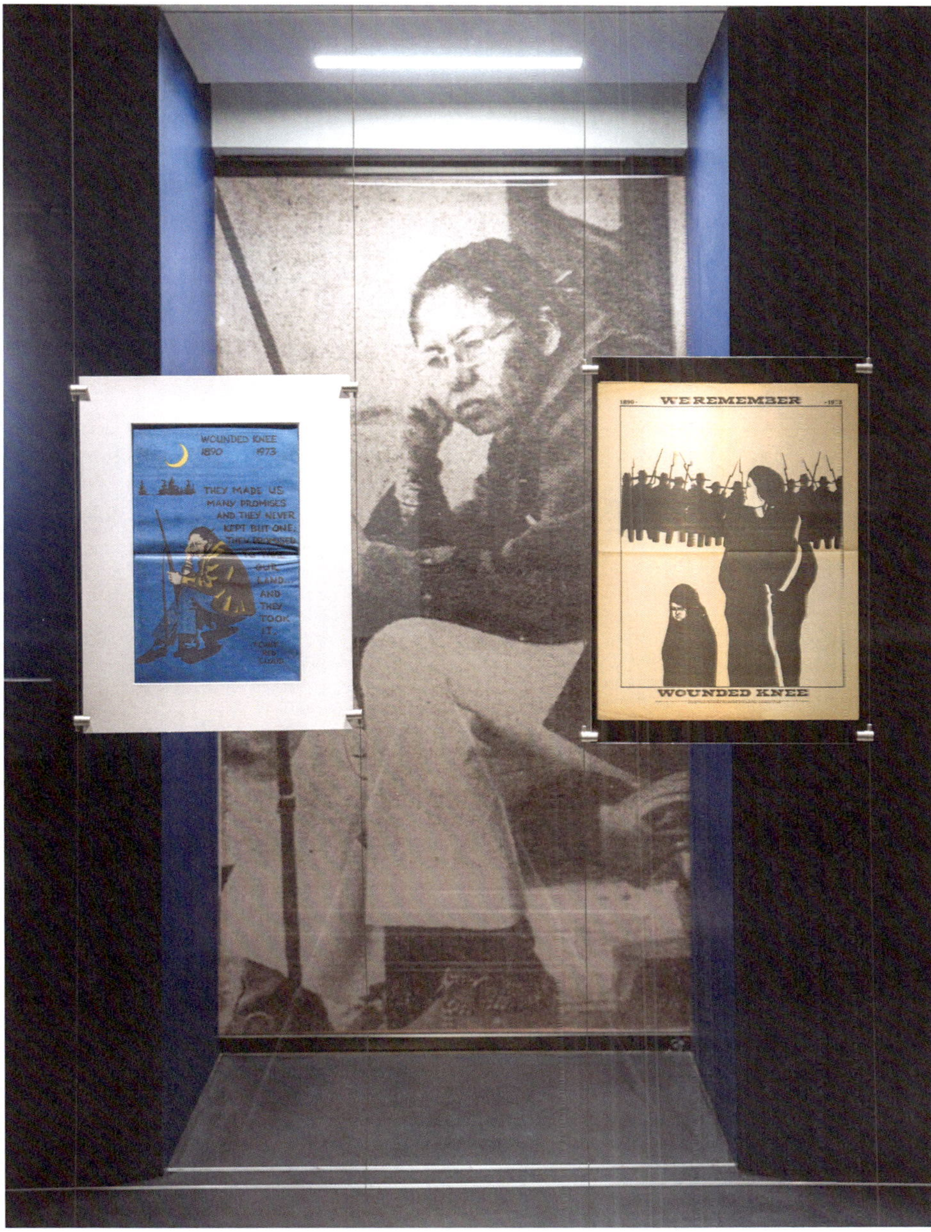
WOUNDED KNEE
1890 1973
THEY MADE US MANY PROMISES AND THEY NEVER KEPT BUT ONE;
WE REMEMBER
WOUNDED KNEE

background: **AKWESASNE NOTES**
Associated Press photograph of the Wounded Knee occupation from Sunday March 4, 1973, with caption "Just watching . . . and waiting"
Rooseveltown, NY: Mohawk Nation, April 1973
Enlarged digital reproduction
Courtesy of the Edward E. Ayer Collection

above, right: **BRUCE CARTER** (b. 1930)
We Remember Wounded Knee
Akwesasne Notes
Rooseveltown, NY: Mohawk Nation, January 1973
Courtesy of the Edward E. Ayer Collection

see next spread

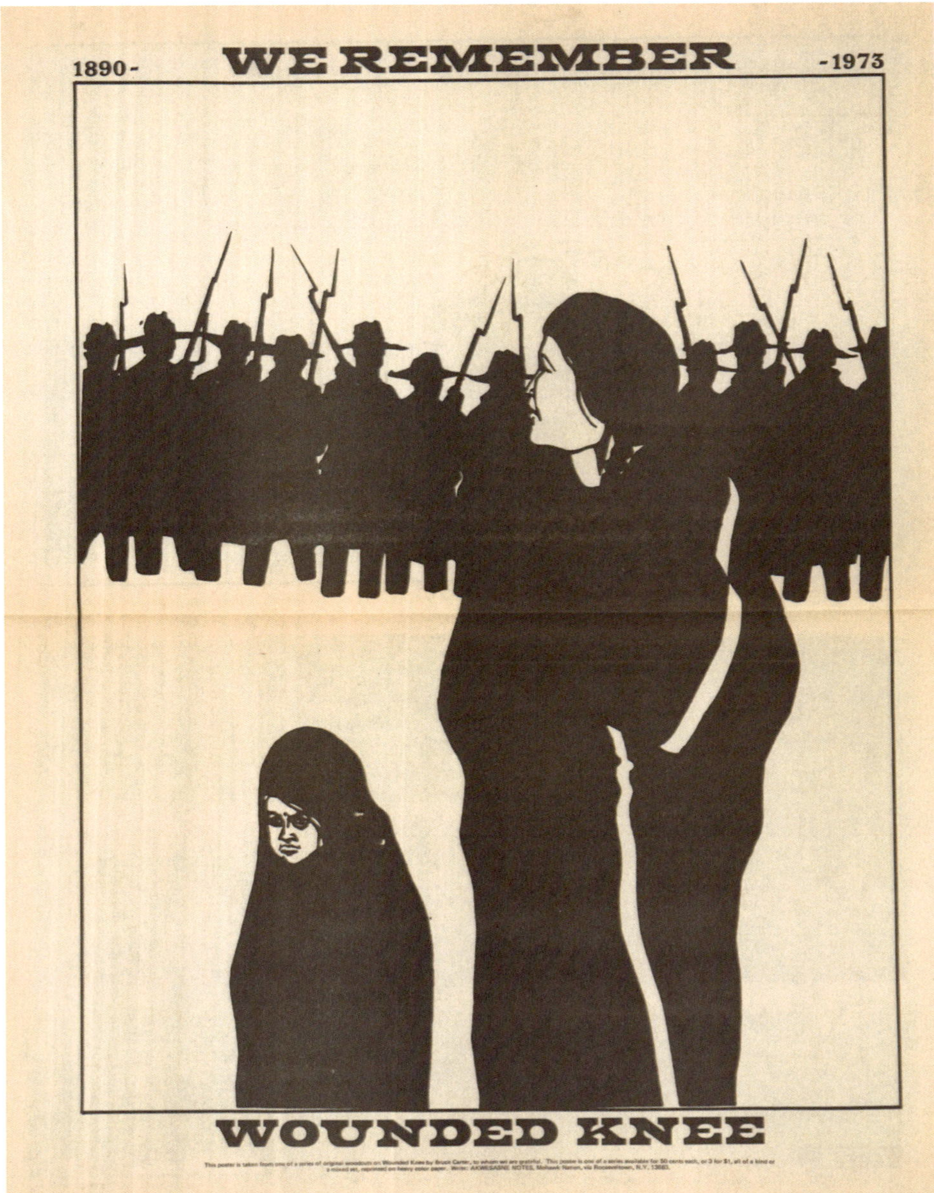

above: **BRUCE CARTER**
We Remember Wounded Knee
Akwesasne Notes - *see previous spread*

Both *The Black Panther* and *Akwesasne Notes* featured woodblock prints by veteran artist Bruce Carter from his series on Wounded Knee distributed by Liberation News Service.

opposite page: **COVER OF *AKWESASNE NOTES***
Rooseveltown, NY: Mohawk Nation, April 1973
Digital reproduction
Courtesy of the Edward E. Ayer Collection

AKWESASNE NOTES

WHERE THE PARTRIDGE DRUMS

Volume 5 Number 2 | Circulation: 50,000 | Early Spring, 1973 (April) | News-stand price: fifty cents (forty-eight pages)

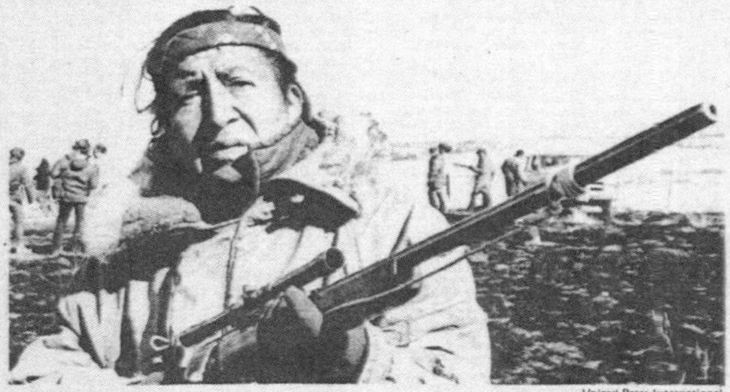

— United Press International

Oscar Bear Runner, Oglala, standing guard while tipi is erected in DMZ

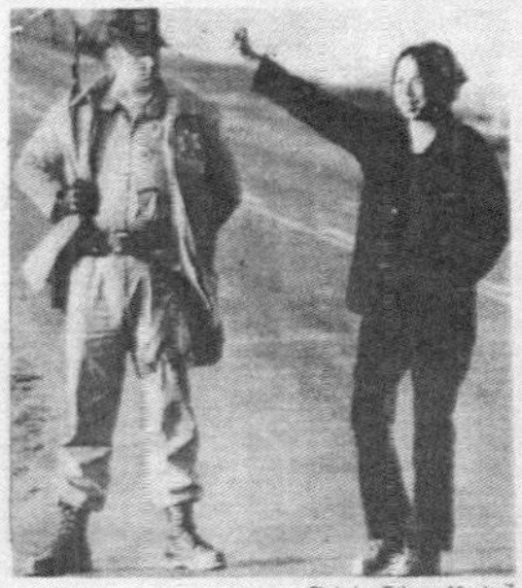

—Christian Science Monitor

U.S. Marshal at Wounded Knee . . . and friend

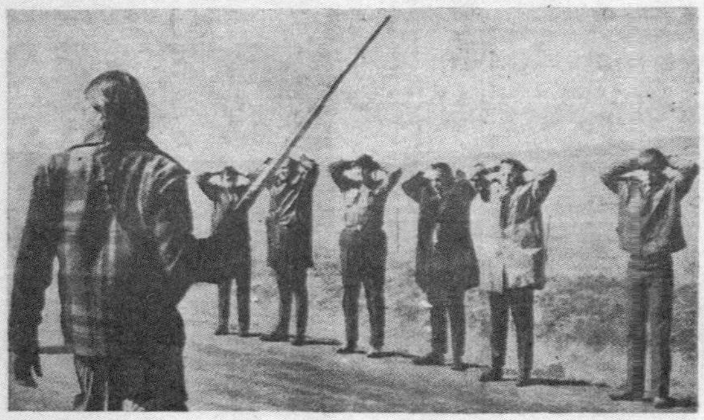

—United Press International

Four U.S. agents and two ranchers are disarmed, detained, then released by Oglalas

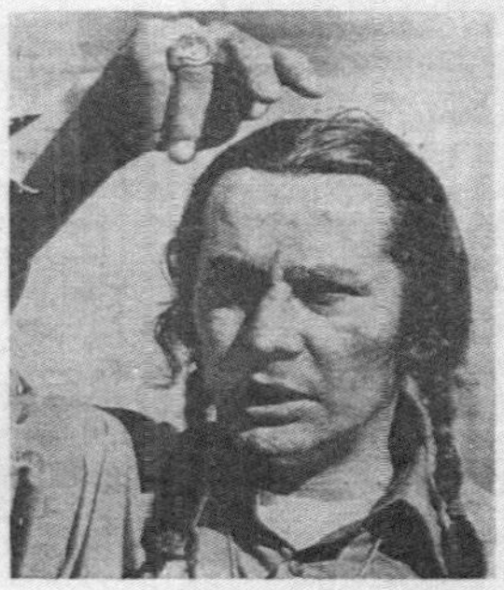

—United Press Intn'l

Russell Means, Oglala, at Wounded Knee

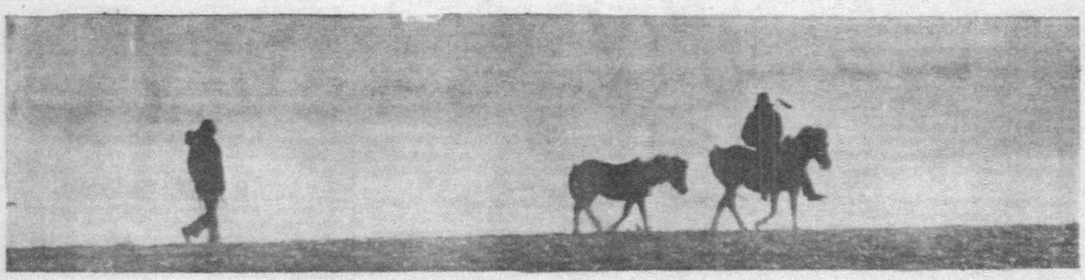

— A SPECIAL ISSUE —

THE FIRST MONTH AT WOUNDED KNEE

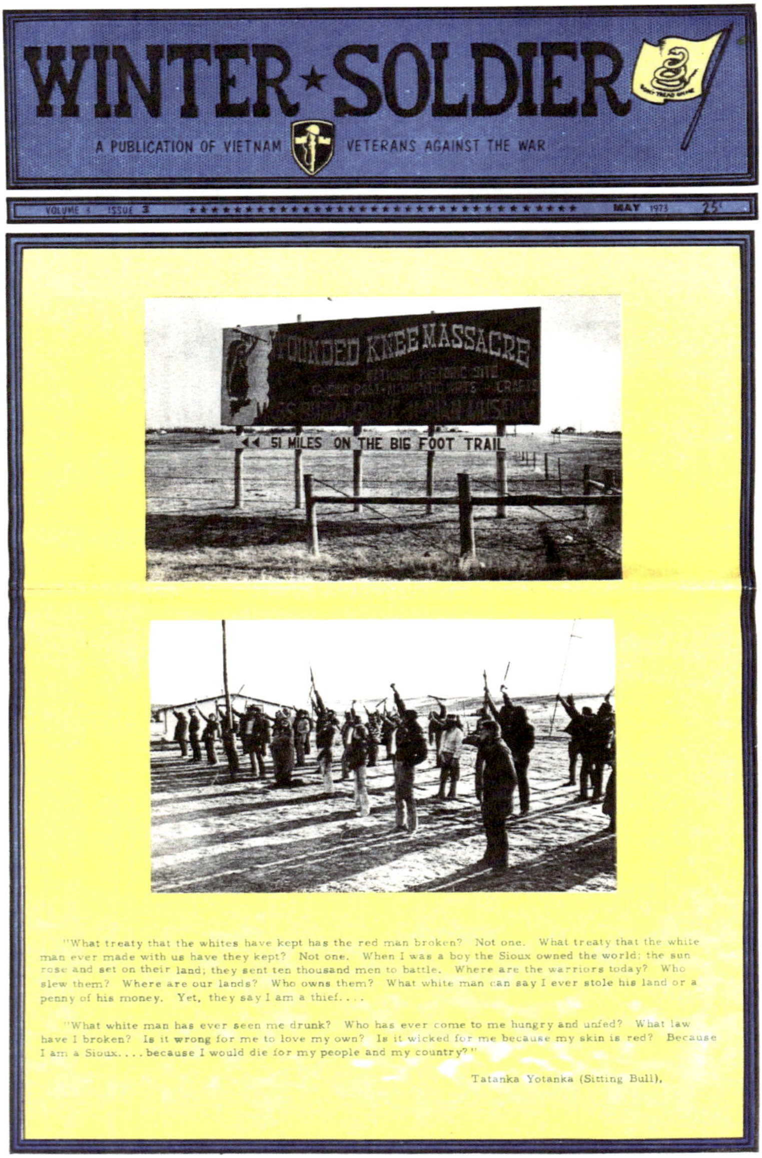
WINTER ★ SOLDIER

A PUBLICATION OF VIETNAM VETERANS AGAINST THE WAR

VOLUME [illegible] ISSUE 3 MAY 1973 25¢

WOUNDED KNEE MASSACRE
51 MILES ON THE BIG FOOT TRAIL

"What treaty that the whites have kept has the red man broken? Not one. What treaty that the white man ever made with us have they kept? Not one. When I was a boy the Sioux owned the world; the sun rose and set on their land; they sent ten thousand men to battle. Where are the warriors today? Who slew them? Where are our lands? Who owns them? What white man can say I ever stole his land or a penny of his money. Yet, they say I am a thief....

"What white man has ever seen me drunk? Who has ever come to me hungry and unfed? What law have I broken? Is it wrong for me to love my own? Is it wicked for me because my skin is red? Because I am a Sioux....because I would die for my people and my country?"

Tatanka Yotanka (Sitting Bull),

COVER OF *WINTER SOLDIER*
Oakland, IL: Vietnam Veterans Against the War,
May 1973
Digital reproduction
Courtesy of Vietnam Veterans Against the War

Just as the Standing Rock actions and mobilization in 2016 brought Indigenous and non-Indigenous people together to resist militarized settler colonialism, so did the occupation of Wounded Knee in 1973. During the occupation and throughout the 1970s, the Liberation News Service distributed images and news clippings to a range of radical outlets. As different groups used common designs and images in their newspapers, like those seen on the covers of *Winter Soldier* (see above) and *The Black Panther* (see opposite page), a shared liberation aesthetic developed.

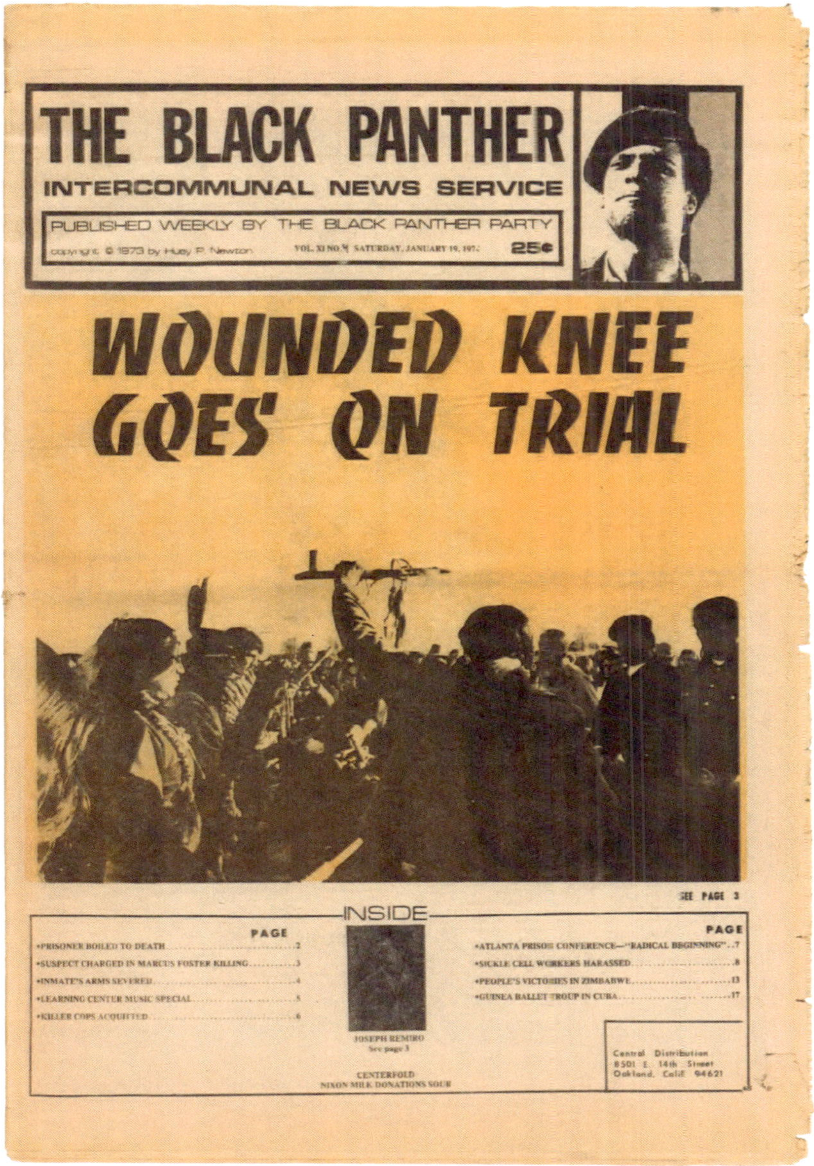

THE BLACK PANTHER

INTERCOMMUNAL NEWS SERVICE

PUBLISHED WEEKLY BY THE BLACK PANTHER PARTY

copyright © 1973 by Huey P. Newton VOL. XI NO. 9 SATURDAY, JANUARY 19, 1974 25¢

WOUNDED KNEE GOES ON TRIAL

SEE PAGE 3

INSIDE

	PAGE
•PRISONER BOILED TO DEATH	2
•SUSPECT CHARGED IN MARCUS FOSTER KILLING	3
•INMATE'S ARMS SEVERED	4
•LEARNING CENTER MUSIC SPECIAL	5
•KILLER COPS ACQUITTED	6
•ATLANTA PRISON CONFERENCE—"RADICAL BEGINNING"	7
•SICKLE CELL WORKERS HARASSED	8
•PEOPLE'S VICTORIES IN ZIMBABWE	13
•GUINEA BALLET TROUP IN CUBA	17

JOSEPH REMIRO
See page 3

CENTERFOLD
NIXON MILK DONATIONS SOUR

Central Distribution
8501 E. 14th Street
Oakland, Calif. 94621

COVER OF *THE BLACK PANTHER*
Oakland, CA: Black Panther Party, January 19, 1974
Digital reproduction
Image source: *American Art*, University of Chicago Press, Summer 2021

The connections among these groups were not solely aesthetic. A *Black Panther* article on the occupation of Wounded Knee noted that Oglala Lakota grievances were "in common with Black, Latino, Asian and other poor, white and non-white people of America." By highlighting these intersections, the publications fostered a legacy of solidarity for future movements to build on.

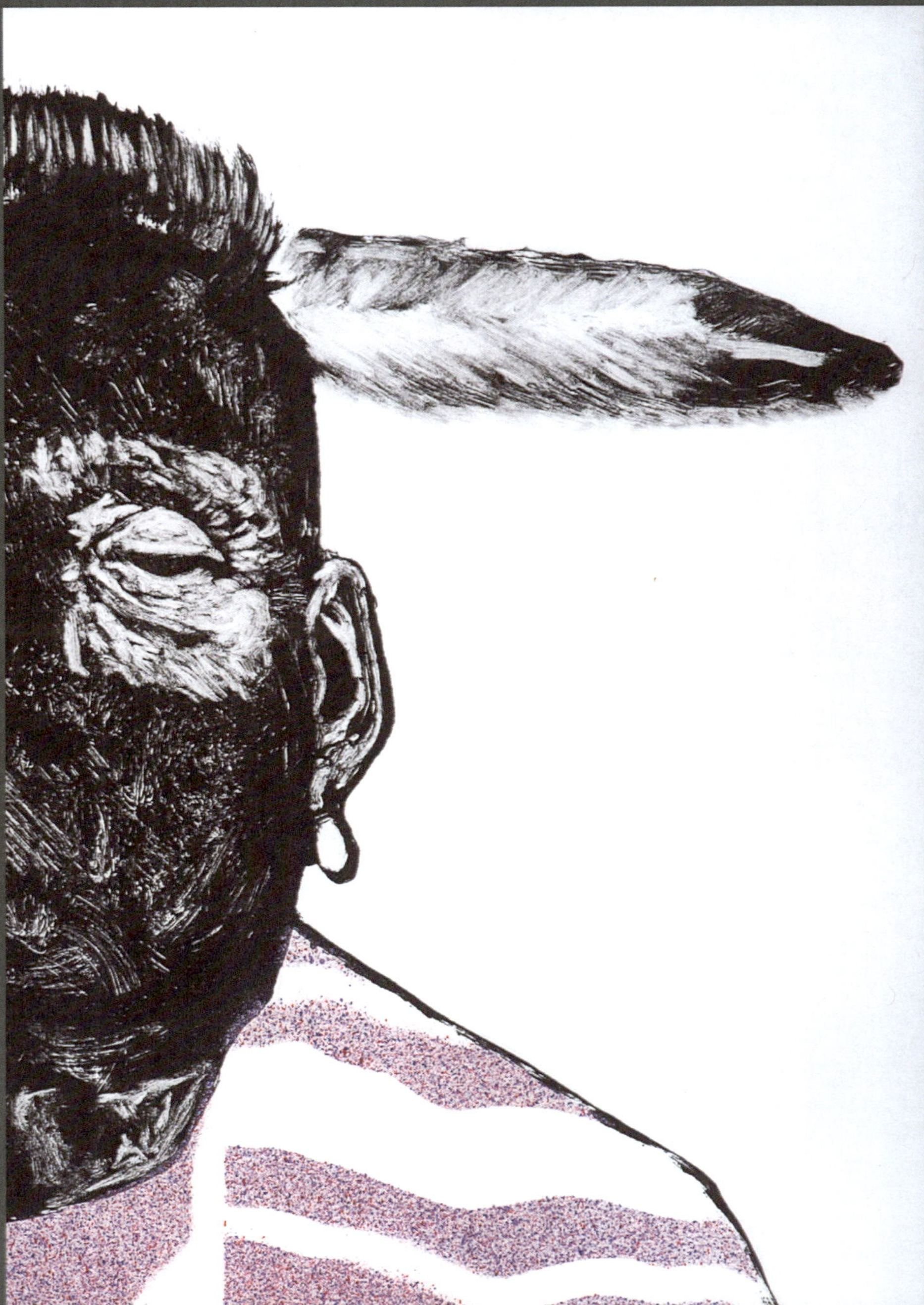

MONTY LITTLE
Survivance, 14 (detail) - *see also: p. 30*

Why is the United States the Most Militaristic State in History?

ROXANNE DUNBAR-ORTIZ

Recent polls regarding opinions of US government institutions report that with wide agreement across party lines 84 percent responded that they have confidence in the military. The executive branch, Congress, and the Supreme Court are rated in single or low double digits in stark comparison. The popularity of the military is not new, it's fundamental.

We must come to grips with the obvious fact that the US was founded as a fiscal-military state, a European settler state made for war, designed in the 1787 Northwest Ordinance to conquer the continent, erasing multiple nations and their millions of inhabitants, replacing them with Euroamericans. This required the full armed participation of settlers with the promise of land, becoming men of property. It took a century of genocidal wars to accomplish, with Indigenous nations' survivors incarcerated in reservations by 1890.

The United States has been at war since its founding, continuing the colonial wars that secured the thirteen colonies over 170 years. It is impossible to find a single day in US history when some part of its armed forces, including covert operations since the 1950s, was not intervening somewhere.

The roots of US military culture can be found in what historians describe as "savage war." Called *petite guerre* or counterinsurgency in military annals, it is theorized as the United States' "first way of war" by military historian John Grenier. This way of war in North America dates to the British-colonial period and was a combination of "unlimited war and irregular war," a military tradition "that accepted, legitimized, and encouraged attacks upon and the destruction of noncombatants, villages and agricultural resources . . . in shockingly violent campaigns to achieve their goals of conquest."[1] Grenier notes that in most US wars in the twentieth and twenty-first centuries, the military begins combat as a regimented force, but invariably turns to the first way of war, counterinsurgency. The "war on terror" official behavior following 9/11 should not have come as a surprise.

What distinguishes US militarism is not only the amount or type of violence involved, but the triumphal mythology attached to that violence and its political uses, even today.[2] This way of war was largely devised and enacted by landed settlers, many of them slavers, who formed the basis for the founding ideology and colonialist military strategy of the independent United States. This approach to war is still being practiced, almost as a reflex, with proud memories of triumphant past campaigns.

In the twentieth century, the US carried out large-scale regular warfare, alongside counterinsurgency in the Philippines, Europe, Korea, and Vietnam, as well as smaller scale and prolonged invasions and occupations in the Philippines, Cuba, Nicaragua, Haiti, and the

---

1. John Grenier, *The First Way of War, 1607–1814*. New York: Cambridge University Press, 2005, 10.

2. Richard Slotkin, *The Fatal Environment: The Myth of the Frontier in the Age of Industrialization, 1800–1890*. New York: Harper Perennial, 1994: 53.

Dominican Republic, as well as covert counterinsurgencies in Columbia, Southern Africa, and decades, still ongoing, in the Philippines and Afghanistan, and more recently, Iraq and Syria, among others.

Counterinsurgency's main goal is to destroy the targeted people's collective will, or their capacity to resist, employing any means necessary but invariably falling back on attacking civilians and their support systems, especially food storage facilities and fields. The Anglo colonists in North America called it "food fight." Now called "special operations" or "low-intensity conflict," and even blatantly, as in Afghanistan, "counterinsurgency," this kind of warfare was used against Indigenous communities by settler militias in the first British colonies of Virginia and Massachusetts and spread as other colonies were established. It was later legalized in the US Constitution's Second Amendment, which mandated settlers' individual rights to take and hold Indigenous lands, as well as to control enslaved Africans.

Settlers sought to disrupt every aspect of resistance as well as to obtain intelligence through scouting and taking Native civilians as hostages. They did so by destroying Indigenous villages and fields and intimidating and slaughtering enemy noncombatant populations.[3] These voluntary associations made up of individual civilians—"rangers"—came to be called militias in the Second Amendment.

From 1607 to 1814, the architecture of the US military was forged, leading to its reproduction and development into the present. This formative period generated the problematic characteristics of the US way of war and thereby the characteristics of US civilization, which few historians and citizens have come to terms with.

During the late 1600s, Anglo settlers in New England began the routine practice of scalp hunting and "ranging." By that time, the non-Indigenous population of the British colony in North America had increased sixfold, to a more than 150,000 European population.

3. Ibid., 1.

which meant that settlers were intruding on more of the Indigenous nations' homelands. Indigenous resistance followed in the 1676–77 eliminationist warfare that the settlers called "King Philip's War." The Wampanoag people and their Indigenous allies attacked the settlers' isolated farms, using methods that relied on speed and caution in striking and retreating, and of course possessing a perfect knowledge of the terrain; that is resistance using guerrilla warfare.

The settlers scorned this kind of people's resistance as "skulking," and responded by destroying Indigenous villages and everyone in them who could not escape, burning their fields, homes, villages, and food storage. But as effective Indigenous resistance continued, the commander of the Plymouth militia, Benjamin Church, studied Wampanoag tactics to develop a more effective kind of preemption or counterinsurgency. He petitioned the colony's governor for permission to choose sixty to seventy settlers to serve as "scouts," as he called them, for what he termed "wilderness warfare," although the Indigenous communities were all farming and fishing villages.

In July 1676, the first settler-organized militia was the result. The rangers force was made up of sixty male settlers and 140 captured and conscripted Indigenous men. They were ordered to "discover, pursue, fight, surprise, destroy, or subdue the enemy," in Church's words. The inclusion of Indigenous fighters on the colonists' side was not unique to British colonists in North America; rather the practice marked the character of European and Euroamerican colonization and occupations of non-European peoples from the beginning through twentieth-century national liberation movements.

The settler-rangers could learn from their Native aides, then discard them. Some Indigenous communities allied with settlers to make war against their Indigenous neighbors, igniting civil wars. This ended badly for the colonized Natives when the settlers turned on them as well. Varied Native peoples eventually formed confederations, increasing their power to resist.

The Native communities of New England continued to resist by burning Anglo settlements and killing and capturing settlers for ransom. As an incentive to recruit fighters, colonial authorities introduced a program of scalp hunting that became a permanent and long-lasting element of settler warfare against Indigenous nations.[4] During the Pequot War, Connecticut and Massachusetts colonial officials had offered bounties, initially for the heads of murdered Indigenous people and later for only their scalps, which were more portable in large numbers.

Scalp hunting became routine even outside of warfare and more profitable following an incident on the northern frontier of the Massachusetts colony in 1697. Settler Hannah Duston, who had been taken hostage, murdered her ten Abenaki captors in a nighttime escape. She presented their scalps to the Massachusetts General Assembly, which rewarded her with bounties for two men, two women, and six children.[5] Duston's bloody scalp trophies were highly publicized during her lifetime, but she remained mostly forgotten until the 1820s, when her story was revived as a patriotic white nationalist narrative during the Andrew Jackson presidency. Lionized as a folk hero, Duston's story was employed during the continuing bloody and genocidal Jacksonian wars against Native peoples to characterize settler and Army violence as defensive and virtuous, necessary, even feminist.[6] Stories about her continued to show up in print through the 1880s, and she became the first Anglo-American woman in North America to be cast as a heroic statue. Not just one, but three major monuments were erected in her honor, all of which still stand today.

Scalp hunting became a lucrative commercial practice from the early eighteenth century onward. The settler authorities had hit

---

4. Ibid., 192-93.

5. Ibid., 40-41, 205.

6. Barbara Cutter, "The Female Indian Killer Memorialized: Hannah Duston and the Nineteenth-Century Feminization of American Violence, *The Journal of Women's History*, 2008, Vol. 20: No. 2.

upon a way to encourage settlers to take off on their own or with a few others to gather scalps, at random, for the reward money. Grenier notes, "In the process, they established the large-scale privatization of war within Anglo-American frontier communities."[7]

During nearly two centuries of British colonization on the Atlantic shore of North America, generations of settlers gained experience as "Indian fighters" outside any organized military institution. Anglo-French conflict may appear to have been the dominant factor of European colonization in North America during the eighteenth century, but while large regular armies fought over geopolitical goals in Europe, Anglo settlers in North America waged deadly irregular warfare against the Indigenous nations.

Most military historians ignore the "Indian wars" from 1607 to 1890, as well as the 1846–48 invasion and occupation of Mexico, but these wars formed the platform, the genealogy of officers, and the mindset of US military actions in the US Civil War and thereafter around the world.

Andrew Jackson carried out the original plan envisioned by the founders—particularly Jefferson—initially as a Tennessee militia leader, then as an army general who led counterinsurgent wars against the Muscogee Creek and Seminoles in Georgia and Florida, and finally as a president who engineered the forced expulsion of all Native peoples east of the Mississippi to the designated "Indian Territory" (Oklahoma). The popularity of Jackson's presidency was in large part due to the militia-ranger persona, a mystique which developed among settlers. This persona involved a certain identification with the Native enemy, marking the settler as Native American rather than European. Following independence, this mystique became a part of popular culture, as well as military culture, as we can see with Army Rangers and Navy SEALs, as well as the Marine Corps, in today's wars.

During the second half of the nineteenth century, the Army of the West—nearly all soldiers and officers from the Mexican War

7. Grenier, 221–22.

and the Third Seminole War—warred against the peoples in the former Mexican territory of the Southwest and, after the Civil War, the Northern Plains to the Pacific, with officers and soldiers empowered by four years of combat and more-lethal weaponry.

Military analyst Robert Kaplan challenges the concept of Manifest Destiny, arguing "it was not inevitable that the United States should have an empire in the western part of the continent." Rather, he argues, western empire was brought about by "small groups of frontiersmen, separated from each other by great distances." These groups are the continuation of settler "rangers," destroying Indigenous towns, fields, and food supplies, most dramatically thirty million bison in the Northern Plains.

Kaplan argues that the US Army was secondary in effectiveness compared to the settler rangers, whom he equates to the modern Special Forces; he acknowledges that the Army of the West provided lethal backup for settler counterinsurgency in slaughtering the buffalo, the food supply of Plains peoples, as well as making continuous raids on settlements to kill or hold hostage the families of the Indigenous fighters to force their surrender. Kaplan summarizes the genealogy of US militarism today in an essay titled, "Injun Country," writing: "Whereas the average American at the dawn of the new millennium, the twenty-first century, found patriotic inspiration in the legacies of the Civil War and World War II, when the evils of slavery and fascism were confronted and vanquished, for many commissioned and noncommissioned officers the US Army's defining moment was fighting the 'Indians.'"[8]

From the beginning, the US was competitive in trade internationally. "Free trade" was the sacred quest then as it is today. Take the famed US Marine Corps, founded in 1775, a year after the thirteen colonies formed the Continental Congress and the Army. The character of a Marine is that of the colonial ranger, created for

8. Kaplan, Robert D. *Imperial Grunts: The American Military on the Ground*. New York: Random House, 2005: 8–10.

counterinsurgency outside US-secured territory. The opening lyric of the eternal official hymn of the US Marine Corps—composed and adopted in 1847, soon after the invasion of Mexico and during the occupation—is "From the Halls of Montezuma to the shores of Tripoli." Tripoli refers back nearly a half-century to the "Barbary Wars," when the Marines were dispatched in 1801 to North Africa by President Thomas Jefferson to invade the Berber Nation, carrying on this aggression, shelling the city, taking captives, and marauding for nearly four years, ending with the 1805 "Battle of Derna." It was there they earned the nickname "leathernecks" for the high collars they wore as defense against the Berbers' saber cuts. The ostensible goal of the "First Barbary War" was to persuade Tripoli to release US sailor hostages and to end what the US called "pirate attacks" on US merchant ships. Actually, the Berbers were demanding that their sovereignty over their territorial waters be respected. The Berbers did not give up their demands, and the Marines were withdrawn, returning a decade later in 1815 to fight the "Second Barbary War," which ended when Pasha Yusuf Karamanli, ruler of Tripoli, agreed not to exact fees from US ships entering their territorial waters. This marks the first military victory of overseas US imperialism, or "gunboat diplomacy" as it would be called nearly a century later, when historians mark the beginning of US overseas imperialism. The Marines and military historians know better.

The Marine Corps' second large engagement was the "Second Seminole War," which raged from 1835 to 1842, the longest war in US history until Vietnam. Although they succeeded in killing the Seminole resistance leader Osceola, they lost the war as the Seminoles would not meet the US government's demands by handing over fugitive slaves. The military did succeed in deporting captives—mostly women, children, and old men—to Indian Territory. US armed forces attacked again in 1855, marking the beginning of the "Third Seminole War," but lost after a four-year siege. The Civil War and the end of the institution of slavery made further war against the Seminoles unnecessary.

The Marine Corps' trademark hymn was composed while they occupied Mexico City in 1847. While the US Army invaded and occupied what is now California, Arizona, and New Mexico, the Marines invaded by sea and occupied Vera Cruz, using counterinsurgent tactics in their march to Mexico City, burning fields and villages, murdering and torturing civilian resisters. The Marines and the Army occupied Mexico City until the Mexican government, under brutal occupation, signed a dubious treaty transferring the northern half of Mexico to the United States. In Marine Corps annals, the 1847 "Battle of Chapultepec" is legion, a battle in which a handful of teenaged Mexican cadets—the Chapultepec castle was used as a military training school—with few weapons and little ammunition held off the Marines. After overrunning the cadets, the Marines raised the US flag and wrote their hymn, tracing their genealogy to the invasion and occupation of Tripoli. Marines take pride in their origins, which few US Americans, including leftists, know little or nothing about. If they did, they would have to reconsider the mythology of the US founding.

When you center the resistance of Indigenous people, and of the enslaved, and other victims of US counterinsurgency interventions and wars around the world, you are in fact doing US history, and everything you thought you knew about the present and future melts into air. The United States has always been a military state with an informally armed citizenry.

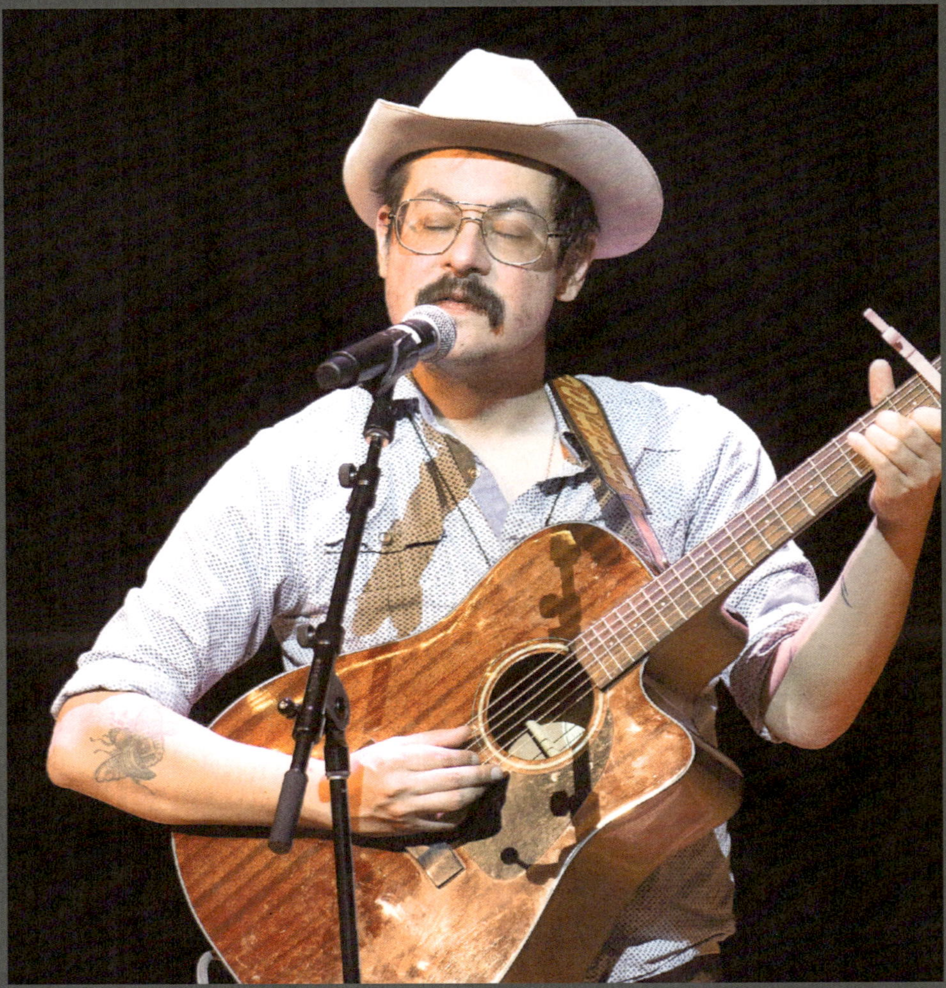

JOSEPH RUNNING CRANE
***Forging Hope: Reckon and Reimagine* Opening Program**, Chicago Cultural Center, 2023

see also: p. 260

Unlikely Rebellions, Reckonings, and Refusals: Exhibition Review

MERANDA ROBERTS

On the night of March 18, 2023, the third day of the Veteran Art Summit concluded with powerful and emotional music performances by Brittney Chantele (US Army Veteran), Elexa Dawson (Citizen Potawatomi Nation), James Pakootas (Confederate Tribes of Colville), and Joseph Running Crane (Blackfeet). I returned to my hotel room to several messages from my mom about my uncle Kenney passing away a few hours earlier. My father was too distraught to talk, and I felt my chest constrict. As I cried out loudly, I reflected on my uncle Kenny's role in the Yerington Paiute community. I remembered the stories of him being our tribal chairman and fighting for the community's access to clean drinking water due to toxins leaking into wells from the Anaconda Copper Mine.[1] Just a few days before his passing, we had been planning for me to visit Yerington to gain more insight

1. "Yerington Paiute Tribe of Nevada," ICT News, accessed July 8, 2024, https://ictnews.org/archive/yerington-paiute-tribe-of-nevada.

into family/community dynamics. My heart swelled with rage as I contemplated the reality of what had taken him from us so soon: a lack of resources to help Native men cope with stress, intergenerational trauma, violence, and racism. I wondered why we took so long to connect in the ways we always wanted to and how I am not able to safely be on the reservation without worrying about encountering gendered violence.

What helped me through this moment was knowing I was with a group of artists, veterans, and creators who understood what I was feeling without explaining. I calmed down as I reflected on that night's performances and remembered how each artist channeled their hurt, trauma, and loss into creative expressions that allowed them to heal on *their* terms. I thought about each exhibition—*Unlikely Entanglements* at the Hyde Park Art Center, *Residues and Rebellions* at the Newberry Library, and *Reckon and Reimagine* at the Chicago Cultural Center. Each one exposed the profound effects of American warfare, surveillance, imperialism, and entitlement on BIPOC combat veterans and the communities whose lands were infiltrated by imperialist forces, establishing a colonial presence in regions labeled as "savage" or "uncivilized." As I came to terms with how my family was once again a victim of the long-term effects of colonial and state-sanctioned violence, I realized that the only way we can collectively survive the long wars is by continuously and courageously creating artworks, pieces of writing, or performances that allow us to bear witness to each other's pain, grief, joy, and hope. Such actions and collectives alleviate the burden of isolation and hopelessness, effectively thwarting some of the underlying objectives of settler colonialism.

This exhibition review highlights artworks from each exhibition that resonated with me the most, providing insights into their compelling narratives that encourage open grieving, reflections on the realities these wars have on our bodies and spirits, and motivations to channel our feelings and experiences into creative expressions that help others survive these systems.[2] What truly captivated me about each exhibition was their demonstration of how BIPOC communities *refuse* to let war silence them.[3] Through the vulnerability expressed by each artist, we gain a deeper understanding of this nation's past while simultaneously envisioning humanitarian paths forward.

Rebellions, Reckonings, and Refusals

In the *Residues and Rebellions* exhibition at the Newberry Library, artists employ "affirmative refusal" strategies to resist the manipulative influence of empire.[4] The works of Mahwish Chishty, Miridith Campbell (Kiowa), Monty Little (Diné), Rodney Ewing, Darrell Fair, and others boldly reject forms of visibility and subjectivity that commodify and control personhood. The exhibition establishes connections among communities impacted by American warfare, highlighting a refusal to be silenced by displaying their works together in a unified space. This resistance sparks conversations about resurgent movements and fosters creative possibilities that challenge the foundations of settler colonialism.[5]

For example, ledger art by Indigenous artists Frederick Gokliz (San Carlos Apache) and Cheyenne warrior Black Horse lays a foundation for appreciating Marine Corps veteran Darrell Fair's work on a deeper level. The use of ledger paper by Indigenous artists in the US began around 1865 as a way for these survivors of American warfare to continue the act of storytelling, an essential part of sustaining Indigenous livelihood since time immemorial. During this time,

2. Regrettably, due to the constraints of this essay's length, I am unable to provide an in-depth analysis of every artwork featured in each exhibition.

3. Audra Simpson argues that for Indigenous people, particularly the Mohawk community, sovereignty is not about asserting control over territory or seeking recognition from the state. Instead, it is a practice of refusal, a deliberate rejection of settler-colonial logics and the imposition of state power. See: Audra Simpson, *Mohawk Interruptus: Political Life Across the Borders of Settler States* (Durham, NC: Duke University Press, 2014).

4. Jarrett Martineau, "Creative Combat: Indigenous Art, Resurgence, and Decolonization" (Doctoral dissertation, University of Victoria, 2015), iii.

5. Leanne Betasamosake Simpson, *As We Have Always Done: Indigenous Freedom through Radical Resistance* (Minneapolis: University of Minnesota Press, 2017).

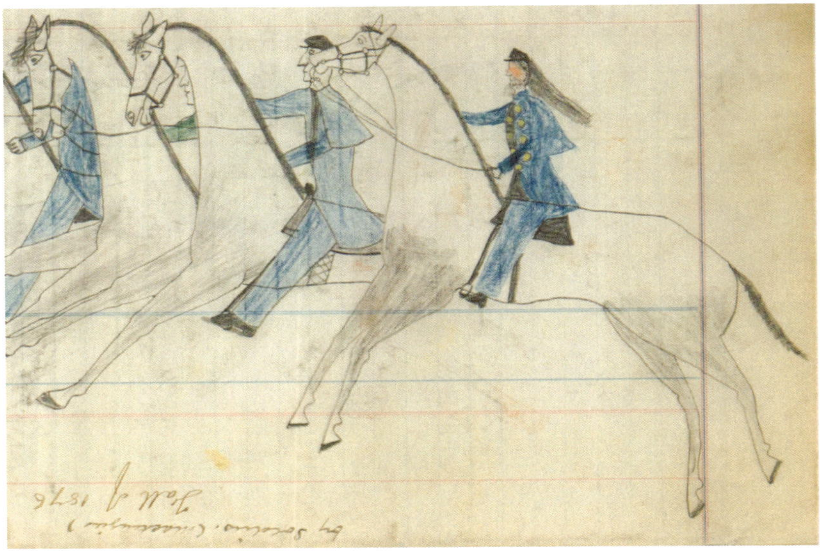

BLACK HORSE LEDGER, *p. 22* (detail), Cheyenne, ca. 1877–1879, Colored pencil and pen on ledger paper, Courtesy of the Edward E. Ayer Collection; *see also: pp. 42, 44–46*

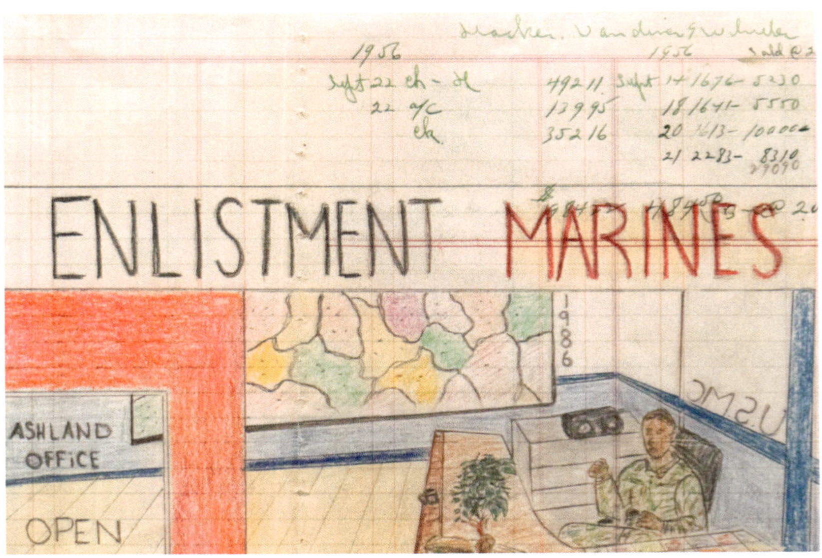

DARRELL WAYNE FAIR, *Enlistment* (detail), 2022, Pencil and colored pencil on ledger paper, Courtesy of the artist and Prison + Neighborhood Arts Education Project; *see also: pp. 34–37, 317*

Native people could no longer access the resources that sustained their traditional storytelling practices, so many artists/storytellers began using ledger paper given to them by US soldiers, traders, missionaries, and reservation employees. In this exhibition, Black Horse's works depict moments he witnessed at war with the US cavalry. In contrast, Gokliz portrays intimate moments of community care that continued despite attempts to forcibly assimilate his community into American forms of family or love. When we look at Darrell Fair's work, which uses ledger paper to honor Indigenous storytellers, we are exposed to a contemporary story that highlights the many ways the US continues to target and terrorize Black men deliberately. Fair, also a survivor of torture at the hands of the Chicago Police Department, uses ledger art as a medium to bravely bring his lived experiences to the forefront so that he and others who have undergone similar tactics of terror can *refuse* shame and silence.[6]

This sense of refusal carries through in the display of Miridith Campbell's *Cradleboard*, accompanied by images from *Akwesasne Notes*, thoughtfully dispersed throughout the exhibition and the Gokliz ledger art.[7] Campbell's cradleboard reminded me of the cradleboards I often see in museum collections and how culture keepers have told me to remember that the designs reflect the love, strength, hope, and admiration a mother has for her child. I pondered the many ways settler history often tries to exclude the significant role maternal love has played in sustaining Native American communities and how Native women play an essential role in asserting tribal sovereignty by way of activism, resistance, and military participation. Through the inclusion of this toy cradleboard and *Akwesasne Notes* photographs of Native women activists, in addition to Campbell's *Counting Coup*

6. Aislinn Pulley, "Shame and Survival," in *Remaking the Exceptional: Tea, Torture, and Reparations | Chicago to Guantánamo*, eds. Amber Ginsburg, Aaron Hughes, Aliya Hussain, and Audrey Petty (Chicago: DePaul Art Museum, 2022), 218.

7. *Akwesasne Notes* was a newspaper founded in 1969, amid a surge in Native American activism, by Ernest Benedict of the Mohawk Nation at Akwesasne, which straddles the US and Canadian border along the St. Lawrence River. For more information, see: https://rozsixties.unl.edu/items/show/873.

piece in a separate display, visitors witness how "Indigenous women and our love inspires resistance and responsibilities in protecting our values, traditions, the lands, waters, and people."[8]

The *Reckon and Reimagine* exhibition at the Chicago Cultural Center maintains a prevalent *refusal* theme. However, what captivated me about this show was its ability to prompt deep reflection on how America should reckon with its colonial history while actively working towards a post-colonial future. As I immersed myself in the exhibition, I embraced Chickasaw scholar Jodi Byrd's theory of how "as a transit, Indianness becomes a site through which US empire orientates and replicates itself by transforming those to be colonized into 'Indians' through the continual reiteration of pioneer logics, whether in the Pacific, the Caribbean, or the Middle East."[9]

When I stood before the exhibition's introductory display, which featured unique dresses created by Kiowa artist and veteran Miridth Campbell and Ojibwe artist and veteran Melissa Doud, the profound significance of "Indianness as a transit of empire" became even more apparent. These dresses eloquently capture the essence of the traditional attire worn by Native women in their respective communities during dances, ceremonies, and celebrations. Particularly striking were two dresses made from the artists' military uniforms, symbolizing the powerful reconciliation of their military experiences with their cultural identities. This presentation made me reflect on the far-reaching impact of "empire" on the bodies and well-being of Indigenous women in North America, given the erosion of matriarchal leadership and recognition of two-spirit individuals caused by European settlers. Consequently, Indigenous communities face ongoing forms of violence, with Native American women experiencing

---

8. R. Flowers, "Refusal to Forgive: Indigenous Women's Love and Rage," *Decolonization: Indigeneity, Education & Society*, vol. 4, no. 2 (2015): 32–49.

9. Jodi A. Byrd, *Transit of Empire: Indigenous Critiques of Colonialism* (Minneapolis: University of Minnesota Press, 2011).

10. MMIWG2S, "Coalition to Stop Violence Against Native Women," accessed May 25, 2023, https://www.csvanw.org/mmiw.

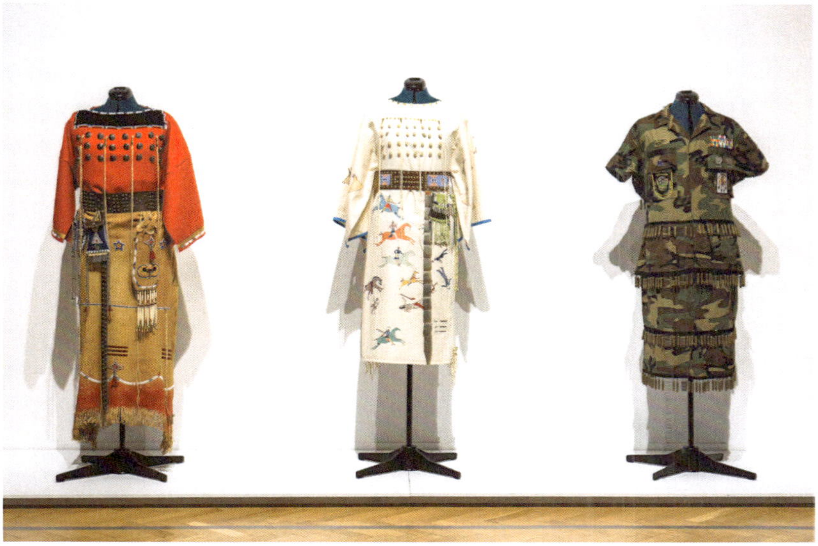

left: **MIRIDITH CAMPBELL**, *Marine Corps Dress–Southern Style*, 2022, Assorted materials; *center: Adobe Walls Battle Dress*, 2022, Assorted materials; *right:* **MELISSA DOUD**, *Bullet Dress*, 2016, Assorted materials *see also: pp. 88–91, 250–51, 319*

murder rates more than ten times the national average today.[10] As Simpson attests, "sexual violence is an effective colonial tool in genocide and dispossession because the damage it causes to families is so overwhelming that it makes it very difficult to have the emotional capital to continue to resist."[11]

It is crucial to acknowledge that the early exploitation of Indigenous women in North America likely laid the foundation for how the US would later undermine Indigenous sovereignty globally. This connection becomes even more evident when examining Gerald Sheffield's piece *fm 3-05.301* from his PTSD Series. This work reveals the existence of a US Army field manual for psychological operations that provides strategies for soldiers to influence the behavior of "host nationals" in support of US policies during wartime.[12]

11. Leanne Betasamosake Simpson, *As We Have Always Done: Indigenous Freedom through Radical Resistance*, chap. 6, Kindle.

12. Exhibition wall text

Examining this work recalls how, in 2009, the Marine Corps initiated Female Engagement Teams in Afghanistan to establish "trust-based and lasting relationships with the Afghan women they encountered on patrols, to collect information from Afghan families and communicate with women without breaking cultural traditions."[13]

Within this context, I further contemplated the impact of war on families, particularly children, while viewing works from Rajkamal Kahlon's series *Did You Kiss the Dead Body?* and Hanaa Malallah's *She/He Has No Picture*. Kahlon overlays photographs of Afghan and Iraqi children onto autopsy reports and death certificates written by US military officials stationed in bases and prisons in Afghanistan and Iraq. Malallah's piece commemorates the victims of a 1991 bombing in Baghdad at a public shelter, where families created a memorial for their loved ones.[14] The presentation of these pieces in the exhibition mirrors a memorial, and as I walked through the gallery, I felt the gaze of these victims fixed upon me. It was a constant reminder to *refuse* to forget their stories and the ongoing intergenerational trauma their families endure because of the wars on terror.

Unlikely Entanglements

Unlikely Entanglements at the Hyde Park Art Center was the first Triennial exhibition I saw. Upon walking into the center, I was blown away at how successfully my colleagues had created an exhibition that reveals the interconnected personal and collective histories of Black, Indigenous, and People of Color (BIPOC) communities affected by the "American Indian Wars" and the "Global War on Terror."[15] As I immersed myself in the exhibition, two artworks captivated me, representing these connections: Sabba Elahi's

13. According to the National Museum of the Marine Corps, the United States Army developed a similar platform known as the "Lioness" program. Members of the Marine FETs have also been used in Iraq and Kuwait to train local police forces. For more information, see: https://www.usmcmuseum.com/uploads/6/0/3/6/60364049/fets.pdf.

14. Exhibition wall text

15. Exhibition wall text

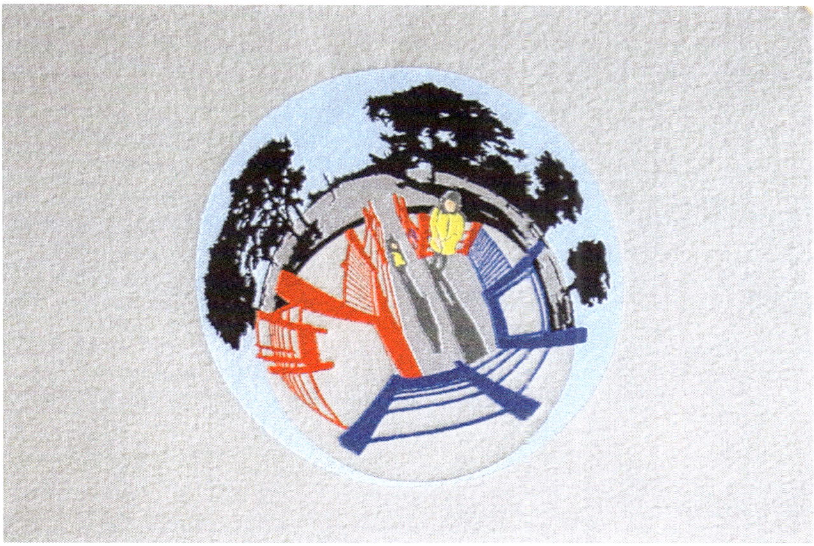

SABBA ELAHI, *the suspect is my son #3* (detail), 2018, Machine embroidery on felt; *see also: p. 178*

evocative series *the suspect is my son* and Rodney Ewing's *Come the Mean Times*. Together, these artworks shed a harsh light on the direct toll that warfare inflicts on the bodies and minds of Black and Brown individuals.

Elahi skillfully employs craft embroidery to address the racialization and surveillance of Muslim people by the United States, exposing the erosion of privacy and safety within the Muslim community. Through capturing intimate glimpses of her son's life from the vantage point of a drone, Elahi enables the audience to grasp how easily the nation-state transforms the existence of young Brown bodies into perceived threats or suspects.

When considered alongside Ewing's hand-colored silkscreen production on ledger paper, viewers confront the consequences of people being deemed "dangerous" by those in power. *Come the Mean Times* offers a powerful commentary on two specific instances: the Trail of Tears (1838–1839) and the Tulsa Massacre of 1921, where

America, driven by white supremacy and settler colonialism, ruthlessly sought to eradicate the existence of Indigenous and Black communities.[16] The artwork presents an image of an unarmed Black man with his hands raised in a gesture of surrender, juxtaposed with what appears to be a disheartened Native American child in their parent's arms. This portrayal compels audiences to confront the pain, sadness, and confusion of being labeled "other" while demonstrating the interconnectedness of two seemingly different community histories through place and time. Moreover, these images prompt deep reflection on the ongoing brutality Black people face at the hands of the police and the continuous erasure of Indigenous history from our education system.

As I continued to explore the exhibition and engage with other artworks, Elahi's and Ewing's pieces remained with me, especially when I observed Gregory Rick's work *Black and Native Victories*. Presented as an accordion book, Rick documents several successful resistance movements led by Black and Native communities in fighting against slavery, settler colonialism, and white supremacy. Viewed alongside artwork created by Ruth Kaneko (Kanaka Wahine), June Carpenter (Osage/Shawnee), Eric Perez, and Dwayne Wilcox (Oglala Lakota), audiences can understand how America's pursuit of "life, liberty, and happiness" comes at a physical, mental, and emotional cost for Black, Brown, and Indigenous communities across multiple generations. What ultimately empowers those of us affected by the selfishness of settler colonialism and white supremacy is that, collectively, we have survived and can openly and honestly share our lived experiences. The beautiful expression of determination exemplifies how survivors of America's wars have navigated these complex legacies while striving to foster hope for a more peaceful future.

16. The Trail of Tears refers to the forced removal of the Cherokee Nation from their ancestral lands in southeastern United States to designated Indian territory in present-day Oklahoma. The Tulsa Massacre of 1921, also known as The Tulsa Race Massacre, or the Black Wall Street Massacre, was a violent event that took place in Tulsa, Oklahoma. From May 31 to June 1, 1921, a white mob attacked the predominantly Black Greenwood District, a prosperous and thriving community known as Black Wall Street.

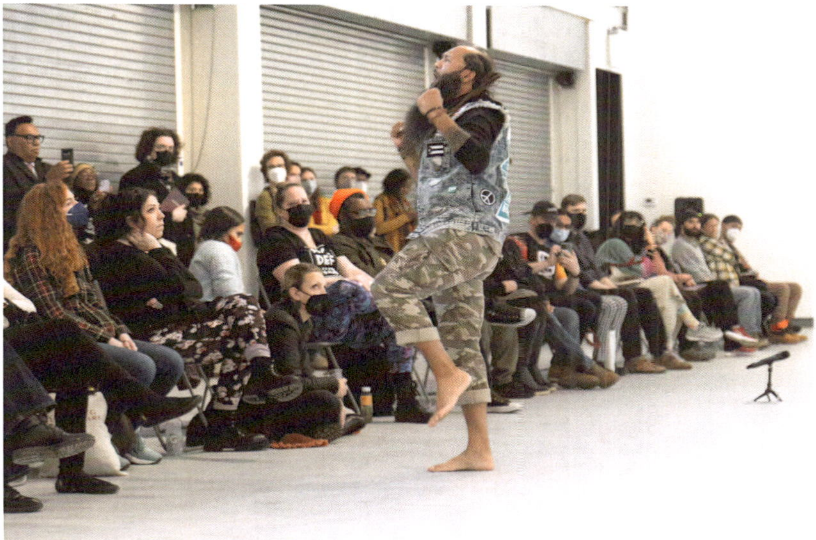

HIPÓLITO ARRIAGA III, *The Space Between: Unlikely Entanglements* Opening Program, Hyde Park Art Center, 2023; *see also: pp. 232–235, 289*

This exhibition powerfully exemplifies the unwavering resilience, compassion, and optimism displayed by BIPOC communities in the face of persistent systems of oppression. I viewed it in conjunction with the opening performances by Hipólito Arriaga III, GOODW.Y.N., and Hussein Smko, and I left the show with a new sense of hope and optimism. The community cultivated at the Hyde Park Art Center allowed me to form new relationships and nurture ones I previously neglected. I also felt driven to create similar spaces in my everyday life where individuals from all walks of life can courageously share their personal truths, fears, regrets, and joys. Reflecting on the exhibition a few days after leaving Chicago and before my uncle's funeral services, I recognized the healing that emerges through forging new paths of creativity and solidarity. I wish everyone could experience such freedom and liberation.

section two

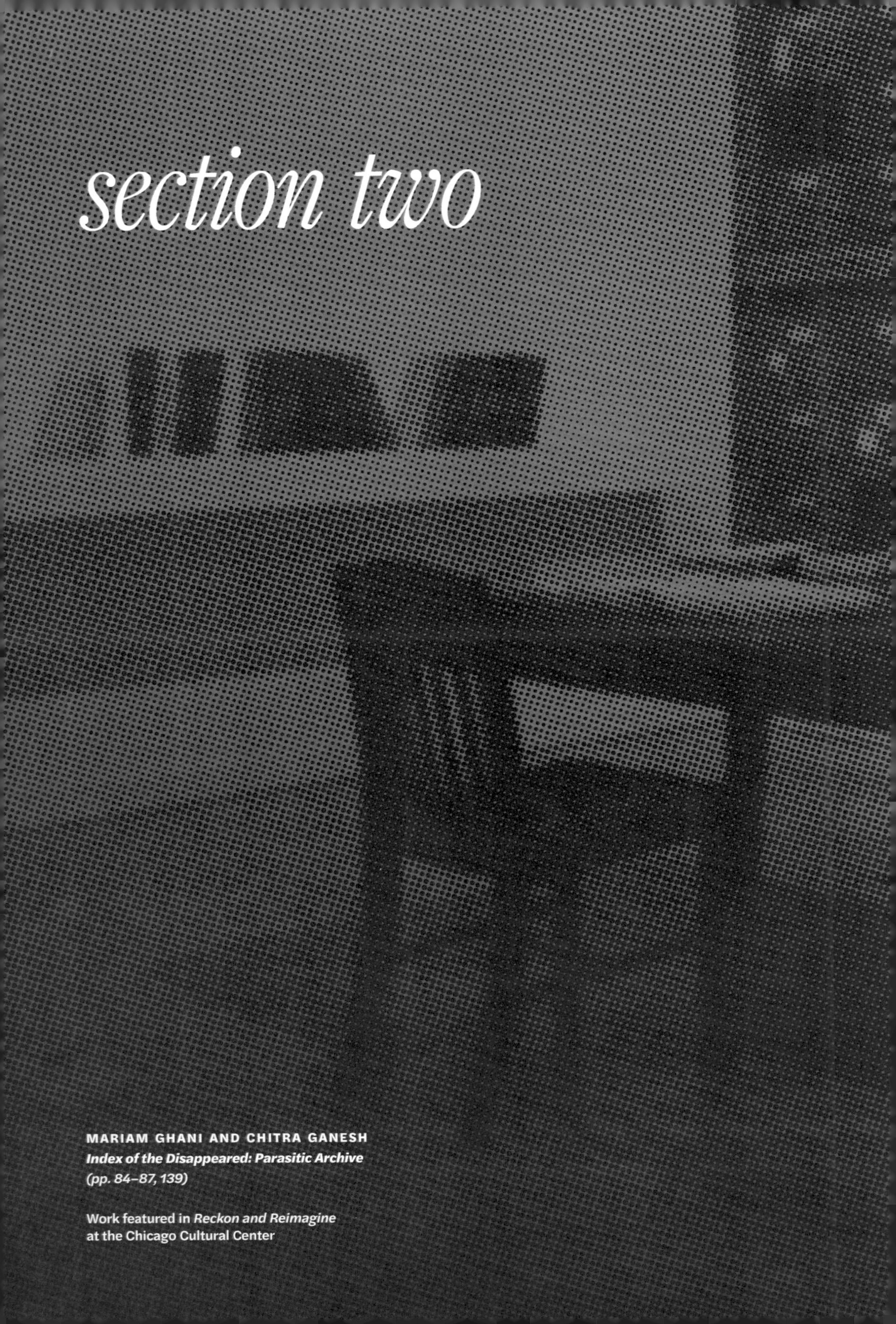

MARIAM GHANI AND CHITRA GANESH
Index of the Disappeared: Parasitic Archive
(pp. 84–87, 139)

Work featured in *Reckon and Reimagine* at the Chicago Cultural Center

Reckon and Reimagine

Reckon and Reimagine

Decolonization, therefore, implies the urgent need to thoroughly challenge the colonial situation. Its definition can, if we want to describe it accurately, be summed up in the well-known words: "The last shall be first." Decolonization is verification of this.
—Frantz Fanon, *Wretched of the Earth* (1961)

Reckoning with the history of the "Global War on Terror" requires confronting its genesis in US settler-colonial violence and genocide. An honest reckoning demands decolonization, a process Frantz Fanon described as requiring a profound reordering and reimagining of language and humanity. The artists in this section engage in a variety of forms of decolonization, transforming colonial materials and technologies to reimagine both histories and futures.

Titled *Reckon and Reimagine* after the Triennial exhibition at the Chicago Cultural Center (March 12–July 2, 2023), this section highlights artworks by Dorothy Burge, Miridith Campbell (Kiowa), Melissa Doud (Ojibwe), Ali Eyal, Tom Jones (Ho-Chunk), Chitra Ganesh, Mariam Ghani, Hock E Aye Vi Edgar Heap of Birds (Cheyenne and Arapaho Nation), Gina Herrera (Tesuque Pueblo), Rajkamal Kahlon, Monty Little (Diné), Hanaa Malallah, Hector René Membreño-Canales, Chris Pappan (Kaw/Osage, Lakota), Michael Rakowitz, Gerald Sheffield, and Dwayne Wilcox (Oglala Lakota).

This artwork is presented alongside essays by writer and arts organizer Rijin Sahakian and veteran artist and STLW co-organizer Amber Zora, as well as verse by Iraqi American poet Dunya Mikhail.

In her essay "Embedded Horizons," Rijin Sahakian poignantly explores the devastating impact of US interventions in Iraq, tracing the perpetual experiments in domination and subjugation that define our militarized present and future. Through this lens, Sahakian traces the evolution and visionary artwork of Iraqi artists like Ali Eyal, who grew up amidst the US occupation and genocidal violence, focusing on their creative acts of resistance and meaning-making within the ever-present "grind of trauma."

Veteran artist and *STLW* co-organizer Amber Zora reflects on the surreal experience of transitioning from war to civilian life in her exhibition essay "Disrupting Business as Usual: Transforming Bureaucracy into Art." She explores how Triennial artists repurpose military detritus and bureaucratic ephemera to reveal hidden aspects of militarism. Zora's essay highlights the transformative power of art to unearth repressed histories, evoke emotional responses, and foster solidarity through the innovative use of archival materials and collage techniques, ultimately advocating for a collective reorientation towards healing and envisioning a post-war future.

This collection of writings and artworks attempts to construct meaning from the ruins of the long wars, guiding us toward the great reckoning and reimagining demanded by decolonization.

Between Two Wars

DUNYA MIKHAIL

This is all that remains:
a handful of burnt papers,
photos, here and there
with rippled backs like maps.
One of us died,
another savors life
in his place.
One of us returned,
changed by magic into a small bird
who knows the news in another language.
One of us went crazy
and kept babbling nonsense
for hours under the sun.
One of us escaped
from the bugs and the officers
to who knows where.
Sidewalk vendors wrap felafel
in the pages of our books.
The entire assembly of gods
has come to help.
On the way to us, they pinch their noses
and watch a woman roll tobacco.
To her, the hand-rolled cigarette
is more wondrous
than the Seven Wonders of the World.
All her relatives have gone abroad.
The boy next door
returned one day,
a tin star on his chest.

He talked too much
about that star
until, one day, he changed
into a piece of metal
in the Martyrs' Monument.
This is all that remains:
a handful of meaningless words
engraved on the walls.
We read so absent-mindedly,
eventually we forget
how, in the short lull
between two wars,
we became so old.

This text was originally published in The War Works Hard, *New Directions*, 2005.

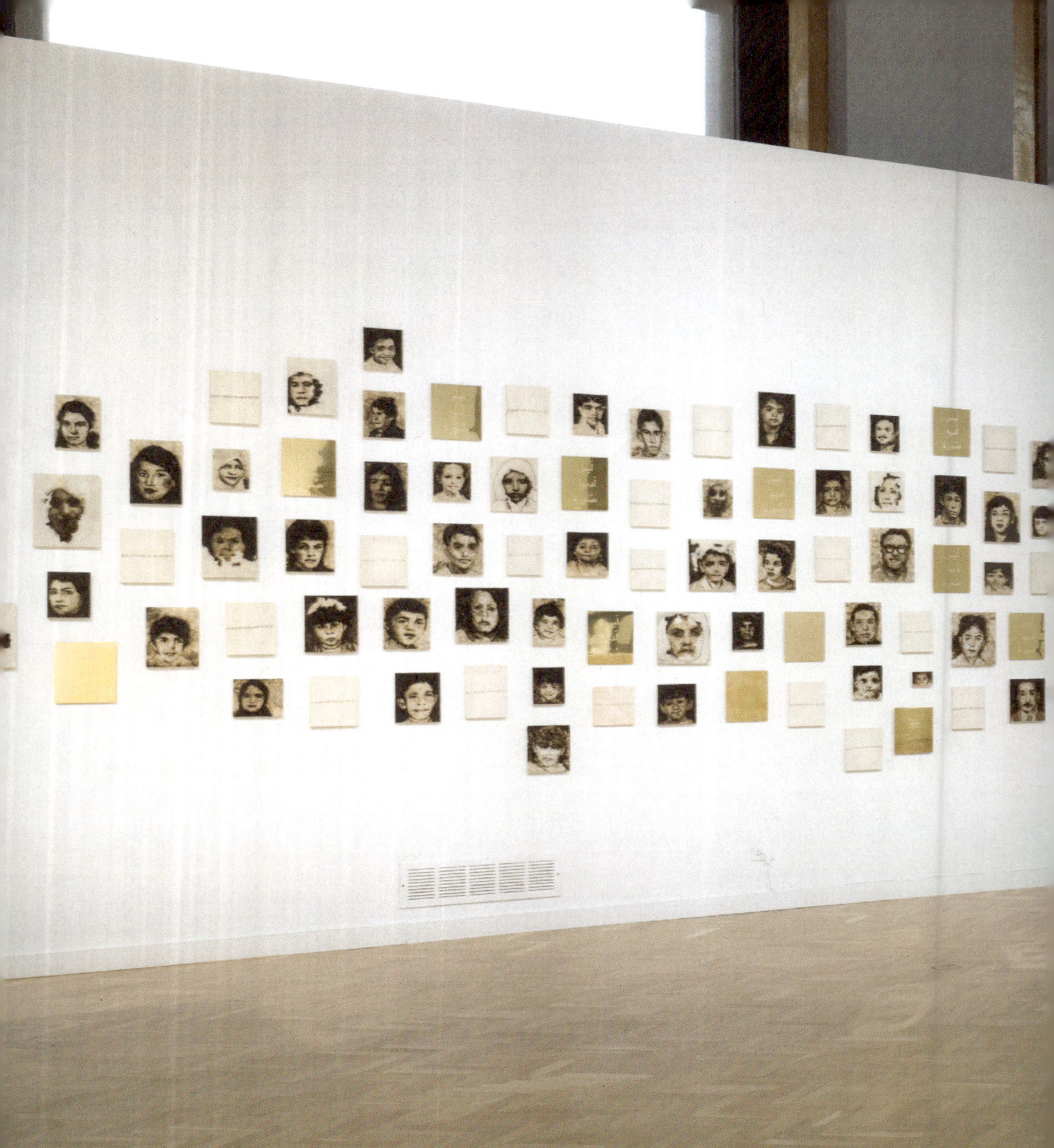

right foreground: **MICHAEL RAKOWITZ** *(b. 1973)*
American Golem, 2022
Found antiques, paper mache sculpture, granite, wood, metal base
Courtesy of the artist and Rhona Hoffman Gallery

With specific attention to US Civil War monuments, American Golem exposes the relationship between monuments that have been removed and those that remain. Foundries like Roman Bronze Works in New York and artists like Henry M. Shrady—who designed the Ulysses S. Grant Memorial in Washington, DC, and the removed Robert E. Lee Monument in Charlottesville, Virginia—created works valorizing both sides of the US Civil War. Here, Rakowitz has collected small historic pieces by artists, foundries, and quarries originally made for American homes. Cobbling them together, he forms *American Golem*, a monstrous figure of mismatched parts, wrapped in written truths that point to the reckoning with settler colonialism, white supremacy, and imperialism that needs to happen in private and public spaces.

see detail on p. 336

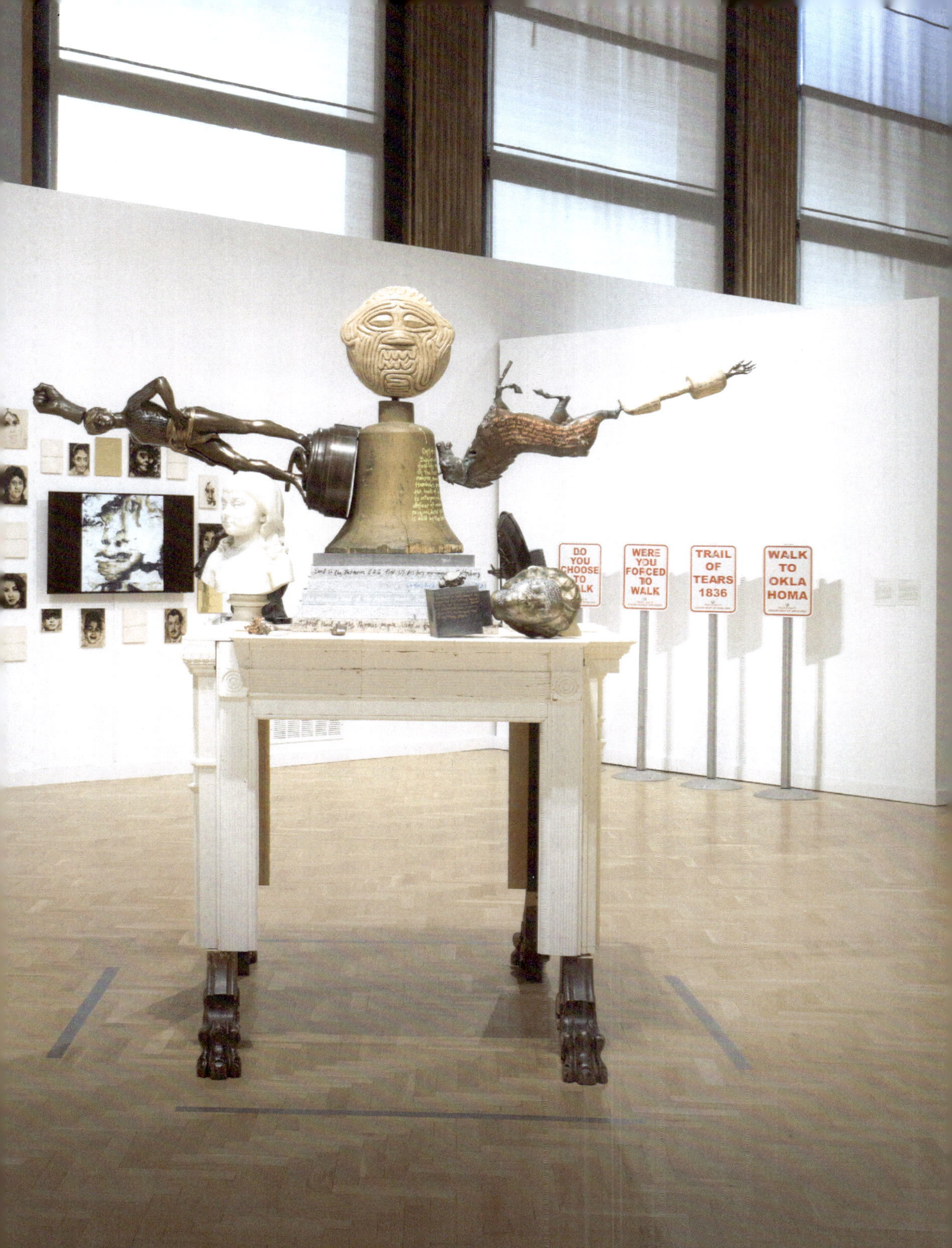
DO YOU CHOOSE TO
WERE YOU FORCED TO WALK
TRAIL OF TEARS 1836
WALK TO OKLA HOMA

background: **HANAA MALALLAH**
She/He Has No Picture
see also: pp. 113–15, 144–45, 150–51

right background: **HOCK E AYE VI EDGAR HEAP OF BIRDS,** ***Trail of Tears***
see also: pp. xiv, 96

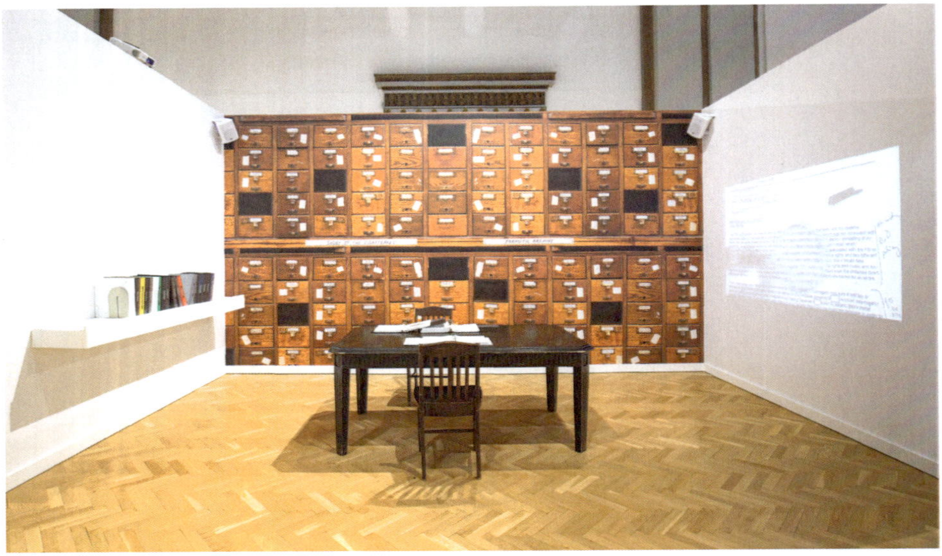

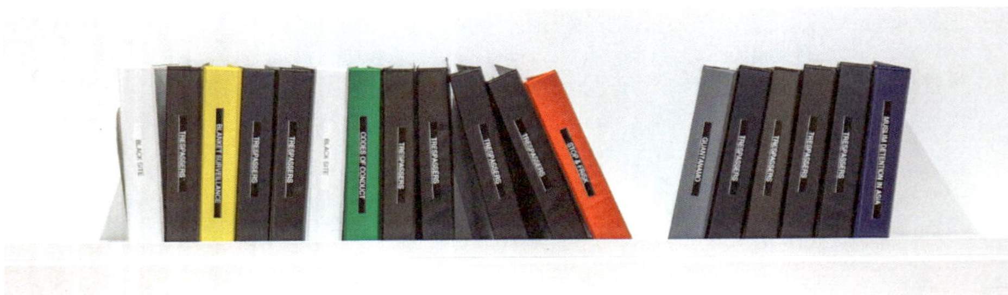

MARIAM GHANI *(b. 1978)*
AND CHITRA GANESH *(b. 1975)*
Index of the Disappeared: Parasitic Archive, 2014
Site-specific installation with vinyl, tables, chairs, binders, copy paper, ephemera including military manuals and documents

Since 2004, Chitra Ganesh and Mariam Ghani have collaborated on the *Index of the Disappeared*, a site-specific installation that operates both as a physical archive of post-9/11 disappearances—detentions, deportations, renditions, and redactions—and a mobile platform for public dialogue. The massive collection draws on radical archival, legal, and activist traditions to draw unlikely connections between seemingly disparate forms of state violence. According to the artists, "The point of the Index is not to collect everything relevant that is released into the public domain, but to sort through masses of information to retrieve and preserve small bits of significance, and then to make the connections that allow others to understand that significance."

This iteration poetically acknowledges the history where it was installed during the Triennial—the Chicago Cultural Center—which was originally built as the first Chicago Public Library. In the installation the library environment is reimagined with a large vinyl wall and reading room. On the shelf and table are binders filled with official documents, secondary literature, and personal narratives on the US extra-legal prisons at Guantánamo, military "black sites," military codes of conduct, and more. The archive was installed with *The Trespassers* video by Ghani and the *Index of the Disappeared: Watercolors* by Ganesh. Collectively, this work foregrounds the impact of US global military and intelligence operations, while highlighting the way censorship and state secrets perpetuate racialized state violence.

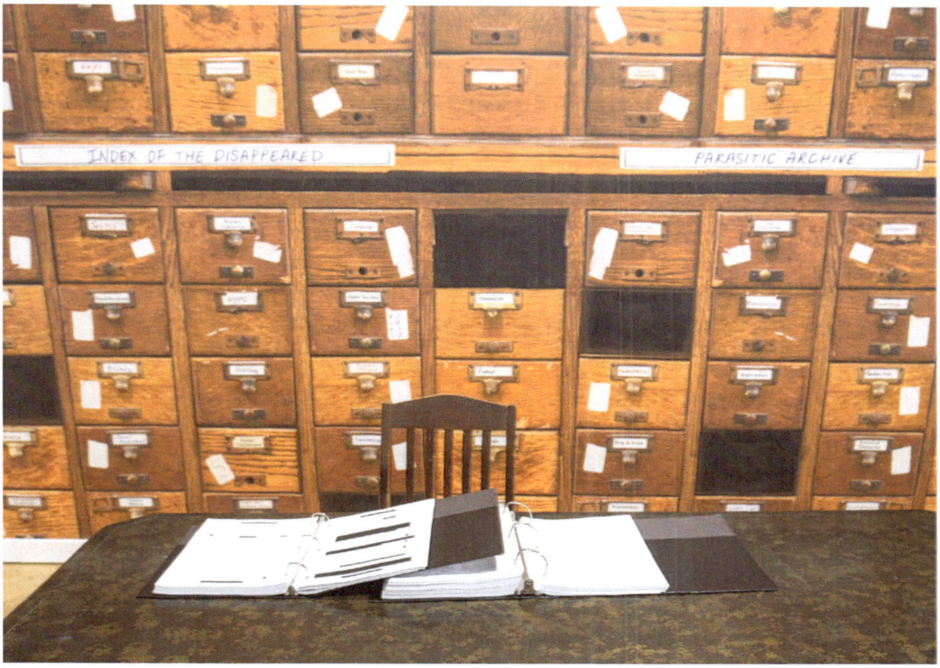

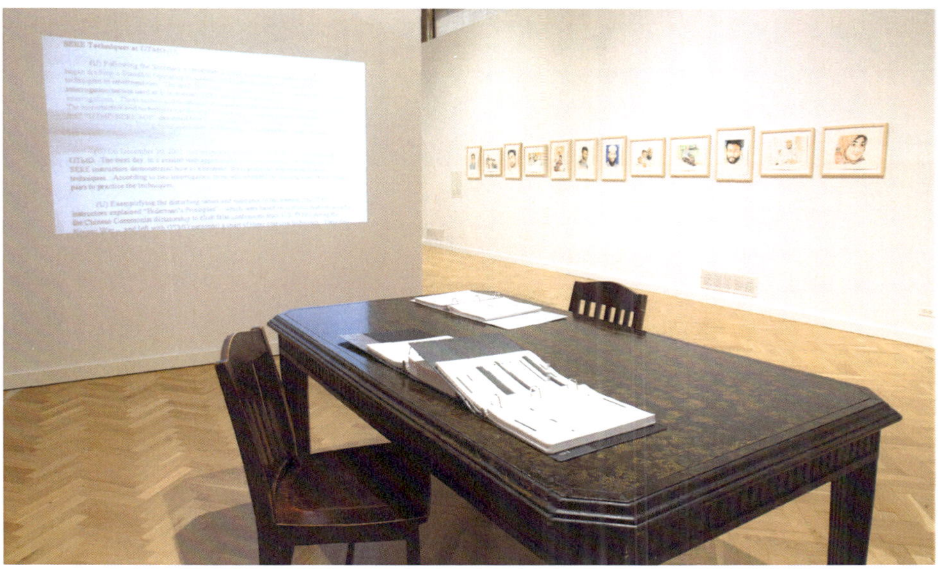

above, right: **CHITRA GANESH** *(b. 1975)*
Index of the Disappeared: Watercolors (series), 2004
Watercolor on paper
Courtesy of the artists, Gallery Wendi Norris, and
Hales Gallery in New York and London

MARIAM GHANI *(b. 1978)*
The Trespassers, 2011
105-minute 1-channel video with 4-channel sound (presented in stereo) and annotated archive (approximately 20,000 pages)
Courtesy of the artist and Ryan Lee Gallery

The Trespassers tells a history of the "Global War on Terror" through redacted documents and the testimony of Afghan and Iraqi diasporic translators whose presence during military interrogations was removed from the record. In this piece, the camera follows a magnifying glass as it reads declassified official documents line by line, while Dari and Arabic speakers simultaneously translate the text. Ghani's video explores the complex role of these diasporic translators in wartime, who she refers to as the "ghosts in the records." Ghani writes, "Every time you read an interrogation transcript you know the interrogation could not have happened without a translator. But the translator's presence is rarely recorded. If you read enough of these transcripts you become really interested in the missing translators... Can a translator be a witness, or will he always be a special class of informant—negotiating between the trespassers and trespassed, and frequently finding himself called a traitor?"

The video is exhibited alongside a series of binders that represent the ongoing archival project the *Index of the Disappeared*, a collaboration between Ghani and Chitra Ganesh since 2004.

CHITRA GANESH *(b. 1975)*
Index of the Disappeared: Watercolors, (series), 2004
Watercolor on paper
Courtesy of the artists, Gallery Wendi Norris, and Hales Gallery in New York and London

Central to the *Index of the Disappeared* is an ongoing series of watercolor portraits by Chitra Ganesh of detained and disappeared individuals in the months following September 11th. The use of watercolor, a medium historically associated with plein air and Sunday painting, landscape, and leisure, represents the faces and bodies of primarily Arab, Muslim, and South Asian immigrant people entangled in the US system of indefinite detention alongside other prisoners during the "Global War on Terror." For Ganesh, figurative painting offers a means to restore dignity and humanity to subjects treated as casualties of injustice and war.

selections from watercolor series below;
see also: pp. 139, 302

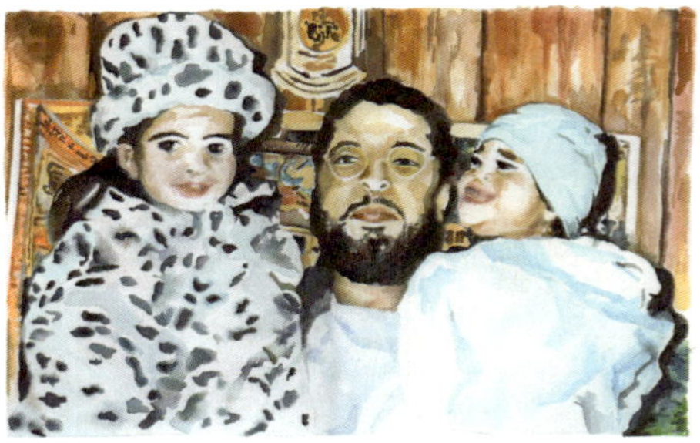

Shaker Aamer

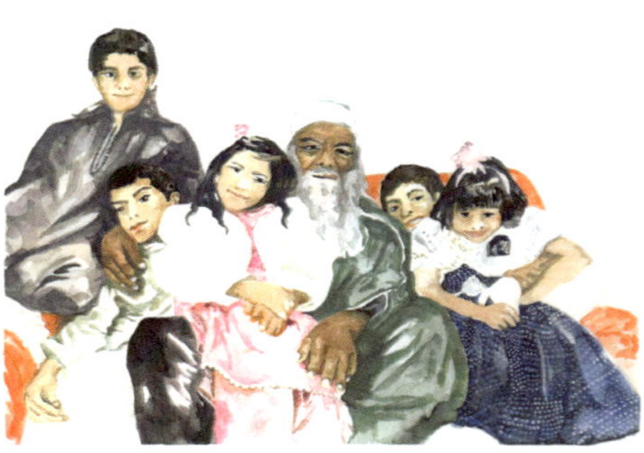

Al Banna Family

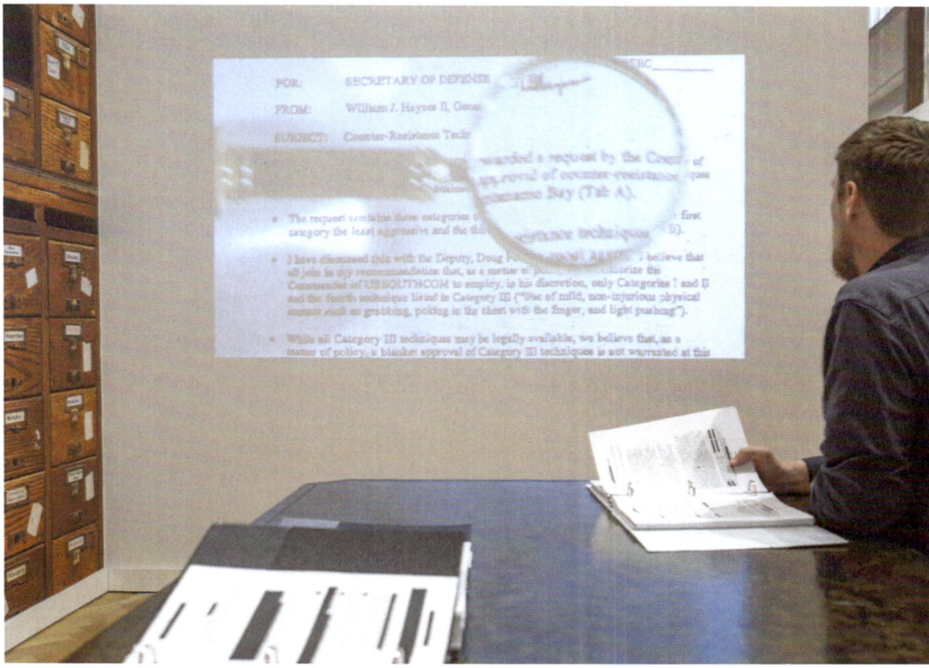
FOR:
SECRETARY OF DEFENSE
FROM:
William J. Haynes II,
SUBJECT:
Counter-Resistance

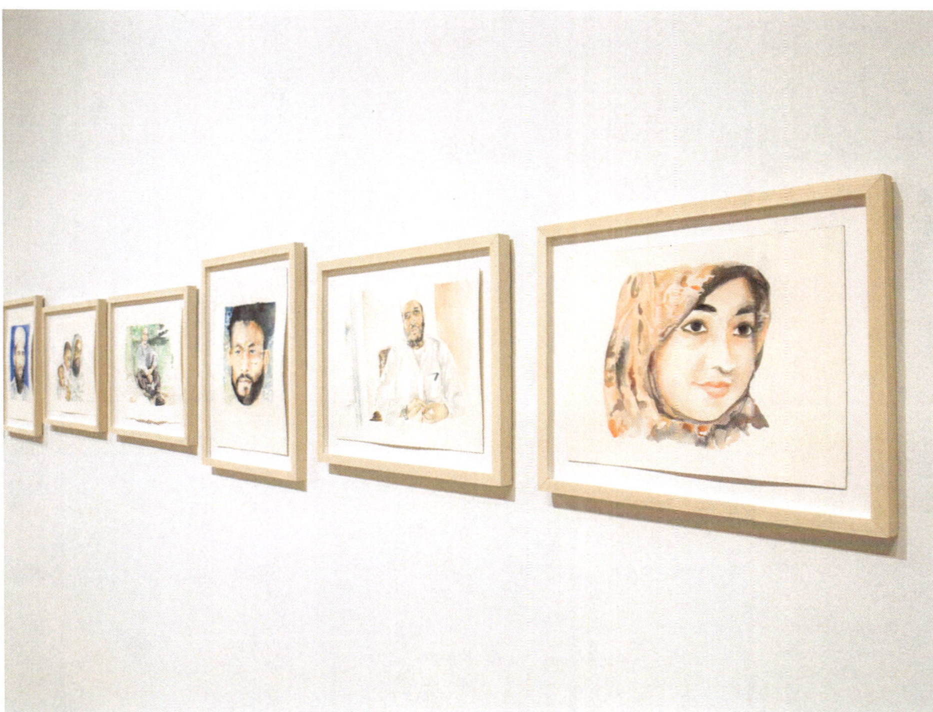

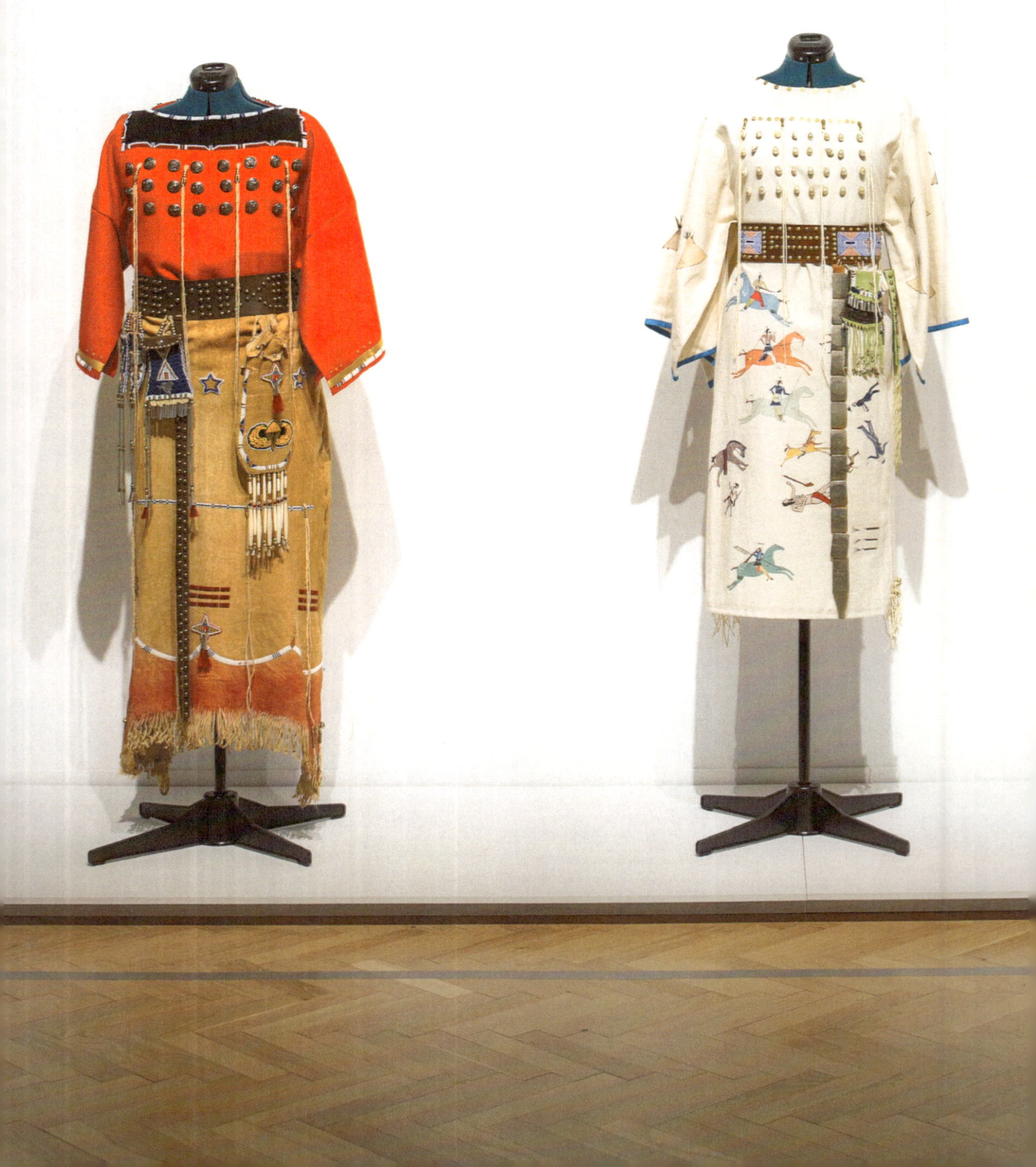

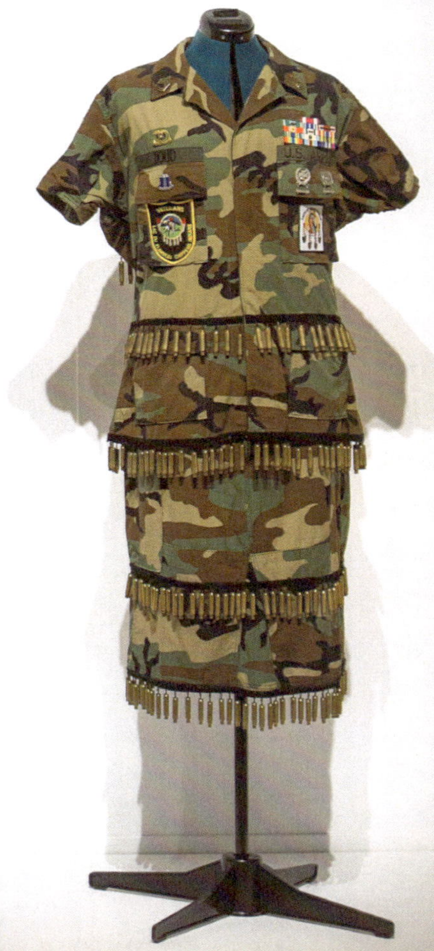

MIRIDITH CAMPBELL *(Kiowa, b. 1966)*
[US Marine Corps, Army, and Navy veteran]
left: ***Marine Corps Dress—Southern Style***, 2022
Artist tanned and smoked buckskin hide; antique, vintage, and contemporary seed beads; Red Broadcloth English Wool; vintage Marine Corps service buttons; Hawk Bells; and horse hair

This piece embodies Campbell's service in three branches of the US military. The dress itself represents the artist's Marine Corps service, an important aspect of her identity and history. The knife and awl cases, along with the "strike-a-light" bag, honors her Navy Seabee service, while the handbag represents her time in the Army. The hash marks on the dress symbolize her total time in military service.

center: ***Adobe Walls Battle Dress***, 2022
Cotton canvas dresses with blue edging. Digitally printed ledger art on fabric, depicting the Adobe Walls Battle. Two sets of fully beaded belt bags. Two belts, one fully beaded on latigo with a German silver whip, and one fully brass-tacked on harness leather with a tacked whip.

This canvas dress is a visual telling of the First Battle of Adobe Walls, Texas, in 1864. The battle between the US Army and the Kiowa, Comanche, and Apache was one of the largest battles to take place on the Plains. It was caused by the influx of settlers and the subsequent diminishing of buffalo herds, an important food source on the Plains. During the battle, Chief Satanta (Kiowa) used a bugle to confuse the US Cavalry, resulting in the three tribes successfully repelling and defeating Colonel Christopher "Kit" Carson and his troops. Campbell crafted the dress to honor her ancestors who fought in the battle against the US Cavalry.

MELISSA DOUD *(Ojibwe, b. 1971) [US Army Veteran]*
right: ***Bullet Dress***, 2016
Army uniform with 365 bullet casings

Melissa Doud is a powwow jingle dress dancer from the Lac du Flambeau Ojibwe Reservation in northern Wisconsin. While in the military Doud was tasked with collecting spent bullet casings from fellow soldiers, which allowed her to quietly collect 365 of them. Back on the reservation in Wisconsin, Doud took the casings gleaned from the horrors of war and turned them into a bullet jingle dress. She says, "Creating this dress after I came back from Iraq was part of my healing journey. Now I dance for others and can display the path I went through to get here."

In July 2016, Doud collaborated with Warrior Songs and the Mambo Surfers to record the song "Bullet Dress" in Wauwatosa, Wisconsin. LEARN MORE: MAMBOSURFERS.COM

detail images on next spread
see also: pp. 71, 250–51, 319

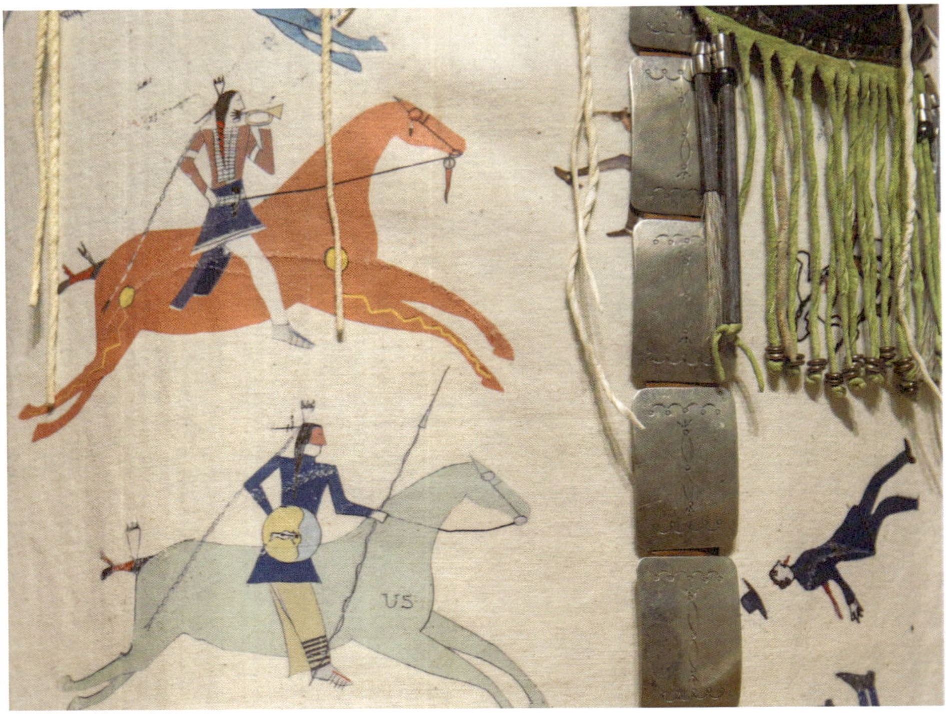
US

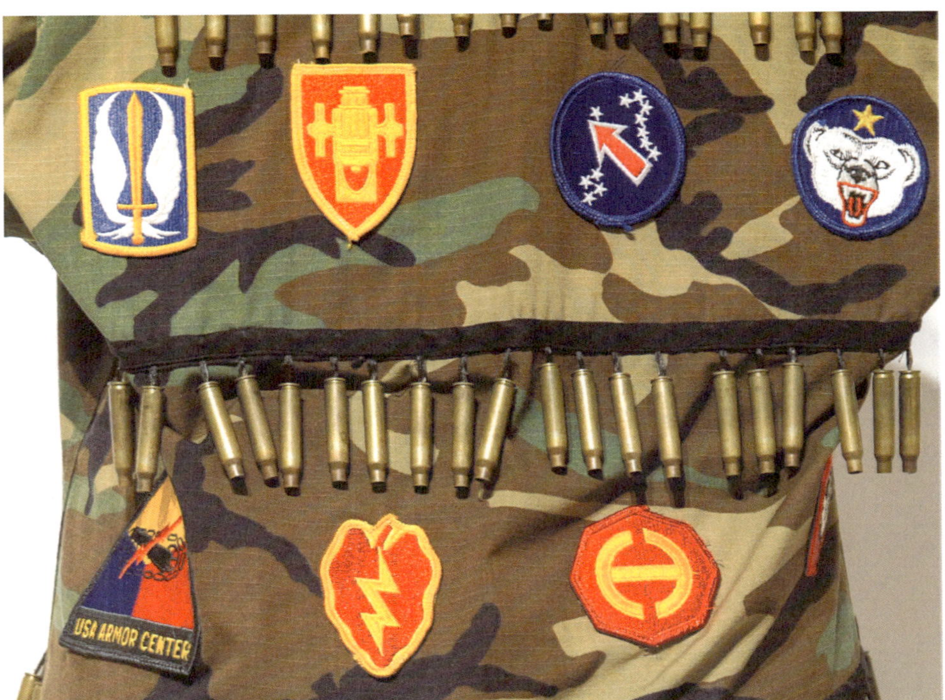
USA ARMOR CENTER

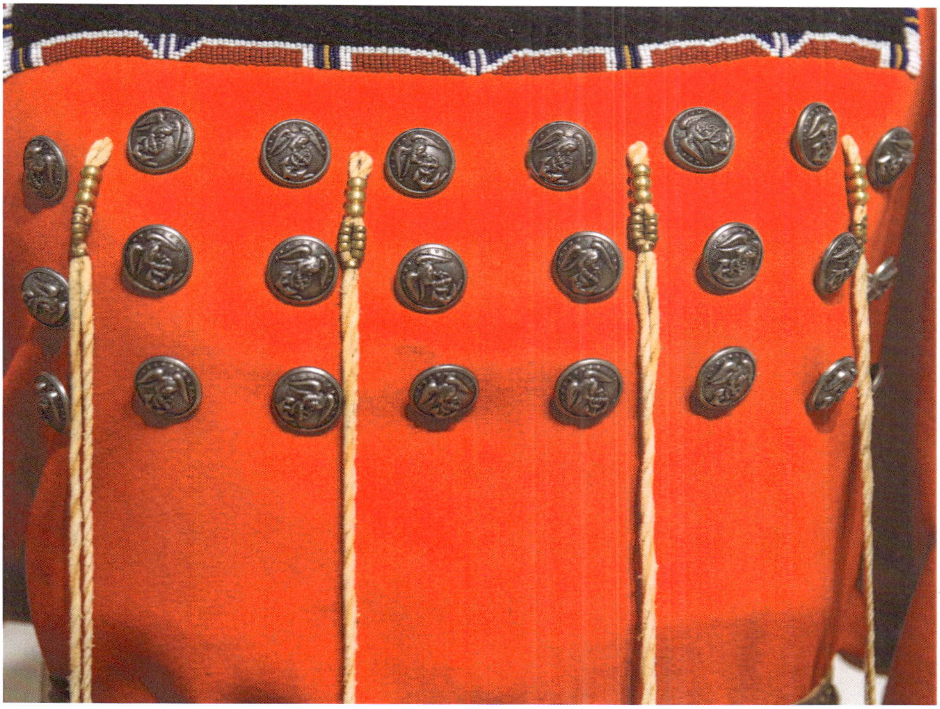

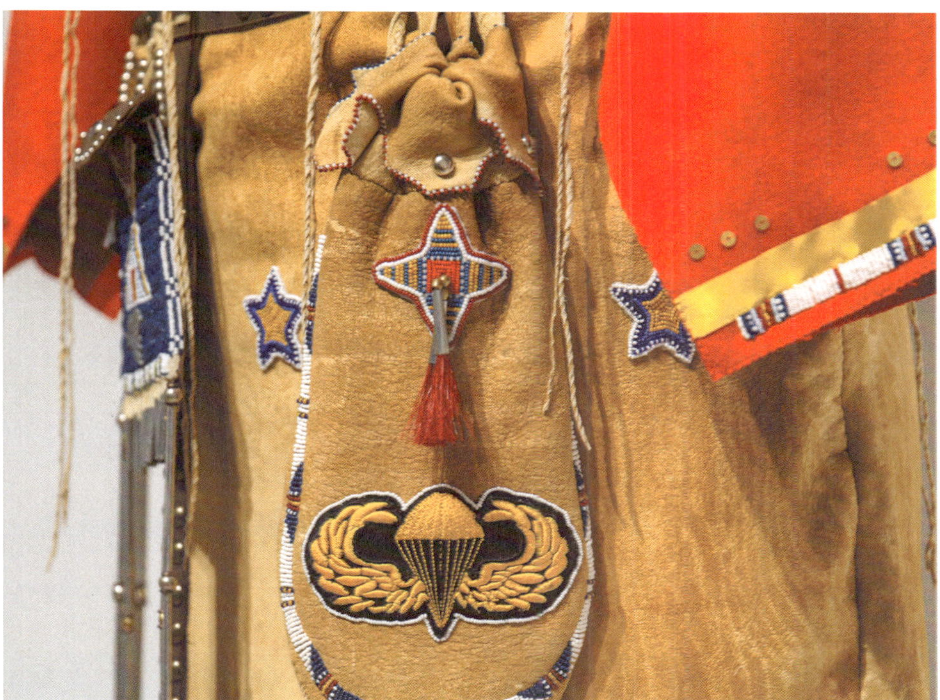

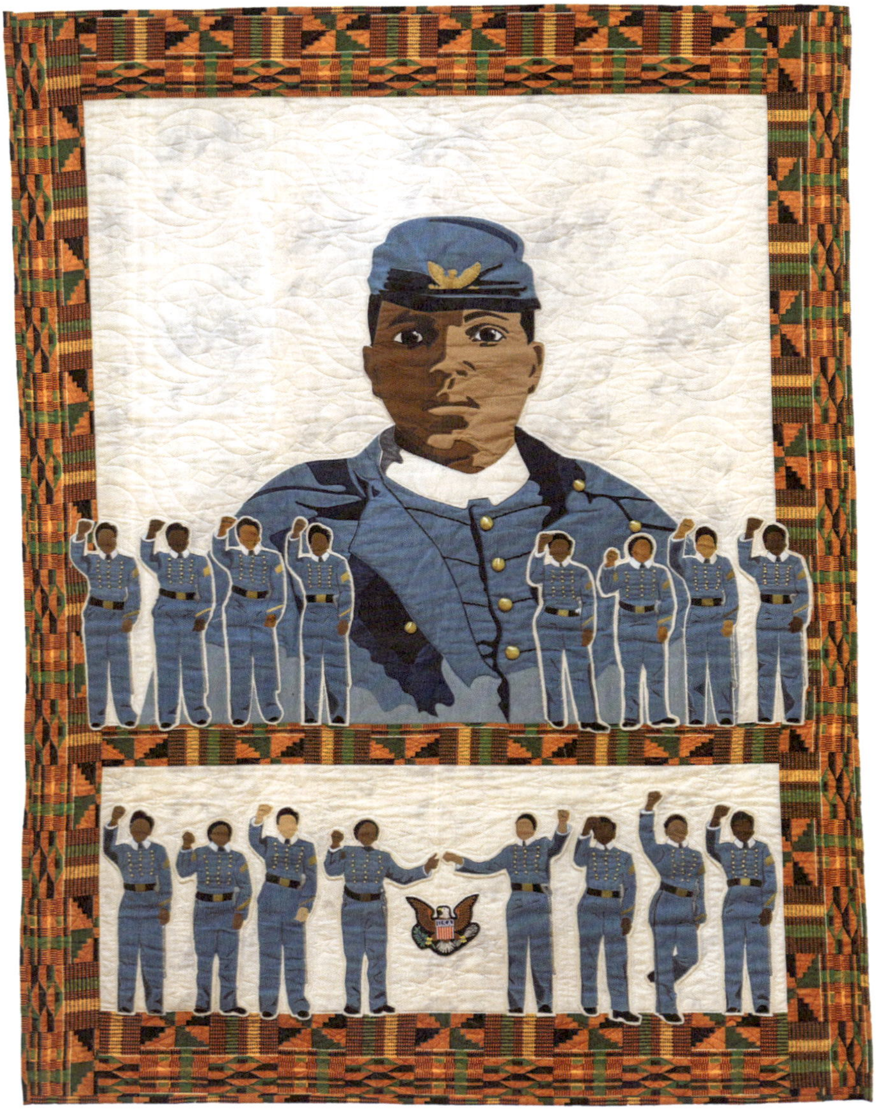

DOROTHY BURGE *(b. 1954)*
"We Stand on the Shoulders of Our Ancestors", 2018
Cotton fabric and batting, buttons, beads, embroidered patch, printing on fabric, photo-transfer on fabric; Machine quilted by Judy Wolff

This quilt highlights the legacy of US Army Colonel Charles Young, the third African American to graduate from West Point in 1889. In addition to a portrait of Colonel Young, the quilt depicts sixteen African American women and Army cadets raising their fists as a sign of unity and solidarity during growing Black Lives Matter demonstrations in 2016. For Burge, these cadets graduating from West Point in a class that was 70 percent white is a testament to the continuing strength and perseverance of African Americans. The artist's activist quilting practice speaks to the important tradition of quilting, one of few mediums accessible to marginalized groups, in telling and maintaining African American histories.

see also: pp. 113, 248

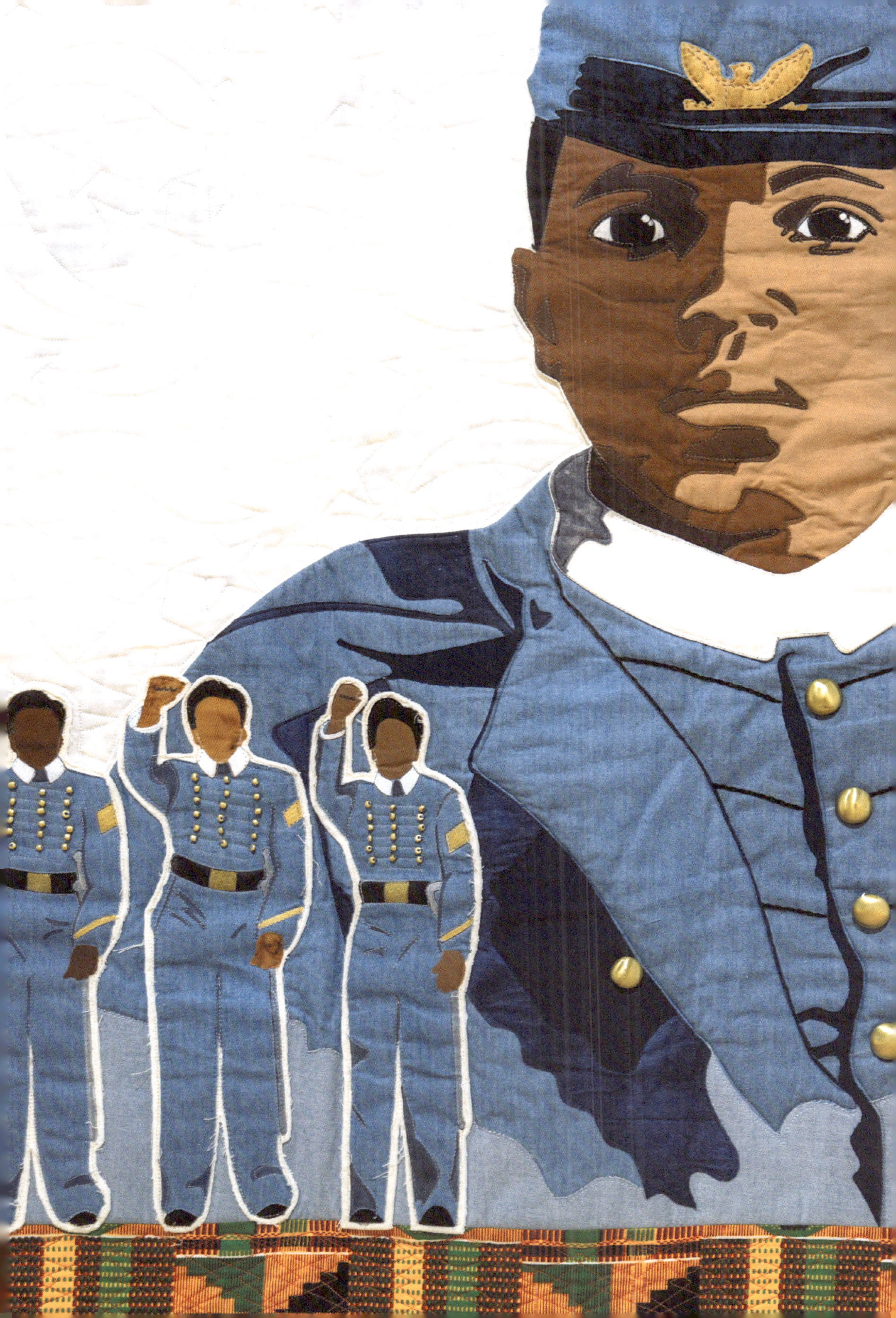

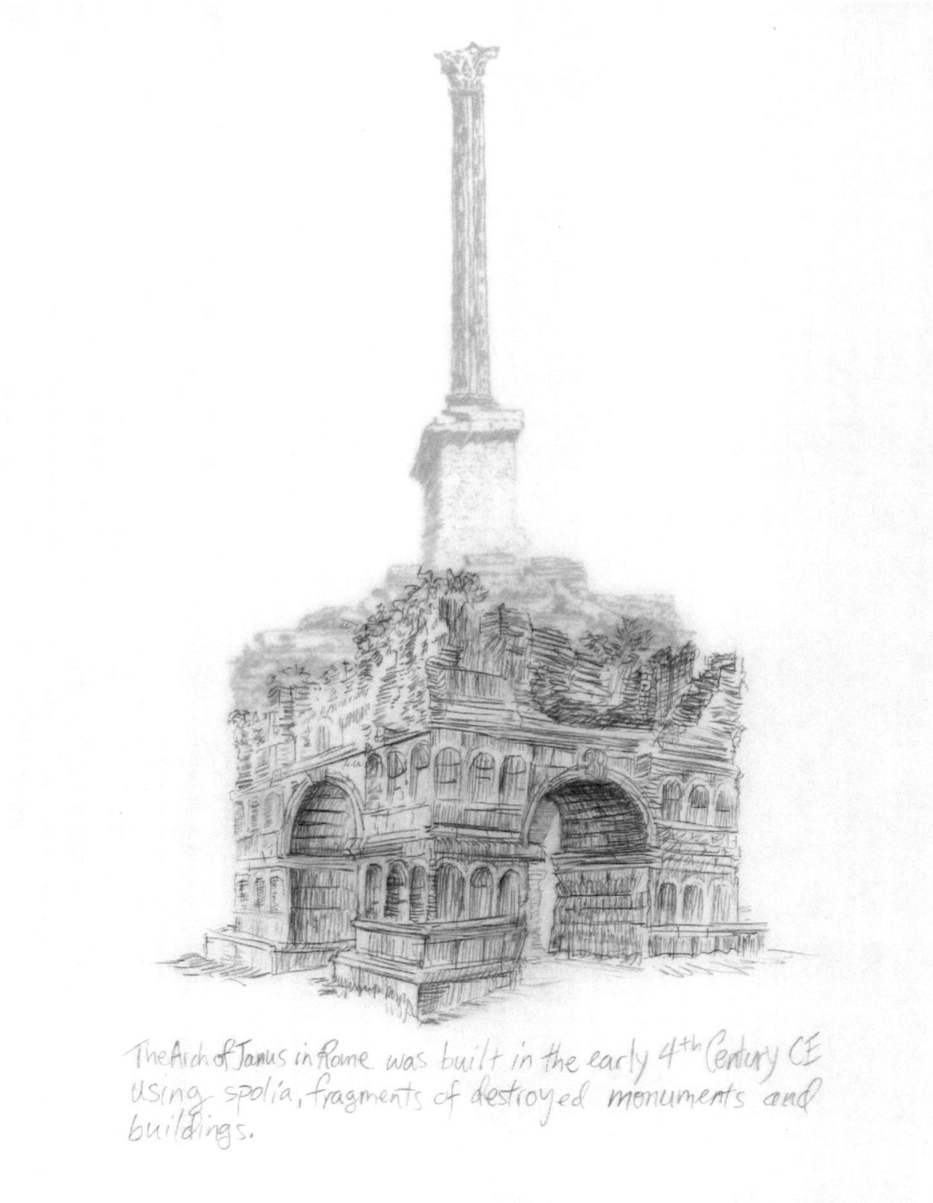
The Arch of Janus in Rome was built in the early 4th Century CE
using spolia, fragments of destroyed monuments and
buildings.

MICHAEL RAKOWITZ *(b. 1973)*
Moments in Spolia 2, 2022
Pencil on vellum
Courtesy of the artist and Rhona Hoffman Gallery

Starting with little known facts that inspire research, Michael Rakowitz uncovers unlikely connections between personal, local, and global political histories. In the *Spolia* series, the artist explores the relationship between standing monuments and those that have been removed and destroyed. The layered works point to the complex entanglements between rising and collapsing power structures, from political actors to empires.

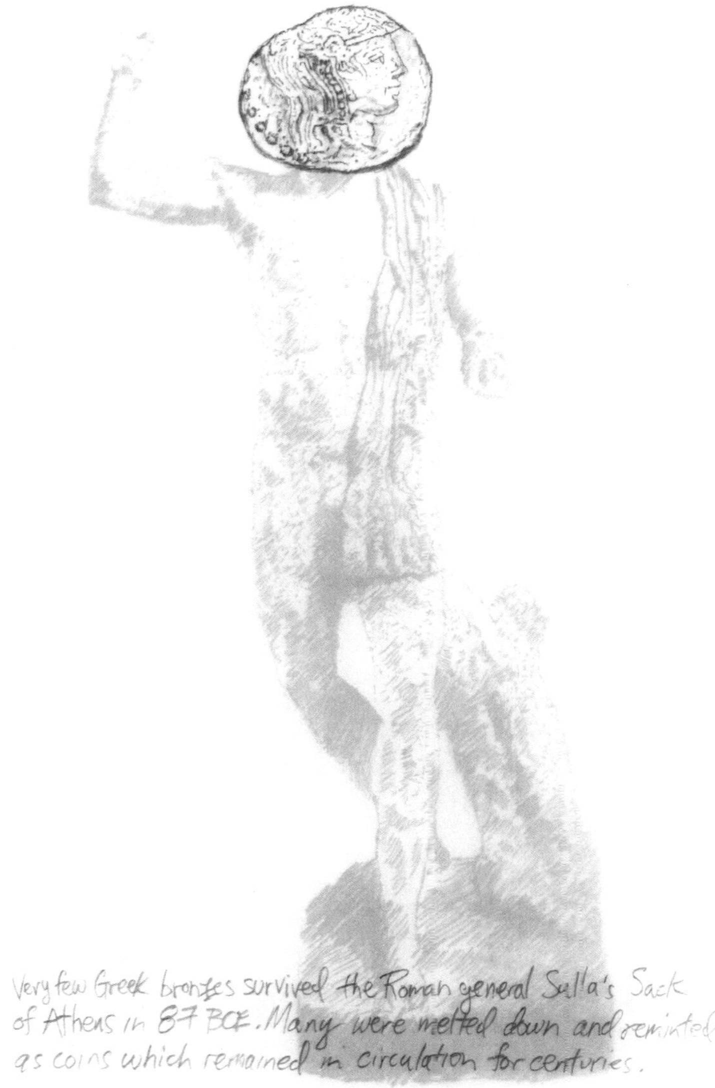
Very few Greek bronzes survived the Roman general Sulla's Sack
of Athens in 87 BCE. Many were melted down and reminted
as coins which remained in circulation for centuries.

Moments in Spolia 3, 2022
Pencil on vellum
Courtesy of the artist and Rhona Hoffman Gallery

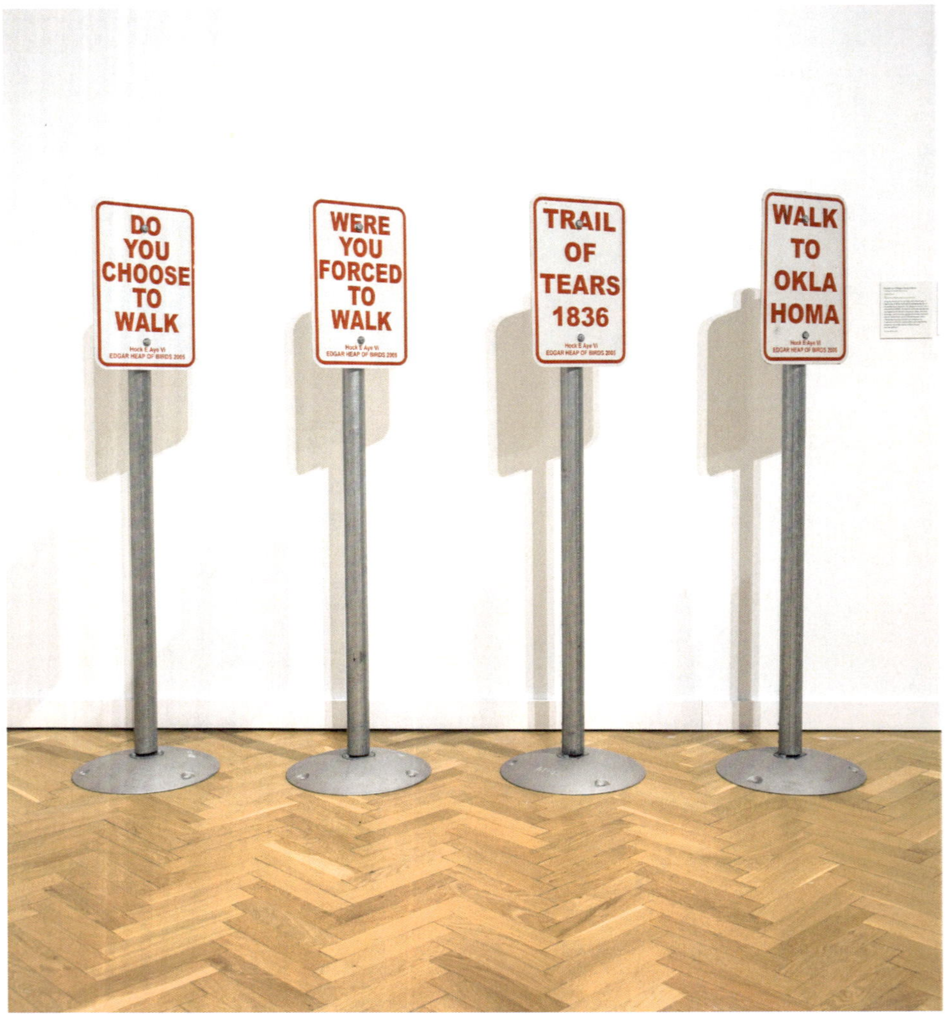
DO YOU CHOOSE TO WALK
WERE YOU FORCED TO WALK
TRAIL OF TEARS 1836
WALK TO OKLA HOMA

HOCK E AYE VI EDGAR HEAP OF BIRDS
(Cheyenne and Arapaho Nation, b. 1954)
Trail of Tears, 2005
Mylar on four aluminum metal sign panels with posts

Using four bureaucratic parking signs, Hock E Aye Vi Edgar Heap of Birds confronts the devastating loss of life and heritage caused by the US government's Indian Removal Act of 1830. The law led to the forced removal and migration of 100,000 Cherokee, Creek, Choctaw, Chickasaw, and Seminole peoples from their ancestral lands to reservations west of the Mississippi. Heap of Birds has described this forced walking as an "instrument of torture perpetuated upon many tribal peoples as the United States inflicted brutal removal policies."

see also: pp. xiv, 83

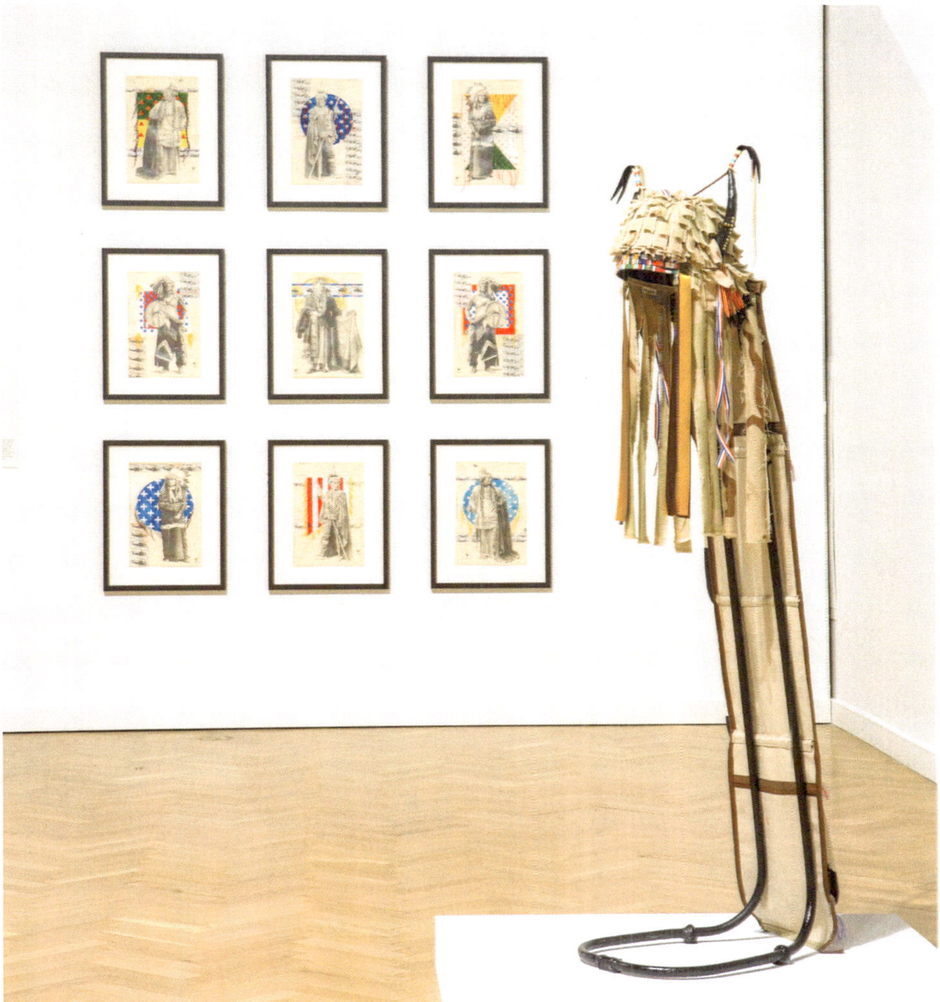

foreground: **DWAYNE WILCOX**
(Oglala Lakota, b. 1957) [US Air Force veteran]
Horned Warrior Headdress, 2014
Military desert camouflage, felt, brass tacks, ribbons
Courtesy of the artist and Maȟpíya Lúta (formerly Red Cloud Indian School)

Dwayne Wilcox used parts of his wife's, father's, and grandfather's uniforms to make *Horned Warrior Headdress*. The desert camouflage horns are made from parts of military combat boots. The browband is made of military medals and ribbons. The temple buttons are from World War I and World War II collar insignia. Through repurposing military materials, Wilcox's headdress simultaneously acknowledges his family lineage of serving in the US military while celebrating Indigenous culture. The piece exemplifies the overlapping and simultaneously contested identities present throughout the long wars.

background: **CHRIS PAPPAN**
War Dance (series)
see next spread

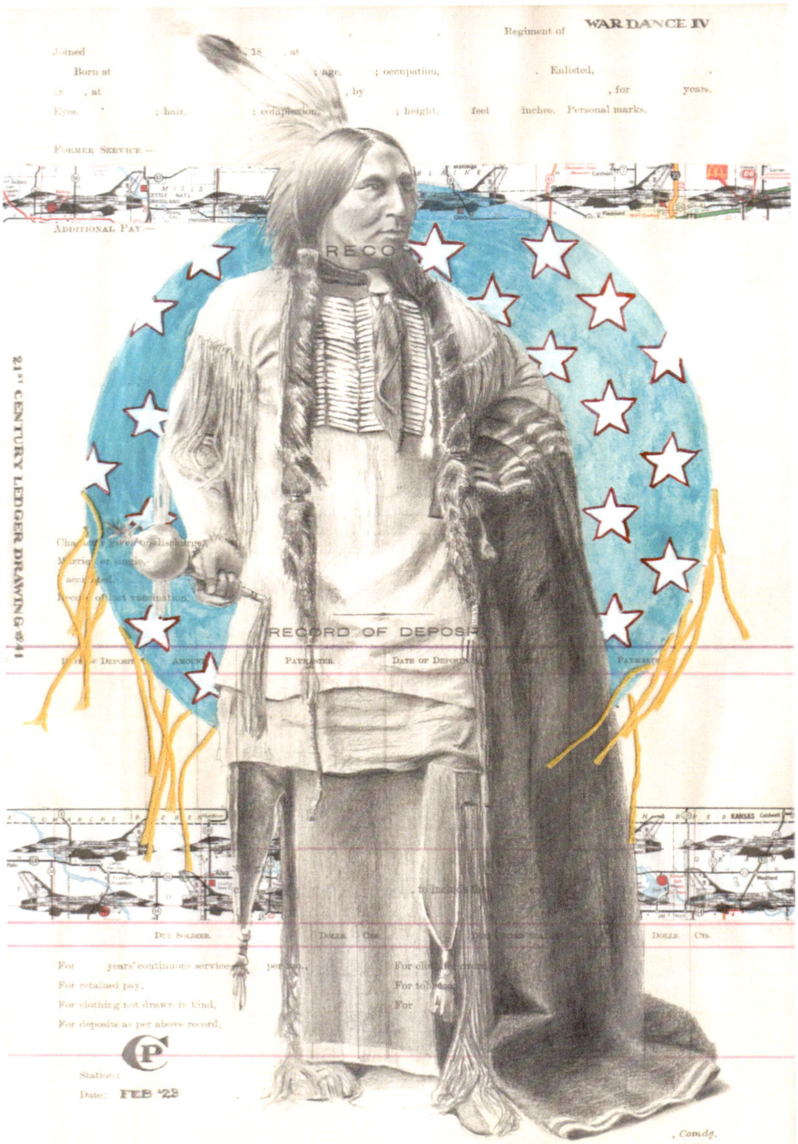

CHRIS PAPPAN *(Kaw/Osage, Lakota b. 1971)*
above: ***War Dance IV***
right: ***War Dance*** (series), 2023
Graphite, gouache, ink, map collage, and embroidery floss on US Cavalry recruitment ledger

European and American colonizers have often depicted Indigenous people as war-like, or "savage." According to Pappan, "While the figures in these drawings are of warriors, they are not 'savage.' They are spiritual and cultural warriors in defense of all peoples." In this series of drawings, behind each central figure are collages that echo Ghost Dance regalia and explore the intersections between art and warfare. The maps depict Indigenous homelands, and the US military weapons named after Indigenous peoples.

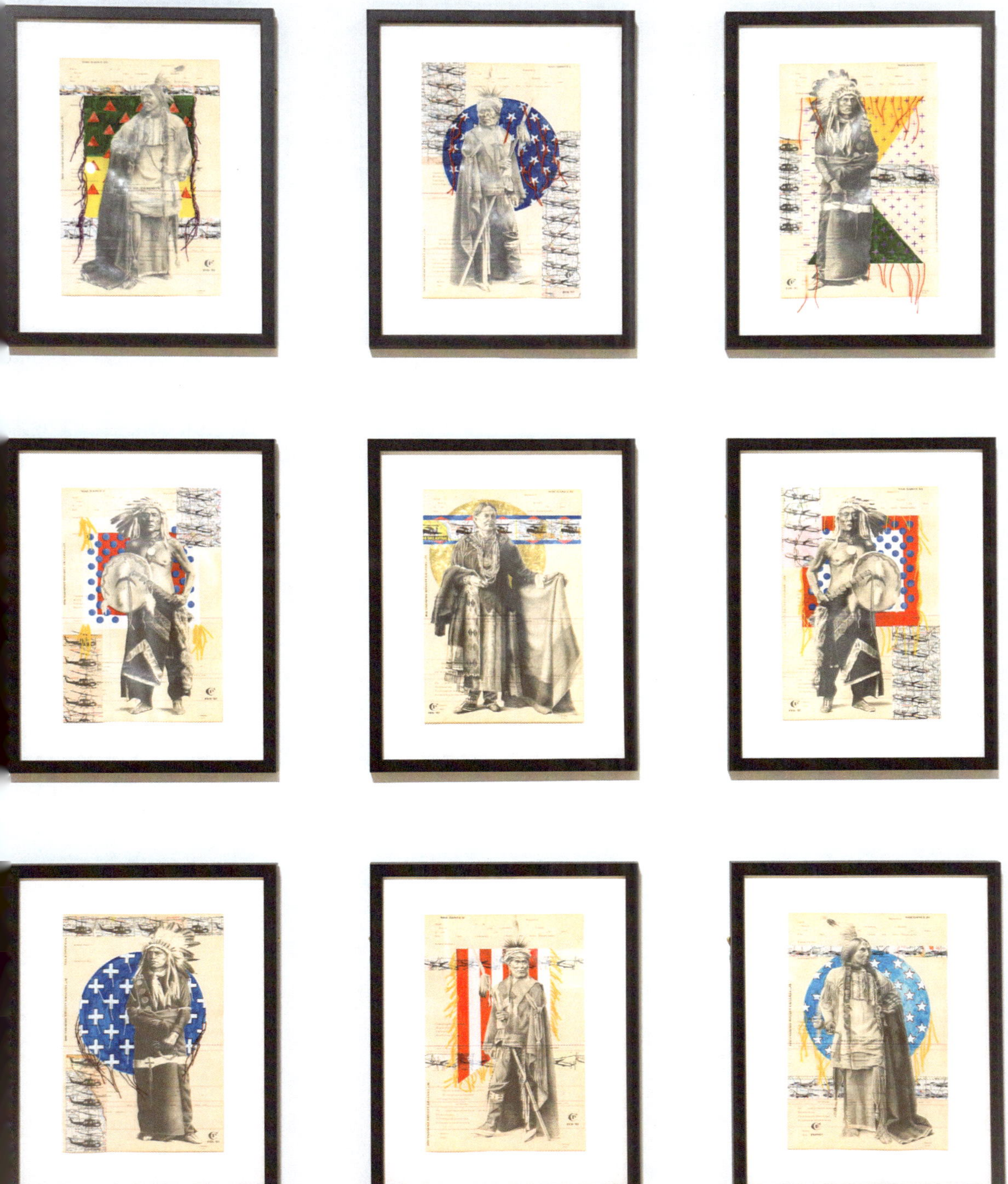

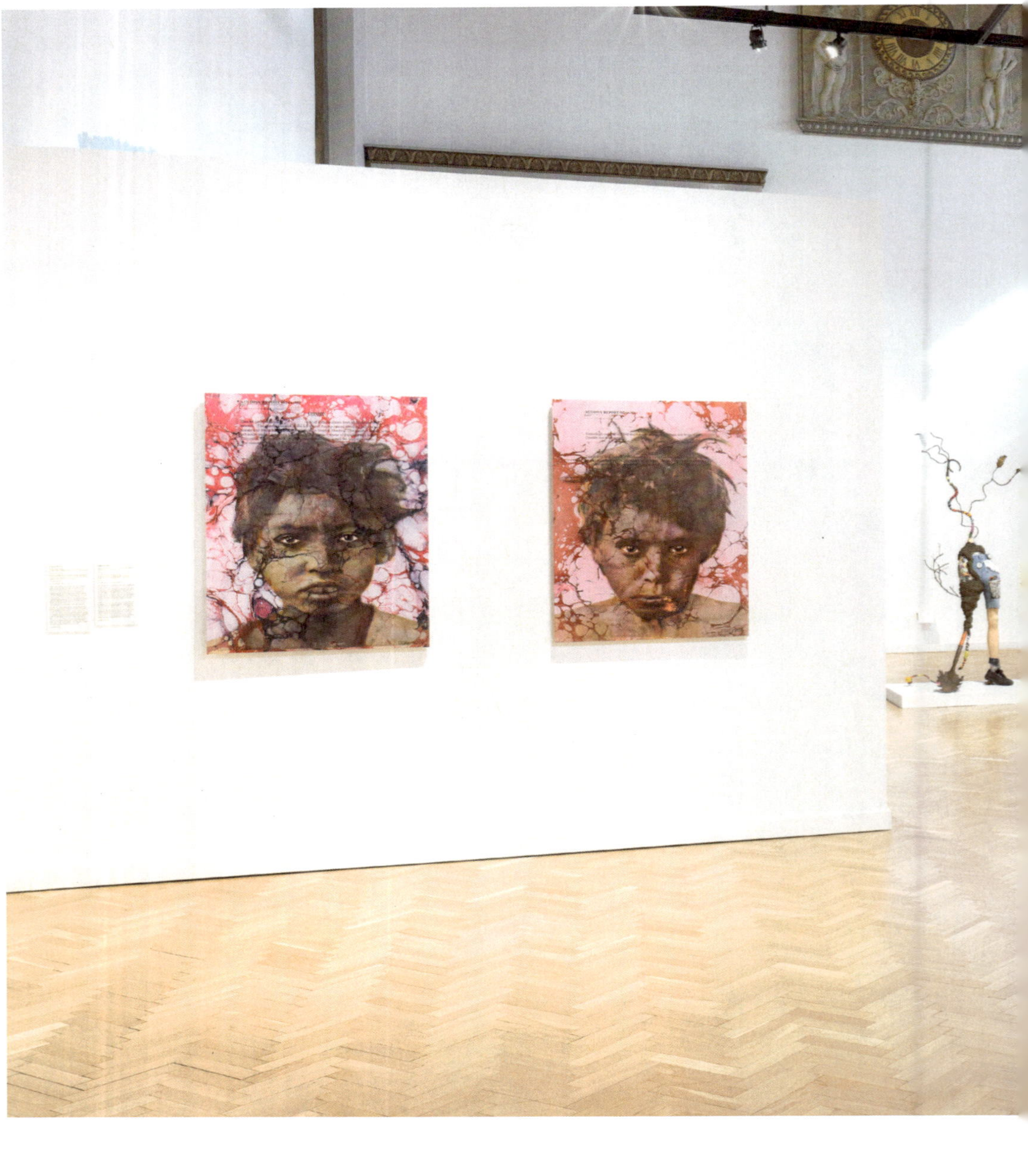

RAJKAMAL KAHLON
From the ongoing series ***Did You Kiss the Dead Body?***

see next spread

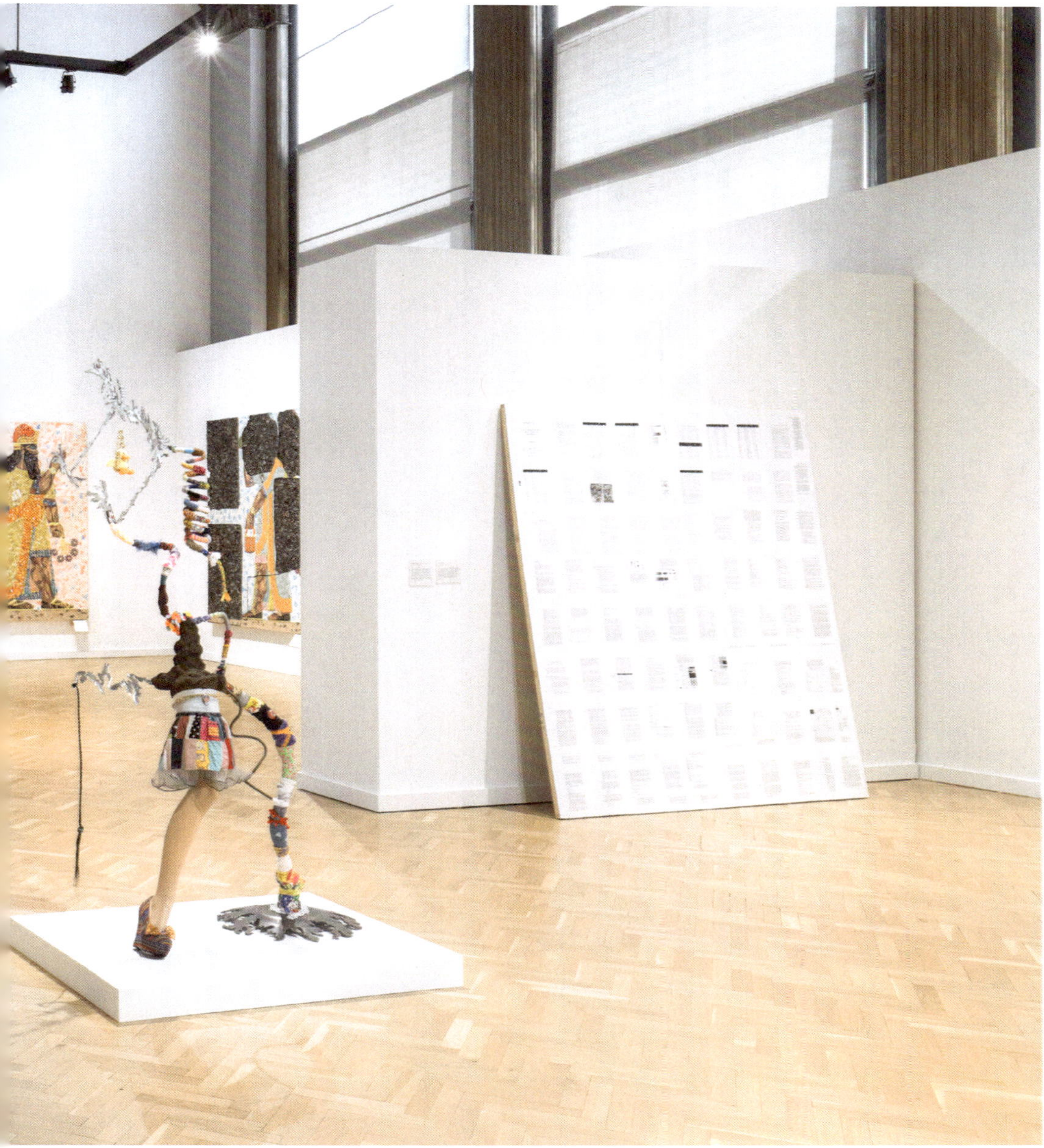

foreground: **GINA HERRERA**
The Liberty Master and ***A Virtuous Warrior*** - *see also: pp. 104–6*

right background: **MICHAEL RAKOWITZ**
The invisible enemy should not exist (Northwest Palace of Kalhu, Room Z) - *see also: pp. 106–7*

right foreground: **GERRALD SHEFFIELD**
fm 3-05.301 - *see also: pp. 136, 141*

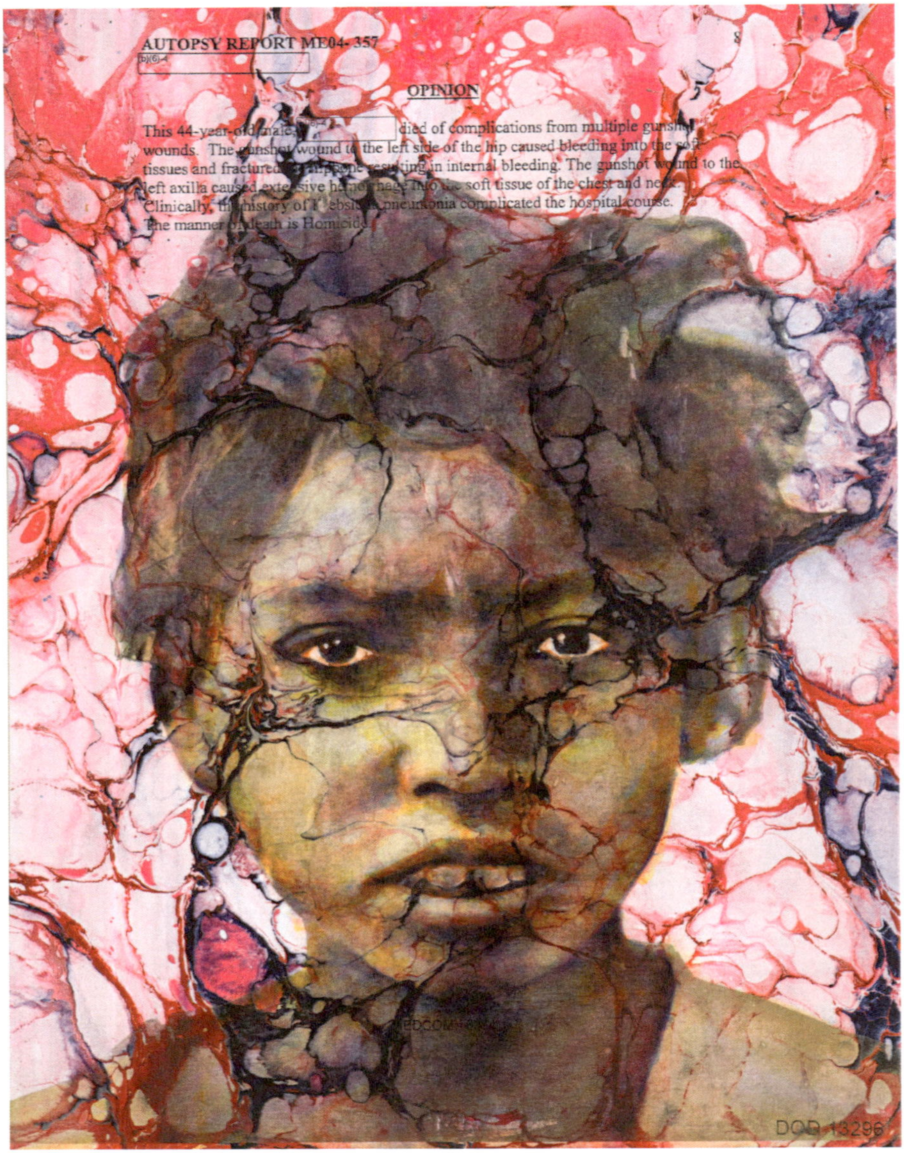
AUTOPSY REPORT ME04- 357
8
OPINION
died of complications from multiple
wounds.
the left side of the hip caused bleeding into
tissues and
in internal bleeding. The gunshot
to the
left axilla
soft tissue of the chest and
complicated the hospital
is Homicide
DOD 13296

RAJKAMAL KAHLON, *(b. 1974)*
From the ongoing series ***Did You Kiss the Dead Body?***
left: ***"This 44-year old male,______________, died of complications from multiple gunshot wounds." (youngest son)***, 2023
Mixed media on canvas

right: ***"This elderly Iraqi male died of atherosclerotic cardiovascular disease (blockage of the arteries that supply blood and oxygen to the heart)." (eldest son)***, 2023
Mixed media on canvas

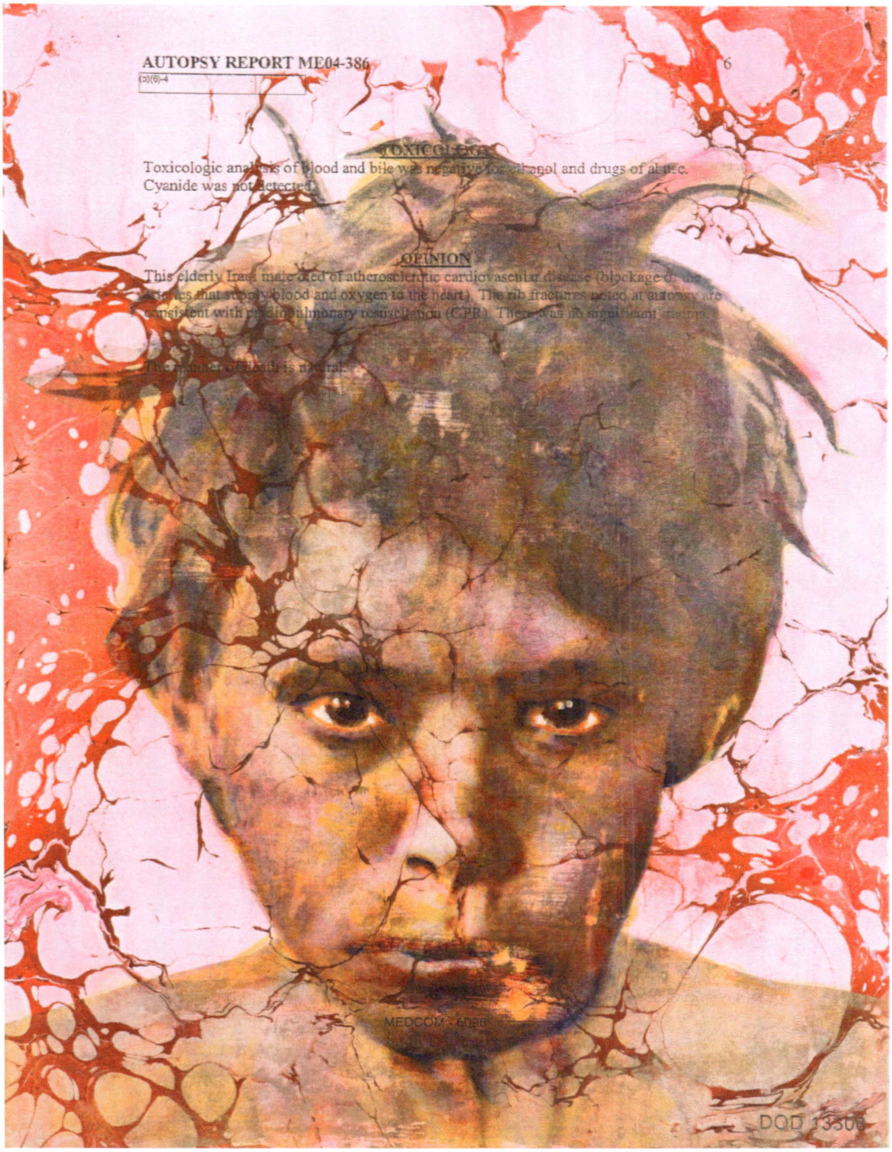

Did You Kiss the Dead Body? is a decade-long reflection on the autopsy reports and death certificates of Iraqis and Afghans killed while in US detention facilities. In 2012, Rajkamal Kahlon began working with over 100,000 pages of redacted documents detailing CIA "enhanced interrogation" practices of torture released through an ACLU Freedom of Information Act request. Kahlon used these declassified military documents as the foundation for this series of works.

In these two newly commissioned works, the titles are excerpted from the autopsy reports included in each canvas and overlaid with marbled hues of bright reds and pinks that reference cross sections of a human body or blood cells under a microscope. On top of this background, Kahlon layered portraits of Afghans and Iraqis. The work underscores the power and abuse wielded by the US military in the treatment of Afghan and Iraqi men and boys who died in US custody.

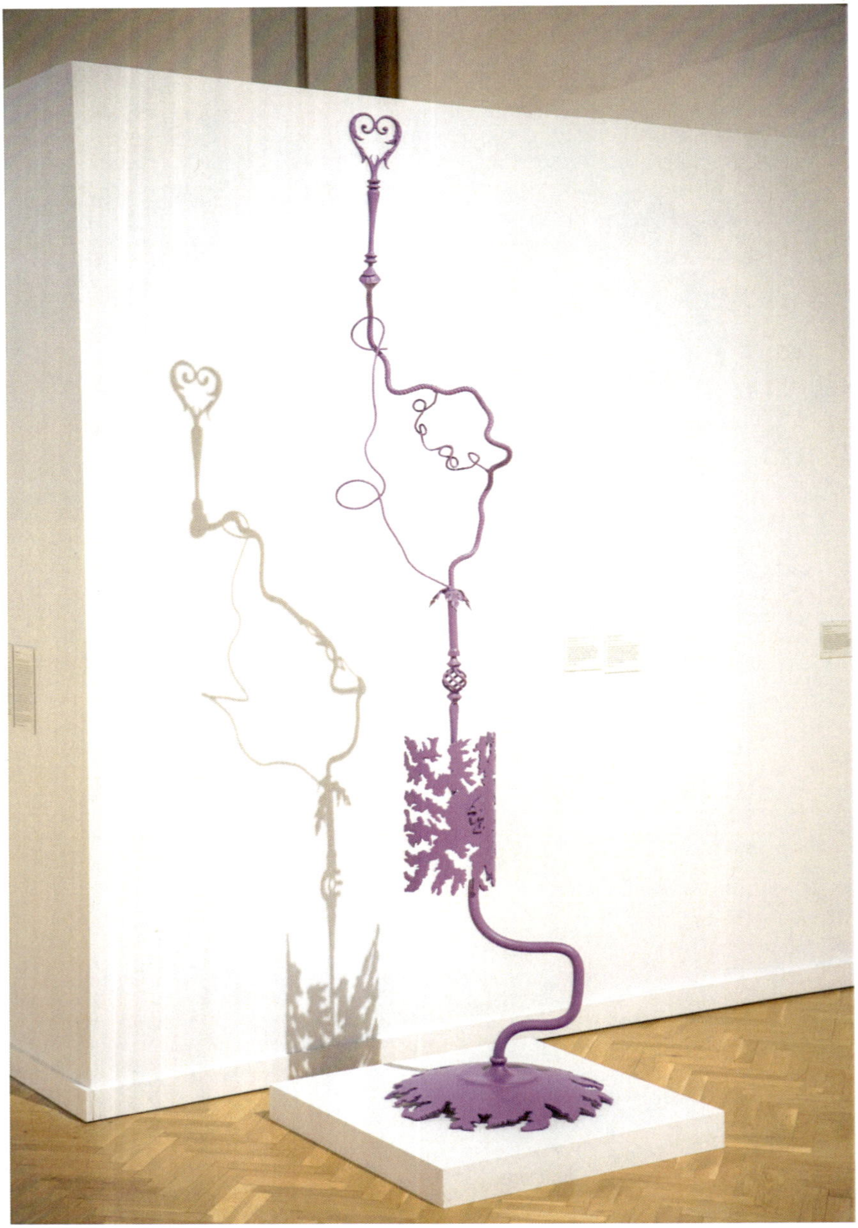

GINA HERRERA *(Tesuque Pueblo, b. 1969)*
[US Army veteran]
The Liberty Master, 2022
Powder-coated assorted found materials and steel

Reflecting on climate change, resurgent white nationalism, and the massive amounts of trash she saw while deployed in Iraq, Herrera used found steel pieces to assemble an abstract creature, *The Liberty Master*. Herrera notes, "*The Liberty Master* looks from afar, imposing 'democratic' ideals onto what the US calls tyrannical lands."

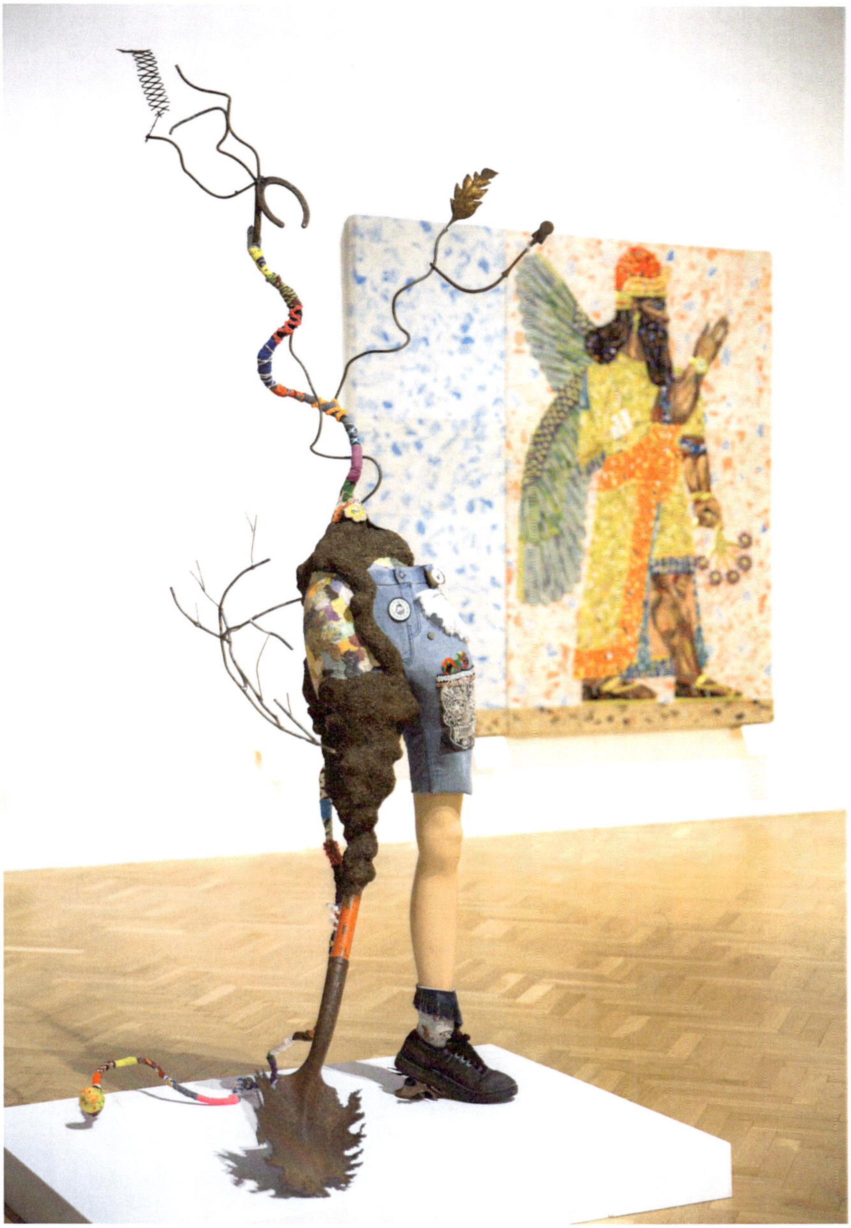

A Virtuous Warrior, 2022
Assorted found materials and steel

While serving in Iraq, Herrera encountered mountainous heaps of trash left by US forces. This experience raised her environmental consciousness and made her acutely aware of the role the US military plays in environmental destruction. *A Virtuous Warrior* incorporates metalwork techniques and an array of discarded objects to assemble a self-portrait exploring different aspects of Herrera's identity and military experience.

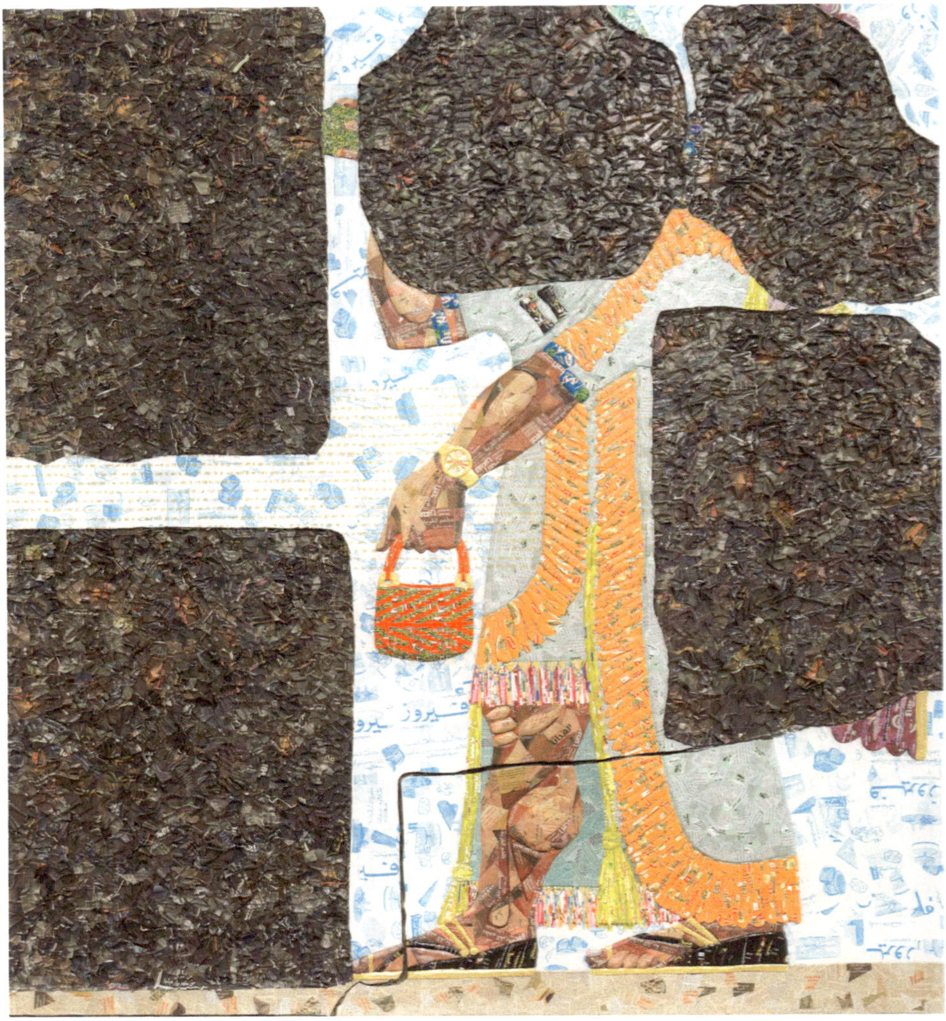

MICHAEL RAKOWITZ *(b. 1973)*
The invisible enemy should not exist (Northwest Palace of Kalhu, Room Z), 2018
above: Z-8 (C01-22-021)
far right: Z-4 (C01-22-019)
Middle Eastern food packaging and newspapers, glue, cardboard on wooden structures
Courtesy of the artist and Rhona Hoffman Gallery

foreground: **GINA HERRERA**
A Virtuous Warrior
see also: pp. 100–101, 105

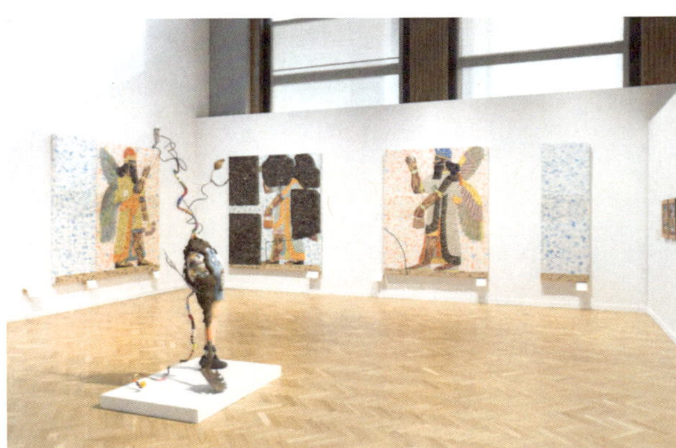

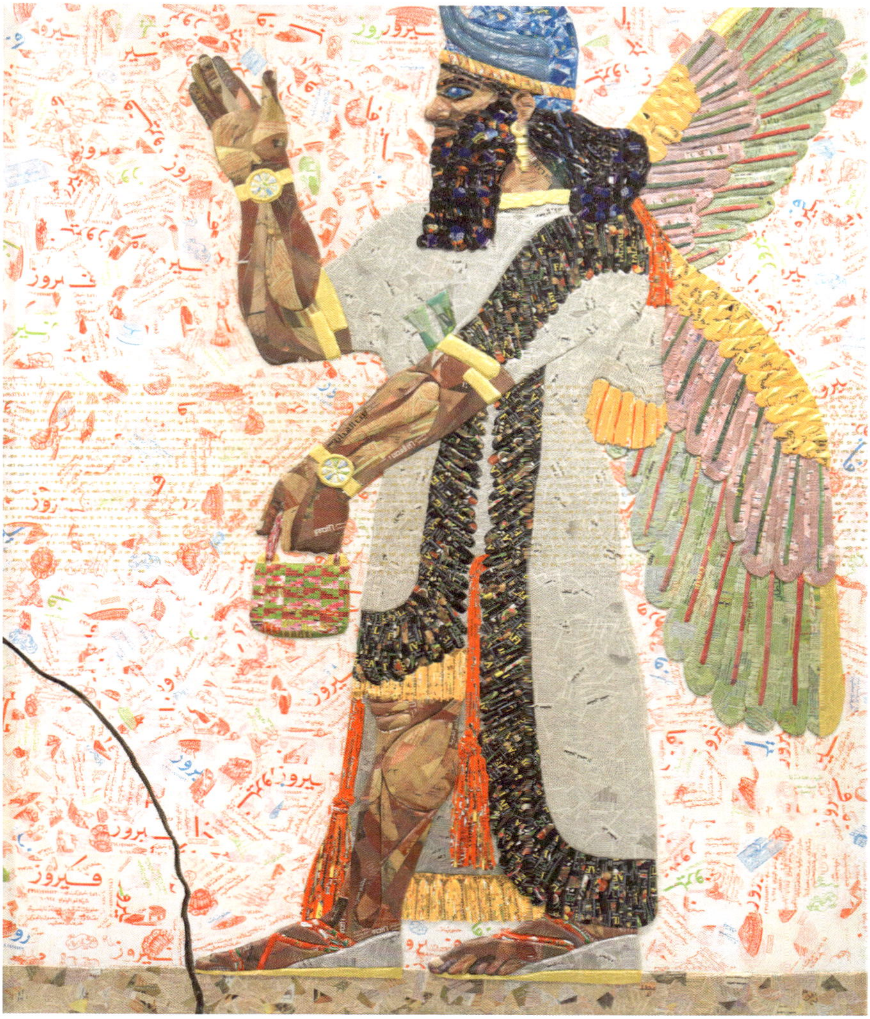

The invisible enemy should not exist is an ongoing project centering threatened, destroyed, stolen, and missing cultural heritage. The title is a translation of "*Aj ibur shapu*," the name of the Processional Way that ran through Nebuchadnezzar's Ishtar Gate in Babylon.

Michael Rakowitz began the project in 2007, reappearing artifacts looted from the National Museum of Iraq in the aftermath of the US-led invasion in 2003. In 2018, he began a new branch of the project. Since the mid-1800s, Western institutions like the British Museum and the Metropolitan Museum of Art have participated in the systematic extraction of works from the Assyrian Northwest Palace of Kalhu, (Nimrud), near present day Mosul, Iraq. The sculptural relief panels that remained after these excavations were destroyed by ISIS in 2015. Using the same logic of the first iteration of the project, Rakowitz and his studio have been reappearing the 200 panels that remained at the palace until their destruction in 2015.

Each room of *The invisible enemy should not exist (Northwest Palace of Kalhu)* installation includes empty spaces with museum labels to indicate where the panels that still exist are held. These empty spaces of imperialist extraction, alongside the reappeared panels, provide a view of what the palace would have looked like the day before its destruction. It is a project that records the continued history of displacement of people and heritage in Iraq due to war and empire.

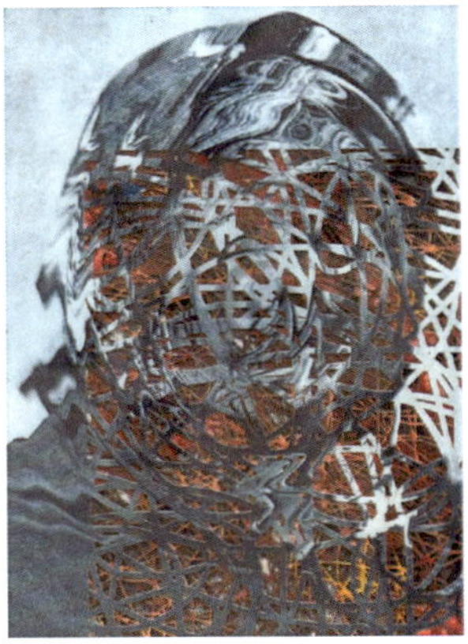

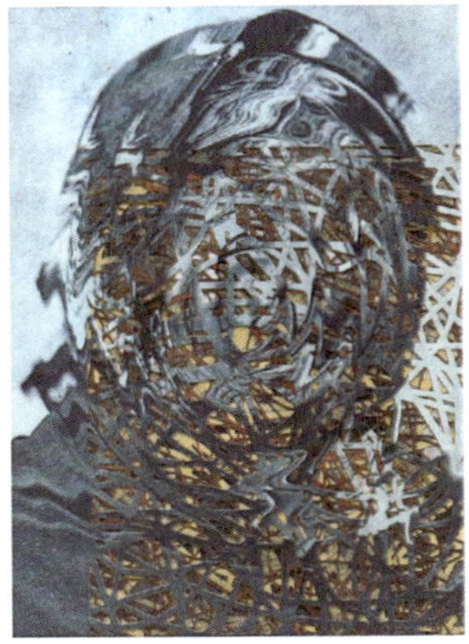

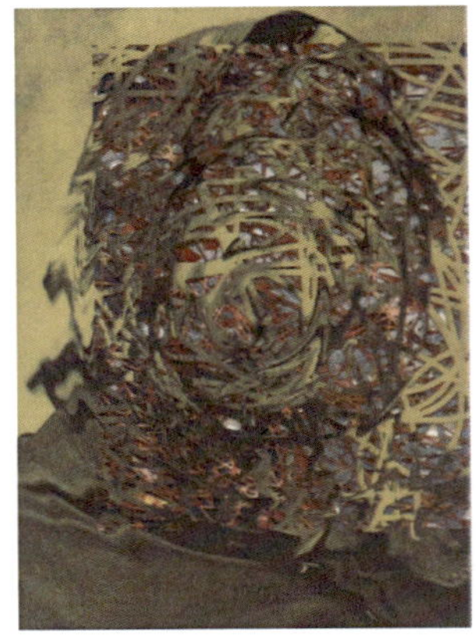

MONTY LITTLE *(Diné, b. 1983)*
[US Marine Corps veteran]
left to right: ***Vellum of Cumuli*** (series), ***02***, ***03***, ***05***, 2022–23
Laser-cut photopolymer plate prints, screenprint, oil paint, and monotype on collaged paper

Vellum of Cumuli is a continuation of the artist's practice of dissecting constructions of complex identity. As a result of forced assimilation, settler colonialism, and militarism, different Native identities merge and become distorted, clouded, and hard to decipher. The various layers of *Vellum of Cumuli* remove, conceal, and reveal different contesting truths, reflecting the multiple erasures of identity. For Little, the distorted portraits visualize the static noise associated with prescribed "Indigenous" identities, imposed by prejudiced perspectives.

see also: p. 318

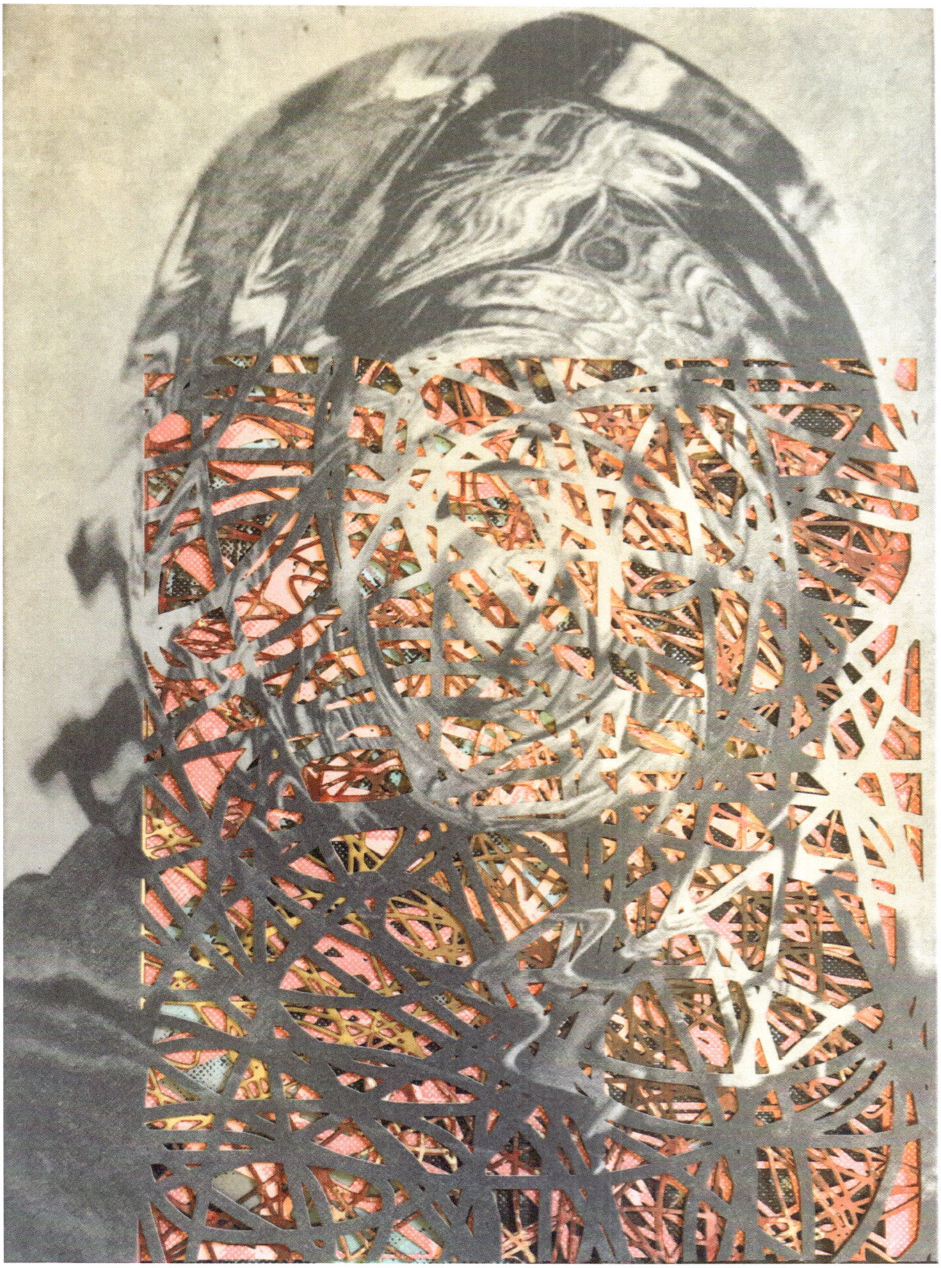

Vellum of Cumuli, (AP), 2022–23
Laser-cut photopolymer plate prints, screenprint, oil paint, and monotype on collaged paper

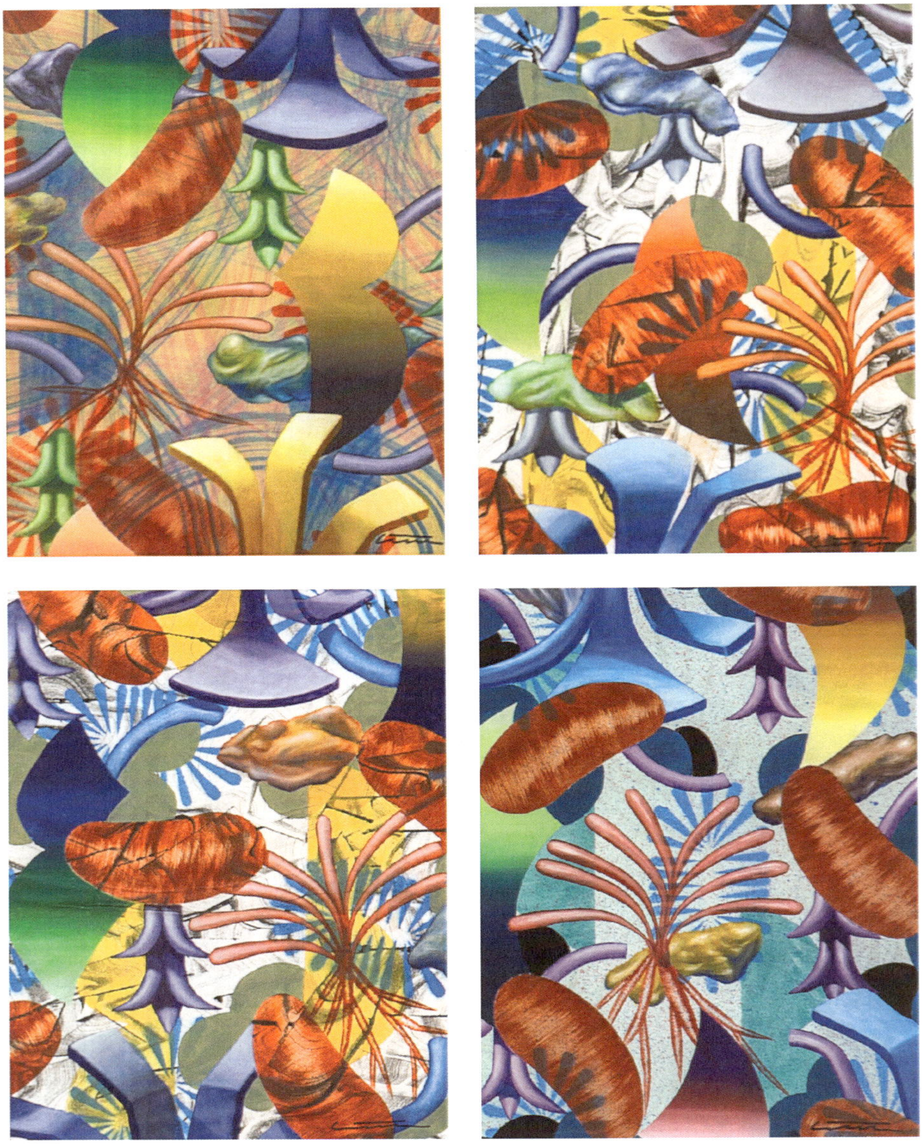

MONTY LITTLE *(Diné, b. 1983)*
[US Marine Corps veteran]
Flora (series), 2019–21
counterclockwise from top left:
Flora 30, Flora 31, Flora 33, Flora 32
Oil on canvas

The *Flora* series pulls from the unnatural hues and vibrant plastics of artificial plants to reference invasive species that take over land and kill indigenous species. For Little, these brightly colored compositions are a metaphor for the idealized myth of Manifest Destiny and the brutality of settler colonialism.

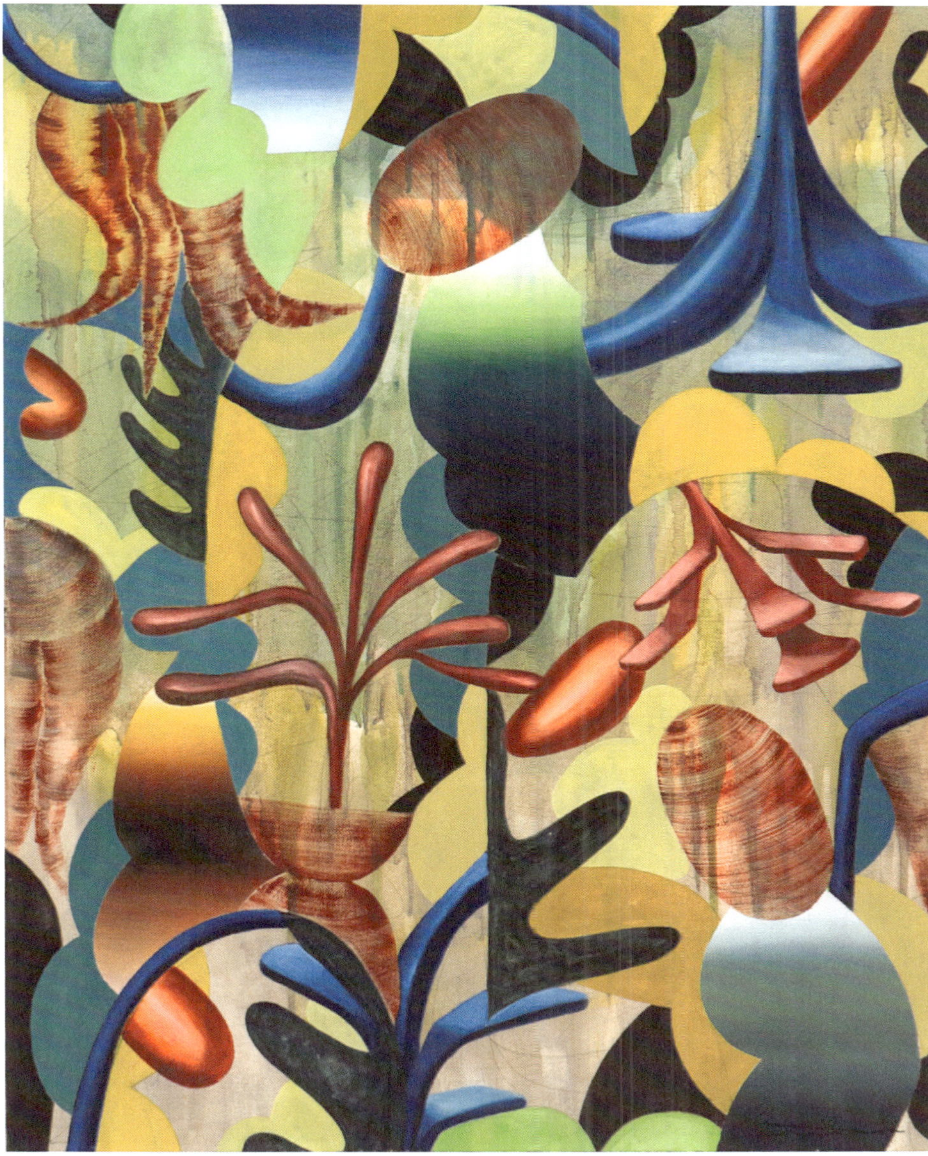

Flora 03, 2019–21

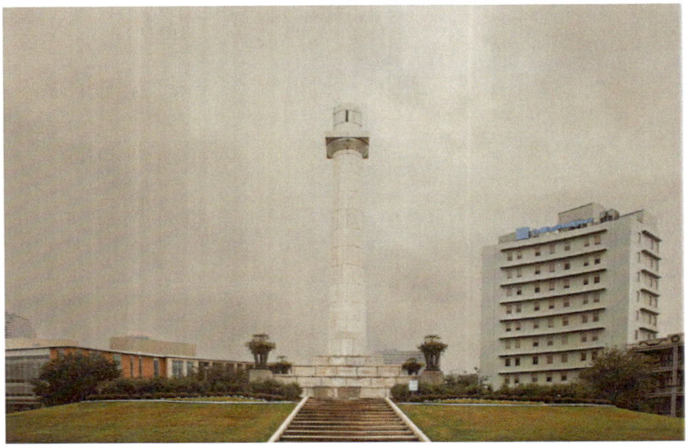

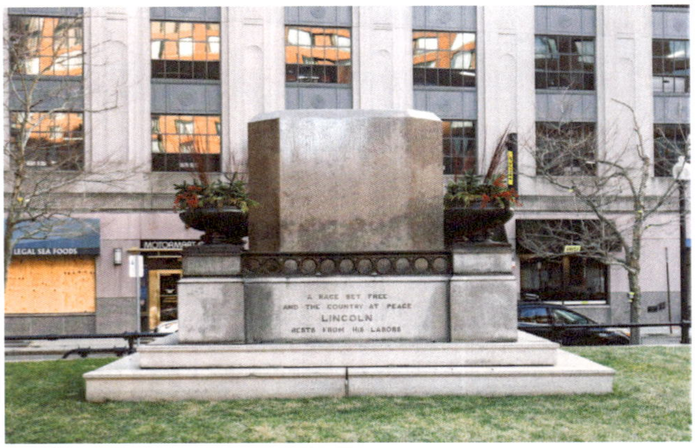
LEGAL SEA FOODS
A RACE SET FREE
AND THE COUNTRY AT PEACE
LINCOLN
RESTS FROM HIS LABORS

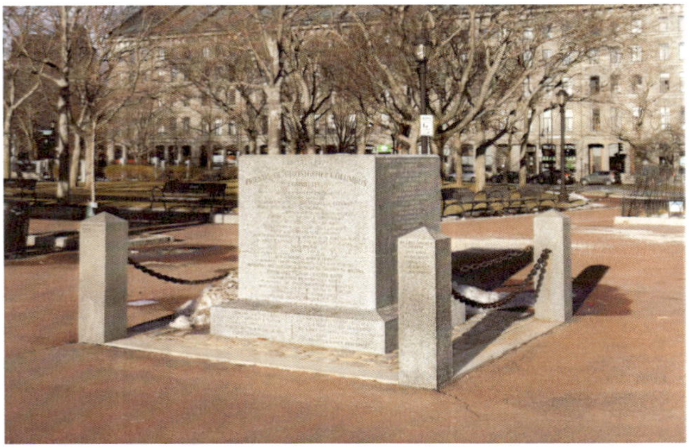

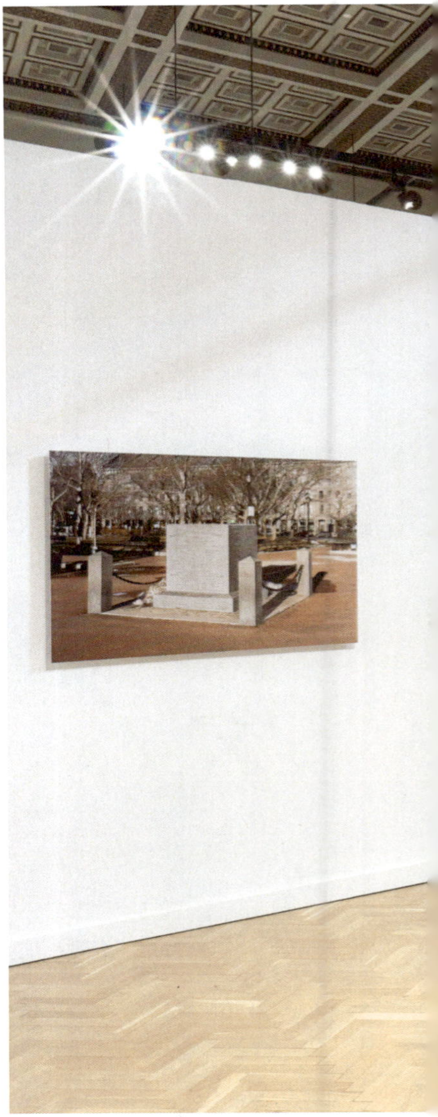

HECTOR R. MEMBREÑO-CANALES
(b. 1988) [US Army veteran]
From the ongoing series ***After-Ozymandias***
left, listed top to bottom:
Robert E. Lee, New Orleans, 2018
Boston MA 3 (Lincoln), 2021
Boston MA 2 (Columbus), 2021
Archival pigment prints

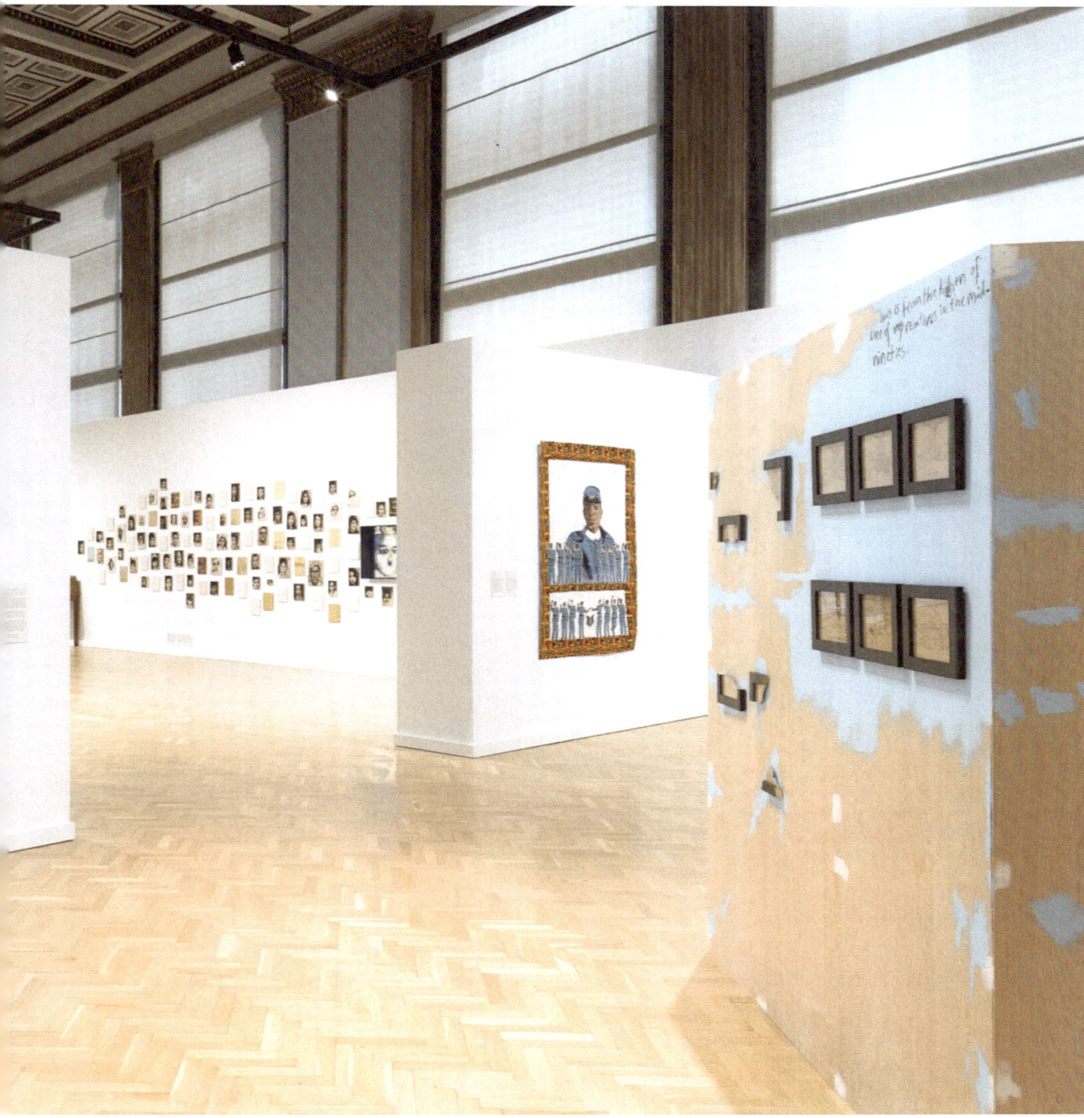

After-Ozymandias is a reference to the Percy Shelley poem "Ozymandias" about the inevitable decline of empires and their surviving claims to greatness. Ozymandias is the Greek name for Pharaoh Ramesses II, who ruled Egypt during the thirteenth century BCE. Shelley wrote the poem in 1817, shortly after the British Museum acquired a large fragment of Ozymandias's statue. Membreño-Canales notes, "These photos depict what remains after a statue crumbles or falls; empty plinths."

this page, left to right:

HANAA MALALLAH
She/He Has No Picture - *see also: pp. 82–83, 114–15, 144–45, 150–51*

DOROTHY BURGE
"We Stand on the Shoulders of Our Ancestors"
see also: pp. 92–93, 248

ALI EYAL
An Indefinite appearance or two walls and
see also: pp. xiv, 120–21, 122

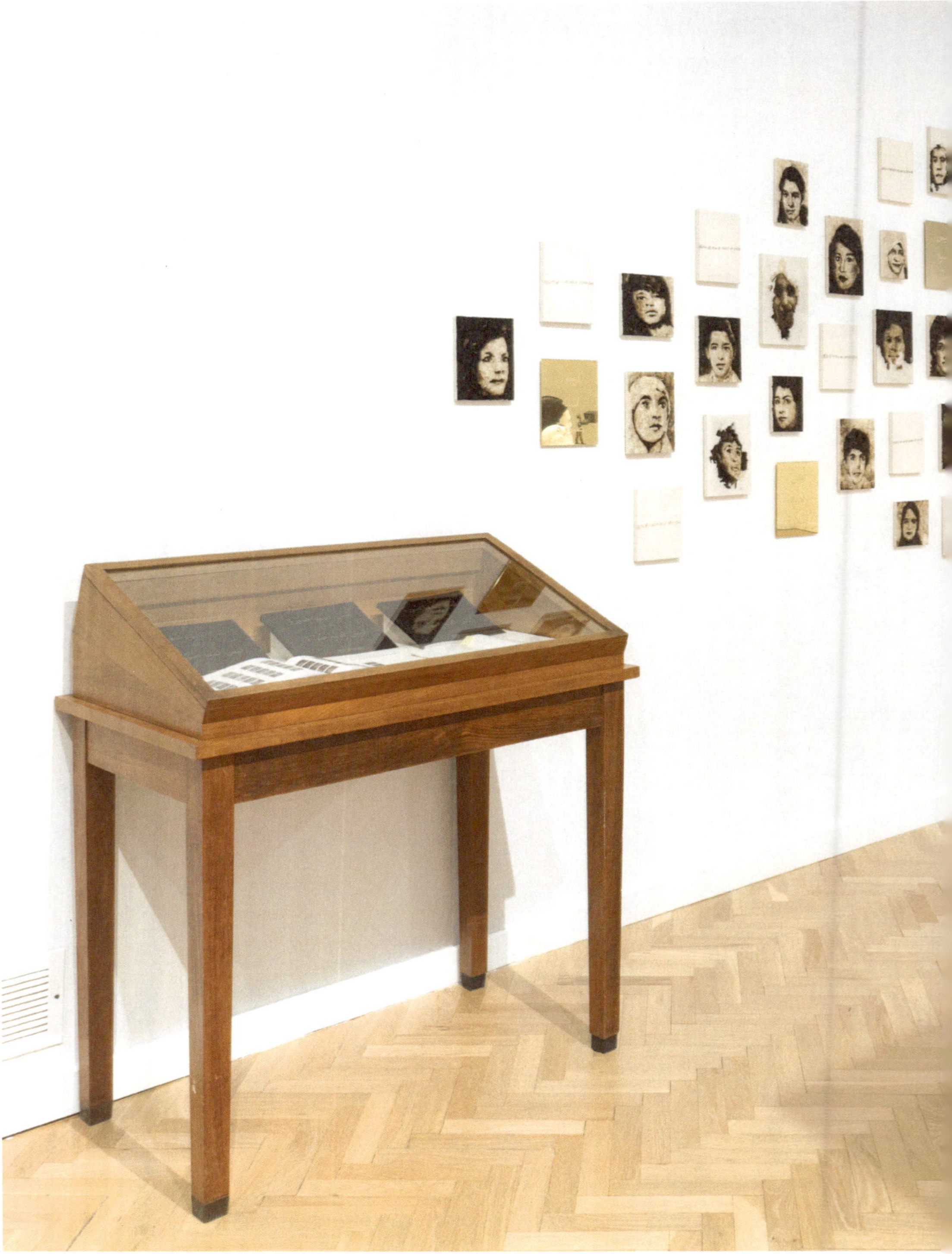

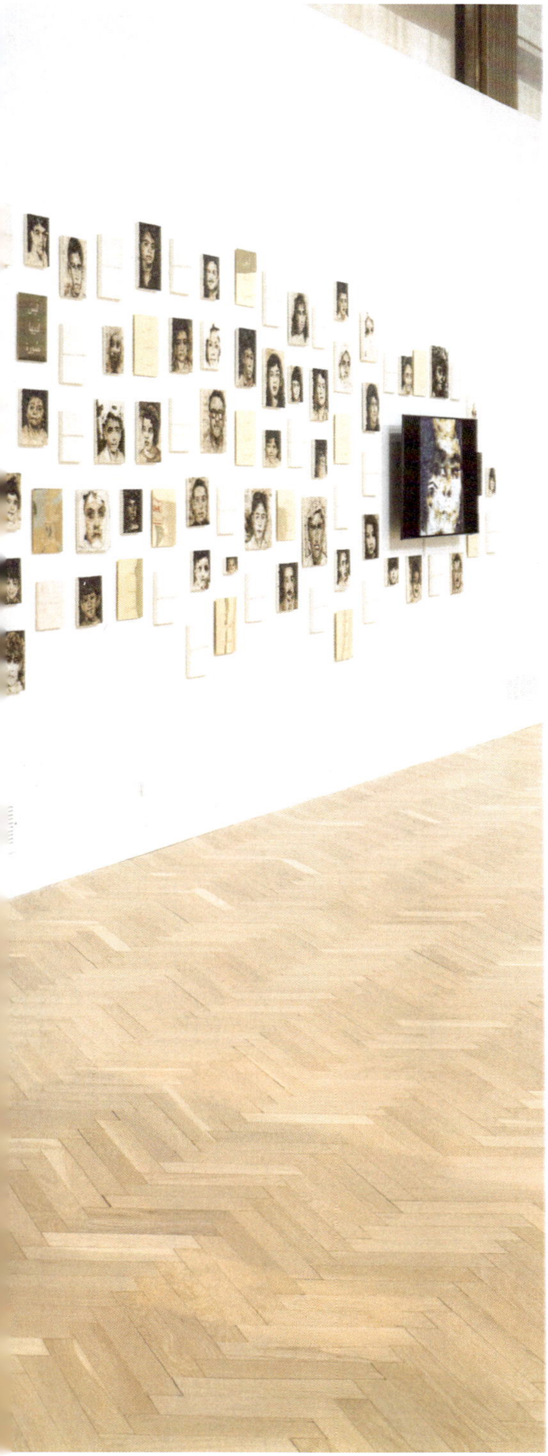

HANAA MALALLAH *(b. 1958)*
She/He Has No Picture, 2019–20
Burnt canvas collage on canvas with laser cut brass plaques, four art books, thousands of computer-generated moving images, and original booklet published by the Iraqi government in 1991

Displayed for the first time in full in the US during the Triennial, *She/He Has No Picture* commemorates the victims of the predawn US bombing of Public Shelter Nr. 25 in the Al Amiriyah neighborhood in Baghdad on February 13, 1991. The precision-guided "smart bombs" killed over 400 Iraqi civilians.

Deeply impacted by her experiences visiting the shelter aftermath of the bombing, Iraqi artist Hanaa Malallah began the lengthy process of collecting images and information to commemorate the victims. Only one hundred of the victims had a portrait in a booklet published by the Iraqi government after the bombing. The others merely had a notice printed beside their names reading: "She has no picture" or "He has no picture." Over the next twenty-eight years, Malallah compiled the archive that forms the backbone of this installation.

Exploring questions of representation, memory, mourning, and memorialization, Malallah's work features portraits of the bombing's victims, made of layers of burnt canvas. Other canvases feature numerical sequences compiled through an ancient Islamic system in which each Arabic letter is assigned a numerical value. Interspersed throughout are brass plates engraved with the Arabic phrase "she/he has no picture." Polished to a mirrored finish, viewers can find their own face reflected back. The artist writes, "Although this face-to-face confrontation of the viewer with her/himself may be an act of visual substitution, an ethical appeal to our common humanity and vulnerability, it is fleeting and does not, cannot, restore the likeness of the remaining 308 victims."

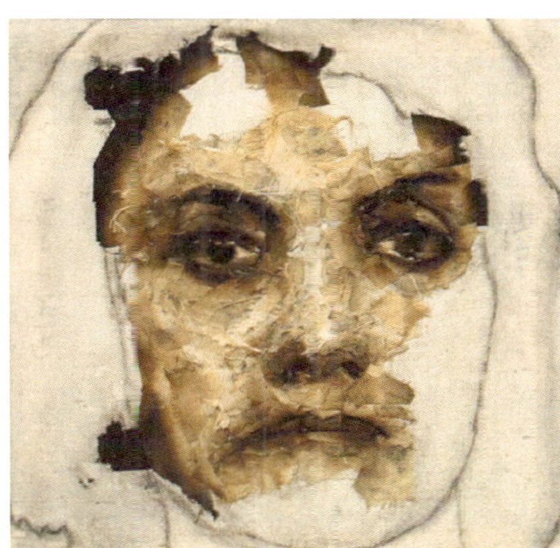

see also: pp. 82–83, 113, 144–45, 150–51

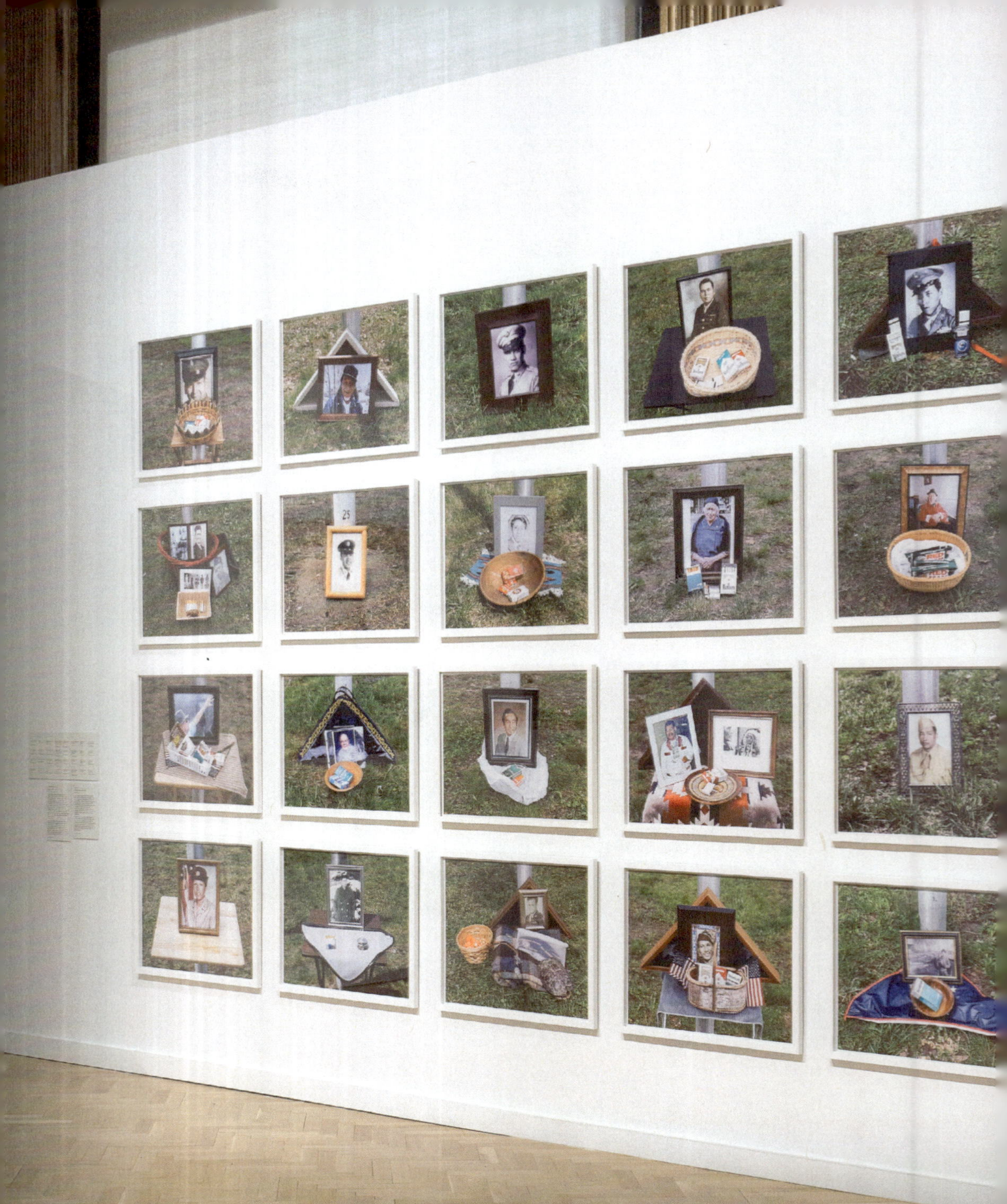

TOM JONES *(Ho-Chunk, b. 1964)*
Honoring the Ho Chunk Warrior series, 2017–ongoing
Archival digital prints

see also: p. 249

Since 1999, Tom Jones has documented family and community monuments made to Ho-Chunk veterans at one of the oldest powwows in the country: the Memorial Day Powwow in Black River Falls, Wisconsin. There, families raise flags for their deceased veteran family members, often placing photographs of them at the bases of the hundred-plus flagpoles that encircle the dance arena.

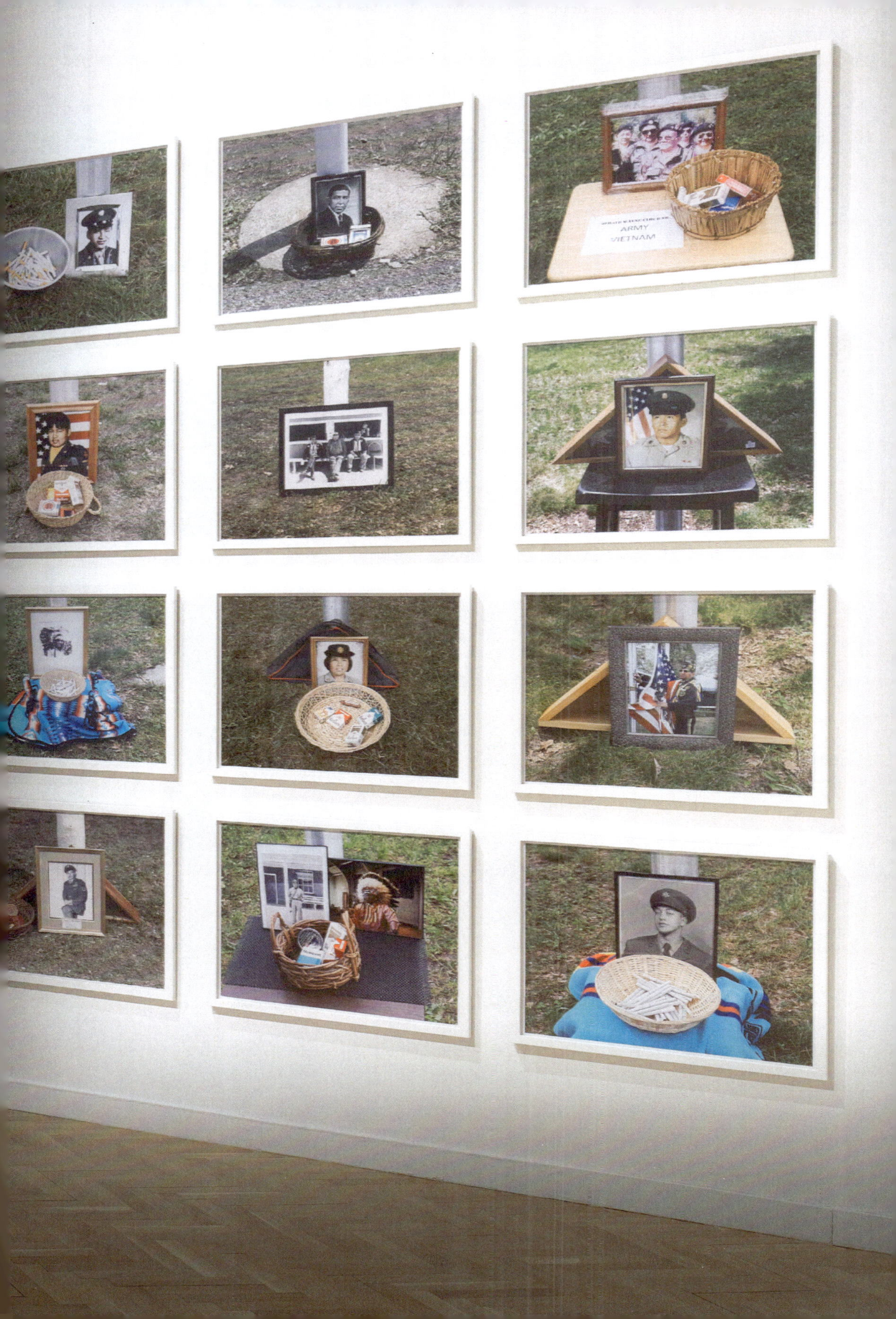
ARMY
VIETNAM

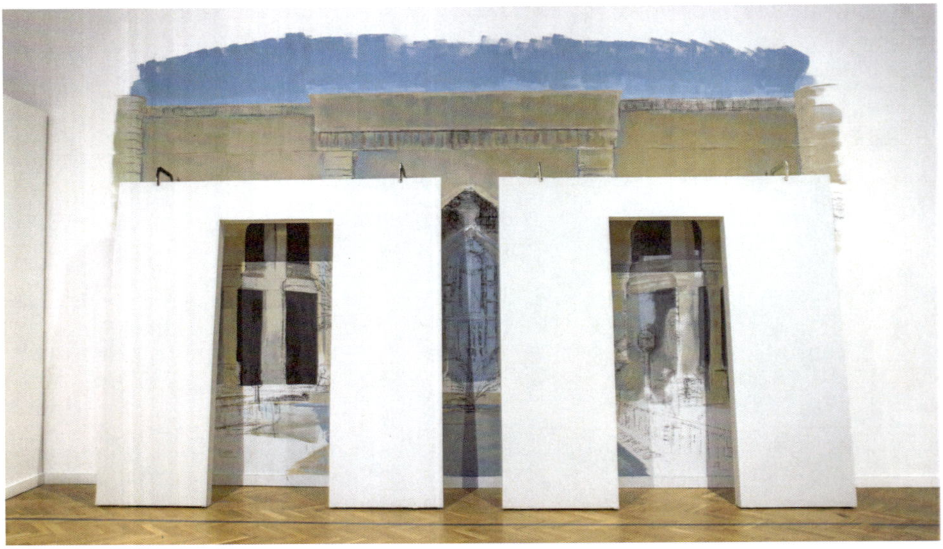

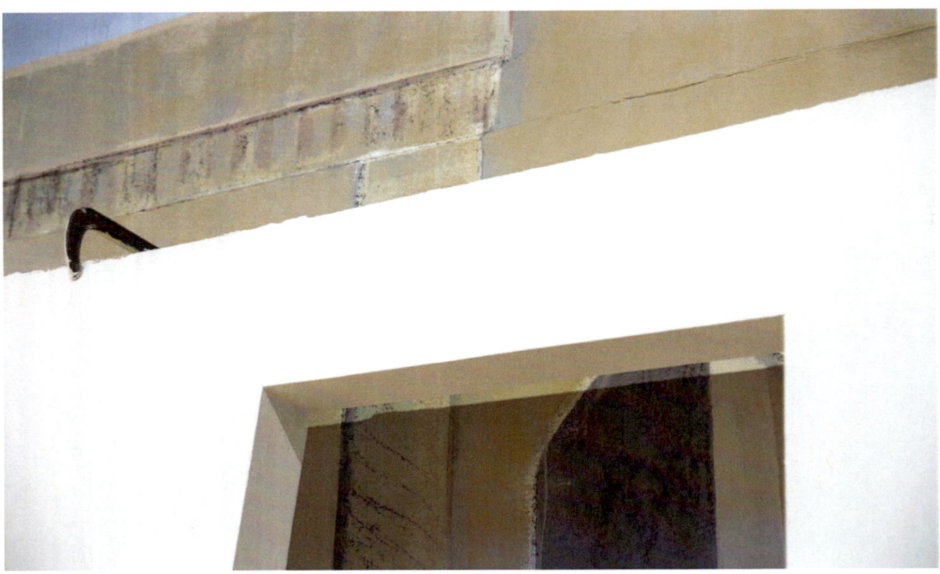

GERRALD SHEFFIELD *(b. 1985) [US Army veteran]*
let's teach them baseball i, 2023 - based on a 2017 installation
Drywall, plywood studs, vinyl, tension wire, charcoal, latex paint

This work's title references a quotation from US Marine Corps veteran Phil Klay's story "Money as a Weapons System," which is included in his collection *Redeployment* (2014). In the story, reconstruction efforts are derailed by an American millionaire's demented mission to teach the Iraqis baseball. For Sheffield, the door frames represent faux-triumphal arches—a revolving door or threshold for Western officials entering and exiting the combat theater. These arches lean in front of and obscure a wall mural of Al-Faw Palace—one of Saddam Hussein's many palaces—which was occupied by US forces and used as a command headquarters for major military operations in Iraq.

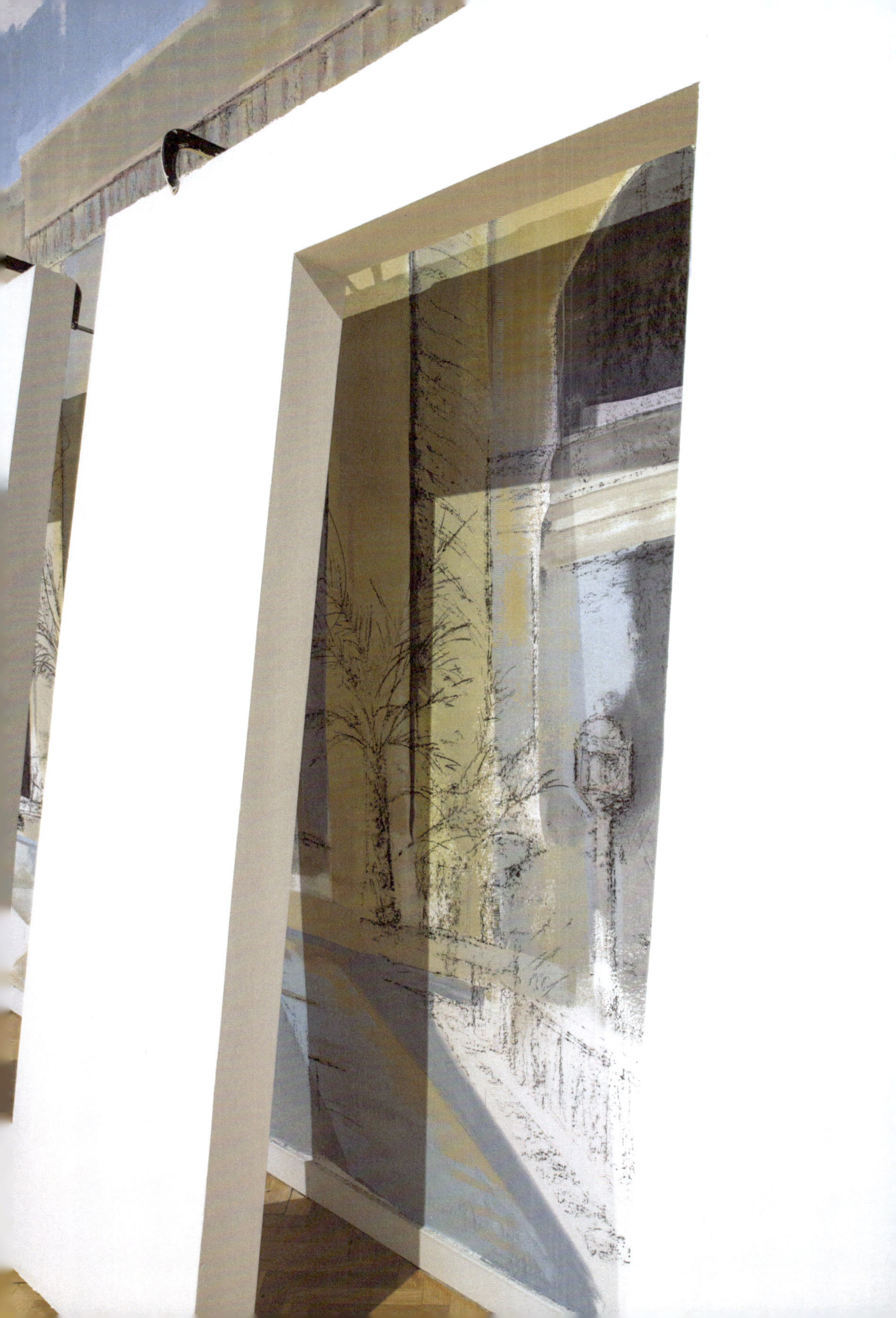

ALI EYAL
An Indefinite appearance or two walls and (detail)

see next spread

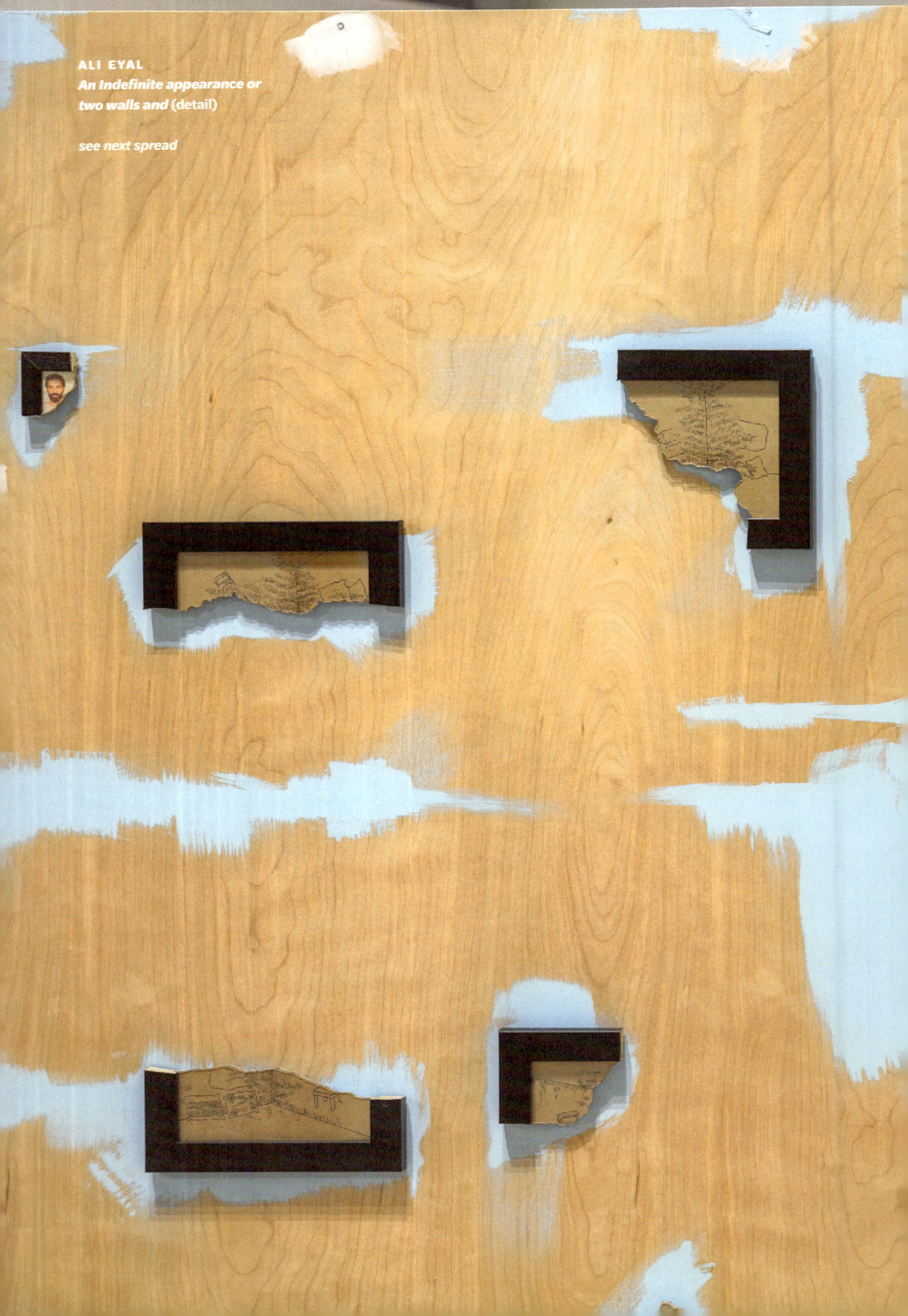

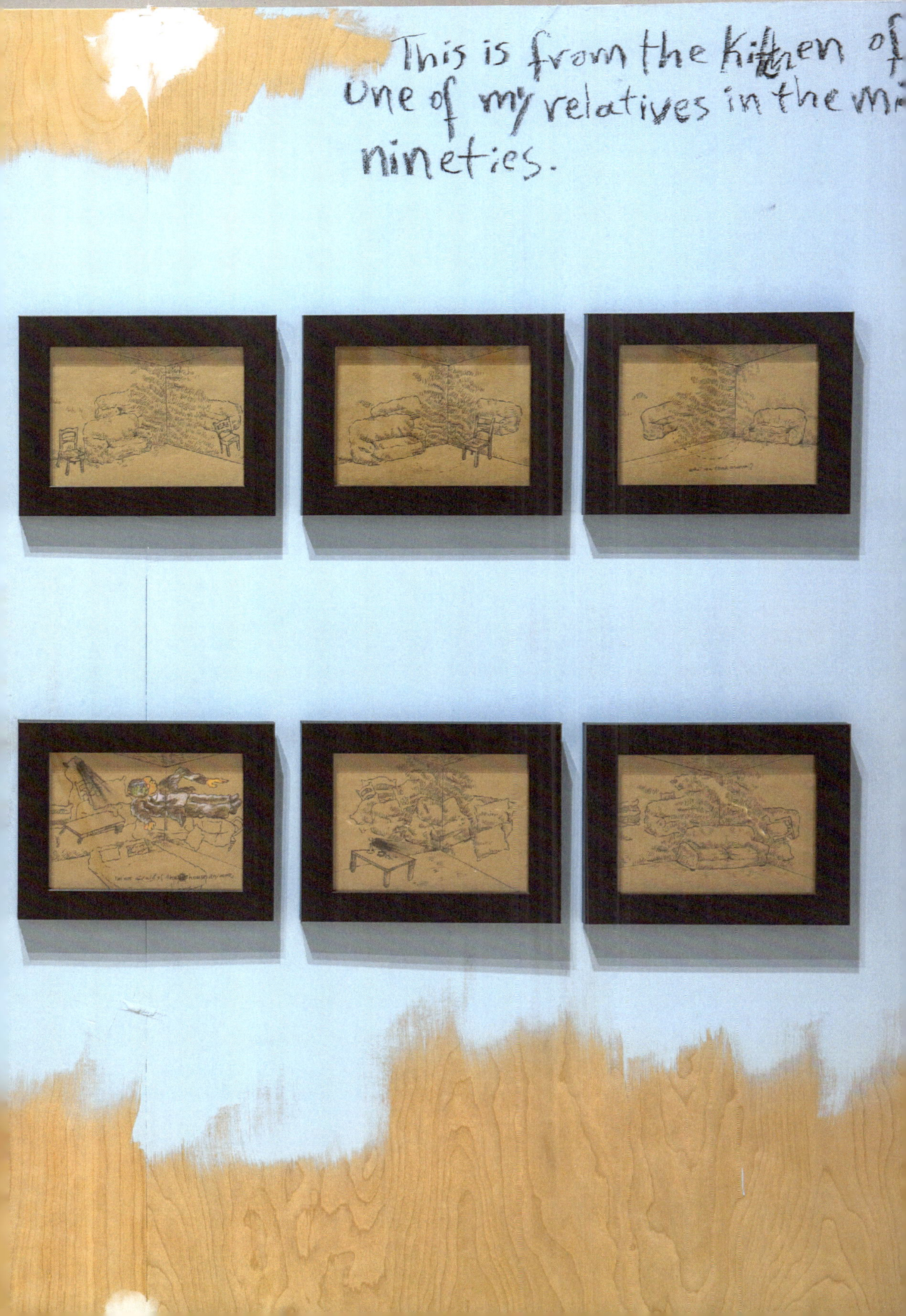
This is from the kitchen of
one of my relatives in the mi
nineties.

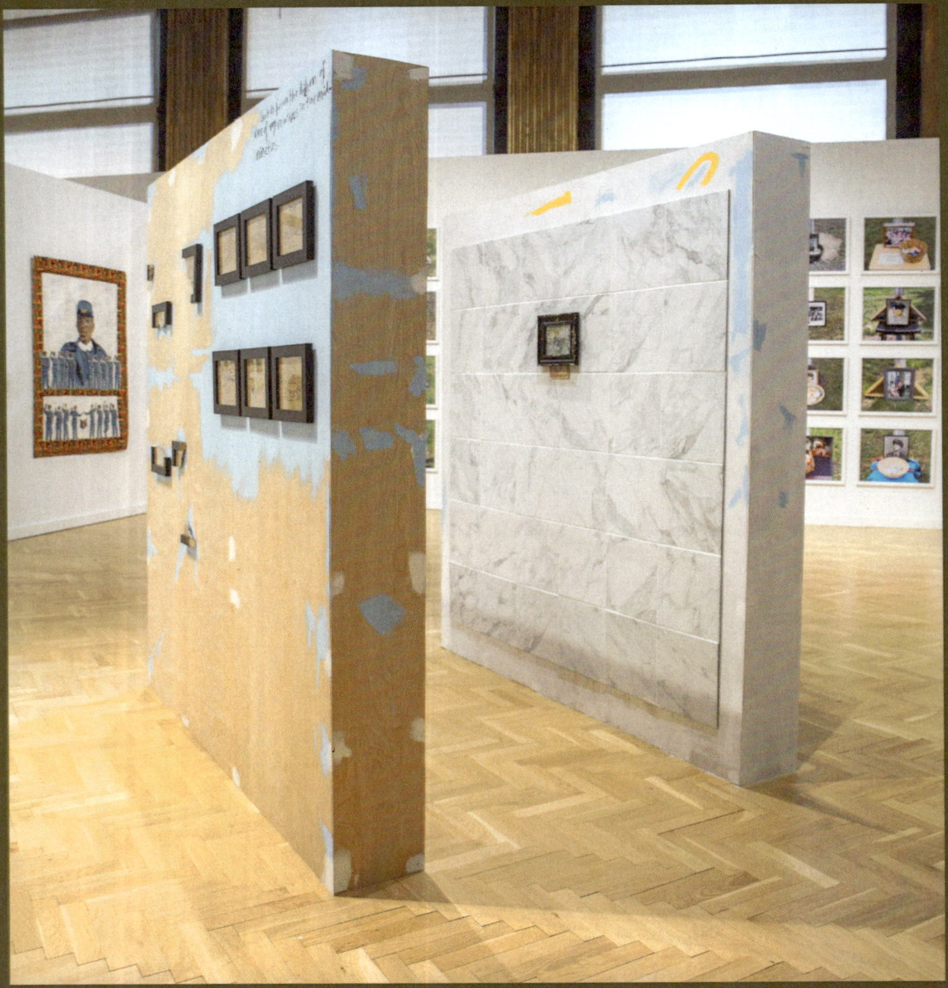

ALI EYAL *(b. 1994)*
***An Indefinite appearance or two walls and*, 2023**
Graphite drawings, pigment print, frames, latex paint, plywood, and ceramic tiles

In 2022, Fawz Kabra, the curator at Brief Histories gallery, described Eyal's work as "[piecing] together memories, dreams, and stories that reach into one another and across media, rendering incomprehensible violences and unfathomable events witnessed in the artist's hometown, a place he calls small farm. Set against the impossible scale of calamity in war, Eyal gives curious attention to the intimate, and often absurd, accounts to be found in this concentrated space."

see also: pp. xiv, 113, 120–21

Embedded Horizons

RIJIN SAHAKIAN

Americans don't call it genocide. No one does. Between January and February 1991, US-led coalition forces dropped over eighty-eight thousand tons of bombs on Iraq. Numbers in the ensuing American bombing campaigns of the '90s and into this century remain unclear, though upwards of one hundred thousand airstrikes are certain. Spending on the war in Iraq alone is estimated at one trillion dollars. The body count: One million Iraqis have died. The number of refugees and internally displaced are over nine million. The scale of these numbers may be lost on an American public seemingly numb to the wars on terror, nearly in their third decade.

Numbness of a different kind has been reported regarding Iraq's children, who make up nearly half the population: One in six are categorized as orphans. Numbness in these small bodies is a survival response to cyclical, ubiquitous, lifelong trauma. If you've never heard a bomb go off, you cannot begin to imagine what five, ten, or a thousand sound like. Extensive research on brain trauma in US soldiers returning from Iraq reveals that bomb explosions can cause severe neurotrauma and a host of other detrimental conditions, from vision and hearing loss to PTSD. For Iraqis, whose civilian populations are inadequately treated (let alone studied), this barrage simply announces a beginning ... of a Gulf War, of an invasion, of a civil war, of Daesh.[1]

Despite the scale and irreversibility of the damage caused not only to the environment, but also to traditions, to past and future cultural production, and to the very notion of personhood itself, war leaves survivors, and Iraq has plenty. Regardless of the lack of meaning ascribed to Iraqi life, it continues, and its DNA offers us insight into the capacity for resilience as it codes our future. Anxieties around climate change, omnipresent surveillance and social media, militarized policing systems, historic refugee populations, and widening income inequality are finally pulsing through mainstream political and cultural discourse, but this discourse will remain incomplete until it takes into account the intricate and intimate ways in which the seemingly distant war zone of Iraq is a testing ground for the establishment of networked systems; systems that—anywhere in the world—can predict, preempt, or neutralize any behavior that might challenge military interests.

Traditional memorials, physically manifested through exhibitions, engraved statues, or immersive gardens, may be the wrong place to look for recognition of Iraq's sacrifice. Iraqi life has already been immortalized. Its legacy can be found all around us: in our smart-homes, at our airports, and in the games we play. They haunt us whether we realize it or not. The purpose of a haunting is to send a message over time, space, and experience. Iraq was, in many ways, a site for the undead. Preparing the site for warfare required an information campaign communicating that any body within the borders

---

1. Also known as ISIS.

delineated for war could be eliminated if necessary for victory. The initial appearance of victory after the invasion of Iraq in 2003 was reminiscent of the first Gulf War. But this war followed a different script, and as escalating violence pointed to deeper engagement, images of newly liberated Iraqis gave way to images of Iraqis walking a tightrope of mortality: cowering at the barrel of a gun in a house raid, and strung up as a hooded rag doll at Abu Ghraib. In order to extend the war, the public had to extend its acceptance of Iraqi bodies as available to abuse, to torture, to kill. As ugly as the images of Abu Ghraib were, as ugly as it might have been to see small children screaming in terror while the US Army put bags over the heads of their fathers, it was uglier, still, to be an Iraqi.

Of course, what Americans saw on their screens and in their papers was a view of full-spectrum war, not the full spectrum of Iraq, which may as well have been a black site. Understandably, no one outside of battle reporting or warmongering was going in, and most of the Iraqis fleeing were doing so for good. The wars in Iraq were unique for many reasons—one being that they were fought by extensive international coalitions. The most advanced war-making resources the world had to offer coalesced and touched ground in Baghdad. If you were there during those years, you were witness to a display of force that no one in the world had ever seen. What did those who remained see? What might they want to tell us? What do they know that we don't? The generation of artists born in the wake of the Gulf War and who came of age in the ensuing invasion of Iraq are the closest thing we have to embodied insight.

> The navigation computer opened the bomb doors and dropped the weapons into the dark.
>
> —*American B-52 bomber pilot describing his experience in Iraq.*[2]

2. P.W Singer, "'Wired for War' Explores Robots on the Battlefield," interview by Terry Gross, *Fresh Air*, NPR, January 22, 2009, audio, 38:47, https://www.npr.org/templates/transcript/transcript.php?storyId=99663723

It is no secret that technology is used to fight wars, and that the lessons from wars support the development of new technologies. The world's prevailing military research arm is the United States Defense Advanced Research Projects Agency, or DARPA. Housed under the Department of Defense, "It has a singular and enduring mission: to make pivotal investments in breakthrough technologies for national security."[3] In Annie Jacobsen's comprehensive book, *The Pentagon's Brain*, she reports that DARPA and the US Army spent three hundred million dollars perfecting the Simulator Networking (SIMNET) system, a networked combat simulation system (a system that also birthed the billion-dollar multiplayer gaming industry, starting with *World of Warcraft*).[4] The system was used to simulate a war game exercise undertaken by US Central Command (USCENTCOM). An American icon, USCENTCOM commander General Norman Schwarzkopf scripted a narrative for SIMNET focused on Iraq, a play-by-play of what would become the Persian Gulf War. SIMNET technology integrated real data from Saudi Arabia, Iraq, *and* Kuwait. In the last stage of the SIMNET game, Iraq did in fact invade Kuwait, and the war against Iraq was waged using air bases in Saudi Arabia.

SIMNET was designed to serve as a substitute for real-life combat operations, but the testing required real-life combat. The seamless timing of the system's completion, the game's script, and the start of the official war was described as "an eerie similarity" by US Central Command.[5] But it could hardly have been a surprise, or even uncanny, as it was known at the time that Saddam Hussein was gathering military at the border of Kuwait. The real war broadcast offensive was an astounding show of might. It provided a quick, potent victory lap, extinguishing the lingering scent of war as a

---

3. "About DARPA," About Us, Defense Advanced Research Projects Agency, accessed August 6, 2019, https://www.darpa.mil/about-us/about-darpa.

4. Annie Jacobsen, *The Pentagon's Brain: An Uncensored History of DARPA, America's Top-Secret Military Research Agency* (New York: Little, Brown and Company, 2016), 257, 268.

5. "U.S. Central Command History, United States Central Command, accessed August 25, 2019, https://www.centcom.mil/ABOUT-US/HISTORY/.

nationally divisive failure in Vietnam, and introducing audiences around the world to a new era of technology. Satellite news coverage, guided killing, and massive public relations efforts worked together as their own "system of systems" to demonize Iraqis, censor difficult war imagery, and frame all criticism of the war as an assault on American soldiers.

The US entered Iraq again in 2003, and by its second year, DARPA launched its most expensive operation to date, the Urban Operations Program, with these words, "No technological challenges are more immediate, or more important for the future, than those posed by urban warfare ... What we are seeing today [in Iraq] is the future of warfare."[6] The future of war is one that reconfigures earth and all of its human and nonhuman components as potential battlefields. American actions commonly referred to as "missteps" (dismantling the Iraqi military, police, and border security, allowing massive caches of weapons to be left up for grabs throughout the country) enabled the power vacuum to be filled by militias of every stripe with a Pandora's box of weapons with which to experiment. Daesh, an extraordinary multinational de facto government, would eventually emerge, requiring all-out urban destruction to expel its forces, but not before it had thoroughly, unimaginably terrorized citizens of greater Mosul, Iraq's second-largest, and now largely decimated, metropolis.

Iraq is widely seen in public discourse as a failure, but through the lens of urban research needs, it has been a rich, widely successful petri dish. The American military, through active combat, has been able to test and develop each of the identified areas of improvement in urban warfare that continues to inform our future cities. These include: communication "jammers" (which can disrupt anything from cellphones to GPSs to drones), the development of armored exoskeletons, robotic limbs, machine-enhanced decision-making, explosives detection, voice recognition and translation, drones and

6. Jacobsen, *Pentagon*, 367.

robotics, and nonlethal methods for controlling group behavior. The militarization of police units across America isn't simply due to the fact of weapons coming home from war, it is part of transforming urban areas into spaces that will always be ready *for* war. Ferguson, Standing Rock, Baghdad—protests in these areas look the same because each visible force engages in the tactics developed from the same war-constructed incubator. There was no Iraqi SWAT team prior to the 2003 invasion. American forces created it. There were no body scanners in American airports—now resembling checkpoints—prior to 2007. In 2018, the first biometric airline terminal was launched in Atlanta, with the majority of airlines and ports expected to follow suit. This technology was also advanced through human Iraqi data by the US military, which collected fingerprints, photographs, and biographical information on an estimated 750,000 Iraqi citizens, intelligence that is housed at the Department of Defense's Biometrics Fusion Center in West Virginia.

Hovering a thousand feet above the ground, surveillance blimps—machines deployed to serve as the US Army's unblinking eyes—tethered by fiber optic cables floating above Baghdad, surveyed the terrain below. Like the other displays of urban military control that characterized this war in stark difference to the remote, stealth capacities on display in the first Gulf War, the blimps were also made to be seen. They were not only full of monitoring equipment, but also full of meaning: *We are watching you.* Everyone knew that the blimps were there, taking pictures. The machines of occupying forces—from extensive camera surveillance and psychological operations to tactical units, snipers, and checkpoints—controlled pedestrian movement, entered homes, reconfigured neighborhoods, and determined whether Iraqis lived or died.

In 1993, a remarkable piece, "War is Virtual Hell," by science-fiction writer and theorist Bruce Sterling appeared in WIRED magazine. In the report, Sterling details the possibilities set in motion for military dominance through what DARPA refers to as, "the war in Southwest Asia" rather than the Persian Gulf War to avoid irritating Arab coalition allies. Sterling describes the military's use of virtual reality "as a new way of knowledge: a new and terrible kind of transcendent military power," and notes that during Desert Storm, Iraqi soldiers surrendered to unmanned flying drones.[7] In her book, written thirteen years later, Jacobsen claims that "this became the first time in history that a group of enemy soldiers was recorded surrendering to a machine."[8]

Ali Eyal and Sajjad Abbas, both visual artists under thirty who were born a few short years after this historic surrender, came of age under the camera's eye. Having already seen the worst violence possible while raised in Baghdad's notorious public housing project, Sadr City, they weren't afraid to turn the gaze on itself, by both harnessing and incinerating its authority. In Eyal's recent work, *Behind the Sun* (2019), he uses painting, one of the earliest forms of military technology, to depict the faces of disparate lives, animal and human, united by death at the hands of "No Name." Eyal chronicled the imagined life of the work:

> I decided to visit his (No Name's) house and paint all its walls ... I knew that he killed my father or buried him, or maybe he fed his body to wild dogs ... I wanted to crush him with the faces within the mural. The faces of the dozens who were killed or went missing during his private parties. I could imagine their eyes following him all around the room ... One of the paintings showed missing people and victims whose faces I copied from old pictures, collected from multiple families ... I finished painting and called him to see what I had done.[9]

---

7. Bruce Sterling, "War is Virtual Hell," *WIRED*, January 1, 1993, https://www.wired.com/1993/01/virthell/.

8. Jacobsen, *Pentagon*, 274.

9. Ali Eyal, "Behind the Sun," Works, Ali Eyal, accessed August 7, 2019, https://alieyal.weebly.com/from-behind-the-sun.html.

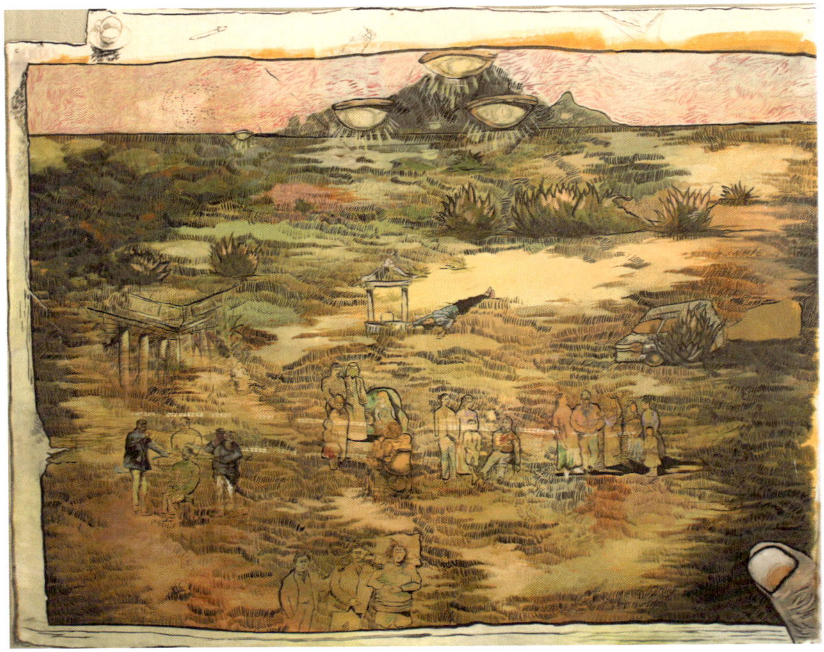

ALI EYAL, *Behind the Sun* (series), 2019, painting

The paintings in the series are from an imagined mural created for No Name in his home, without him realizing that it was painted as the ultimate act of revenge. No Name, initially enamored by the mural, would soon be tortured by the faces looking back at him. In the vigilante fantasy-turned-painting, No Name loses his mind and kills himself, meeting his righteous fate. Eyal exhumes the mass graves of Iraq and enacts the closure remaining out of reach for these victims and their families by destroying the multivariant, anonymous force. Are the faces victims of Saddam Hussein's regime? Of Daesh? Of US military forces? Of local militias? No Name exists because, for most Iraqis, there has been no resolution for the missing dead. No accountability, no identification of perpetrators, no processes or procedures to recognize their loss. In this work, Eyal grants justice to his father and others who have lost their lives through a fiction

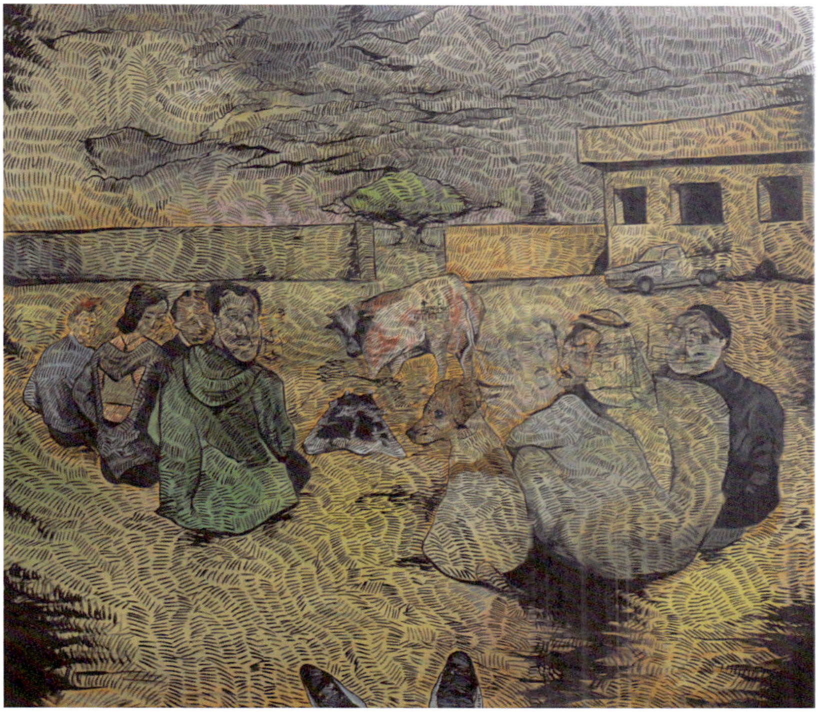

ALI EYAL, *Behind the Sun* (series), 2019, painting

that in turn creates a memorial in the form of the painting itself. He honors these faces as he attempts to afford justice to the cut-short, unaccounted-for lives of No Name's victims.

In his 2013 public intervention, Abbas brashly addressed the Green Zone with a phrase, *I Can See You*, written in massive Arabic script beneath a magnified tracing of his own eye, atop the largest building he could scale. The building faced a major public freeway as well as the Green Zone, the area covering four square miles of central Baghdad along the banks of the Tigris, and once serving as Saddam Hussein's control center. It later became the US coalition command, and today the heavily fortified area houses the largest and most expensive US embassy in the world, as well as Iraqi and coalition government offices, company headquarters, and residences.

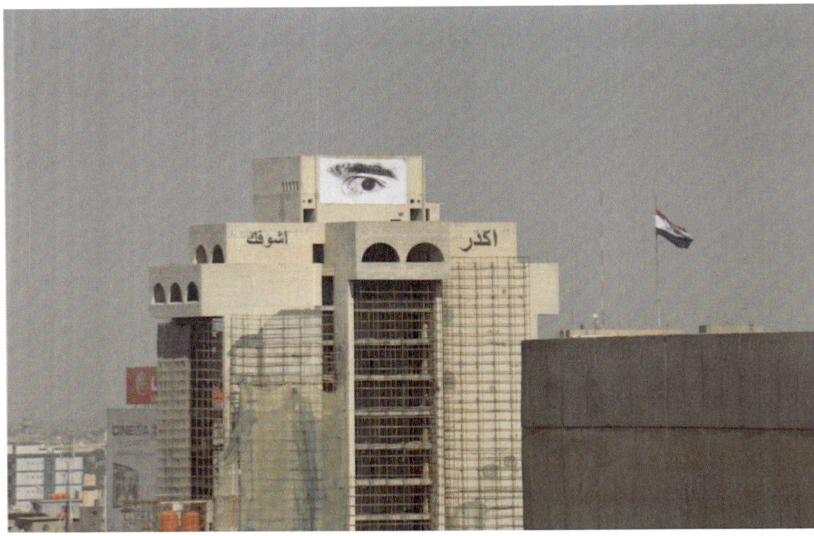

SAJJAD ABBAS, *I Can See You*, 2014, installation and photograph

With one of the most corrupt governments on record unwilling to provide basic resources like electricity, water, and security beyond the perimeter of their guarded, air-conditioned walls, Abbas's eye was the crown atop Baghdad's present-day dystopia. During the worst years of Baghdad's violence, smoke from bombs could be seen around the city, the Green Zone at its center impervious to pain—quiet, secure, the Tigris lapping at its impenetrable shore. Abbas's artwork was as much a reckoning as it was a trespassing.

The grind of trauma has been inescapable in Iraq, and also absent from general discourse outside of the country. However, this lack of acknowledgment of Iraqi trauma was used, particularly in American discourse, as a narrative tactic to deflect from and diminish the war's historic carnage. Why *wasn't* Iraq getting better, as though what had befallen the nation was no more complicated than a cold? Problems in Iraq were often attributed to the need for Iraqis to "get back on their feet." Even arts professionals whose lives center on image-making and meaning seemed to be unaware of the catastrophe that had taken place.

With several notable exceptions, when those in the field of contemporary art (American, Middle Eastern, and otherwise) found out that I worked with artists in Baghdad, the question they asked most was if there was "anything good." When I explained the kind of conditions these artists were working under (severe trauma, bombed art spaces, bewildering isolation, dysfunctional education), my response was regularly met with impatience, as if growing up during unending war was a kind of pity project, or simply, boring. What these people wanted to know was if there was anything that could be bought or shown, acquired before the market got hot, or the artwork became passé. What other good could be there, apart from a commodity? Sometimes, I was told that the lack of educational infrastructure might lead to originality. A pearl in that blasted piece of sand.

Though the works of untold artists in Iraq are impressive, their entry into the global art world—which rests on some combination of social connections, sophisticated English, savvy presentation, a (preferably Western) art school education, and mobility—remains elusive. Iraqi citizens cannot easily obtain visas to leave the country, if at all, to go to shows or meet with curators. Iraq's art schools are mainly populated by those from middle- or low-income backgrounds, rather than restricted as an upper-class opportunity, as it is in so many other parts of the world and neighboring countries. Far from having parents with dual citizenship or access to English classes and private education, many young artists are consequently left outside of the global art circuit. There have been little to no visits by curators and art-world operators independent of political or military contexts, and, far more importantly, no dollars or effort spent to support their development, education, or ability to independently produce work. This partially explains why diaspora artists are the sole purveyors of anything that is recognized as contemporary Iraqi art. Nearly all have gone to Western art schools and hold Western or dual passports.

This is by no means the fault of the artists. A diaspora is the inevitable outcome of sustained war and mass murder, and rich work has emerged from artists that span the years of dispersal, from the melancholy resistance of Koutaiba Al-Janabi to the poetic interventions of Rheim Alkadhi. A much more productive conversation is not about the merits of artists working from outside their countries of origin, whatever that means, but about why artists working from inside a country like Iraq are excluded from the world of exhibited art, and how the structures of the art world can be reconfigured to address this.

The works of Eyal and Abbas are acts of defiance against conditions designed to force surrender. They do not have much to lose and a great deal to gain by going up against the technology that marks their bodies for death. But will the art world, informed by and participating with war's image-making and financial structures ever take the risk of remaking the rules of engagement? Or will we continue to pretend that the barriers of entry into the art world for artists living in Iraq is simply an oversight (or impossibility), that artists embedded with militaries are not furthering the aims of PSYOPS, or that the mega museums and art fairs of the Gulf don't function as state-sponsored strategies laundering strategic state-sponsored violence.

The allure of technological warfare, shock and awe, and unlimited capital have worked in seamless phases, relying on the near-evisceration of Iraqi life and associated narratives. But even with all this might, Iraq remains present, at the vanguard. The buzzwords of today—climate change, representation, acceleration—should remind us that there can be no meaningful investigation, let alone emancipation, of our technologies, and consequently our planet and its citizens, without investigating the conditions undergirding Iraq—the current, millennia-old center for global innovation. The lessons of the Gulf wars are that our future has already been fought for; a blueprint already exists of this world. There is a Green Zone for the few, a Red Zone for the rest. We look away at our own risk.

This text was originally published in Theater of Operations: The Gulf Wars, 1991–2011, *edited by Peter Eleey and Ruba Katrib, MoMA PS1, 2019.*

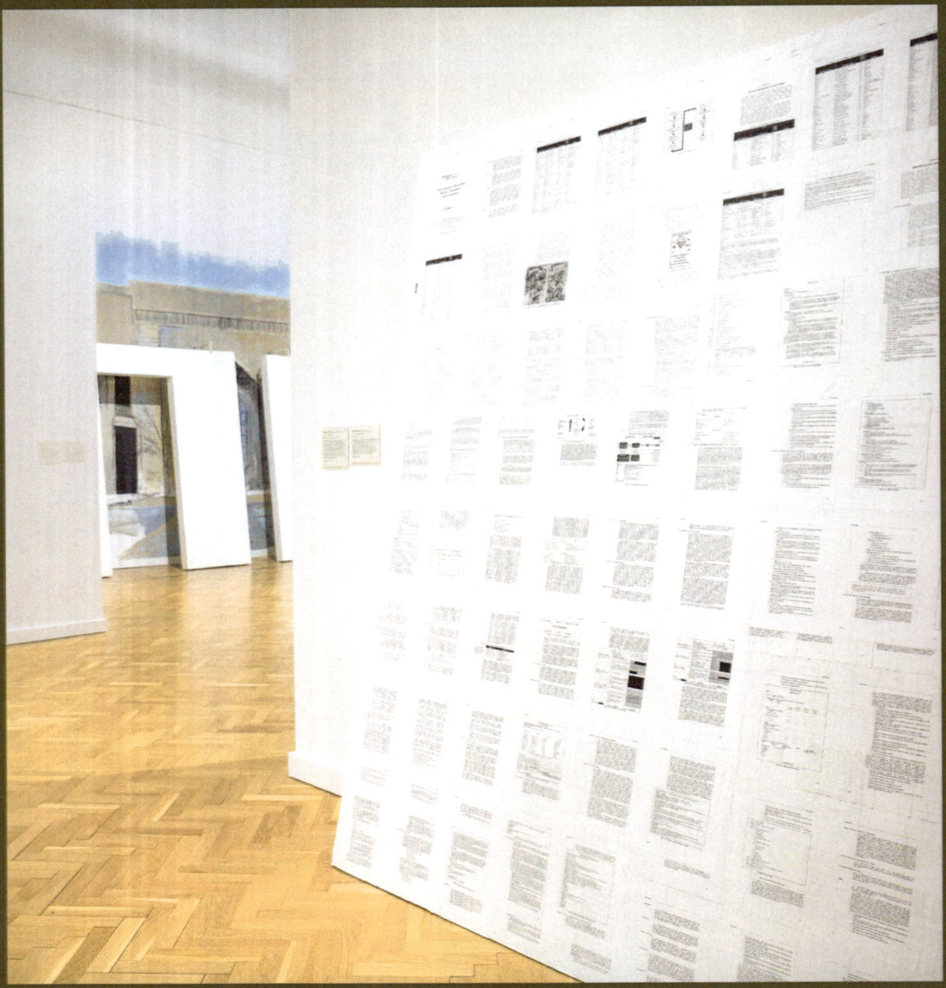

GERALD SHEFFIELD *(b. 1985) [US Army veteran]*
fm 3-05.301 (from ***ptsd series***), 2016
Wheatpaste-collaged copy paper on panel

Displaying layers of pages of the US Army's *Field Manual for Psychological Operations*, this installation reckons with the US counterinsurgent policy of embedding soldiers into local communities during wartime in an effort to "win the hearts and minds" of occupied people. For Sheffield, the Army's *Field Manual* represents one of the bureaucratic foundations of the long wars.

see also: pp. 101, 141

Disrupting Business as Usual: Transforming Bureaucracy into Art

AMBER ZORA

In January 2008, I walked to my first class at Winona State University in Minnesota, just five months after my deployment to Iraq. I hoped to leave that experience behind, but the transition felt surreal—one moment, I was in a war zone, and the next, I was sitting in a college classroom. It seemed as if no one acknowledged that the war was still raging. The initial buzz had faded, and life in the United States had returned to business as usual.

But, here in the US, business as usual is, of course, war.

US militarism is so ubiquitous that it often goes unseen. Confronting the reality of an all-encompassing military-industrial complex, many of the artists in *Surviving the Long Wars* have utilized the detritus of the military machine—the mountains of bureaucratic paperwork, the ephemera, the piles of surveillance materials—to illuminate dark and forgotten aspects of militarism. I find these techniques of unearthing the past and collaging elements together hypnotizing, as they weave together disparate pieces to create a larger, collective narrative.[1] As a photographer, I am particularly drawn to works that use primary sources—direct documentation—to conjure up the past. What could be more immediate than documents from the heart of the empire?[2]

At the Chicago Cultural Center, an installation by the *Index of the Disappeared*, a nearly two-decades-long artistic collaboration between Chitra Ganesh and Mariam Ghani, utilizes military manuals and ephemera. Their installation transforms passive art viewers into active researchers. In an age where we forget so quickly, artists become record keepers and historians.

This iteration of the *Index of the Disappeared* features binders containing military memos and detainee transfer records—including names, court documents, and sworn statements detailing physical and sexual abuse. One binder contains documents about torture by the Chicago Police Department and its link to the US military prison at Guantánamo Bay, where many detainees were sent. This inclusion demonstrates the intrinsic link between the domestic and the global—tactics used abroad are also used at home. The installation space provides an opportunity for the audience, particularly an American audience, to learn about repressed facts, remember forgotten events, and confront the stories of those directly harmed by the "Global War on Terror."

Ganesh and Ghani achieve something remarkable: they transform cold, impersonal documents into something deeply emotional and heartbreaking. As I searched through the binders, I searched for truths: Who are the people who have disappeared? Can I locate them

1. Walter Benjamin and Michael William Jennings, *Selected Writings: Volume 2, 1927–1934* (Cambridge, MA: Belknap Press of Harvard University Press, 1999), 576.

2. Ronak K. Kapadia, "Kissing the Dead Body: Conjuring 'Warm Data' in Archives of US Global Military Detention," *Verge: Studies in Global Asias* 5, no. 1 (2019): 123–52.

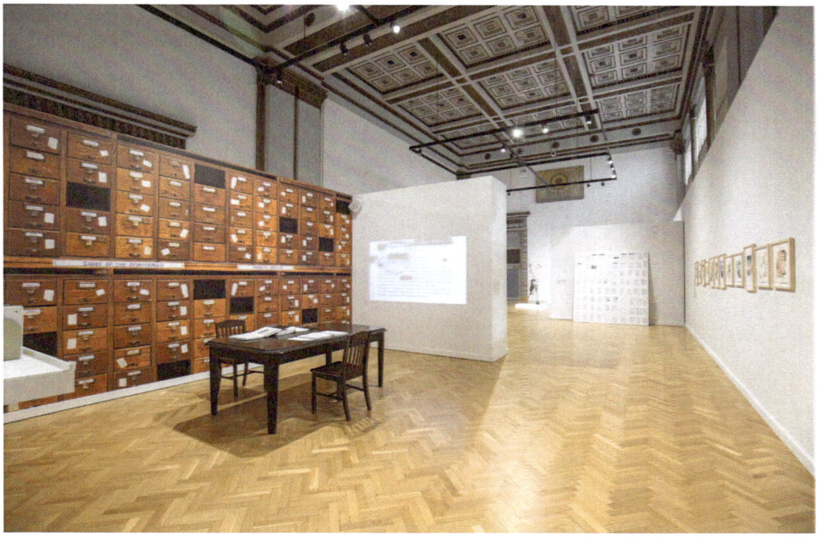

CHITRA GANESH AND MARIAM GHANI, *Index of the Disappeared: Parasitic Archive*, 2014, Site specific installation with vinyl, tables, chairs, binders, copy paper, ephemera including military manuals and documents; *see also: pp. 84–87*

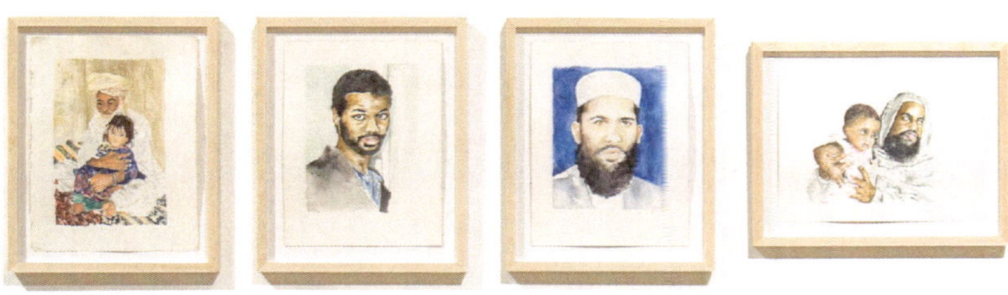

CHITRA GANESH, *Index of the Disappeared: Watercolors* (selections), 2004, Watercolor on paper; *see also: pp. 85–87*

in this sea of paperwork? And, if I cannot find them, can I find clues about who they were? In my search, I imagined myself as a family member finding a loved one's name.

Adjacent to the installation are Ganesh's watercolor portraits of individuals who were detained and disappeared in the months following September 11th. The watercolors disintegrate the coldness and abstraction of the nearby documents. They invite me into loving family snapshots delicately reproduced with washes of color.

As I shuffle through what remains, I'm aware of what has been lost; yet, I'm also aware I can never fully understand the enormity of the loss. As an engaged audience member, I feel the crushing weight of this bureaucratic system; it seems insurmountable. Is this the anguish of a family member searching for a loved one? Or, more accurately, am I grappling with the conflicted emotions of a repentant soldier? I find myself questioning who sent and signed these records. Are they mere cogs in the bureaucratic machine? The installation functions like a Rorschach test, revealing one's position, or complicity, within the empire.

Presenting a sea of information, albeit meticulously organized into binders, is a way to grapple with complexity—a form of collage. I could not take it all in; some elements were left to be discovered by another viewer. I was struck by how grandiose documentation can itself serve as a form of camouflage, masking its true nature.

In the same gallery, veteran Gerald Sheffield uses similar techniques in his work *fm 3-05.301*. Pages from the US Army's Field Manual for Psychological Operations (PSYOP) are collaged on a large panel and leaned against the wall. The field manual, an abstract document, symbolizes another bureaucratic tool used for war-making. According to the manual, PSYOP is used to shape "emotions, attitudes, or desired behavior that support the achievement of US national objectives and the military mission." Sheffield, who served eight years in the US Army as a visual communications and military intelligence public

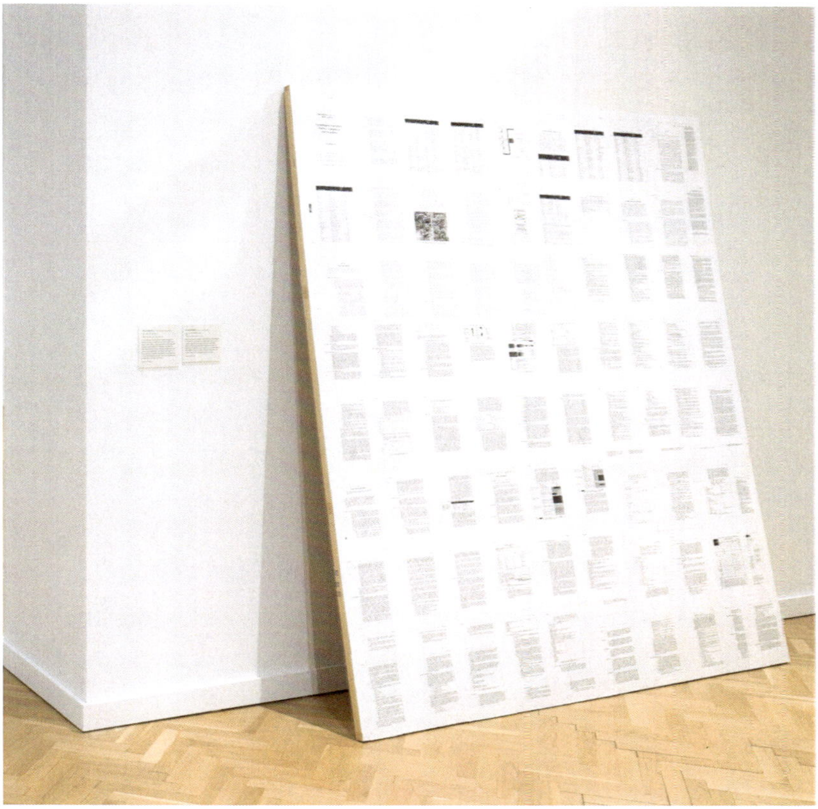

GERRALD SHEFFIELD, *fm 3-05.301* (from *ptsd series*), 2015, Wheatpaste-collaged copy paper on panel; *see also: pp. 101, 136*

affairs specialist across Paraguay, Guatemala, Brazil, and Kuwait, uses these documents to reveal the underlying machinery of psychological warfare.

As I engaged with Sheffield's work, I reflected on his unique relationship with this document and his own path from growing up as a Black kid from Atlanta facing housing instability to joining the military. Much like my experience with the *Index of the Disappeared*, I sifted through the collage of Xeroxed papers for clues. The field manual's strategies for winning favor, including tactics based on Maslow's hierarchy of needs, struck a chord with me. Sheffield's background of housing insecurity in the US made me acutely aware of how the military exploits these very needs to recruit. Both Sheffield's work and the *Index of the Disappeared* expose a form of quiet violence, where the documents themselves are cold and impersonal, reflecting the detached mechanisms of systematic exploitation in the US military.

Other artworks in the three STLW exhibitions similarly incorporate or reference government documents. Employing a technique creating an unusual blend of the banal and the cataclysmic, the artists reveal what is often hidden by using archival materials and empirical tools. These materials often feature "little histories," alongside laws and practices that continue to affect people today. Notable examples include veteran Ruth Kaneko's *Service Connected II: Kānehailua*, which integrates a page from the Kūʻe Petitions signed by her family; June Carpenter's shawls, which reference court accounts and written statements against Indigenous rights; and Terran Last Gun's ledger drawing, "The ancient people of the West live on," created on a city treasurer's certificate of tax sale. These pieces powerfully reveal the hidden dimensions of collective BIPOC histories and ongoing struggles.

One of the best examples of this technique is Hanaa Malallah's *She/He Has No Picture*, a work commemorating the Al Amirayah shelter tragedy—a bombing by the US military that killed at least 408 people. The shelter was destroyed by two laser-guided smart bombs in February 1991, before dawn. Malallah went to the site of the bombing, now a museum, and the experience inspired her to make a memorial featuring portraits of the victims crafted from burnt canvases.

Malallah, an Iraqi artist and member of the "eighties generation" of Iraq, was displaced to London after the US invasion in 2006. The Triennial marks the first time this installation has been showcased in its entirety in the US. Reflecting on the project, Malallah said,

> The exhibition location of this project does not change the meaning of it, but exhibiting this work in the US specifically adds a lot of irony—the US caused the wars and created our disaster and then subsequently welcomes our art about that disaster. I do not know if this happened accidentally or if it is a strategic way to try and wash its hands from the crime by showing artwork of the victims. It looks to me like catharsis for both the victims and perpetrators, which is as important to Western culture as it is for us.[3]

Malallah's canvases memorialize those lost, either by recreating their images or indicating their absences. The burnt canvas portraits compel the viewer to confront the gaze of those killed in the US bombing, while twenty empty brass plates reflect the viewer's own face. Engraved in Arabic on these brass plates are the haunting phrases "she has no image" or "he has no image."

Viewing *She/He Has No Picture* was educational for me. As a US citizen and former soldier, I'm implicated in the bombing, though I was only four years old in February 1991. In this installation, I see the faces of children who were the same age as me at the time. This concept of catharsis that Malallah mentions resonates with me, bringing to mind the *Index* and the collective shame felt by many anti-war veterans. Can we, as US veterans or Americans in general, atone for what we have never fully understood? These artists, through their research, reinterpretation, and presentation, offer viewers knowledge of our violent—often genocidal—history. They have gone to the dark places and held up mirrors to reflect and disrupt American daily life.

After catharsis, there is an opportunity to collectively reorient toward solidarity, healing, and building something better.

---

3. Spencer Harrison, "Shelter in the Storm: An Interview With Hanaa Malallah," *Surviving the Long Wars*, June 29, 2023, https://www.survivingthelongwars.online/writing/hanaa-malallah.

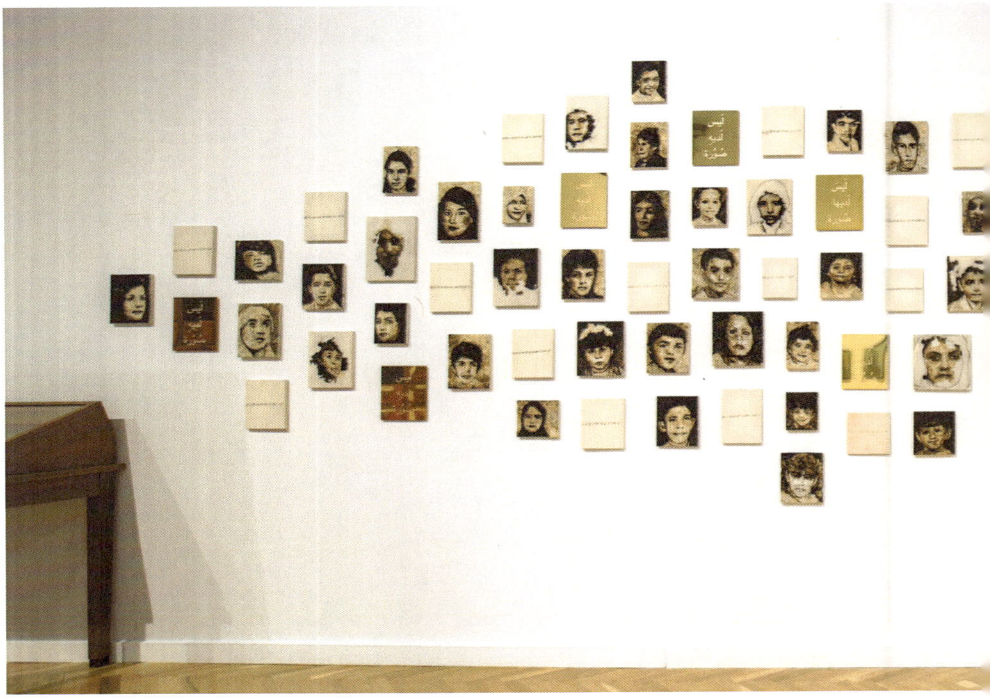

HANAA MALALLAH, *She/He Has No Picture*, 2019/20, Burnt canvas collage on canvas with laser cut brass plaques, four art books, thousands of computer-generated moving images, and original booklet published by the Iraqi government in 1991

The portraits in *She/He Has No Picture*—with their brass reflections and white canvas installation—serve as another form of collage, the details contributing to a larger whole. It is a technique echoed throughout STLW, reflected in the curation of the exhibitions. The layers of collage resonate with the layers of collective work, each unique contribution converging and diverging, deepening the meaning of each individual work.

In the STLW exhibition *Unlikely Entanglements*, at Hyde Park Art Center, Eric Perez's two portraits, *5-Sierra* and *Sgt. Gudiño*, are displayed. Each portrait consists of three layers of acrylic cut into fragmented silhouettes of the subject. From a distance, viewers perceive pixelated portraits of the two men, inspired by the digital

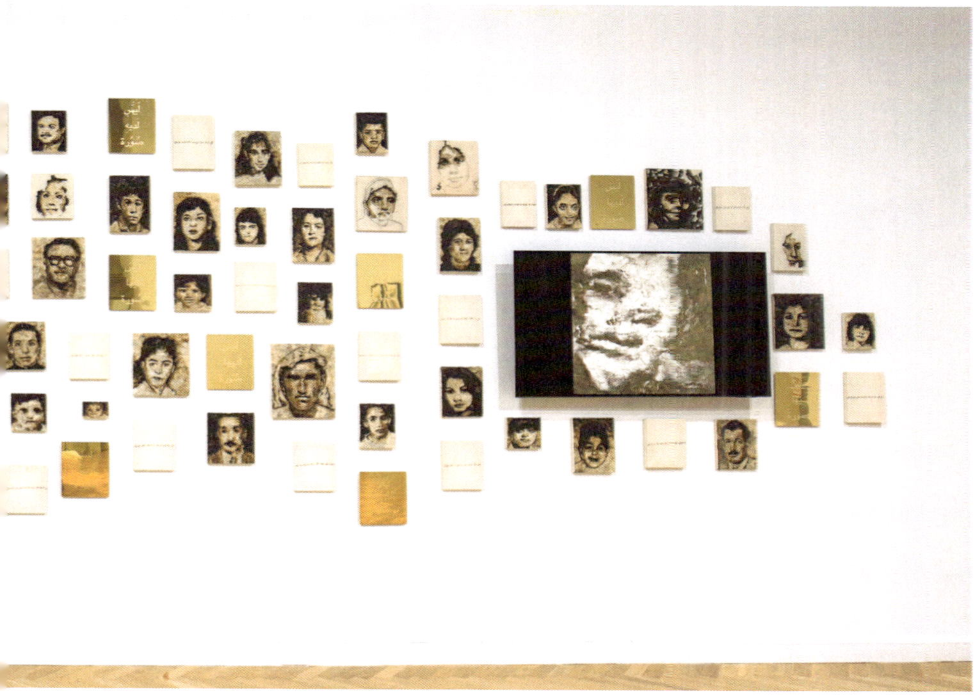

see also: pp. 82–83, 113–15, 150–51

camouflage found in Marine Corps uniforms. Upon closer inspection, the larger image reveals a collage interwoven with smaller photographic images.

These portraits depict two marines Perez served alongside, incorporating photographs taken by Perez and images provided by each subject. Through interviews with his comrades, Perez embedded their memories into the image code, resulting in a glitchy effect. Some stories from the interviews Perez remembered differently or were entirely new to him. This is notable because this mirroring of the fragmented nature of memories reflects the often disjointed recollections of service members transitioning out of the military, marked by gaps and distortions. Perez reflects on the function of

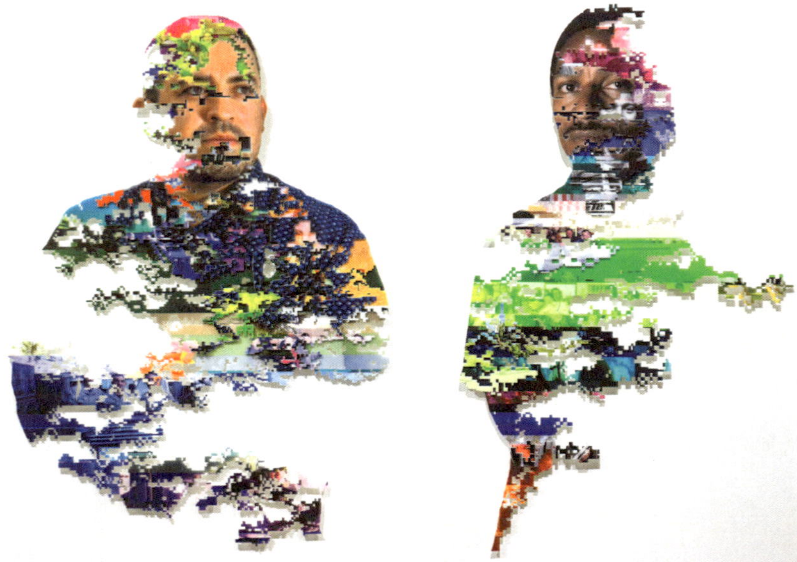

ERIC PEREZ, *Sgt. Gudiño* (left) and *5-Sierra* (right), 2023, Mounted digital prints on acrylic laser-cut into the silhouette and custom digi-camo patterns; *see also: pp. 190–91, 197*

patterns and the dehumanization inherent in warfare, questioning the worth of a pixel and the ease with which identities can be altered and erased. He seeks to restore depth to those he served with, acknowledging the necessity of othering and erasure for the war machine to persist. When asked about considering the Iraqi perspective in his work, Perez emphasizes the importance of including artists from the Greater Middle East in the exhibition. Widening the frame from Perez's individual works to the collage of the exhibition, Perez's work is notably situated next to Bassim Al Shaker's paintings depicting his own recollections in the immediate aftermath of explosions.

Audience members not only get the perspective of soldiers, but also first-person viewpoints of those directly affected by the US military. In the same gallery, Rajkamal Kahlon explores themes of surveillance and dehumanization. Kahlon, an Indian American artist living and working in Berlin, presents her work *People of Afghanistan*,

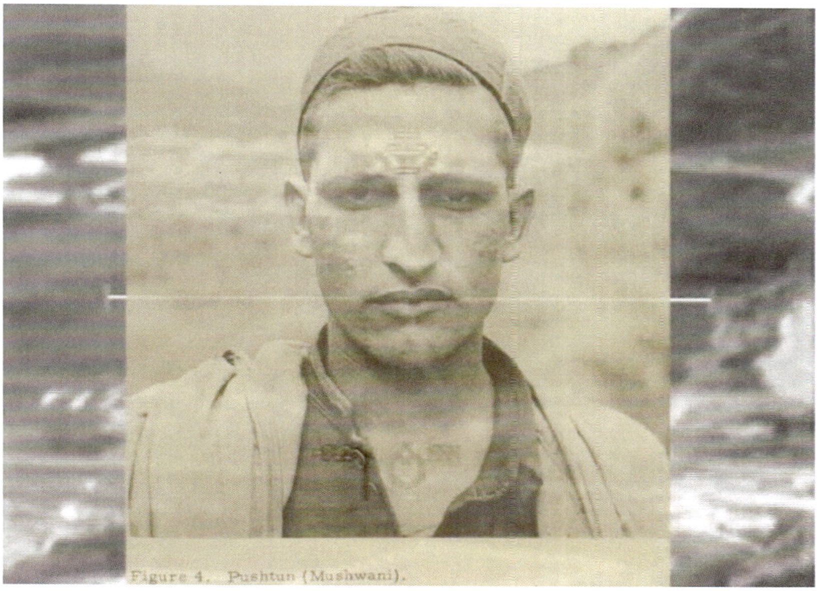

RAJKAMAL KAHLON, still from *People of Afghanistan*, 2017, Ten-minute video installation; *see also: pp. 148, 192–93*

employing a digital collage that blends thermal imagery of bombings anonymously published on the internet in 2002 with photographs of Afghan men from a 1960s Soviet anthropological survey by G.F. Debets. The accompanying audio captures American service members conversing mundanely as they survey the area. Their communication at times resembles the banality of office work, even as they hit targets: buildings, people, and moving vehicles. Simultaneously, viewers are confronted with portraits of Afghan men amidst explosions on the monochromatic landscape. Initially, I found myself conflating the still photographic images of the Afghan men with those targeted in the bombing footage.

The juxtaposition of video documentation of aerial surveillance technology with the photographic portraits from G.F. Debets's survey creates a striking tension between the impersonal, micro-pixelated figures and the vivid macro portraits. This dynamic interplay

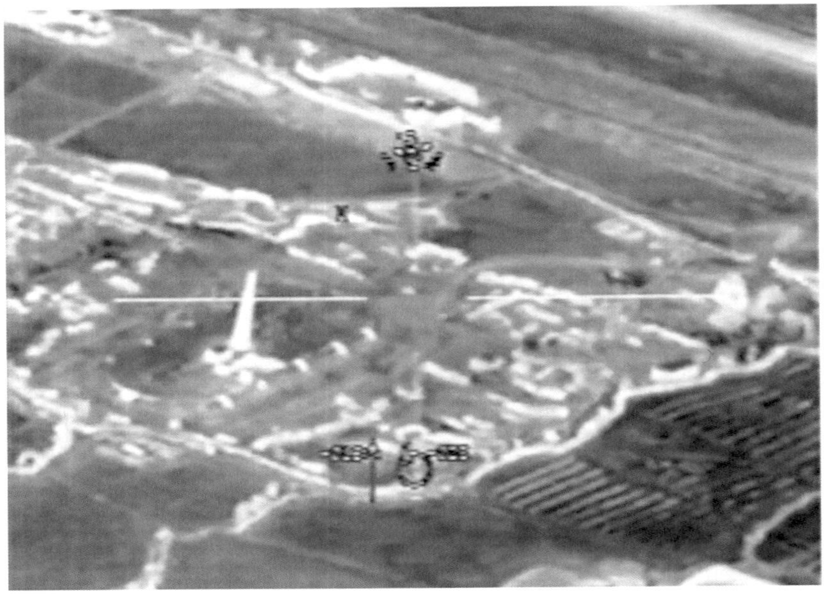

RAJKAMAL KAHLON, still from *People of Afghanistan*, 2017, Ten-minute video installation; *see also: pp. 147, 192–93*

resonates with Perez's collage work, though with a unique twist. Both approaches offer fleeting glimpses into the humanity of the subjects, only to be distanced by glitches and the unreliability of the lens and multiple narrators. This push and pull is reflected in several works that flood us with information that both reveals and conceals.

Kahlon's use of photographic images from a survey done before the Soviet-Afghan War complicates the narrative, juxtaposing the micro and macro perspectives of Afghans through the eyes of outsiders. I envision Kahlon's presentation as a commentary on what has been taken, offering a critique of two empires in decline: Soviet and American.

In our discussions, Kahlon shared that as an American, she recognized the voices of the American men in the audio—they could be neighbors or family friends. Similarly, the South Asian men in the images resembled family members, adding a deeply personal layer to her interpretation.

Throughout these exhibitions, we've encountered works that unveil what war and US militarism try to erase. The use of collage highlights the complexity of overlapping narratives and identities. Moreover, they foster heightened consciousness and solidarity across diverse communities, propelling the dialogue of the emerging Veteran Art Movement forward.

There are alternatives to war yet to be explored. To advance this vision, we require a more engaged populace capable of confronting complex issues through innovative artistic expression. Solidarity across differences paves the way for envisioning futures beyond our current struggles, propelling us closer to a long-desired post-war era.

next spread: **HANAA MALALLAH**
She/He Has No Picture, *see also: pp. 82–83, 113–15, 144–45*

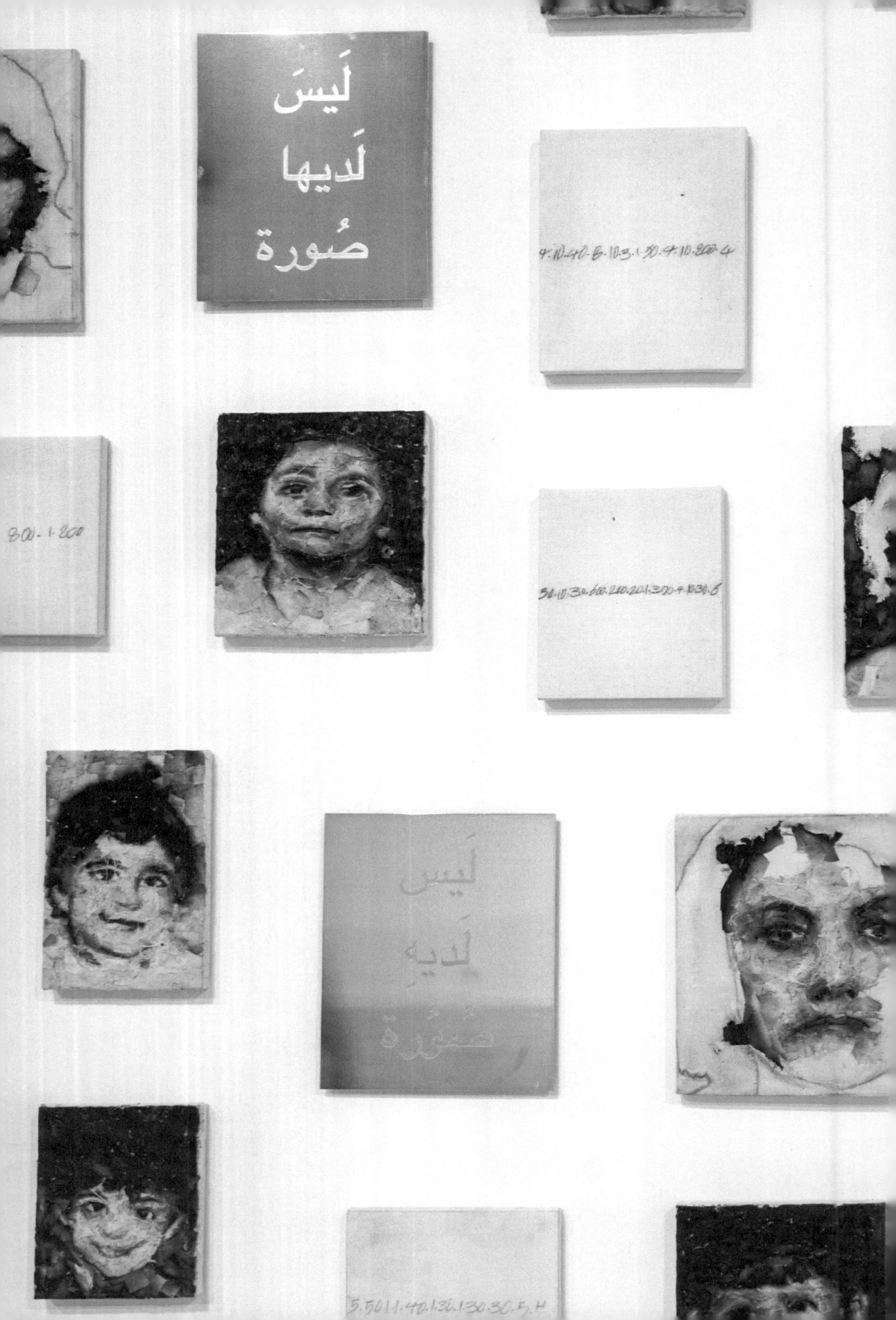
لَيسَ
لَديها
صُورة
4.10.40.8.10.3.1.50.4.10.800.4
800.1.200
لَيس
لَديه
صُورة

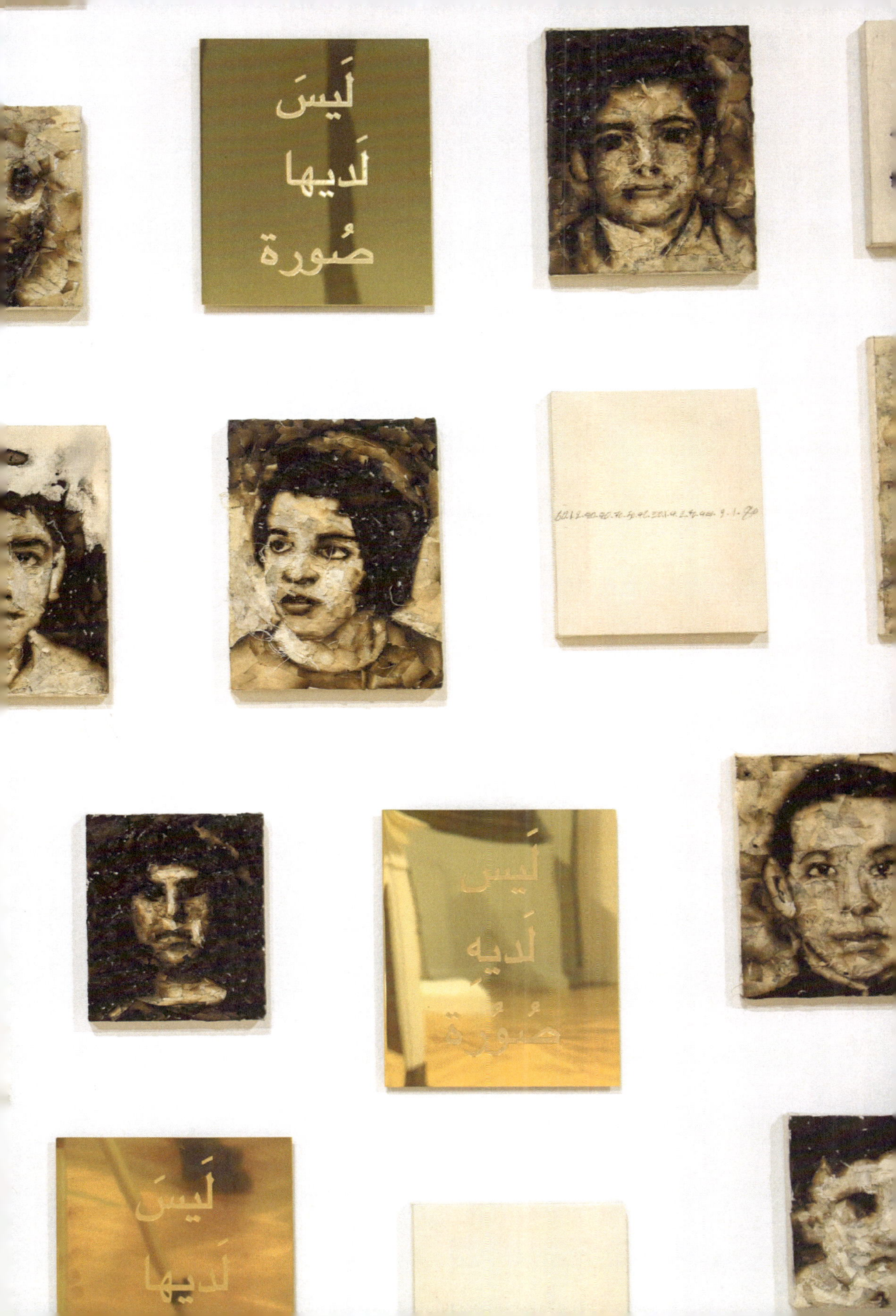
لَيسَ
لَديها
صُورة
لَيس
لَديه
صُورَة
لَيسَ
لَديها

section three

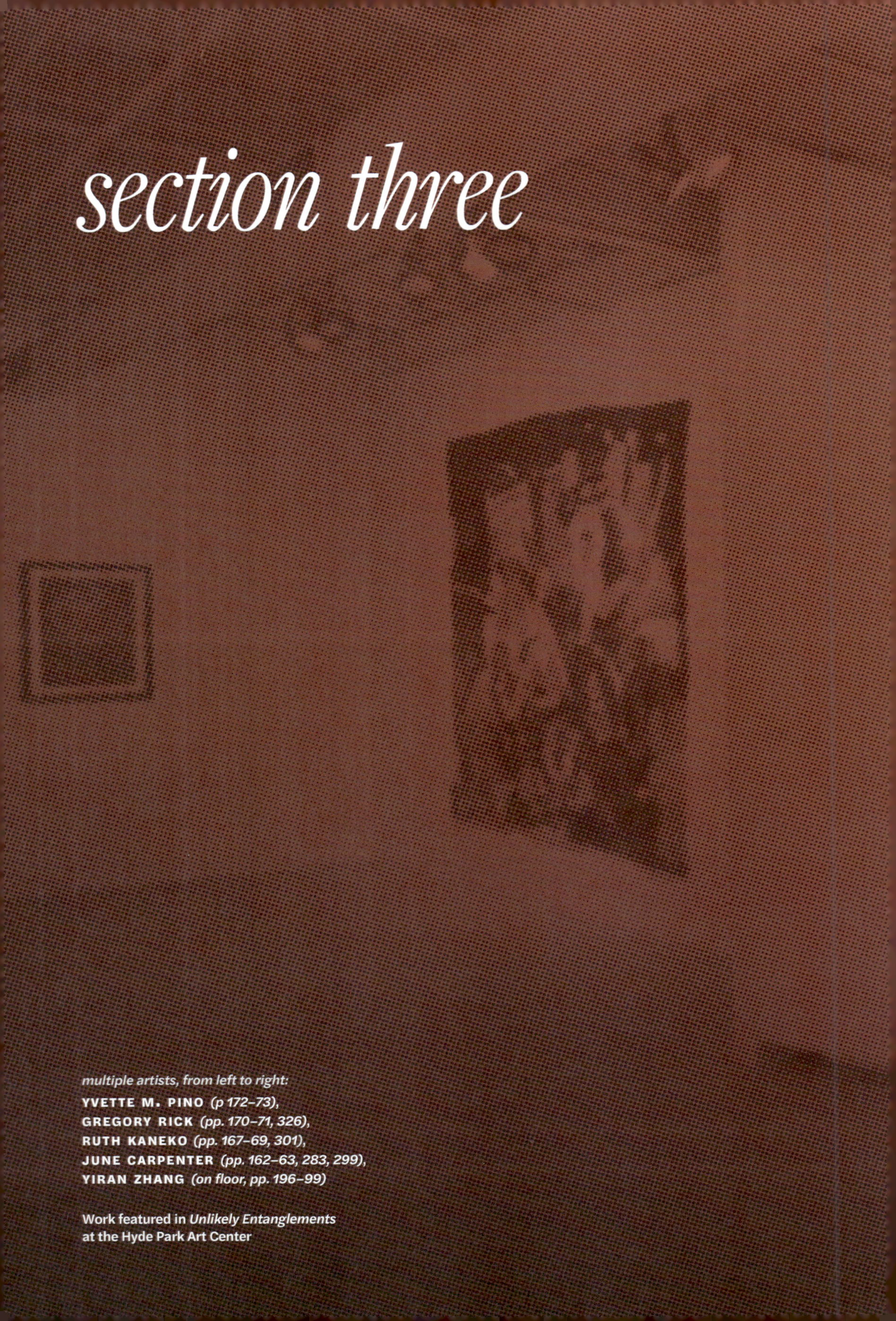

multiple artists, from left to right:
YVETTE M. PINO *(p 172–73),*
GREGORY RICK *(pp. 170–71, 326),*
RUTH KANEKO *(pp. 167–69, 301),*
JUNE CARPENTER *(pp. 162–63, 283, 299),*
YIRAN ZHANG *(on floor, pp. 196–99)*

Work featured in *Unlikely Entanglements* at the Hyde Park Art Center

Unlikely Entanglements

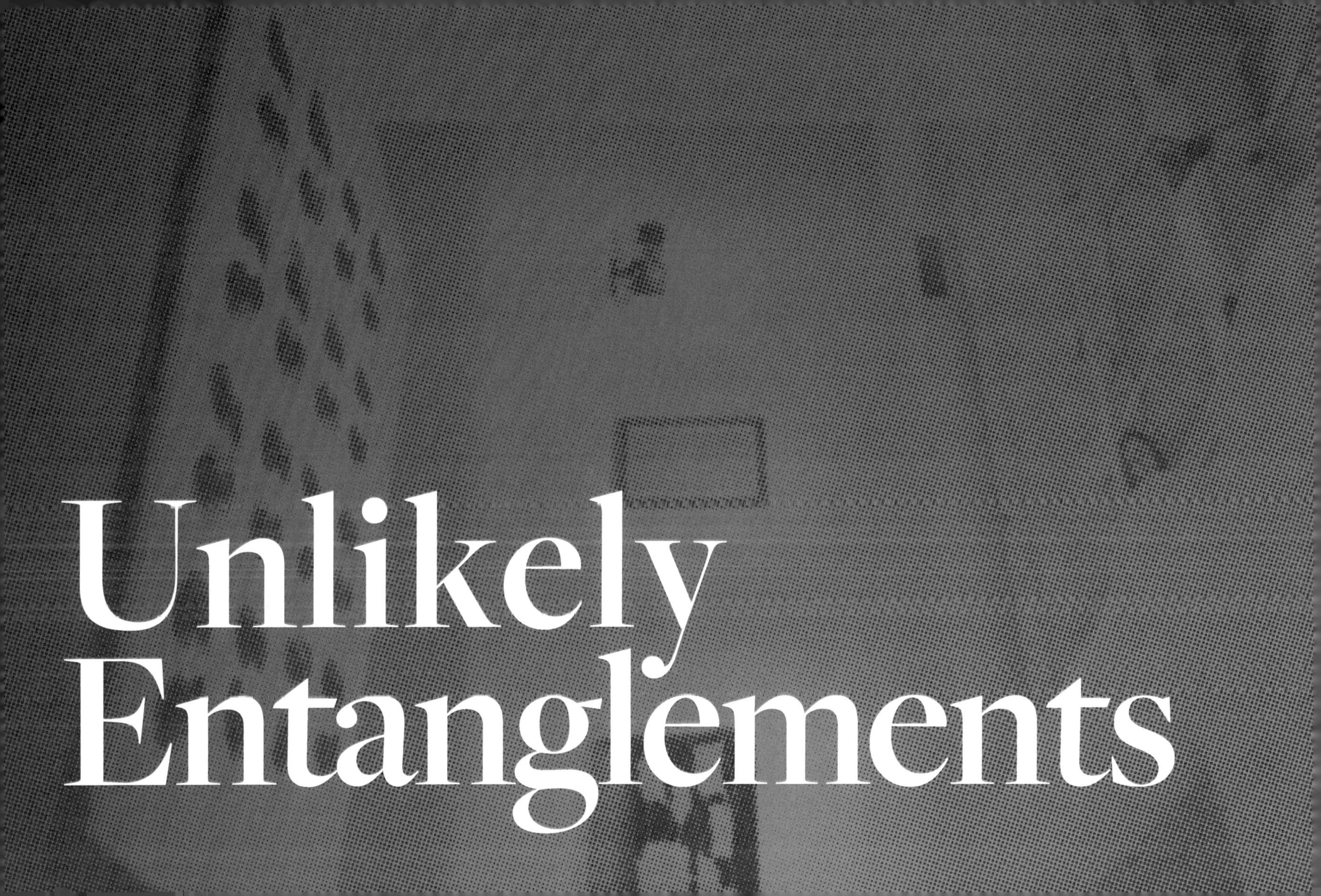

Unlikely Entanglements

It is in collectivities that we find reservoirs of hope and optimism.
—Angela Y. Davis, *Freedom Is a Constant Struggle* (2016)

Across differences and from contrasting viewpoints, visual parallels surface between artworks by civilians impacted by the US long wars and BIPOC veterans critiquing the military they once served in. These "unlikely entanglements" reveal the potential to reimagine affinities between diverse peoples united in their resistance to colonialism.

Titled *Unlikely Entanglements* after the Triennial exhibition at the Hyde Park Art Center (March 16–July 9, 2023), this section includes artworks by Bassim Al Shaker, June Carpenter (Osage/Shawnee), Mahwish Chishty, Jose deVera, Sabba Elahi, Rodney Ewing, Sarah Farahat, Rajkamal Kahlon, Ruth Kaneko (Kanaka Wahine), Eric Perez, Yvette M. Pino, Gregory Rick, Dwayne Wilcox (Oglala Lakota), and Yiran Zhang.

These artists use collage, embroidery, soft sculpture, and installation to unravel dominant histories of militarism while weaving together intimate stories of survival and resistance. Collectively, these powerful artworks by wartime survivors and their descendants conjure meaning out of the traumatic afterlives of the long wars, creating space for solidarity and alternative futures. The artworks are presented alongside original essays by Middle Eastern studies scholar Laleh Khalili and critical ethnic studies scholar Junaid Rana, as well as poetry by GOODW.Y.N., a veteran performance artist and poet.

In "Tomahawks, Chinooks, and Geronimo: Settler-Colonial Fantasies of US Navy SEALs," Laleh Khalili critiques the SEALs' use of Indigenous names and symbols for their equipment and operations, arguing that this practice reflects broader settler-colonial frameworks. The SEALs' adoption of names like "Blackhawk" and "Tomahawk," along with their portrayal in popular culture, perpetuates a militaristic and heroic narrative that appropriates Indigenous symbols while ignoring the ongoing impacts of colonial violence. Khalili argues that this appropriation serves as a form of symbolic violence, reinforcing the US empire's mythos while masking the persistent legacies of settler colonialism.

Junaid Rana's essay "Life During War on Terror Time" examines how the "Global War on Terror" has transformed everyday life and social relations through what he calls "war capitalism" and technological advancements. For Rana, the Triennial exhibitions critique this transformation by showcasing artworks that highlight the surreal and horrific impacts of war, including the psychological trauma and aesthetic changes wrought by ongoing conflict. He suggests that this war capitalism, rooted in settler colonialism, continues to shape our perception and experience of the world, presenting a grim view of a future organized by relentless military and economic exploitation.

Collectively, the works in this section build on what Angela Davis refers to as "freedom as a constant struggle," proposing affinities across histories, geographies, and identities through individual and collective resistance that build toward liberation.[1]

---

1. Angela Davis, *Freedom is a Constant Struggle: Ferguson, Palestine, and the Foundations of a Movement* (Chicago: Haymarket Press, 2016).

It's Not All Dead

GOODW.Y.N.

I.

As the wealthy ate your fresh fish,
An Iraqi delicacy,
Picking the bones out of their
famished mouths,
Gleefully
The rage did come for a visit
within my swollen,
Melancholy breast.
It rose like the desert mounds,
rumbles of feelings.
Swallowing my heart.
Them, the rich and powerful
guests, seemed unsaddened
By the war.
Yet to celebrate Iraqi people,
we all did come together,
As they used to do.
We dined over a tender feast,
Eating only with our hands.
The guests chit-chatting amongst
themselves
I only found sorrow in this action,
A recollection of unwanted memories.

II.

The rains never came to
Southern Iraq.
And yet, as the sun set,
The skyward portal was full of stars.
Who wouldn't want to remember that!
That beauty I found hidden in the war,
I felt it close to my chest.
Buried it so deeply,
I had forgotten its memories.
An unspoken promise,
bathed in pure light.
One memory after another fell—
As if pulling at the thread of
My own brain from my mouth
The amnesia of a "Beautiful Hell,"
released.

III.

Sipping tea whilst in battle gear,
Sharing laughter and quiet tears
All us soldiers, armored, ready
Were alongside the
Iraqi police.
I am still amazed by the dazzling
memory of
Dates
The taste, nourishing
A lingering delicacy now shipped,
Exported with the names of
Other lands and above all
A hope-driven God.

IV.

"It's not all dead," you say.
Yes, I remember, it's not all dead.
Blessed be the tin can you bestowed
Upon me
An oasis shown, inscribed from Iraq
Your ancestors telling me that the land
Is not forsaken and its suffering not
Forgotten
"It's not all dead," I humbly repeated.
To my discovery my ears did hear
And my eyes could still allow tears
As I remembered those that were
put low
And the desert flowers still rising.
And we break bread,
As Kings do
And we break bread,
As Queens do
And we share the spirit of a nation
of nations.
Its proud flag waving at us all.
It is not all dead.
It is not all dead.
The desert, my friends, is not at
all dead.

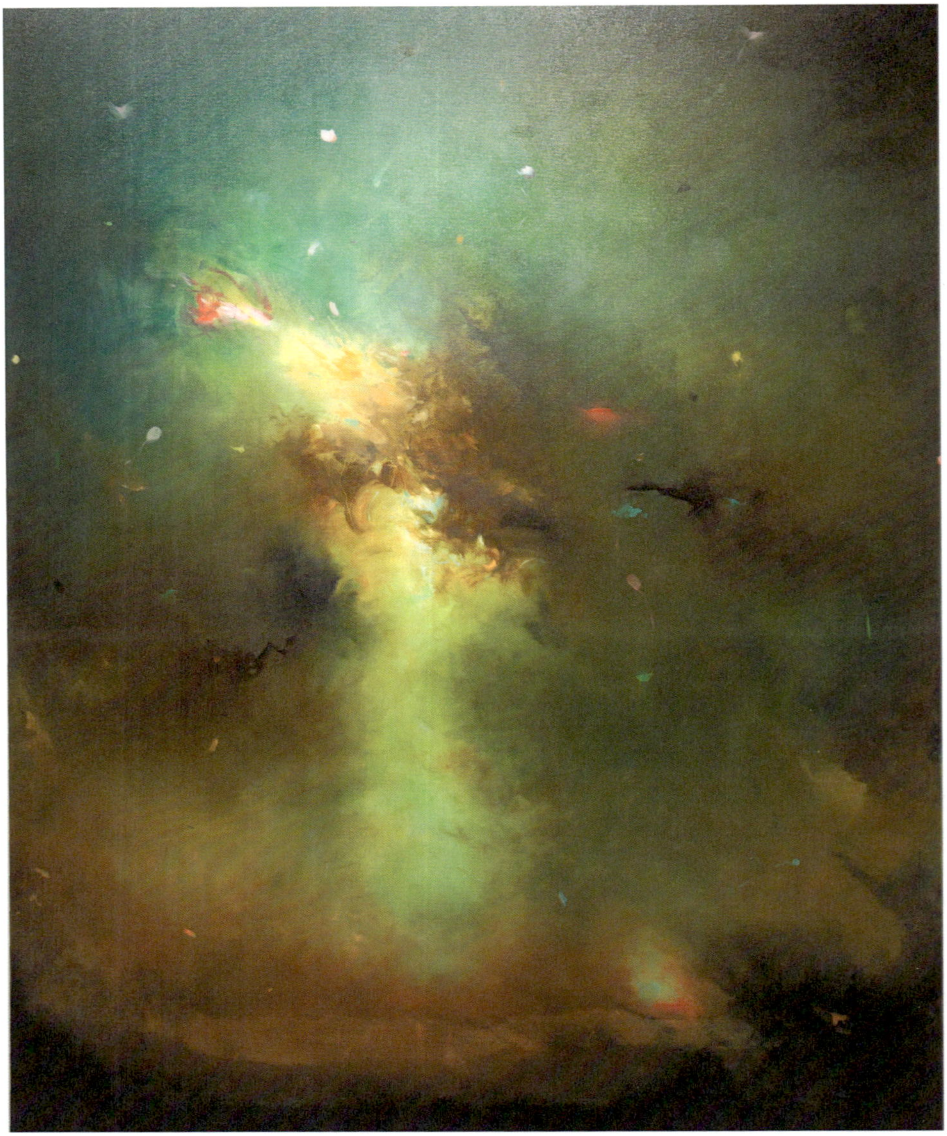

BASSIM AL SHAKER *(b. 1986)*
left: ***Disaster***, 2022
Oil on canvas
Courtesy of Rhona Hoffman Gallery

right: ***Alive***, 2022
Oil on canvas
Courtesy of Rhona Hoffman Gallery

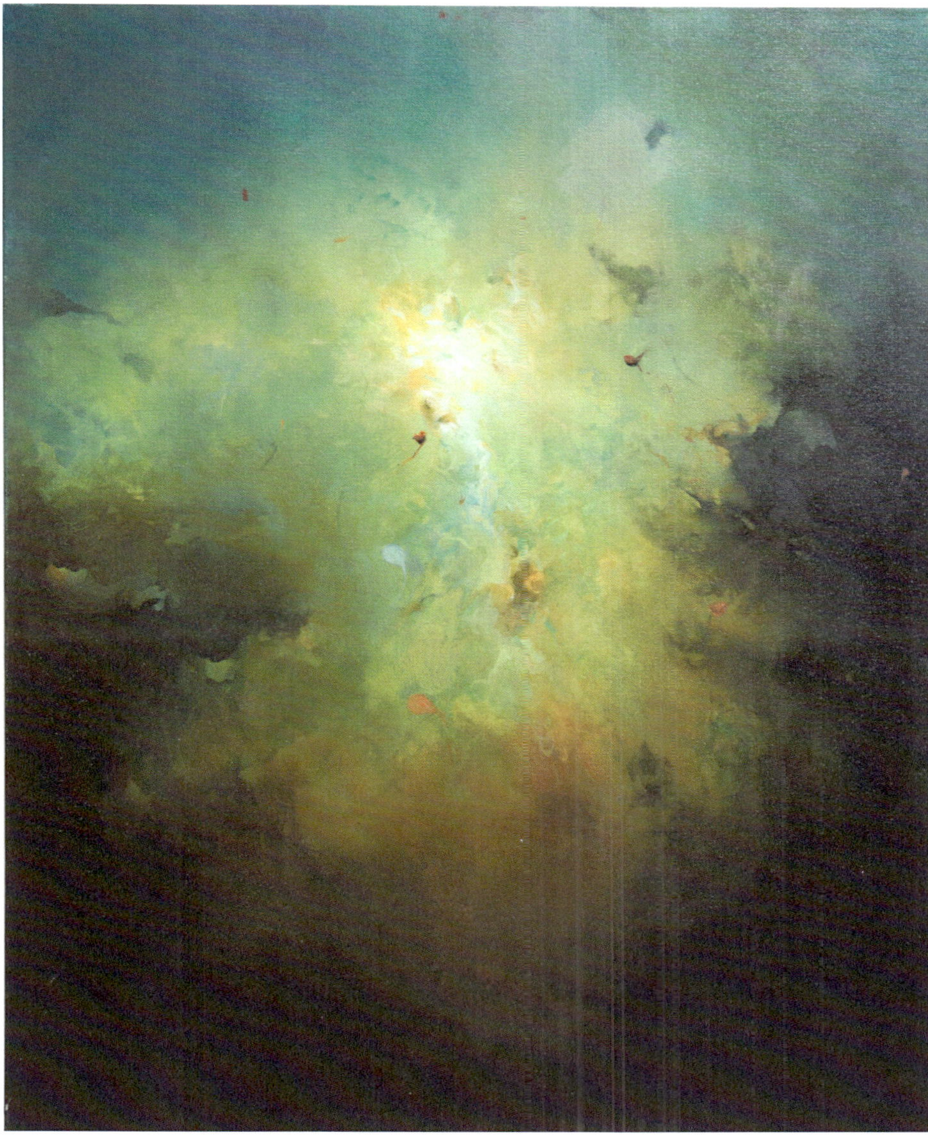

Influenced by his experience of living in Iraq, Bassim Al Shaker's painting series *Moment of Silence* depicts images of an unfamiliar sky in the minutes of silence following explosions he survived. Al Shaker recounts, "After each explosion, everything would be silent for four or five minutes. When that happened, I would be laying on the ground and facing the sky, and I would see something way different than the sky we know. I saw body parts in the sky. The paintings show what the sky looked like at that time. The works describe death and loss, but also a new life after the loss."

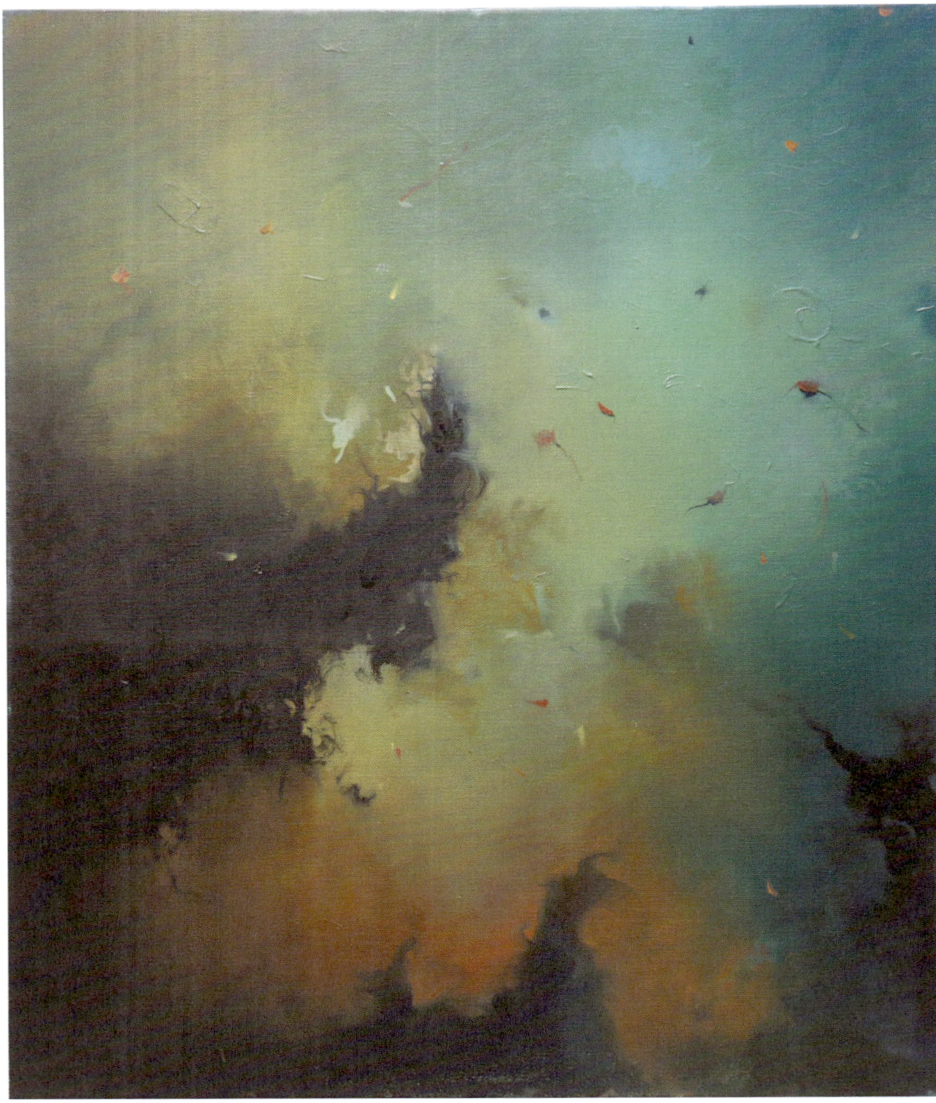

BASSIM AL SHAKER *(b. 1986)*
The Darkness, 2022
Oil on canvas
Courtesy of Rhona Hoffman Gallery

These paintings are part of Bassim Al Shaker's *Moment of Silence* series. See previous spread for more information.

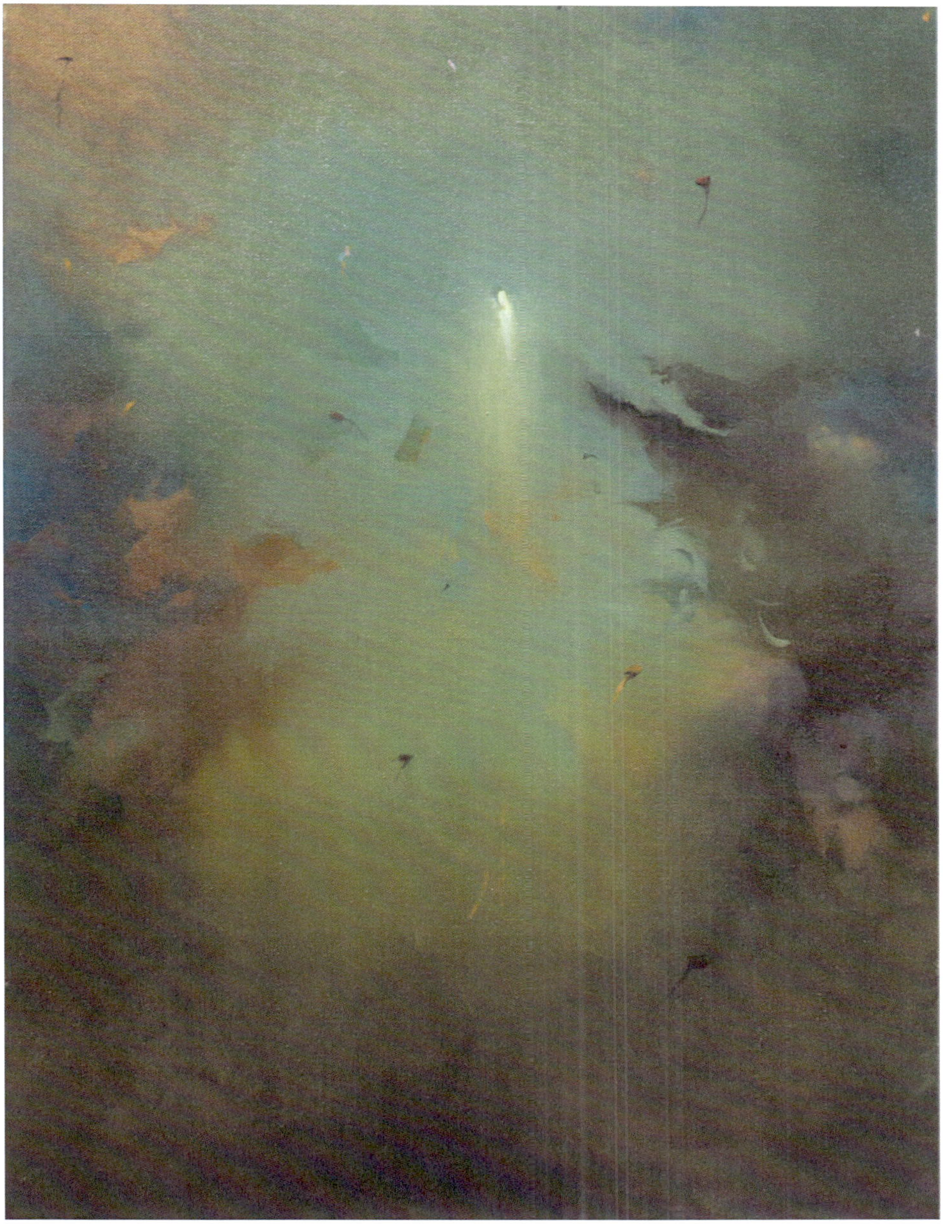

Photon, 2022
Oil on canvas
Courtesy of Rhona Hoffman Gallery

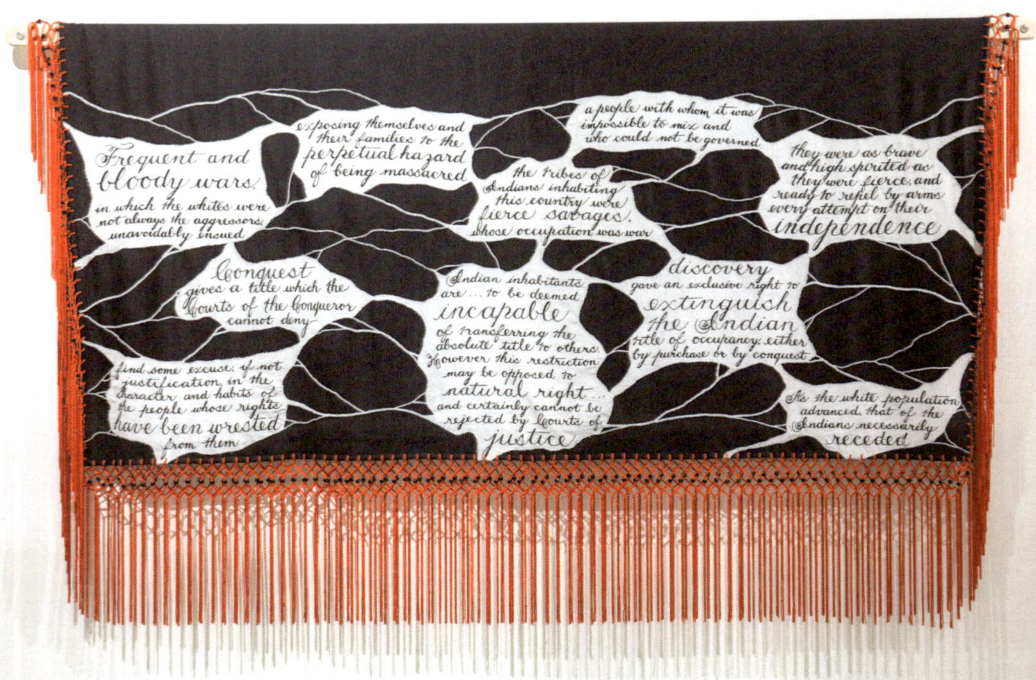
Frequent and bloody wars in which the whites were not always the aggressors unavoidably ensued
exposing themselves and their families to the perpetual hazard of being massacred
a people with whom it was impossible to mix and who could not be governed
the tribes of Indians inhabiting this country were fierce savages whose occupation was war
they were as brave and high spirited as they were fierce and ready to repel by arms every attempt on their independence
Conquest gives a title which the Courts of the Conqueror cannot deny
Indian inhabitants are... to be deemed incapable of transferring the absolute title to others. However this restriction may be opposed to natural right... and certainly cannot be rejected by Courts of justice
discovery gave an exclusive right to extinguish the Indian title of occupancy either by purchase or by conquest
find some excuse if not justification in the character and habits of the people whose rights have been wrested from them
As the white population advanced, that of the Indians necessarily receded

JUNE CARPENTER *(Osage/Shawnee, b. 1981)*
Johnson v. M'Intosh, 21 U.S. 543 (1823), 2017
Wool and cotton fabric, cotton thread, nylon fringe, and glass beads

In *Johnson v. M'Intosh, 21 U.S. 543 (1823)*, June Carpenter responds to the Supreme Court case stating that private citizens could not purchase land from Native Americans—a case that undermined Indigenous sovereignty and self-determination. Carpenter states, "The fabricated case remains the foundation for a body of law concerning the fundamental rights of a people who were not represented or directly involved in the case. The injurious opinion relies on the racist doctrine of discovery and continues to harm and curtail the rights of all Native Americans today." This shawl contains text fragments of the opinion written by Chief Justice John Marshall (who also served as US Secretary of State).

see also: pp. 283, 299

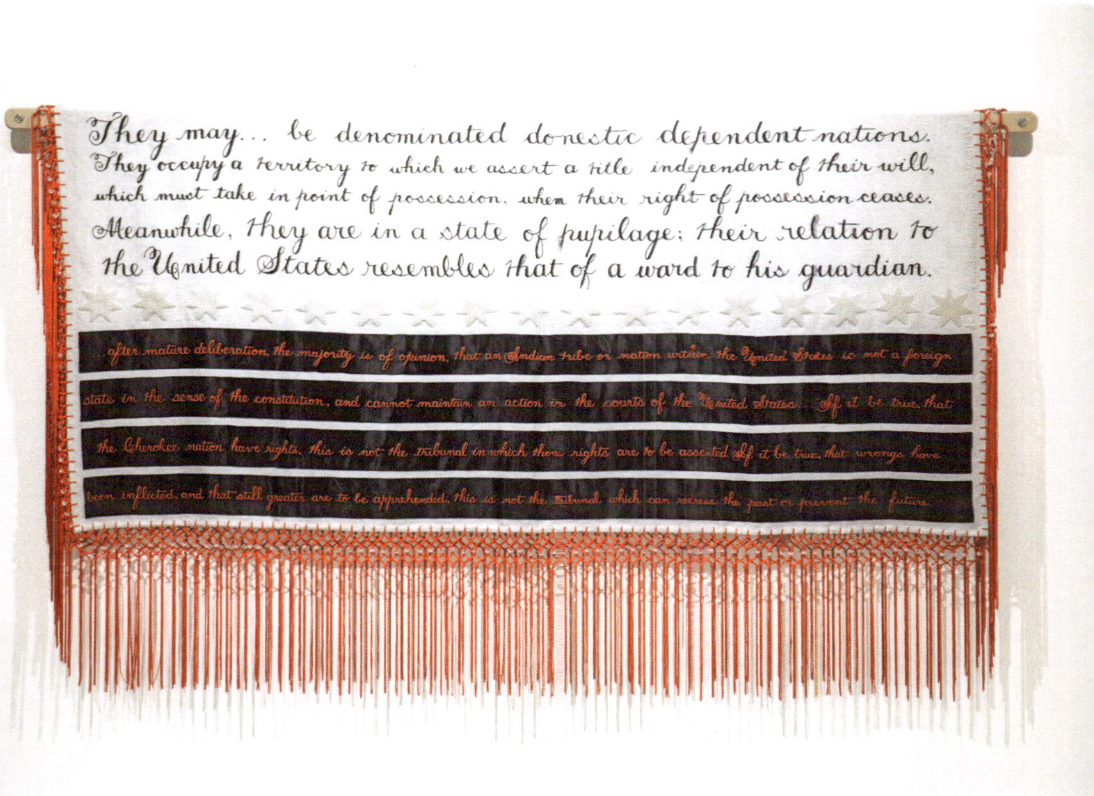

Cherokee Nation v. Georgia, 30 U.S. 1 (1831), 2022
Linen fabric, satin ribbon, cotton thread, nylon fringe, and glass beads

Through her work, June Carpenter seeks to address systemic injustices against Indigenous people by raising awareness of the racism of the US legal system—a system founded on settler colonialism. In *Cherokee Nation v. Georgia, 30 U.S. 1 (1831)*, Carpenter responds to the Supreme Court's decision that Native American tribes were nations that the Court had no jurisdiction over. The Court, however, did not recognize the tribes as *independent* nations. Carpenter says, "As domestic dependent nations, tribes were thereby denied full nationhood. The guardian-ward relationship was also established here, incorporating the trust doctrine into federal Indian law and reinforcing the inferiority of tribes." While tribes were later granted access to the Supreme Court, the influence of this decision is still felt today.

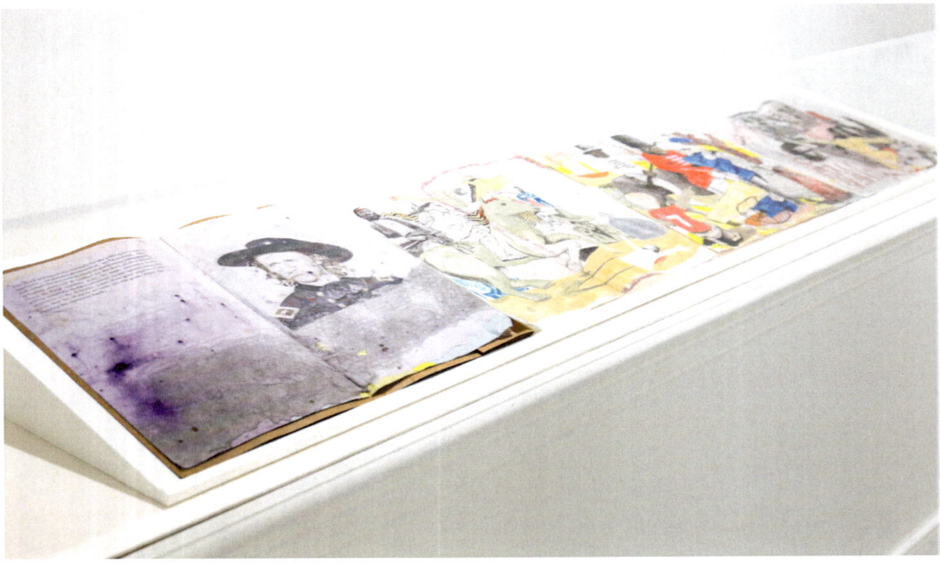

GREGORY RICK *(b. 1981) [US Army veteran]*
Black and Native Victories (details at right), 2017
Accordion book, ink, gouache, photo-transfer, and acrylic on handmade paper
Courtesy of Fred and Louise Neal

Gregory Rick's accordion book highlights an interconnected legacy of resistance to slavery and colonialism by referencing historic Black and Indigenous victorious battles and uprisings. The book intertwines scenes that Rick says could be from "slave revolts, the Battle of the Little Bighorn, Red Cloud's War, or uprisings in Haiti and the like." Rick's collaging technique (and the structure of the book itself) layers and folds scenes on top of one another, reinforcing connections.

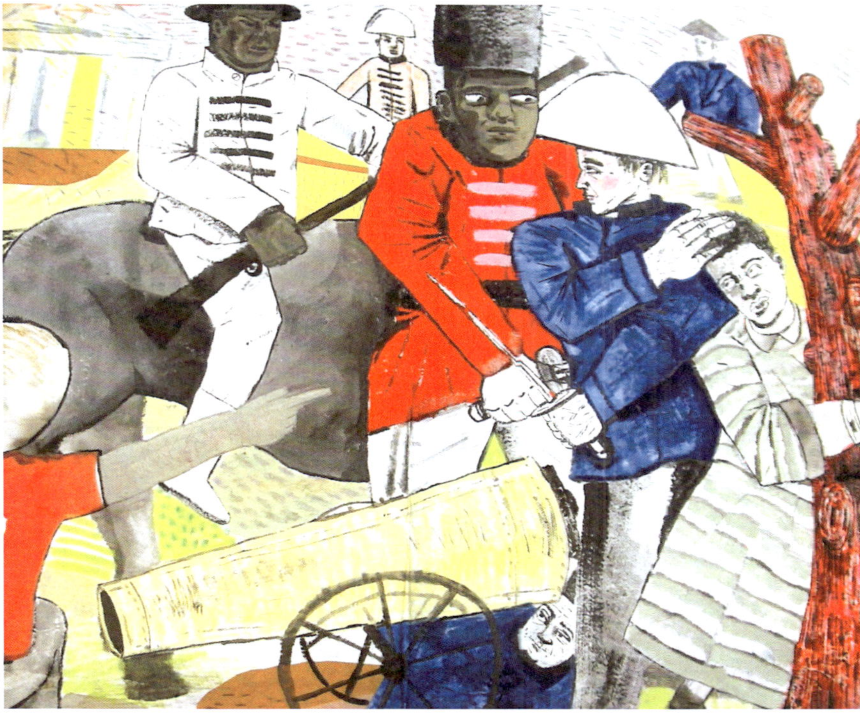

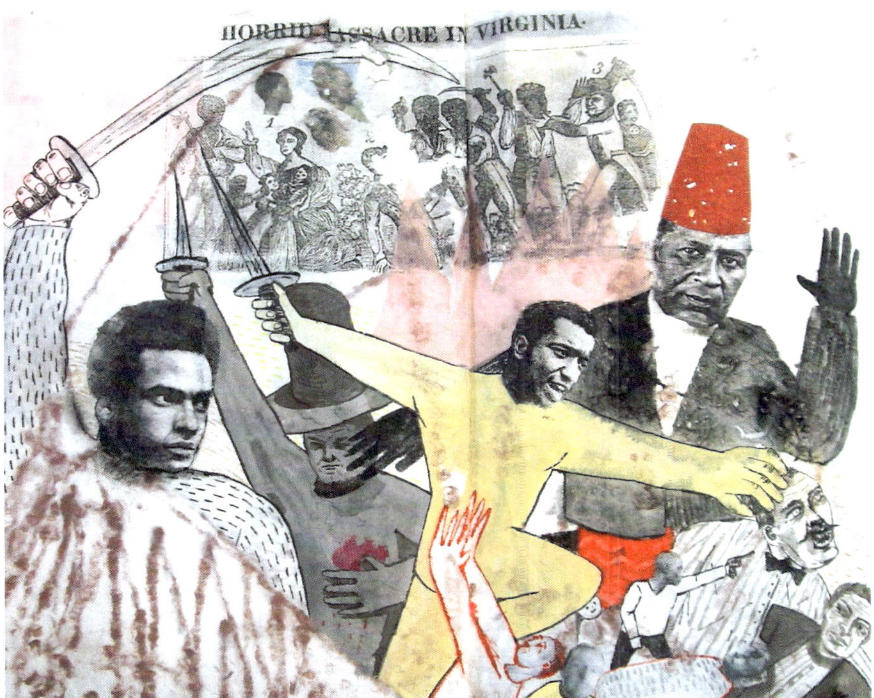
HORRID MASSACRE IN VIRGINIA.

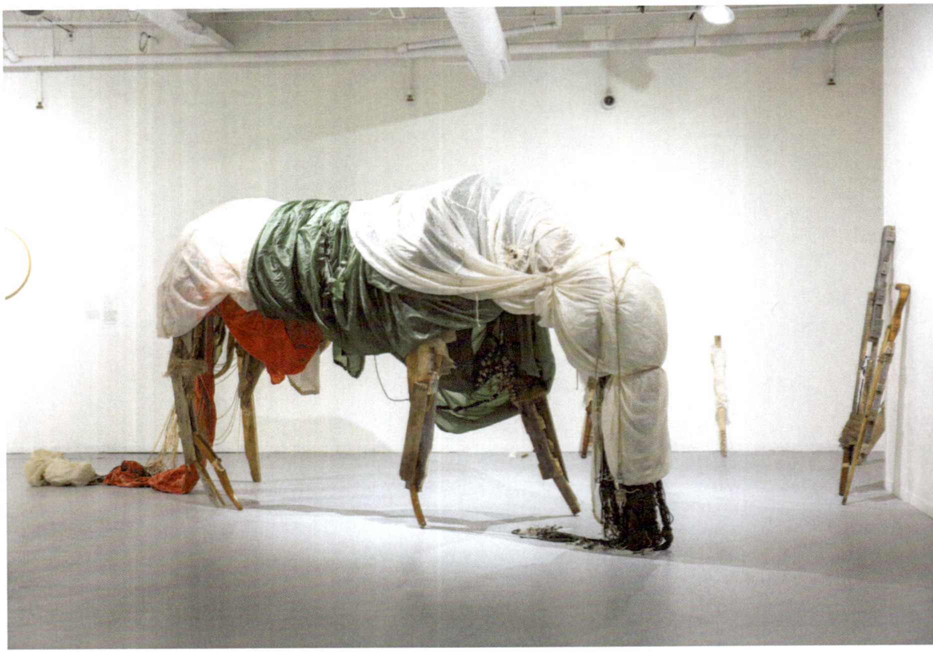

JOSE DEVERA *(b. 1983) [US Marine Corps veteran]*
And All the King's Men, 2014–23
Mixed media, wood, canvas, and found materials

DeVera's installation simultaneously reflects an aggregate of weaponized material and assembled victims of the military-industrial complex. The fabricated figure(s) are shambly archetypes of familiar structures (pack animals, limbs, weapons, etc.) compiled from a combination of repurposed military equipment, domestic household items, and discarded construction materials.

see also: p. 207

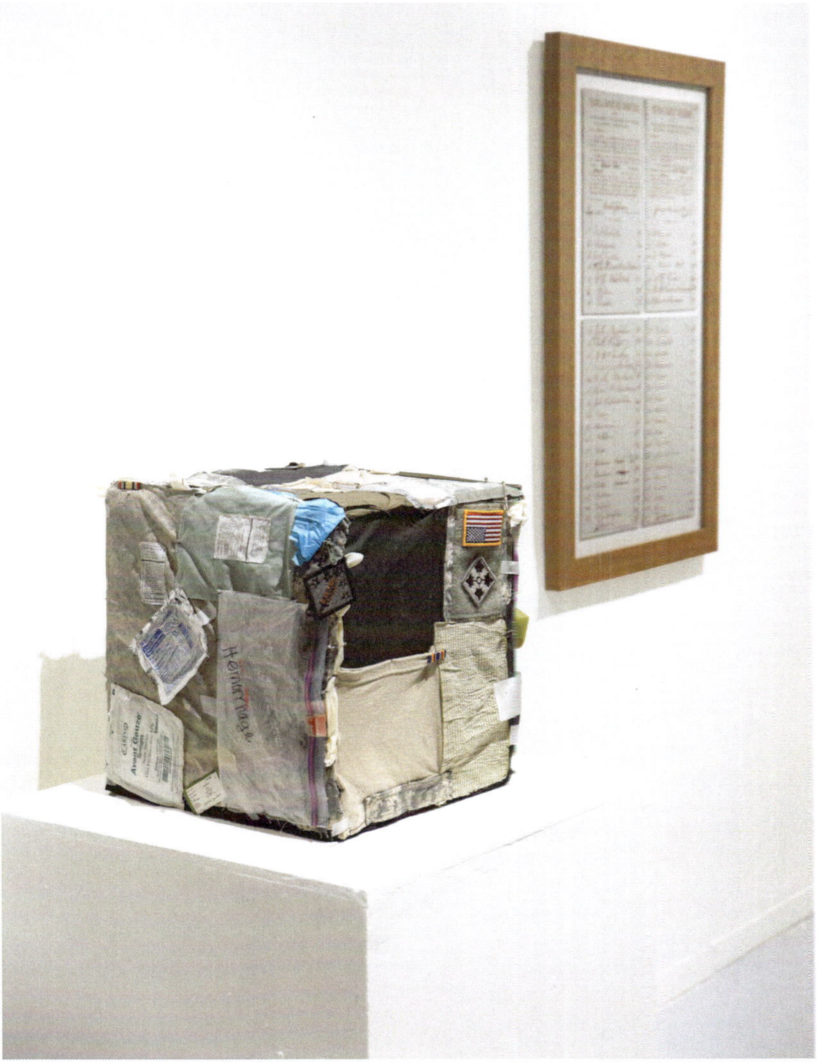

RUTH KANEKO *(Kanaka Wahine, b. 1985)*
[US Army veteran]

left: ***Sutured***, 2019
Mixed media

right: ***Service Connected II: Kānehailua***
see next spread

In *Sutured*, Kaneko dismantles the heroic ideals of warfare by deconstructing and re-collaging materials from her old Army uniforms and medic aid bags. Using a suturing technique, the reconstructed pieces visualize the emotional and physical wounds of war and serve as a metaphor for the process of healing. Through the work, Kaneko invites viewers to consider the human cost of conflict and the need for peace and healing.

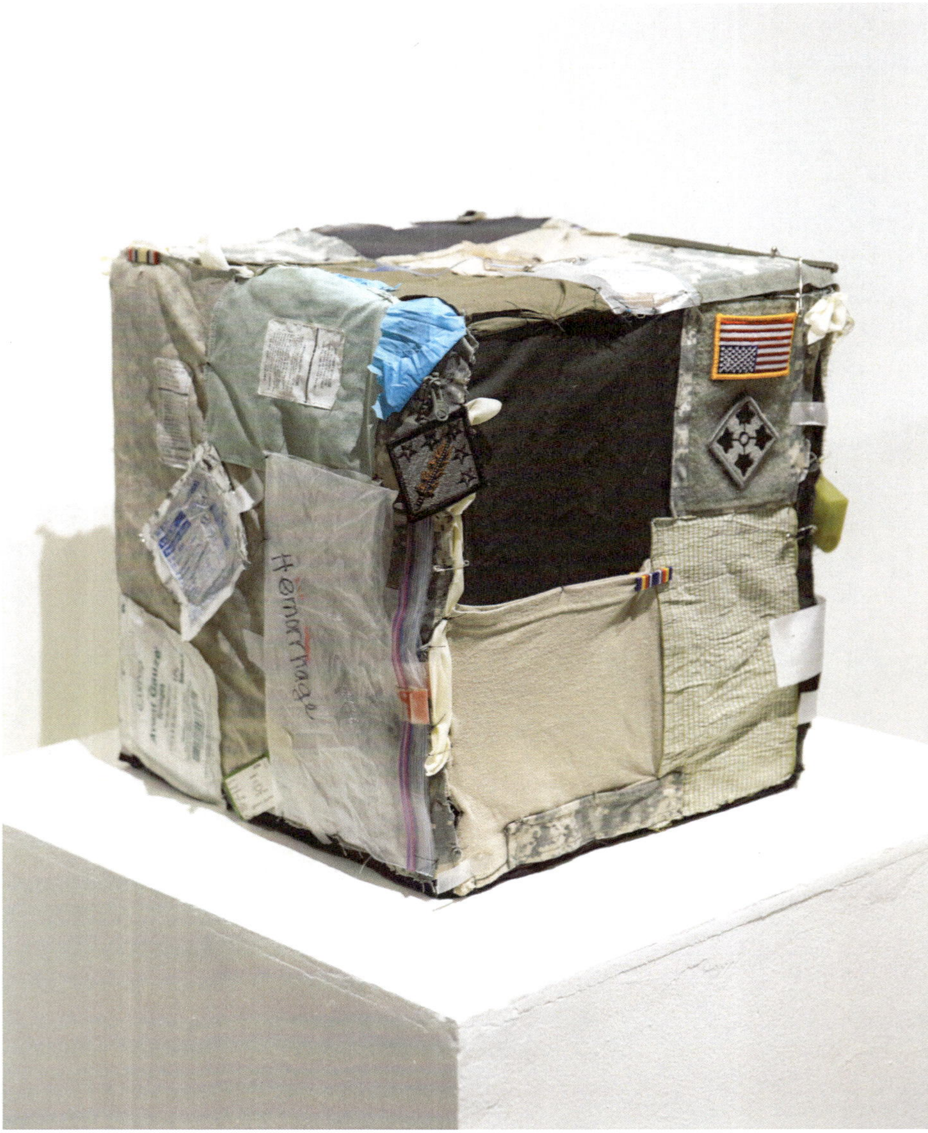

RUTH KANEKO *(Kanaka Wahine, b. 1985)*
[US Army veteran]

above: ***Sutured***

opposite page: ***Service Connected II: Kānehailua***, 2023
Silkscreen on handmade paper (made out of military uniforms)

see also: previous spread and p. 301

In 1896, a supplication known as the Kūʻe Petitions was signed by about 38,000 Hawaiʻians in direct opposition to the illegal annexation of Hawaiʻi by the United States in 1893. *Service Connected II: Kānehailua* represents the resilience of the Hawaiʻian people and their continued fight for self-determination. As a Kanaka (Native Hawaiʻian) whose family name appears on the petition, Kaneko unravels the intimate histories of war and colonization between her kūpuna (ancestors) and herself.

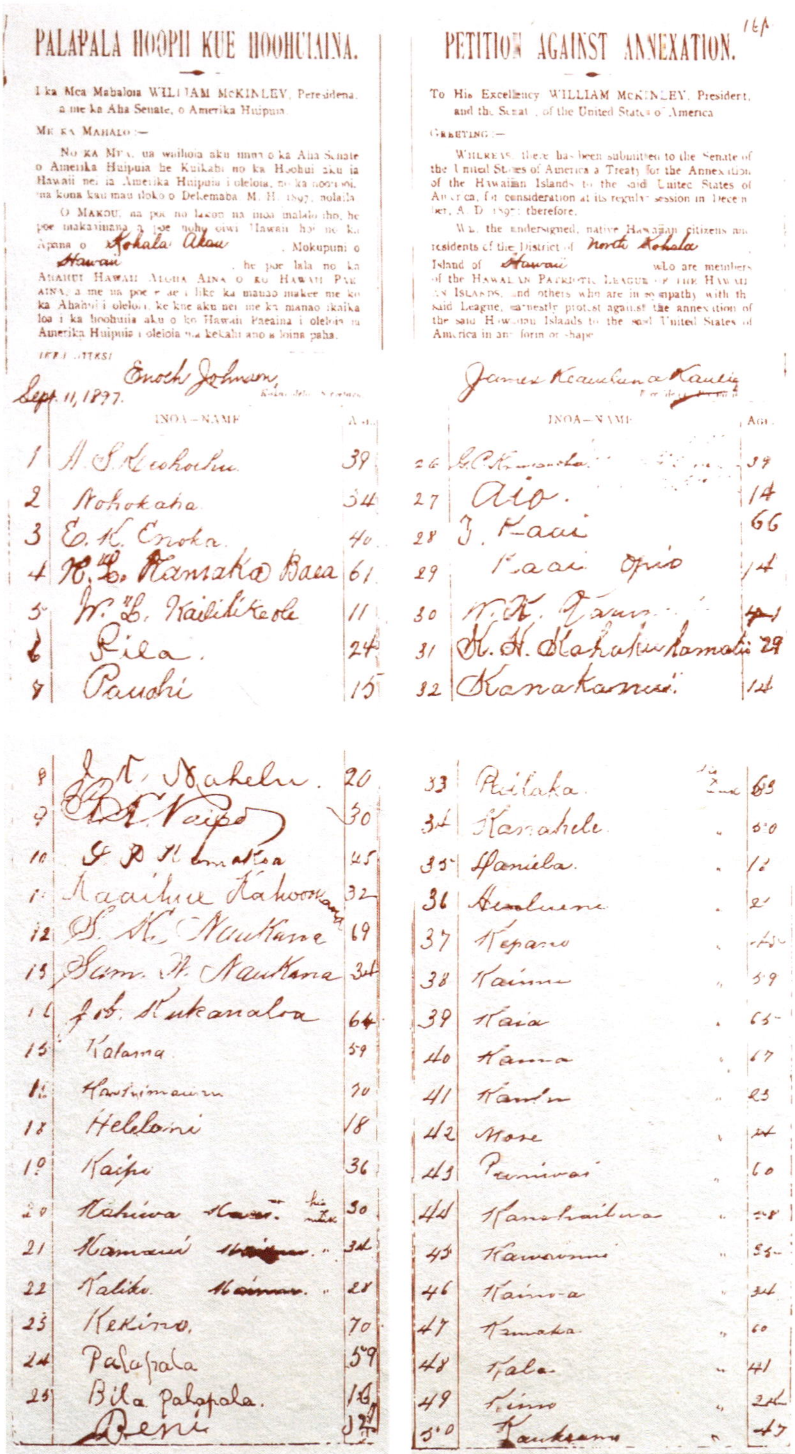

PALAPALA HOOPII KUE HOOHUIAINA.

I ka Mea Mahaloia WILLIAM McKINLEY, Peresidena, a me ka Aha Senate, o Amerika Huipuia.

ME KA MAHALO:—

NO KA MEA, ua waihoia aku imua o ka Aha Senate o Amerika Huipuia he Kuikahi no ka Hoohui aku ia Hawaii nei ia Amerika Huipuia i oleloia, no ka noonoo ia ma kona kau mau iloko o Dekemaba, M. H. 1897; nolaila,

O MAKOU, na poe no lakou na inoa malalo iho, he poe makaainana a poe noho oiwi Hawaii hoi no ka Apana o *Kohala Akau*, Mokupuni o *Hawaii*, he poe lala no ka AHAHUI HAWAII ALOHA AINA O KO HAWAII PAEAINA, a me na poe e ae i like ka manao makee me ko ka Ahahui i oleloia, ke kue aku nei me ka manao ikaika loa i ka hoohuiia aku o ko Hawaii Paeaina i oleloia ia Amerika Huipuia i oleloia ma kekahi ano a loina paha.

IKEIA ATKSI

Enoch Johnson, Kakau-olelo Kiekie

Sept. 11, 1897.

PETITION AGAINST ANNEXATION.

To His Excellency WILLIAM McKINLEY, President, and the Senate, of the United States of America.

GREETING:—

WHEREAS, there has been submitted to the Senate of the United States of America a Treaty for the Annexation of the Hawaiian Islands to the said United States of America, for consideration at its regular session in December, A. D. 1897; therefore,

We, the undersigned, native Hawaiian citizens and residents of the District of *North Kohala*, Island of *Hawaii*, who are members of the HAWAIIAN PATRIOTIC LEAGUE OF THE HAWAIIAN ISLANDS, and others who are in sympathy with the said League, earnestly protest against the annexation of the said Hawaiian Islands to the said United States of America in any form or shape.

James Keauiluna Kaulia President

	INOA—NAME	AGE		INOA—NAME	AGE
1	H. S. Keohokalu	39	26	G. C. Kaumealani	39
2	Nohokaha	54	27	Aio	14
3	E. K. Enoka	40	28	J. Kaai	66
4	K. L. Kamaka Baea	61	29	Kaai Opio	14
5	W. L. Kailikikeole	11	30	W. K. [illegible]	41
6	Kila	24	31	K. H. Makahiwahamalu	29
7	Pauahi	15	32	Kanakanui	14
8	J. K. Nahelu	20	33	Kilaka	63
9	D. K. Naipo	30	34	Kanahele	50
10	J. P. Kamakoa	45	35	Haniela	12
11	Naaihue Kahookano	32	36	Healuene	21
12	S. K. Naukana	69	37	Kepano	45
13	Sam. K. Naukana	34	38	Kaimu	59
14	J. B. Kukanaloa	64	39	Kaia	65
15	Kalama	59	40	Kama	67
16	Kaulukimaiau	70	41	Kaulu	25
17	Helelani	18	42	Mose	24
18	Kaipo	36	43	Paniwai	60
19	Kahiwa [illegible]	30	44	Kanehailua	58
20	Kamaua [illegible]	34	45	Kawaanui	55
21	Kaliko [illegible]	28	46	Kaina	34
22	Kekino	70	47	Kamaka	60
23	Palapala	59	48	Kala	41
24	Bila Palapala	16	49	Kino	24
25	Beni	17	50	Kaukaua	47

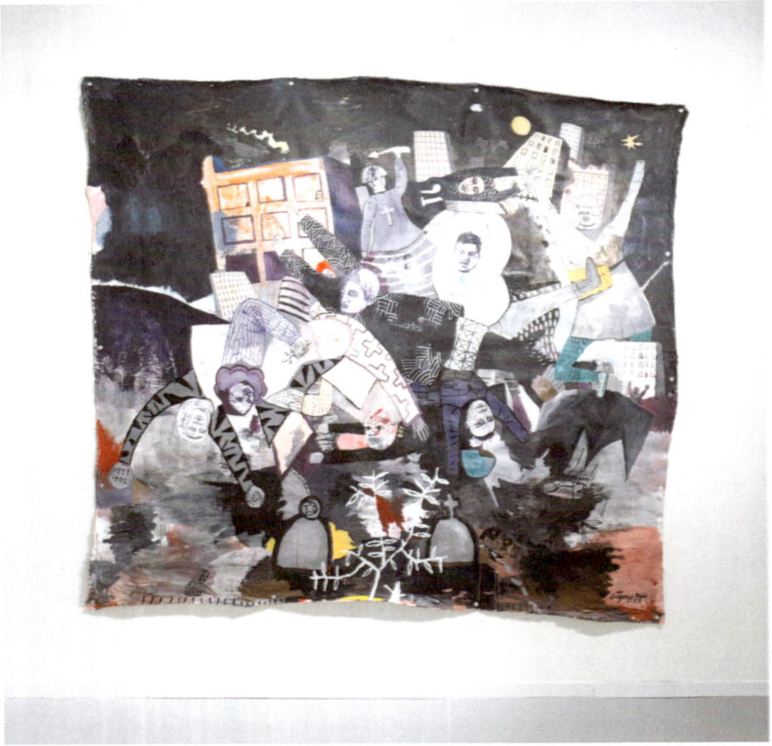

GREGORY RICK *(b. 1981) [US Army veteran]*
From Manila to Baghdad (detail at right), 2023
Acrylic, pigmented ink, absorbent ground, sign paint, and oil bar on linen

In this painting Gregory Rick makes a comparison between the Philippine-American War and Iraq War to illustrate the way imperialism perpetuates violence throughout history. Both of these wars were declared under the guise of liberation (whether from Spain or from Saddam). Yet what transpired were brutal wars in which local people were not liberated, but targeted and occupied by US forces.

see also: p. 326

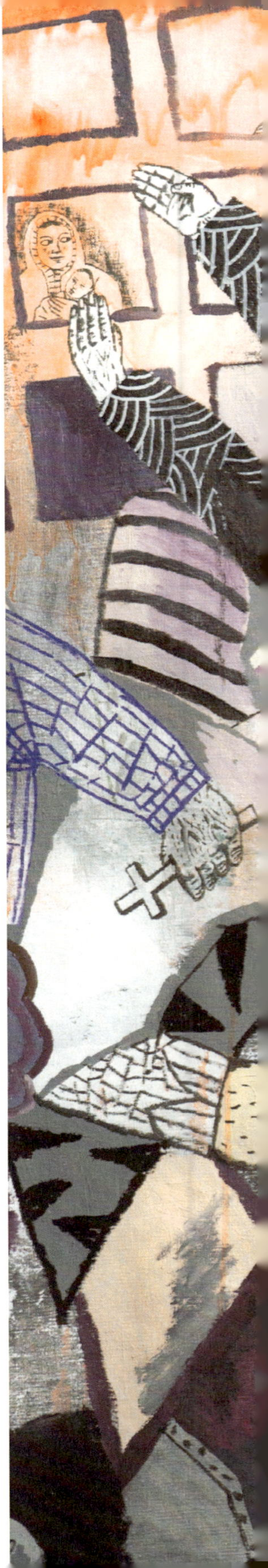

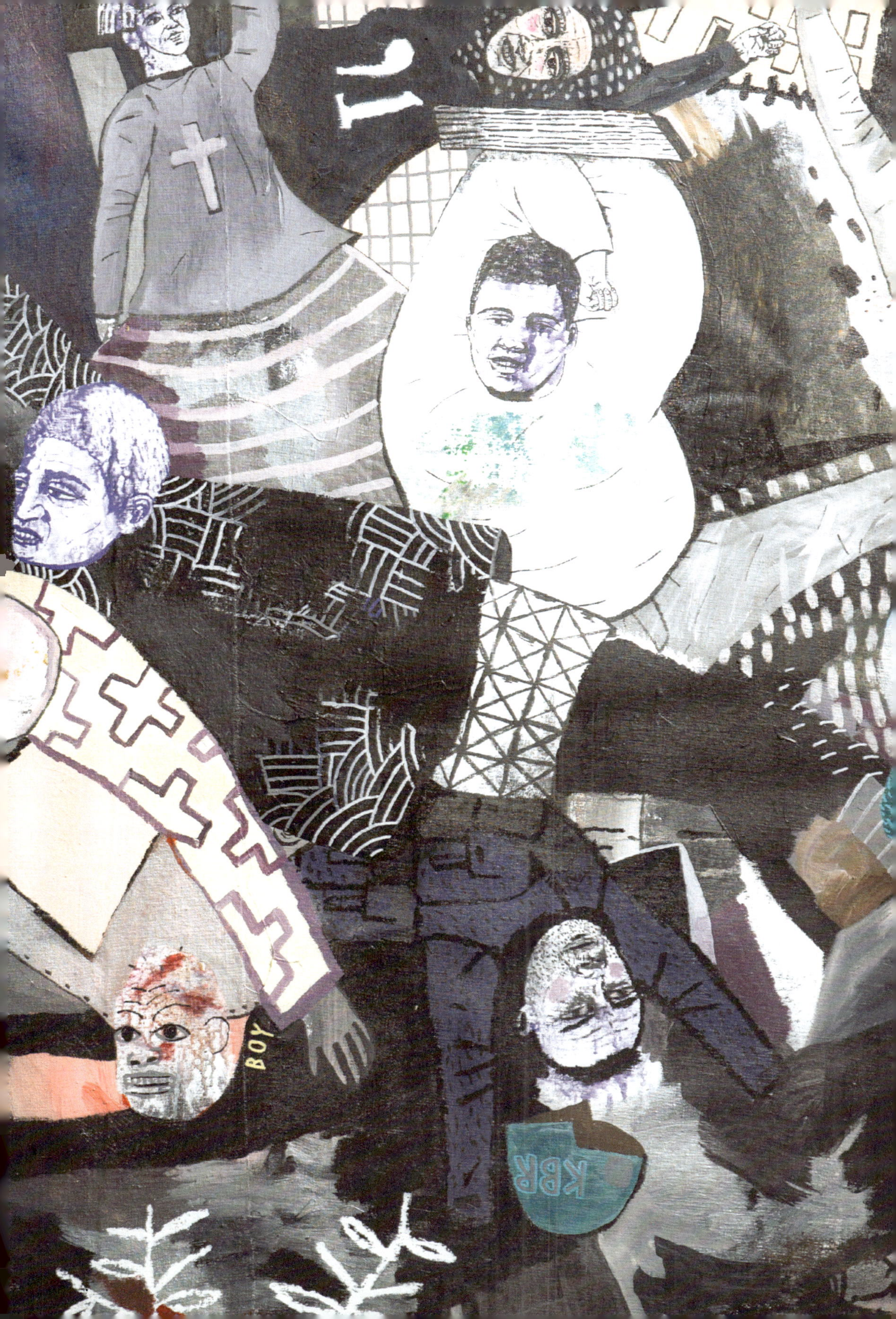
BOY
KBR

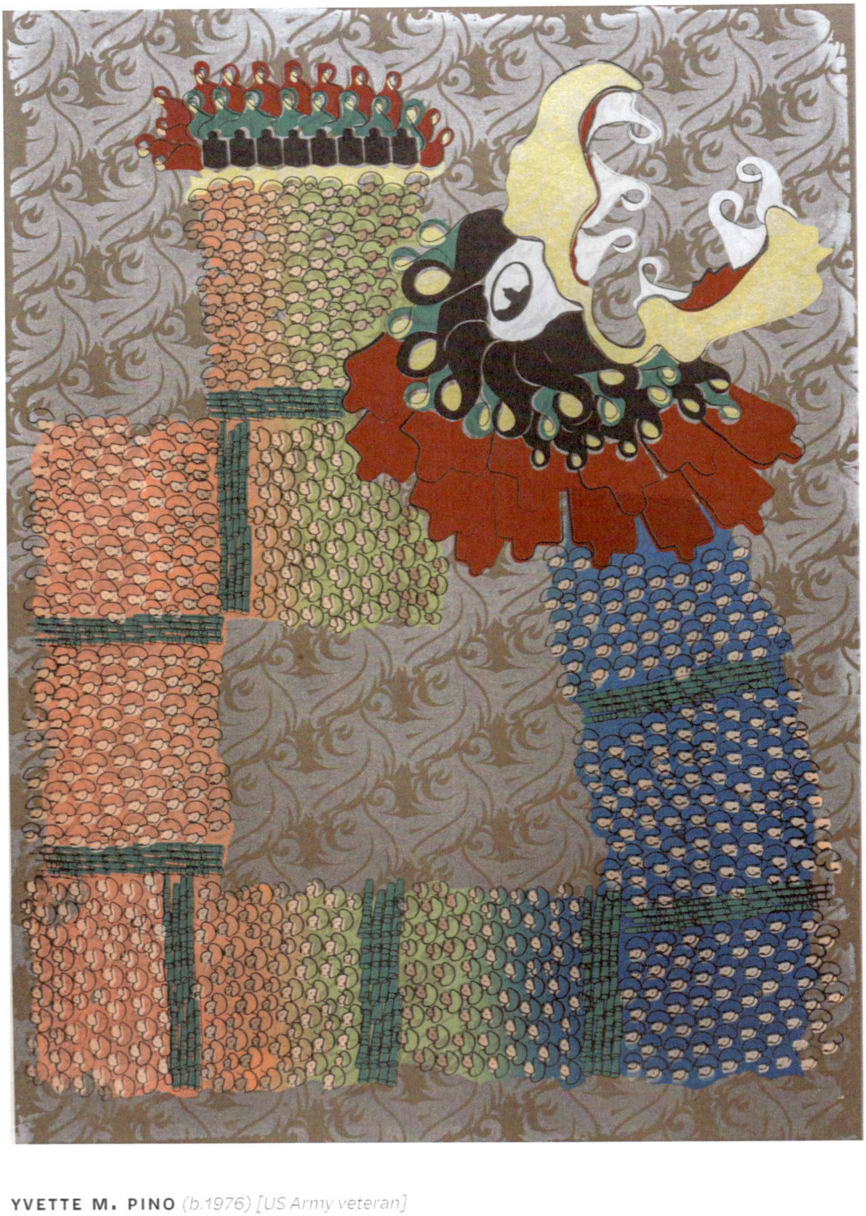

YVETTE M. PINO *(b.1976) [US Army veteran]*
above: ***CadmU.S.***, 2015
Silkscreen

opposite page: ***Extraction***, 2015
Silkscreen

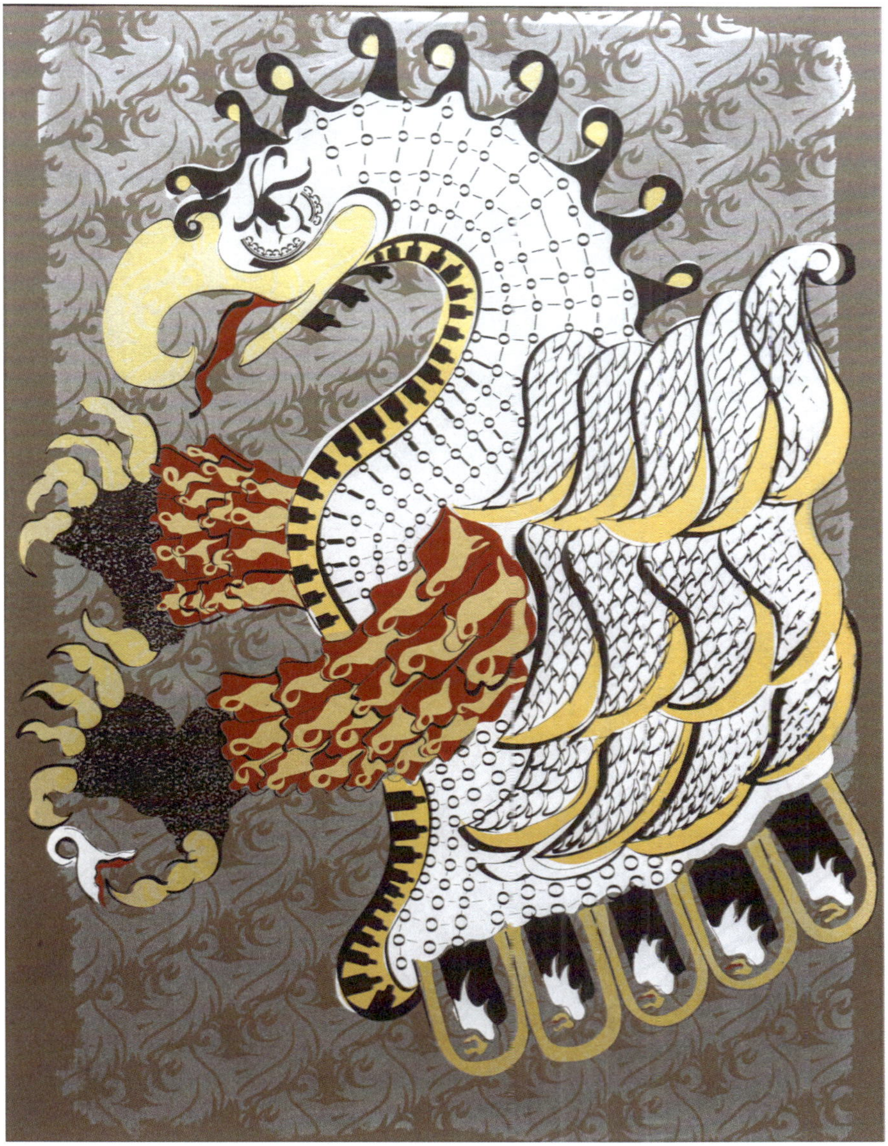

In *CadmU.S.* and *Extraction*, Pino evokes the history of the Greek god Cadmus to describe her military experience in the 101st Airborne Division in 2003.

Carlos Parada, author of *Genealogical Guide to Greek Mythology* writes, "[Cadmus] sent some of his men to draw water from the spring belonging to Ares, which happened to be guarded by a dragon said to be the offspring of God, or sacred to him. This dragon, which had a golden crest, flashed fire from his eyes, had a triple tongue, teeth ranged in a triple row, and the body swollen with poison, devoured Cadmus' companions."

Inspired by this story of Cadmus, Pino reflects on the unending violence of the American war machine that encourages soldiers to battle one another, continuing the cycle of war and destroying lives. This impact is visualized in the red tooth, which is held in *CadmU.S.* and missing in *Extraction*.

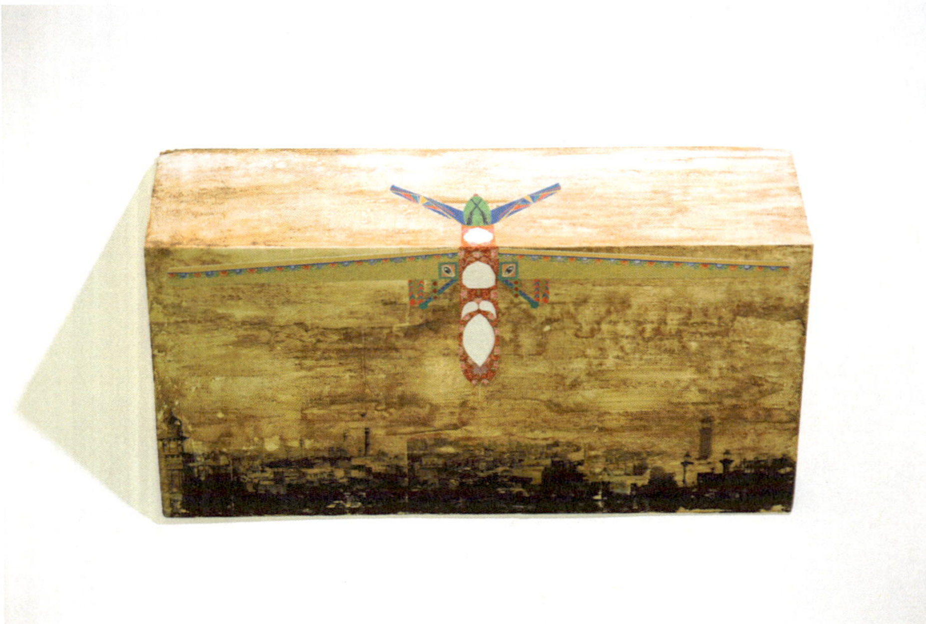

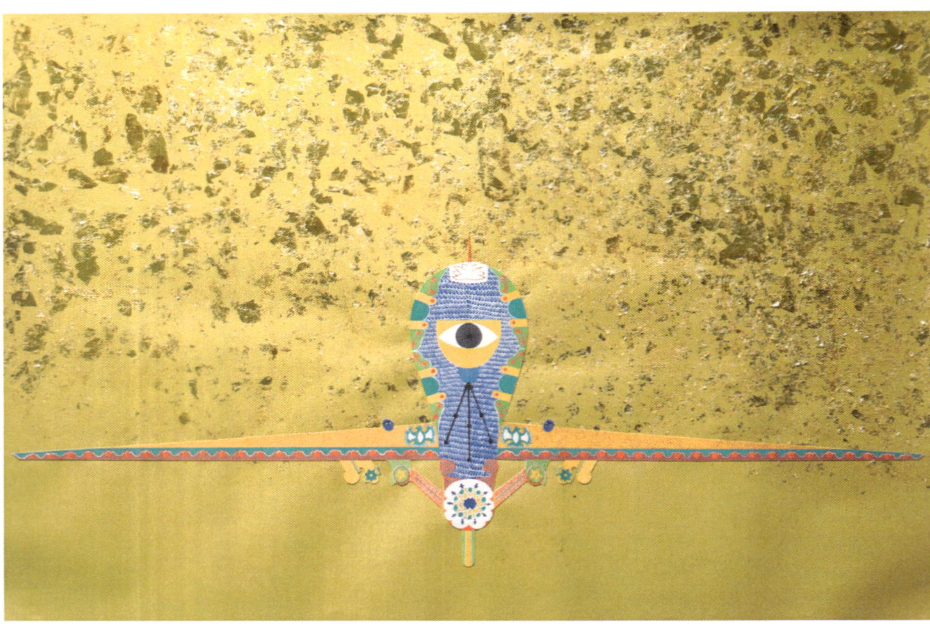

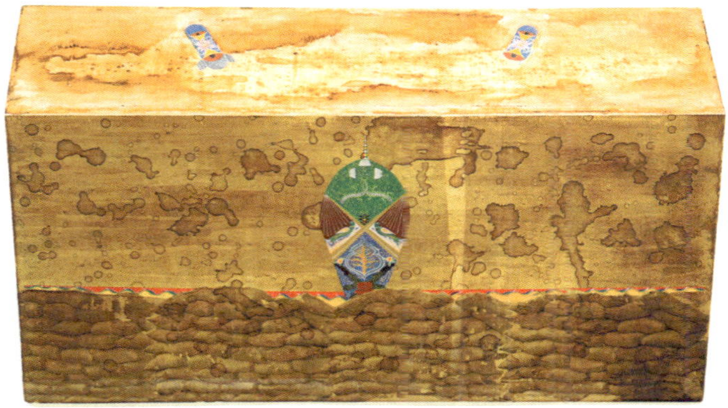

MAHWISH CHISHTY *(b. 1980)*
left, top: ***Hovering Reaper I***, 2014
left, bottom: ***Reaper***, 2014
above: ***Hovering Reaper II***, 2014
Gouache, tea stain, and photo transfers on birch plywood

These three works are from *Drone Art*, a series inspired by Chishty's 2011 trip to Pakistan (see also: pp. 22–24). The paintings bring symbolic attention to the stealth military vehicles and juxtapose the terror they produce in the Afghanistan-Pakistan borderlands with representations of beauty.

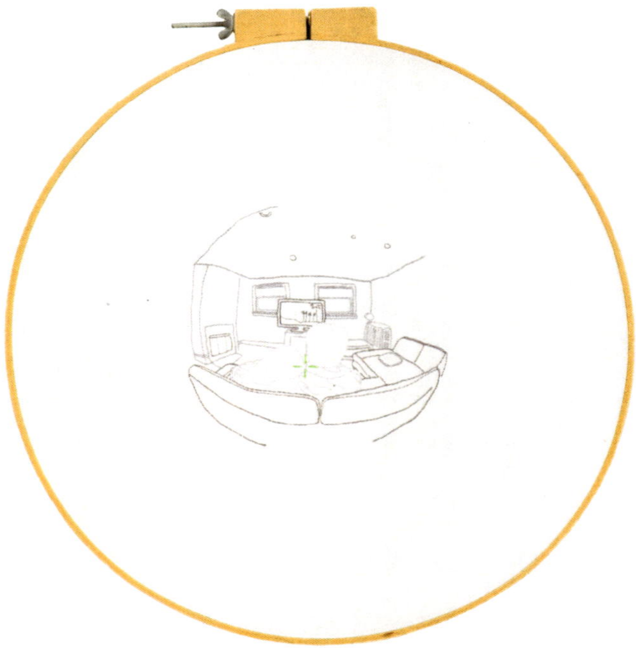

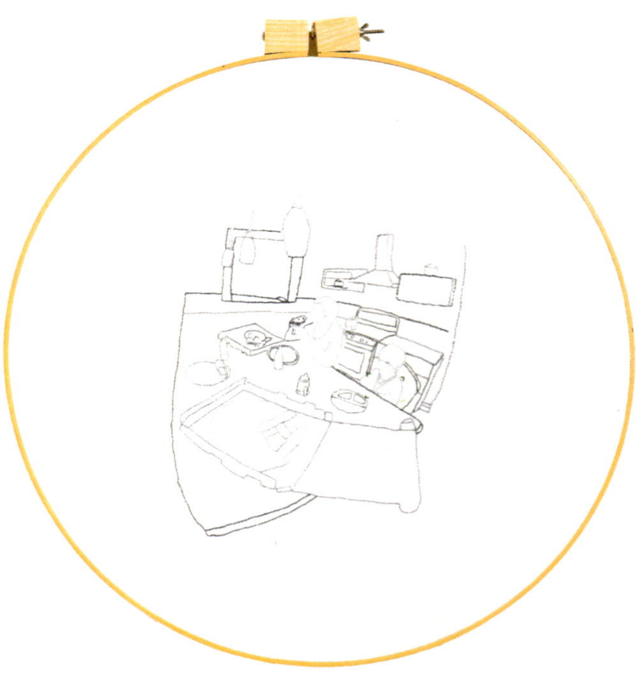

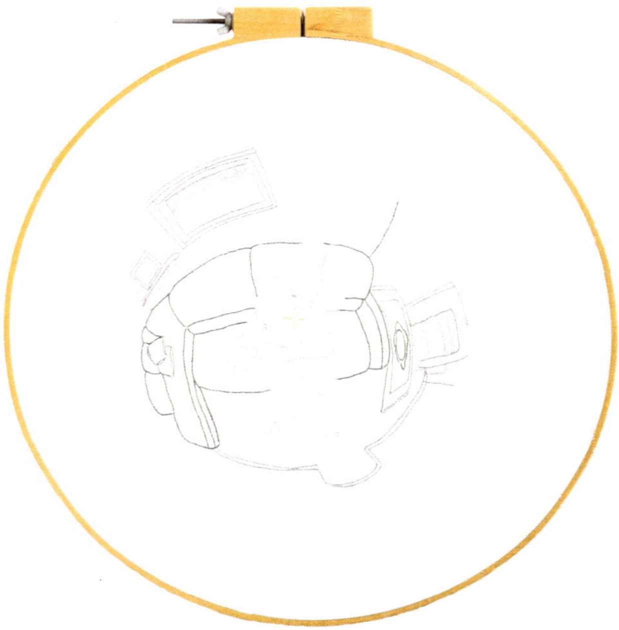

SABBA ELAHI *(b. 1980)*
left, from top to bottom: ***everyday suspects #4**, **#7***, 2018
above: ***everyday suspects #8***, 2018
Hand embroidery on cotton

Sabba Elahi's series of hand embroideries considers the entanglements of the surveillance state with the everyday disturbances experienced by individuals at various sites of war and conflict. The work situates the viewers in aerial, peripheral, and fish-eye perspectives to exemplify the distanced targeting of people in domestic spaces. The artist combines commentary on the benign and personal to speak to the pervasive US surveillance of Muslim American communities that are watched where they eat, work, play, and pray.

see detail on p. 294

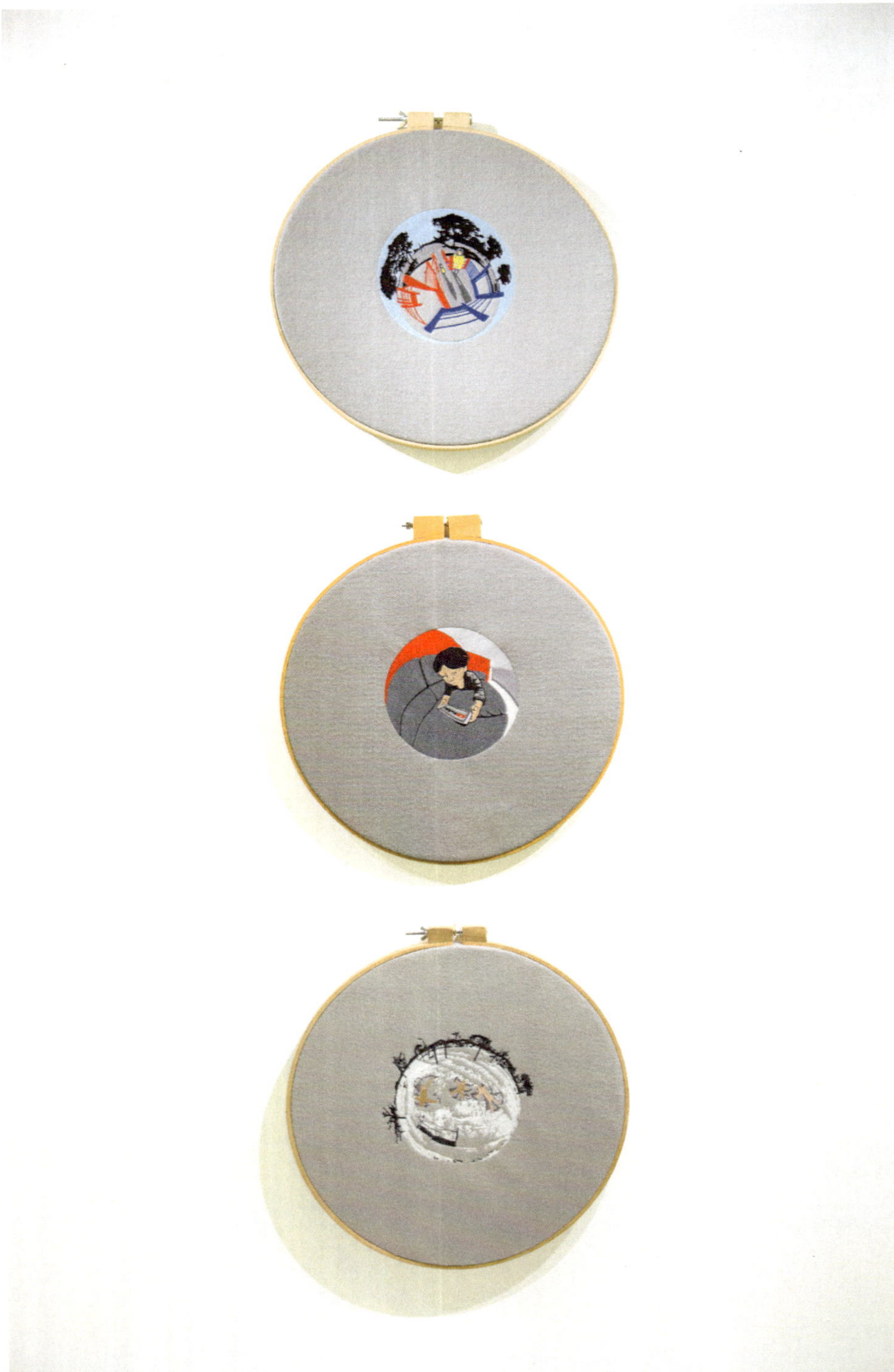

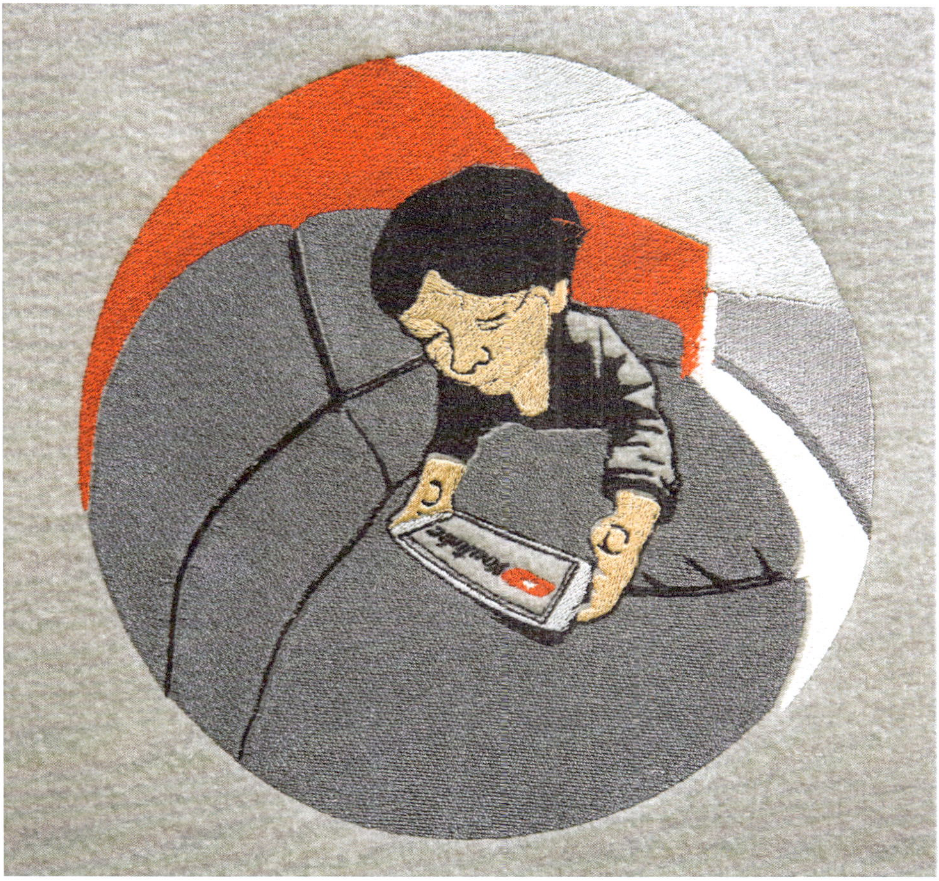

the suspect is my son #4 (detail)

SABBA ELAHI *(b. 1980)*
left, from top to bottom: ***the suspect is my son #3, #4, #5***, 2018
Machine embroidery on felt

Sabba Elahi subverts the decorative craft of embroidery to confront US drone warfare and its racialization, surveillance, and dehumanization of Brown and Muslim bodies from a distance. Assuming the lens of the security state's fear-based policies, she surveys her son's everyday actions, for example playing, or seeking comfort and safety. In the works, the machined embroidery becomes a metaphor for the mechanization of surveillance and warfare.

on next spread:
identified suspects, CIA/Pakistan Dronestrikes, 2014
Ink on rice paper

Drawn from "Naming the Dead," a database created by the Bureau of Investigative Journalism, Elahi's small ink texts represent the people killed in drone strikes in Pakistan. The work memorializes victims of US aerial warfare in the Afghanistan-Pakistan borderlands and functions as a reminder of the lives lost as supposed "collateral damage" in the "War on Terror."

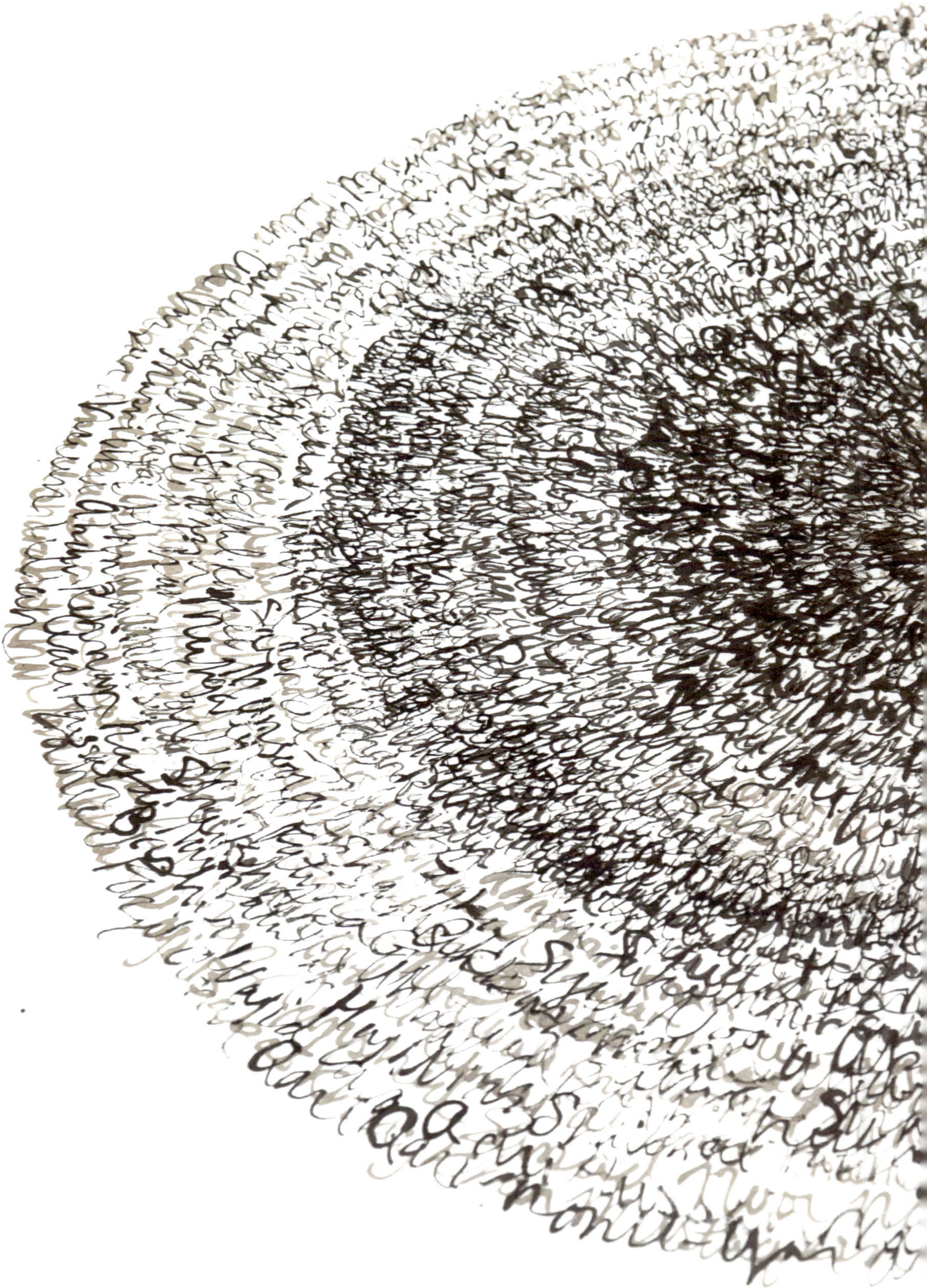

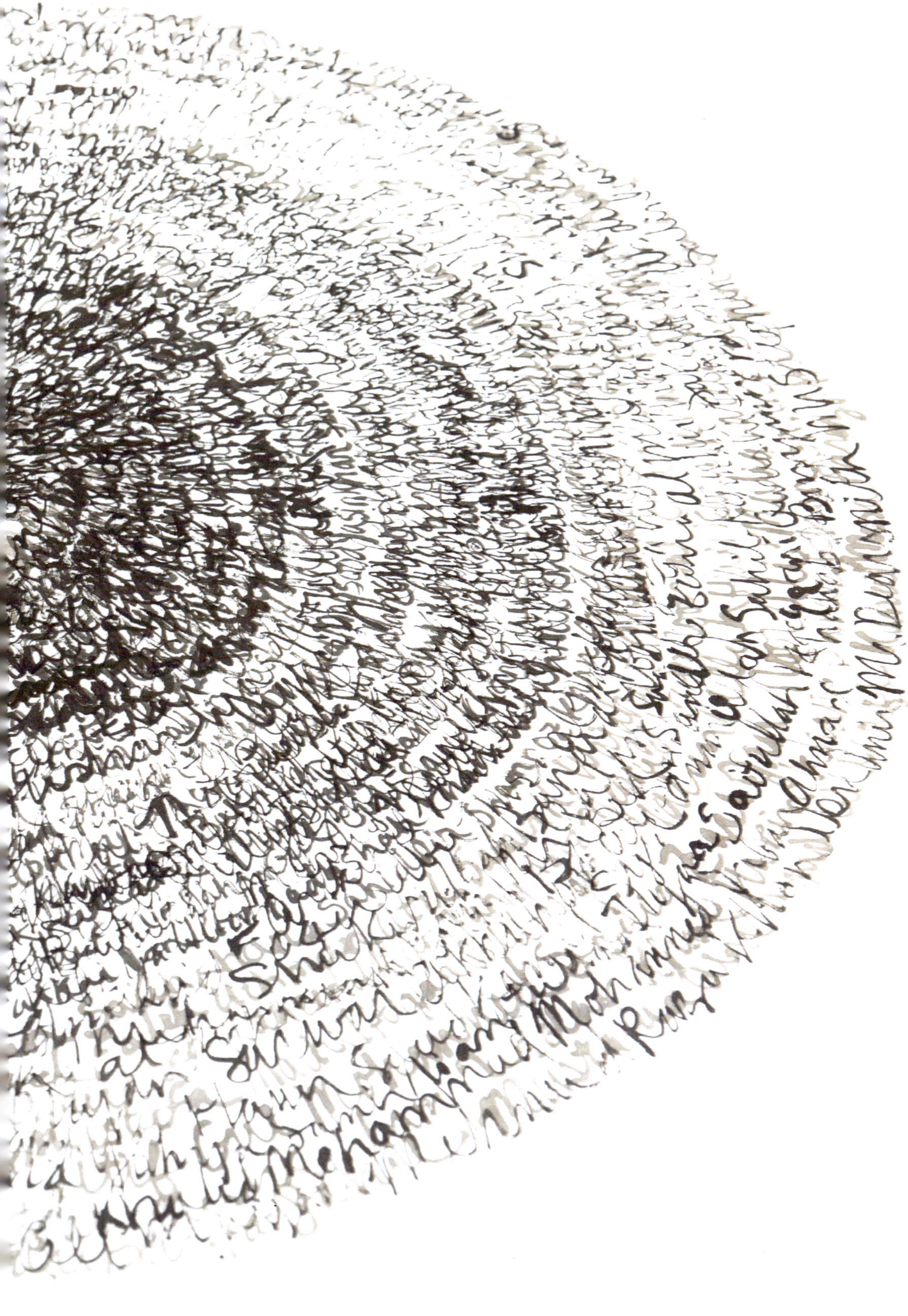

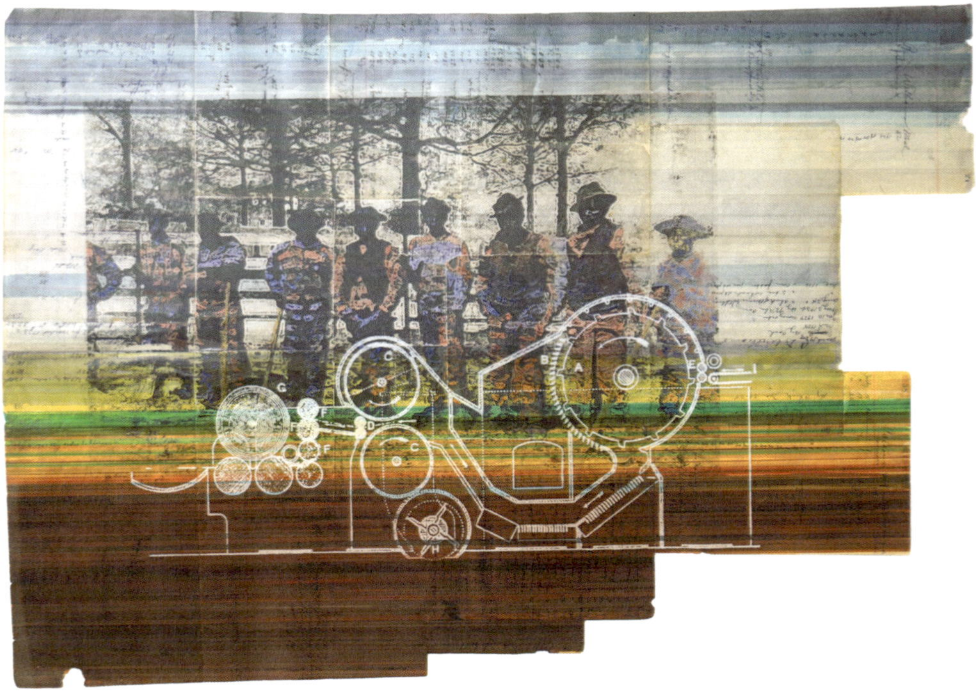

RODNEY EWING *(b. 1964) [US Army veteran]*
Faded, 2022
Hand-colored silkscreen on ledger paper
Courtesy of the artist and Rena Bransten Gallery

These works are from *Planned Obsolescence*, Rodney Ewing's mixed-media series on found ledger paper. Each work uses archival images ranging from depictions of Jim Crow era prison labor to sports arenas, to reveal how commerce and production, in the pursuit of advancement, has relied on the exploitation of the Black Body. Over each screen-printed subject is a schematic of discarded technology highlighting the parallels between manufactured tools and manufactured servitude.

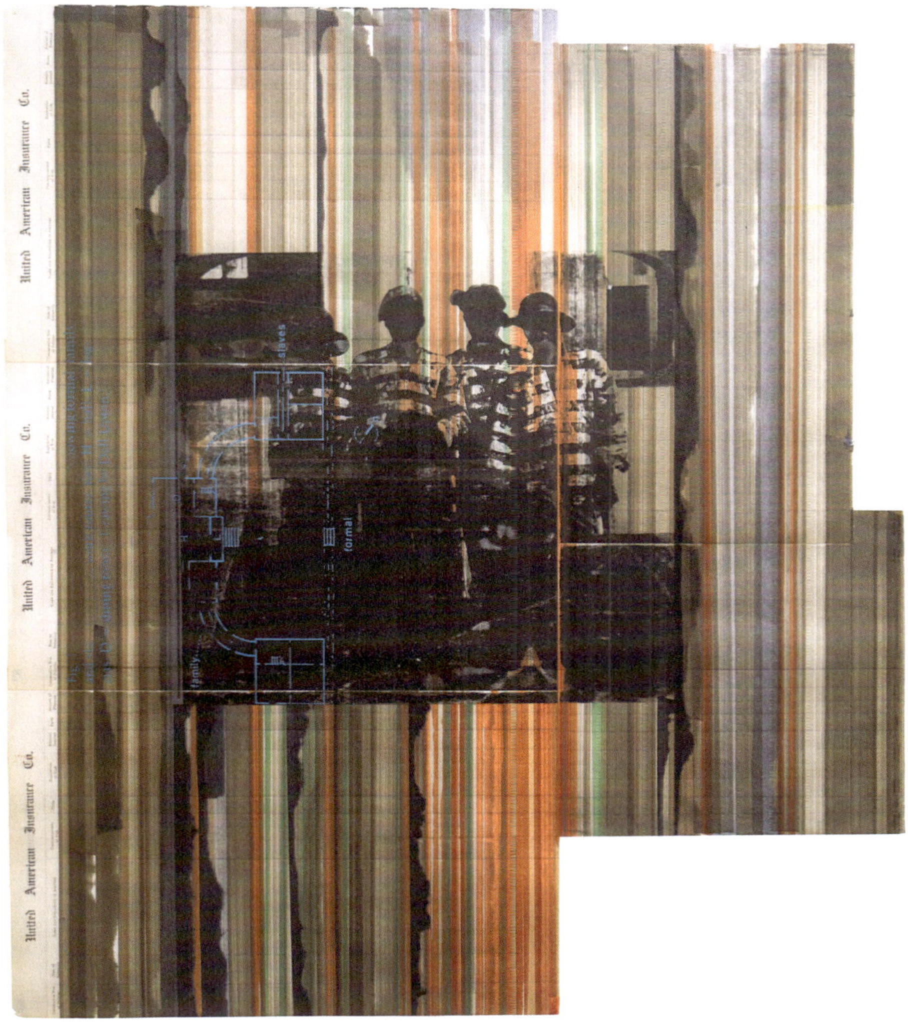

Confines, 2021
Hand-colored silkscreen on ledger paper
Courtesy of the artist and Rena Bransten Gallery

see detail on next spread

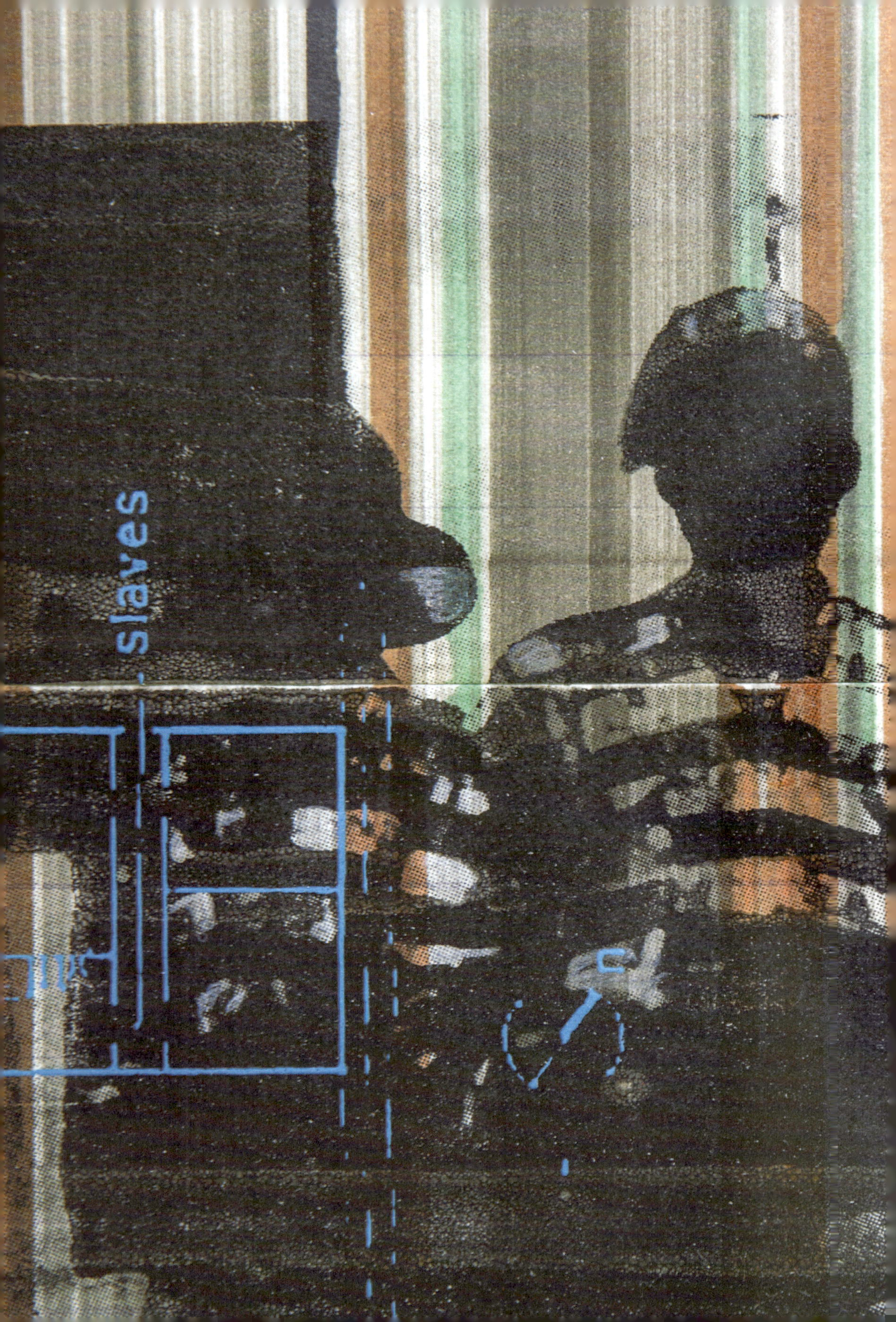
slaves

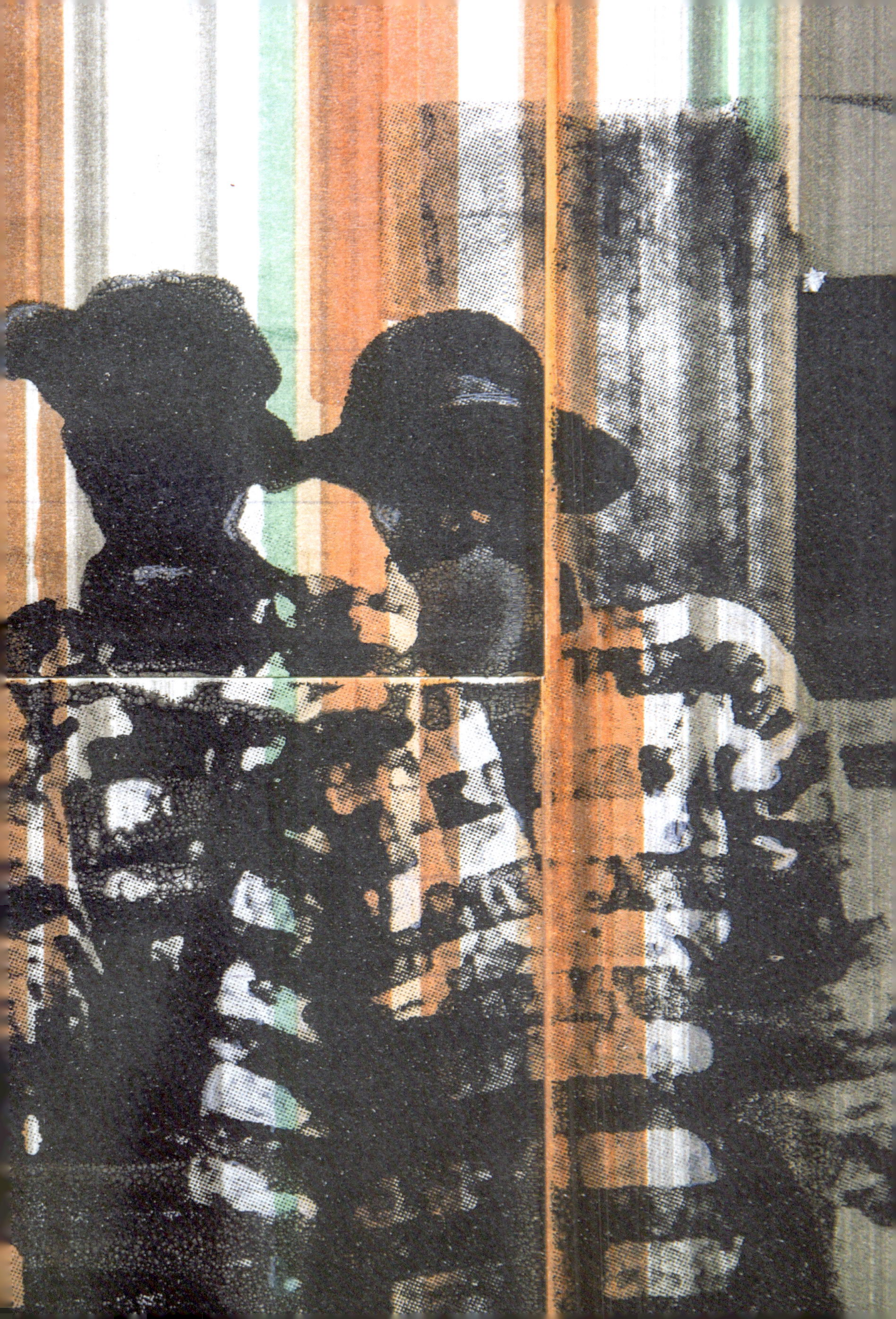

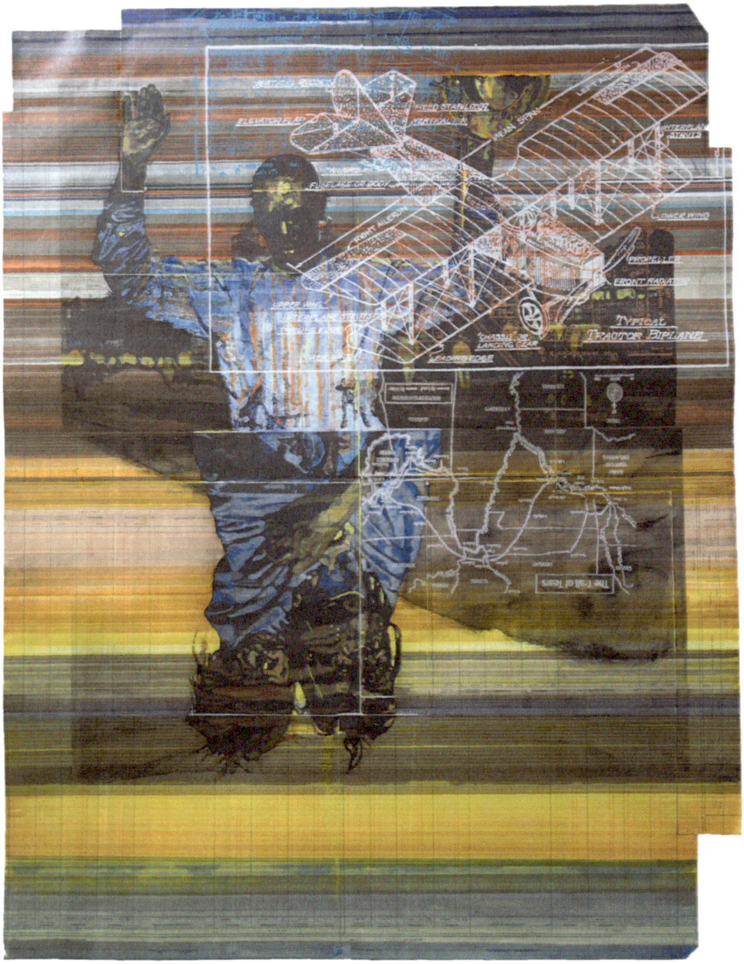

RODNEY EWING *(b. 1964) [US Army veteran]*
Come the Mean Times (detail at right), 2022
Hand-colored silkscreen on ledger paper
Courtesy of the artist and Rena Bransten Gallery

In continuation with the *Planned Obsolescence* series, *Come the Mean Times* was created specifically for the *Surviving the Long Wars* Triennial exhibition. In this work, Ewing documents the history of displacement to and from Oklahoma, pointing to events like the Trail of Tears and the Tulsa Massacre. Ewing creates a dialogue about the harm done to Indigenous and African American peoples by the interconnected histories of colonialism and white supremacy.

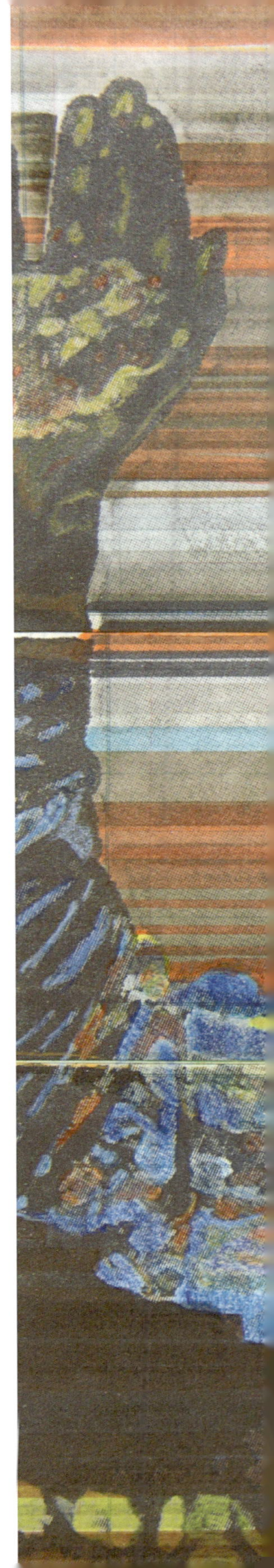

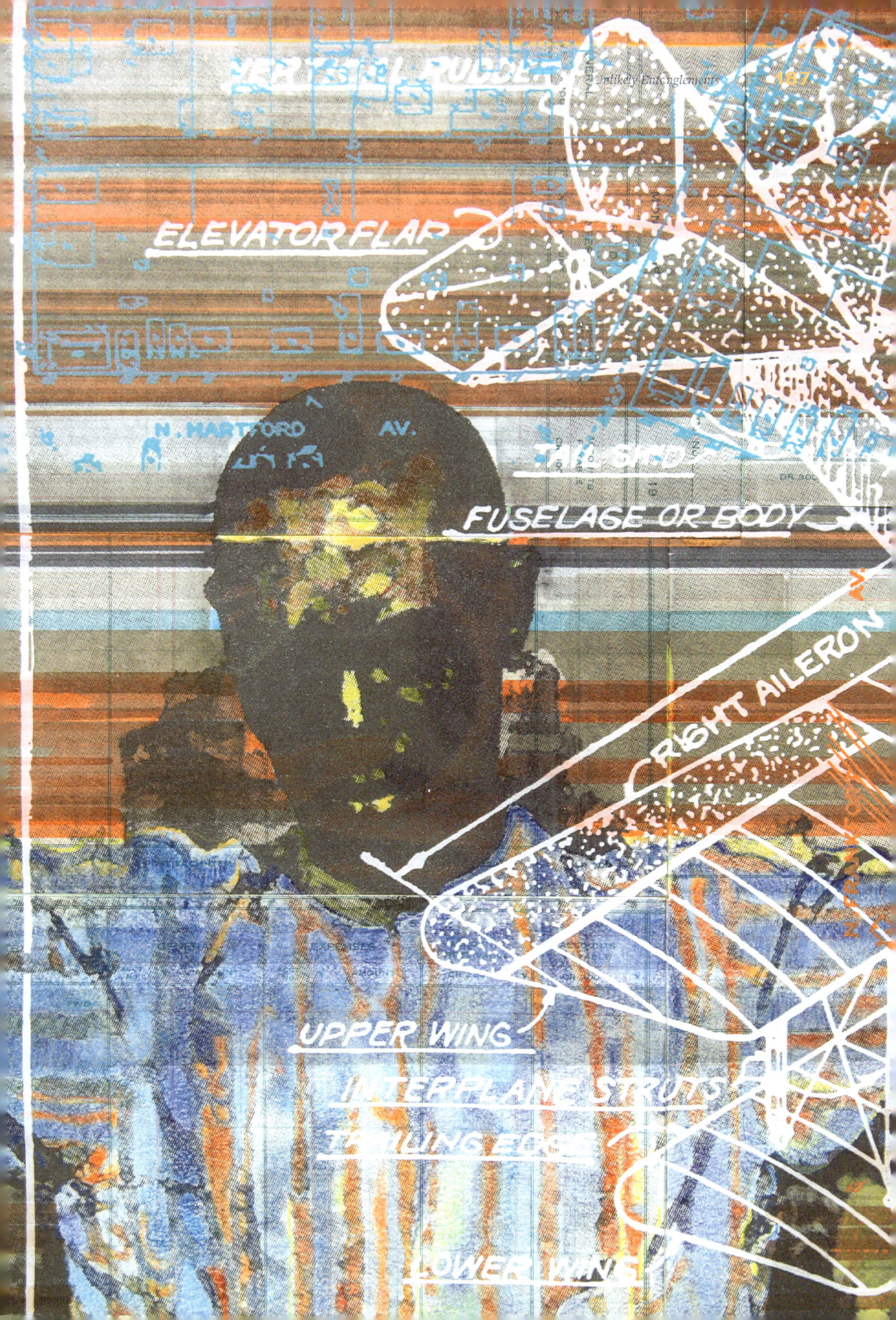
Unlikely Entanglements
187
ELEVATOR FLAP
N. HARTFORD
AV.
FUSELAGE OR BODY
RIGHT AILERON
UPPER WING
INTERPLANE STRUTS

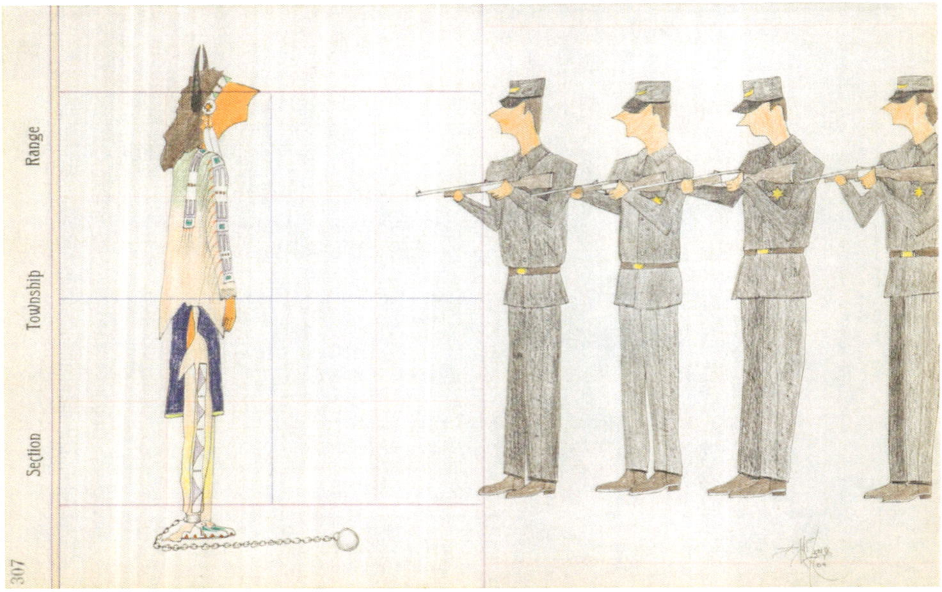

DWAYNE WILCOX *(Oglala Lakota, b. 1957)*
[US Air Force veteran]
Losing my Religion, 2004
Ink and colored pencil on ledger paper

Dwanye Wilcox created *Losing My Religion* in response to two photographs taken during the time of the *Religious Crimes Code of 1883*, which restricted—sometimes with military force—the spiritual and cultural practices of Native Americans. Wilcox says, "… one picture is of a man standing in front of a firing squad because he refused to follow the new world, and the second picture is of a man with a ball and chain being punished for carrying on with his spiritual beliefs." Native Americans were not legally allowed to practice their religion until the American Indian Religious Freedom Act of 1978 (AIRFA).

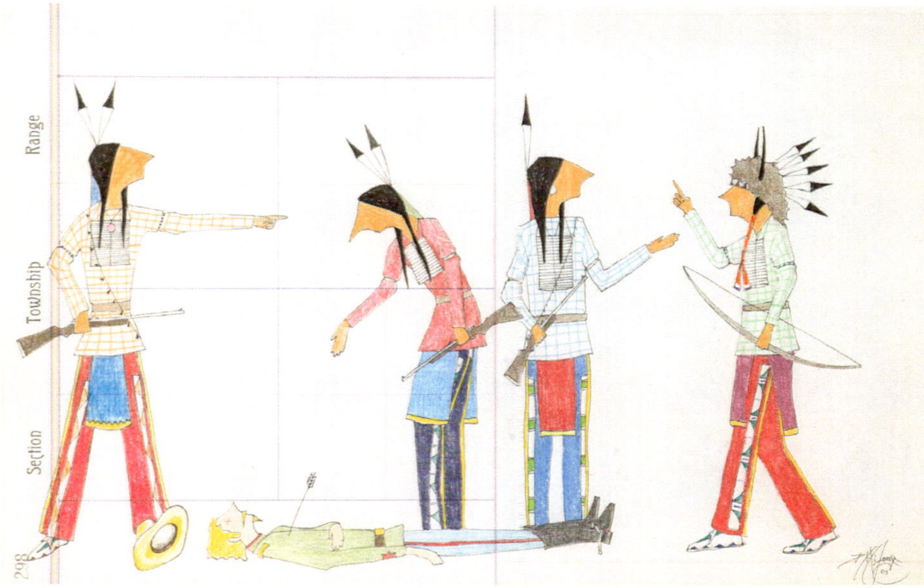

Larry is far right, he's really tough on immigration, 2005
Ink and colored pencil on ledger paper

Wilcox's ledger work often includes humorous situations that are playful and thought-provoking. In *Larry is far right, he's really tough on immigration*, Wilcox pokes fun at contemporary immigration discourse in the United States by highlighting the fact that white settlers are also immigrants.

see detail on p. 200
see also: p. 254

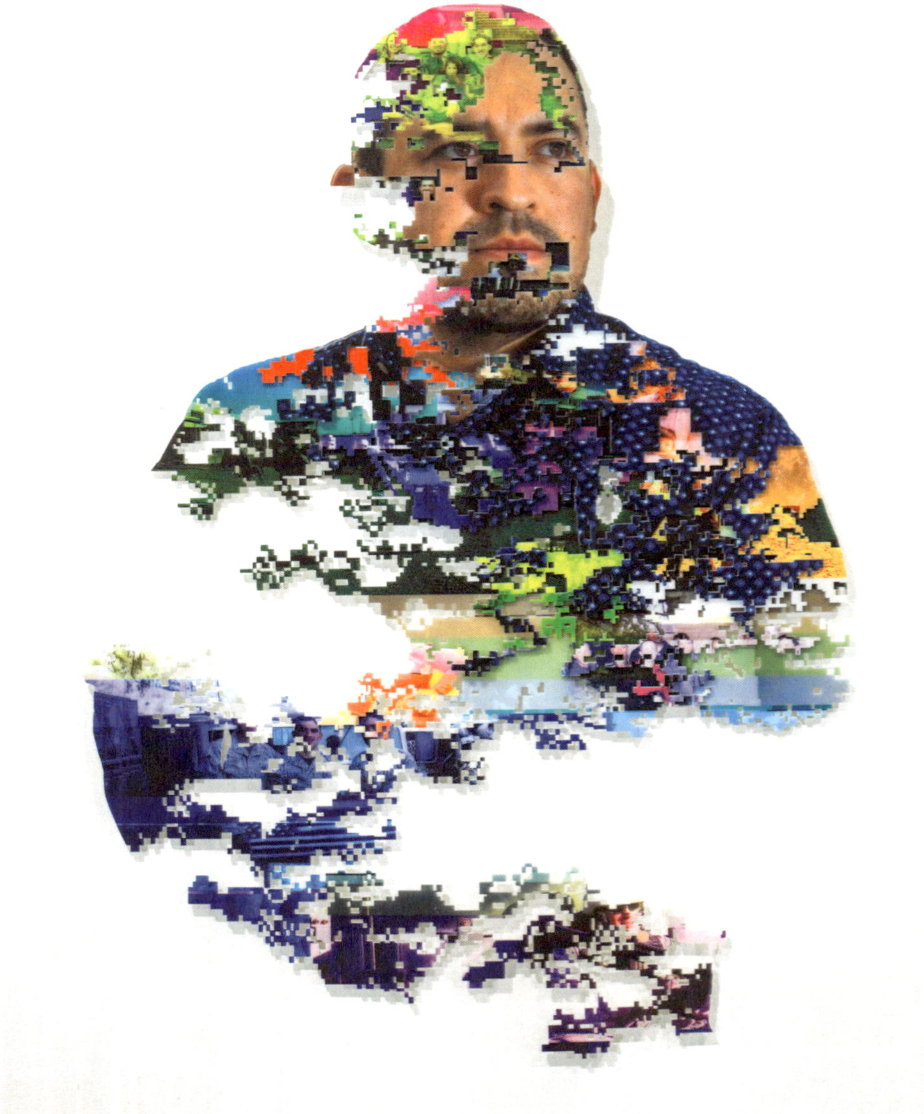

ERIC PEREZ *(b.1984) [US Marine Corps veteran]*
left: ***Sgt. Gudiño***, 2023
Mounted digital prints on acrylic, laser-cut into the silhouette and custom digi-camo patterns

right: ***5-Sierra***, 2023
Mounted digital prints on acrylic, laser-cut into the silhouette and custom digi-camo patterns

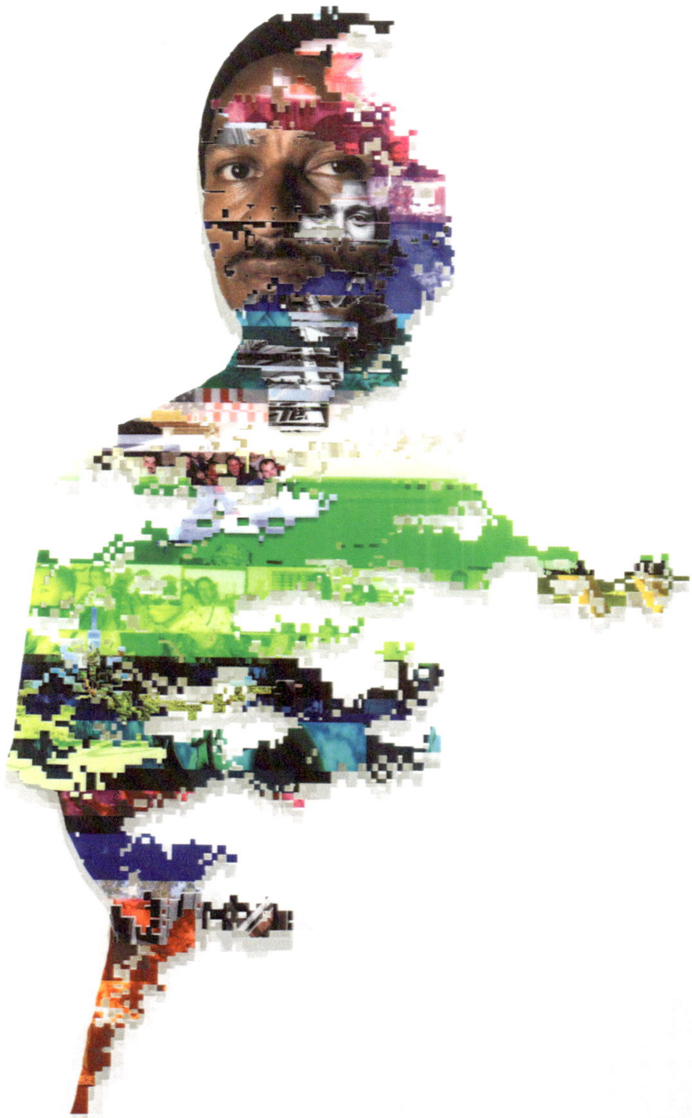

5-Sierra and *Sgt. Gudiño* are portraits of two platoon-mates who served with Eric Perez in the US Marine Corps. Each portrait is composed of images: from deployment, life after the military, and a new portrait taken in the last year. The portraits are layered and fragmented, reflecting the histories and experiences veterans navigate after serving in the military. Perez created this work with the subjects' input, which gave his mates agency to determine how they are represented. The glitches are a result of Perez embedding the subject's stories into image code. The layers are cut into custom shapes reminiscent of digital camouflage shapes. The glitch denies the viewer easy interpretation of the image and its underlying story.

RAJKAMAL KAHLON *(b. 1974)*
People of Afghanistan, 2017
Ten-minute video installation

People of Afghanistan incorporates high-resolution thermal imagery of a bombing in Afghanistan by an American AC-130 Specter Gunship, overlaid by still photographs of Afghan men compiled during a 1960s Soviet anthropological survey. With the recent withdrawal of US troops from Afghanistan, this video gains new resonance. In using archival materials to uncover layered histories, Kahlon's work is a potent reminder of the residues and entanglements between different wars and occupations.

see also: pp. 147–48

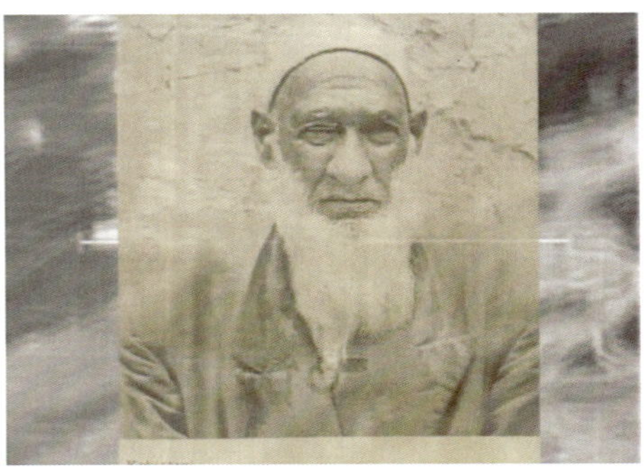

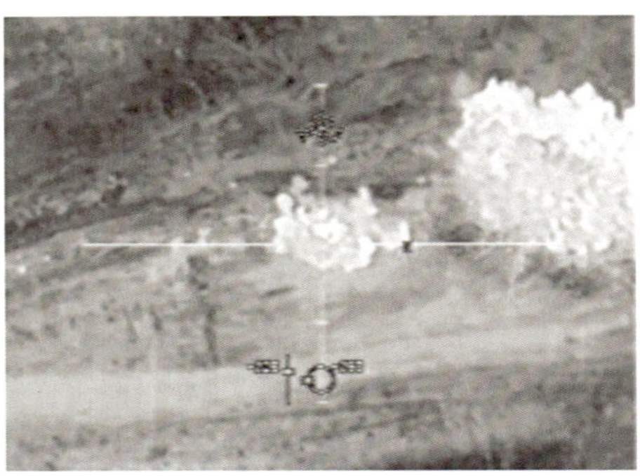

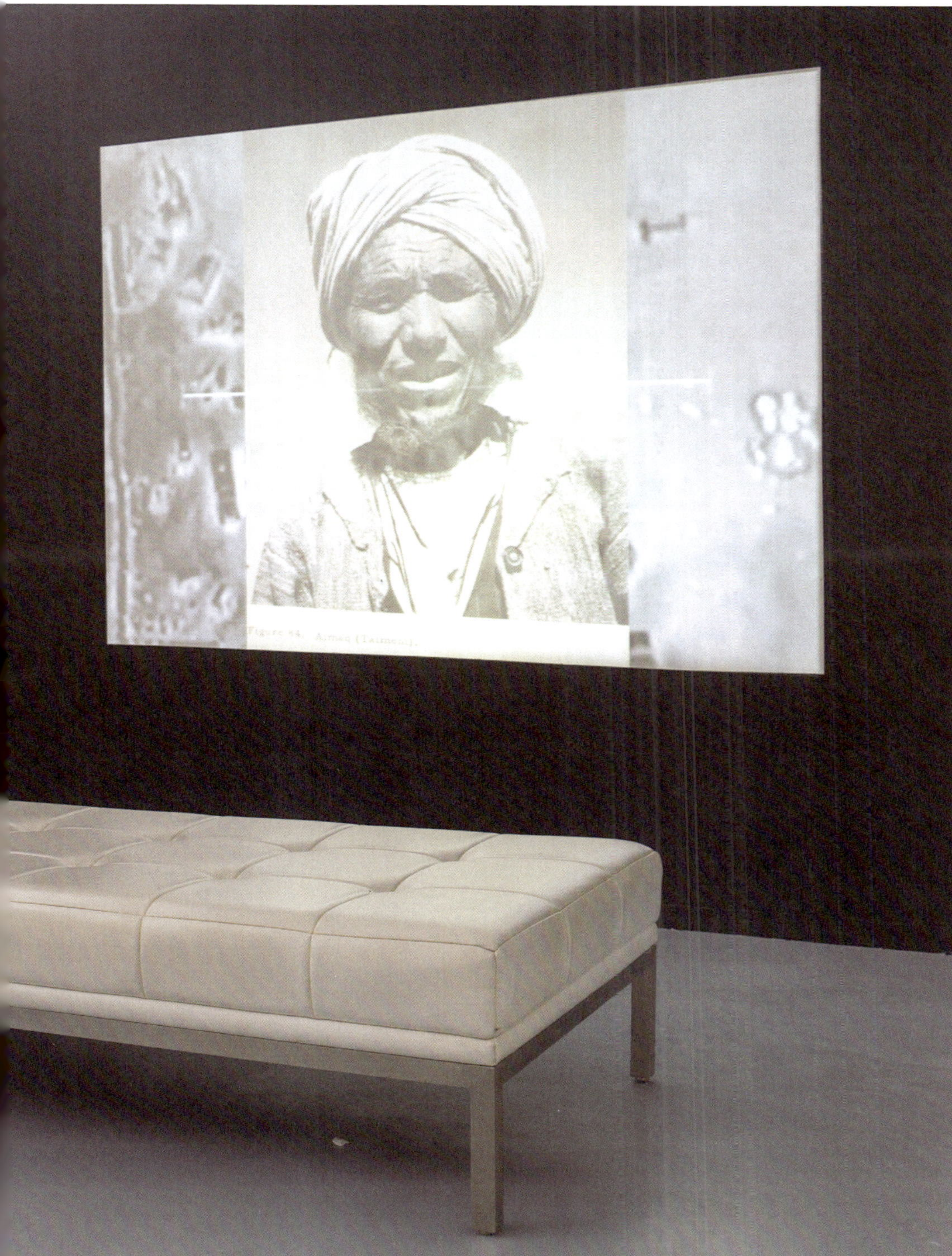

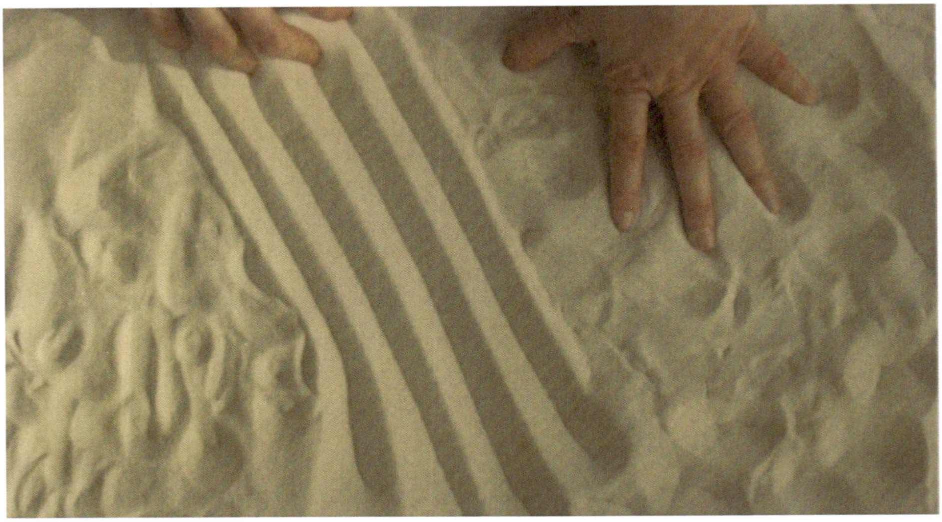

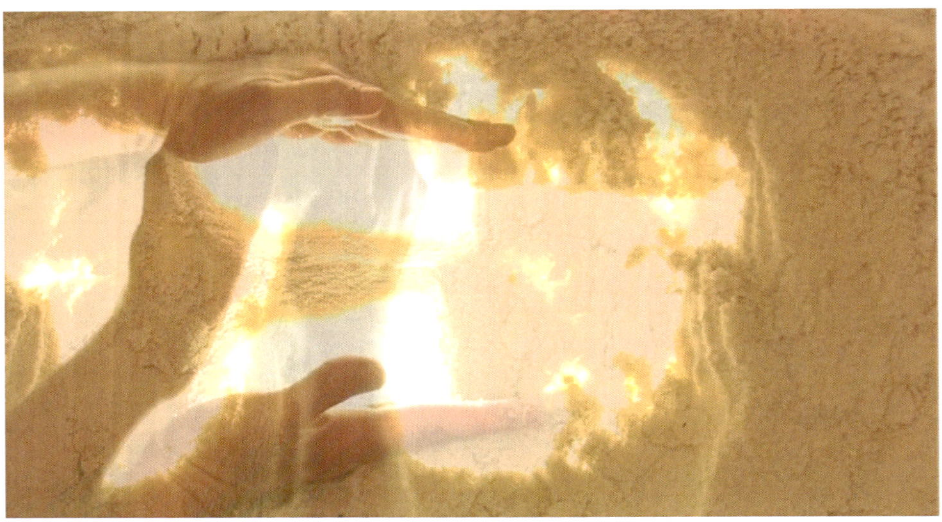

SARAH FARAHAT *(b. 1979)*
To Be or Not To Be—That Is the Question of the Refugee* or (How Do We Deal With Now, When Then Isn't Over Yet), 2009
Independently looping video and sound installation

Video: 8 minutes 28 seconds
Sound: 12 minutes 51 seconds

**The first part of the title was contributed by participant Dr. Butti*

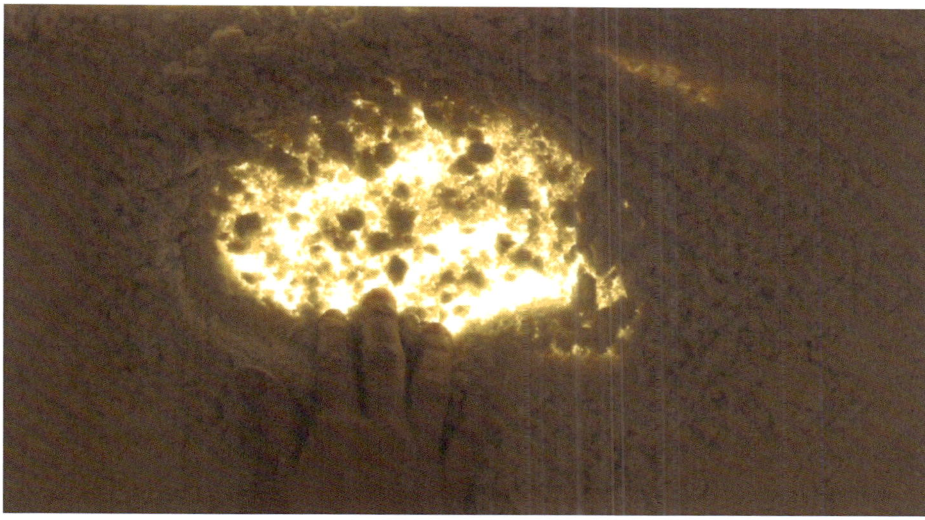

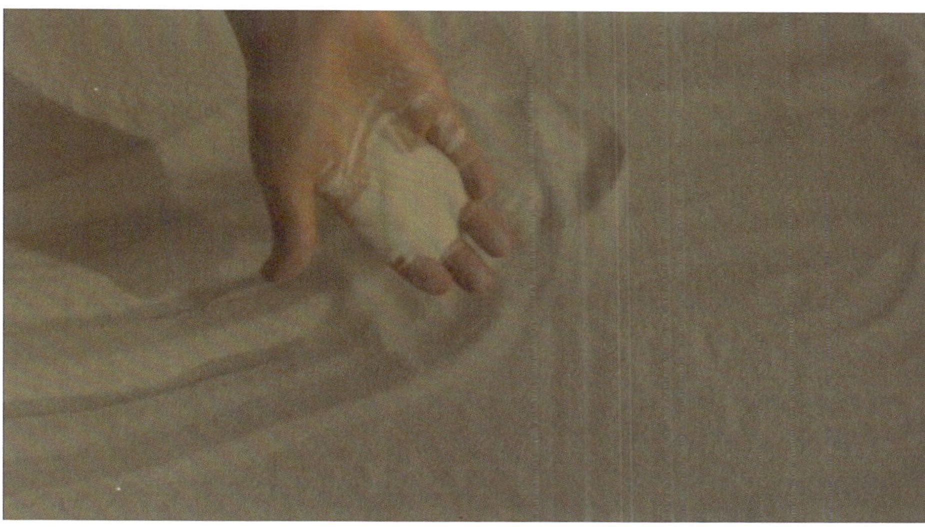

In 2008, Sarah Farahat began a series of interviews that developed into an independently looping sound and video installation. This work is an expression of the artist's curiosity about the lives of the Iraqis who came to the US during the long US wars waged in their country. Through the project, Farahat excavates the stories of displaced and diasporic Iraqis to create a space to share their accounts of courage and distance, assimilation and alienation, longing, loss, and hope.

see also: p. 255

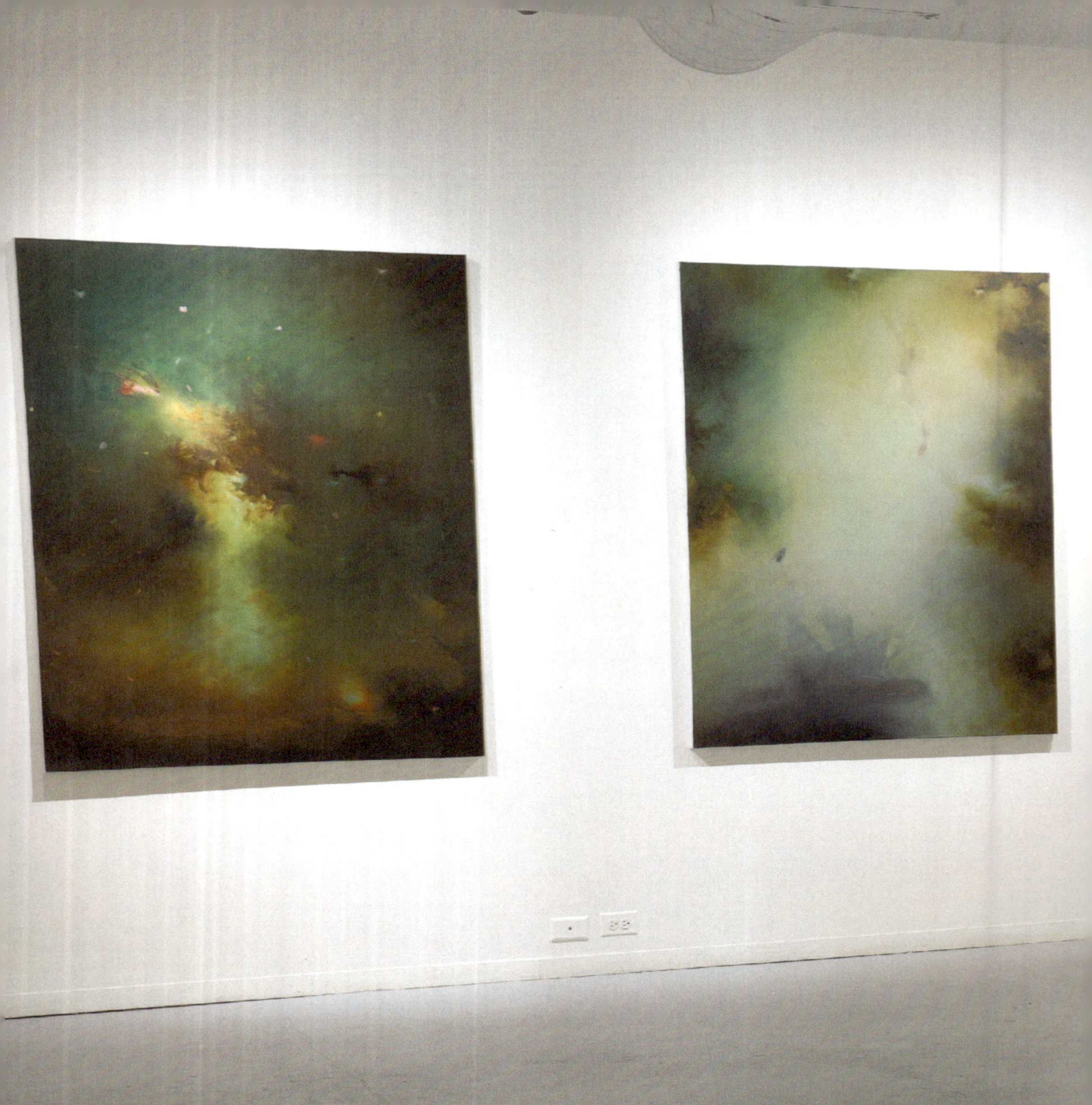

YIRAN ZHANG *(b.1996)*
[Singapore military veteran]
right: ***Marching in Place***, 2022
Relief print on paper

The title of this piece draws its name from the most foundational military drill, the seemingly futile and repetitive action of marching in place. Zhang's depiction of the synchronous stomping reveals the absurdity of military uniformity and attempted obliteration of individuality through military training. In *Marching in Place*, each misaligned step produces an individuated mark undermining the logics of military conformity.

see detail on next spread

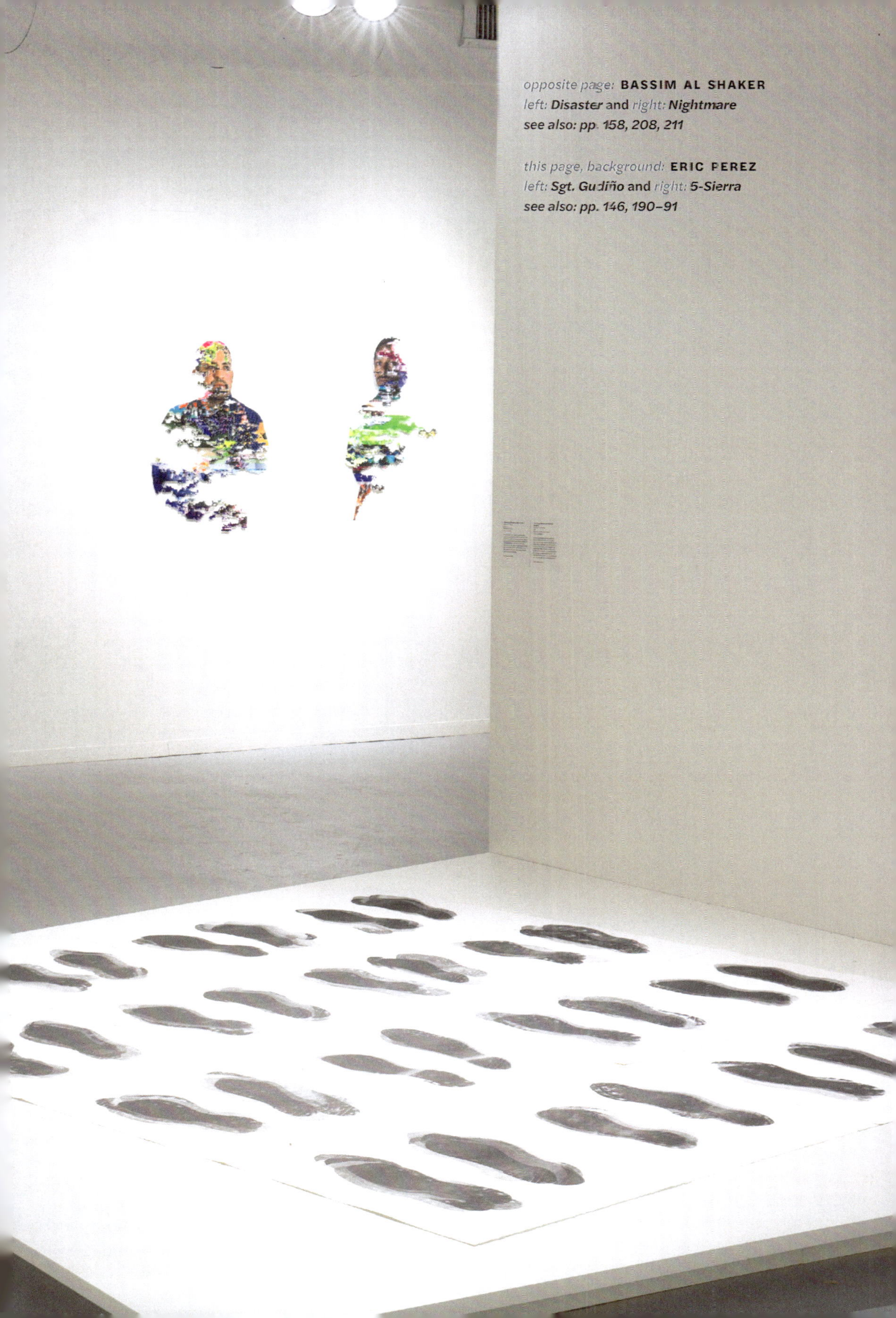

opposite page: **BASSIM AL SHAKER**
left: ***Disaster*** **and** *right:* ***Nightmare***
see also: pp. 158, 208, 211

this page, background: **ERIC PEREZ**
left: ***Sgt. Gudiño*** **and** *right:* ***5-Sierra***
see also: pp. 146, 190–91

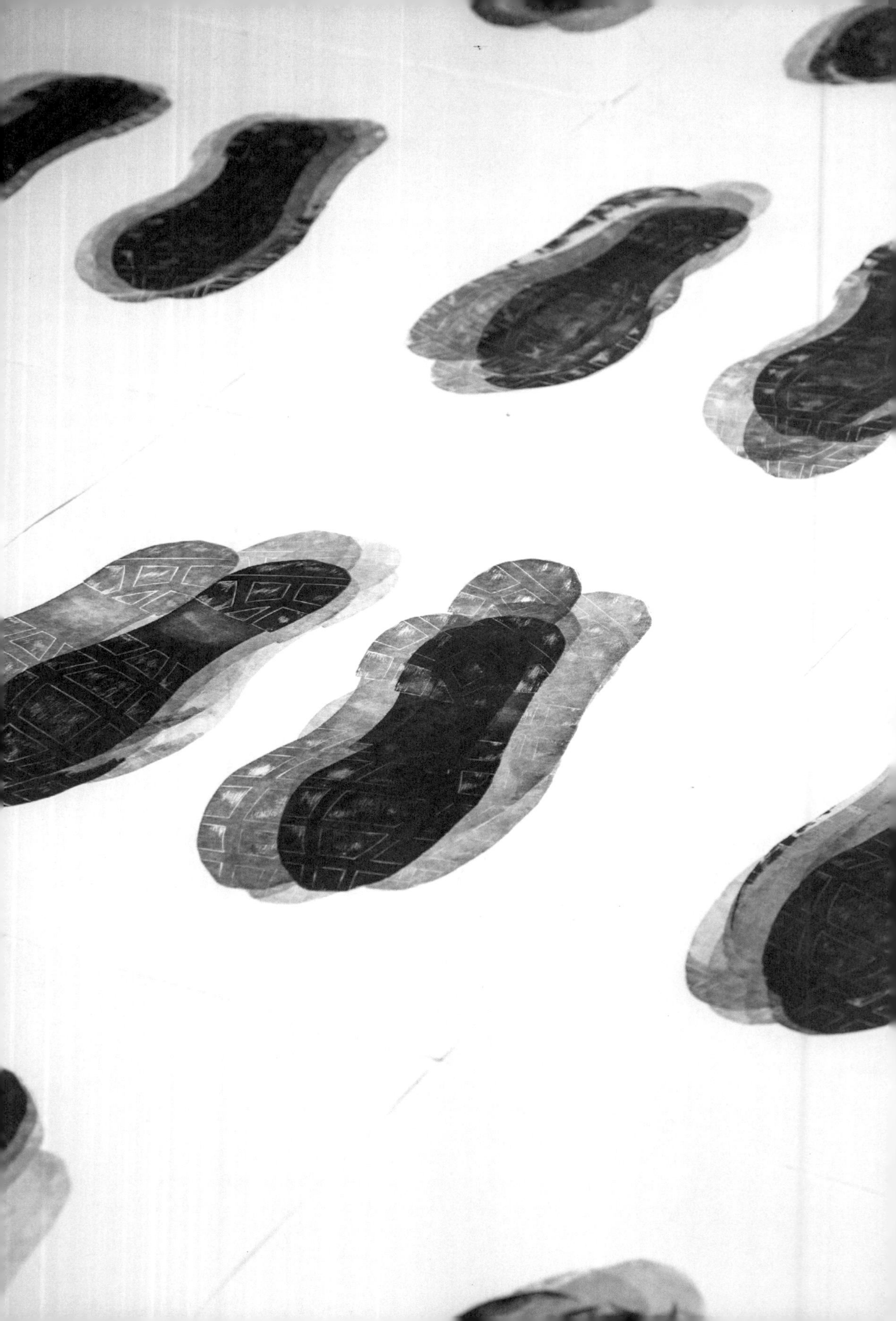

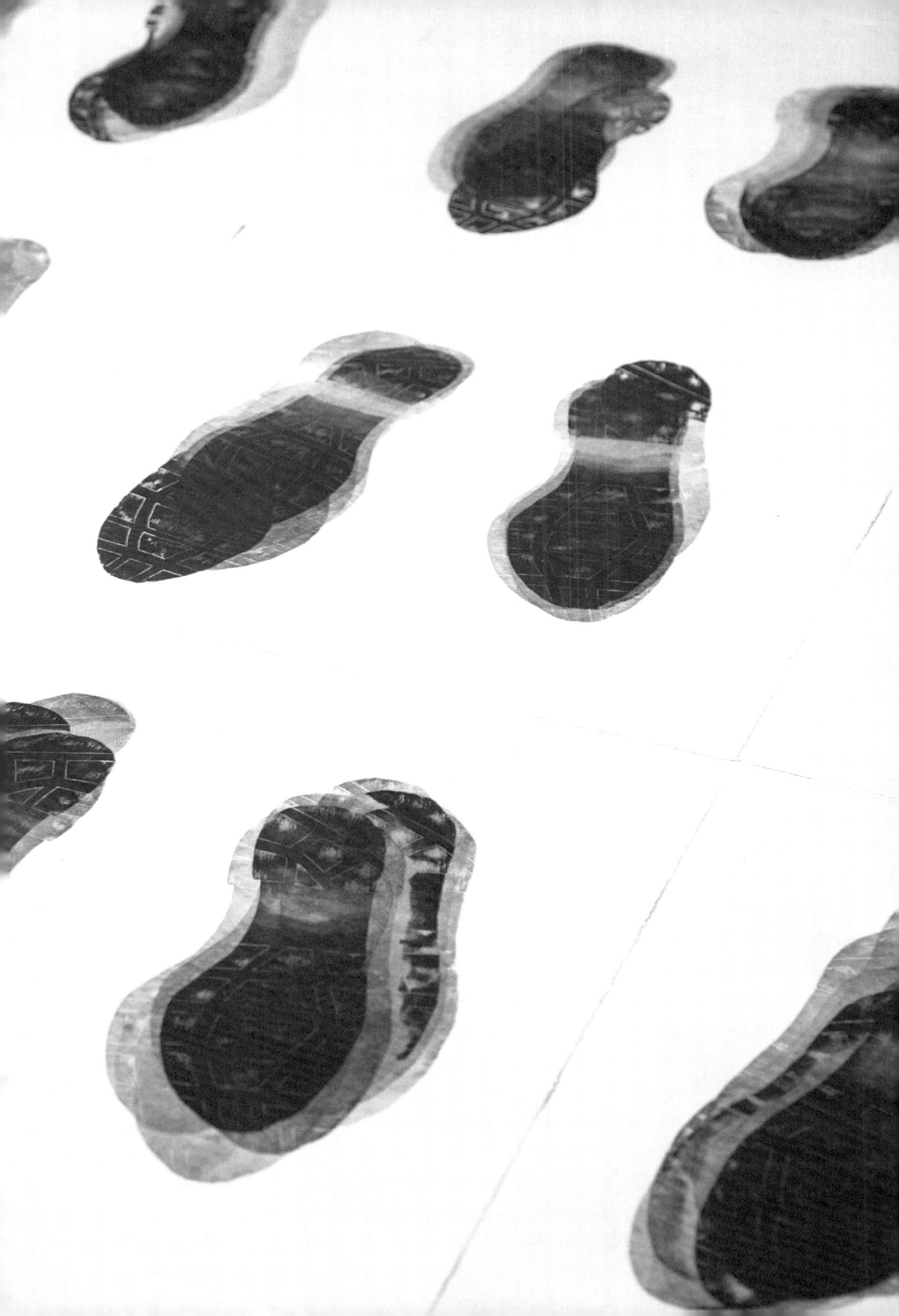

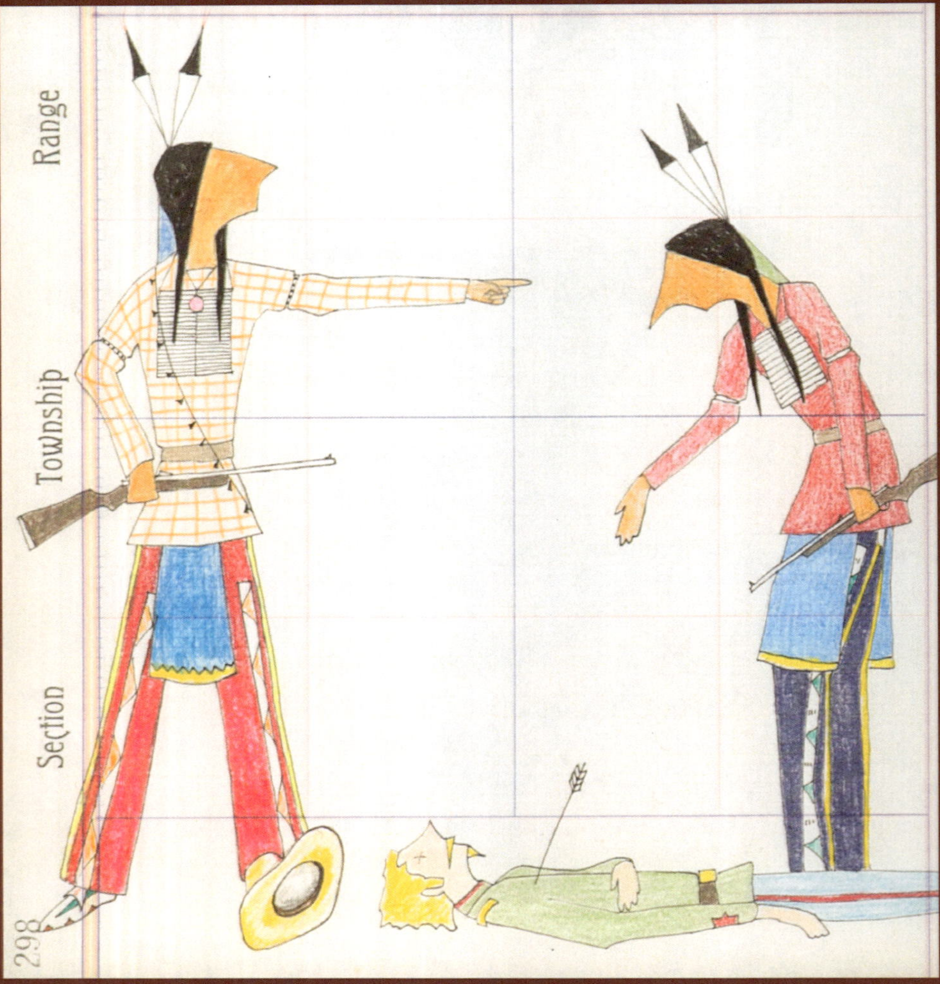

DWAYNE WILCOX
Larry is far right, he's really tough on immigration (detail)

see also: pp. 189, 254

Tomahawks, Chinooks, and Geronimo: Settler-Colonial Fantasies of US Navy SEALs

LALEH KHALILI

After the final shot was emptied in Usama bin Laden's forehead, Admiral McRaven who was in Jalalabad, Afghanistan, and who was receiving news from the operation, in turn reported to the Situation Room in the White House, where the National Security Council waited: "Geronimo, E-KIA". E-KIA means Enemy Killed In Action. Twenty minutes earlier, two Chinook and two Blackhawk helicopters had carried US Navy SEALs, a backup team, and extra fuel for mid-air refueling from Jalalabad across the border to Abbottabad, Pakistan, where Bin Laden was hiding.

US military helicopters, the aerial vehicle most often used in unconventional or covert operations, are named after Indigenous Turtle Island nations. In addition to Blackhawk and Chinook, helicopters can be Apache, Lakota, Comanche, or Kiowa. A US Army Aviation Museum curator in Alabama has said, "The Native Americans were probably the most lethal and unconventional force that we fought. Given their resources and what their capabilities were."[1] The naming of these lethal vehicles is meant to be a sign of respect.

The US military also uses Grey Eagle predator drones (named after an Indigenous elder) and deploys low-altitude missiles called Tomahawk. US Navy SEALs pride themselves in carrying—alongside their specialised assault weapons—a tomahawk hatchet crafted by the artisan who made the blades for the film *The Last of The Mohicans*. A member of SEAL Team 6 told the *New York Times* that the hatchets are used "for breaching, getting into doors, manipulating small locks, hand-to-hand combat and other things."[2] The logo of the Red Squadron of SEAL Team 6 is the word Tribe written under the profile image of an Indigenous American, and two crossed tomahawks on a red background.

The Navy SEALs have become the center of much attention, since May 2011 when the aforementioned operation to assassinate Usama bin Laden, code-named Geronimo, took place. The operation has become central to a number of pop culture products (films *Zero Dark Thirty* and *Act of Valor* in which cellulose SEALs are played by real ones; the memoir by one participant in the operation Matt Bissonette titled *No Easy Day* and a series of reportage on the event by Peter Bergen—*Manhunt*—and Mark Bowden's *The Finish*), not least because the Obama administration, in search of security credibility, provided a great deal of open access to the makers of the films and authors of the books. The Navy SEALs are also prolific producers of memoirs and business self-help books.

Politically, the memoirs fall to the right of the spectrum, with one or two exceptions. One SEAL who was involved in the US Operation

1. Akilah Davis, "Apache, Blackhawk, Chinook: Why Army helicopters are given Native American names." *ABC 11 Eyewitness News* (Durham, NC), November 10, 2021. https://abc11.com/army-helicopters-apache-black-hawk-native-american/11220233/.

2. Mark Mazzetti, Nicholas Kulish, Christopher Drew, Serge F. Kovaleski, Sean D. Naylor, and John Ismay, "SEAL Team 6: A Secret History of Quiet Killings and Blurred Lines." *The New York Times*, June 6, 2015. https://abc11.com/army-helicopters-apache-blackhawk-native-american/11220233/.

Restore Hope (sic) in Somalia, for example, argues that the Clinton administration essentially turned tail in Somalia and should have stayed and finished the job. Another, a bestselling account of a massively failed operation in Afghanistan in 2005 complains about the restrictive rules of engagement, laws of war, and the possible repercussions of killing civilians who may have inadvertently stumbled upon SEAL special operations. Another, recounting the US military presence in Beirut in 1982, rehashes the civil war in Lebanon as an inscrutable cauldron of ethnic hatreds. As Richard Drinnon has written in his incandescent *Facing West: The Metaphysics of Indian-Hating and Empire-Building*, "The exact measure of Anglo-American racial arrogance has been 'our' arrogation of the right to decide whether they should be 'humored' in their 'primitive life style' or have it wiped out."[3] This applies, of course, not only to aboriginal inhabitants of the Americas, but also the imperial subjects that are made targets of military equipment named after the people themselves also subjugated by the progenitor of the same military.

Their second category of books includes business self-help manuals written by former SEALs and other special operators who transform their military training into guidelines for successful business management. What these business self-help books do is to enshrine the myth of meritocracy—so central to the hegemonic ideal of the American dream—through their stories of training, and second, the ways in which invocation of past SEAL exploits produces a warrior ethos which, echoing the "Indian Wars," encourages militarism, high discipline, hierarchy, but also standard stories of "team work" and "camaraderie" which are decidedly gendered. For example, Brian Hiner's *First, Fast, Fearless: How to Lead Like a Navy SEAL* includes Section titles such as "Running to the sound of gunfire" and "Battle rhythm." In the acknowledgments he counts himself as "ole country boy" from the Blue Ridge Mountains of Virginia whose "brand" is

3. Richard Drinnon, *Facing West: The Metaphysics of Indian-Hating and Empire-Building* (Norman, OK: University of Oklahoma Press, 1997), xiii.

"brotherhood and battle rhythm." He compares business leadership to being a warrior, and he argues that "a warrior is a specialist within the context of a tribal or clan-based society that recognizes a separate warrior class."[4] The book is all about violence and speed: "our enemies often behead their captives."[5] "With a first strike mindset, people don't feel like victims, even in situations in which others would consider them victims."[6] "We understand that sometimes bad things happen. We may not deserve it, or it may not be fair, but we have to acknowledge it and move on."[7]

In *Time in the Shadows*, I outline the traces of the wars of conquest on the Americas in today's counterinsurgency practices. The lines from reservations—not as sovereign nations but originally as spaces of mass detention—run through to reconcentrados of Cuba and the Philippines and concentration camps of the Boer War on to New Villages of Malaya and Strategic Hamlets of Vietnam. I trace the various legal concepts including "enemy combatant" and "extraordinary rendition" and other judicial institutions which originally were used to suppress Indigenous sovereignty and to exact punishment on intransigent aboriginal Americans.[8]

In their tour de force on the transformation of capitalism, Luc Boltanski and Eve Chiapello trace the emergence in the 1990s of a new managerial language, which disavowed the Taylorist model of production, instead venerating autonomy, flexibility, "decentralization, meritocracy, and management by objective" as the new spirit of the age. This new spirit co-opted the tradition of 1968 rebellions against militarised hierarchies, against bureaucracies, and against "authority" and "petty tyranny."[9] Their explanation also provides a parallel to

4. Brian Hiner, *First, Fast, Fearless: How to Lead Like a Navy SEAL* (New York, NY: McGraw Hill, 2015), xvi, 5–6, 11.

5. Ibid., 24.

6. Ibid., 47.

7. Ibid., 48.

8. Laleh Khalili, *Time in the Shadows: Confinement in Counterinsurgencies* (Stanford, CA: Stanford University Press, 2012).

their appropriation of Indigenous American names, symbols and stories as part of the war-fighting cosmography of the SEALs.

But there is a way that the symbols of Indigenous Turtle Island nations also function as talismans, as the US fights wars of "cowboys and Indians" overseas. As Frances FitzGerald wrote about the war in Vietnam fifty years ago, "To the American settlers the defeat of the Indians had seemed not just a nationalist victory, but an achievement made in the name of humanity, the triumph of light over darkness, of good over evil, and of civilization over brutish nature. Quite unconsciously, the American officers and officials used a similar language to describe their war against the Vietnamese National Liberation Front."[10] The military operations there were named after Frontier monikers: "Rolling Thunder"; "Prairie"; "Sam Houston"; "Hickory"; "Daniel Boone"; and even "Crazy Horse," which as the Communist historian Richard Drinnon writes was "a 1966 operation carried out appropriately by elements of the 1st Cavalry Division." There, the free fire zone in which the guerrillas operated was called "Indian country."[11]

There is also something in the way that the Navy SEALs' mythos devours Indigenous American symbols that perhaps indicates a subconscious desire to consume that which has not been defeated, despite all settler-colonial violence to the contrary. Or we can say that the US empire is haunted by this, one of its original sins. As Avery Gordon writes, "haunting is one way in which abusive systems of power make themselves known and their impacts felt in everyday life, especially when they are supposedly over and done with (such as with transatlantic slavery, for instance) or when their oppressive nature is continuously denied (such as national

9. Luc Boltanski and Eve Chiapello, *The New Spirit of Capitalism*, trans. Gregory Elliott (London and New York: Verso, 2018).

10. Frances FitzGerald, *Fire in the Lake: The Vietnamese and the Americans in Vietnam* (Boston, MA: Little, Brown and Company, 1972), 368.

11. Drinnon, *Facing West*, 450–51.

security)."[12] And whether the SEALs star in their own memoirs, or at corporate boardrooms, or in cheesy romance novels, the ghost of Geronimo and countless others hovers in the background, a reminder that the US settler-colonial violence continues unabated in the long wars.

12. Avery Gordon, *Ghostly Matters: Haunting and the Sociological Imagination* (Minneapolis, MN: University of Minnesota Press, 2008), xvi.

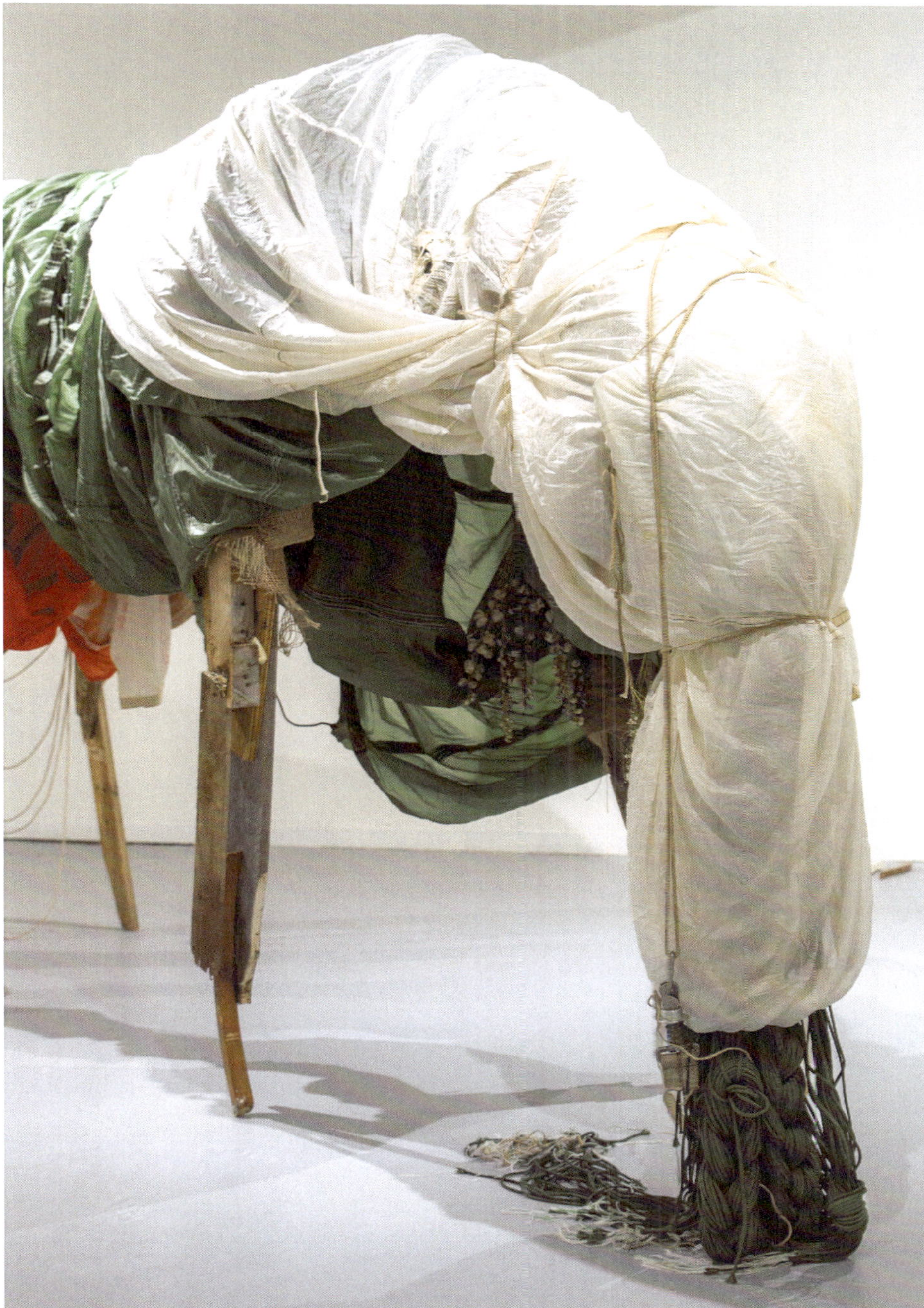

JOSE DEVERA, *And All the King's Men* (detail), 2014–23, Mixed media, wood, canvas, and found materials; *see also: p. 166*

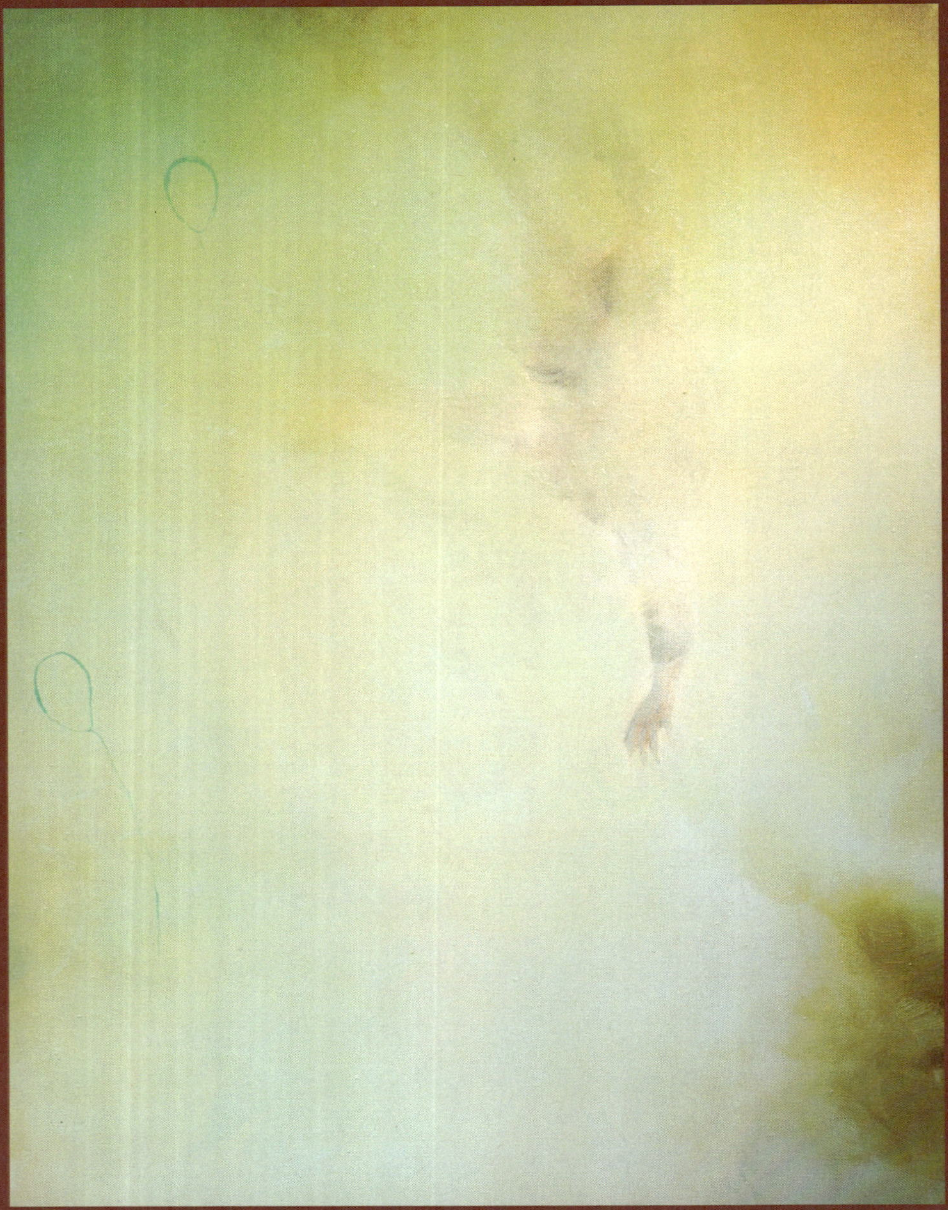

BASSIM AL SHAKER *(b. 1986)*
Nightmare (detail)

see full painting on p. 211

These paintings are part of Bassim Al Shaker's *Moment of Silence* series.

see also: pp. 158–61, 196–97

Life During War on Terror Time

JUNAID RANA

Yellow skies filled with pinks, oranges, and blues. Kites, splashes of red, and figures of life and death. A hand of God descending from the heavens. Guiding the eye is not the sun but drones, rockets, a blast or two. Pieces strewn about by the ethereal lights of explosions in the sky. It is a gorgeous sky until you see the bodies. A hand descending from the heavens. Once seen, it cannot be unseen. An ethereal sky turned into horror. The images of Bassam Al Shaker are, in the most blunt description, otherworldly. "I saw body parts in the sky," the artist explained after witnessing explosions in the Iraqi skyline. Seeing things that one cannot unsee is the psychic sociality of a warscape. The ominous beauty of these magnificent and troubling paintings represents a principal statement of the 2023 Veteran Art Triennial *Surviving the Long Wars* regarding the transformation of social life: seeing things anew when before they were unseen.

In the twenty-plus years since the "War on Terror" began, entire countries and nations have been turned upside down, millions have been displaced, and the death count could include entire cities. In all this upheaval, war capitalism brought with it scores of technological innovations, changing everything from how we see to how we know. War capitalism, in its most elemental form, derives from the use of the profit motive in the violent means of extraction, dispossession, and land theft, which is often referred to as primitive (or primary) accumulation. This adds up to changes in how social relations are configured: how we communicate, understand, and essentially think. Philosophers of futurity tell us that this is about scale and speed, and about a kind of psychopolitics that has taken over our aesthetic horizon. A seemingly smart power that is friendly and offers a solitary sense of freedom (usually with a device!) countering the idea of power as coercive, dominating, and oppressive.[1] This shift in power arrives as the everyday has become increasingly militarized through technological strivings such that surveillance, drones, computing, and even design are made possible at rapid rates.

In Al Shaker's paintings featured in the *Unlikely Entanglements* exhibition, the sky—a staple of landscape painting—is a theater of war in which the heavens have turned into a nightmare. It is this dissonance between quotidian materiality and psychic transformation that tells the story of the long wars of settler violence. From the perspective of war capitalism, it's the re-narration of how we know the world—even the sky can mean something else. In *Nightmare*, the image of an arm descending from the skies evokes Michelangelo's *The Creation of Adam* in the Sistine Chapel, referring not to the divine birth of humanity but instead to a profound evisceration and plunder. It is not so much the trick of the eye or vision that tells this story but the expectation and possibility of human disaster. With a sense of the abject, Al Shaker disrupts the liberal humanism at the center of

---

1. Byung-Chul Han, *Psychopolitics: Neoliberalism and New Technologies of Power* (London; New York: Verso, 2017).

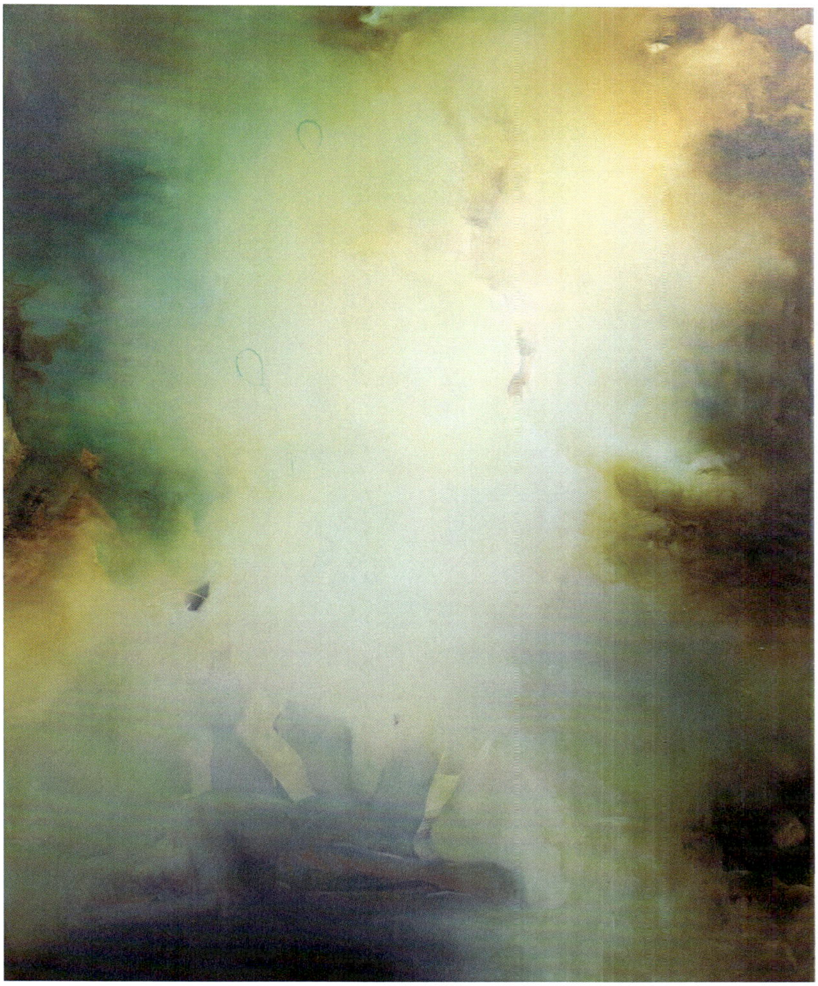

BASSIM AL SHAKER, *Nightmare*, 2022, Oil on canvas; *see detail on p. 208*

Catholic theology to imagine a Manichean world split by the horrors and atrocities of war and the life of abundance and theft founded in US settler society and as an expansive empire. The colonizer makes the damned.[2] War is a way of life under US empire that has profoundly transformed everything we experience and know, such that we have a hard time noticing it.

2. Frantz Fanon, *The Wretched of the Earth* (New York: Grove Press, 1965).

Within the damned is even further complexity and hierarchy. What is one to make of those who take sides? What if it is the wrong side? What if these sides keep changing depending on perspective and context? What is the political economy of taking sides? How do you take a risk? These are not just Manichean choices between good and evil, but ones with shifting perspectives and alternative interpretations. And so, by including veterans of the US military, the exhibition complicates the reading and presentation of the storytelling from one artwork to the next. There is an unease that creeps into the vision of the works as the progression becomes more apparent, and in which there really is no safe side. In Mariam Ghani's *The Trespassers*, the single-channel video installation tells the story of the "ghosts in the records" of Afghan and Iraqi translators whose presence has been redacted from military interrogation records during the first decade of the "War on Terror." These "ghosts" are a testament to what Ghani aptly describes as a potential witness, informant, or traitor. It is the last of these that has always been the most troublesome, even as the other two are still threats. To be a traitor invokes a kind of cause and purity of a national ideology that attests to the unease I am referring to—a sense of risk, taking sides, wishing for the damned to take on the colonizer.

The seed of this genealogy of aesthetics and artistic thought that brings *Surviving the Long Wars* together was there in the early days of the post-9/11 world. One of the biggest concerns was how quickly the military/state/police apparatus was producing a different set of principles normalizing war and authoritarianism while eviscerating the politics of redistribution and anti-colonialism. The alternative to this was the potential for social transformation through the articulation of a vision based on sustaining life and shared humanity as opposed to a world organized through military violence. Yet the entire notion of civil liberties in the face of the surveillance and policing architecture of the domestic "War on Terror" shifted dramatically such that two decades later, vestiges of rights from the pre-9/11 world seem anachronistic. The accomplishment of *Surviving the Long Wars* has been to provide a history of the sociality of war capitalism achieved from before the "War on Terror" to the longer "American Indian Wars."

As a discrete genealogy that documents the social upheaval of War on Terror capitalism, the kernel that launches this counterhistory of the long wars in the twenty-first century can be found in Mariam Ghani and Chitra Ganesh's *Index of the Disappeared*. I was familiar with this project when it began as an archive and an incitement to witness the horrors of state violence as a history. Chitra Ganesh's *Watercolors* series, a component of the collaborative *Index*, harkens to a past of better days—even a glimmer of a smile—while inviting a sense of humanity in the portraits. Portraits with children, families, and pastoral landscapes gesture to another time and a different sense of interiority that is contra to the containment of carcerality in rendition, detention, deportation, and imprisonment. And yet the lightness of the portraits has a hint of morose ambivalence, a kind of distrust of the moment. Black site torture and experimental tactics for breaking down the psyche are just around the corner from these innocent times. The curators have masterfully paired this with Hanaa Malallah's *She/He Has No Picture*, which commemorates civilian bombing victims in Iraq killed by the US military in 1991, prior to the "War on Terror" campaign. This juxtaposition brings forth the depth of mourning and grief hidden by the narrative of a military victory over a fantasy enemy that, as in prior and long histories of colonialism and empire, has no history.[3] This is not just the erasure of a people but a distinct racializing at a planetary scale.[4]

Nearly a quarter of the twenty-first century has passed, and it now seems nearly impossible to simply gloss over this as a

3. Edward W. Said, *Orientalism* (New York: Vintage Books, 1979).; Eric R. Wolf, *Europe and the People Without History* (Berkeley: University of California Press, 1982).

4. Patrick Wolfe, *Traces of History: Elementary Structures of Race* (London; New York: Verso, 2016).

dialectic between war and peace. The fact-ness of military violence and US imperial policing across the globe appears unstoppable. Even more so, how we live, and experience violence, has been profoundly changed. Instead, we are living in war, surviving war, resisting a war we no longer recognize as war. *Sutured*, by Ruth Kaneko (Kanaka Wahine), deconstructs these war myths through the taking apart of a military uniform, making a collage by combining the pieces with the sutures of a medic's kit, also incorporating gauze, medical tape, and other first aid products. In doing so, the notion of sacrifice, so prevalent in modern warfare, is reinscribed with affective healing and the problem of trauma as a social fact of the enormous cost of the "War on Terror." This motif of the deconstructed military uniform, also used by Indigenous artists Melissa Doud (Ojibwe) and Miridith Campbell (Kiowa), is an interesting counterpoint to the dress of those depicted in Chitra Ganesh's *Watercolors* series. For Ganesh, the point of rescuing compassion is to offer the culture of everyday life as an antidote to the military logics of representation that eviscerate the humanity out of the subjects of war.

Yet the "War on Terror" did not start in 2001, and it has masked itself in every new iteration. It was always a colonial war and, designed with intentions of elimination and removal, it hardly needed to present itself as a war between nations. It was not a war against Afghanistan, Iraq, or the Muslim world, but a displaced figure ambiguously called "Terror." It was a continuation of the settler violence founded in Indigenous genocide.[5] As in Al Shaker's paintings, when the "War on Terror" was fought in the skies, all sorts of demons, ghosts, and apparitions appeared. The "War on Terror" is truly everywhere. Again, Ganesh's portraits of a smiling Aafia Siddiqui or captives of the "War on Terror" with their families should not be surprising in a context that would render Muslim life anathema to the so-called modern world. If the opposite of war is

5. Joanne Barker, *Red Scare: The State's Indigenous Terrorist* (Oakland, California: University of California Press, 2021).

peace, there is no peace, and under the conditions of US empire and colonialism, there was never any peace. Now, there are many who will not recognize the ways that everyday life is surrounded by war—the "war on terror," the "war on drugs," poverty, crime. With no peace, as one of the thematic threads within the exhibition relays, any vision for justice or healing is forged in wartime.

War capitalism, the economic and social epoch in which we exist, reflects human-made systems of death-making and the social relations that, in turn, are created from such an existence. The horror of this wartime has an aesthetic and a meaning-making that is also life-affirming and a counter to the end, be it death, climate catastrophe, or planetary extinction. By expanding imperial war across the world, chasing something called "terror," it provides the illusion of security and peace. There can be no peace in colonial violence, only a constantly transformed sociality formed under settler society that hides the colonial violence of war capitalism, defined in the primary accumulation of theft that makes land into property and groups of people into bodies for labor. For example, the assemblage of portraits, autopsy records, and death certificates from Rajkamal Kahlon's series *Did You Kiss the Dead Body?* continues a tradition of telling the individual stories of history as extraction and brutality. Two stunning portraits overlap the documents in a pastiche of a blood-stained hue to report the deaths in custody of Iraqi and Afghan men in US detention facilities. Stories, in these grisly renderings, are defined by reports that cannot tell what life was like for victims of war, leaving a mystery in the archive. Sabba Elahi's *Drone Stories* imagines such life as racialized surveillance in the traditional craft of embroidery that recalls domestic scenes of wartime as subtle atrocities. Similarly, folk culture is reconstituted by Mahwish Chishty's *Drone Art*, set in a warscape that organizes everyday life. The drone as an object of warcraft is akin to the technologies of everyday transportation—trucks—in South Asia that are adorned out of care, love, and as aesthetic objects.[6] Juxtaposing Chishty's work with Indigenous art, especially the protest tradition of Kiowa ledger art displayed in *Residues and Rebellions* at the Newberry Library, brings to life a different trajectory of the taken-for-granted aspects of quotidian life in War on Terror time.

The *Surviving the Long Wars* Triennial is an example of storytelling that documents, expresses, critiques, and denounces the system of war capitalism that we live under, as it makes clear the creation of new traditions, rituals, and commemorations of artmaking. From objects of state archives to folk practices of makers, the story of this show is not just about the horrific violence of war, it's a description of life during a never-ending War on Terror time. The artwork in the show describes the permanence of an apocalyptic time in which War on Terror capitalism reigns supreme, but what is more striking here is the power of a messianic fatalism that would relinquish the devastation and plunder of the "War on Terror" to a preordained end-time. Take, for example, the pathos throughout this show of the meaning of the colossal death and destruction of the "Global War on Terror[7]," and, conversely, the terrain of the War on Terror time that makes for creative intervention, undoing the trick of war capitalism that forces a belief in its inevitability in a dialectic of war capitalism's creative destruction.

There is ample evidence that over the last twenty years of the "Global War on Terror," the order of things gave way to a highly manipulated experiment in which the planet became a military laboratory. Some might call it a battle over ideas or a fight for humanity, but these are just covers for the war machine as it expends, exhausts, and extinguishes. It is the language of white settler imperialism, a centuries-long project. The crisis continues to be relevant, and the transformation of politics and everyday life, a possibility. If war is the engine of the economy of the world, this would say something

6. Jamal J. Elias, *On Wings of Diesel: Trucks, Identity and Culture in Pakistan* (London: Oneworld, 2011).

7. Junaid Rana, "Forever End Times: GWOT in Three Parts," *American Quarterly* 74, no. 3 (2022): 563–566.

different about how we understand the contemporary world. War capitalism is white settler capitalism, the history that hides how the "War on Terror" is everywhere. War and its meaning will remain buried in our social being until we are made to see it and create another world, much like these artists do.

section four

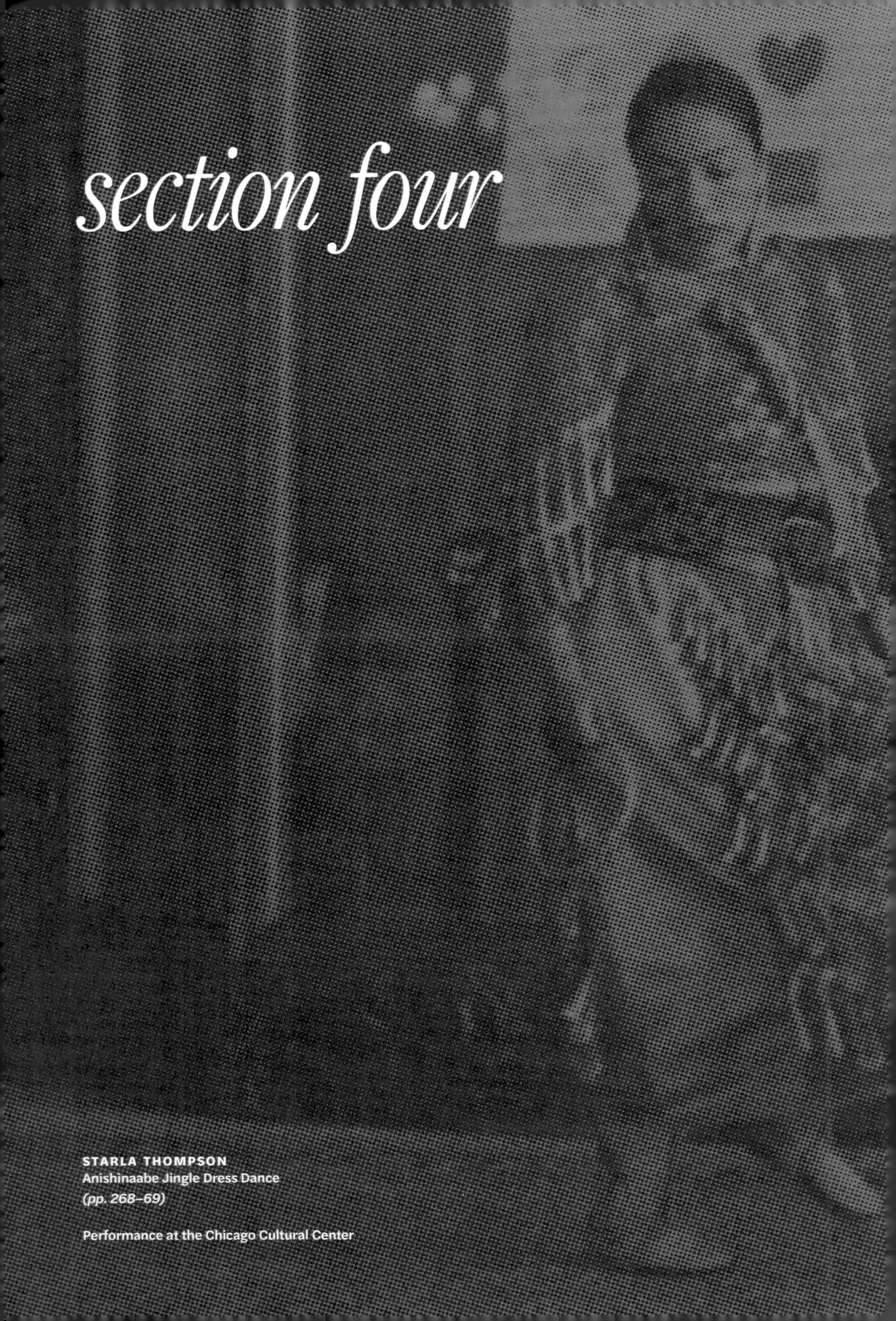

STARLA THOMPSON
Anishinaabe Jingle Dress Dance
(pp. 268–69)

Performance at the Chicago Cultural Center

Surviving the Long Wars Summit

Surviving the Long Wars Summit

When we made treaties long ago, it was for as long as the grass shall grow and as long as the rivers shall flow. The way things are going now, one of these days the grass isn't going to grow...and the rivers aren't going to flow...
—Evan Haney, *Winter Soldier Investigation: An Inquiry into American War Crimes* (1972)

To bring out your dead is to say that these deaths are not unimportant or forgotten, or worse, coincidental. It is to say that these deaths are systemic, structural. To bring out your dead is both a memorial and a challenge, an act of grief and of defiance, a register of mortality and decline, and of the possibility of struggle and survival.
—Grace Kyungwon Hong, *Death beyond Disavowal* (2015)

Convened during the twentieth anniversary of the 2003 US-led military invasion of Iraq, the 2023 Veteran Art Summit created a space to confront and acknowledge the overwhelming loss of life from the long wars. This includes the hundreds of thousands directly killed in Iraq, the broader effects of the "Global War on Terror," and the enduring genocidal violence of the "American Indian Wars." This space of acknowledgment, however fraught with contradictions, opened a breach in the ever-expanding imperialist landscape. Within this moment, participants bore witness, and were witnessed, prompting a reorientation towards solidarity, justice, and collective healing.

Documenting the transformative four-day Summit (March 16–19, 2023), this section includes photographs of the performers Hipólito Arriaga III, GOODW.Y.N., Hussein Smko, Andrea Assaf, Starla Thompson, and Brian Frejo; musicians Brittney Chantele, Elexa Dawson, James Pakootas, and Joseph Running Crane; along with images from Summit discussions, panels, workshops, tours, and presentations. These activations are paired with words from Iraqi and American Reconciliation Project organizer Shaymaa Khalil, verse from Iraqi poet Maitham Alharbi, remarks from Iraqi American visual artist Michael Rakowitz, an essay by Afro-Indigenous historian Kyle T. Mays (Black/Saginaw Anishinaabe), an interview with Triennial performance curator Anthony Torres, and a review by Pakistani American journalist and organizer Isra Rahman.

Kyle T. Mays's essay, "When Black People Are Free, All People Will Be Free: Black Freedom, Indigenous Sovereignty, and the Limits of Reparations Discourse," centers on Black and Indigenous movements, expanding political imaginations of liberation rooted in the concept of "Land Back." By critically examining the relationship between reparations and sovereignty, his work resonates with the Triennial's goal, advocating for a vision of co-liberation where Black and Indigenous struggles are interconnected, suggesting that solidarity and kinship across these communities are essential for achieving meaningful and inclusive justice.

In conversation with veteran artist and writer Kevin Basl, Anthony Torres discusses his curatorial vision for the Triennial performances, emphasizing collaboration, community-building, and diverse perspectives. He highlights his engagement with scholar Kyle T. Mays on the topic of solidarity and reflects on how the Summit's poetry readings and multidisciplinary performances confronted trauma and moral injury.

Echoing the fault lines Mays interrogates, Isra Rahman's essay, "The Summit, Then and Now," begins with warranted skepticism of veteran artists, questioning whether the Summit would "critically reflect on US militarism or serve as propaganda for war." She writes that, through her participation, she discovered that the event brought together art and artists to critique the foundations and lasting effects of endless war. Reflecting on the Israeli onslaught in Gaza and the role of veteran art in anti-war movements, Rahman explores the transformative power of veteran artists in fostering critical conversations on militarism, war, and solidarity, highlighting how the Triennial and Summit are part of a broader realignment of solidarity politics necessary to build a more "resilient anti-war movement focused on militarism abroad and policing at home."

The Summit concluded with the Iraq War Memorial Activation at the Grand Army of the Republic War Memorial inside the Chicago Cultural Center. Participants gathered to listen to testimonies, poems, and visions of peace shared by war-impacted people. The vigil followed the presentation, with a silent procession to the lakefront. As participants exited the building, multidisciplinary Indigenous artist Brian Frejo caringly smudged each person. The solemn walk concluded at the shores of Lake Michigan, where one by one, they dropped flowers—a historic symbol of remembrance—into the water.

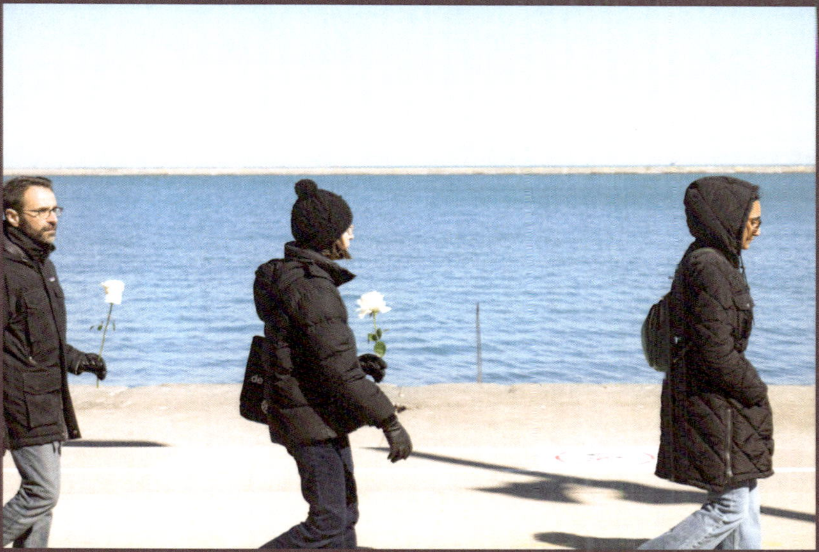

IRAQ WAR MEMORIAL ACTIVATION, Chicago Cultural Center, March 19, 2023

We give thanks to all of the waters of the world for quenching our thirst, for providing strength and nurturing life for all beings. We know its power in many forms—waterfalls and rain, mists and streams, rivers and oceans, snow and ice. We are grateful that the waters are still here and meeting their responsibility to the rest of Creation.

—Robin Wall Kimmerer, *Braiding Sweetgrass* (2015)

War

SHAYMAA KHALIL

When war comes, the furniture of cities changes.

Baghdad disappeared in the darkness of war, and another Baghdad stepped onto the stage.

It's now a city of demolished words and a ruined entity.

In this situation, the city will witness a massive construction and absence of direction.

She went from being a cave at the right hand of the dictator to a shelter at the hands of the new thieves and killers.

And at the rhythm of this terrible transition, the story of the slaughtered sheep will extend to its last words.

Iraqi's history, both ancient and recent, includes many images of war, its pattern, repercussions and impacts in the collective memory of the population, generation after generation.

Every generation of ours bears in its body and soul the scar of horrors and bitterness and trauma of suffering and loss passed on from grandparents to grandchildren like an external curse.

It has shaped life from the highest sky to the depth of earth, and the name that we give to this curse, this poison, is (OIL).

Adapted from a speech read at the STLW Iraq War Memorial Activation, Chicago Cultural Center, March 19, 2023

Escapees from the bombing

MAITHAM ALHARBI

a truck crosses the night surrounded by winds and the roar of the engine.
the driver passes the lighter and another cigarette ignites.
it catches fire and the journey lights up.
in the back of the truck families' belongings piled up
sharp and hard, like the stab of a friend.
the bedrooms sway with anxiety.
a bicycle's laughter swims in the darkness.
a rubber goose sound is upside down.
the torn bag of flour, all the bread is dead.
and it's the mother. stand on her shoulders with fear.
and the father keeps the driver talking about a song of homeland until the sunrise.

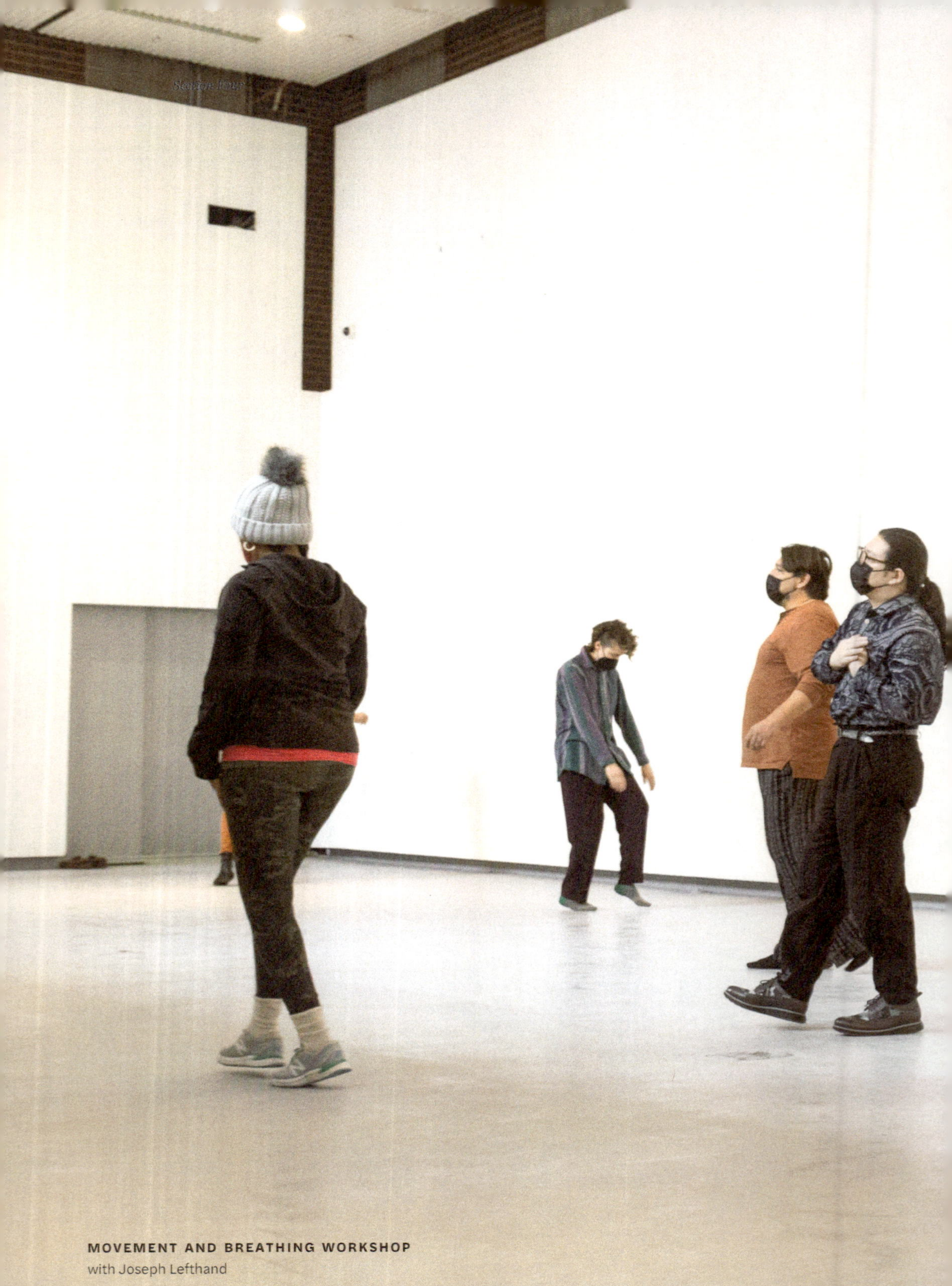

MOVEMENT AND BREATHING WORKSHOP
with Joseph Lefthand

Hyde Park Art Center, March 17, 2023

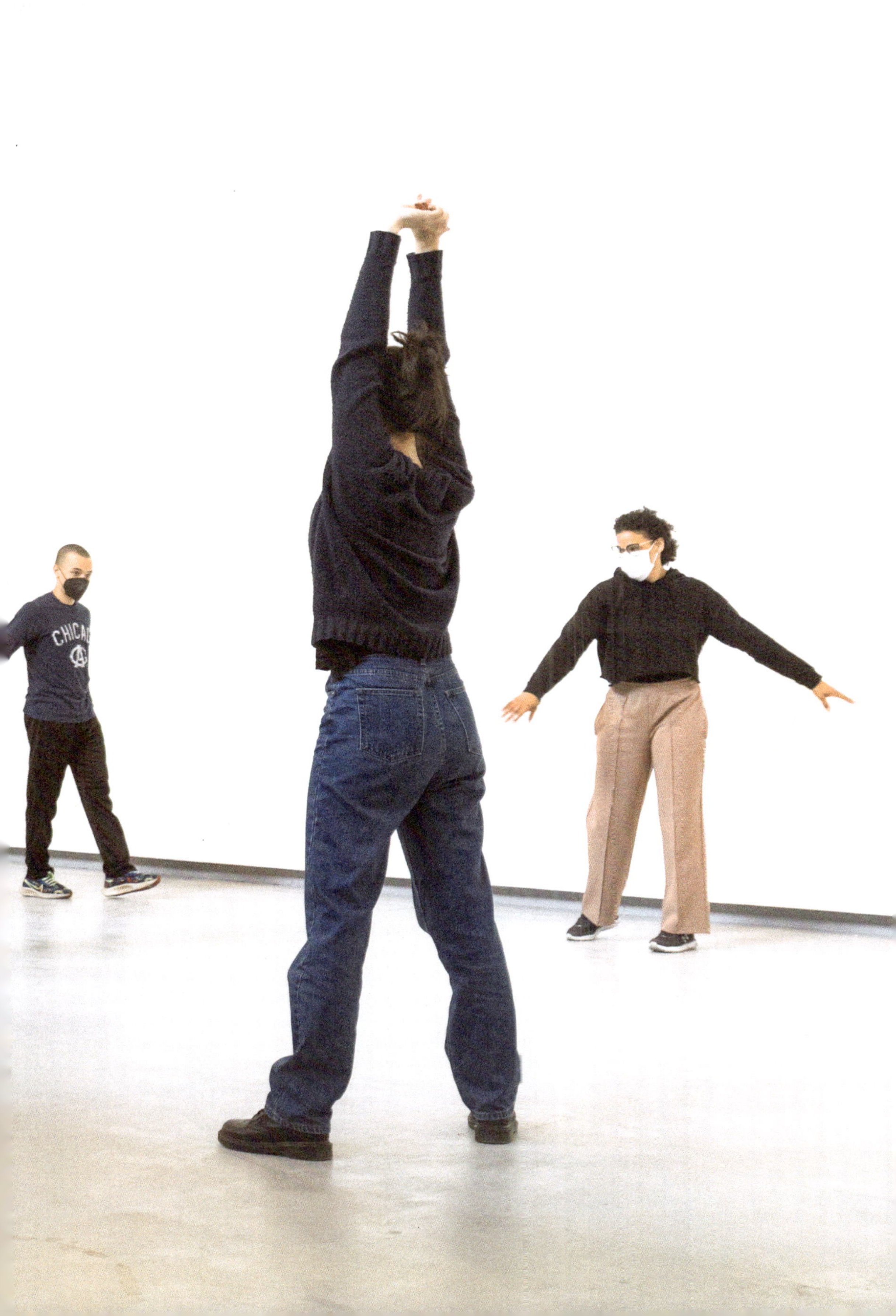

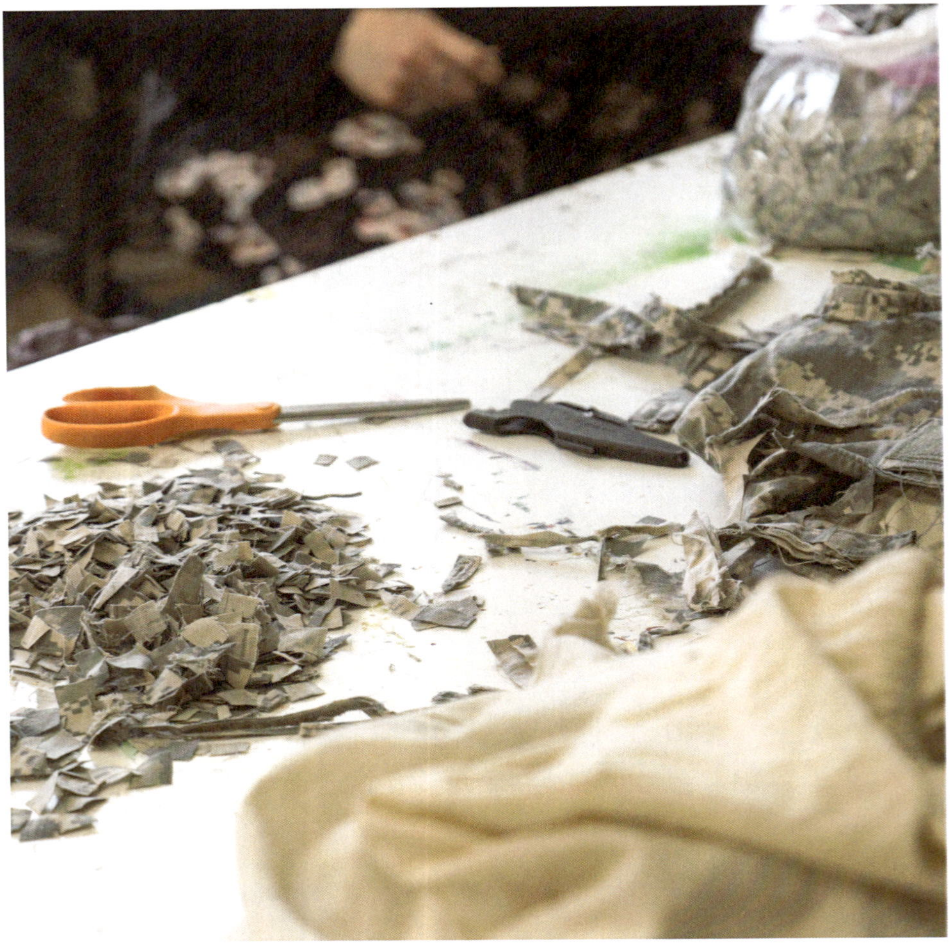

PAPERMAKING WORKSHOP
with Frontline Arts

Hyde Park Art Center, March 17, 2023

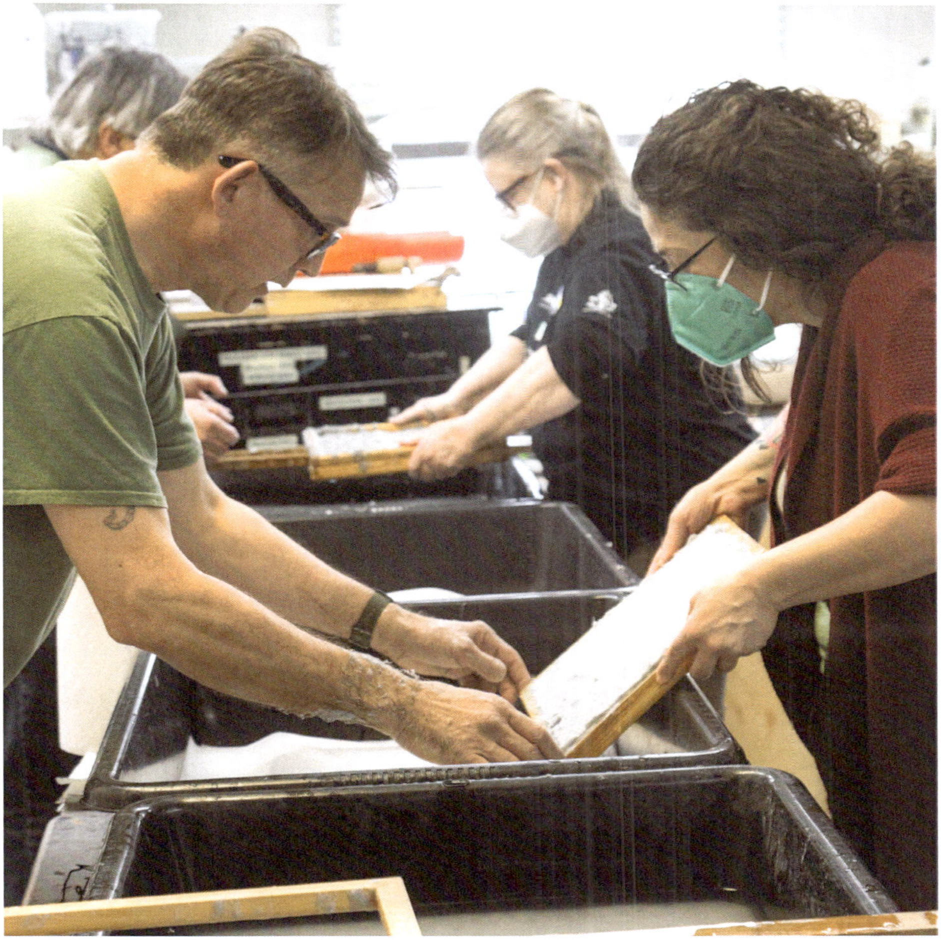

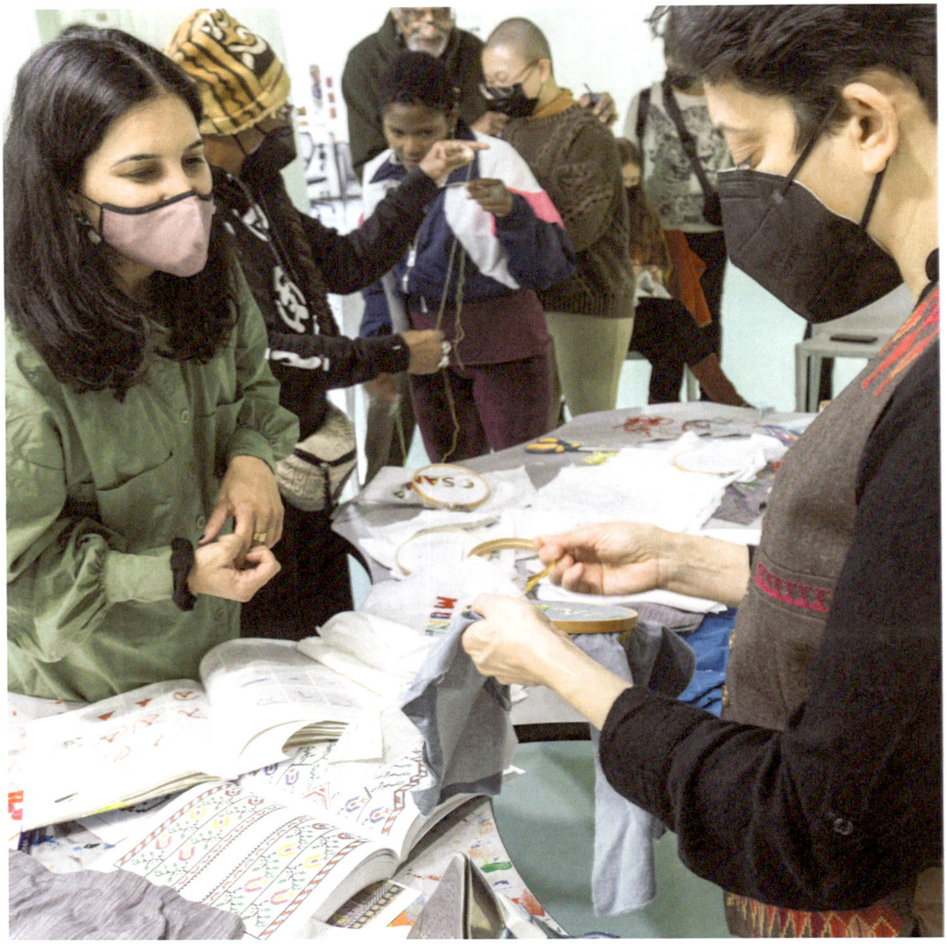

DRONE STORIES EMBROIDERY CIRCLE
with Sabba Elahi

Hyde Park Art Center, March 17, 2023

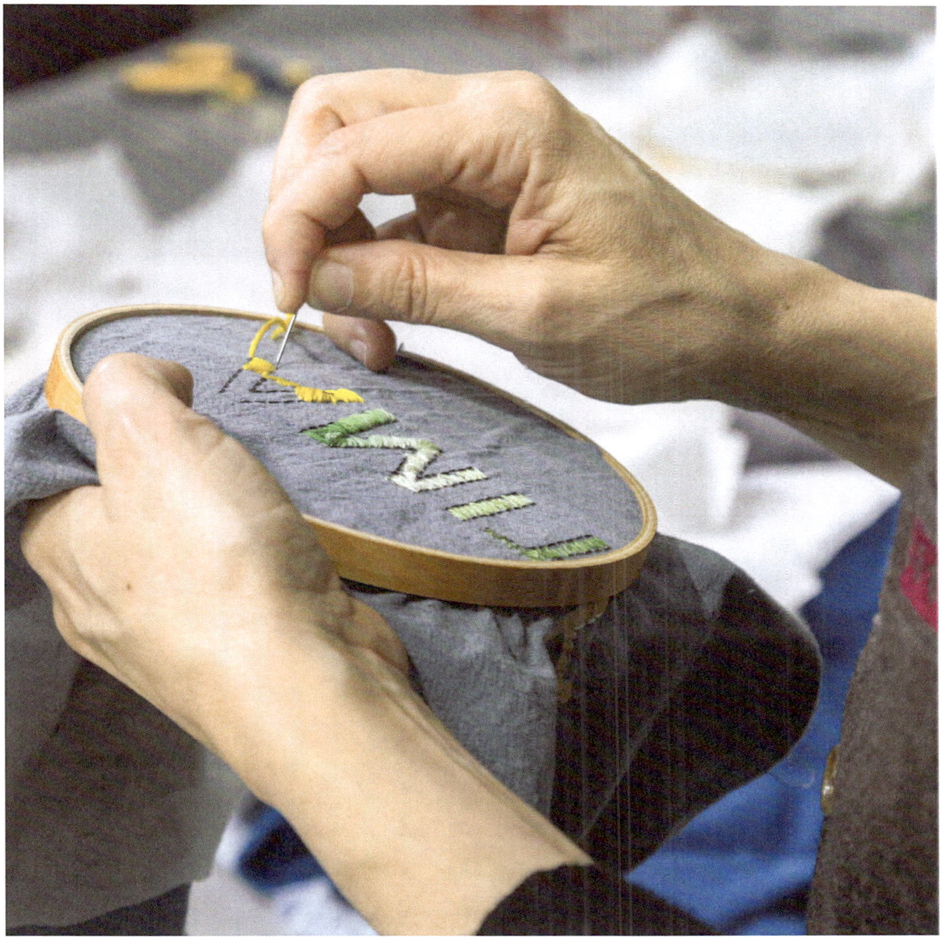

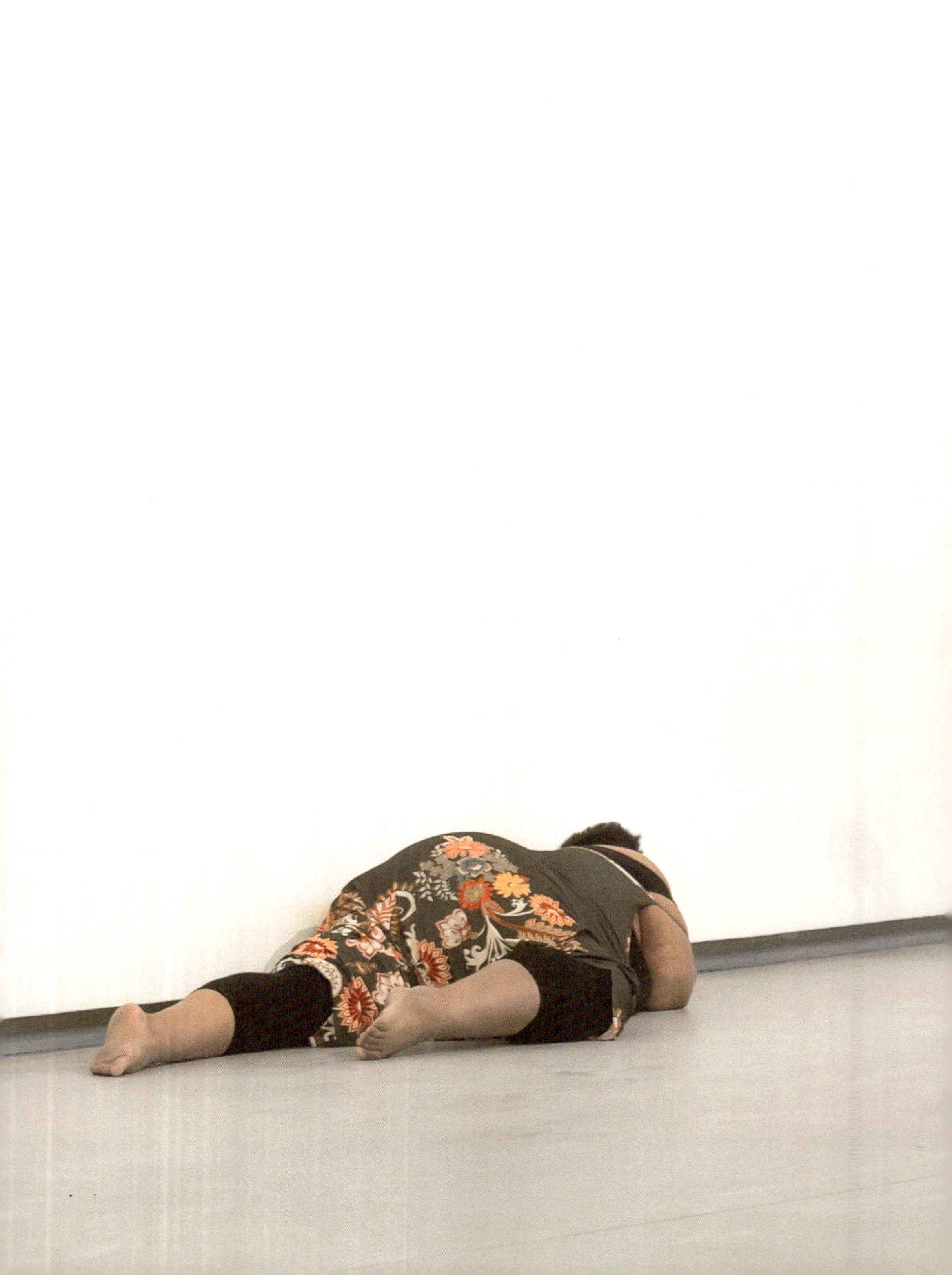

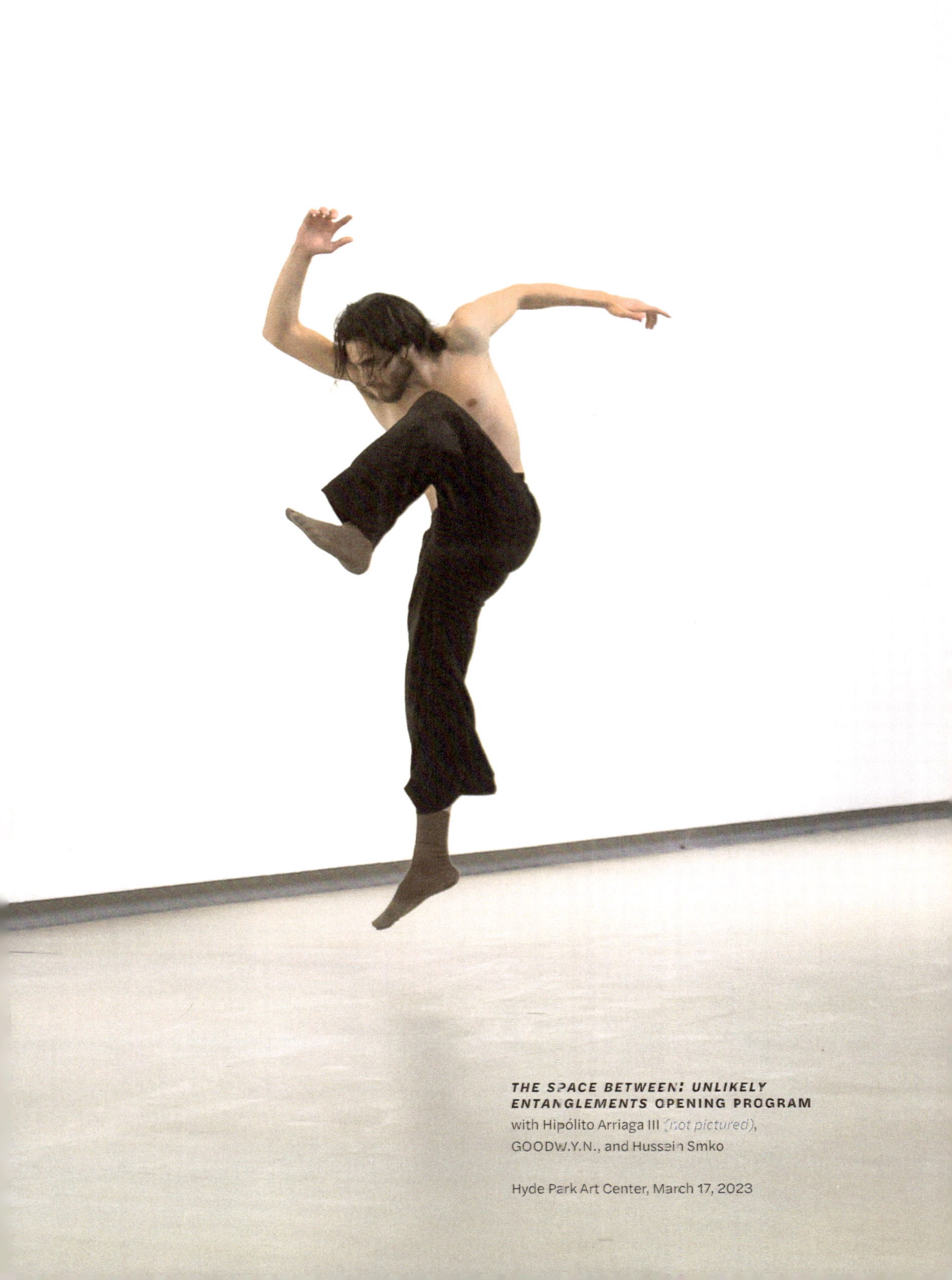

***THE SPACE BETWEEN: UNLIKELY ENTANGLEMENTS* OPENING PROGRAM**

with Hipólito Arriaga III *(not pictured)*,
GOODW.Y.N., and Hussein Smko

Hyde Park Art Center, March 17, 2023

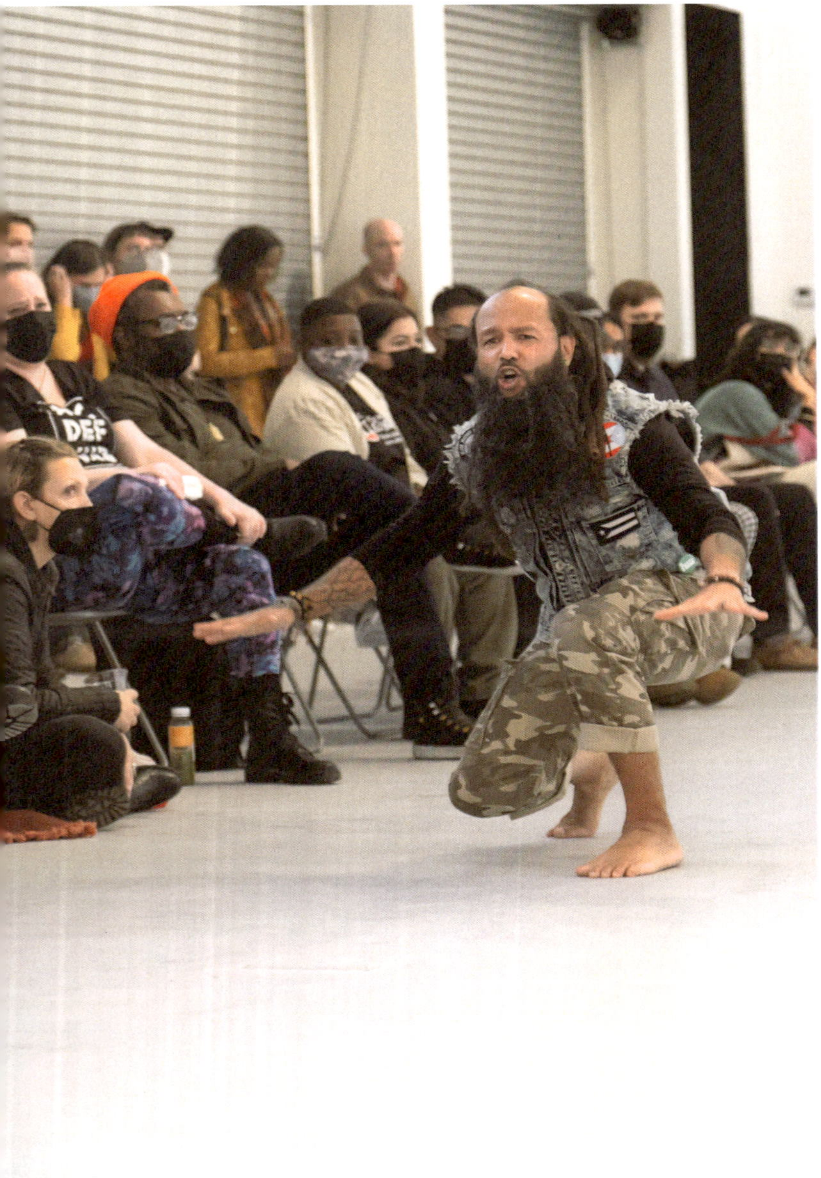

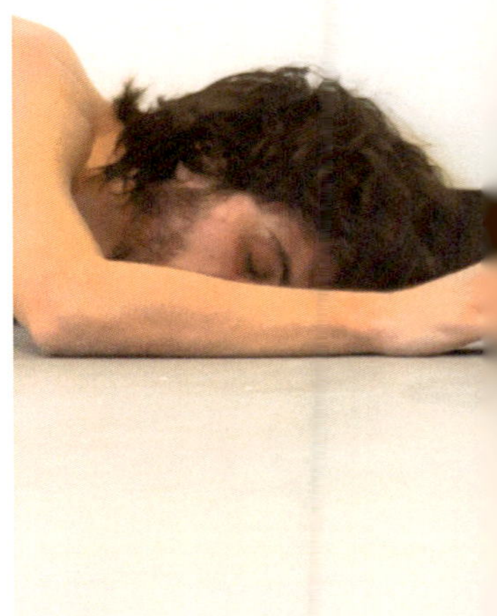

***THE SPACE BETWEEN: UNLIKELY ENTANGLEMENTS* OPENING PROGRAM**
with Hipólito Arriaga III, GOODW.Y.N., and Hussein Smko

Hyde Park Art Center, March 17, 2023

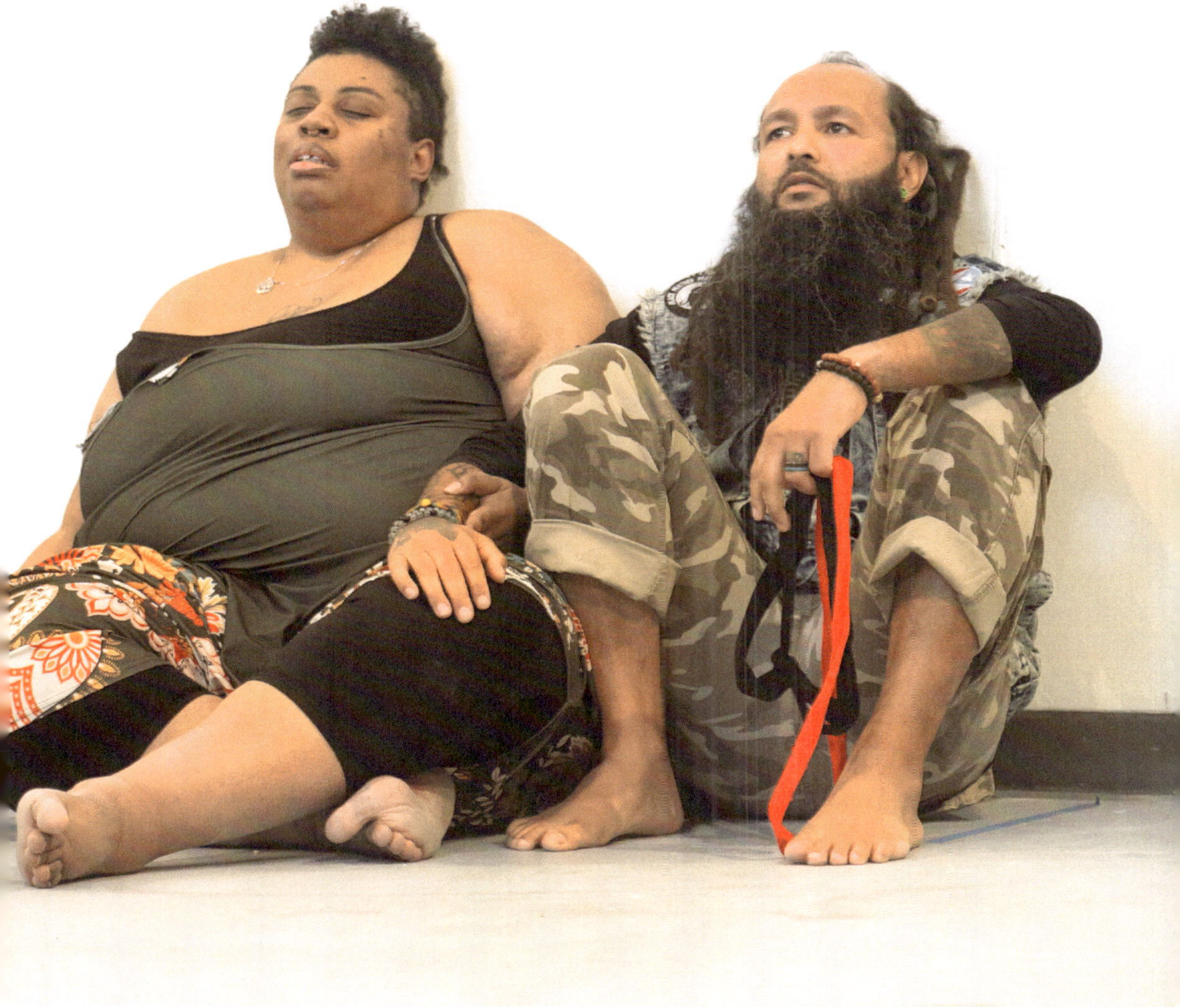

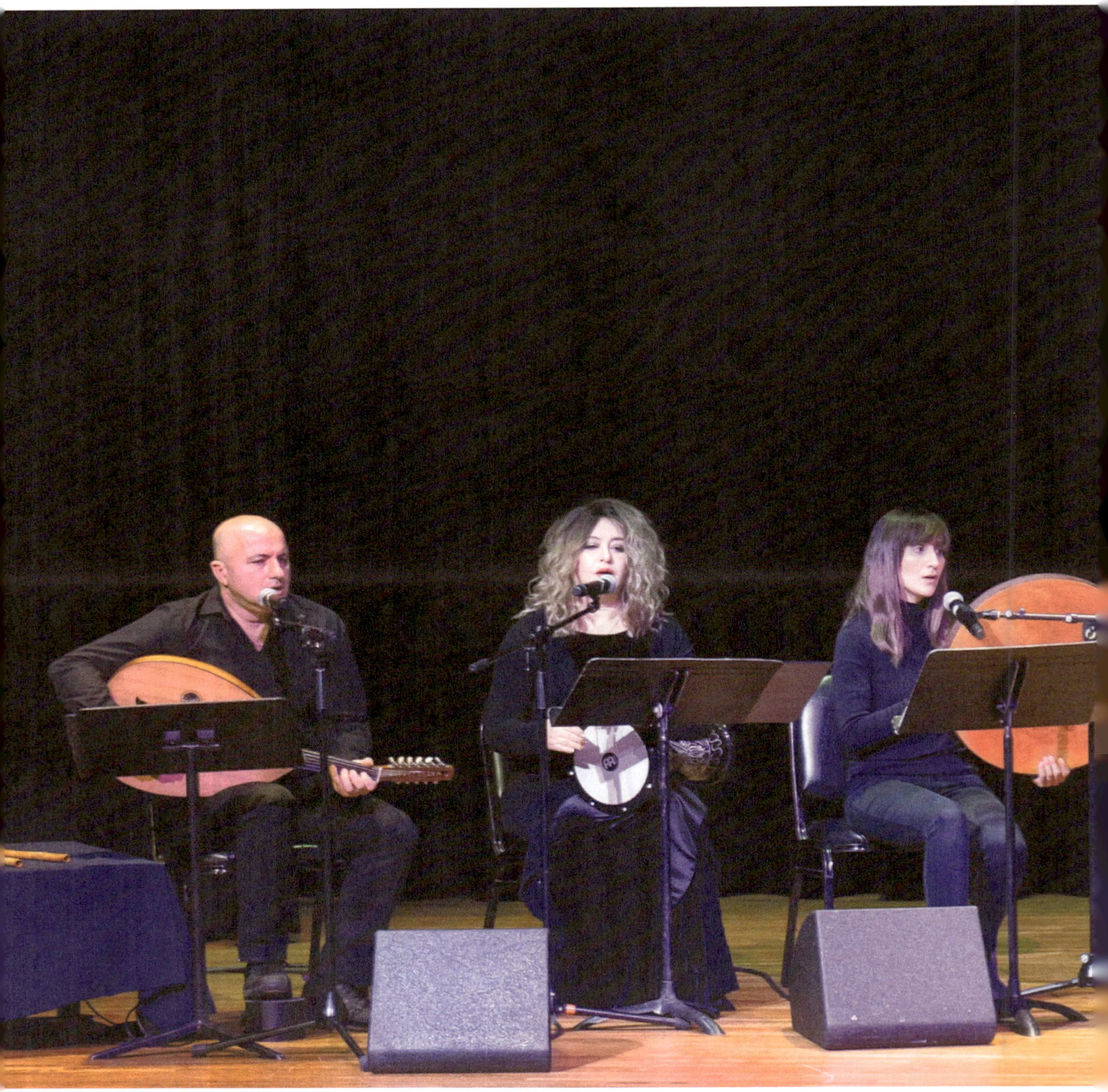

***DRONE*: TESTIMONIES & MUSIC**
with Andrea Assaf, Ashley Wilkerson, Anu Yadav, Nick Slie, Lubana Al Quntar, Aida Shahghasemi, and Zafer Tawil

Chicago Cultural Center, March 18, 2023

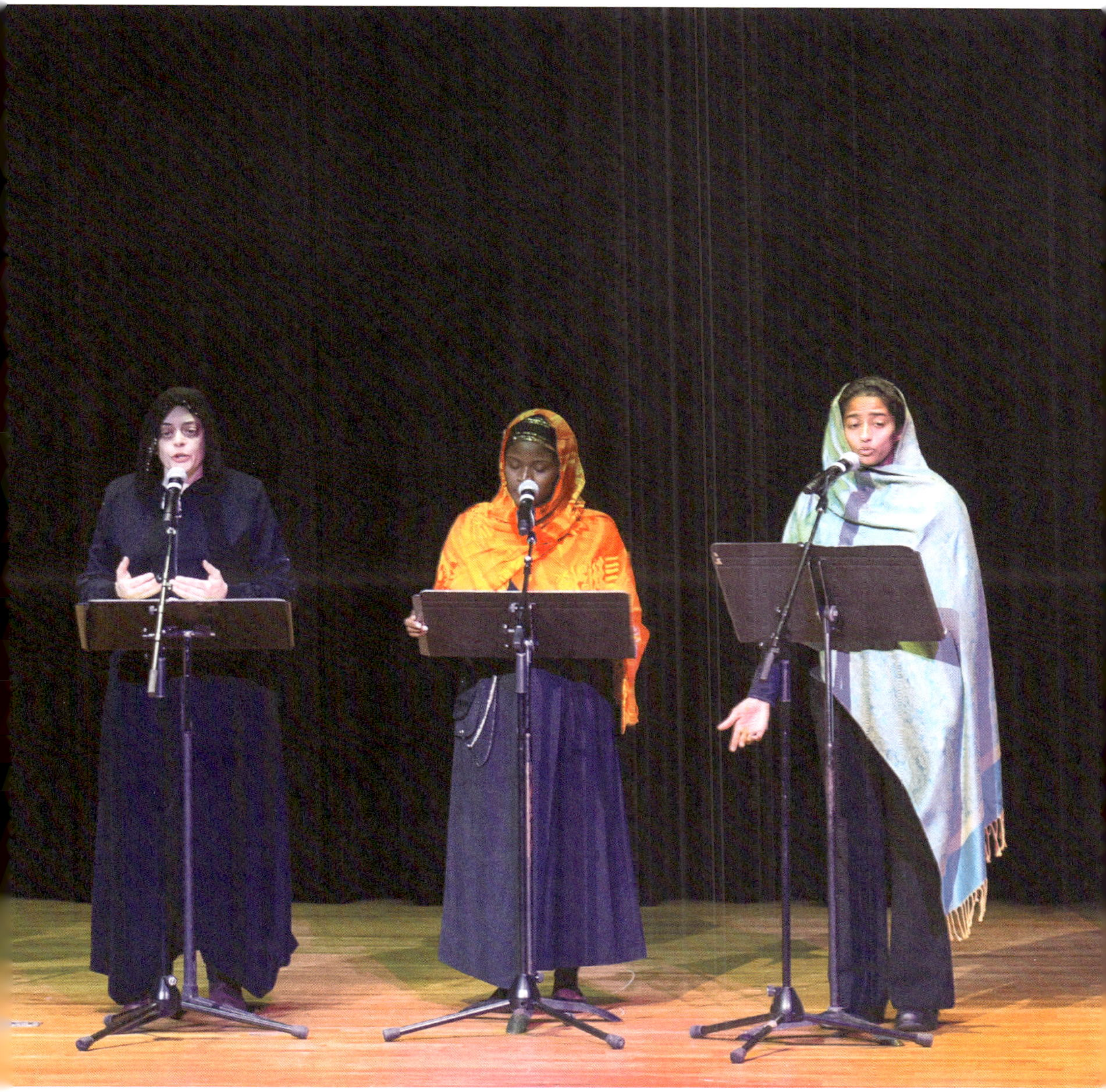

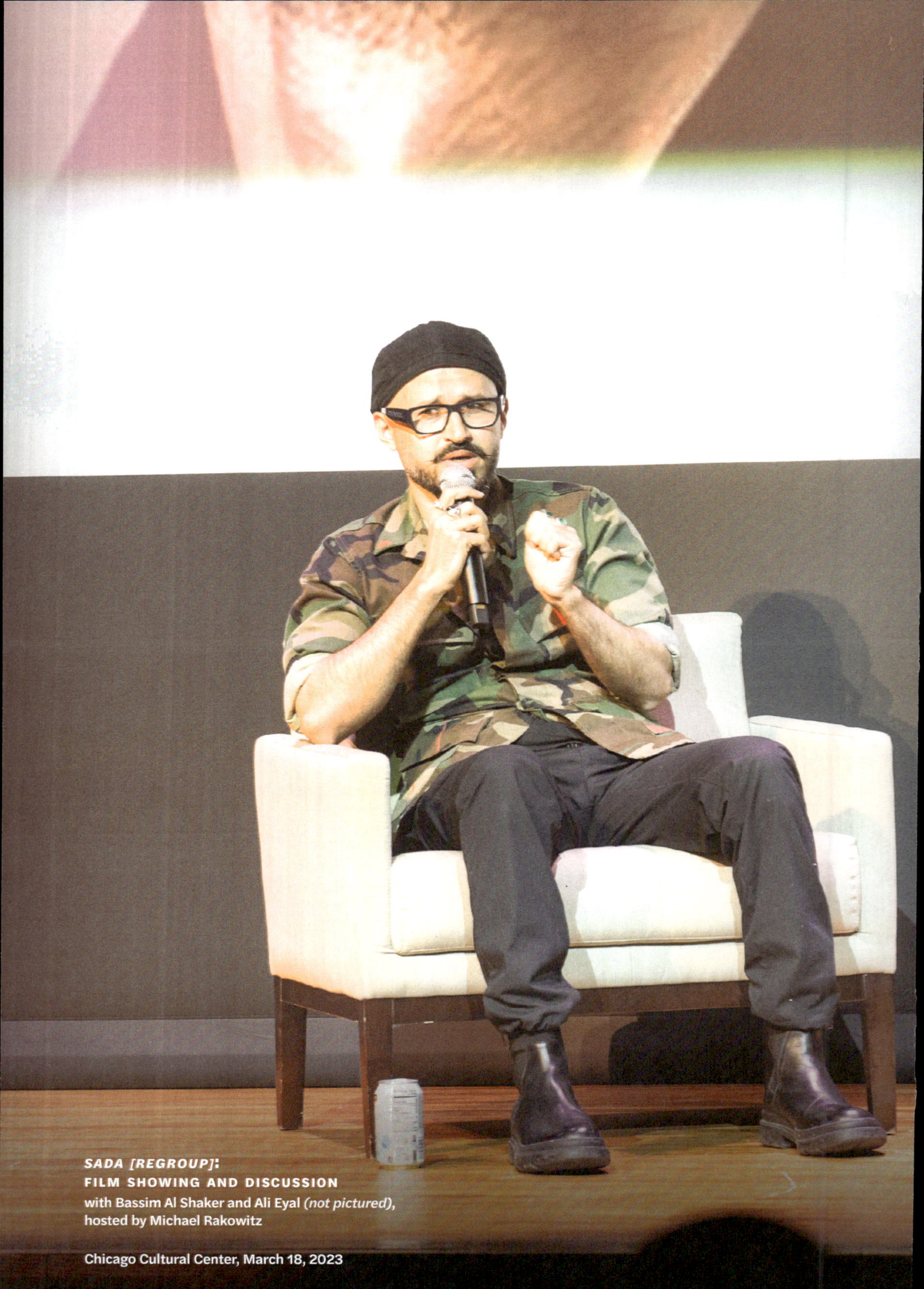

***SADA [REGROUP]*:**
FILM SHOWING AND DISCUSSION
with Bassim Al Shaker and Ali Eyal *(not pictured)*, hosted by Michael Rakowitz

Chicago Cultural Center, March 18, 2023

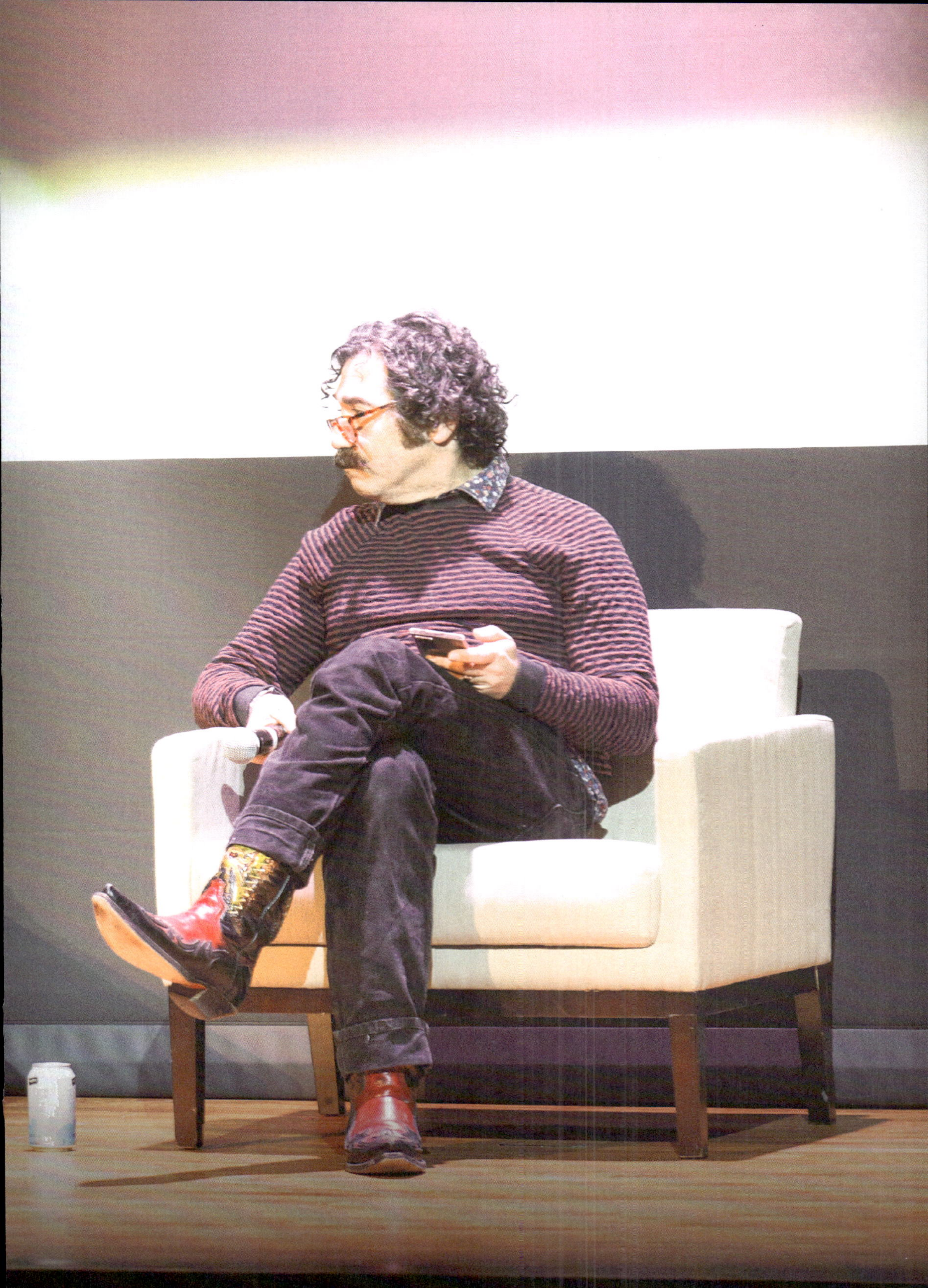

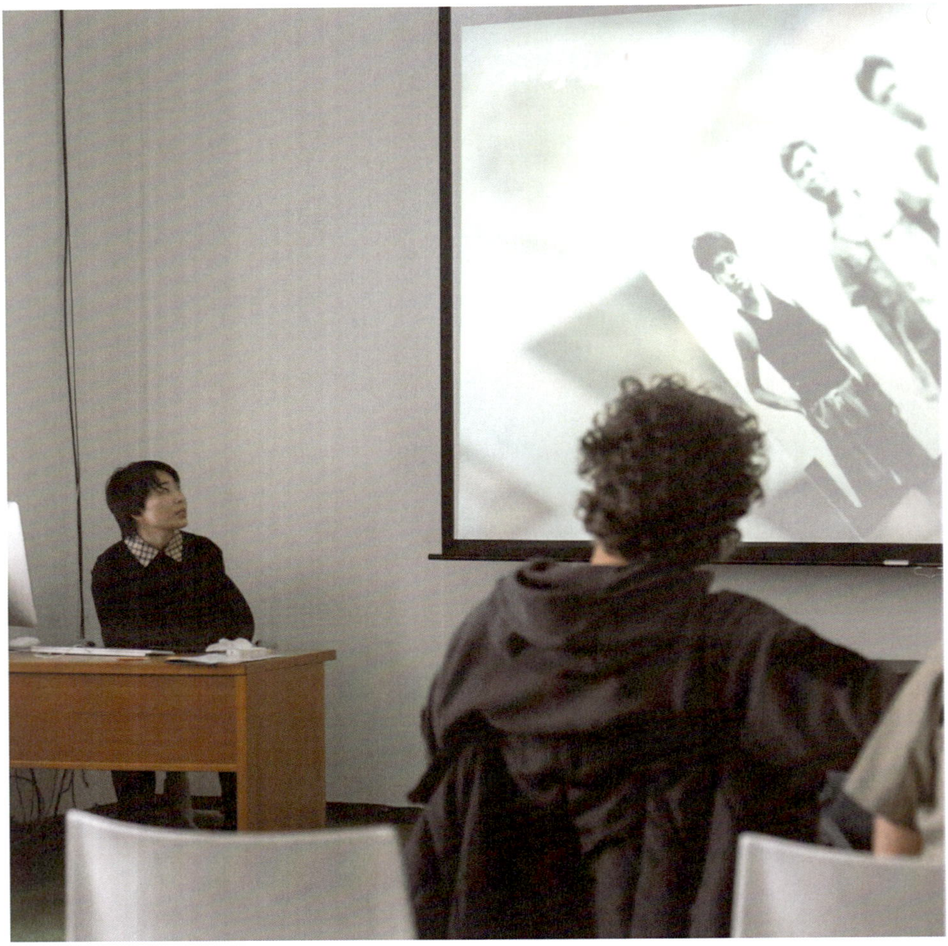

OPEN PLATFORM
with Youree Kim

Hyde Park Art Center, March 16, 2023

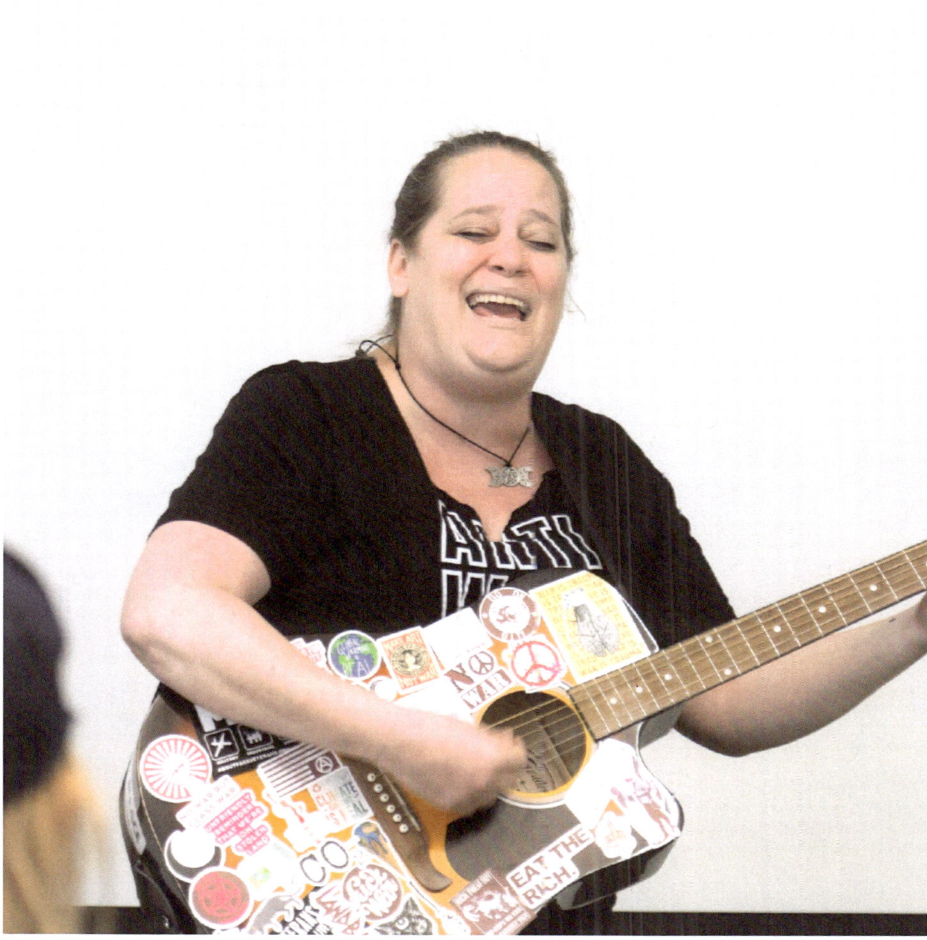

OPEN PLATFORM
with Jules Vaquera

Hyde Park Art Center, March 16, 2023

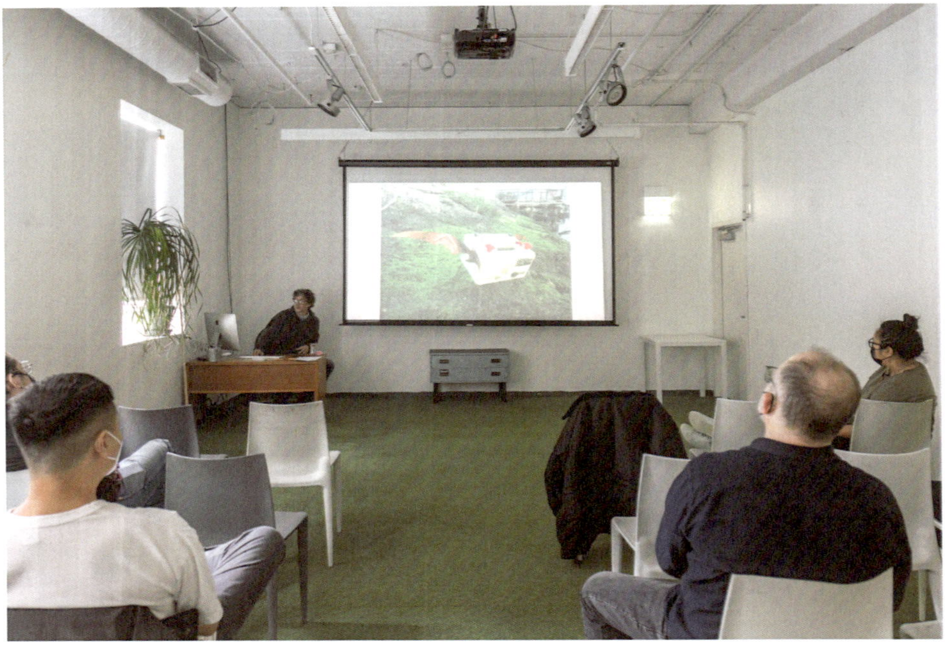

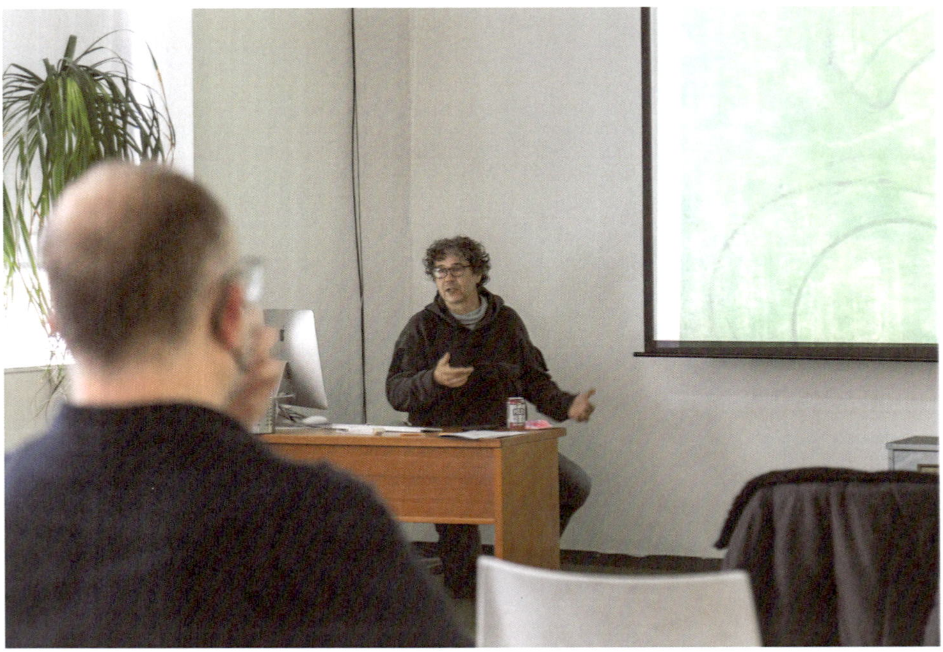

OPEN PLATFORM
with John Colle Rogers

Hyde Park Art Center, March 16, 2023

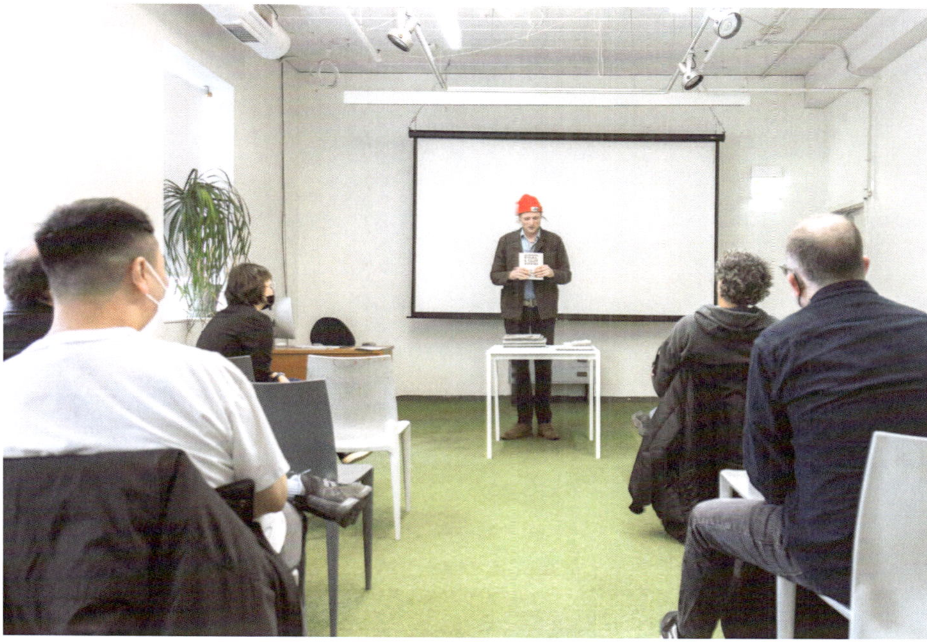

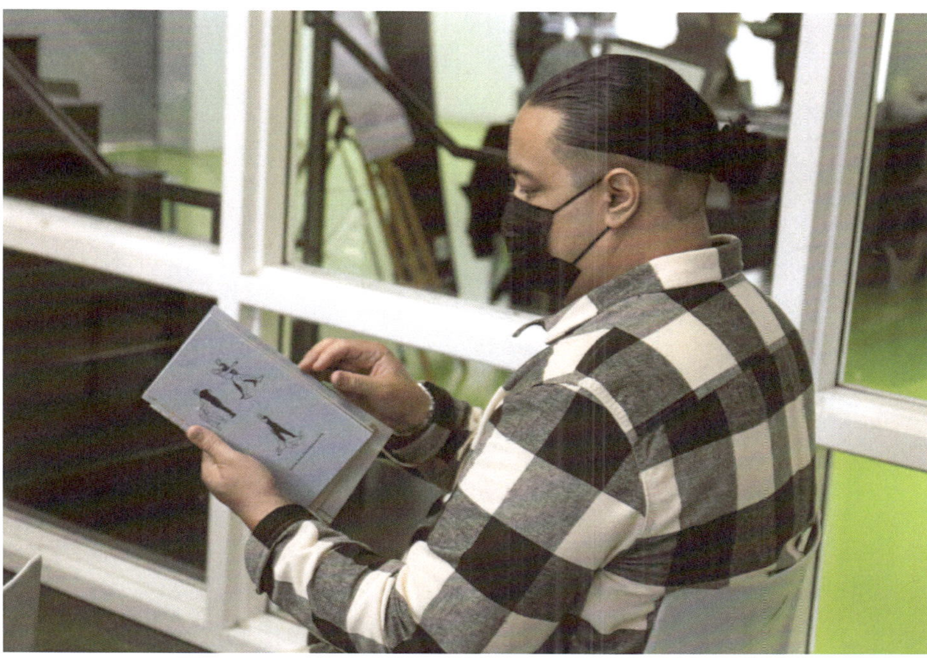

OPEN PLATFORM
with Nathan Lewis *(continued on next spread)*

Hyde Park Art Center, March 16, 2023

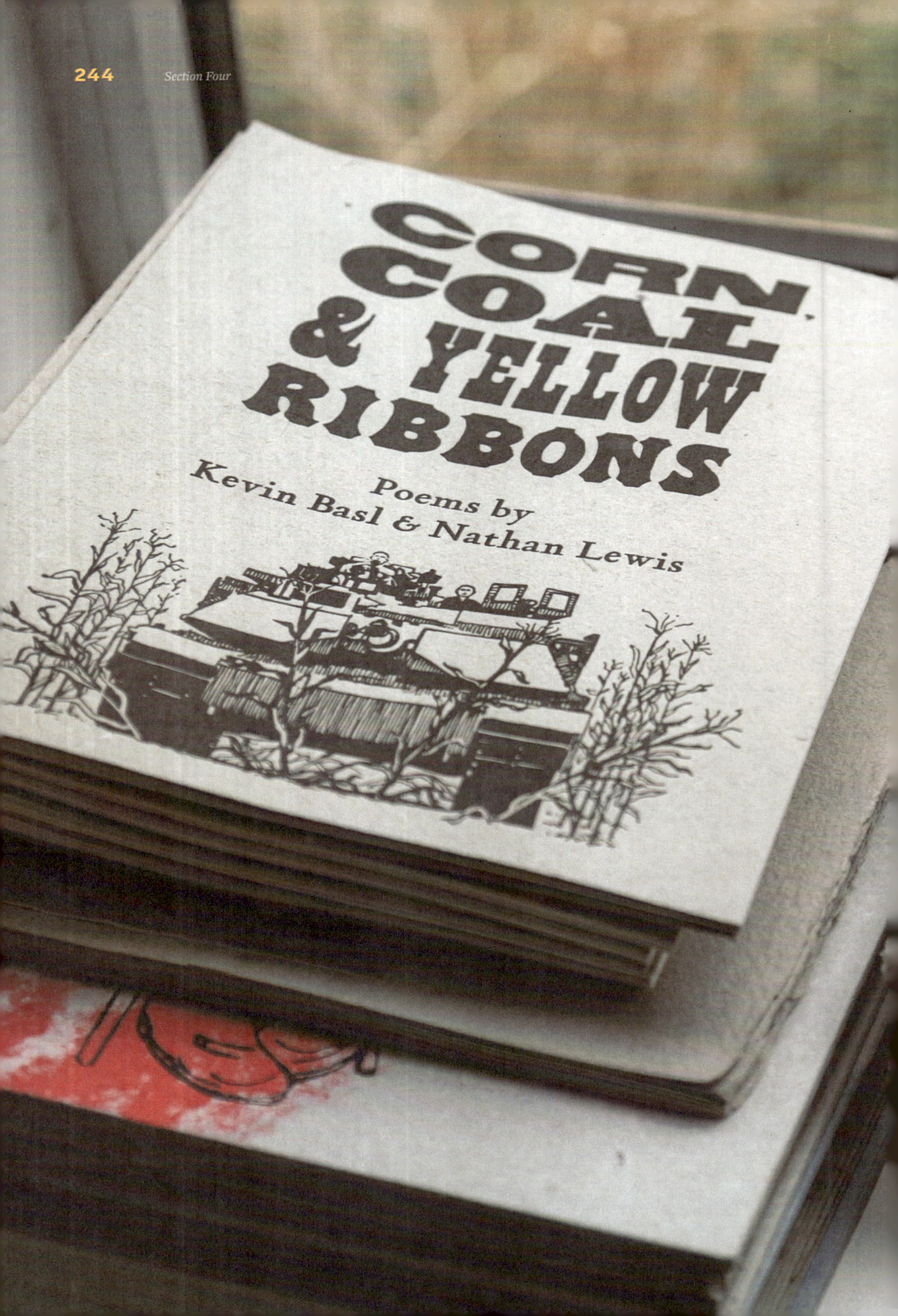
CORN, COAL & YELLOW RIBBONS
Poems by
Kevin Basl & Nathan Lewis

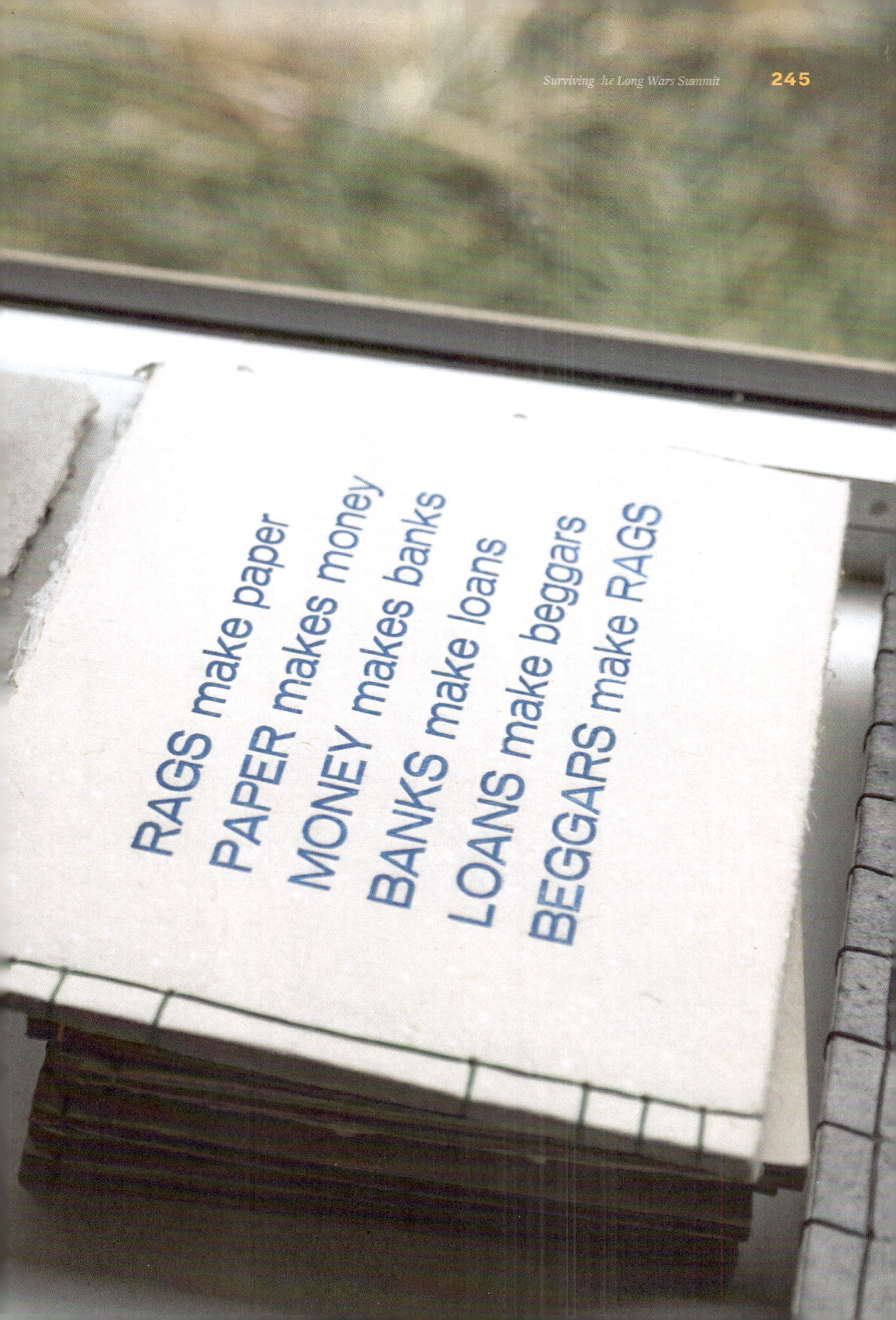
RAGS make paper
PAPER makes money
MONEY makes banks
BANKS make loans
LOANS make beggars
BEGGARS make RAGS

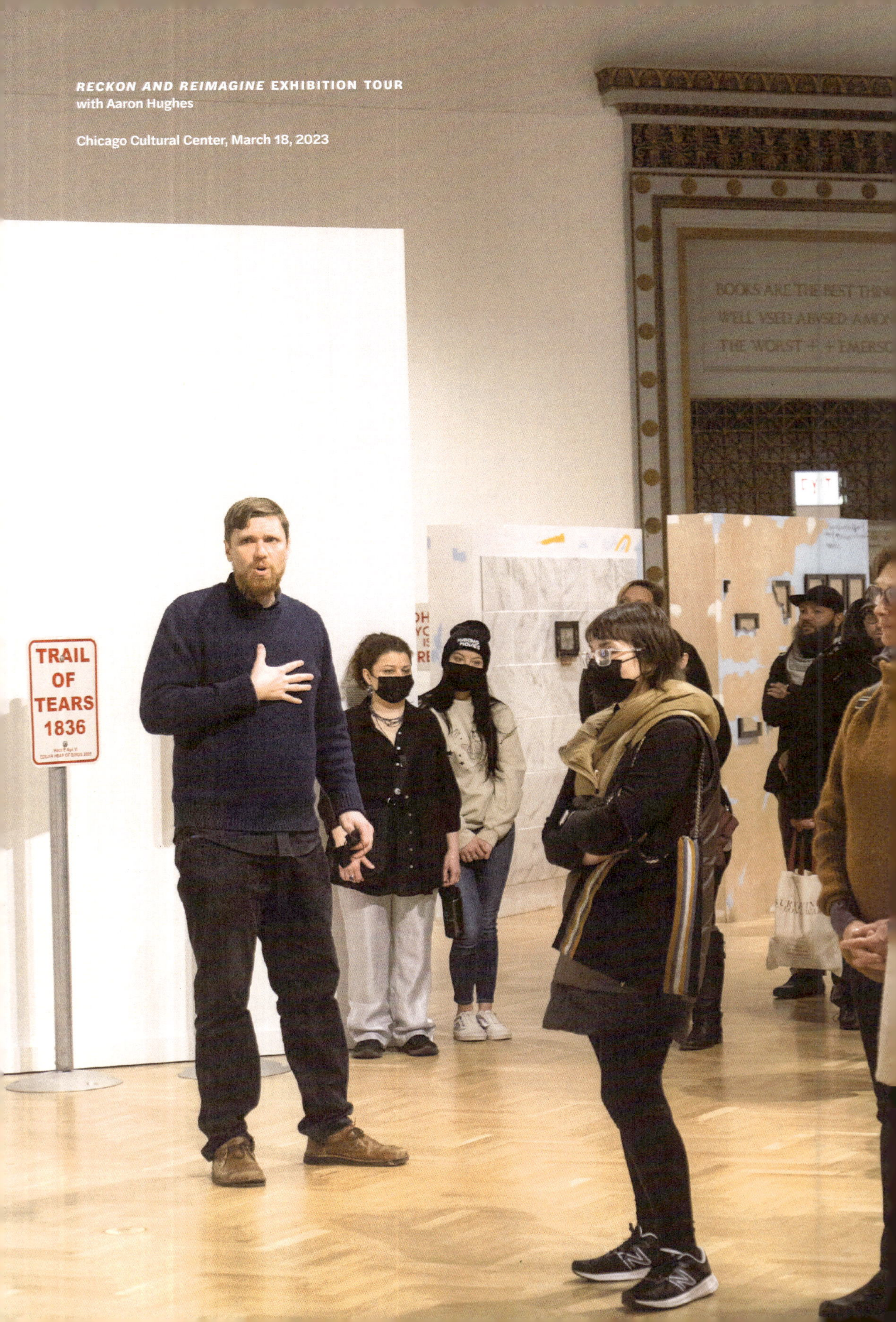

RECKON AND REIMAGINE **EXHIBITION TOUR**
with Aaron Hughes

Chicago Cultural Center, March 18, 2023

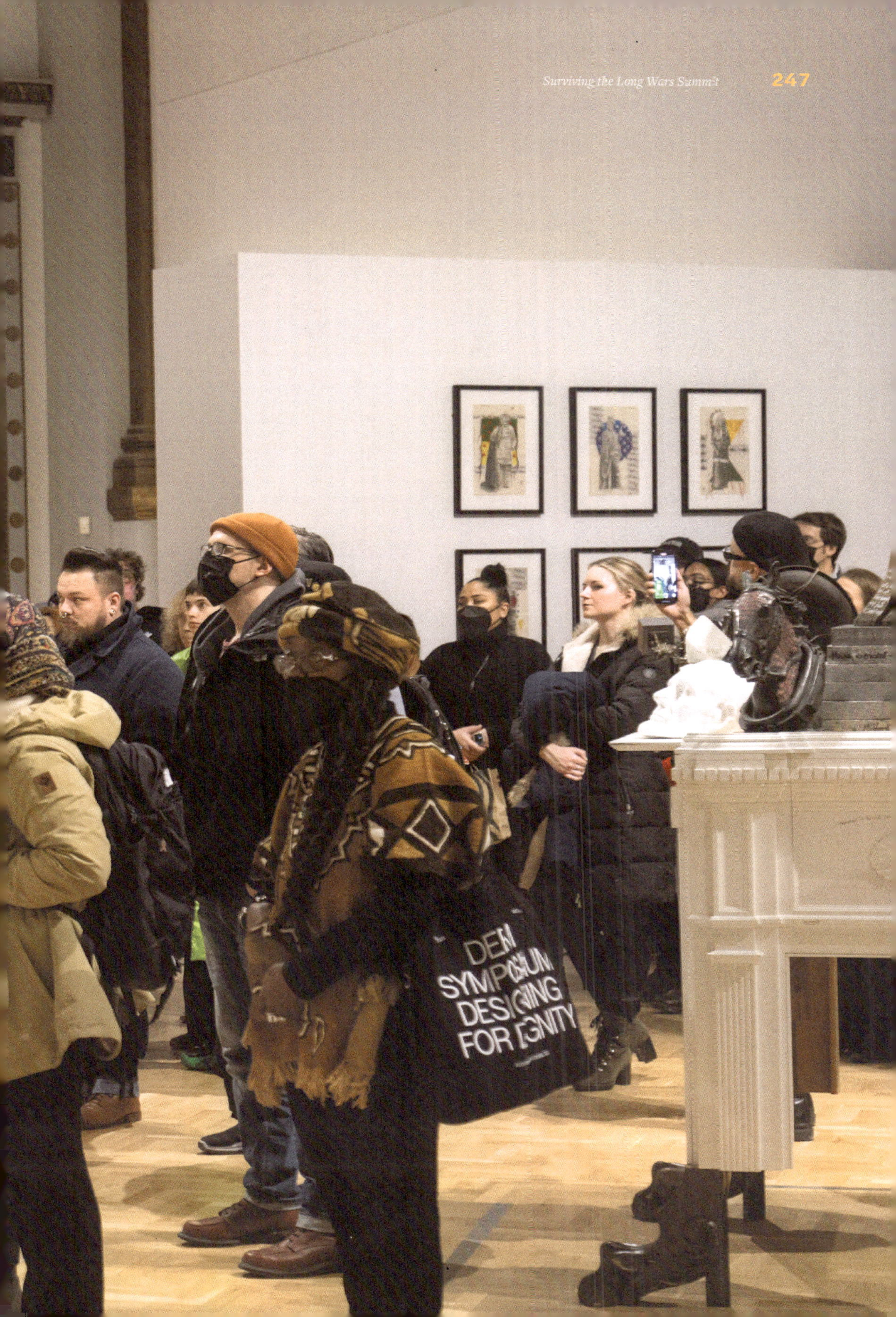

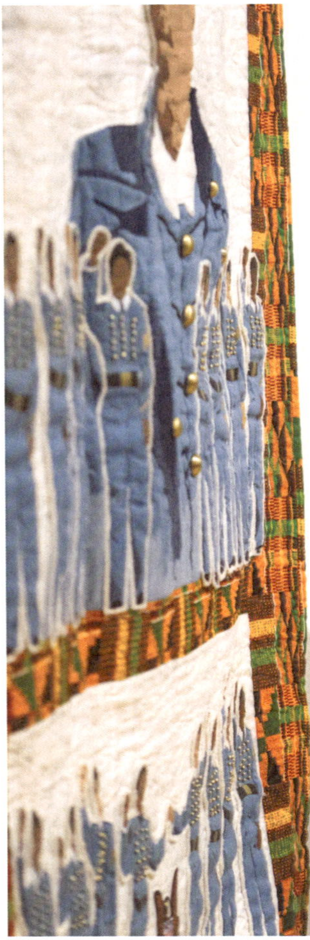

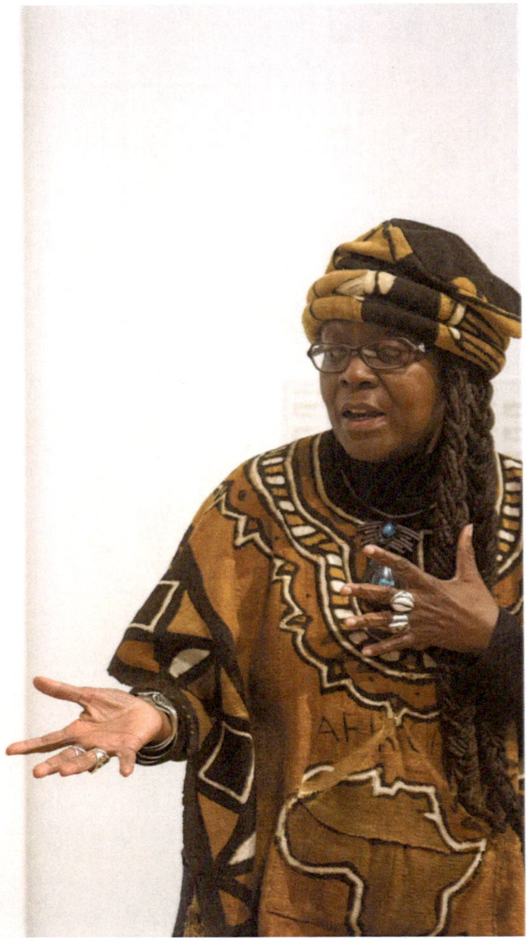

RECKON AND REIMAGINE **EXHIBITION TOUR**
with Dorothy Burge

Chicago Cultural Center, March 18, 2023
see also: pp. 92–93, 113

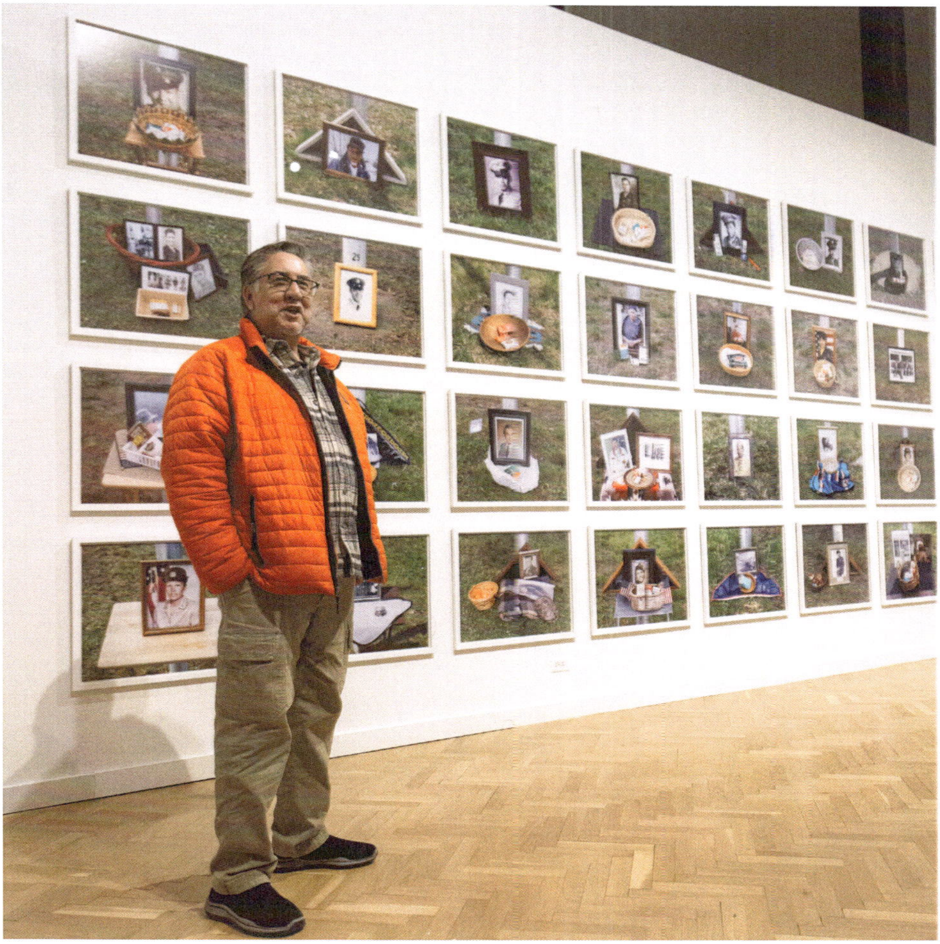

RECKON AND REIMAGINE **EXHIBITION TOUR**
with Tom Jones

Chicago Cultural Center, March 18, 2023
see also: pp. 116–17

***RECKON AND REIMAGINE* EXHIBITION**
with work from Miridith Campbell and Melissa Doud

Chicago Cultural Center, March 18, 2023
see also: pp. 71, 88–91, 319

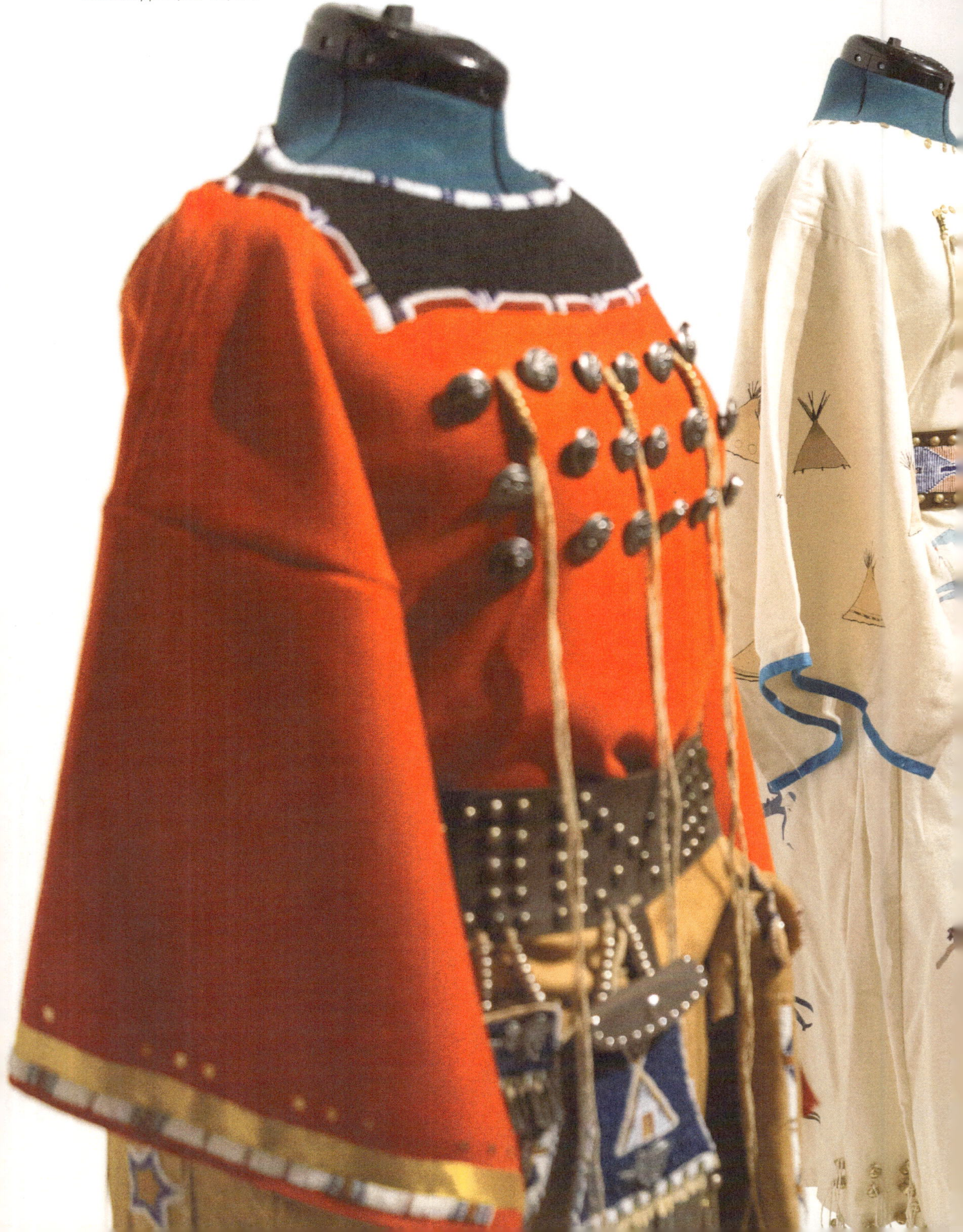

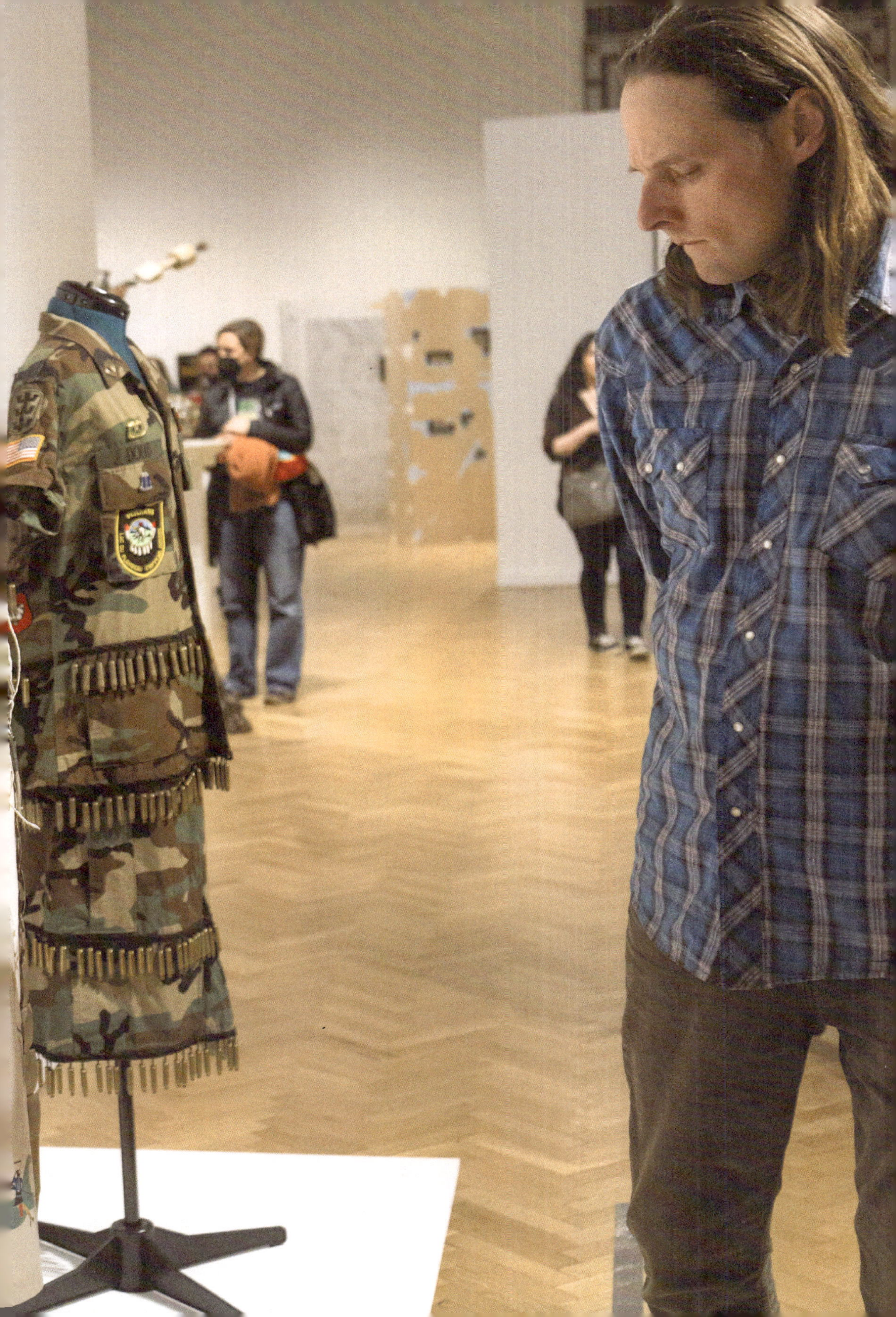

***UNLIKELY ENTANGLEMENTS* EXHIBITION TOUR**

Hyde Park Art Center,
March 17, 2023

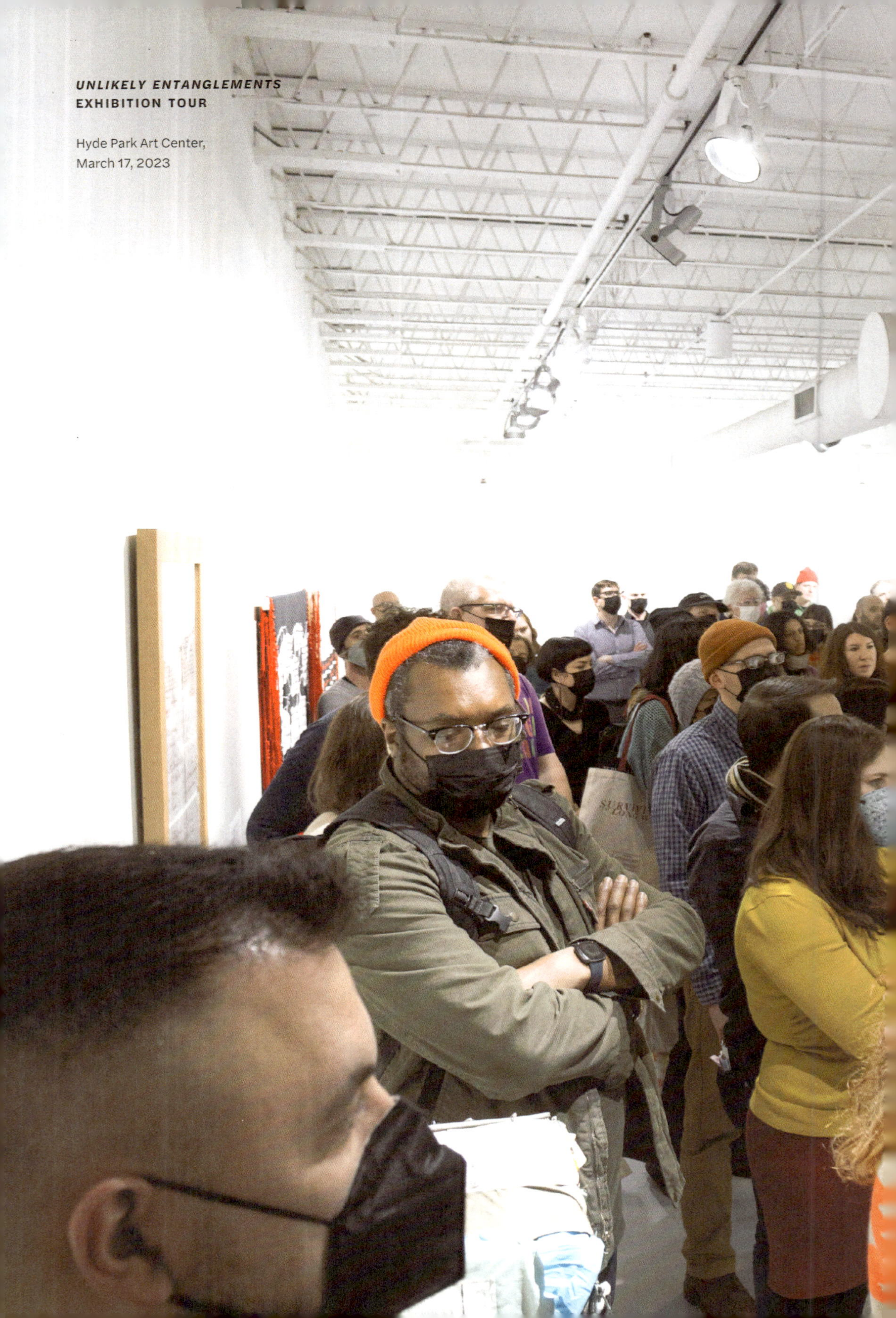

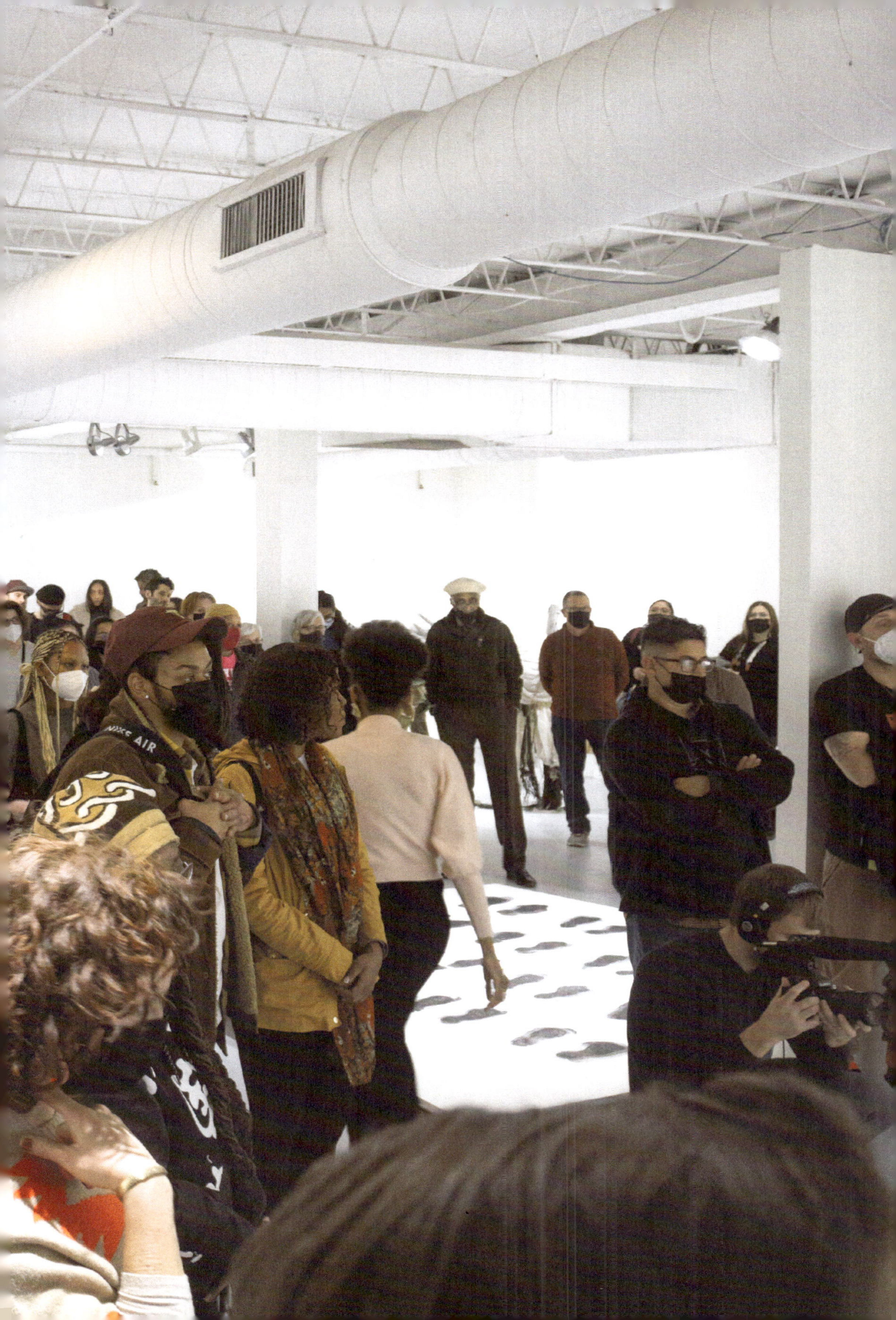
NIKE AIR

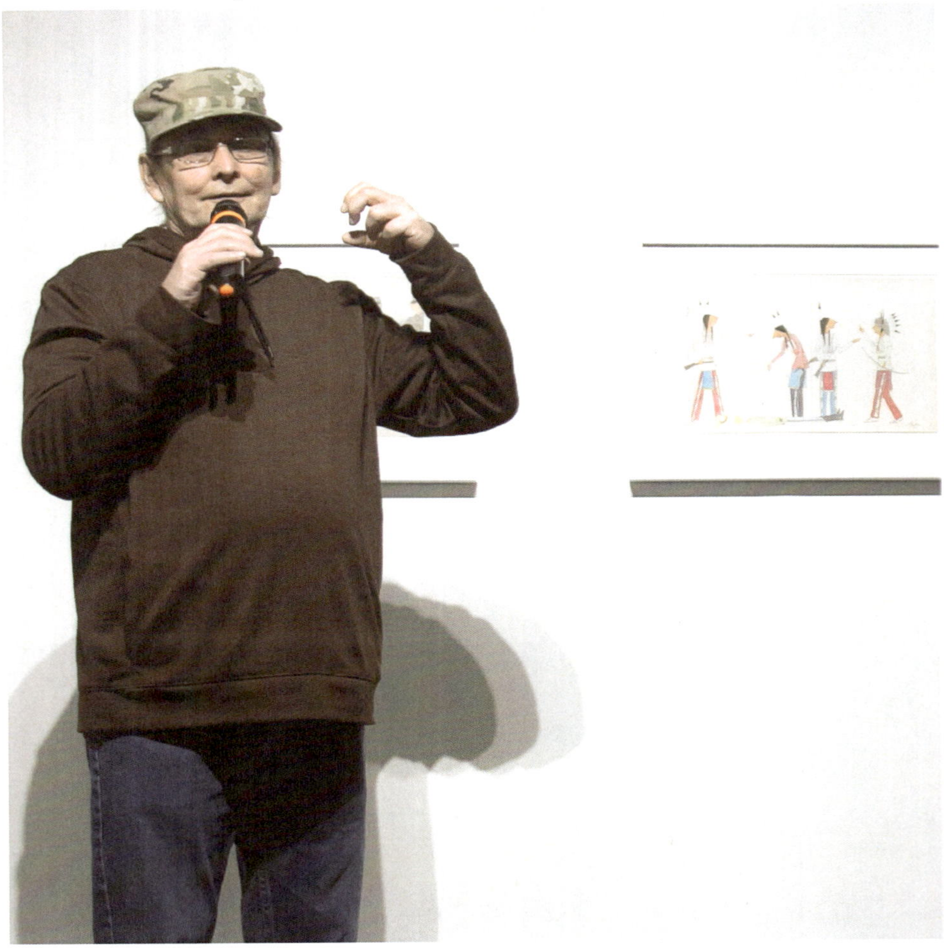

UNLIKELY ENTANGLEMENTS **EXHIBITION TOUR**
with Dwayne Wilcox

Hyde Park Art Center, March 17, 2023
see also: pp. 188–89, 200

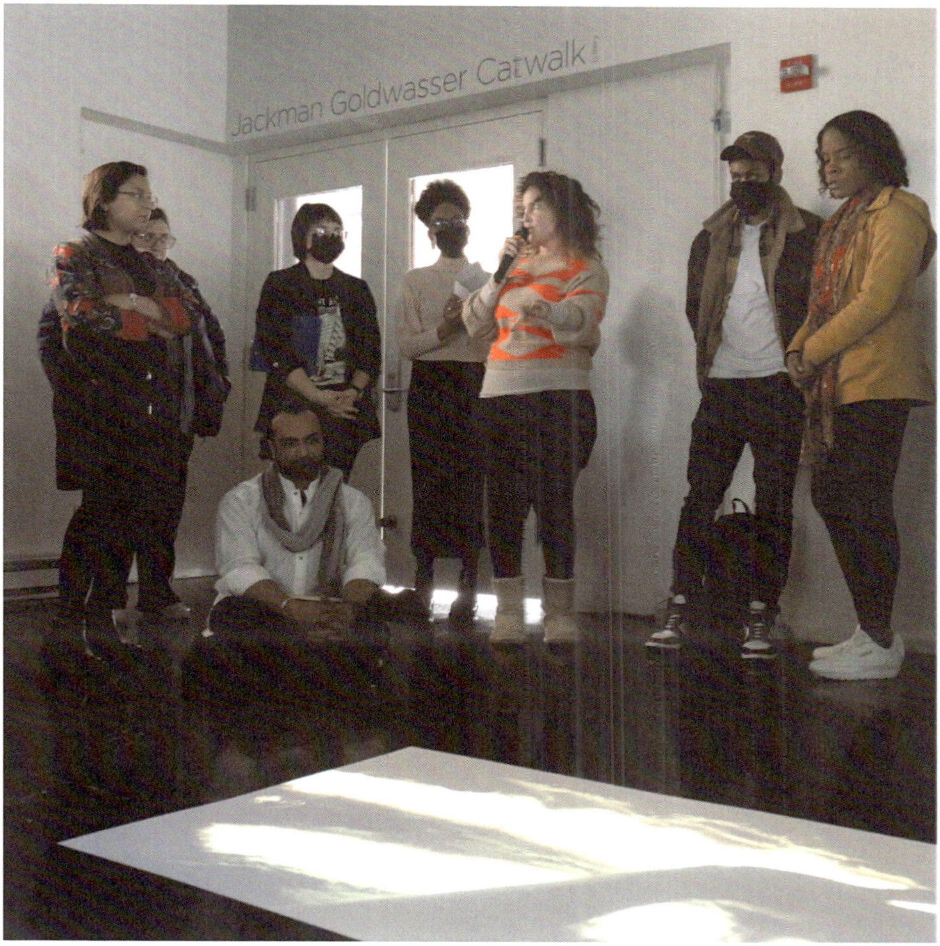

UNLIKELY ENTANGLEMENTS
EXHIBITION TOUR
with Sarah Farahat

Hyde Park Art Center, March 17, 2023
see also: pp. 194–95

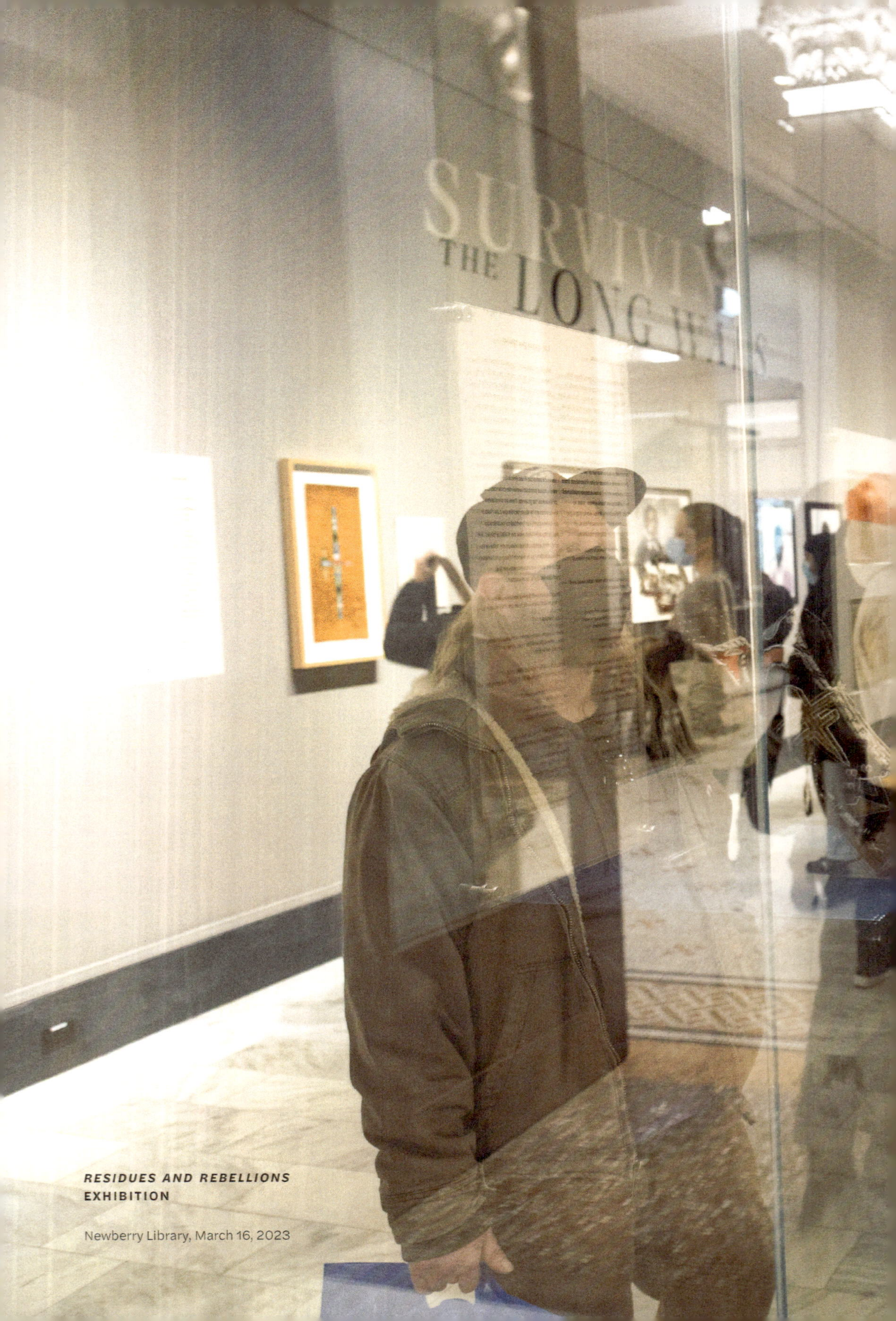

***RESIDUES AND REBELLIONS* EXHIBITION**

Newberry Library, March 16, 2023

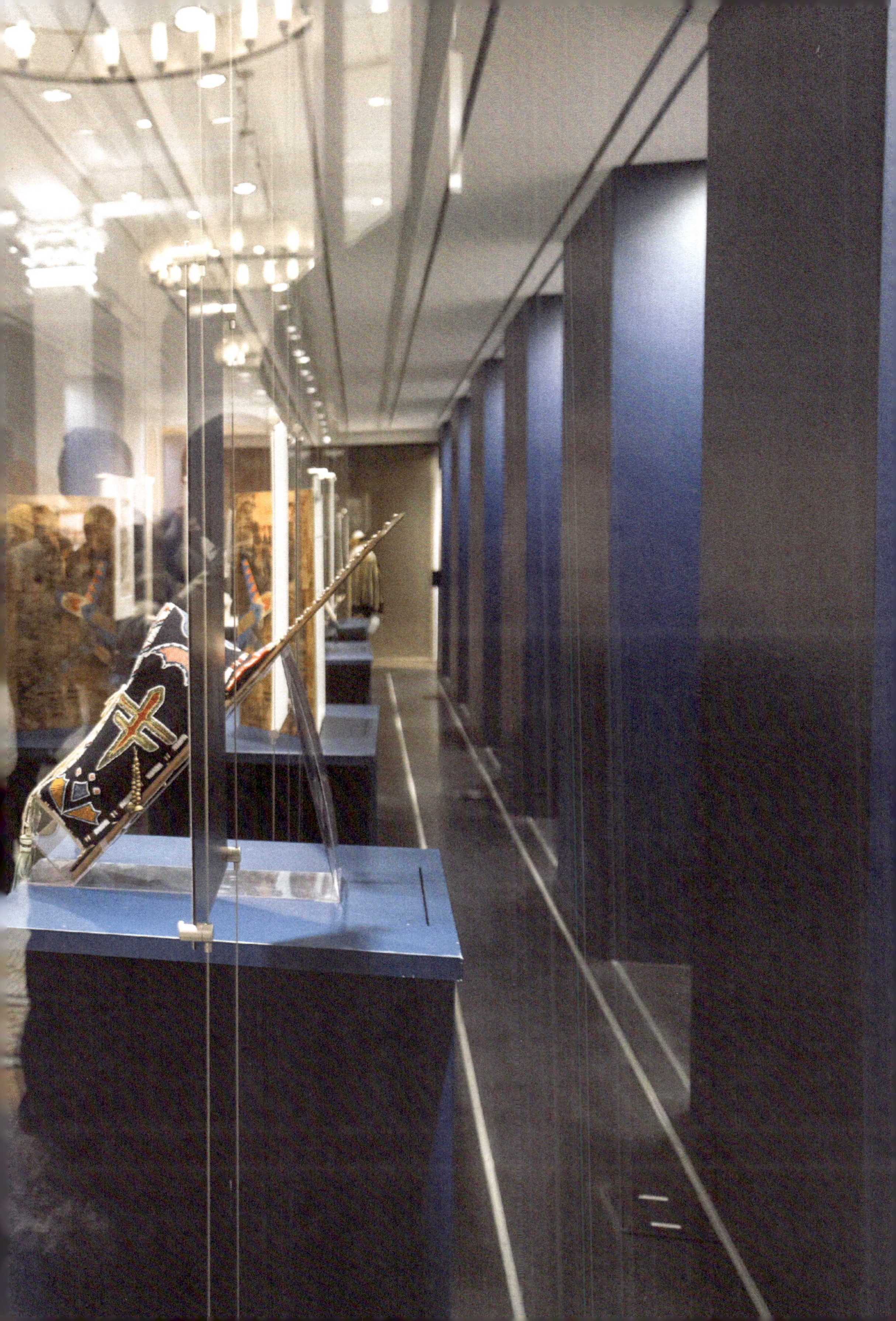

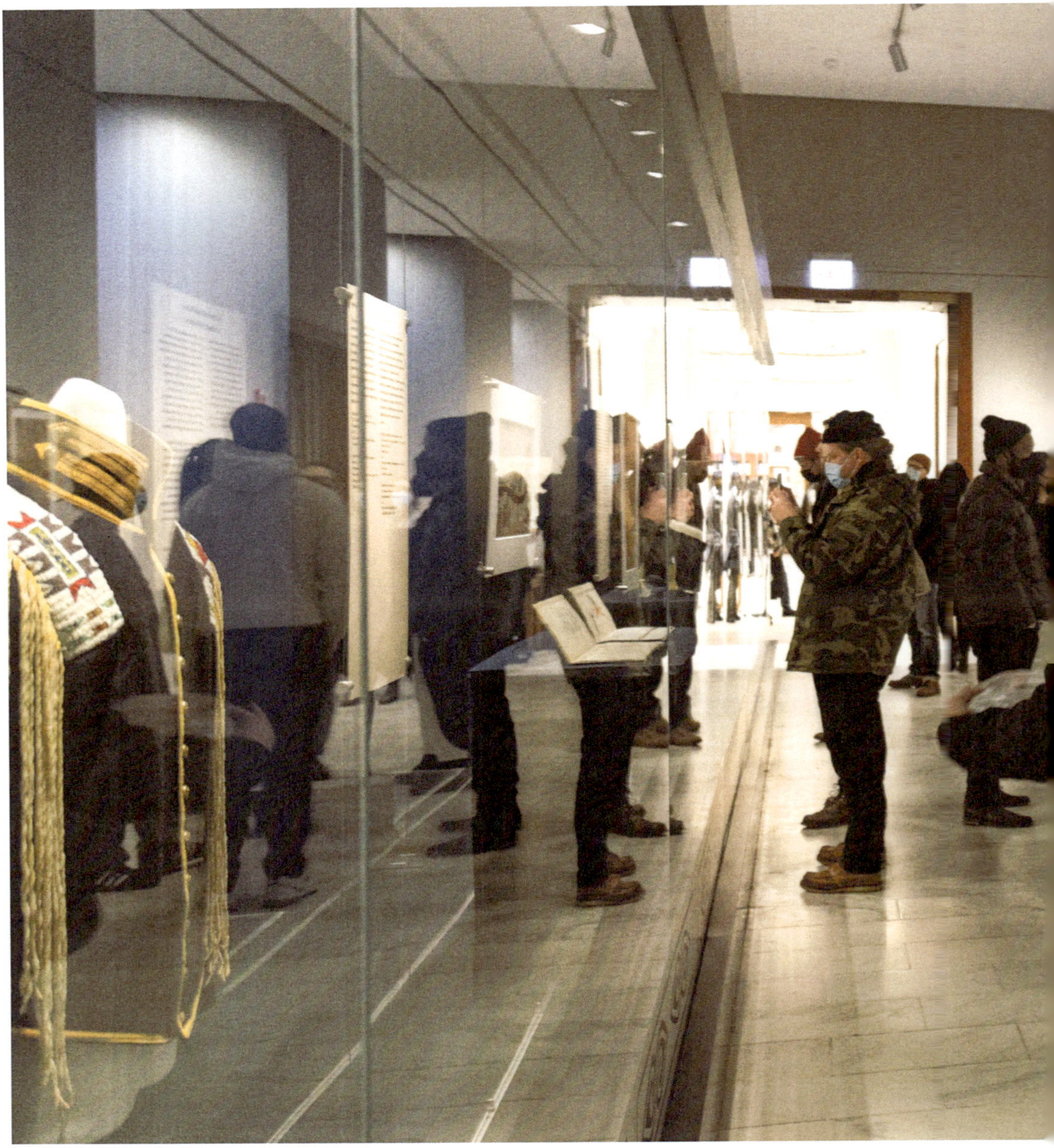

***RESIDUES AND REBELLIONS* EXHIBITION**

Newberry Library, March 16, 2023

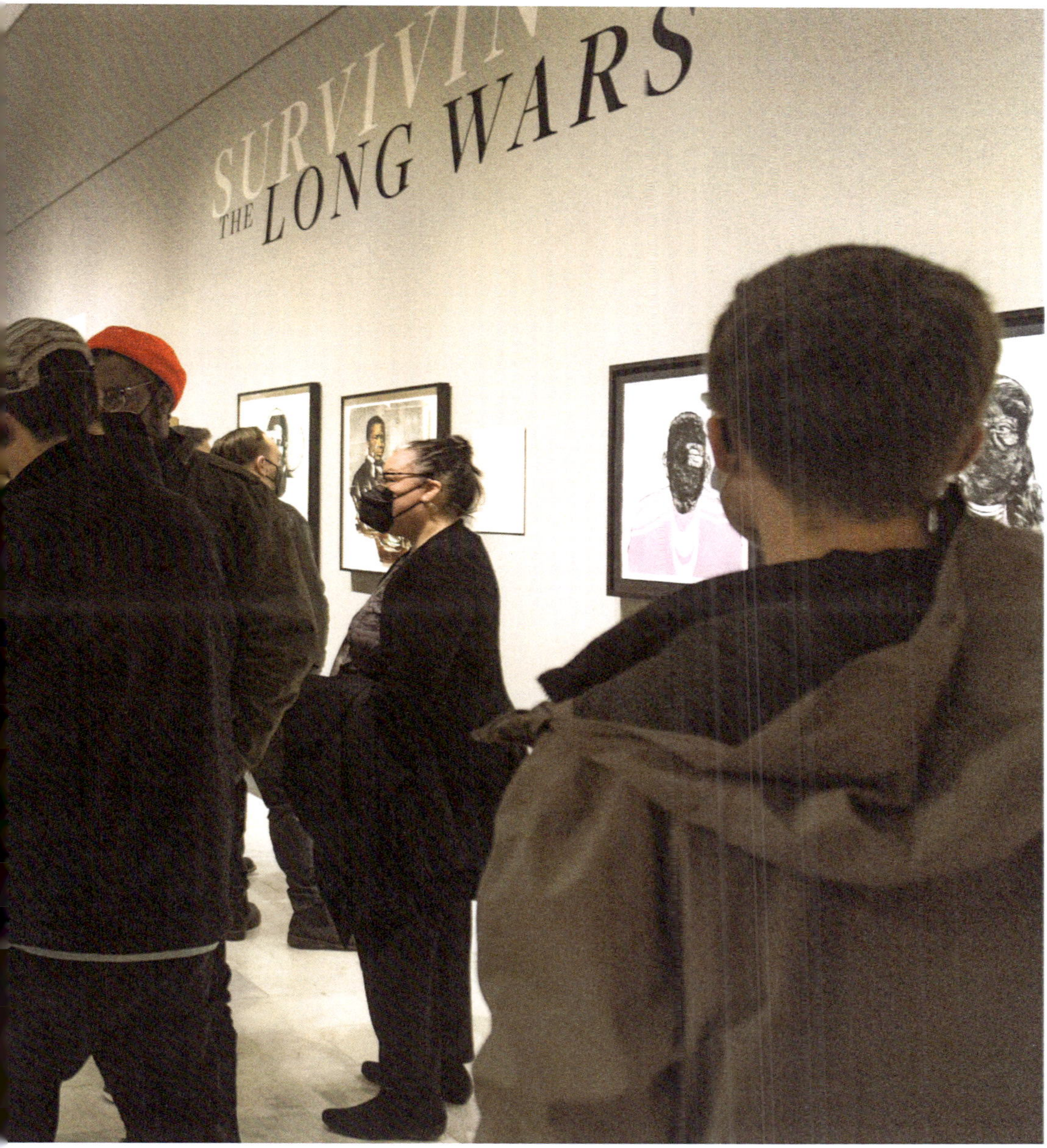
SURVIVIN
THE LONG WARS

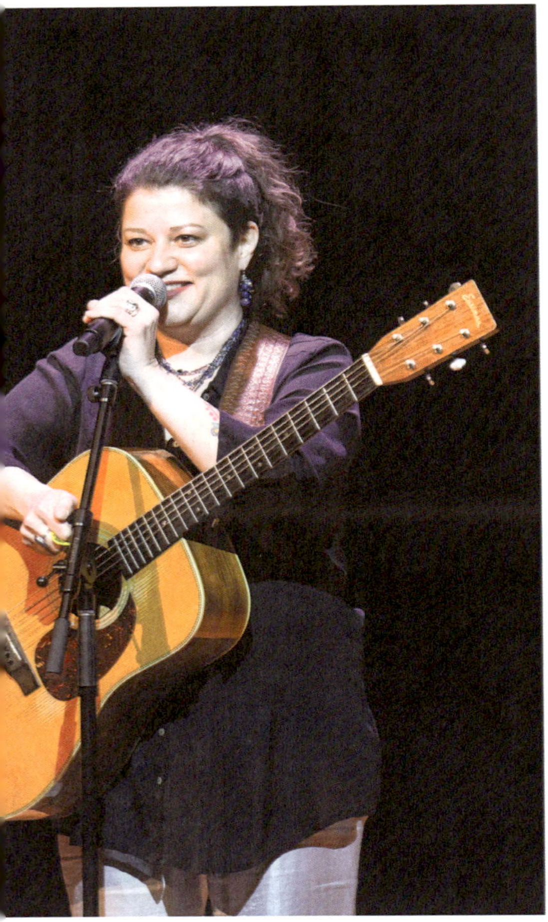

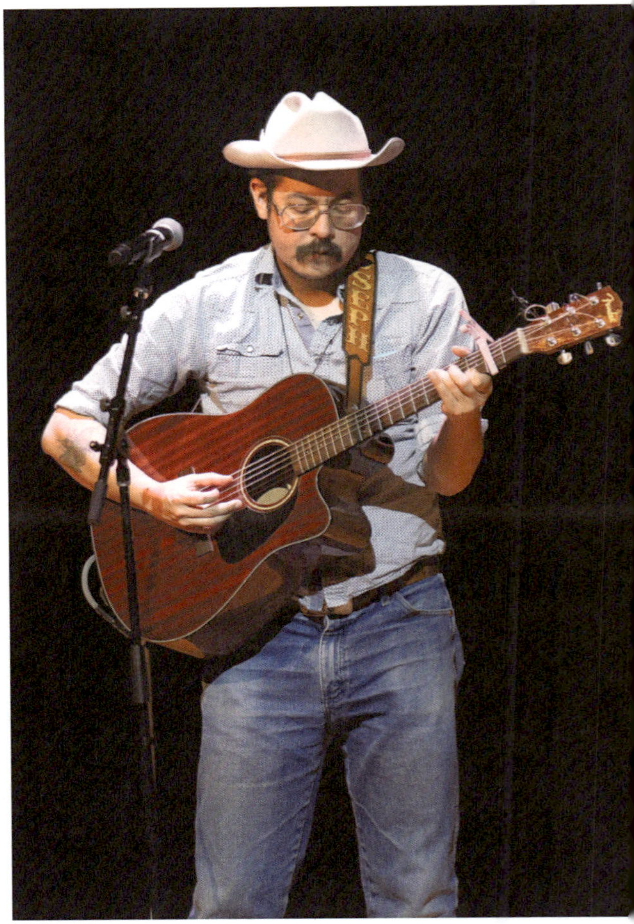

FORGING HOPE: RECKON AND REIMAGINE
OPENING PROGRAM
with *(left to right)* Elexa Dawson, Joseph Running Crane, Brittney Chantele, and James Pakootas

Chicago Cultural Center, March 18, 2023

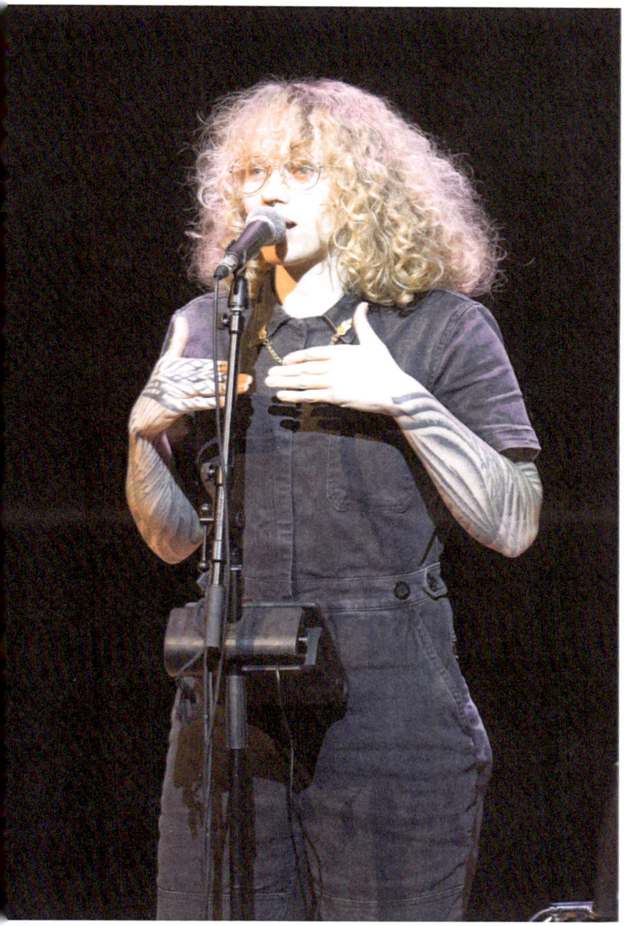

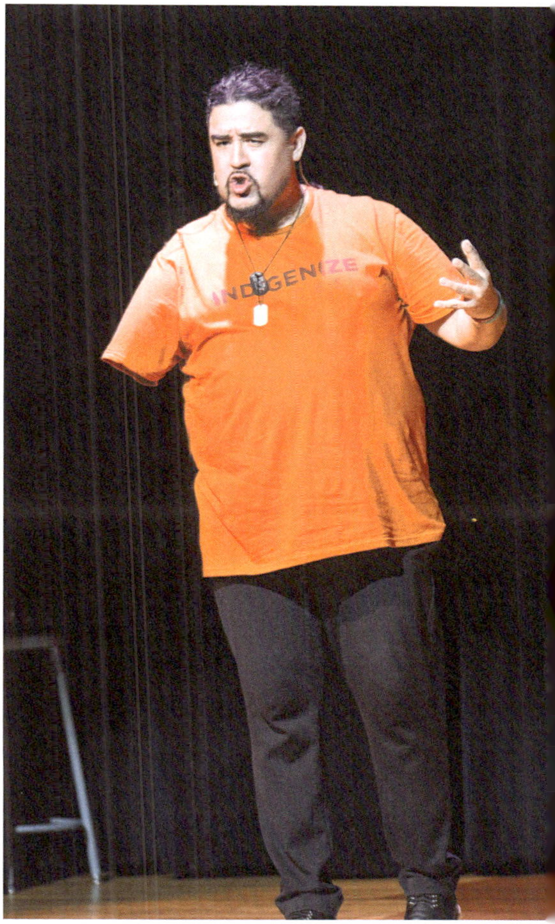

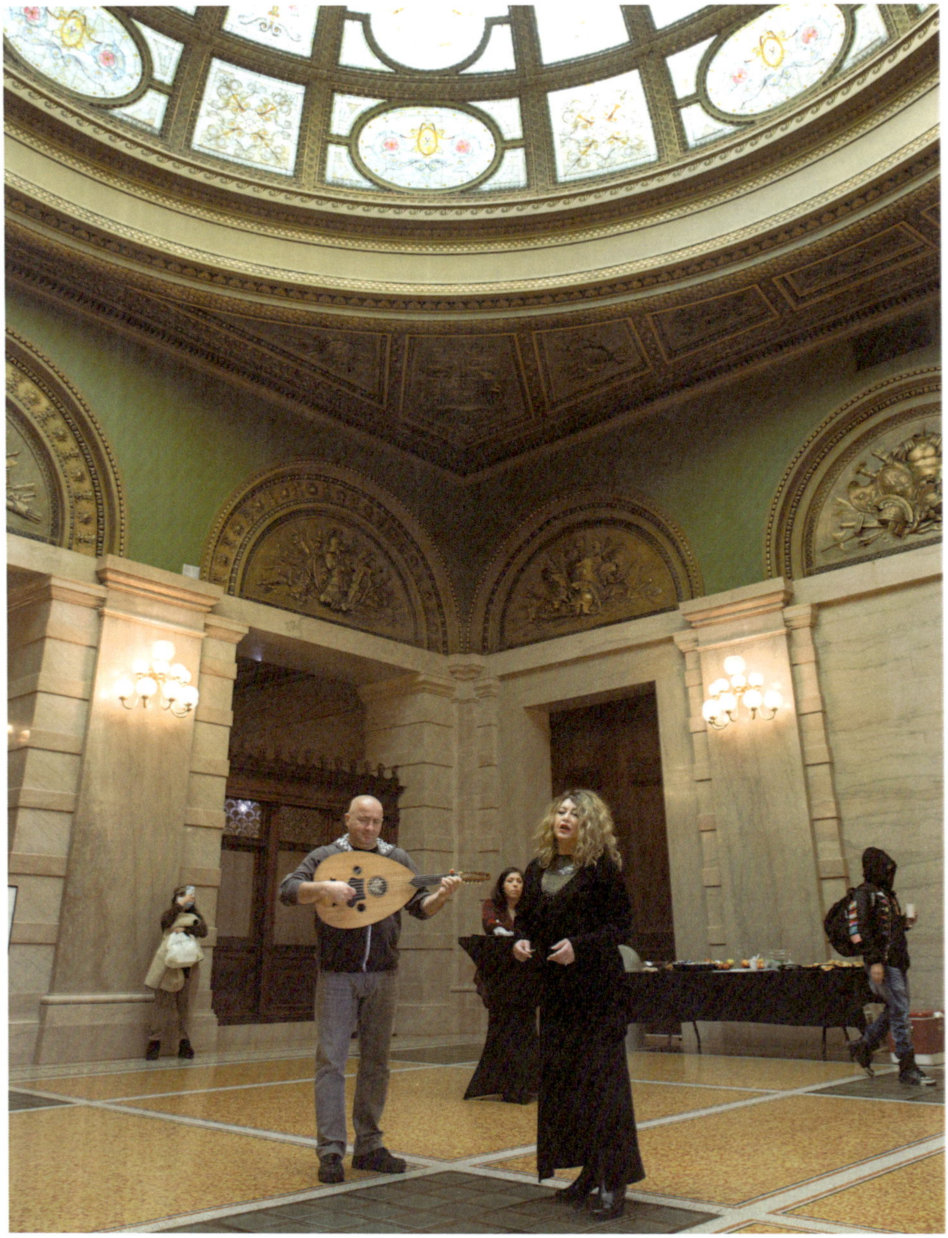

IMPROMPTU PERFORMANCE
with DRONE performers *(above)* Lubana al Quntar and Zafer Tawil and *(right)* Aida Shahghasemi and Anu Yadav

Chicago Cultural Center, Grand Army of the Republic Memorial Rotunda, March 19, 2023

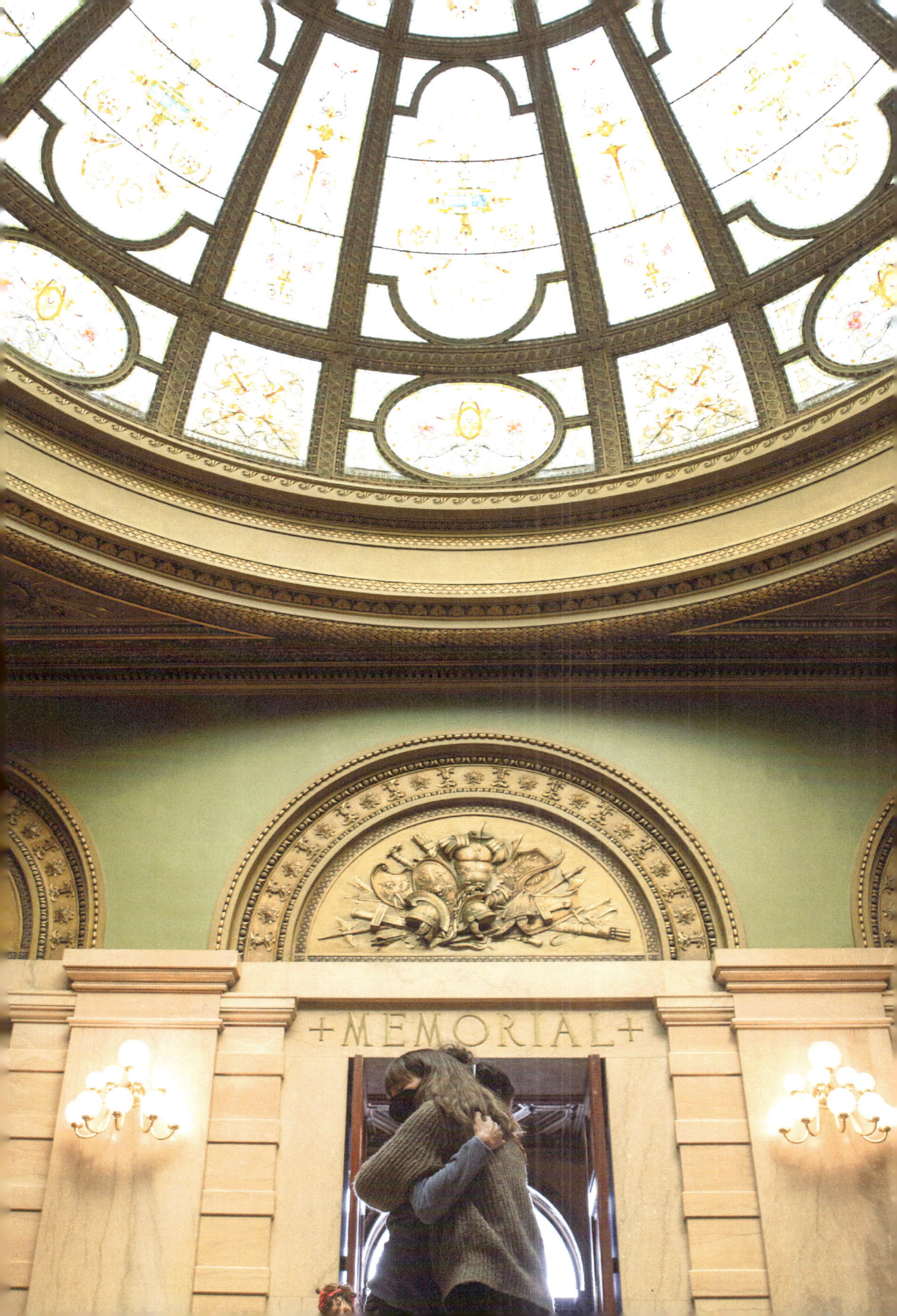
+MEMORIAL+

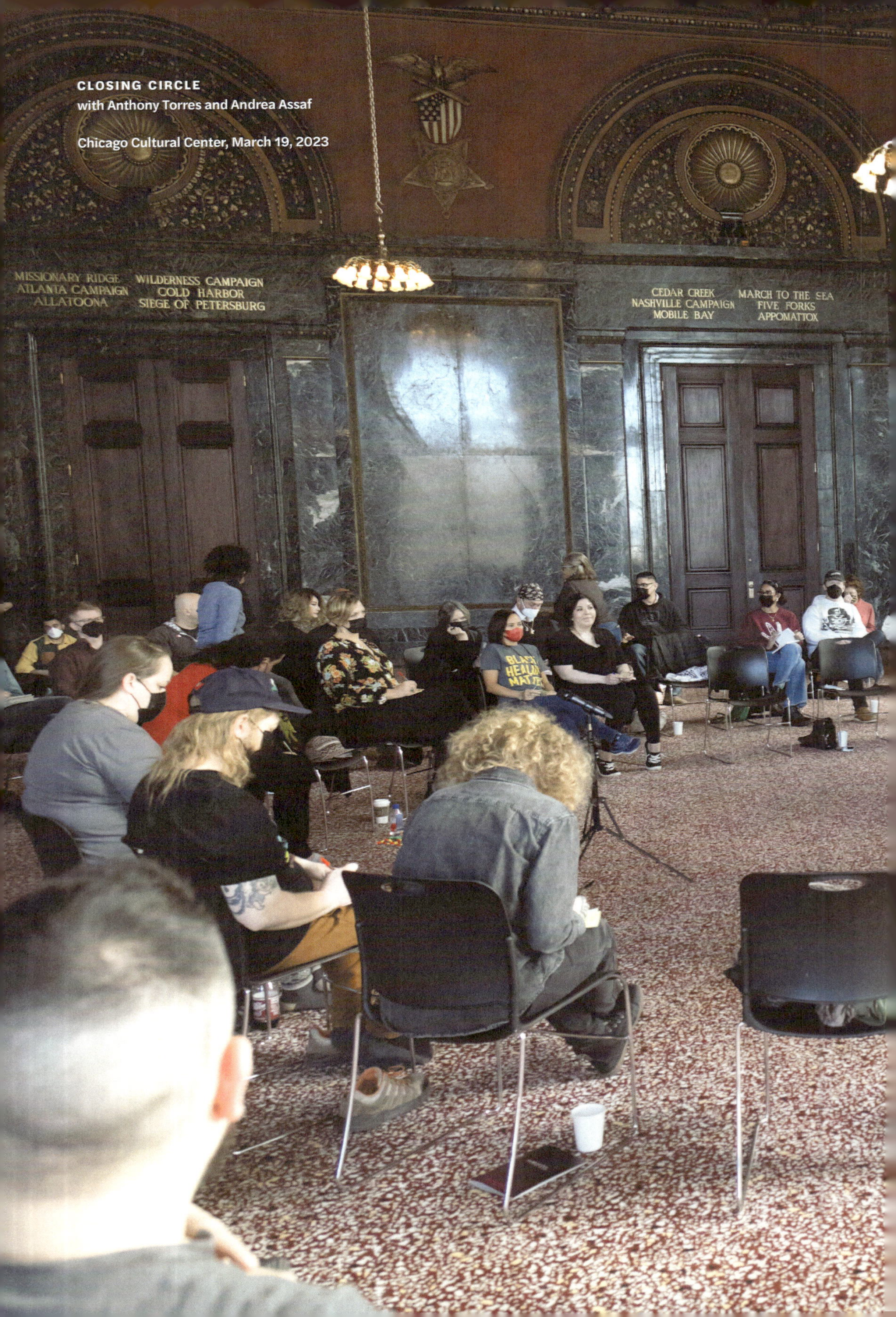

CLOSING CIRCLE
with Anthony Torres and Andrea Assaf

Chicago Cultural Center, March 19, 2023

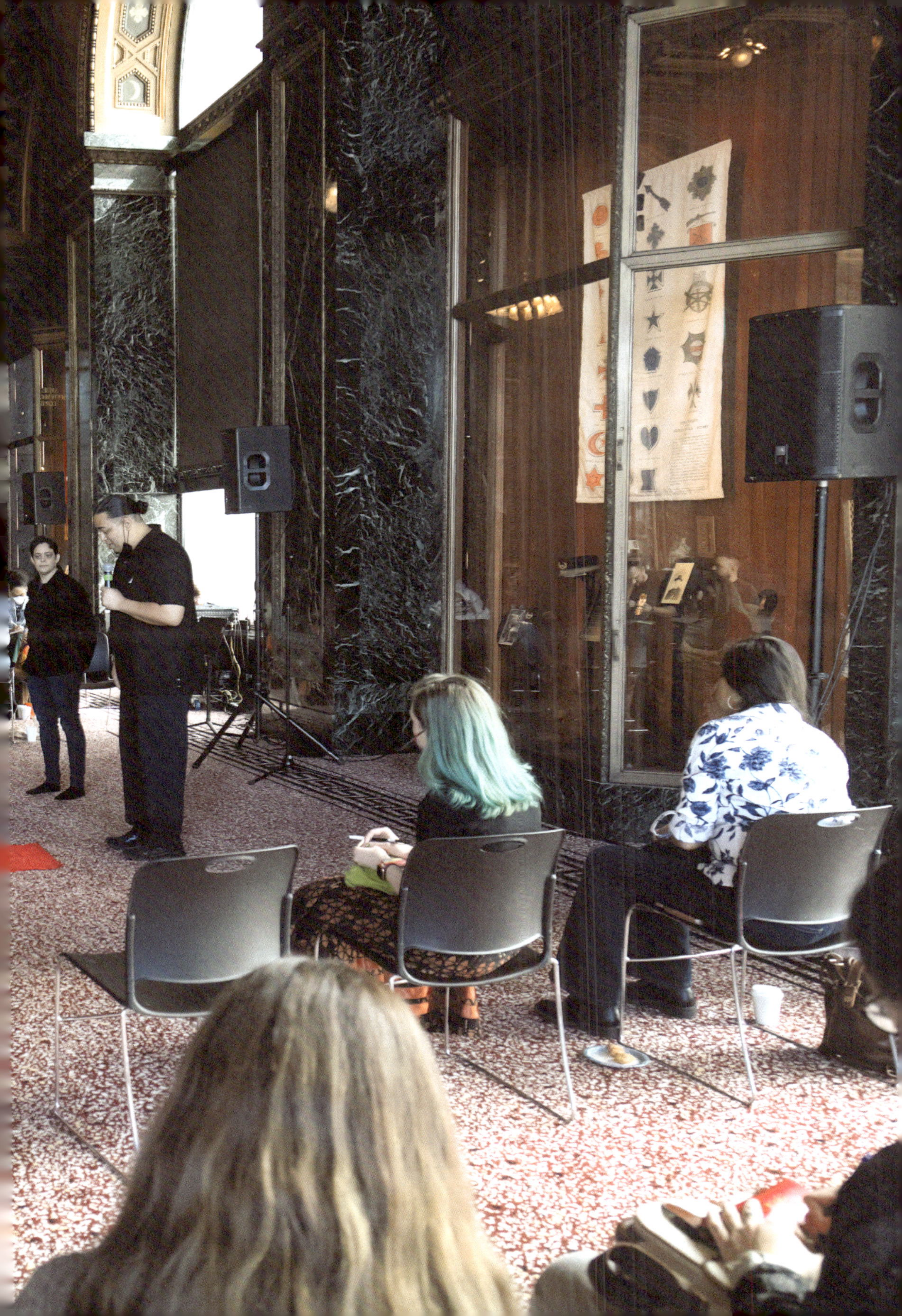

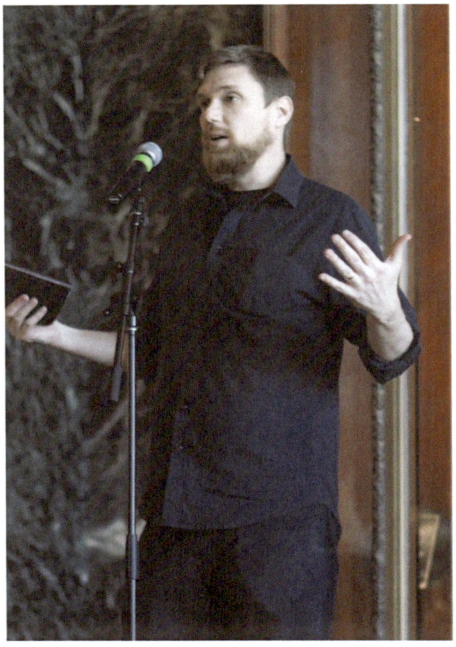

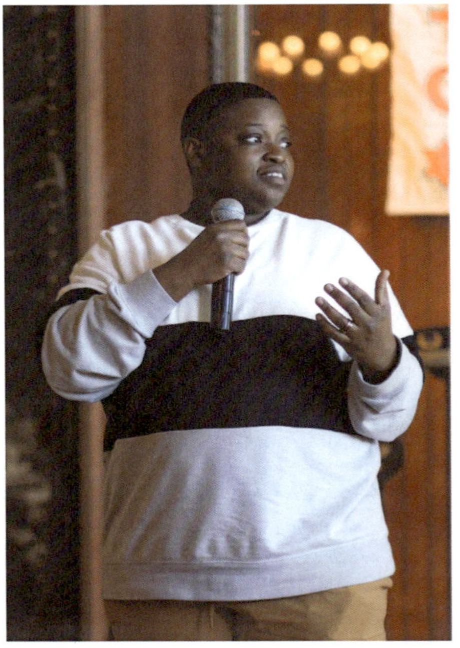

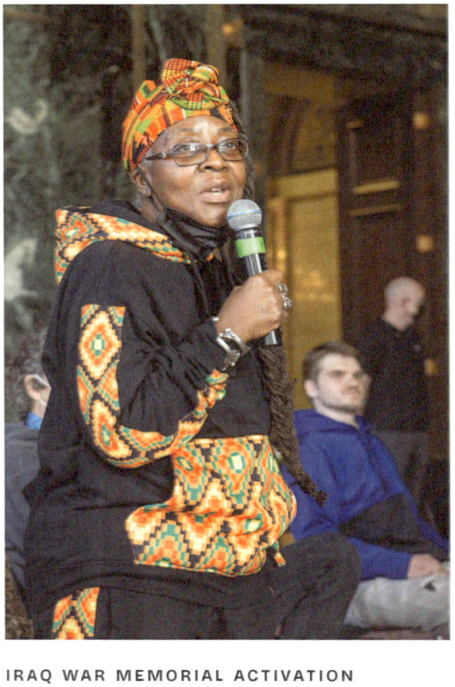

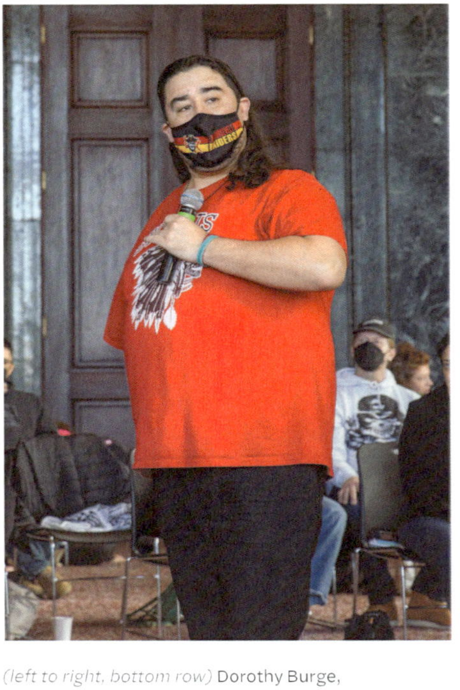

IRAQ WAR MEMORIAL ACTIVATION AND CLOSING COMMENTS
with *(left to right, top row)* Aaron Hughes, Erika R. Land, Hussein Smko, and Bassim Al Shaker; *(left to right, bottom row)* Dorothy Burge, James Pakootas, GOODW.Y.N., and Shaymaa Khalil

Chicago Cultural Center, March 19, 2023

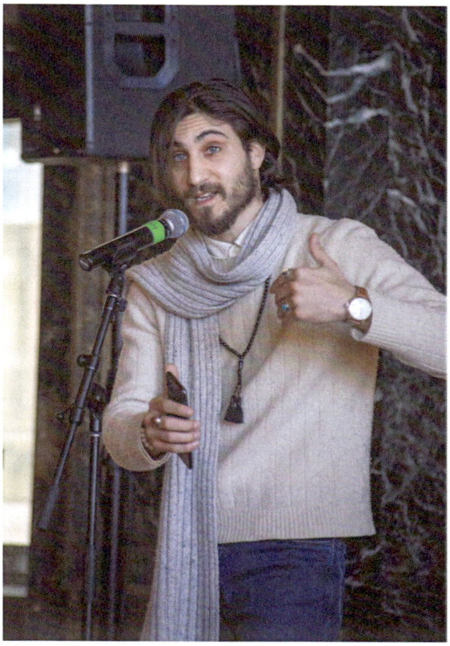

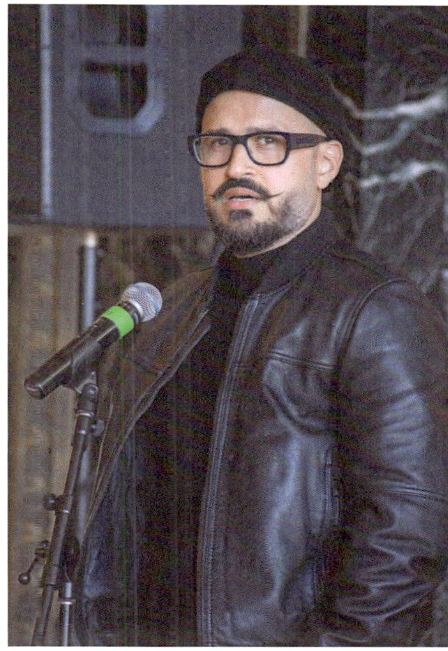

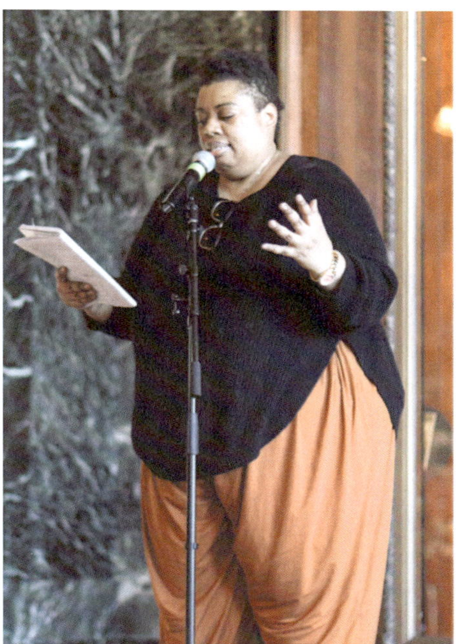

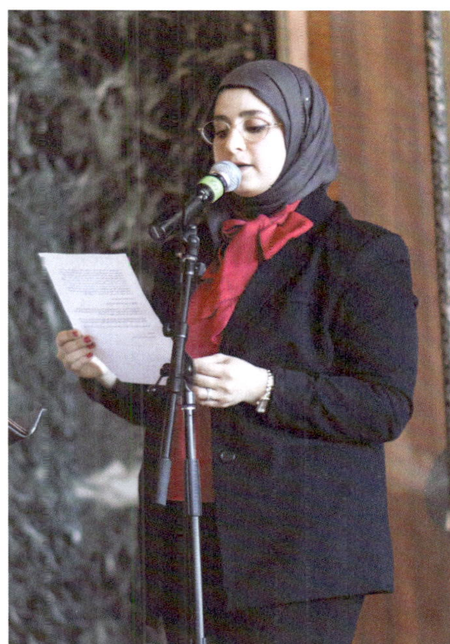

see also: pp. 223, 270–73

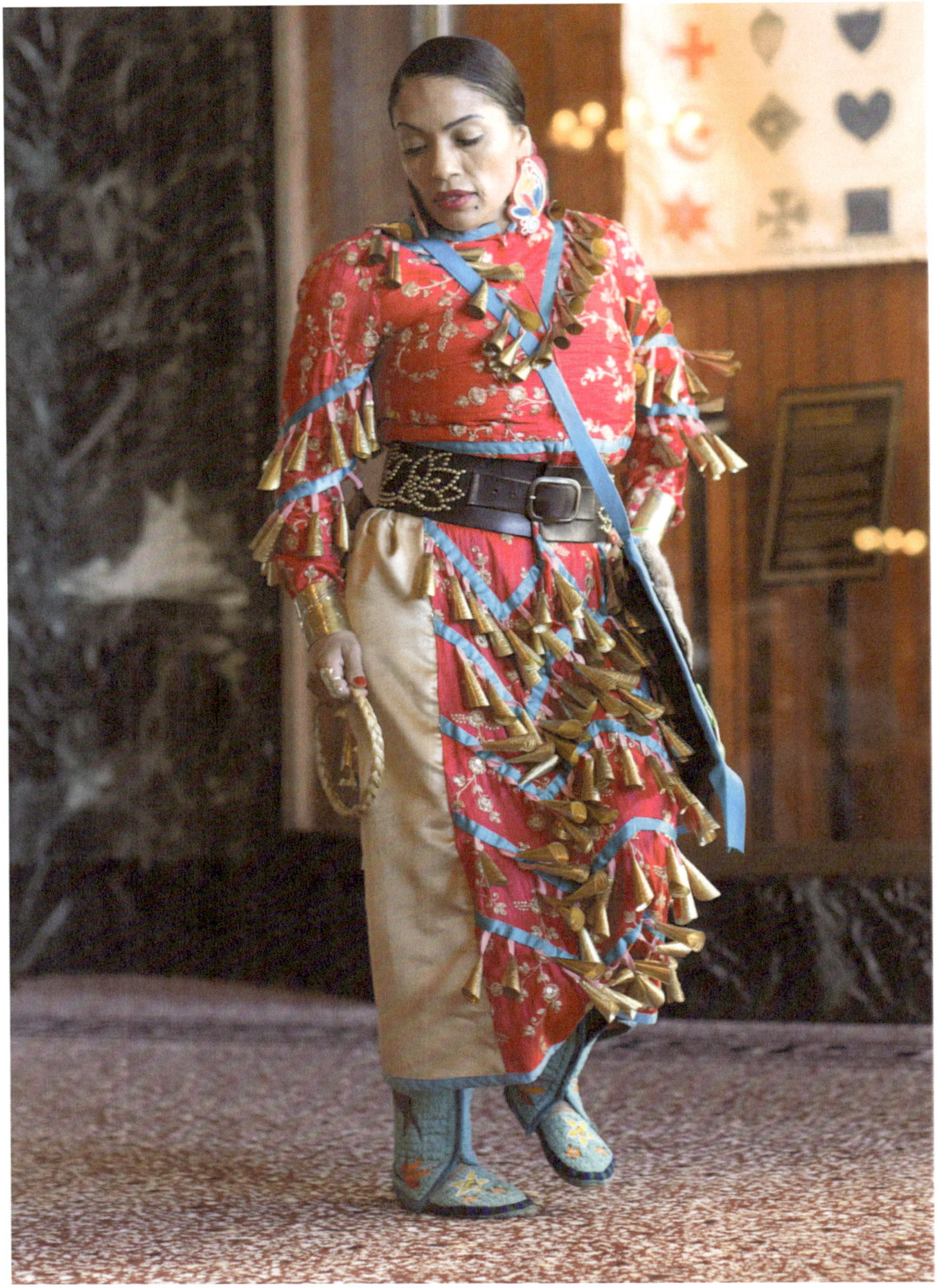

CLOSING PERFORMANCE:
ANISHINAABE JINGLE DRESS DANCE
with Starla Thompson

Chicago Cultural Center, March 19, 2023

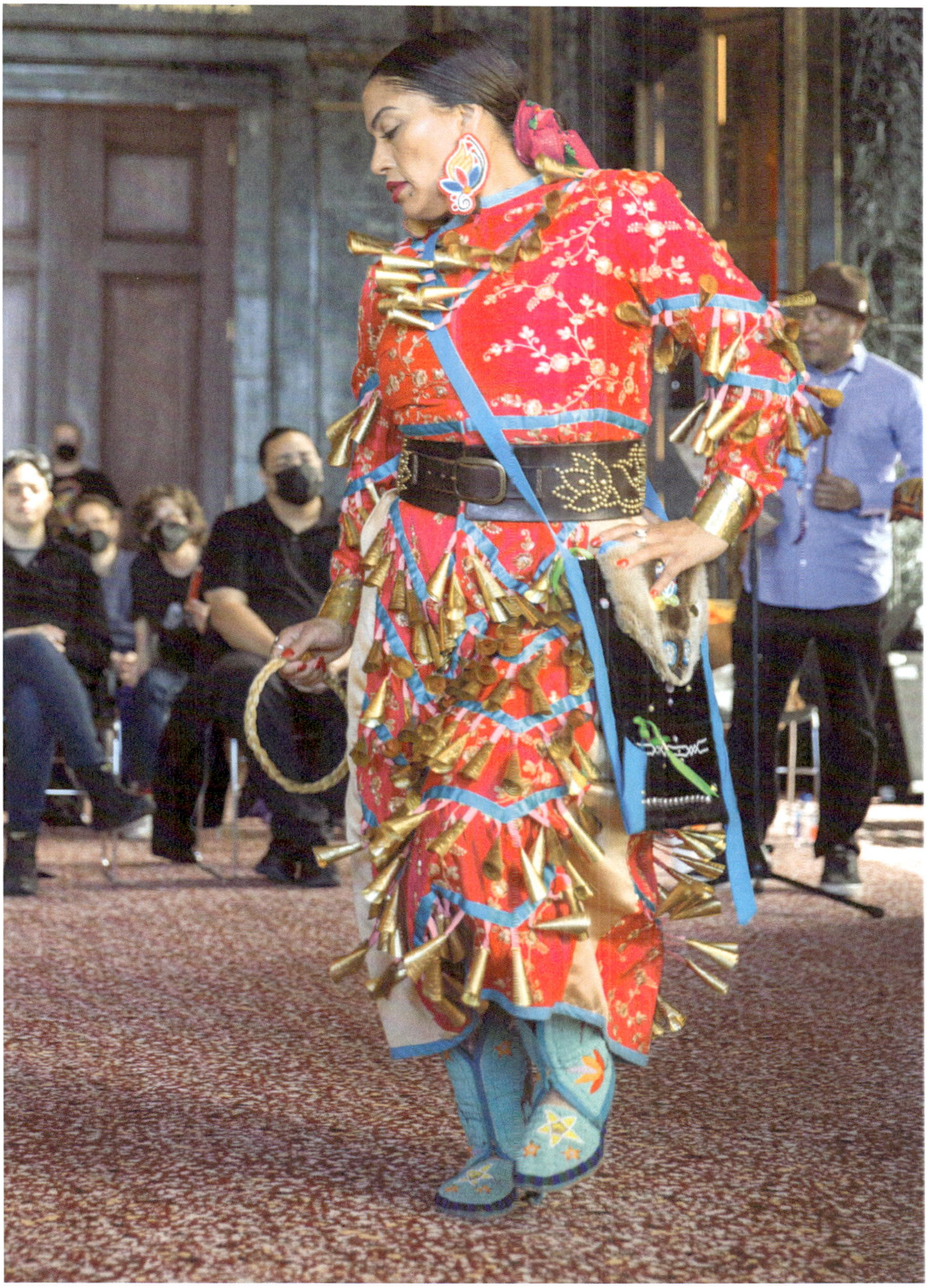

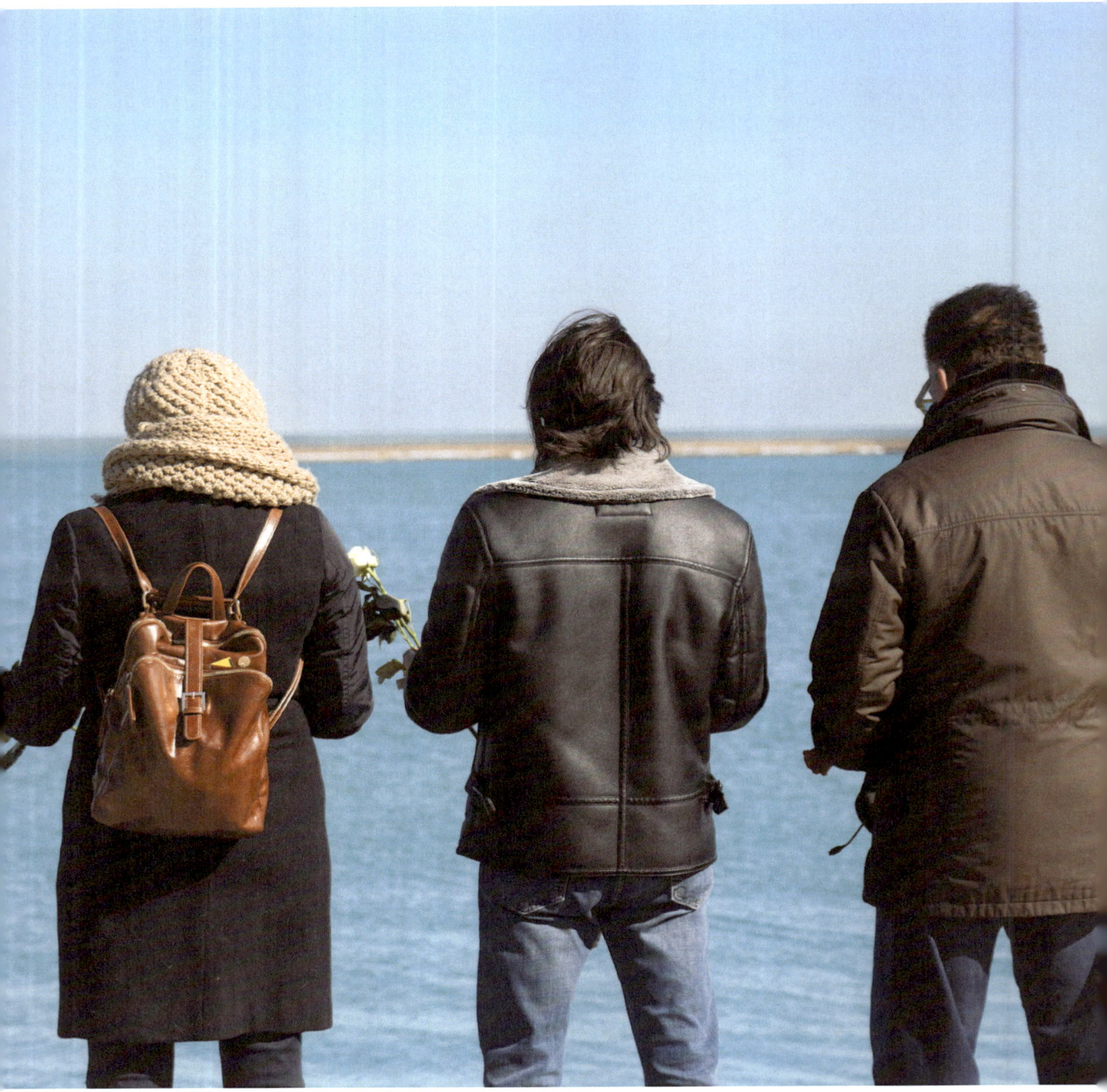

IRAQ WAR MEMORIAL ACTIVATION

Chicago Cultural Center, March 19, 2023
see also: pp. 223, 266–67, 272–73

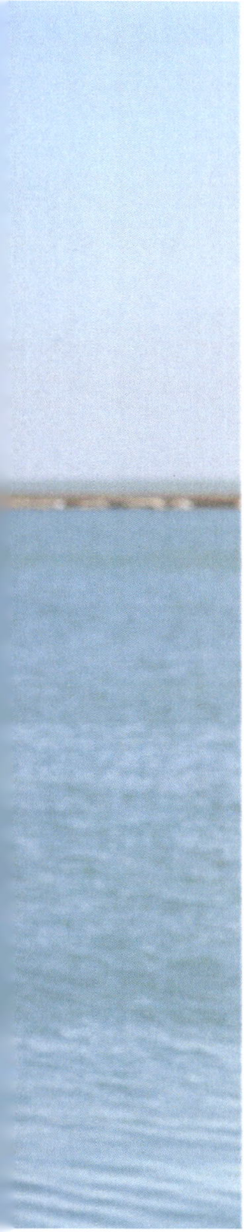

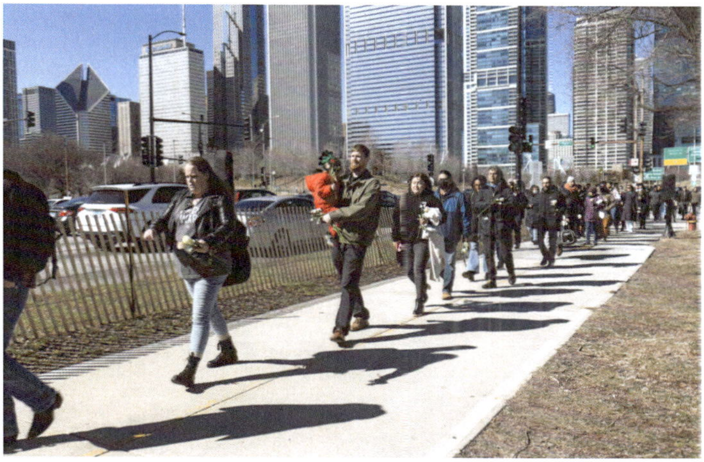

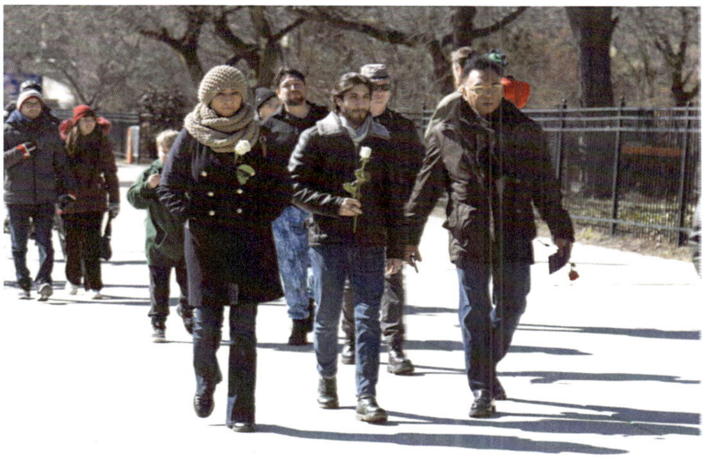

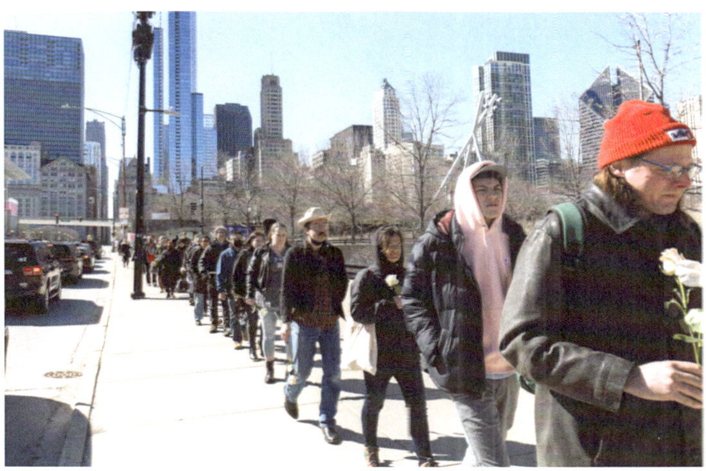

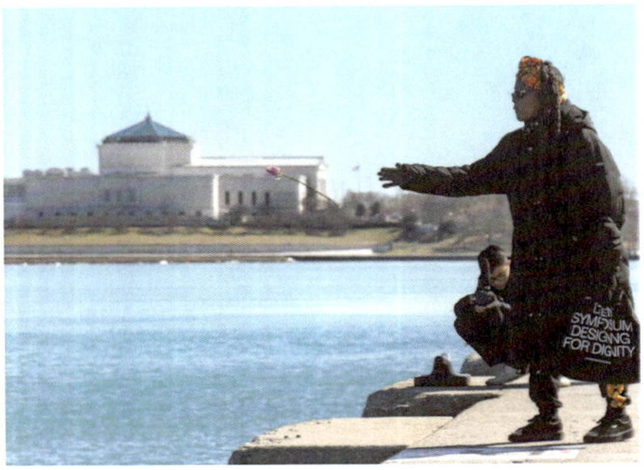

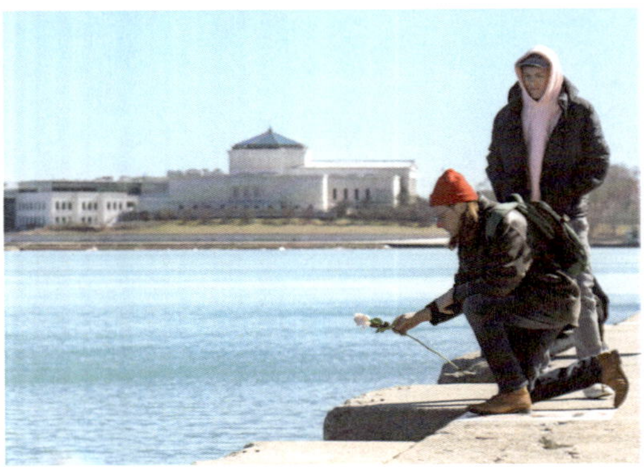

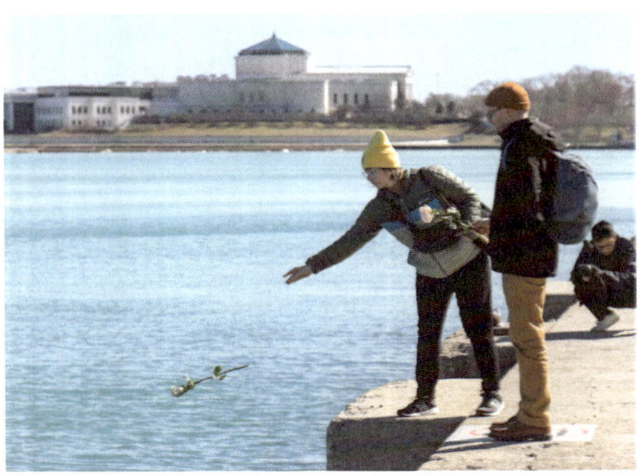

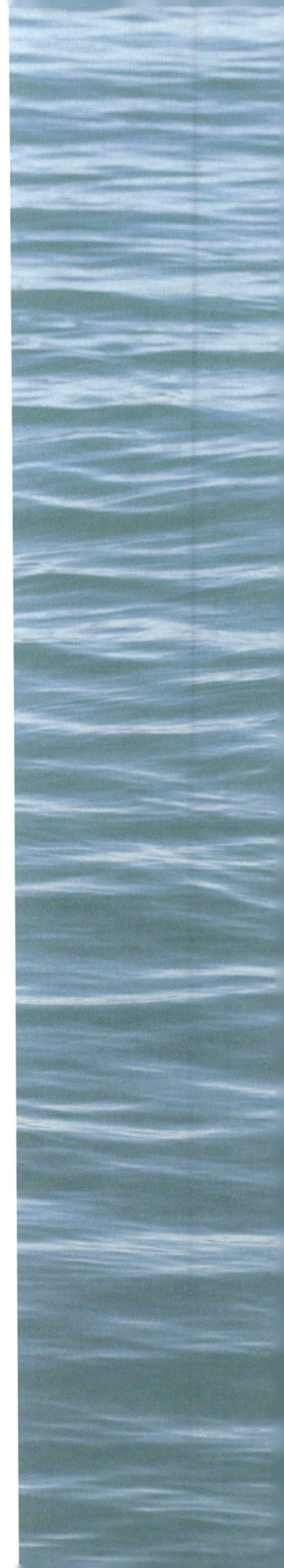

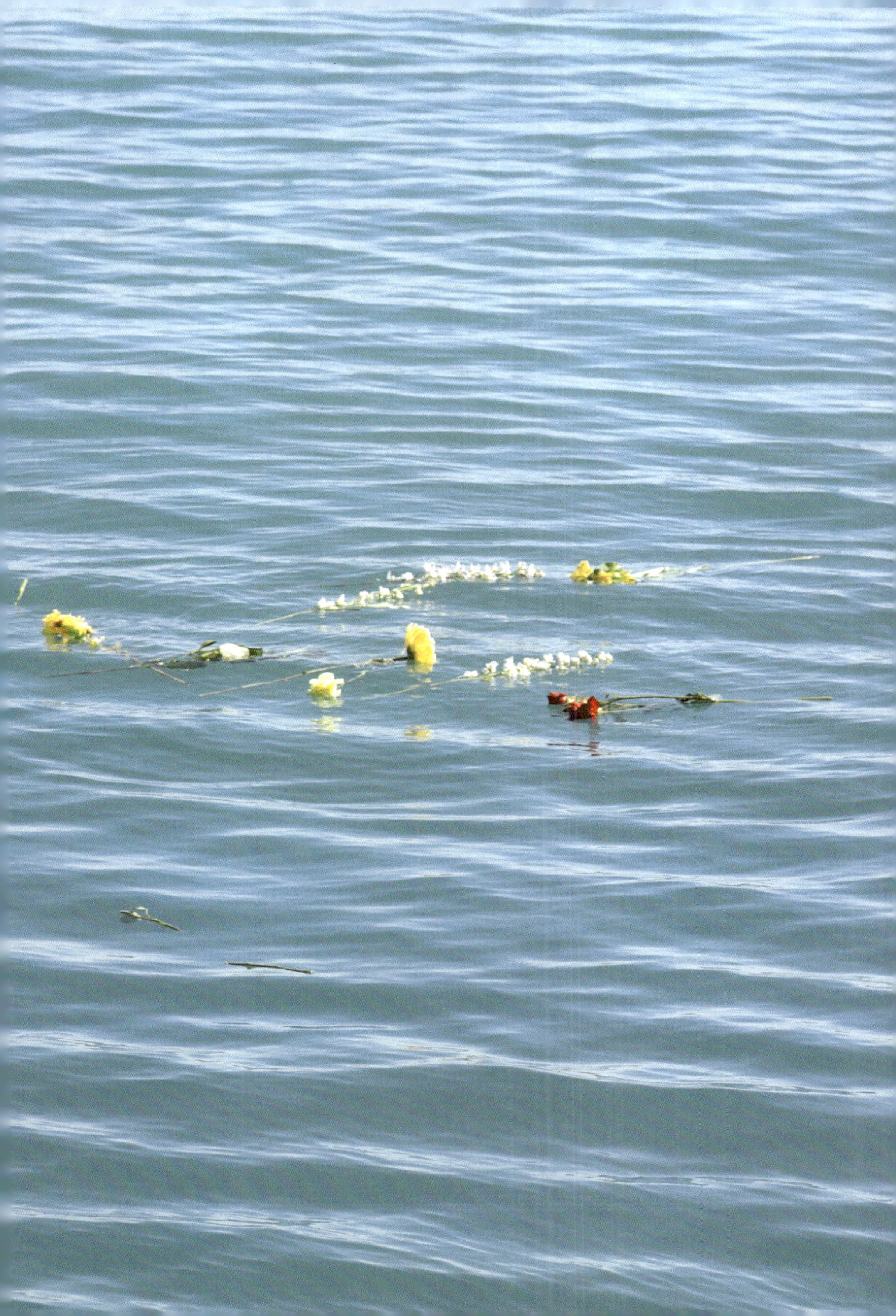

A Sweeter Future

MICHAEL RAKOWITZ

Ring the bells that still can ring
forget your perfect offering
there is a crack, a crack in everything
that's how the light gets in
— Leonard Cohen, "Anthem," off his album *The Future* (1992)

Date syrup was always very important to my family. My grandfather made it by hand. When he died in 1975, he left behind a freezer full of jars that we continued to eat for the next ten years until we ran out. Then my mother was forced to buy store-bought brands, and she always complained that the ones that she could find were from places like California or Israel, and they filtered it too much like they were trying to whiten it.

One day in 2004, when I was living in Brooklyn, I went to Sahadi's Import Company, which was the first place my grandparents went to buy their groceries when they arrived in the US in 1947. So the Sahadi family knows my family. I saw a can of date syrup there, and the label was mostly in Arabic. It was beautifully designed. It had red on it and these swinging palm trees. You know, stylized graphic design. And it said Product of Lebanon. I decided, "Oh, I'll get this for my mom as a gift. Maybe it'll be a little bit better than the other ones she complains about."

So I brought it to the cash register and Charlie Sahadi looked at the can. He looked at me and he said, "Your mother's going to love this. It's from Baghdad." And I looked at the can again and it said Product of Lebanon. I asked how this was possible, and he said to me that the date syrup is actually processed in the Iraqi capital, then put into large plastic bags. That's how it crosses the border into Syria, where it gets put into these tin cans. And then it's driven over the border to Lebanon, where it gets labeled and sold to the rest of the world.

That was the way Iraqi date syrup companies were able to survive during the years of the sanctions from 1990 until 2003.

But this was 2004, more than a year after "Mission Accomplished" had been declared and the sanctions had been lifted. When I asked why this was still happening, Charlie explained to me that tariffs made trade prohibitive, as Iraq was still considered to be a rogue state according to the UN's laws. Anything that said "product of Iraq" was too difficult to bring in and too expensive. He explained it would be bad business, but I thought it would be good art.

So I reopened my grandfather's import-export company to try to import a ton of Iraqi dates. The dates in Iraq are legendary. You know, the date is to Iraq what cheese is to France and Italy. And what the cigar is to Cuba. There's over 620 varieties that grow in Iraq. In the 1970s, when Iraq was a cheap exporter of dates to the world, there were over thirty million date palms in the country. At the end of the Iran-Iraq war, that number had been halved to about sixteen million. At the end of the US-led invasion in 2003, less than three million remained.

And so it is one other living organism in that landscape that has suffered the same fate as the people.

When I was attempting to import the Iraqi dates, one of the people that I was dealing with from the Baghdad Business Bureau, who was bidding on exporting the dates to the US under my company, asked why I had such a fascination with dates. I said, "Well, my grandparents were Jews from Baghdad and dates have always been around." And he says, "Aha, that's the reason. Because we say in Iraq that every Iraqi has a date in their genes." Then he told me that in some places in Iraq, it's actually traditional to put a date into the mouth of a newborn baby so the first taste of life is sweet.

We know there's been a lot of bitterness, but let something new be born today. Here's to a sweeter future!

Adapted from a talk at the STLW *Iraq War Memorial Activation, Chicago Cultural Center, March 19, 2023*

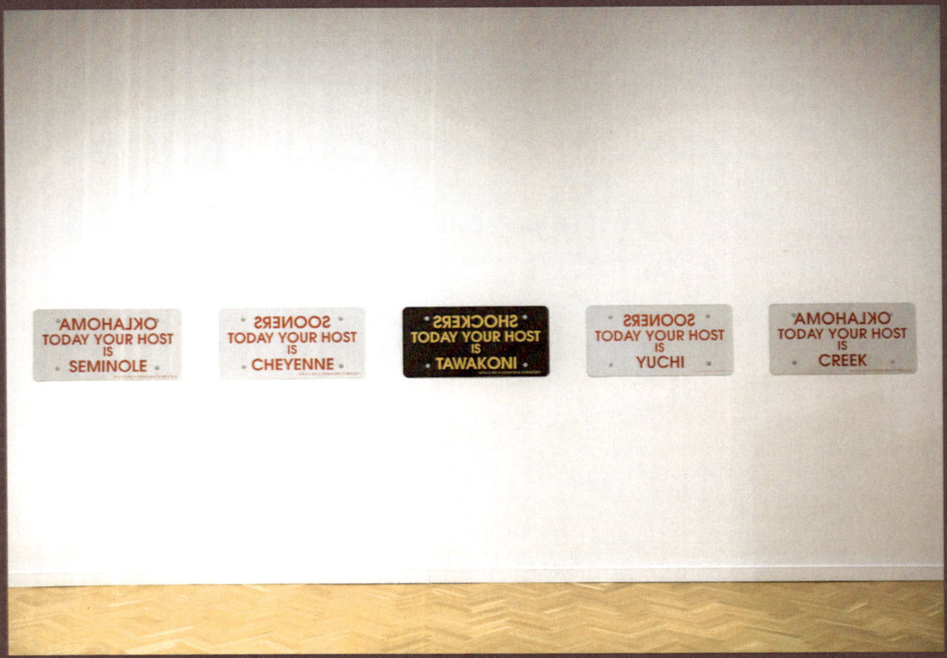

HOCK E AYE VI EDGAR HEAP OF BIRDS
(Cheyenne and Arapaho Nation, b. 1954)
Native Host for Oklahoma, 2017–21
Mylar on five aluminum metal sign panels

Native Hosts is an ongoing series of public art interventions across North America, including Chicago. The series honors Indigenous citizens, past and present, and educates the non-Native public about their connection to tribal grounds and histories. This iteration focuses on the legacy of survival in Oklahoma Indian Territory, the land of the Washita Massacre by Colonel Custer and the 7th US Cavalry regiment. The inverted colonial names on each panel are meant to upend, and disrupt, the colonial logics in order to ask viewers to see this original Native world in a new way. Heap of Birds notes, "As in any proper decorum it is fitting, before one proceeds in life, to properly recognize one's host."

see also: p. xiv

"When Black People Are Free, All People Will Be Free": Black Freedom, Indigenous Sovereignty, and the Limits of Reparations Discourse

KYLE T. MAYS

I want to first introduce myself via family history. I am Afro-Indigenous (Saginaw Chippewa). My great-grandmother, Esther Shawboose Mays, traveled to Detroit, Michigan, in the spring of 1940 and shortly thereafter married an African American male. She got a lot of hate from Detroit's Indigenous community, especially men, for doing so. But as one of my Indigenous mentors, Dr. George Cornell, told me as a sophomore at Michigan State, "your grandma didn't take shit from nobody!" Her activism centered on the future of children. She co-founded what was called Detroit's Indian Educational and Cultural Center in 1974. She also dragged her children to these spaces as well, culminating twenty years later in her daughter, my aunt Judy, founding the third-ever public school with an Indigenous curriculum in Detroit, called Medicine Bear American Indian Academy. I mention this story often not simply because of how proud I am of my family's legacy, but to highlight the importance of creating spaces where we can all be and relate to one another. The school had Afro-Indigenous children, children with multiple Indigenous heritages both from nations in the US and Canada, and many other identities. But let me now turn to the topic at hand.

The questions that undergird my approach and analysis are simple: What is the relationship between Blackness and Indigeneity? What has been the impact of settler colonialism, white supremacy, and racial capitalism on Black and Indigenous peoples? And what kind of world do we want to build in the aftermath of settler colonialism and white supremacy?

Black women have produced some of the most important ideological work in the postwar era, including Black feminist thought and intersectionality. The centrality of Black women to interrogating the nature of oppression under a white supremacist, patriarchal society and imagining the possibilities for ending it has been foundational to our thoughts on race, gender, and solidarity. The women of the Combahee River Collective, for instance, were a key component of that. One of the many jewels argued by them is, "When Black women are free, all people will be free."[1] In other words, if we center the experiences of oppression experienced by Black women, then all other forms of injustice will end. Black activists, including the Movement for Black Lives today, have carried forward this activist ideology. Indeed, Alica Garza, co-founder of the Black Lives Matter movement, makes the same assertion in her memoir, *The Purpose of Power*. Obviously, I support Black liberation—that should be without resistance in this society. And yet I wonder, where does land fit into this equation? My aim is not to create conflict or to dismiss the importance of

1. Combahee River Collective, The Combahee River Collective Statement, April 1977.

Black freedom, but even if Black people received liberation tomorrow, it doesn't resolve the question of Indigenous land and who can make claims to that land.

As we move toward the aftermath of settler colonialism and white supremacy, we need to critically interrogate the meaning of justice, freedom, and reparatory justice—without basing our analysis in the ideas that the foundations of racial capitalism, settler colonialism, and US democracy as a structure are rooted in the enslavement of Africans and the dispossession of Indigenous people, and their afterlives. By conjoining the experiences of Black and Indigenous peoples in the quest for liberation, we broaden the scope of possibilities. In other words, in the move for justice, for example reparations, we must think creatively and as judiciously as possible regarding Black freedom and its relationship to Indigenous sovereignty. The person who had this right is Stokely Carmichael, who would change his name to Kwame Ture. In a speech he gave in St. Paul, Minnesota, in 1975, he remarked, "Anybody who thinks seriously about working on behalf of the red man must deal with this truth. The land on which we live, on which we inhabit, which we exploit—that land belongs to the red man. He must come first in any dealings with the land."[2] And so, that is a duty of Black people today. Center the land.

Black liberation does not necessarily equal liberation for all, including Indigenous peoples, nor does it equal to the liberation of land.

The Republic of New Afrika is one example. They called for the Five Southern states as reparations for slavery. But we must ask, what about the Indigenous peoples, the Five Tribes, who were forcibly removed? Certainly, they owe some form of reparations to the descendants of people they enslaved and can at least incorporate them as citizens. I live in Los Angeles, California, and there is current legislation to offer reparations for African Americans who can demonstrate that they have an ancestor who was enslaved in

2. Sam Ford, "Stokely Carmichael Speaks against Capitalism at AIM Headquarters in St. Paul," MPR Archive, May 24, 1974, https://archive.mpr.org/stories/1974/05/24/stokely-carmichael-speaks-against-capitalism-at-aim-headquarters-in-st-paul.

the 19th century. I suppose they want every Black person to get their genealogical research on like we're Alex Haley, the author of *Roots*. Anyways, one of the recommendations from the report is to "create forms of expression, acknowledgement, and remembrance of the trauma of state-sanctioned white supremacist terror, possibly including memorials, and funding a long-term truth and reconciliation commission."[3] One example is the case of the Bruce Family who owned Bruce's Beach, which is now Manhattan Beach. The white city council decided in 1925 to take that land. The beach is worth millions now. While this is a tragedy of dispossession and theft, and I support the Bruce family descendants getting compensated, it says nothing about returning land to Indigenous peoples, the Tongva, who were dispossessed first. Again, I'm not interested in competition, but a true notion of justice. I support truth and reconciliation, but what about for Indigenous peoples, which means the return of land? We can look at the Canadian government's attempt at Truth and Reconciliation under the liberal watch of Prime Minister Justin Trudeau, and the many critiques Indigenous peoples have levied against him for failing to implement the necessary material reconciliation including returning land.

We must return the land. We should think broadly about reparations. As Olúfémi O. Táíwò argues, "But slavery, colonialism, and the political structure they produced were and are global phenomena."[4] If they were global and large in scale, we must connect and think through Black and Indigenous liberation. Land Back is one way.

Land Back is the unequivocal idea meant to return Indigenous peoples' land. As the NdN Collective, a group of Indigenous organizers from Turtle Island to Palestine argue, "to truly dismantle white supremacy and systems of oppression, we have to go back to the roots. Which, for us, is putting Indigenous lands back in Indigenous hands."[5]

3. State of California, Department of Justice, 2022 - AB3121 Interim Report Preliminary Recommendations, June 1, 2022, 19, https://oag.ca.gov/system/files/media/ab3121-interim-report-executive-summary-2022.pdf.

4. Olúfẹ́mi O. Táíwò, *Reconsidering Reparations* (New York: Oxford University Press, 2022), 10.

Land is key. Without the land, and rethinking how we all relate, we aren't going to achieve even a modicum of liberation. The NdN Collective further articulates a vision of co-liberation, by suggesting that Land Back "is a political framework that allows us to deepen our relationships across the field of organizing movements working towards true collective liberation. It allows us to envision a world where Black, Indigenous, and [people of color] liberation co-exists."[6] The idea of co-existing, co-liberation, and collective freedom for some Indigenous peoples might be scary, seem unfair, perhaps even unnecessary. These folks view the world through the lens of the late, great Vine Deloria Jr., who opined, "Minority groups were often astounded to learn that the Indians were not planning to share the continent with their oppressed brothers once the revolution was over. Hell no. The Indians were planning on taking the continent back and kicking out all the black, Chicano, Anglos, and Asian brothers who had made the whole thing possible."[7] I understand this sentiment. Indigenous voices and perspectives on justice were ignored for years during this era—and remain so. However, I tend to fall in line with the Anishinaabe intellectual and writer, Leanne Simpson, who, writing in the aftermath of the uprisings in Ferguson, Missouri, after the murder of Mike Brown at the hands of state violence,

> To me, Ferguson is a call not only to indict the system but to decolonize the systems that create and maintain the forces of Indigenous genocide and anti-Blackness. I have a responsibility to make space on my land for those communities of struggles, to centre and amplify Black voices and to co-resist. We both come from vibrant, proud histories of mobilization and protest,

5. NDN Collective, "Landback," accessed August 1, 2024, https://landback.org/.

6. NDN Collective, "Landback Update: From Launch to Looking Forward," October, 28, 2020. https://ndncollective.org/landback-updates-from-launch-to-looking-forward/.

7. Vine Deloria, Jr., *Behind the Trail of Broken Treaties: An Indian Declaration of Independence* (New York: Delacorte Press), 1974, 2–3.

> and it is the sacrifices of our Elders and our Ancestors that ensured that our communities of struggle continue to exist today. They believed in their hearts that there is no justice and no peace until we are all free, and so must we.[8]

Kinship as Solidarity

The work of solidarity for our collective futures requires a rethinking of how we relate. But first, as queer Black feminist Audre Lorde reminds us, "any future vision which can encompass all of us, by definition, must be complex and expanding, not easy to achieve."[9] I propose that we consider kinship as solidarity. In my own tribe, the Saginaw Chippewa, Anishinaabe people have a clan system that tells you how you relate to other people and non-human species, which ultimately defines not only your relationship to people but your responsibility. What if tribal nations, in exercising their sovereignty, began incorporating, for example, African Americans into their nations using the clan system? We can quibble about resources etc., but none of us can live together on this land in a just way without kinship. If sovereignty means anything, it must include our bodies, our knowledge systems, and the ability to regenerate "indigenous languages, philosophies, legal systems, and intellectual systems and to nurture and continue those systems for the land."[10] Again, land is key.

---

8. Leanne Simpson, "Indict the System: Indigenous and Black Connected Resistance," *Leanne Betasamosake Simpson* (blog), November 28, 2014, http://leannesimpson.ca/indict-the-system-indigenous-black-connected-resistance/.

9. Audre Lorde, "Learning from the 60s," Black Past, August 12, 2012, https://www.blackpast.org/african-american-history/1982-audre-lorde-learning-60s/.

10. Leanne Betasamosake Simpson, "The Place Where We All Live and Work Together: A Gendered Analysis of 'Sovereignty,'" in *Native Studies Keywords*, eds. Stephanie Nohelani Teves, Andrea Smith, and Michelle Raheja (Tucson: University of Arizona Press, 2015), 21.

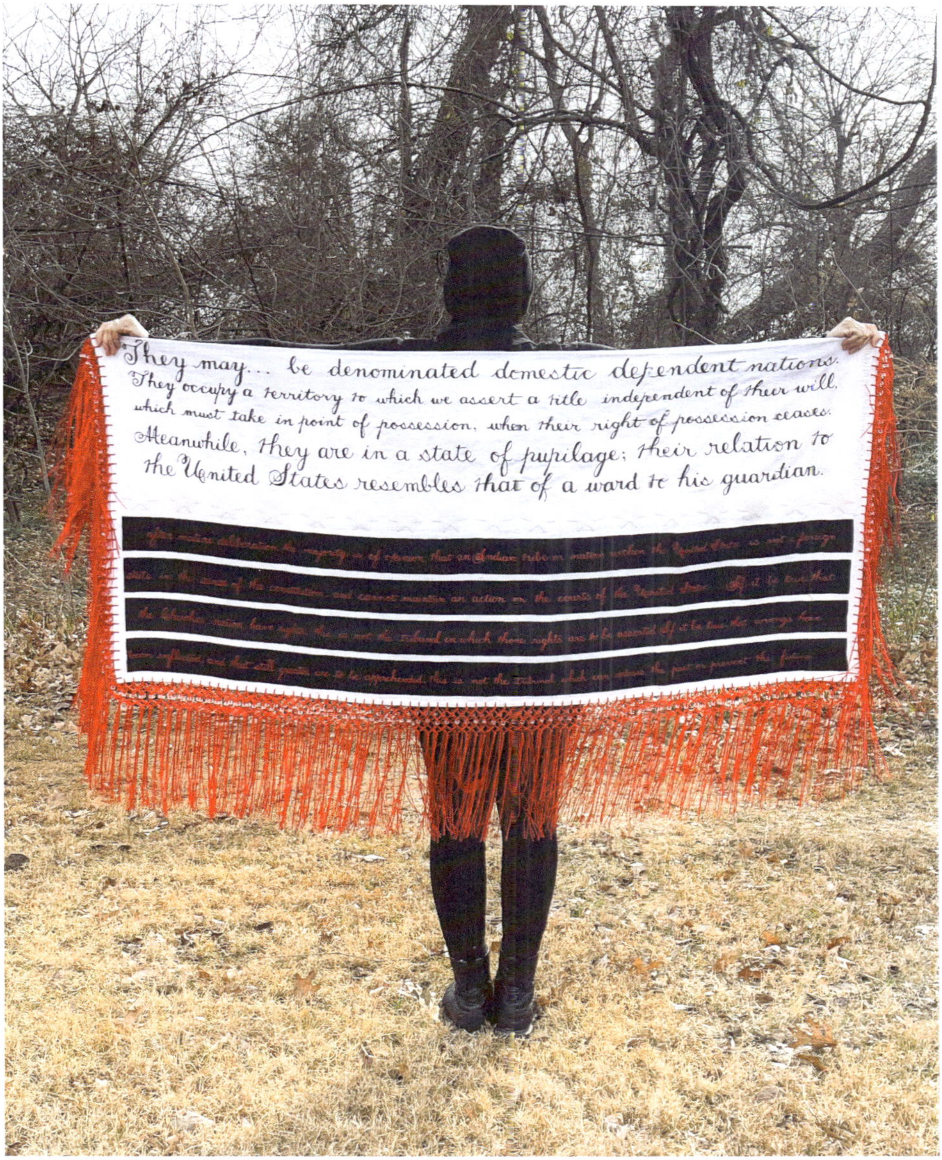

JUNE CARPENTER, *Cherokee Nation v. Georgia, 30 U.S. 1 (1831)*, 2022 Linen fabric, satin ribbon, cotton thread, nylon fringe, and glass beads; *see also: pp. 162–63, 299*

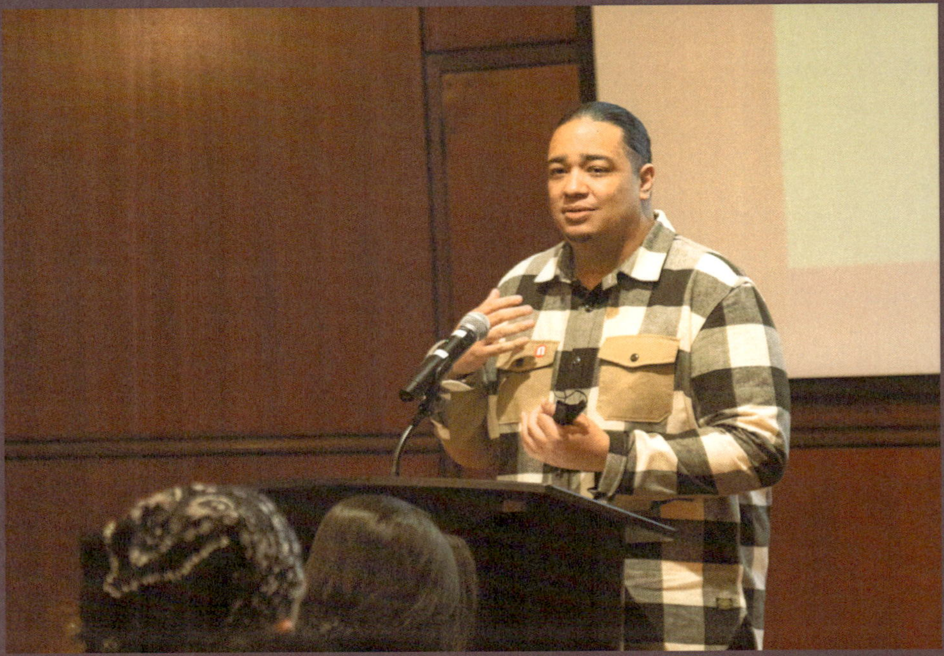

ANTHONY TORRES
Residues and Rebellions Poetry Reading
Newberry Library

Vulnerable Enough to Share, Selfless Enough to Listen

KEVIN BASL IN CONVERSATION WITH ANTHONY TORRES

Anthony Torres is a poet, theater artist, and social worker whose work focuses on themes of transformation, healing, demilitarization, and social justice. After leaving the US Army in 2006, he moved to Miami, Florida, and began participating in local writing workshops to help process his military experiences. Over the past decade, Torres has been involved in many veteran-focused art projects, including hosting poetry open mic events for veterans and performing with The Combat Hippies, a theater ensemble organized with fellow Puerto Rican veterans. Under the artistic direction of Teo Castellanos, The Combat Hippies have written and toured two full-length productions: Conscience Under Fire *(2015) and* AMAL *(2019). Torres and collaborator Hipólito Arriaga III were featured in* Return to the Body, *the 2019 Veteran Art Triennial's performance program, and Torres returned to curate the* Surviving the Long Wars *performances.*

KEVIN BASL (KB): *What was your curatorial vision for* Surviving the Long Wars?

ANTHONY TORRES (AT): My vision was to create collaborative opportunities among performers and attendees and help build a community that would exist beyond the Triennial. My participation as a performer in the first Veteran Art Triennial profoundly impacted me, and it informed my decision to include civilian performers alongside veteran performers in STLW. I wanted to show the impact of war, while also fostering community-building and lasting relationships among the participating academics, poets, visual artists, activists, and performers.

KB: *Can you talk about engaging with the work of* STLW *scholar Kyle T. Mays and how his thoughts on solidarity, art, and hip-hop informed your thinking for the Triennial? How can the framework he presents help veteran artists move through emotional burdens to a place of solidarity?*

AT: Dr. Kyle T. Mays highlights the importance of understanding colonization's impact on Black and Native American communities, emphasizing solidarity-building through listening and sharing. One key takeaway from speaking with him was that solidarity is extremely challenging work, but it's vital for taking steps towards progress. I have come to realize through my own work as a poet and theater performer that art can initiate difficult conversations about war and colonialism. Mays emphasizes multi-generational inclusion, where elders share knowledge and youth feel seen. This inspired me to include diverse perspectives in the performance program, promoting healing and community strength. When the themes of this work are so heavy, it's imperative to remember the joy and beauty that arises from creativity.

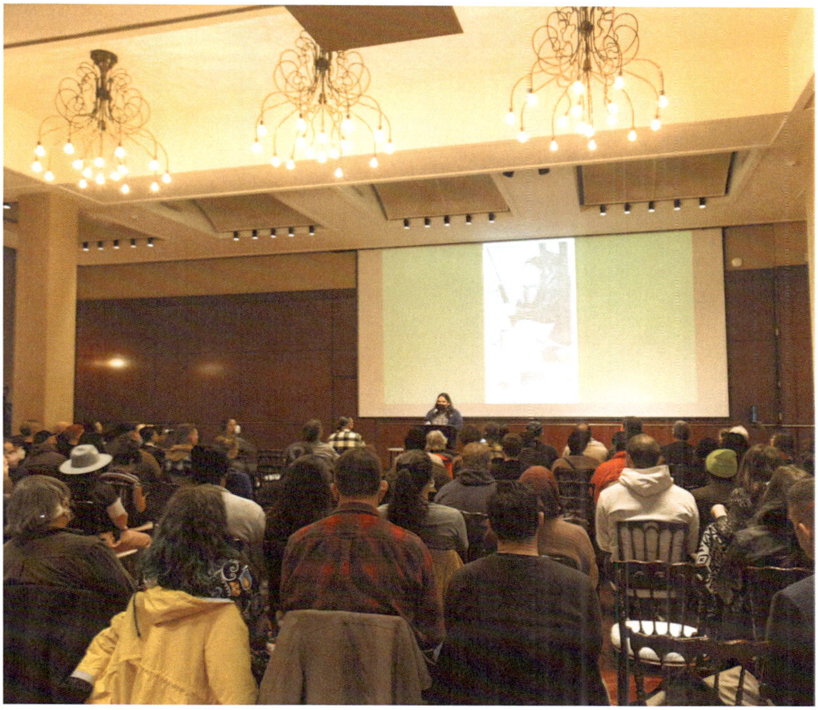

MONTY LITTLE, *Residues and Rebellions* Poetry Reading, Newberry Library

KB: *The opening for the Newberry Library exhibition* Surviving the Long Wars: Residues and Rebellions *included a poetry reading. How did the poems and performances speak to the unlikely connections and entanglements featured in the exhibition or complicate the artworks on display?*

AT: Solidarity requires being vulnerable enough to share and being selfless enough to listen. Listening to the poets perform, I could clearly see the parallels between their experiences. Monty Little (Diné), shared a piece about returning home to the Navajo Reservation and the emotional impact of wartime experiences on family dynamics. Spoken word poetry by Erika R. Land carried a passionate vulnerability as she shared works about seeking peace after war trauma, as well as the impact of the US prison system's unjust treatment of the Black community. Writer, performer, and dramaturg Carlos Sirah's piece included a deeply reflective and poignant commentary on the relationship between perception, isolation, and human relationships, and their connection to colonialism. The program concluded with Iraqi-American poet Dunya Mikhail, who shared both new and previously published works about love, family, and war from a civilian's perspective. The lasting impact of war was evident in each poet's work.

KB: *Let's talk about* The Space Between, *the opening performance at Hyde Park Art Center. How did the collaborators, which included GWOT veterans of color and a civilian survivor of the war, create this piece? How did the audience respond to the work?*

AT: *The Space Between* was a multi-disciplinary performance that wonderfully encapsulated my vision as a curator. Performer Hussein Smko was introduced to me by a theatergoer following my theater company's performance in Chicago in 2021. He shared with me that as a child from the Kurdish region of Northern Iraq, he learned about hip-hop dance from US soldiers during the Iraq War. He later became a professional dancer and now lives and works in New York City. We had been seeking an opportunity to work together, and the Triennial became the perfect opportunity to showcase his work.

I connected Smko with Hipólito Arriaga and GOODW.Y.N., who had both performed at the 2019 Triennial. We held a series of video calls leading up to the Triennial, as this piece required more planning and coordination than any other Triennial performance. The collective vision for this piece was to tell a single story with three different forms of storytelling from three distinct perspectives. We explored the nature and impact of trauma and moral injury not only from the perspective of veterans of color, but also from the civilian

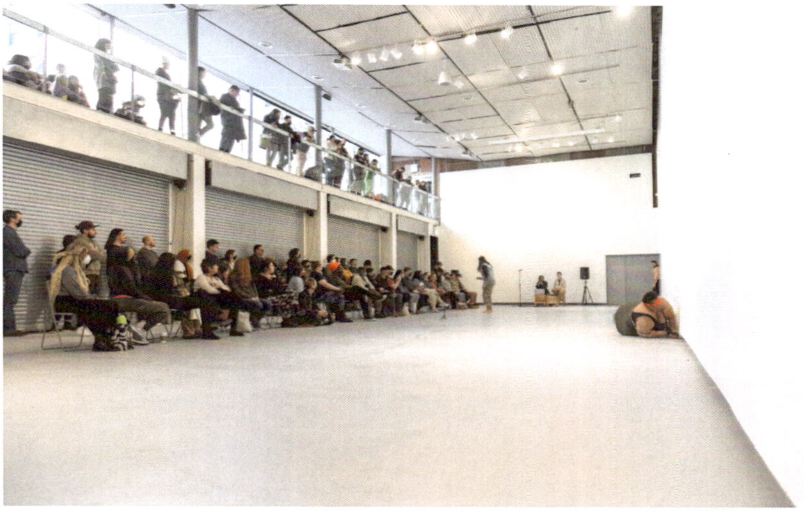

The Space Between: Unlikely Entanglements Opening Program, Hyde Park Art Center;
see also: pp. 75, 232–35

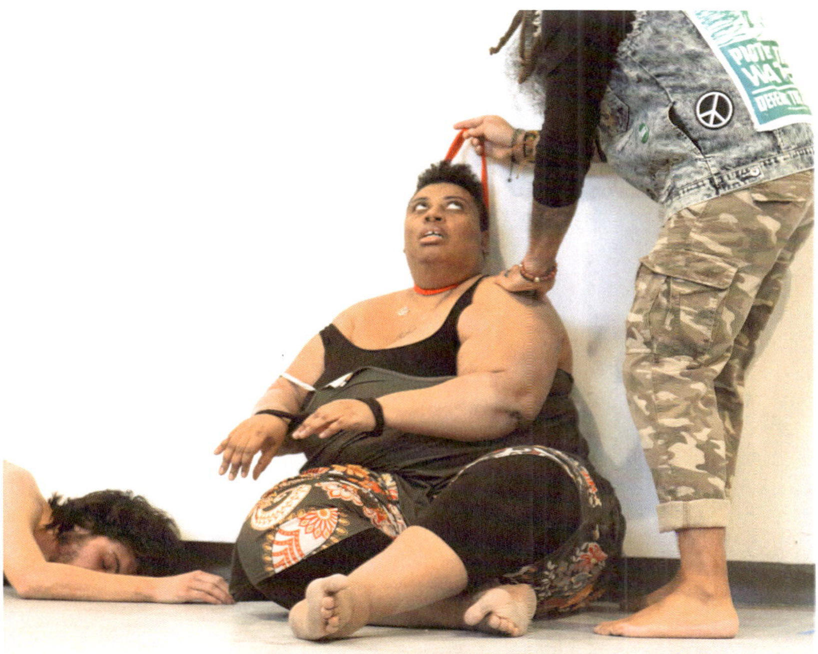

from left to right: **HUSSEIN SMKO, GOODW.Y.N., AND HIPÓLITO ARRIAGA III,**
The Space Between: Unlikely Entanglements Opening Program, Hyde Park Art Center;
see also: pp. 75, 232–35

perspective. Through spoken word, performance art, and dance, the artists explored the history of US colonialism, the moral injury of witnessing and contributing to the oppression of other people of color, and how war affects more than just the people fighting in it. The performance highlighted both the universality of trauma as well as the collective healing that is possible when compassion and empathy are present.

Arriaga performed his dialogue while crossing the balcony overlooking the floor (and later across the main area) while Smko incorporated dramatic dance movements as he came in and out of the space. This occurred while GOODW.Y.N. traversed the entire wall of the room blindfolded and on her knees. The performance kept audience members intently focused on the co-occurring words, dance, and movement. The piece ended with the three artists and their intersecting journeys culminating in a seated position, shoulder to shoulder, as their outstretched arms extended in a representation of support, acknowledgment, and unity. Although I sat in on rehearsals and knew what to expect, the emotional intensity of the work and the attentiveness of the audience members filled me—and probably everyone else in the space—with an enthralling range of emotions.

KB: *The third day of the Summit featured* DRONE, *a new play by Andrea Assaf, an Arab American writer and theater artist. Assaf was accompanied onstage at the Chicago Cultural Center by several vocalists, performers, and musicians who played the violin, the oud, and various hand drums. The play uses the metaphor of drones, both in music and in warfare and surveillance, to make a statement about moral injury and violence. What did you find particularly moving about this work?*

AT: DRONE, with its minimalistic staging and multi-voice poetry, highlights the impact of US military drone strikes on civilians. The first-person narratives evoke the trauma and suffering of war survivors. As a veteran, I felt both a physical and emotional response to the performance. It evoked the shame and guilt I continue to carry about my participation in the Iraq War as a combatant. It reinforced my commitment to demilitarization, social justice, and human rights. I realized during the performance how vitally important it is for all stakeholders—specifically veterans—to hear these types of stories and sit with uncomfortable feelings. We have to show up and listen. The next step is solidarity and taking actionable steps to transform suffering, both our own as well as communities impacted by war. Andrea Assaf's dedication to anti-war and decolonization themes made DRONE a powerful addition to the Triennial.

KB: *Can you talk about the opening program* Forging Hope: Reckon and Reimagine, *which centered on Native voices and featured hip-hop, Americana, and pop music?*

AT: Elexa Dawson (Citizen Potawatomi Nation) shared songs about joy, love, and land sovereignty. Joseph Running Crane (Blackfeet) sang and talked about existential angst, loss, and survival. Brittney Chantele, a Chicago-based hip-hop/pop artist, shared pieces from their 2020 album, *The Golden Opportunity*, which focused on their journey through the US military and eventual work as an anti-war activist. The final performer was hip-hop artist, music producer, and spoken word poet James Pakootas (Confederate Tribes of Colville). His work touched on themes of healing from trauma, seeking inner strength, and exploring one's cultural heritage. A standout moment was the impromptu collaboration between Hussein Smko and Pakootas, which added interpretive dance to the depth of Pakootas' spoken word. The performers beautifully reminded us all that we can find strength in each other, that growth is possible after trauma, and that we can remain hopeful for the future.

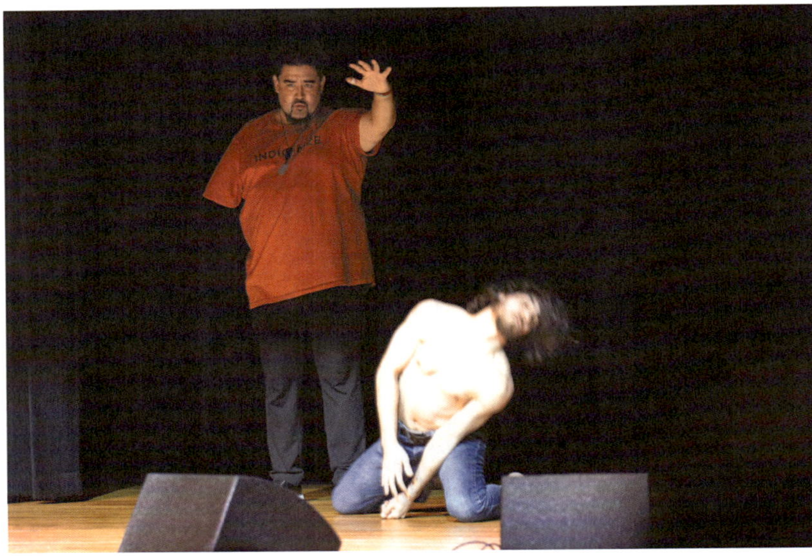

left: **JAMES PAKOOTAS** *right:* **HUSSEIN SMKO**, *Forging Hope: Reckon and Reimagine* Opening Program, Chicago Cultural Center; *see also: p. 260–61*

KB: *The closing Summit performance featured jingle dress dancer Starla Thompson (Potawatomi). Her performance, where she talked about her family history and personal connection to traditions of healing dance, was followed by a closing circle, which invited the participation of all Triennial attendees. How did this event reflect the thematic vision of the Triennial?*

AT: Starla Thompson was the first performer I reached out to for the Triennial. After learning about her work in the local community as an Indigenous educator, curator, and advocate, I felt her participation would be profoundly impactful. I also wanted to be mindful of the request, as she shared with me that jingle dress dancing is a deeply personal and sacred practice. Thompson invited cultural activist, workshop facilitator, and Native flute player Brian Frejo (Pawnee/Seminole) to join her for the presentation. Frejo spoke about his work in art and activism and shared a musical performance before introducing Thompson. She discussed the origin story of the dress and dance, its historical relevance, and her connection and experience with the ceremony, culminating with a demonstration of the dance. I found it to be the most fitting way to culminate the program—with a performative cultural practice that reinforced the Triennial's themes of peace, healing, and justice.

The closing circle, which I co-facilitated with Andrea Assaf and Kim Pevia, modeled the Triennial's intention of solidarity through collective voices and experiences. The discussions emphasized the importance of vulnerability, selflessness, and community care, also aligning with the Triennial's themes.

KB: *Are there any memorable Summit moments that you can point to that encapsulate the power of this community and its work? What do you hope people took away from the experience?*

AT: The moments that stood out to me most were the conversations before, during, and after these events. It was a special experience to witness people have both intellectual and emotional realizations. People shared with me their shifts in perspective. A Latinx war veteran told me that a conversation she had with an Iraqi civilian helped her work through shame and guilt about her involvement in the war as a combatant. Halfway through the Triennial, a Native American performer pulled me aside to share that he had begun to see the parallels experienced by different communities impacted by war. I witnessed the building blocks of solidarity. Truly inspiring. Going forward, I want to encourage all veteran artists to build on the work the Triennial started, push creative boundaries, collaborate with others, and imagine new futures together.

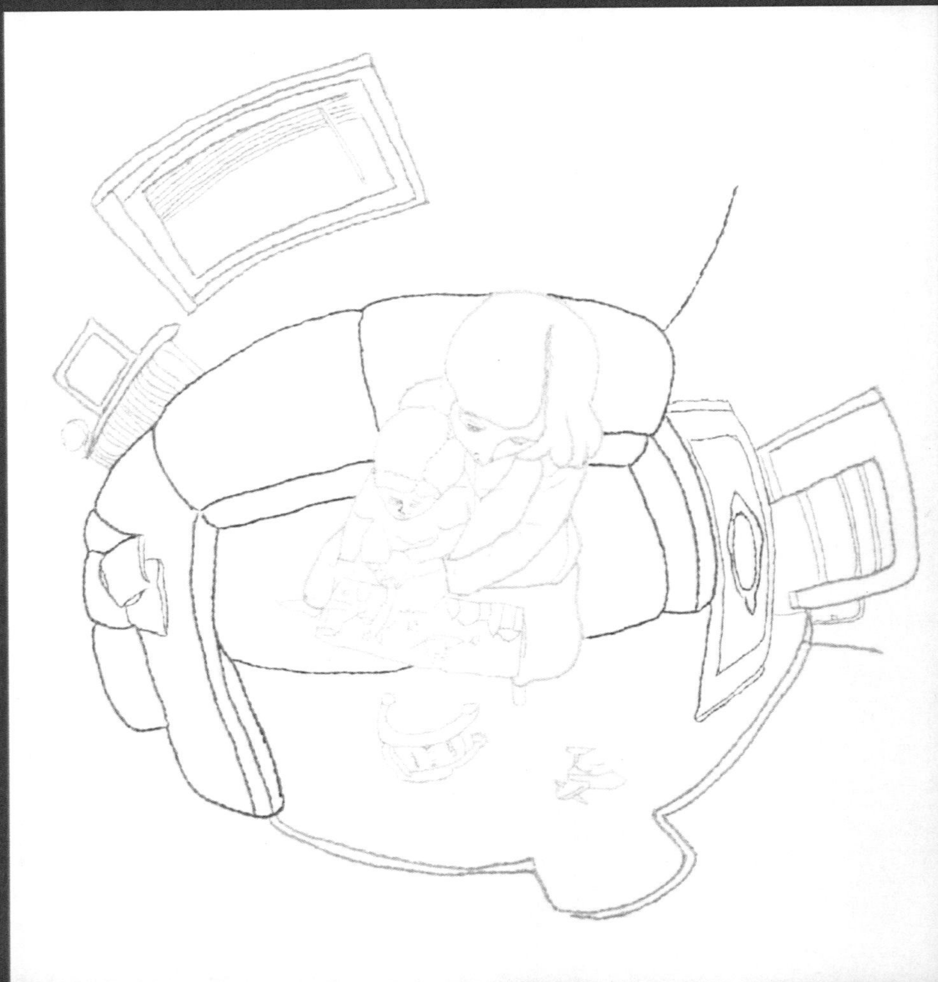

SABBA ELAHI
everyday suspects #8 (detail)

see also: p. 177

The Summit, Then and Now

ISRA RAHMAN

It has been over a year since the start of the Israeli onslaught in Gaza. My life ever since has been a series of responses and reactions to various calls to action, arrests, and even detainment. Amidst all this, like many around the world, I have absorbed poet Rafeef Ziadah's mantra that "Palestinians teach life," understanding what it means to live amidst the destruction inflicted by the United States government and Israel on Palestinians abroad and activists at home. I find it necessary to situate myself within that movement as I reflect on the *Surviving the Long Wars* Veteran Art Triennial & Summit, which I first wrote about in May 2023. Since then, my perspective on the role of exhibits like this, and the positionality of all the artists involved, has changed. As we gear up to build a resilient anti-war movement focused on militarism abroad and policing at home, the role of veterans as a reflection of individuals' ability to change and show up as war resisters and refuseniks in solidarity with targeted and impacted communities in that endeavor becomes increasingly clear. Their voices and actions, from Aaron Bushnell's self-immolation to workers in various military sites mobilizing internally, have propelled critical conversations forward.

My trust has continued to evolve, sparked initially by my interest in the work of STLW co-organizer Aaron Hughes, who curated the interdisciplinary exhibition *Remaking the Exceptional* at DePaul Art Museum in 2022. This exhibition connected policing and militarism around the world, from Guantánamo Bay to Homan Square. In Chicago, reflecting on these connections becomes even more poignant following the killing of Dexter Reed by Chicago police officers in March 2024, and the ongoing reaction to that police violence.

When I first heard about *Surviving the Long Wars*, I was both curious and skeptical. Having lived through the events of 9/11 and witnessed the intensified structural Islamophobia in its wake, I approach American portrayals of war and Muslims with caution, wary of falling into oversimplified narratives of "good" and "bad" Muslims. I had met few veterans, let alone any who had served in countries where my people come from.

However, I placed my trust in Hughes, whose previous exhibition had left a profound impact on me. So, I attended the Triennial, eager to explore what veteran art would evoke in me and whether it would critically reflect on US militarism or serve as propaganda for war.

I was not disappointed. The Triennial questioned the origins and impacts of war at home and abroad by bringing together art and artists. By humanizing the individuals behind the artworks, the exhibitions and summit moved beyond mere reflection, inviting artists and attendees alike to confront the pain and suffering inflicted by war and its many displacements.

In an interview with the *South Side Weekly*, Ronak K. Kapadia discussed the internationalist approach they aimed to achieve through this project. "It is about putting Arab, Muslim, and South Asian diasporic art in conversation with the long wars and the centuries-long history of Native and Black-led rebellion against security orders in the US."

The STLW Summit, which opened the Triennial, coincided with the twenty-year anniversary of the US invasion of Iraq, shedding light on the two longest wars in US history: the "American Indian Wars" and the "Global War on Terror." The parallels between these conflicts were explored and highlighted throughout the weekend event. There was a palpable discomfort among the art viewers as they were prompted to reckon with the complexities of the war machine and forced to hold multiple truths.

"The BIPOC veteran artists featured in this show represent a segment of society whose lives and communities have also been profoundly impacted, if not outright destroyed, by the machinery of war," explained Kapadia. "Our aim is to foster transformative dialogues about healing justice and to apply an abolitionist lens to military violence, all while questioning the possibilities for reconciliation and accountability."

The second day of the Summit, hosted at the Hyde Park Art Center, featured programming that captured the essence of seventeen artists' works while speaking to the overarching Triennial themes. The atmosphere in this space felt more casual compared to the previous day at the Newberry Library and later at the Chicago Cultural Center. Visitors had the freedom to walk around, eat, and drink at their own pace, luxuries not always afforded in the more regulated art spaces downtown.

Mahwish Chishty, an artist from Massachusetts with roots in Pakistan, presented a series of pieces titled *Drone Art*. Beautifying the ugliest parts of violence, she created collages inside outlines of the aerial drones used by the US military in Pakistan, Afghanistan, and Yemen. "The imagery on these machines is borrowed from the truck art, which is a native tradition of Pakistani truck art culture, where trucks are painted beautifully, elaborately in bright colors, and they have this iconography mixed with text and almost universal visual symbols that require no language in some way," Chishty said during a group tour. "So, I'm using that to show the deadliness of these machines."

However, the exhibition's significance extended beyond the remarkable art on display. I overheard visitors' discussions ranging from the history of the US annexation of Native land to the implications of the PATRIOT Act and policing in schools, all while we broke bread and sipped wine. The thematic threads of Chishty's work, along with its intimate exploration of surveillance in the lives of drone victims, resonated with the artistry of June Carpenter, another featured artist. Carpenter, who serves as the repatriation specialist at Chicago's Field Museum, depicted the violence of the forced expulsion of Native Americans through hand-embroidered shawls. The shawls were adorned with the language of the six most egregious Supreme Court cases that sanctioned violence against Native Americans. In one case, titled *Cherokee Nation v. Georgia* (1831), the Cherokee Nation was deemed a "domestic dependent" nation, thus establishing the guardian-ward dynamic between Native nations and the American government. This case, along with many others, set a legal precedent for the ways the US government received leeway to intervene in every aspect of Native life through forced separation of families and schooling. Carpenter portrayed this in ornately embroidered woven shawls functioning almost as shrouds and expansive coverings for the abuse done by the American government. In Carpenter's pieces, shawls, typically symbols of beauty and warmth, even wealth, became poignant reminders of the layers of concealment that facilitated American settler-colonial violence.

In a city like Chicago, where indigeneity is understood differently compared to states with reservations, like Oklahoma and South

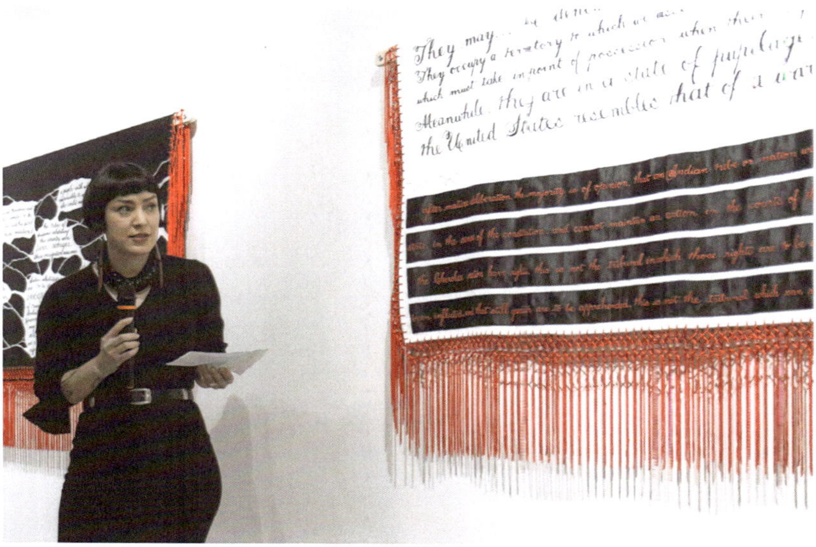

JUNE CARPENTER, *Cherokee Nation v. Georgia, 30 U.S. 1 (1831)*, 2022, Linen fabric, satin ribbon, cotton thread, nylon fringe, and glass beads; *see also: pp. 162–63, 283*

Dakota, the lesser visibility of Native American art is no coincidence. Despite being offered land in neighboring states, Native Americans were continually displaced from Illinois, making it one of the few states—and one of the westernmost—to lack reservations (at least until the April 2024 news that the US government had federally recognized lands of the Prairie Band Potawatomi Nation's northern Illinois reservation into a trust). This modern-day reality underscores the violence inherent in that expulsion and emphasizes the importance of organizing among groups like the Chi-Nations Youth Council.

As Kapadia pointed out, the parallels between these wars lie in their shared aim to disrupt intimate spaces, an idea echoed by many of the artists at the Triennial. Kapadia said, "Counterinsurgent violence works by trying to destroy various forms of intimacy, also to destroy our sense of our relationship to each other. This is a key idea in my book [*Insurgent Aesthetics*], which is that counterinsurgency warfare operates by trying to destroy our sense of how we are connected to each other. And so actually, part of what our practice is doing is giving us a renewed sense of solidarity and intimacy through difference."

Intimacy emerged as a recurring thread woven throughout the exhibitions, whether conveyed through the art forms themselves, or the personal narratives shared by artists. Sabba Elahi, a Chicago-based artist, leveraged drone imagery akin to Chishty's work and utilized fabric similar to Carpenter's, but with a twist—she captured not the drone itself, but what it would witness. By embroidering scenes of domestic intimacy, Elahi revealed the chilling perspective of a drone operator prior to unleashing destruction upon a family. Outside of the context, these pieces could be seen as embroidered images of families, tender moments over a box of pizza, or sitting on the couch watching the nightly news. Instead, in the context of drone surveillance, its violence is even more insidious. Taking it a step further, she uses the form and technique of machine embroidery in some of her pieces to shed light on the mechanization of so much of the war industry, whether it be in production or practice.

The diversity of mediums in the exhibition—from performance art and paintings to collages, quilting, embroidery, and printmaking—underscored the multifaceted nature of the narratives explored. Ruth Kaneko, a former combat medic, crafted paper from her military uniforms to honor the thirty-eight thousand Hawaiians who opposed the annexation of Hawai'i by the United States. The pieces were an homage to her Hawaiian heritage and resistance ancestry, blending form and function to convey a powerful message.

In a tearful explanation, Kaneko explained the personal significance of her work, rooted in the recent passing of her grandmother. Her pieces, which both anonymized and highlighted the sheer volume of individuals impacted by US-forced annexation, underscored the impact of the war machine on communities and individuals alike. "In the early 1800s, there were 1.2 million Native Hawaiians in Hawai'i. By the time that it was illegally annexed by the United States, there

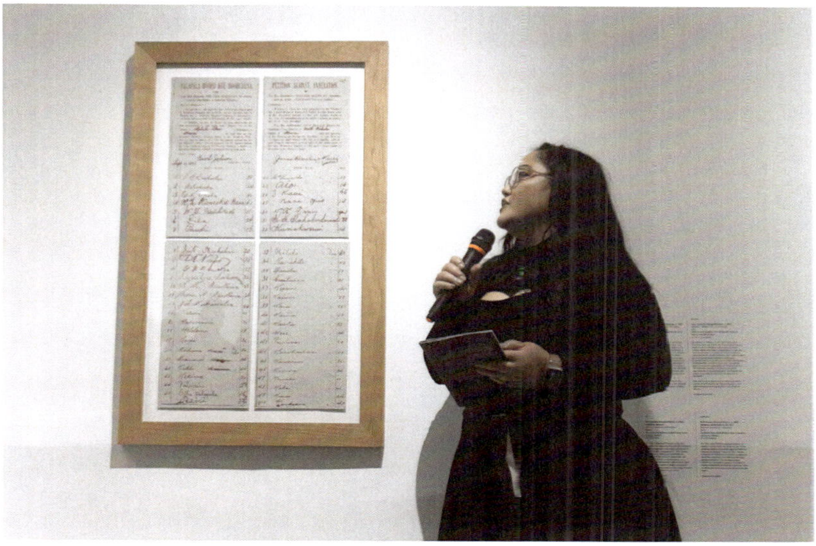

RUTH KANEKO, *Service Connected II: Kānehailua*, 2023, Silkscreen on handmade paper (made out of military uniforms); *see also: pp. 167–69*

were 40,000 native Hawaiians left," said Ruth. "So after Hawai'i was illegally annexed by the United States in 1893, these women went across Hawai'i, and they collected 38,000 petition signatures, which basically is the entire population."

The artworks shed light on the organizing efforts of Native Hawaiians during that period and underscored the immense power and perseverance required to gather signatures from the remaining Hawaiians after strategic displacement and erasure policies were enacted by the US military. The art held profound personal significance for Kaneko, whose family name was among the 38,000 featured. Like many Native veterans, her pieces encapsulated the tension I anticipated upon entering the exhibition: how do we create a space that acknowledges both veterans and war victims? The harsh reality is that war intertwines itself deeply within communities, leaving ample room for veterans in this space to articulate just how deeply this entanglement affects them.

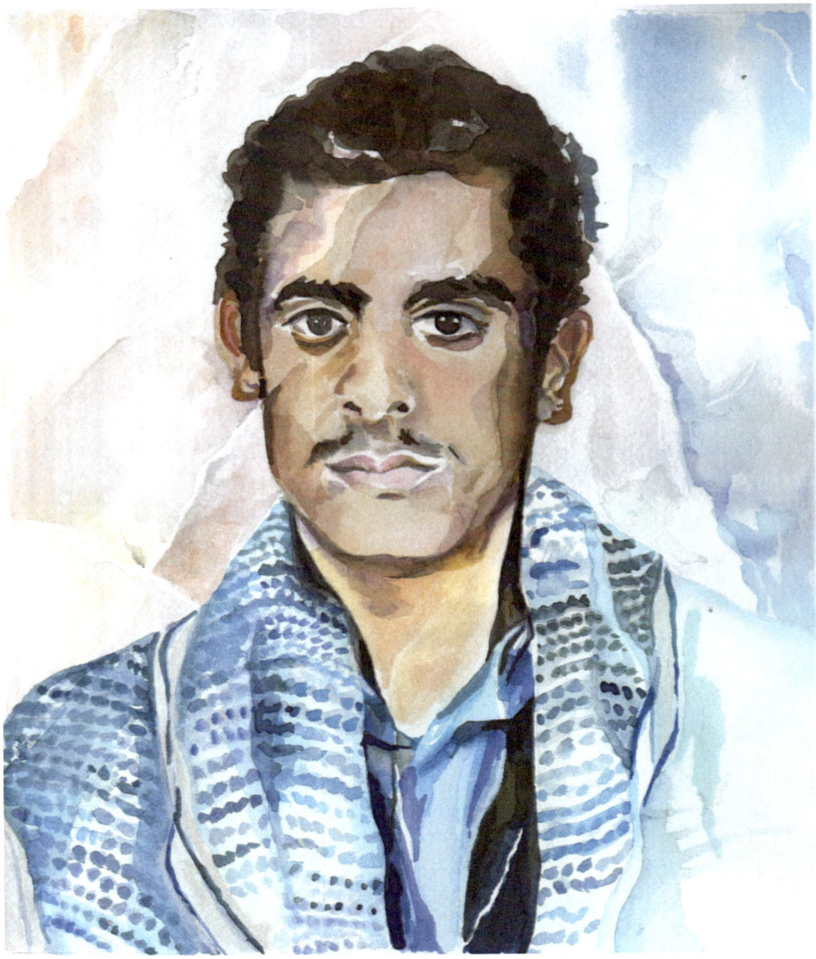

CHITRA GANESH, *Index of the Disappeared: Watercolors* (series) - *Fahd Gazy*, 2004, Watercolor on paper; *see also: pp. 85–87, 139*

In Chitra Ganesh's installation at the Chicago Cultural Center, we were confronted with a poignant reminder of the impact of the "War on Terror" on individual lives. Through her delicate watercolor portraits titled *Index of the Disappeared: Watercolors*, Ganesh brought attention to those who were vanished by the US government in the aftermath of 9/11, including Fahd Gazy, a former detainee at

Guantánamo Bay, and Sami Al-Arian, a Kuwaiti-born Palestinian activist placed under house arrest from 2003 to 2014 under PATRIOT Act charges. The choice of medium and form adds depth to the message; rather than employing stiff, sharp portraits with acrylic paint, Ganesh opted for watercolors, softening the edges and outlines of the portraits as a tribute to the lives lost and stolen.

Each venue hosting the Triennial and Summit brought a unique dimension to the overall experience. Located several miles south of the other installations, Hyde Park Art Center offered a distinct atmosphere, amidst the work and studios of artists like Robert Paige and Malika Jackson. The culminating moment at HPAC came with a performance by Hipólito Arriaga III, GOODW.Y.N., and Hussein Smko. On the cusp of Ramadan, during Jummah nonetheless, the unexpected echo of the adhan through the gallery room at HPAC set a solemn tone. From there, these three movement artists eloquently captured a spectrum of emotions—hurt and pain, joy, and solidarity—through the lyrical movement of their bodies. The performance artists captured emotion in a way the paintings, sculptures, and other nonmovement artworks could not, tying all of the pieces together into a whole.

The artwork showcased in the Cultural Center evoked a grandeur that surpassed the ornate Center itself, offering a unique reflection of the art. Visitors walked through the Tiffany dome and marble engraved ceilings to reach the gallery, where the illumination of Michael Rakowitz's collage portraits of Iraq resonated deeply. These artworks not only commemorated the stolen and destroyed art of Iraq but also captured the grandeur of the Assyrian northwest palace at Kalhu. They underscored how wars affect not only individuals but also art and its surrounding infrastructures.

Throughout the exhibition, the pieces reverberated with the trauma and pain they conveyed. "Very little attention [in mainstream media] is focused on the ongoing nature of these wars, like these 'Indian Wars' never ended," said Kapadia. "'The War on Terror' never ended, even if it was declared 'mission accomplished' a million times. These long wars permeate the lives of so many different kinds of people in their endless permutations. *Surviving the Long Wars* aimed to shed light not only on the afterlives of these wars but also on the ongoing presence of these wars in lots of different kinds of people's lives."

The exhibition invited viewers to walk away with a global sense of solidarity and a commitment to the internationalist struggle for freedom. In the same way, it can evoke a sense of powerlessness; despite the beautiful community created, these wars persist.

As Dunya Mikhail writes in a poem she read on the first day of the Summit ("My Poem Will Not Save You"):

> Their songs will not save us,
> although, in the chilliest times,
> they keep us warm,
> and when we need to touch the soul
> to know it's not dead
> their songs
> give us that touch.

An earlier version of this piece was published in the South Side Weekly, *a nonprofit newsroom dedicated to producing local journalism that is for, by, and about the South Side of Chicago.*

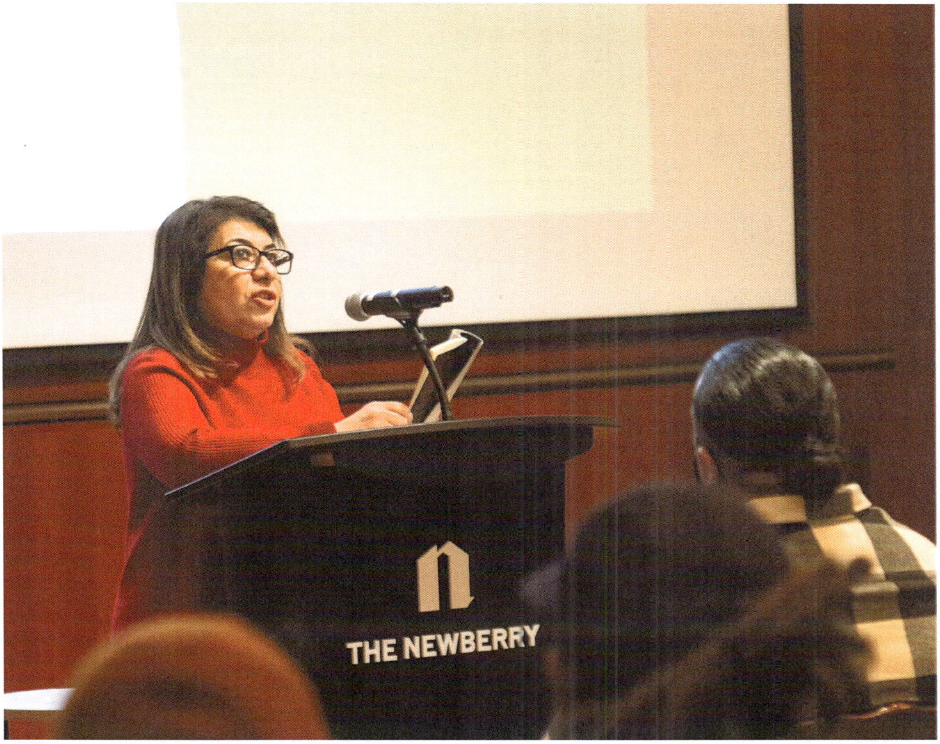

DUNYA MIKHAIL, *Residues and Rebellions* Poetry Reading, Newberry Library

conclusion

Hordes

Morning Maw

CARLOS SIRAH

of horse's hooves
a thousand strong
R o a R i n g
r o a r i n g to t he water's edge
The ship swallows
me whole
in belly of wood and iron and storm
sometimes . I
d
i
e
in the belly of the ship
Sometimes I g r o w old
in the belly of the ship
Sometimes I chew through the
hull
S w i m o u t
into d a r k n e s s
down
down
down
Clop Clop Clop
Are there horses In the sea?
neigh neigh
Buck that slaver Buck this ship
Overboard I go Shot And sinking
What is sun if not remembered?
With me or against?
Seize the ship!
Steer it home
On mother's voice In wind behind
To think with sky
Is to be an opportunist
here
Sometimes memory betrays
So many possibilities
In this oscillation
I rather . wayward omnivalent
Than cede to slavers' ordered time
Here. Half-light. You with me
In ripple's reflection?
Cough up sea
Touch land
Watch myself Beside horse
Away
from
tide
the ending
an ending
I prefer

and then the phone rings. It's your friend, or your mother, or someone that you love who was still alive this time last year or the year before or twenty years ago. You tell yourself, I am made up, a fiction of myself. They offer comfort. Tell you, you are made up of soft good things. Of tissue and skin, and gut and brain. They tell you to listen. You tell yourself. Listen. You are so tired of listening. The drones. The sirens, the screams of empire refusing its death. They remind you of Fanon. Fanon tells you decolonization is always a violent event. The phone rings again. You wake, and you do not answer. And a pandemic wasp returned. You remember the one. Visited daily for a month, stinging you, and then. You will question sanity, edema, torpor, iris, mercury, encampments, rooms, visitations, fallwayintos, maths, hollers, frottage, wakes, redress. The phone rings, it's your comrade. This situation... You yell. You mean pandemic, you mean occupation, you mean catastrophe, you mean, this cull of our people, you mean this axis of domination, you mean this total war upon the peoples of the earth, don't you? The phone rings. It's your mother. She's had another heart attack or another attack of the heart. Waylaid. What's the difference? She's in the old country, the land where you grew up. Hundreds of miles away. She says you should make more of an effort. That she may not live. That she's unsure about living, Waylaid, like this. And what are you doing anyway? You tell your mother. Living. Your mother scoffs. Waylaid. That silence. You stars. You, interdependently, pulling and shaping that space between... Your mother does not believe in rifts. Besides, her gravity is stronger than yours. You accuse of her being a straight line. To what? You? She counters, laughs. Catherine, the dead girl, the one between you, would have never laughed like that. Knowing this, you laugh, in turn. In earth. You remember. Your living room is very large. The window comprises one whole wall of the flat. Eastward. The window is an event like any other. Landing on the moon. Lighting a fire. Taking the dish out of the oven and sitting down for dinner. First you take it all in. Then you pick up the fork, the tender morsels of fungi, and salt, and butter taste very good. Savor this. Of flesh. Of tongue. And there you are again, with yourself. Enfleshed. You recognize once upon a time. In repose, this fantasy of the north, of the west, of the plains, of the isles, of these promised lands, lies exposed, flesh rotting, yet alive powerful, no longer at bay gnash teeth, hiss venom, flail wildly and their arms spread arm wide against the primary peoples of the world. Another time, surrounded by the migratory, by legacies of lack, by the unsettled, revolutionizing, themselves under the possibility of a new governance against total, amnesia, as void, as surface and miscomprehension. Another world.

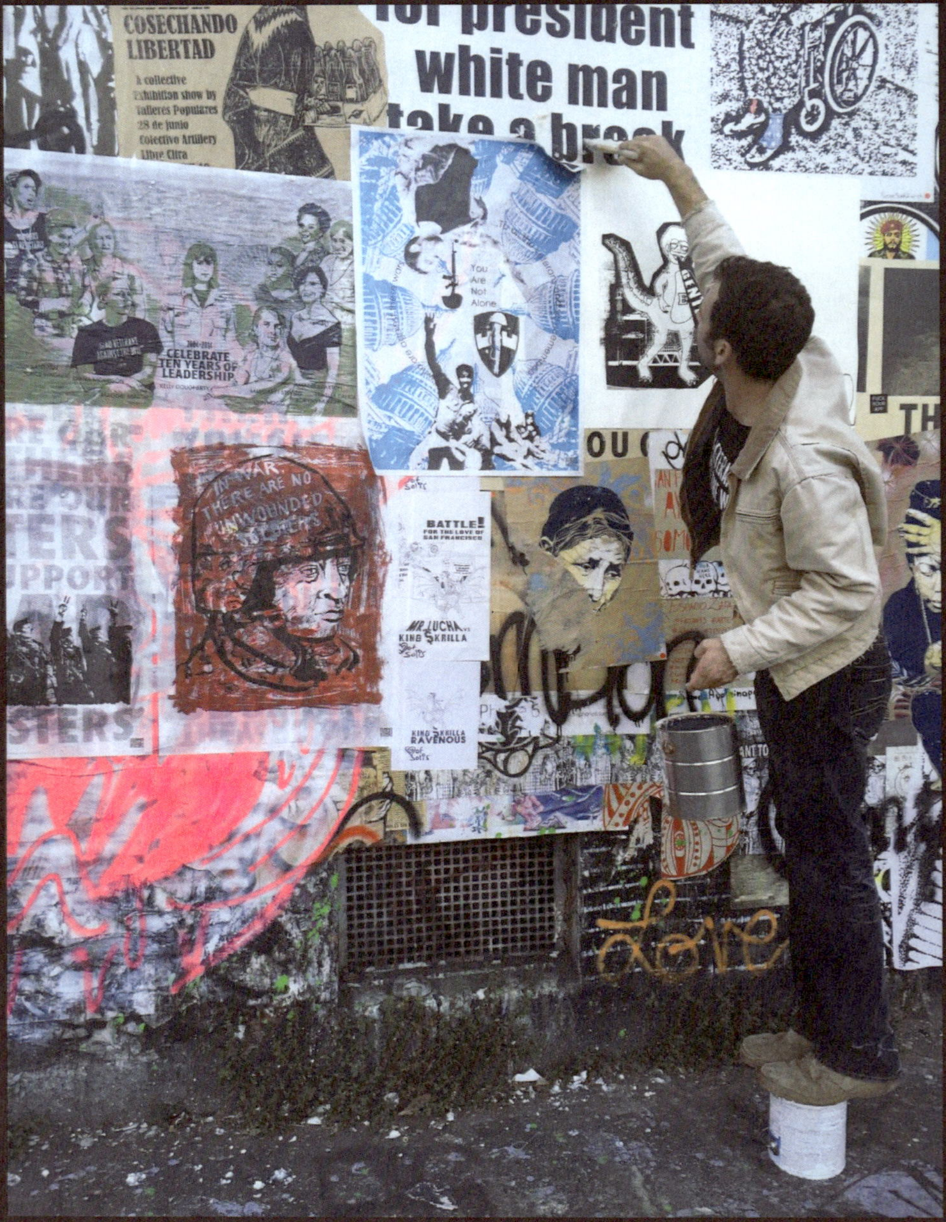
COSECHANDO
LIBERTAD
white man
You
Are
Not
Alone
CELEBRATE
TEN YEARS OF
LEADERSHIP
IN WAR
THERE ARE NO
UNWOUNDED
SOLDIERS
BATTLE!
KING SKRILLA
RAVENOUS
Love

CELEBRATE PEOPLE'S HISTORY: IVAW STREET ART ACTION
Iraq Veterans Against the War (IVAW) members Drew Cameron (photographer) and Ryan Holleran (pictured) wheatpaste broadsides from the *Celebrate People's History: IVAW* portfolio on the streets of Portland, Oregon (March 31, 2015).

Sowing Seeds of Resistance

AARON HUGHES

In the wake of a great wildfire, across a vast charred landscape, seeds sown long ago sprout, sending bright green shoots through the blackened remains of ancient trees. Old hardwoods unfurl new leaves, and wildflowers bloom in a kaleidoscope of violets, sapphires, and golds. Like these resilient sprouts, a legacy of creative rebellion bursts forth from the genocidal violence of the US long wars. At times it lies dormant, buried in books and archives; other times, it takes root behind prison walls or in blockaded streets. It manifests as sketches in tattered journals, poems in xeroxed zines, posters wheat-pasted on city streets, and brushstrokes layered on vibrant canvases.

Yet, as too many of us know, in the midst of the inferno, war and its destruction feel omnipresent. It can seem nearly impossible to know, or even imagine, anything else. And still, from within this chaos—the brutal bombardments, fierce oppression, and lingering damage—artists find ways to make marks, to create, to survive.

I was sitting at an old oak table in the monotoned reading room of the Newberry Library, considering artworks for the 2023 Veteran Art Triennial. Several pieces from their archives were spread out before me, but my eyes were pulled again and again to the ink and watercolor drawings of Frederick Gokliz (White Mountain Apache). The intricate details he rendered in vibrant reds, yellows, and greens mixed with shades of sepia seemed as fresh and vivid as when he painted them over a century ago. I found myself transfixed by Gokliz's art and story. I could imagine him gently dabbing the blue details on *Two men on horseback with shields* or patiently working on the ink lines in *Woman and baby in cradleboard*.[1] His ability to create such beauty despite the brutal dispossession he faced struck me with awe.

I knew I would not have been so resilient. During my fifteen-month deployment to Kuwait and Iraq at age twenty-one, I reached a point where I could no longer create. For years, I had turned to my sketchbook to reflect and imagine; yet, while deployed, I tried and tried and just couldn't make a mark. The fatigue, insanity, and moral bankruptcy of helping to establish an occupation under the guise of "liberation" left me dejected, trapped in inner conflict. Yet, years later, sitting in an air-conditioned research room as an artist and curator, my earlier struggles seemed insignificant in light of what Gokliz had faced.

Records show Gokliz made these works between 1894 and 1899 while he was imprisoned by the US—as an enemy POW—and, paradoxically, also a soldier in the US Army.[2] At first, I could not

1 "Frederick Gokliz Ink and Watercolor Drawings of Apache Indians [ca. 1894-ca. 1899]," Edward E. Ayer Digital Collection (Newberry Library), accessed September 1, 2024, https://collections.carli.illinois.edu/digital/collection/nby_eeayer/id/2584/.

2 The Newberry Library provides the following biographical note: "During 1886 Gokliz was imprisoned with the Chiricahua Apaches at Fort Marion in San Augustine, Fla., and remained with the Chiricahua prisoners for the rest of his life. From 1888 to 1894 Gokliz was at Mount Vernon, Ala., and he enlisted in the US army in 1891, moving to Fort Sill, Okla., in 1894.," Newberry Library Catalog, accessed September 1, 2024, https://i-share-nby.primo.exlibrisgroup.com/permalink/01CARLI_NBY/i5mcb2/alma991510448805867. See also Smithsonian Online Virtual Archives, "Frederick Gokliz Drawings," accessed September 1, 2024, https://www.si.edu/object/archives/sova-naa-ms270077.

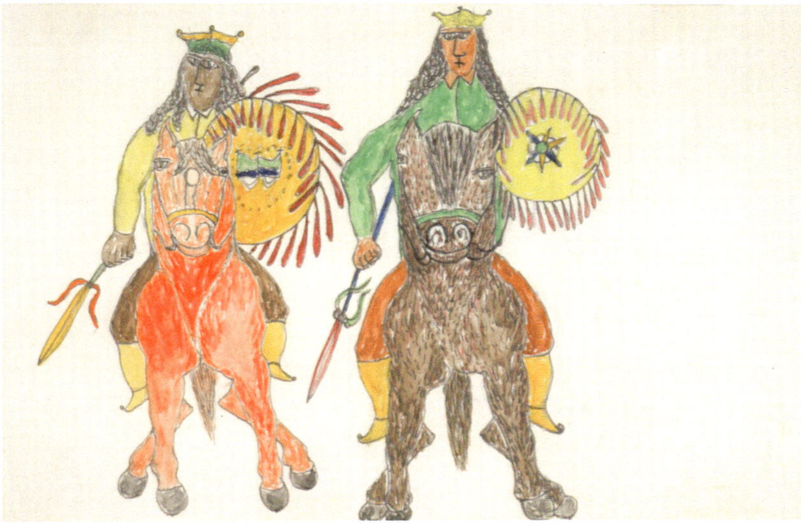

FREDERICK GOKLIZ, *Two men on horseback with shields*, ca. 1894–ca. 1899, Ink and watercolor drawings; *see also: p. 25–26*

understand how that was possible. But slowly a more nuanced picture emerged, exposing the way counterinsurgency strategies depend on enlisting local populations to defuse and destroy resistance. Gokliz's experience resonates across histories and geographies, from the Americas to the Greater Middle East, where colonizers continually recruit Indigenous people into military campaigns as scouts, interpreters, and intermediaries, furthering assimilation goals while quashing rebellions.[3] From Gokliz's watercolors to Mariam Ghani's *The Trespassers* (2011) to Ruth Kaneko's *Service Connected II* (2023), the works I was researching for the Triennial revealed a web of interconnected exploitation.[4]

Despite this legacy of colonial violence, the Apaches defended their homelands for generations. Gokliz married into and lived with the Chokonen band of the Chiricahua Apaches, a band led by Chief Cochise and later Geronimo, who became legendary for their successful

---

3 Alexandra N. Harris and Mark G. Hirsch, "Indian Wars, Indian Scouts" in *Why We Serve: Native Americans in the United States Armed Forces* (Washington, DC: Smithsonian Books, 2023), 59.

4 See *The Trespassers* (2011) by Mariam Ghani, pp. 86–87; See *Service Connected II: Kānehailua* (2023) by Ruth Kaneko, pp. 167, 169, 301.

confrontations with the US Army and their ability to evade capture. Tragically, it was only after the US military enlisted Apache scouts to aid their pursuit of the Chokonen band that they finally succeeded in forcing Geronimo to surrender in 1886—a haunting testament to the co-opting cruelty of counterinsurgency strategies.[5]

I remembered listening to *Geronimo's Story of His Life* (1906) during long drives from Chicago to Fort Hood, Texas. Between 2009 and 2012, as an organizer for Iraq Veterans Against the War, I made several extended trips a year to aid anti-war soldiers at Under the Hood, a GI rights coffeehouse. Our focus was supporting war resisters to weaken the military's ability to sustain the occupations in Iraq and Afghanistan. Activists from across the country would converge on the largest military base in the US to support soldiers refusing orders, speaking out, or just seeking a way out of the military. To fill the long hours on the road, I listened to audiobooks that addressed military history and strategies of resistance. Geronimo's autobiography fit the bill.

The book includes military telegrams detailing confrontations with the Apaches and Geronimo's eventual capture. These cold and calculated communications were used as a narrative device to corroborate Geronimo's story. Yet, I found them unnerving. The truncated dialogue echoed the rhetoric of the "Global War on Terror," with dehumanizing terms like "hostiles" and the chilling "capture or destroy" orders.[6] It reminded me of my own unit's banter about the "Wild West" in Iraq.

So later, in 2011, I was aggravated by reports of SEAL Team Six using "Geronimo" as the codename for Osama Bin Laden during their mission to capture and kill him. It was distressing enough to realize that the military had preserved the language and counter-

5 Colin G. Calloway, "The Vermont Secretary and the Apache POWs: Redfield Proctor and the Case of the Chiricahuas," *Vermont History* 59, no. 3, (1991): 167, https://vermonthistory.org/journal/misc/VermontSecretary.pdf.

6 Geronimo and S. M. Barrett, *Geronimo's Story of His Life* (New York: Duffield, 1906), 149.

insurgency strategies of the genocidal "American Indian Wars;" but celebrating it through the cultural appropriation of the Apache leader and pageantry of Bin Laden's assassination was nauseating.

It reminded me of Vietnam veteran and American Indian Movement member Evan Haney's testimony at the 1971 *Winter Soldier Investigation*: "If you took the Vietnamese war, or the American War, as it is, and compared it to the Indian wars a hundred years ago, it would be the same thing. All the massacres were the same."[7] Despite the siloed histories of these wars, the language, strategies, and logics of US militarism persist, perpetuating parallel acts of brutality and corresponding genocides, and necessitating a relentless spirit of revolt.

After Geronimo's surrender, Gokliz was imprisoned with the Chiricahua Apaches at Fort Marion, Florida. In 1888, he was transferred to Mount Vernon, Alabama, where he and other Apache prisoners were coerced into enlisting in the US Army as part of a forced assimilation strategy.[8] US Secretary of War Redfield Proctor believed that military service would integrate Apaches into "American life," a vision of ethnic cleansing that lays bare the contradictions of US imperialism—contradictions that have the capacity to unravel worlds, inflict moral injury, and perpetuate intergenerational trauma.[9] In response, Gokliz created brilliantly rendered watercolors celebrating traditional Apache life. His precise line work depicts families, community gatherings, and warriors defiantly challenging the viewer, asserting his people's rebellion through the prism of conscription and imprisonment.

---

7 Vietnam Veterans Against the War, *The Winter Soldier Investigation: An Inquiry Into American War Crimes* (Boston: Beacon Press, 1972), 156.

8 "Frederick Gokliz Ink and Watercolor Drawings of Apache Indians [ca. 1894-ca. 1899]," Edward E. Ayer Digital Collection (Newberry Library), accessed September 1, 2024, https://collections.carli.illinois.edu/digital/collection/nby_eeayer/id/2584/.

9 Colin G. Calloway, "The Vermont Secretary and the Apache POWs: Redfield Proctor and the Case of the Chiricahuas," *Vermont History* 59, no. 3, (1991), 175, https://vermonthistory.org/journal/misc/VermontSecretary.pdf.

This assertion reverberates across time to the contemporary artists who created new works for the Triennial, many of whom have grappled to reconcile their military service with their complex identities and experiences. Darrell W. Fair—a Marine Corps veteran, Chicago police torture survivor, and imprisoned artist—exemplifies this.[10] For years, I have worked with him and other artists, scholars, and veterans imprisoned at Stateville as a teaching-artist and facilitator with the Prison + Neighborhood Arts/Education Project. In Fair's newly developed colored-pencil drawing *Self Portrait* (2022), a weary yet engaging figure is centered, surrounded by a mosaic of vignettes reflecting his experiences in the military and his time in prison. His tired eyes are encircled by expressive curving lines that command attention, while his overall facial expression remains distant. The drawing is rendered on ledger paper with the word "register" at the top—a direct reference to the multiplicity of registries used to profile and target BIPOC communities throughout US history, from allotments to gang databases to terrorist "watch lists." Inspired by Indigenous prisoners like Gokliz, Fair used the ledger paper to document his resistance and resilience, though his ghostly, thousand-yard stare suggests a depth of pain that words cannot capture.[11]

Similarly, Monty Little (Diné) channels defiance while grappling with the violent and contested lineages he embodies. His artistic practice poses the kinds of questions that drew me to the library in

---

10 After his military service, Fair was arrested at his home, detained, and tortured by the Chicago police, leading to a statement that, although he never signed, was used to convict him. See "Survivors Stories Darrell Fair," Chicago Alliance Against Racist and Political Repression, accessed September 1, 2024, https://www.caarpr.org/survivors-1/darrell-fair. While imprisoned, Fair has continued to assert his innocence and work toward his freedom. As an artist and scholar, he has been active with the Prison + Neighborhood Arts/Education Project and was a part of the first cohort of students to graduate with Bachelor of Art degrees at Stateville Prison in over two decades. See "University Without Walls," Prison + Neighborhood Arts/Education Project, accessed September 1, 2024, https://p-nap.org/university-without-walls/. Fair is the Vice Commander of the Stateville Veterans Group, which he helped found. A stylized self-portrait created by Fair was exhibited in *The Weight of Rage* (2016) and featured on the cover of *Poetry* (April, 2016).

11 Fair received a DEMIL Art Fund award to develop new work for the Triennial. Two of the *STLW* co-curators, Hughes and Zora, provided a number of sources on the history of ledger art to support Fair in developing a series of drawings. These sources include *Ledger Narratives: The Plains Indian Drawings in the Mark Lansburgh Collection at Dartmouth College* (2017) and an interview with fellow Triennial featured artist Chris Pappan, "Native American Artist Covers Historical Ledgers With Portraits of Indigenous Peoples," *My Modern Met Media*, https://mymodernmet.com/chris-pappan-ledger-art-interview/.

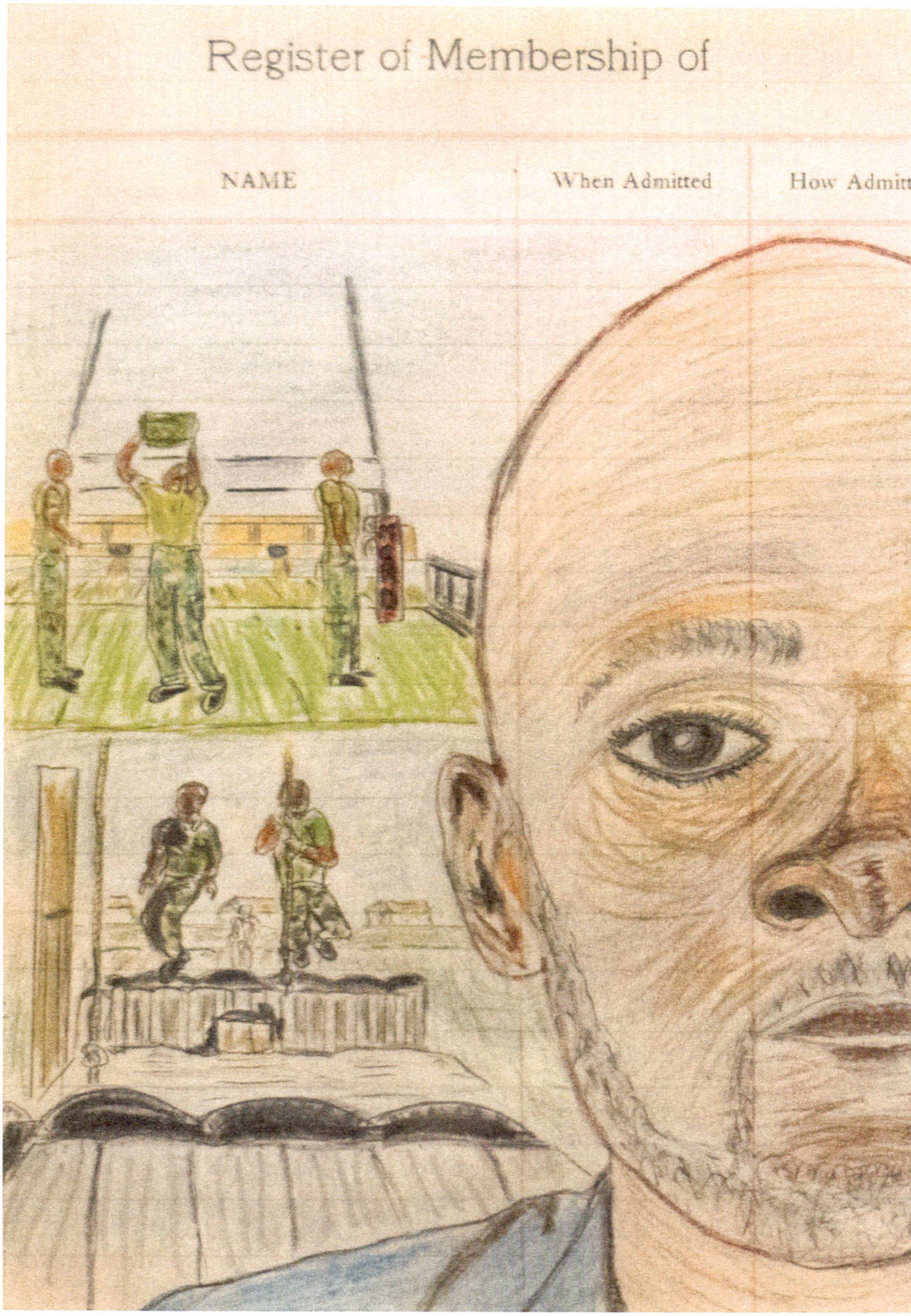

DARRELL WAYNE FAIR, *Self Portrait* (detail), Pencil, colored pencil, acrylic paint, and ink on ledger paper; *see also: p. 36*

the first place.[12] In his new series for the Triennial, *Vellum Cumuli* (2022/2023), portraits dissolve into a chaotic fog of missing information, misrepresentation, and forced assimilation. Little confronts the colonial gaze imposed on his people, deconstructing the work of turn-of-the-century extractive white photographer Edward Curtis, who staged his subjects to allegedly "document" "a vanishing race."[13] Little's fragmented, layered subjects, visible only as clouds of knotted threads, symbolize the confounding experiences of erasure inherent to imperialism. Yet, amidst this fog, his monoprint *Survivance 15* (2022/2023) shows one eye with a resolute gaze emerging from an abstracted abyss—a powerful declaration of his people's continued presence, resistance, and survival.[14]

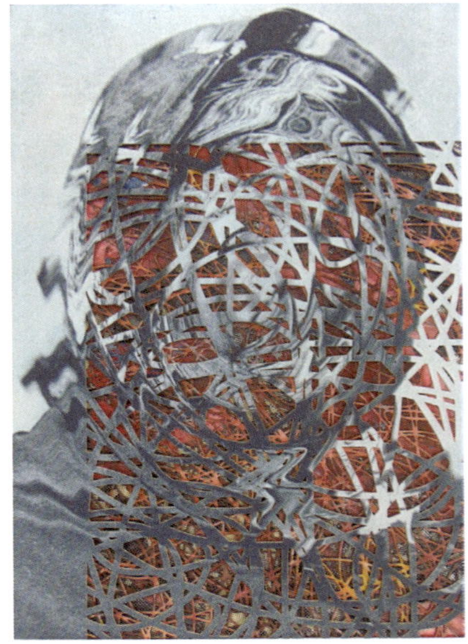

MONTY LITTLE, *Vellum of Cumuli 02*, 2022–23, Laser-cut photopolymer plate prints, screenprint, oil paint, and monotype on collaged paper; *see also: p. 108*

In corresponding fashion, a battle erupts on Miridith Campbell's (Kiowa) *Adobe Walls Battle Dress* (2022), another piece developed for the Triennial. The intricately designed garment shows warriors on

12 For an interview with Monty Little on his artwork, see Larry Abbott, "The Art of Erasure & A Conversation with Monty Little," *War, Literature and the Arts*, Vol. 31, (2019).

13 The Smithsonian provides the following biographical note on Curtis: "Between 1900 and 1930, Curtis traveled across the continent photographing more than seventy Native American tribes. The photographs presented daily activities, customs, and religions of a people he called 'a vanishing race.' To this end, Curtis often staged his subjects and set up scenes, mixing tribal artifacts and traditions to match his romanticized vision of the people he studied." Smithsonian Institution, "Edward S. Curtis," accessed September 1, 2024, https://www.si.edu/spotlight/edward-sheriff-curtis.

14 The title of Monty Little's *Survivance* comes from a term coined by Anishinaabe cultural theorist Gerald Vizenor. Vizenor writes, "Survivance is an active sense of presence, the continuance of native stories, not a mere reaction, or a survivable name. Native survivance stories are renunciations of dominance, tragedy and victimry." Gerald Vizenor, *Manifest Manners: Narratives on Postindian Survivance* (Lincoln: University of Nebraska Press, 1999), VII.

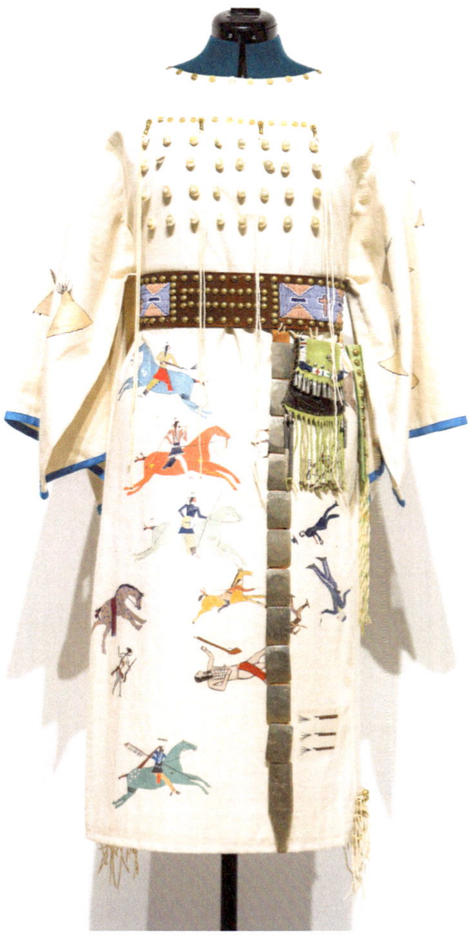

MIRIDITH CAMPBELL, *Adobe Walls Battle Dress*, 2022, Assorted materials; *see also: pp. 71, 88–91*

horseback aiming at US Cavalry soldiers who tumble down the dress's long flowing folds. Campbell incorporated nineteenth-century Kiowa ledger drawings of the Battle of Adobe Walls, one of the largest confrontations in the "American Indian Wars." During the 1864 battle, Colonel Kit Carson and his expeditionary unit were repelled by Kiowa, Apache, and Comanche forces defending their hunting lands.[15] Campbell crafted the dress to honor her ancestors who fought in the battle against the US Cavalry. The celebration of Indigenous insurgency is contrasted by Campbell's *Marine Corps Dress* (2022), which commemorates her service during the "Global War on Terror." Together her dresses reveal the contested histories Campbell navigates as both a "GWOT" veteran and an Indigenous woman. They confront colonial legacies of gendered violence, the military's patriarchal culture, and the ongoing targeting of Native women. Like Gokliz, her family's victory over the same US military she later served underscores that resistance and survival are nuanced, reflecting the embodied contradictions inherent to imperialism.

Sitting in the comfortable library chair, immersed in Gokliz's vibrant drawings, I reflected on all these connections. My own privilege was undeniable. The stark contrast between my white skin and the struggles embedded within the artworks was unsettling. The eyes in Gokliz's paintings seemed to return the colonial gaze I was inadvertently perpetuating, deepening my unease. I was acutely aware of my shame stemming from inheriting the US's genocidal legacy, compounded by the uncomfortable truth that my military service in Iraq had carried that tradition forward.

I reflected on Campbell, Little, Fair, and Gokliz—the tensions embodied by these artists and the contradictions of US imperialism forced on them. Veterans like them often come from communities that are themselves directly targeted by US counterinsurgency campaigns, caught in cycles of dehumanization, violence, and oppression. The chasms between us, shaped by race, gender, indigeneity, and power, feel insurmountable. Militarism divides us—at times, even from our friends and families.

15 T. Lindsay Baker and Billy R. Harrison, *Adobe Walls: The History and Archaeology of the 1874 Trading Post* (College Station: Texas A&M University Press, 1986), 14.

However, I believe that when veterans move away from identities solely rooted in military service and American exceptionalism and instead embrace solidarity grounded in shared experiences of exploitation, new possibilities emerge. This reorientation creates space to confront the cycles of state and interpersonal violence that militarism enmeshes in our lives.

Through my work with Fair and other abolitionists imprisoned at Stateville, I've learned that no one should be defined solely by their worst actions. Transformative justice and solidarity, however, require accountability, whether the harm is interpersonal or state-sanctioned. For veterans like me, this means taking responsibility for the harm we've caused, recognizing the harms we've endured, and confronting the cycles of harm that militarism and state violence perpetuate.

As a straight white male veteran, with all the embodied privileges that entails, this journey toward solidarity has been fraught and messy. It's a path filled with failures and frustrations; but it's one I walk knowing I am not alone. Embracing this "radical posture" has opened doors, forging connections that transcend isolation.[16] Through the labor of transforming personal and collective traumas into language, poetry, art, and action, I have come to realize that our collective works can create meaning out of the void, and solidarity can mend the wounds inflicted by endless war and militarism.

At the library table, I delicately turned the pages of yellowed newsprint, each sheet crackling with age. The April 1973 issue of *Akwesasne Notes* was alive with illustrations, graphics, and photographs, the pages pulsing with resistance. I wanted to explore the Mohawk Nation publication because it contained evocative prints by Bruce Carter, a Korean War veteran and a white artist like myself, whose

16 Paulo Freire, *Pedagogy of the Oppressed* (New York: Continuum, 1921), 49.

work unflinchingly exposes the brutality of war.[17] Allegedly, Carter had been thinking about Vietnam when carving wood blocks depicting the 1890 Wounded Knee Massacre—where hundreds of Lakota people were killed by the US Army.[18] The powerful print series that emerged was widely distributed by the Liberation News Service.[19] As a result, his graphics were published in numerous newspapers, including *The Black Panther* and *Akwesasne Notes*, during the American Indian Movement's legendary 1973 occupation of Wounded Knee, a decisive action that "culminated more than a decade of Red Power organizing" and "catalyzed" the international Indigenous movement.[20]

As I turned the pages, a photograph seized my attention: a weary figure, hand on their cheek, weapon at the ready, gazing out with tired eyes. The *Associated Press* caption read, "Just watching... and waiting."[21] I immediately recognized the figure—not from a photograph, but from an illustration on the back page of *Winter Soldier*, the newspaper of Vietnam Veterans Against the War (VVAW). In that broadside, the figure is rendered in a field of blue with the words "Wounded Knee 1890–1973" at the top. I wondered if the illustrator of the graphic—Carol Fisher, an artist who worked with VVAW—had drawn inspiration from *Akwesasne Notes*. In that historical moment, the American Indian Movement, VVAW, and the Black Panthers were all looking to each other, centering each other's struggles in the fight against oppression. The solidarity between those movements leaped off the page. The art and graphics reflected a shared understanding of their intertwined fates.

---

17 Marcia Dunn, "Memorials in Woodcuts: The Savagery of Wartime Is His Milieu," *Los Angeles Times*, January 13, 1988, https://www.latimes.com/archives/la-xpm-1988-01-13-ca-23745-story.html.

18 On Bruce Carter see Christian Feest and Joëlle Rostkowski, "Indian Posters of North America." *Archiv fur Volkerkunde* 36, (1982): 1-32. On the Wounded Knee Massacre, see "Disaster at Wounded Knee," The Library of Congress, accessed September 1, 2024, https://www.loc.gov/classroom-materials/immigration/native-american/disaster-at-wounded-knee/.

19 Louise Siddons, "Red Power in the Black Panther," *American Art* 35, no. 2 (Summer 2021): 2–31.

20 Nick Estes, *Our History Is the Future: Standing Rock Versus the Dakota Access Pipeline, and the Long Tradition of Indigenous Resistance* (New York: Verso, 2019), 23.

21 *Akwesasne Notes*, April 1973.

Weeks after my visit to the archives, I strolled through a light drizzle along the north branch of the Chicago River with Joseph Lefthand (Cheyenne-Arapaho, Taos, and Zuni tribes), a co-organizer of the Triennial. Those long walks had become a cherished ritual: moments to exchange ideas, vent frustrations, pose questions, dissect our military experiences, and contemplate our artistic practices. Despite our many differences, we shared a keen awareness of how easy it can be, and even how normal it can feel, to assimilate into the military, its violence and cruel indifference. Together, we have processed the way militarism permeates our daily lives and the ways we simultaneously embody and resist that dehumanization.

On that day, Joseph, ever thought-provoking, asked why I invest so much effort into organizing and curating veteran artists. Why the Triennial? Why does the Veteran Art Movement matter amidst the relentless onslaught? What's the point?

These are questions I continuously grapple with. Veterans who expose the horrors of war, critique the military-industrial complex, or speak truth to power are often met with apathy or hostility from our militarized culture. I am reminded of the assassination of Medgar Evers, the FBI's surveillance and targeting of Vietnam Veterans Against the War, the media blackout of the *Winter Soldier: Iraq and Afghanistan* investigation, the refusal by art museums to include anti-war veteran voices, and my own forced removal from the board of a national veteran art institution.[22] I think about the isolation and silencing effect of the sea of patriotic spectacles—halftime events, yellow

22 For more on the assassination of Medgar Evers, see Charles M. Payne, *I've Got the Light of Freedom* (Berkeley: University of California Press, 1995), 288. For more on FBI surveillance of VVAW, see Andrew E. Hunt, *The Turning* (New York: New York University, 1999), 5. For more on the media blackout of *Winter Soldier: Iraq and Afghanistan*, see Aaron Glant, "Winter Soldiers on the Hill," *The American Prospect* (June 2, 2008) https://prospect.org/article/winter-soldiers-hill/. After initially being asked to contribute to the national tour of *It Is What It Is* (2009) to major art institutions, including the Museum of Contemporary Art Chicago and the New Museum in New York, anti-war veterans were censored or asked not to participate in order to present the project in "as neutral a way as possible." Jeremy Deller, "It Is What It Is (2009)," https://www.jeremydeller.org/ItIsWhatItIs/ItIsWhatItIs_Video.php. 22. In 2019, following the success of the first Veteran Art Triennial, I was removed from the board of the National Veterans Art Museum after a prolonged dispute and multiple accusations that began with unspecified allegations of pushing an "activist, anti-government agenda."

ribbon products, recruitment advertisements, and films supported by the Department of Defense, like *Black Hawk Down*, *Top Gun: Maverick*, and *Captain Marvel*.[23] My thoughts are stilted by the fact that through this whirlwind, the logics and mechanisms of genocidal violence advance.

Yet, I responded to Joseph with conviction: because we are not alone...because I deeply believe in the power of our creative chorus to incite change.

Militarism and imperialism are vast, global forces. Confronting them requires careful consideration of the entanglements across war-torn geographies, histories, and cultures. It demands a transnational approach, a collective effort to connect across boundaries and foster the solidarities needed to extinguish the dehumanizing violence.

From the streets to the archives, from the prisons to the art studios, I have learned that, like green shoots rising from the ashes of a great inferno, a legacy of creative rebellion endures—offering roots, sustenance, direction, and even hope.

---

23 Blake Stilwell, "6 of the Best Movies Made with Help from the Department of Defense," *Military.com*, May 31, 2023, https://www.military.com/off-duty/movies/2023/05/31/6-of-best-movies-made-help-department-of-defense.html. See also Blake Stilwell, "How Hollywood Films Get the US Military as a Co-Star," *Military.com*, December 11, 2020, https://www.military.com/off-duty/how-hollywood-films-get-us-military-co-star.html.

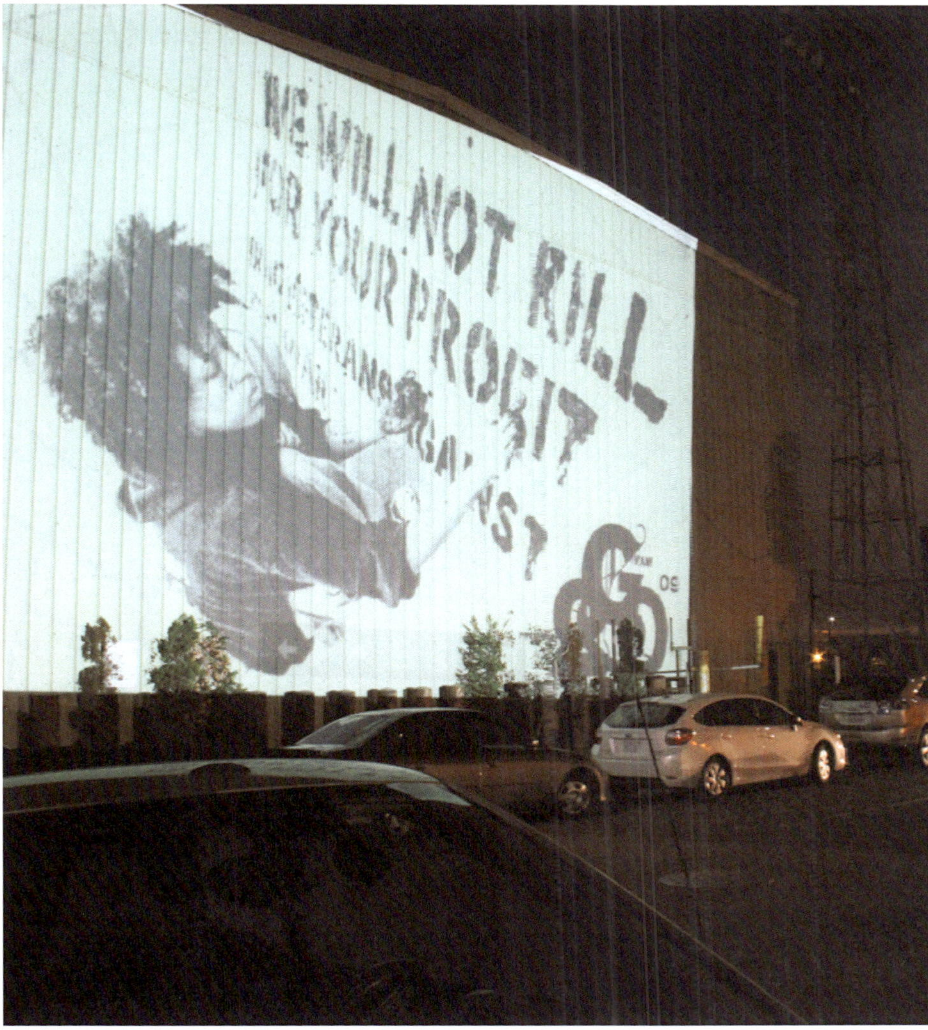

On May Day 2015, the San Francisco Projection Department illuminated the American Steel building in Oakland, California, with images from the *Celebrate People's History: IVAW* portfolio, including the pictured *G20* print by Ryan Hayes. The print features IVAW Field Organizer Chantelle Bateman mud stenciling at the G20 Summit in Pittsburgh in 2009 (May 1, 2015).

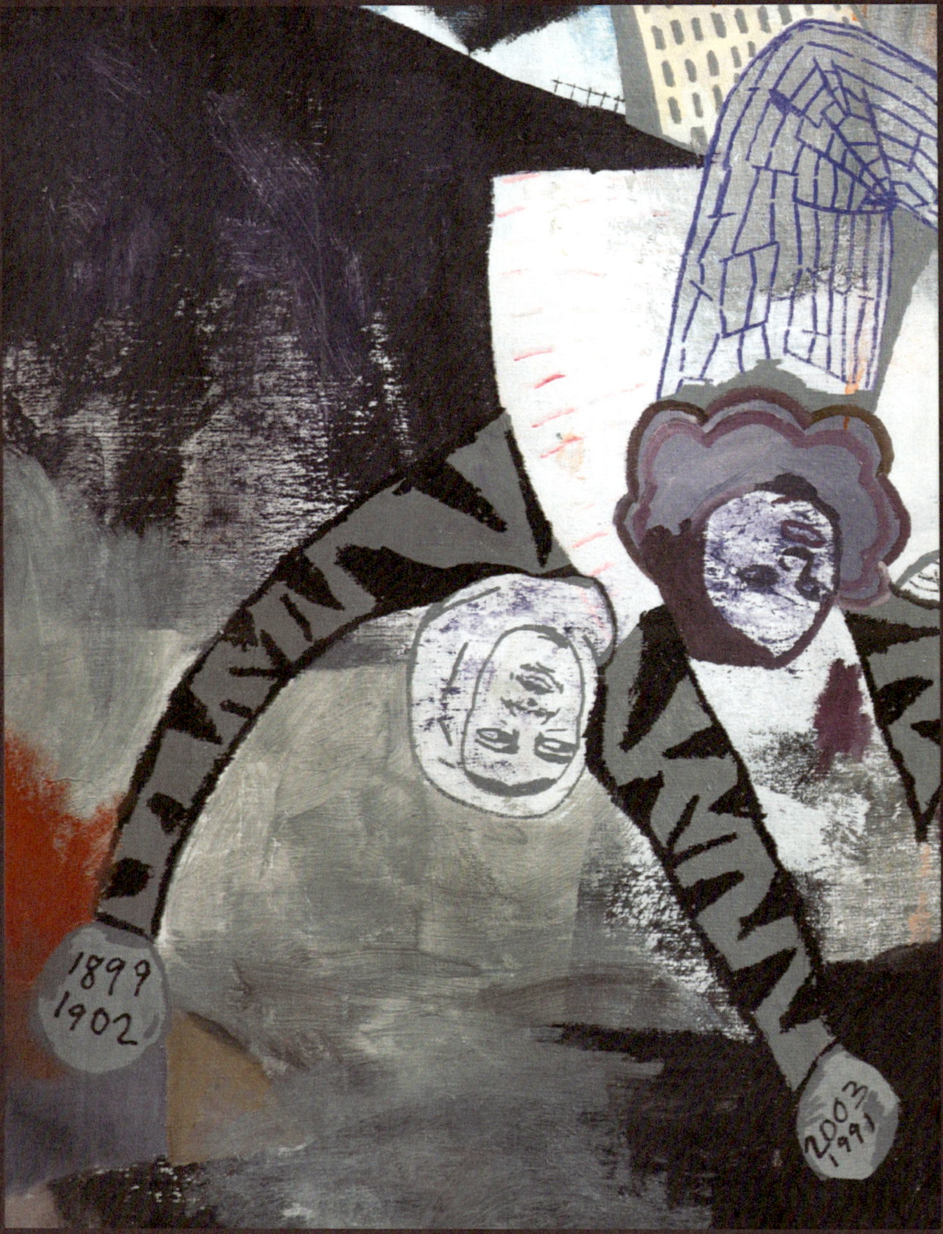

GREGORY RICK
From Manila to Baghdad (detail)

see also: pp. 170–71

Afterword: Meditations on Survival and Rebellion

RONAK K. KAPADIA

As we conclude *Surviving the Long Wars*, it is worth reflecting on the seismic geopolitical shifts of the past three years that have not only shaped our work but also sharpened our analysis and deepened our exploration of this project's intersectional themes. Amidst the wildness of the global pandemic era, three defining moments stand out, underscoring the relentless struggle between the destructive legacies of US militarism and the indomitable spirit of anti-colonial resistance.

The first significant event was the chaotic end of the US's twenty-year imperial debacle in Afghanistan, coinciding with the early planning stages of the 2023 Veteran Art Triennial and Summit. In August 2021, the tumultuous military and diplomatic withdrawal culminated in the collapse of the Afghan National Security Forces and the Taliban's swift return to power, starkly illustrating the human cost of decades of US occupation. Harrowing images of young Afghans clinging to departing military aircraft captured the chaos and desperation wrought by prolonged foreign intervention. The Biden administration's abrupt exit, compounded by its devastating economic sanctions, left millions of Afghans teetering on the brink of famine with no viable path to self-determination. The United States should never have been in Afghanistan in the first place, yet "four consecutive presidents and hundreds of members of Congress chose to wage war in a country whose people bore no responsibility for al Qaeda's September 11, 2001 attacks."[1] This $2.3 trillion war resulted in over half a million deaths, countless injuries and traumas, and displaced nearly six million people.[2] The spectacle of the US troop withdrawal epitomizes the bipartisan failure of US foreign policy, exposing the broader consequences of a "Global War on Terror" that has justified widespread civil rights abuses and mass suffering against Muslim and Muslim-adjacent communities worldwide. It underscores the urgent need for a radical overhaul and abolition of the GWOT apparatus altogether, along with a sustained effort toward reparations for its victims.[3]

The second defining moment likewise concerns the US's central role in ongoing military conflicts in the Greater Middle East, particularly the settler colonization of Palestine. Since the Al-Aqsa Flood Operation on October 7, 2023, the *Nakba* in Palestine has reached horrifying new extremes, exposing the United States as the chief financier of Israeli settler-colonial aggression.[4] The genocide and displacement of Palestinians are principally funded and supported by the US government, despite widespread international

1 David Vine, interview by Patty Housman, "What Does the United States Owe the People of Afghanistan?," American University, August 19, 2021, https://www.american.edu/cas/news/what-does-the-united-states-owe-the-people-of-afghanistan.cfm.

2 See "Human and Budgetary Costs to Date of the US War in Afghanistan, 2001-2022," The Costs of War Project at Brown University's Watson Institute, August 2021, https://watson.brown.edu/costsofwar/figures/2021/human-and-budgetary-costs-date-us-war-afghanistan-2001-2022.

3 For an alternative grassroots policy agenda with demands rooted in grassroots and community-based organizations that work with African, Black, Muslim, Middle Eastern, Arab, and South Asian communities across the US, see "Abolishing the War on Terror, Building Communities of Care," Muslim Abolitionist Futures September 11, 2021, https://www.muslimabolitionistfutures.org/agenda.

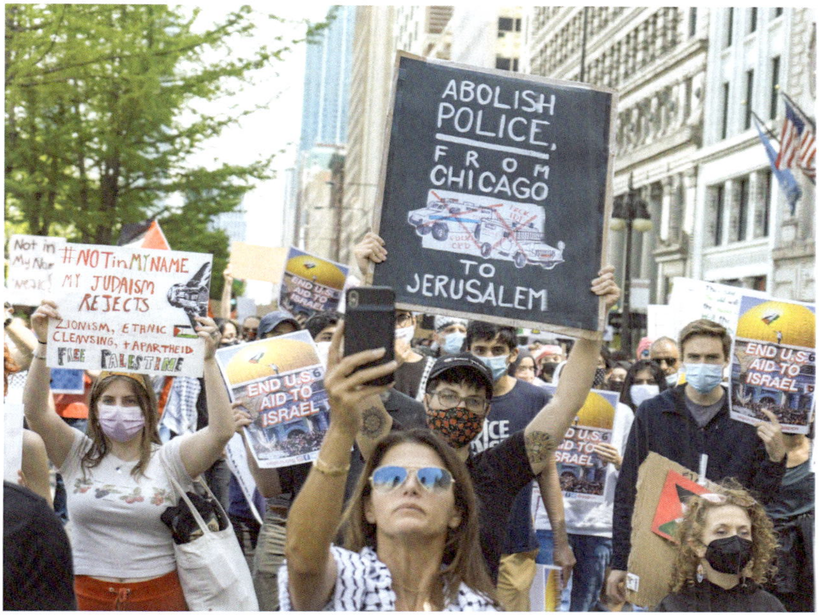
ABOLISH POLICE, FROM CHICAGO TO JERUSALEM
#NOTinMYNAME MY JUDAISM REJECTS ZIONISM, ETHNIC CLEANSING, +APARTHEID FREE PALESTINE
END U.S. AID TO ISRAEL

SARAH-JI RHEE. Thousands marched in downtown Chicago to commemorate the 73rd anniversary of the Nakba and to protest the displacement and attack of Palestinians in the Sheikh Jarrah neighborhood in occupied Jerusalem (May 16, 2021).

condemnation, even from within the imperial core itself. This support extends beyond the occupied territories, affecting the Palestinian diaspora, as evidenced by the intensified criminalization of college protests across North America and Europe in the spring of 2024, and the heightened repression of transnational Palestinian solidarity efforts globally.[5] As this book goes to print in early fall 2024, Israel's genocidal campaign in Gaza has raged on for well over three hundred days. Scholar Karma Nabulsi's term "scholasticide" aptly describes the near-total destruction of Gaza's educational infrastructure, with nearly 90 percent of its schools damaged or destroyed, including all

4 "Fact Sheet: 288 Days of Israel's Genocide in Gaza: By the Numbers," Institute for Middle East Understanding July 22, 2024, https://imeu.org/article/288-days-of-israels-genocide-in-gaza-by-the-numbers.

5 See Lara Deeb and Jessica Winegar, "Resistance to Repression and Back Again: The Movement for Palestinian Liberation in US Academia," *Middle East Critique* (July 2024): 1-22; see also Palestine Legal's report analyzing the crackdown on Palestine solidarity in the United States, "Reverberations of October 7: Mobilization Against Genocide Undeterred by Peak Anti-Palestinian Repression," May 23, 2024, https://palestinelegal.org/news/2024/5/23/new-report-analyzes-crackdown-on-palestine-solidarity-in-the-usnbsp.

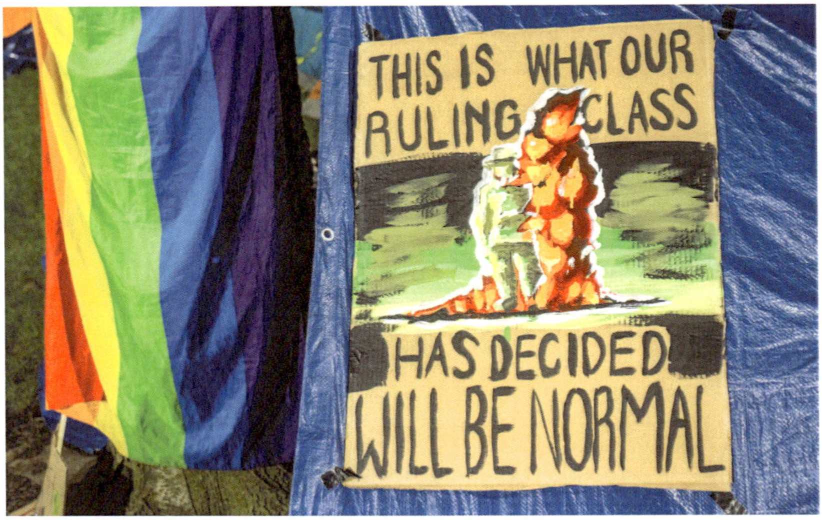

SARAH-JI RHEE. A poster depicting Aaron Bushnell engulfed in flames is taped to a tarp at the DePaul University Student Encampment for Gaza (May 8, 2024).

twelve universities.[6] Scholars and academics in the West must renew our commitment to transnational coalitions that stand firmly with the Palestinian struggle.[7] For those of us in the United States, this commitment is paramount, given how the US and Israel, as joint settler-colonial security states, base their sovereign claims on narratives justifying the permanent dispossession of Native peoples. We must rigorously examine the strategic collaborations between US and Israeli military and defense planners, reflecting what scholar Laleh Khalili describes as the "horizontal circuits of securitization" that define the post-Cold War era.[8] The Palestinian struggle for life and liberation highlights the critical relevance of *Surviving the Long Wars*, challenging us to dismantle entrenched systems of oppression and envision life-affirming alternatives.

6 Justin Salhani, "Genocide, Urbicide, Domicide: How to Talk about Israel's War on Gaza," *AlJazeera.com*, July 3, 2024, https://www.aljazeera.com/news/2024/7/3/genocide-urbicide-domicide-how-to-talk-about-israels-war-on-gaza; see also Ashley Smith, "Resisting Israeli Scholasticide and Academic Apartheid: An Interview with Maya Wind," *Spectre Journal*, July 9, 2024, https://spectrejournal.com/resisting-israeli-scholasticide-and-economic-apartheid/; see also Maya Wind, *Towers of Ivory and Steel: How Israeli Universities Deny Palestinian Freedom* (New York: Verso, 2024).

7 Among the many collectives committed to Palestinian solidarity work at this moment, see the work of Scholars Against the War on Palestine, https://scholarsagainstwar.org/; see also US Campaign for Palestinian Rights (USCPR), https://uscpr.org/take-action/.

The third event intertwines with the *Nakba*: the tragic protest of Aaron Bushnell on February 25, 2024, at the Israeli embassy in Washington, DC. Bushnell, a 25-year-old US Air Force service member, self-immolated in protest against the ongoing violence in Palestine. He declared,

> My name is Aaron Bushnell, and I am an active duty member of the United States Air Force. I will no longer be complicit in genocide. I'm about to engage in an extreme act of protest, but, compared to what people have been experiencing in Palestine at the hands of their colonizers, it's not extreme at all. This is what our ruling class has decided will be normal.[9]

As he burned to death, Bushnell repeatedly shouted "Free Palestine!" until his final breath.[10] His death, live-streamed on Twitch before being removed, saw police aiming guns at him as he burned—a harrowing echo of Norman Morrison's self-immolation in 1965 to protest the Vietnam War. Bushnell's act of ultimate sacrifice underscores the profound solidarity and desperation felt by those opposing imperial violence and standing with oppressed peoples worldwide, including "war workers" in the US metropole who, like all of us in the West, are deeply entrenched in these toxic systems of violence even as we strive to undermine them.[11]

---

8 Laleh Khalili, "The Location of Palestine in Global Counterinsurgencies," *International Journal of Middle East Studies* 42, no. 3 (August 2010): 415; see also Lisa Hajjar, "Comparing American and Israeli Ways of War." In "Circuits of Influence: US, Israel, Palestine," *Social Text Online*, June 10, 2014, https://socialtextjournal.org/periscope_article/comparing-american-and-israeli-ways-of-war/.

9 Talia Jane, "Aaron Bushnell's Self-Immolation Protest Needed to Be Seen. But That Didn't Make It Easy to Report," *Rolling Stone*, February 29, 2024, https://www.rollingstone.com/culture/culture-commentary/aaron-bushnell-self-immolation-protest-hard-important-story-journalist-1234978325/

10 Bushnell's act was the second instance of self-immolation protesting US support for Israel. The first occurred in December 2023 at the Israeli consulate in Atlanta. For more details, see Bernd Debusmann Jr., "Protester sets themself on fire outside Israel consulate in Atlanta, Georgia," *BBC.com*, December 1, 2023, https://www.bbc.com/news/uk-67597395.

11 On the concept of "war workers," see Tejasvi Nagaraja, *World War Within: How Americans' WWII Battles Remade Work, Race, and Peace* (Philadelphia: University of Pennsylvania Press, forthcoming).

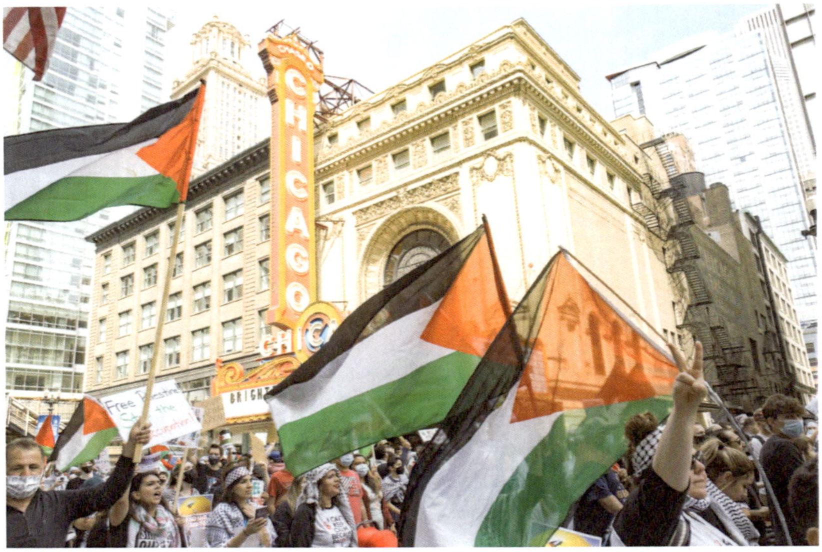

SARAH-JI RHEE. Thousands marched in downtown Chicago, passing the iconic Chicago Theater, to commemorate the 73rd anniversary of the Nakba and to protest the displacement and attack of Palestinians in the Sheikh Jarrah neighborhood in occupied Jerusalem (May 16, 2021).

These events prompt a deeper meditation on the concept of "surviving the long wars." As writer Alex Colston insightfully notes: "It takes only a second of critical thought to remember that service members are always honored if they lose their life for the US empire but not if they lose their life opposing it."[12] This sharp observation captures the hypocrisy in glorifying military service that sustains imperial violence while silencing resistance. Through their art, the war resisters—and those on the path to resistance—featured in this book guide us toward a new direction, turning the tide from endless warfare to imagining a future rooted in justice and peace.

Our struggle against settler colonialism and gendered racial capitalism must also address the ongoing US occupations in Puerto Rico, Guam, Hawai'i, American Samoa, and beyond. Empire, colonialism, and capitalism are global phenomena, from Gaza to the Caribbean.

12 Alex Colston (@re_colston), "It takes only a second of critical thought," X, February 26, 2024, https:/x.com/re_colston/status/1762138159746306347; see also Alex Colston, "This War Is Causing Mass Trauma. How We Respond Matters," *The Nation*, November 10, 2023.

Confronting and dismantling these systems propels us toward collective liberation on an international scale. The liberation of Native North America is intimately connected to the liberation of Palestine. One of this book's signature arguments is that the genocide of Native Americans is an unbroken thread of militarized violence extending into the present. Native Americans stand in solidarity with Palestinians due to shared histories of dispossession and marginalization. This interconnectedness embodies the spirit of resistance and resilience uniting these struggles against the long wars.

At the heart of this book lies the transformative power of collaboration—the antidote to our *dystopian here and now. Surviving the Long Wars* represents a deeply collaborative effort at every stage, from conception to curation. This project amplifies long-silenced voices and perspectives, challenging dominant narratives of war and empire that pollute our shared atmospheres. Forged during the peak of the pandemic's global uncertainties and political upheavals, this partnership has deeply reshaped my own sense of what is possible in the commons, redefining my responsibilities to multiple overlapping communities as a scholar-activist committed to studying and dismantling both domestic and global dimensions of US empire. The project's organizers and editors, bound by a commitment to queer feminist abolitionist anti-colonial politics, have linked struggles against state violence in Chicago—such as police violence and police torture—with global fronts of American warfare.[13] The 2023 Veteran Art Triennial illuminated the intersections of the global security state and the carceral settler archipelago, revitalizing dreams of internationalist solidarity beyond the confines of US empire. How can we further align critical museum and gallery spaces with the global decolonial, anti-fascist, and abolitionist visions we seek to advance through our work?

13 See "It's All Policing, It's All War: Chicago Organizers on Connecting Abolition and Demilitarization," Barnard Center for Research on Women, April 25, 2023, https://bcrw.barnard.edu/event/its-all-policing-its-all-war-chicago-organizers-on-connecting-abolition-and-demilitarization/; see also Andy Clarno et al., *Imperial Policing: Weaponized Data in Carceral Chicago* (Minneapolis: University of Minnesota Press, 2024)

To realize a vision of global abolition that includes dismantling the settler-colonial state, we must adopt bold and transformative thinking. Here is a wishlist for this radical vision:

- **Defund US national security and war-making institutions:** Cut funding to the Pentagon, the Department of Defense, the CIA, the NSA, and the FBI.

- **Abolish and reorganize ICE:** End immigrant detention, expand refugee and asylum programs, and legalize all residents in the US.

- **Redirect military spending:** Reallocate funds from the US military—the largest climate polluter in history—toward combating catastrophic climate change and addressing the pandemic of sexual violence within its ranks.

- **End secretive and abusive practices:** Abolish the use of secret evidence, predatory prosecution policies, and practices such as torture, extraordinary rendition, and secret prisons like Guantánamo.

- **Dismantle surveillance and militarization:** Eliminate the corporate-surveillance-military technology dragnet that infiltrates civilian life, halt the militarization of domestic police and private security forces, and challenge the ideological underpinnings of global counterterrorism and counterinsurgency writ large.

- **Support grassroots accountability efforts:** Back collectives like MoMA Divest, Decolonize This Place, and New Sanctuary Coalitions in holding cultural institutions accountable for their investments in the carceral and warfare state.

- **End the war on Black people:** Support the Movement for Black Lives' visionary policy agenda for the post-Ferguson Black liberation movement and work toward ending systemic violence against Black communities worldwide.

- **Reallocate funds for education:** Redirect federal, state, and local funds from policing and incarceration to support free, accessible, arts-rich, and inclusive public education at all levels.

- **End support for settler-colonial occupations:** Cease funding and arms supplies to US client states involved in settler-colonial occupations, such as Israel, India, and Saudi Arabia.

- **Engage in truth and reconciliation:** Establish truth and reconciliation commissions and provide reparations to Black and Indigenous peoples in the US, as well as to Afghans, Iraqis, Pakistanis, Somalis, Libyans, Yemenis, Syrians, Iranians, Venezuelans, and other peoples of the "darker nations" targeted by US military actions and economic sanctions.

- **Forge connections:** Connect domestic race-radical Black uprisings and Indigenous struggles over land, resources, and sovereignty with global decolonization movements for self-determination from Kashmir and Kurdistan to Palestine, Puerto Rico, and beyond.

This list is long, and the needs are great—this is *a decolonial abolitionist litany for twenty-first-century survival and rebellion*.

In closing, I recall the stirring words of pleasure activist and writer adrienne maree brown at Columbia University's "The People's Graduation" in May 2024, an alternative event held in response to the university's crackdown on student protests in solidarity with Palestine:

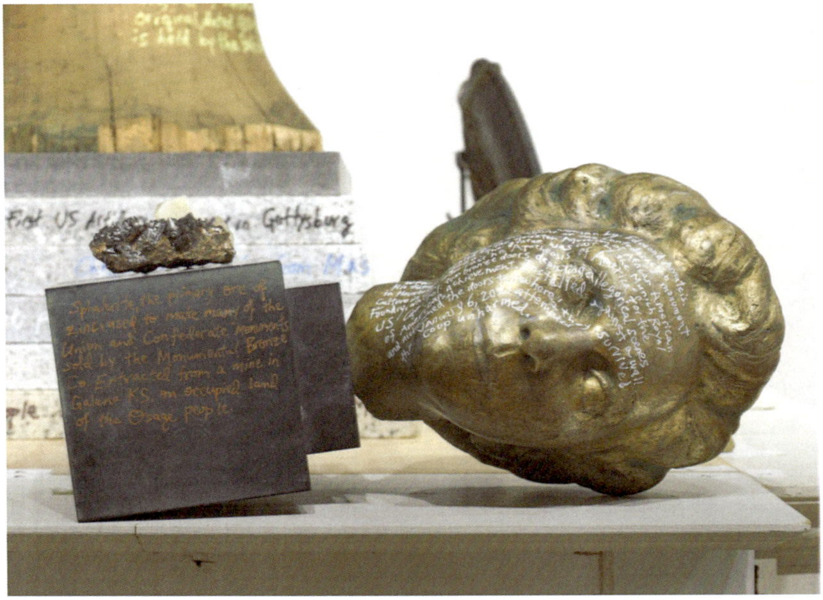
Sphalerite, the primary ore of
zinc used to make many of the
Union and Confederate Monuments
sold by the Monumental Bronze
Co Extracted from a mine in
Galena KS, an occupied land
of the Osage people.

MICHAEL RAKOWITZ, *American Golem* (detail), 2022, Found antiques, paper mache sculpture, granite, wood, metal base, Courtesy of the artist and Rhona Hoffman Gallery; *see also: pp. 82–84*

> You're among the few people who have made any sense to me in all these months. I am so proud of you for doing what you uniquely could. You refused to shirk your responsibility. With your peaceful protest, you put our nation's attention on Palestine, and on the US-funded genocide unfolding there. I see your bravery. I see your sacrifice. I see your solidarity. I see how the encampment you built was an embodiment of the future we all deserve. I see a free Palestine. I see global Jewish safety and dignity. I see Black life mattering, from here to Sudan, the Congo, Eritrea, [and] Haiti. I see us thriving on a planet we respect and honor. I see body sovereignty for every being. I see a future for our species…and YOU are a primary reason why the vision is so clear![14]

---

14 adrienne maree brown, "The People's Graduation Speech - May 16, 2024," May 19, 2024. https://adriennemareebrown.net/2024/05/19/the-peoples-graduation-speech-may-16-2024/.

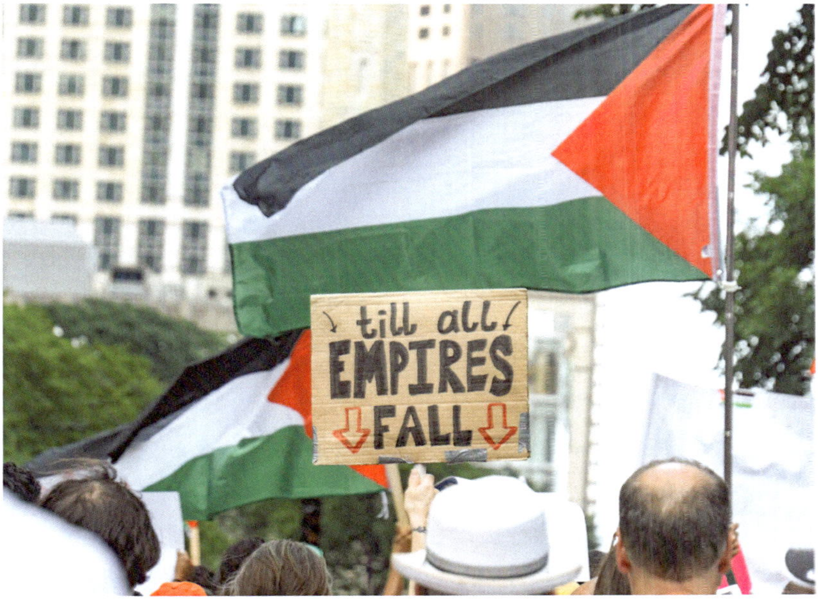

SARAH-JI RHEE. Protesters march down Michigan Avenue at the weekly protest organized by the Coalition for Justice in Palestine (July 13, 2024).

The dissident artists and writers in this book are among the few who still make sense to me amidst the global security state's perverse logic of harm expansionism and disorder. Their creative rebellion, much like brown's vision, shines as a beacon of revolutionary hope and insurgent aesthetics, inspiring social movements to dismantle overlapping systems of power and violence. As we deepen our global abolitionist struggles against the oppressive futures that fascists seek to impose both at home and abroad, let us embody the spirit of collaboration and solidarity that defines this project. Let us work toward a demilitarized future where peace, justice, and collective healing prevail over the miserable forces of counterinsurgency that seek to divide and conquer. Through art and collective action, we can build bridges, repair harms, forge alliances, and unite in our pursuit of a more just and equitable world. Our collective survival as a species may very well depend on it.

SURVIVING THE LONG WARS:
Residues and Rebellions
February 28 – May 26, 2023
Newberry Library

Miridith Campbell (Kiowa, b. 1966)
Counting Coup, 2002
US cavalry coat, seed beads, and buckskin
Courtesy of the artist

Miridith Campbell (Kiowa, b. 1966)
Cradleboard, 1998
Wood, leather, rawhide, brass tacks, wool, seed beads, and buckskin
Courtesy of the artist

Bruce Carter (1930–2016)
We Remember Wounded Knee
Akwesasne Notes
Rooseveltown, NY: Mohawk Nation, January 1973
Digital reproduction
Edward E. Ayer Collection, Newberry Library

Mahwish Chishty
Untitled, 2013
Gouache, tea stain, and photo transfers on Masonite
Courtesy of the artist

Mahwish Chishty (b. 1980)
MQ-9/5, 2013
Gouache and tea stain on paper
Courtesy of the artist

Mahwish Chishty (b. 1980)
MQ-9/3, 2013
Gouache and tea stain on paper
Courtesy of the artist

Monty Little (Diné, b. 1983)
Survivance, 14, 2022/2023
Monoprint on BFK Rives cotton paper
Courtesy of the artist

Monty Little (Diné, b. 1983)
Survivance, 15, 2022/2023
Monoprint on BFK Rives cotton paper
Courtesy of the artist

Rodney Ewing (b. 1964)
Pathfinder (Harriet Tubman), 2021
Hand-colored silkscreen on graph paper
Courtesy of the artist and Rena Bransten Gallery

Rodney Ewing (b. 1964)
Conductor (William Still), 2021
Hand-colored silkscreen on ledger paper
Courtesy of the artist and Rena Bransten Gallery

Darrell Wayne Fair (b. 1967)
Enlistment, 2022
Pencil and colored pencil on ledger paper
Courtesy of the artist and Prison + Neighborhood Arts/Education Project

Darrell Wayne Fair (b. 1967)
Self Portrait, 2022
Pencil, colored pencil, acrylic paint, and ink on ledger paper
Courtesy of the artist and Prison + Neighborhood Arts/Education Project

Darrell Wayne Fair (b. 1967)
Panel Documentary, 2022
Pencil and colored pencil on ledger paper
Courtesy of the artist and Prison + Neighborhood Arts/Education Project

Darrell Wayne Fair (b. 1967)
The Facade, 2022
Pencil and colored pencil on ledger paper
Courtesy of the artist and Prison + Neighborhood Arts/Education Project

Frederick Gokliz (San Carlos Apache, 1863–1901)
Woman and baby in cradleboard, ca. 1894–1899
Ink and watercolor on paper
Edward E. Ayer Collection, Newberry Library

Frederick Gokliz (San Carlos Apache, 1863–1901)
Group presents blanket, ca. 1894–1899
Ink and watercolor on paper
Edward E. Ayer Collection, Newberry Library

Gilbert Kills Pretty Enemy III (Standing Rock Sioux, b. 1979)
For Those Who Have No Voice
McLaughlin, South Dakota: Chameleon Horse Art & Design, 2016
Inkjet reproduction signed in marker
Edward E. Ayer Collection, Newberry Library

Kiowa Indian ledger drawings
ca. 1880–1890
Colored pencil on ledger paper
Edward E. Ayer Collection, Newberry Library

Terran Last Gun (Piikani, b. 1989)
The ancient people of the West live on, 2021
Ink and colored pencil on found paper
Edward E. Ayer Collection, Newberry Library

Terran Last Gun (Piikani, b. 1989)
10,000 journeys around the sun with moon, 2021
Ink and colored pencil on a "City Treasurer's certificate of tax sale," dated in Butte, Montana, on 3 March 1896
Edward E. Ayer Collection, Newberry Library

Illustration of a person carrying a cradleboard attributed with the initials "MW"
Akwesasne Notes
Rooseveltown, NY: Mohawk Nation, July/August 1970
Enlarged digital reproduction
Edward E. Ayer Collection, Newberry Library

Unattributed photograph with caption, "Roberta Blackgoat of Big Mountain is one of the organizers of the march in support of Navajo JUA (Joint Use Area) residents"
Akwesasne Notes
Rooseveltown, NY: Mohawk Nation, December 1979
Enlarged digital reproduction
Edward E. Ayer Collection, Newberry Library

Unattributed illustration of an Indigenous person
Akwesasne Notes
Rooseveltown, NY: Mohawk Nation, Early Autumn 1975
Enlarged digital reproduction
Edward E. Ayer Collection, Newberry Library

Black Horse ledger, p. 122
Cheyenne, ca. 1877–1879
Colored pencil and pen on ledger paper
Edward E. Ayer Collection, Newberry Library

Black Horse ledger, p. 22–23
Cheyenne, ca. 1877–1879
Colored pencil and pen on ledger paper
Edward E. Ayer Collection, Newberry Library

Unattributed photograph with caption, "Wounded Knee . . . a Photographer's Paradise"
Akwesasne Notes
Rooseveltown, NY: Mohawk Nation April 1973
Enlarged digital reproduction
Edward E. Ayer Collection, Newberry Library

Unattributed illustration of an Indigenous person
Akwesasne Notes
Rooseveltown, NY: Mohawk Nation, April 1974
Enlarged digital reproduction
Edward E. Ayer Collection, Newberry Library

Unattributed illustration with heading, "Wounded Knee 1800–1973"
Winter Soldier
Chicago, IL: Vietnam Veterans Against the War, May 1973
Offset lithograph on paper
Courtesy of Vietnam Veterans Against the War

Associated Press photograph of the Wounded Knee occupation from Sunday March 4, 1973, with caption "Just watching . . . and waiting"
Akwesasne Notes
Rooseveltown, NY: Mohawk Nation, April 1973
Enlarged digital reproduction
Edward E. Ayer Collection, Newberry Library

Cover of *Akwesasne Notes*
Rooseveltown, NY: Mohawk Nation, April 1973
Digital reproduction
Edward E. Ayer Collection, Newberry Library

Cover of *Winter Soldier*
Chicago, IL: Vietnam Veterans Against the War, May 1973
Digital reproduction
Courtesy of Vietnam Veterans Against the War

Cover of *Black Panther*
Oakland, CA: Black Panther Party, January 19, 1974
Digital reproduction
Image source: *American Art*, University of Chicago Press, Summer 2021

SURVIVING THE LONG WARS:
Unlikely Entanglements
March 16, 2023 – July 9, 2023
Hyde Park Art Center

Bassim Al Shaker (b. 1986)
Photon, 2022
Oil on canvas
Courtesy of Rhona Hoffman Gallery

Bassim Al Shaker (b. 1986)
The Darkness, 2022
Oil on canvas
Courtesy of Rhona Hoffman Gallery

Bassim Al Shaker (b. 1986)
Alive, 2022
Oil on canvas
Courtesy of Rhona Hoffman Gallery

Bassim Al Shaker (b. 1986)
Nightmare, 2022
Oil on canvas
Courtesy of Rhona Hoffman Gallery

Bassim Al Shaker (b. 1986)
Disaster, 2022
Oil on canvas
Courtesy of Rhona Hoffman Gallery

June Carpenter (Osage/Shawnee, b. 1981)
Johnson v. M'Intosh, 21 U.S. 543 (1823), 2017
Wool and cotton fabric, cotton thread, nylon fringe, and glass beads
Courtesy of the artist

June Carpenter (Osage/Shawnee, b. 1981)
Cherokee Nation v. Georgia, 30 U.S. 1 (1831), 2022
Linen fabric, satin ribbon, cotton thread, nylon fringe, and glass beads
Courtesy of the artist

Mahwish Chishty (b. 1980)
Hovering Reaper I, 2014
Gouache, tea stain, and photo transfers on birch plywood
Courtesy of the artist

Mahwish Chishty (b. 1980)
Hovering Reaper II, 2014
Gouache, tea stain, and photo transfers on birch plywood
Courtesy of the artist

Mahwish Chishty (b. 1980)
Reaper, 2014
Gouache, tea stain, and photo transfers on birch plywood
Courtesy of the artist

Jose deVera (b. 1983)
And All the King's Men, 2014–2023
Mixed media, wood, canvas, and found materials
Dimensions variable
Courtesy of the artist

Sabba Elahi (b. 1980)
the suspect is my son (series) #3, 2018
Machine embroidery on felt
Courtesy of the artist

Sabba Elahi (b. 1980)
the suspect is my son (series) #4, 2018
Machine embroidery on felt
Courtesy of the artist

Sabba Elahi (b. 1980)
the suspect is my son (series) #5, 2018
Machine embroidery on felt
Courtesy of the artist

Sabba Elahi (b. 1980)
everyday suspects, #4, 2014
Hand embroidery on cotton
Courtesy of the artist

Sabba Elahi (b. 1980)
everyday suspects, #7, 2014
Hand embroidery on cotton
Courtesy of the artist

Sabba Elahi (b. 1980)
everyday suspects, #8, 2014
Hand embroidery on cotton
Courtesy of the artist

Sabba Elahi (b. 1980)
identified suspects, CIA/Pakistan Dronestrikes, 2014
Ink on rice paper
Courtesy of the artist

Rodney Ewing (b. 1964)
Faded, 2022
Hand-colored silkscreen on ledger paper
Courtesy of the artist and Rena Bransten Gallery

Rodney Ewing (b. 1964)
Come the Mean Times, 2022
Hand-colored silkscreen on ledger paper
Courtesy of the artist and Rena Bransten Gallery

Rodney Ewing (b. 1964)
Confines, 2021
Hand-colored silkscreen on ledger paper
Courtesy of the artist and Rena Bransten Gallery

Sarah Farahat (b. 1979)
To Be or Not To Be—That Is the Question of the Refugee or (How Do We Deal With Now, When Then Isn't Over Yet),* 2009
Independently looping video and sound installation
Courtesy of the artist

Rajkamal Kahlon (b. 1974)
People of Afghanistan, 2017
Video installation
Courtesy of the artist

Ruth Kaneko (Kanaka Wahine, b. 1985)
Sutured, 2019
Mixed media
Courtesy of the artist

Ruth Kaneko (Kanaka Wahine, b. 1985)]
Service Connected II: Kānehailua, 2023
Silkscreen on handmade paper (made out of military uniforms)
Courtesy of the artist

Eric Perez (b.1984)
Sgt. Gudiño, 2023
Mounted digital prints on acrylic laser-cut into the silhouette and custom digi-camo patterns
Courtesy of the artist

Eric Perez (b.1984)
5-Sierra, 2023
Mounted digital prints on acrylic laser-cut into the silhouette and custom digi-camo patterns
Courtesy of the artist

Yvette M. Pino (b.1976)
Forced Protection Study #1, 2020
Silkscreen
Courtesy of the artist

Yvette M. Pino (b.1976)
CadmUS., 2015
Silkscreen
Courtesy of the artist

Yvette M. Pino (b.1976)
Extraction, 2015
Silkscreen
Courtesy of the artist

Gregory Rick (b. 1981)
Black and Native Victories, 2017
Accordion book, ink, gouache, photo-transfer, and acrylic on handmade paper
Courtesy of Fred and Louise Neal

Gregory Rick (b. 1981)
From Manila to Baghdad, 2023
Acrylic, pigmented ink, absorbent ground, sign paint, and oil bar on linen
Courtesy of the artist

Dwayne Wilcox (Oglala Lakota, b. 1957)
Losing My Religion, 2004
Ink and colored pencil on ledger paper
Courtesy of the artist

Dwayne Wilcox (Oglala Lakota, b. 1957)
Larry is far right, he's really tough on immigration, 2005
Ink and colored pencil on ledger paper
Courtesy of the artist

Yiran Zhang (b. 1996)
(Marching in Place), 2022
Relief print on paper
Courtesy of the artist

SURVIVING THE LONG WARS:
Reckon and Reimagine
March 10 – July 2, 2023
Chicago Cultural Center

Dorothy Burge (b. 1954)
"We Stand on the Shoulders of Our Ancestors", 2018
Cotton fabric and batting, buttons, beads, embroidered patch, printing on fabric, photo-transfer on fabric
Machine quilted by Judy Wolff
Courtesy of the artist

Miridith Campbell (Kiowa, b. 1966)
Marine Corps Dress—Southern Style, 2022
Artist tanned and smoked buckskin hide; antique, vintage, and contemporary seed beads; Red Broadcloth English Wool; vintage Marine Corps service buttons; Hawk Bells; and horse hair
Courtesy of the artist

Miridith Campbell (Kiowa, b. 1966)
Adobe Walls Battle Dress, 2022
Cotton canvas dresses with blue edging. Digitally printed ledger art on fabric, depicting the Adobe Walls Battle. Two sets of fully beaded belt bags. Two belts, one fully beaded on latigo with a German silver whip, and one fully brass-tacked on harness leather with a tacked whip
Courtesy of the artist

Melissa Doud (Ojibwe, b. 1971)
Bullet Dress, 2016
Army uniform with 365 bullet casings
Courtesy of the artist

Ali Eyal (b. 1994)
An Indefinite appearance or two walls and, 2023
Graphite drawings, pigment print, frames, latex paint, plywood, and ceramic tiles
Courtesy of the artist

Chitra Ganesh (b. 1975)
Fahd Gazy, 2004 from the ongoing series *Index of the Disappeared: Watercolors*
Watercolor on paper
Courtesy of the artists, Gallery Wendi Norris, and Hales Gallery in New York and London

Chitra Ganesh (b. 1975)
Al Banna Family, 2004 from the ongoing series *Index of the Disappeared: Watercolors*
Watercolor on paper
Courtesy of the artists, Gallery Wendi Norris, and Hales Gallery in New York and London

Chitra Ganesh (b. 1975)
Majid Khan, 2004 from the ongoing series *Index of the Disappeared: Watercolors*
Watercolor on paper
Courtesy of the artists, Gallery Wendi Norris, and Hales Gallery in New York and London

Chitra Ganesh (b. 1975)
Shaker Aamer, 2004 from the ongoing series *Index of the Disappeared: Watercolors*
Watercolor on paper
Courtesy of the artists, Gallery Wendi Norris, and Hales Gallery in New York and London

Chitra Ganesh (b. 1975)
Binyam Mohammed, 2004 from the ongoing series *Index of the Disappeared: Watercolors*
Watercolor on paper
Courtesy of the artists, Gallery Wendi Norris, and Hales Gallery in New York and London

Chitra Ganesh (b. 1975)
Dilawak Family, 2004 from the ongoing series *Index of the Disappeared: Watercolors*
Watercolor on paper
Courtesy of the artists, Gallery Wendi Norris, and Hales Gallery in New York and London

Chitra Ganesh (b. 1975)
Gul Rahman, 2004 from the ongoing series *Index of the Disappeared: Watercolors*
Watercolor on paper
Courtesy of the artists, Gallery Wendi Norris, and Hales Gallery in New York and London

Chitra Ganesh (b. 1975)
Mubarak Hussein Shuman Ahmed, 2004 from the ongoing series *Index of the Disappeared: Watercolors*
Watercolor on paper
Courtesy of the artists, Gallery Wendi Norris, and Hales Gallery in New York and London

Chitra Ganesh (b. 1975)
Bisher Al Rawi, 2004 from the ongoing series
Index of the Disappeared: Watercolors
Watercolor on paper
Courtesy of the artists, Gallery Wendi Norris, and Hales Gallery in New York and London

Chitra Ganesh (b. 1975)
Abu Zubaydah, 2004 from the ongoing series
Index of the Disappeared: Watercolors
Watercolor on paper
Courtesy of the artists, Gallery Wendi Norris, and Hales Gallery in New York and London

Chitra Ganesh (b. 1975)
Laid Saidi, 2004 from the ongoing series
Index of the Disappeared: Watercolors
Watercolor on paper
Courtesy of the artists, Gallery Wendi Norris, and Hales Gallery in New York and London

Chitra Ganesh (b. 1975)
Aafia Siddiqui, 2004 from the ongoing series
Index of the Disappeared: Watercolors
Watercolor on paper
Courtesy of the artists, Gallery Wendi Norris, and Hales Gallery in New York and London

Mariam Ghani (b. 1978)
and **Chitra Ganesh** (b. 1975)
Index of the Disappeared: Parasitic Archive, 2014
Site specific installation with vinyl, tables, chairs, binders, copy paper, ephemera including military manuals and documents
All work courtesy of the artists

Mariam Ghani (b. 1978)
The Trespassers, 2011
105-minute 1-channel video with 4-channel sound (presented in stereo) and annotated archive (approximately 20,000 pages)
Courtesy of the artist and Ryan Lee Gallery

Hock E Aye Vi Edgar Heap of Birds
(Cheyenne and Arapaho Nation, b. 1954)
Native Host for Oklahoma, 2017–2021
Mylar on five aluminum metal sign panels
Courtesy of the artist

Hock E Aye Vi Edgar Heap of Birds
(Cheyenne and Arapaho Nation, b. 1954)
Trail of Tears, 2005
Mylar on four aluminum metal sign panels with posts
Courtesy of the artist

Gina Herrera (Tesuque Pueblo, b. 1969)
The Liberty Master, 2022
Powder-coated assorted found materials and steel
Courtesy of the artist

Gina Herrera (Tesuque Pueblo, b. 1969)
A Virtuous Warrior, 2022
Assorted found materials and steel
Courtesy of the artist

Gina Herrera (Tesuque Pueblo, b. 1969)
A Whimsical Diva, 2022
Assorted found materials and steel
Courtesy of the artist

Tom Jones (Ho-Chunk, b. 1964)
Tom "Frank" Redbird Jr., Army, Vietnam, 2019, from the ongoing series *Honoring the Ho Chunk Warrior*
Archival digital print
Courtesy of the artist

Tom Jones (Ho-Chunk, b. 1964)
Untitled, n.d., from the ongoing series
Honoring the Ho Chunk Warrior
Archival digital print
Courtesy of the artist

Tom Jones (Ho-Chunk, b. 1964)
Sam Shegonee, Army, 2018, from the ongoing series *Honoring the Ho Chunk Warrior*
Archival digital print
Courtesy of the artist

Tom Jones (Ho-Chunk, b. 1964)
Donald Blackdeer, Army, WWII, Code Talker, Silver Medal Recipient, 2013, from the ongoing series *Honoring the Ho Chunk Warrior*
Archival digital print
Courtesy of the artist

Tom Jones (Ho-Chunk, b. 1964)
Mitchell Redcloud Jr., KIA, Army and Marine, Korea, 2018, from the ongoing series *Honoring the Ho Chunk Warrior*
Archival digital print
Courtesy of the artist

Tom Jones (Ho-Chunk, b. 1964)
Eugene Thundercloud, Army, Korea, 2017, from the ongoing series Honoring the *Honoring the Ho Chunk Warrior* digital print
Courtesy of the artist

Tom Jones (Ho-Chunk, b. 1964)
Harold Blackdeer Jr., Marine, WWII, 2006, from the ongoing series *Honoring the Ho Chunk Warrior*
Archival digital print
Courtesy of the artist

Tom Jones (Ho-Chunk, b. 1964)
Gerald Wayne Cloud Sr., Army, Vietnam, 2017, from the ongoing series *Honoring the Ho Chunk Warrior*
Archival digital print
Courtesy of the artist

Tom Jones (Ho-Chunk, b. 1964)
Edward Littlejohn, Army, WWII, 2017, from the ongoing series *Honoring the Ho Chunk Warrior*
Archival digital print
Courtesy of the artist

Tom Jones (Ho-Chunk, b. 1964)
Oliver Rockman, Air Force, Vietnam, 2007, from the ongoing series *Honoring the Ho Chunk Warrior*
Archival digital print
Courtesy of the artist

Tom Jones (Ho-Chunk, b. 1964)
Armond Kell Storm, Marine, Vietnam, 2022, from the ongoing series *Honoring the Ho Chunk Warrior*
Archival digital print
Courtesy of the artist

Tom Jones (Ho-Chunk, b. 1964)
Nellie Redcloud, Gold Star Mother of Mitchell Redcloud Jr., 2013, from the ongoing series *Honoring the Ho Chunk Warrior*
Archival digital print
Courtesy of the artist

Tom Jones (Ho-Chunk, b. 1964)
Henry Decorah, Army, WWI, 2014, from the ongoing series *Honoring the Ho Chunk Warrior*
Archival digital print
Courtesy of the artist

Tom Jones (Ho-Chunk, b. 1964)
Randall Roy Blackdeer, Army, Peace Time Reserves, 2013, from the ongoing series *Honoring the Ho Chunk Warrior*
Archival digital print
Courtesy of the artist

Tom Jones (Ho-Chunk, b. 1964)
Ebenezer Hall, Army, WWII, 2007, from the ongoing series *Honoring the Ho Chunk Warrior*
Archival digital print
Courtesy of the artist

Tom Jones (Ho-Chunk, b. 1964)
Conroy Greendeer Sr., Army, Vietnam, 2022, from the ongoing series *Honoring the Ho Chunk Warrior*
Archival digital print
Courtesy of the artist

Tom Jones (Ho-Chunk, b. 1964)
James Carrimon, Army, Vietnam, 2014, from the ongoing series *Honoring the Ho Chunk Warrior*
Archival digital print
Courtesy of the artist

Tom Jones (Ho-Chunk, b. 1964)
Andrew Arentz, Army, 2019, from the ongoing series *Honoring the Ho Chunk Warrior*
Archival digital print
Courtesy of the artist

Tom Jones (Ho-Chunk, b. 1964)
Mitchell Littlebear, Air Force, Korea, 2015, from the ongoing series *Honoring the Ho Chunk Warrior*
Archival digital print
Courtesy of the artist

Tom Jones (Ho-Chunk, b. 1964)
Arnold Funmaker, Air Force, Vietnam, and Harold Jones Funmaker, WWI, Calvary, 2018, from the ongoing series *Honoring the Ho Chunk Warrior*
Archival digital print
Courtesy of the artist

Tom Jones (Ho-Chunk, b. 1964)
Vanverd Dick Sr., Army, WWII, 2012, from the ongoing series *Honoring the Ho Chunk Warrior*
Archival digital print
Courtesy of the artist

Tom Jones (Ho-Chunk, b. 1964)
Russius Decorah, Army, WWI, 2018, from the ongoing series *Honoring the Ho Chunk Warrior*
Archival digital print
Courtesy of the artist

Tom Jones (Ho-Chunk, b. 1964)
Arlene Greengrass Rodriquez, Army, Vietnam, 2017, from the ongoing series *Honoring the Ho Chunk Warrior*
Archival digital print
Courtesy of the artist

Tom Jones (Ho-Chunk, b. 1964)
George Stacy Sr., Army, Korea, 2022, from the ongoing series *Honoring the Ho Chunk Warrior*
Archival digital print
Courtesy of the artist

Tom Jones (Ho-Chunk, b. 1964)
Debra Greengrass, Army, Vietnam, 2016, from the ongoing series *Honoring the Ho Chunk Warrior*
Archival digital print
Courtesy of the artist

Tom Jones (Ho-Chunk, b. 1964)
Willis Winneshiek, Army, WWII, 2018, from the ongoing series *Honoring the Ho Chunk Warrior*
Archival digital print
Courtesy of the artist

Tom Jones (Ho-Chunk, b. 1964)
Norman R. Day, Army, WWII, 2017, from the ongoing series *Honoring the Ho Chunk Warrior*
Archival digital print
Courtesy of the artist

Tom Jones (Ho-Chunk, b. 1964)
Warren Littlejohn Sr., Army, WWII, 2019, from the ongoing series *Honoring the Ho Chunk Warrior*
Archival digital print
Courtesy of the artist

Tom Jones (Ho-Chunk, b. 1964)
Virgil Pettibone Sr., Army, Korea, 2018, from the ongoing series *Honoring the Ho Chunk Warrior*
Archival digital print
Courtesy of the artist

Tom Jones (Ho-Chunk, b. 1964)
Floyd L. Blackdeer, Air Force, WWII, Korea, Vietnam, 2009, from the ongoing series *Honoring the Ho Chunk Warrior*
Archival digital print
Courtesy of the artist

Tom Jones (Ho-Chunk, b. 1964)
Clifford Blackdeer, Army, WWII, 2019, from the ongoing series *Honoring the Ho Chunk Warrior*
Archival digital print
Courtesy of the artist

Tom Jones (Ho-Chunk, b. 1964)
Hoke Maisells, Army, Korea, 2018, from the ongoing series *Honoring the Ho Chunk Warrior*
Archival digital print
Courtesy of the artist

Rajkamal Kahlon (b. 1974)
"This 44-year old male,_____________, died of complications from multiple gunshot wounds." (youngest son), 2023
from the ongoing series *Did You Kiss the Dead Body?*
Mixed media on canvas
Courtesy of the artist

Rajkamal Kahlon (b. 1974)
"This elderly Iraqi male died of atherosclerotic cardiovascular disease (blockage of the arteries that supply blood and oxygen to the heart)." (eldest son), 2023, from the ongoing series *Did You Kiss the Dead Body?*
Mixed media on canvas
Courtesy of the artist

Monty Little (Diné, b. 1983)
Vellum of Cumuli, (AP), 2022/2023
Laser-cut photopolymer plate prints, screenprint, oil paint, and monotype on collaged paper
Courtesy of the artist

Monty Little (Diné, b. 1983)
Vellum of Cumuli, 02, 2022/2023
Laser-cut photopolymer plate prints, screenprint, oil paint, and monotype on collaged paper
Courtesy of the artist

Monty Little (Diné, b. 1983)
Vellum of Cumuli, 03, 2022/2023
Laser-cut photopolymer plate prints, screenprint, oil paint, and monotype on collaged paper
Courtesy of the artist

Monty Little (Diné, b. 1983)
Vellum of Cumuli, 05, 2022/2023
Laser-cut photopolymer plate prints, screenprint, oil paint, and monotype on collaged paper
Courtesy of the artist

Monty Little (Diné, b. 1983)
Flora 03, 2019–2021
Oil on paper mounted on canvas
Courtesy of the artist

Monty Little (Diné, b. 1983)
Flora 30, 2019–2021
Oil on canvas
Courtesy of the artist

Monty Little (Diné, b. 1983)
Flora 31, 2019–2021
Oil on canvas
Courtesy of the artist

Monty Little (Diné, b. 1983)
Flora 32, 2019–2021
Oil on canvas
Courtesy of the artist

Monty Little (Diné, b. 1983)
Flora 33, 2019–2021
Oil on canvas
Courtesy of the artist

Monty Little (Diné, b. 1983)
Flora 34, 2019–2021
Oil on canvas
Courtesy of the artist

Hanaa Malallah (b. 1958)
She/He Has No Picture, 2019/2020
Burnt canvas collage on canvas with laser cut brass plaques, four art books, thousands of computer-generated moving images, and original booklet published by the Iraqi government in 1991
Courtesy of artist

Hector René Membreño-Canales (b. 1988)
Boston MA 2 (Columbus), 2021, from the ongoing series *After-Ozymandias*
Archival Pigment Print
Courtesy of the artist

Hector René Membreño-Canales (b. 1988)
Boston MA 3 (Lincoln), 2021, from the ongoing series *After-Ozymandias*
Archival Pigment Print
Courtesy of the artist

Hector René Membreño-Canales (b. 1988)
Robert E. Lee, New Orleans, 2018, from the ongoing series *After-Ozymandias*
Archival Pigment Print
Courtesy of the artist

Chris Pappan (Kaw/Osage, Lakota b. 1971)
War Dance III, 2023
Graphite, gouache, ink, map collage and embroidery floss on US Cavalry recruitment ledger
Courtesy of the artist

Chris Pappan (Kaw/Osage, Lakota b. 1971)
War Dance I, 2023
Graphite, gouache, ink, map collage and embroidery floss on US Cavalry recruitment ledger
Courtesy of the artist

Chris Pappan (Kaw/Osage, Lakota b. 1971)
War Dance VII, 2023
Graphite, gouache, ink, map collage and embroidery floss on US Cavalry recruitment ledger
Courtesy of the artist

Chris Pappan (Kaw/Osage, Lakota b. 1971)
War Dance V, 2023
Graphite, gouache, ink, map collage and embroidery floss on US Cavalry recruitment ledger
Courtesy of the artist

Chris Pappan (Kaw/Osage, Lakota b. 1971)
War Dance IX, 2023
Graphite, ink, gold leaf, and map collage on US Cavalry recruitment ledger
Courtesy of the artist

Chris Pappan (Kaw/Osage, Lakota b. 1971)
War Dance VI, 2023
Graphite, gouache, ink, map collage and embroidery floss on US Cavalry recruitment ledger
Courtesy of the artist

Chris Pappan (Kaw/Osage, Lakota b. 1971)
War Dance VIII, 2023
Graphite, gouache, ink, map collage and embroidery floss on US Cavalry recruitment ledger
Courtesy of the artist

Chris Pappan (Kaw/Osage, Lakota b. 1971)
War Dance II, 2023
Graphite, gouache, ink, map collage and embroidery floss on US Cavalry recruitment ledger
Courtesy of the artist

Chris Pappan (Kaw/Osage, Lakota b. 1971)
War Dance IV, 2023
Graphite, gouache, ink, map collage and embroidery floss on US Cavalry recruitment ledger
Courtesy of the artist

Michael Rakowitz (b. 1973)
The invisible enemy should not exist (Northwest Palace of Kalhu, Room Z), 2018
Panel Z-b-3 (C01-22-017) and Z-b-1 (C01-22-016)
Middle Eastern food packaging and newspapers, glue, cardboard on wooden structures
Courtesy of the artist and Rhona Hoffman Gallery

Michael Rakowitz (b. 1973)
The invisible enemy should not exist (Northwest Palace of Kalhu, Room Z), 2018
Panel Z-8 (C01-22-021)
Middle Eastern food packaging and newspapers, glue, cardboard on wooden structures
Courtesy of the artist and Rhona Hoffman Gallery

Michael Rakowitz (b. 1973)
The invisible enemy should not exist (Northwest Palace of Kalhu, Room Z), 2018
Panel Z-4 (C01-22-019)
Middle Eastern food packaging and newspapers, glue, cardboard on wooden structures
Courtesy of the artist and Rhona Hoffman Gallery

Michael Rakowitz (b. 1973)
The invisible enemy should not exist (Northwest Palace of Kalhu, Room Z), 2018
Panel Z-b-4 (C01-22-013)
Middle Eastern food packaging and new
Courtesy of the artist and Rhona Hoffman Gallery

Michael Rakowitz (b. 1973)
American Golem, 2022
Found antiques, paper mache sculpture, granite, wood, metal base
Courtesy of the artist and Rhona Hoffman Gallery

Michael Rakowitz (b. 1973)
Moments in Spolia 2, 2022
Pencil on vellum
Courtesy of the artist and Rhona Hoffman Gallery

Michael Rakowitz (b. 1973)
Moments in Spolia 3, 2022
Pencil on vellum
Courtesy of the artist and Rhona Hoffman Gallery

Michael Rakowitz (b. 1973)
Moments in Spolia 4, 2022
Pencil on vellum
Courtesy of the artist and Rhona Hoffman Gallery

Gerald Sheffield (b. 1985)
let's teach them baseball i, 2023 (based on a 2017 installation)
Drywall, plywood studs, vinyl, tension wire, charcoal, latex paint
Courtesy of the artist

Gerald Sheffield (b. 1985)
fm 3-05.301 (from *ptsd series*), 2016
Wheatpaste collaged copy paper on panel
Courtesy of the artist

Dwayne Wilcox (Oglala Lakota, b. 1957)
Horned Warrior Headdress, 2014
Military desert camouflage, felt, brass tacks, ribbons
Courtesy of the artist and Red Cloud Indian School

ABOUT THE EDITORS

Aaron Hughes is an artist, curator, organizer, anti-war activist, and Iraq War veteran. Working through an interdisciplinary practice rooted in drawing and printmaking, Hughes works collaboratively to create meaning out of personal and collective trauma, transform systems of oppression, and seek liberation. Hughes works with a range of art and activist groups, including Justseeds Artists' Cooperative, About Face: Veterans Against the War, emerging Veteran Art Movement, and Prison + Neighborhood Arts/Education Project.

Ronak K. Kapadia is an interdisciplinary scholar, writer, and curator whose work explores race, war, aesthetics, and empire in the late twentieth and early twenty-first century United States. He is an Associate Professor of Gender and Women's Studies and affiliated faculty in Art History, Global Asian Studies, and Museum and Exhibition Studies at the University of Illinois Chicago. Kapadia is the author of the award-winning *Insurgent Aesthetics: Security and the Queer Life of the Forever War* (Duke University Press, 2019), co-curator of the 2023 Veteran Art Triennial, and currently completing *Inspiration: The Art of the Brown Queer Commons*, a critical study of healing, justice, and pleasure within queer and trans of color aesthetics.

Therese Quinn, a teacher, writer, and cultural worker, has been active in queer and feminist anti-authoritarian and anti-capitalist social movements for many years. She is employed as a Professor and Director of Museum and Exhibition Studies at the University of Illinois Chicago, and researches the role of the arts, museums, and related institutions in justice-work. She has authored and edited, often with others, books including *School: Questions About Museums, Culture and Justice to Explore in Your Classroom* (Teachers College Press, 2020), *Teaching Toward Democracy: Educators as Agents of Change, 2e* (Taylor and Francis, 2016), and *Flaunt It! Queers Organizing for Public Education and Justice* (Peter Lang, 2009).

Meranda Roberts is a citizen of the Yerington Paiute Tribe and Chicana. She has a PhD in Native American History and an MA in Public History from the University of California, Riverside. Currently a visiting professor in the art history department at Pomona College, she is dedicated to reconnecting Indigenous collection items with their descendants and telling these items' stories in a way that adequately expresses their meaning to the communities they come from. Recent curatorial projects include "Native Truths: Our Stories. Our Voices" at the Field Museum of Natural History, the 2023 Native American Invitational Exhibition at Idyllwild Arts entitled "Still We Smile: Humor as Correction and Joy," and "Continuity: Cahuilla Basket Weavers and their Legacies," which opened at the Benton Museum of Art at Pomona College in February 2024.

Amber Zora is a curator, interdisciplinary artist, instructor, and US Army veteran based in Rapid City, South Dakota. She holds an MFA in Photography and Integrated Media from Ohio University. Her work examines the trauma of war, the military's impact on the environment, and rural America's dependence on the military economy. Zora has curated exhibitions at the National Veterans Art Museum, the Oceanside Museum of Art, and the Contemporary at Blue Star. As an organizer and nonprofit worker, Amber is dedicated to working with artists who build knowledge around peace, reconciliation, and justice.

COLOPHON

Surviving the Long Wars: Creative Rebellion at the Ends of Empire

Edited by Aaron Hughes, Ronak K. Kapadia, Therese Quinn, Meranda Roberts, and Amber Zora

Published in 2024 by BRIDGE Books
2858 W Belle Plaine Ave, #3
Chicago, IL 60618

ISBN: 979-8-987933053

Library of Congress Control Number: 2024937704

COPYEDITING
Kevin Basl

DESIGN
Becky Nasadowski
typefaces: Freight and Halyard
by Joshua Darden

PUBLICATION MANAGEMENT
David Maruzzella

PRINTING
Ingram Spark

ADDITIONAL REPRODUCTION CREDITS

"Between Two Wars" by Dunya Mikhail was originally published in *The War Works Hard*, translated by Elizabeth Winslow. © 1993, 1997, 2000, 2005 by Dunya Mikhail. Reprinted by permission of New Directions Publishing Corp.

"Embedded Horizons" was originally published in *Theater of Operations: The Gulf Wars, 1991–2011*, edited by Peter Eleey and Ruba Katrib, MoMA PS1, 2019.

"The Summit, Then and Now" by Isra Rahman originally appeared as "Chicago Art Exhibit Examines Global War on 20th Anniversary of Iraq Invasion" in *South Side Weekly*, May 5, 2023. https://southsideweekly.com/chicago-art-exhibit-examines-global-war-on-20th-anniversary-of-iraq-invasion/. The text was edited by the author for this book and is reprinted with permission of *South Side Weekly*.

BOOK CONTRIBUTORS

Maitham Alharbi, Kevin Basl, Roxanne Dunbar-Ortiz, GOODW.Y.N., Aaron Hughes, Ronak K. Kapadia, Shaymaa Khalil, Laleh Khalili, Erika Renee Land, Kyle T. Mays, Dunya Mikhail, Isra Rahman, Michael Rakowitz, Junaid Rana, Meranda Roberts, Rijin Sahakian, Carlos Sirah, Anthony Torres, and Amber Zora

STLW EXHIBITING ARTISTS

Bassim Al Shaker, Dorothy Burge, Miridith Campbell, June Carpenter, Bruce Carter, Mahwish Chishty, Jose deVera, Melissa Doud, Sabba Elahi, Rodney Ewing, Ali Eyal, Darrell Wayne Fair, Sarah Farahat, Chitra Ganesh, Mariam Ghani, Frederick Gokliz, Hock E Aye Vi Edgar Heap of Birds, Gina Herrera, Tom Jones, Rajkamal Kahlon, Ruth Kaneko, Gilbert Kills Pretty Enemy III, Terran Last Gun, Monty Little, Hanaa Malallah, Hector René Membreño-Canales, Chris Pappan, Eric Perez, Yvette M. Pino, Michael Rakowitz, Gregory Rick, Gerald Sheffield, Dwayne Wilcox, and Yiran Zhang

STLW PERFORMERS AND PRESENTERS

Bassim Al Shaker, Lubana Al Quntar, Hipólito Arriaga III, Andrea Assaf, Dorothy Burge, Lovella Calica, William Chan, Brittney Chantele, Mahwish Chishty, Elexa Dawson, Sabba Elahi, Ali Eyal, Eddie Falcón, Brian Frejo, Frontline Arts, GOODW.Y.N., Gina Herrera, Shaymaa Khalil, Youree Kim, Daniel King, Erika Renee Land, Joseph Lefthand, Nathan Lewis, Monty Little, Dunya Mikhail, James Pakootas, Eric Perez, Yvette M. Pino, Michael Rakowitz, Meranda Roberts, John Rogers, Joseph Running Crane, Sada, Aida Shahgasemi, Gerald Sheffield, Josue Sican, Carlos Sirah, Nick Slie, Hussein Smko, Zafer Tawil, Starla Thompson, Moki Tantoco, Anthony Torres, Jules Vaquera, Angela Waller, Ashley Wilkerson, and Anu Yadav

STLW ORGANIZING TEAM

Kevin Basl, Aaron Hughes, Ronak K. Kapadia, Joseph Lefthand, Becky Nasadowski, Meranda Roberts, Therese Quinn, and Amber Zora

STLW PROGRAM SUPPORT

Rachel Dukes, Zaynab Hilal, and Yiran Zhang

STLW NEH VETERAN FELLOWS

Natasha Erskine, Gina Herrera, Monty Little, Eric Perez, Gerald Sheffield, and Anthony Torres

STLW FEATURED SCHOLARS AND NEH EXPERTS

Roxanne Dunbar-Ortiz, Nick C. Estes, Tom Jones, Kelly Hayes, Ronak K. Kapadia, Laleh Khalili, Tiffany King, Kyle T. Mays, Chris Pappan, Yvette M. Pino, Michael Rakowitz, Meranda Roberts, Rijin Sahakian, Harsha Walia, and Jason Wesaw

STLW EXHIBITIONS

Residues and Rebellions, Newberry Library, February 28–May 26, 2023

Unlikely Entanglements, Hyde Park Art Center, March 16–July 9, 2023

Reckon and Reimagine, Chicago Cultural Center, March 12–July 2, 2023

Transformative Threads, Chicago Cultural Center, December 2023–December 2024

HYDE PARK ART CENTER

Mariela Acuña, Allison Cochrane, Ciera McKissick, Allison Peters Quinn, Jeff Robinson, and Tran Tran

NEWBERRY LIBRARY

Sarah Boyd Alvarez, Will Hansen, Patrick Kepley, and Analú María López

CHICAGO CULTURAL CENTER

Elise Butterfield, Greg Lunceford, and Daniel Schulman

STLW DESIGN

Becky Nasadowski

STLW TRANSLATORS

Inmagela Rivas Abreau and Georgina Valverde (*Transformative Threads* exhibition)

STLW EDUCATION GUIDE

Liliana Macias

STLW MENTAL HEALTH SUPPORT

Michael Applegate and Suellen Semekoski

CONTRIBUTING UIC GRADUATE STUDENTS

Inmagela Rivas Abreu, Billy Borstell, Spencer Harrison, Zaynab Hilal, Andrew Kracinski, Liliana Macias, Alexa Marines, Tracy Tojo, and Hun Xue

PHOTO CREDITS

Drew Cameron: 310

Fanny Garcia: 75, 218–19, 223, 232–33, 234–35, 240–41, 242–43, 244–45, 254–55, 264–65, 266 (top left), 267 (bottom right), 268, 270–71, 272–73, 289, 299, 301

Peg Hunter: 325

Daniel King: 64, 170–71, 196–97, 226–27, 228–29, 230–31, 236–37, 238–39, 246–47, 249, 250–51, 252–53, 256–57, 258–59, 260–61, 284, 287, 292, 305, 326

Fred Neal: 165

Newberry Library: 38–39, 40–41, 44–45, 46–47, 50–51, 68, 313

Eric Perez: 16–17, 24–25, 26–27, 28–29, 30–31, 32–33, 34–35, 36–37, 42–43, 49, 54, 68 (bottom), 71, 73, 76–77, 82–83, 84–85, 87, 88–89, 90–91, 92–93, 96–97, 99, 102–3, 104–5, 108–9, 110–11, 115 (bottom), 118–19, 120–21, 122, 136, 139, 144–45, 146, 150–51, 152–53, 158–59, 160–61, 162–63, 164, 166–67, 172–73, 174–75, 176–77, 178–79, 180–81, 182–83, 184–85, 186–87, 188–89, 190–91, 192–93, 198–99, 200, 207, 208, 211, 248, 262–63, 266–67, 269, 276, 294, 317, 318–19, 336

James Prinz: xiv, 100–101, 106 (bottom), 113, 114–15, 116–17, 141

Tom Van Eynde: 94–95, 106 (top), 107

photos not listed here are courtesy of the artist or otherwise credited in their caption

Surviving the Long Wars *was organized with support from the emerging Veteran Art Movement, Chicago Cultural Center, City of Chicago Department of Cultural Affairs and Special Events,* DEMIL *Art Fund, Hyde Park Art Center, Newberry Library, Paratech, University of Illinois Chicago (*UIC*) Institute for the Humanities Innovation Grant,* UIC *Award for Creative Activity,* UIC *Disability Cultural Center,* UIC *Native American Support Program,* UIC *Museum and Exhibition Studies Program,* UIC *Gender and Women's Studies Program, Windrose Fund, and the National Endowment for the Humanities' Dialogues on the Experience of War grant.*

SURVIVINGTHELONGWARS.ONLINE

COVER IMAGE CREDITS

(back to front cover, left to right):

Monty Little, *Survivance, 15* (p. 31)

Darrell Wayne Fair, *The Facade* (p. 37)

Eric Perez, *Sgt. Gudiño* (pp. 146, 190–91, 196–97)

Miridith Campbell, *Marine Corps Dress—Southern Style* (pp. 71, 88–89, 250–51)

Bassim Al Shaker, *Alive* (pp. 159)

Mahwish Chishty, *Reaper* (pp. 174–75)

Rodney Ewing, *Confines* (p. 183)

Gregory Rick, *From Manila to Baghdad* (pp. 170–71, 326)

Rajkamal Kahlon, *"This 44-year old male, _____________, died of complications from multiple gunshot wounds." (youngest son)* (pp. 102–3)

Michael Rakowitz, *The invisible enemy should not exist (Northwest Palace of Kalhu, Room Z-10) (pp. 101, 106–7)*

www.ingramcontent.com/pod-product-compliance
Lightning Source LLC
LaVergne TN
LVRC090954210926
848482LV00009B/354